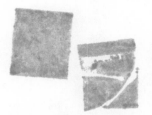

At the time of his death in 1928, Alexander A. Maximow left an unfinished manuscript of a *Textbook of Histology*. This was completed by Dr. William Bloom with the help and advice of some of his colleagues and friends, C. Judson Herrick, George Bartelmez, Clayton Loosli, J. Walter Wilson, Edward A. Boyden, and W. H. Taliafero. The book went through seven editions as Maximow and Bloom's *Textbook of Histology* — 1930, 1934, 1938, 1942, 1948, 1952, 1957. There have been translations into Spanish, Polish, and Italian.

In the eighth and ninth editions (1962, 1968), Don W. Fawcett joined William Bloom as co-author of the book. In 1972, Dr. William Bloom died after nearly fifty years of devoted service to the University of Chicago. His long experience and wisdom have been greatly missed in the preparation of the tenth edition, which has been largely the work of Don Fawcett, with helpful suggestions from a number of his colleagues and with important contributions by Dr. J. Angevine on the nervous system and Dr. Elio Raviola on the immune system and lymphoid organs.

Tenth Edition

A TEXTBOOK OF
HISTOLOGY

WILLIAM BLOOM, M.D.

Late Charles H. Swift Distinguished Service Professor
of Anatomy, The University of Chicago

DON W. FAWCETT, M.D.

Hersey Professor of Anatomy
Harvard Medical School

W. B. SAUNDERS COMPANY *Philadelphia* • *London* • *Toronto* •

W. B. Saunders Company: West Washington Square
                          Philadelphia, Pa.   19105

                          12 Dyott Street
                          London, WC1A   1DB

                          833 Oxford Street
                          Toronto, Ontario M8Z 5T9, Canada

Library of Congress Cataloging in Publication Data

Bloom, William, 1899–1972.

A textbook of histology.

Includes bibliographies.

1. Histology.   I. Fawcett, Don Wayne, 1917–
   joint author.   II. Title.

QM551.B56 1975   611'.018   73–77935

ISBN 0–7216–1757–3

A Textbook of Histology   ISBN 0-7216-1757-3

Print No.:   9   8   7   6   5   4   3   2

Preface

In the six years since publication of the ninth edition of the *Textbook of Histology* our knowledge of the microscopic structure of the body has continued to expand at a remarkable rate, while the time devoted to this subject in the medical curriculum has steadily diminished. Despite the current trend toward superficiality in basic science instruction we have chosen not to produce a book that would present only the prerequisites for an understanding of pathology; or the least information needed to pass the National Board Examinations; or the minimum required safely to practice medicine. There would be little satisfaction in writing a book with such limited and short-range goals. Histology is a fascinating and important branch of biomedical science that deserves more thorough treatment. Nevertheless, we have endeavored to be selective and to keep the book within reasonable limits of size by adding only the more significant new findings and by deleting many passages considered obsolete or of interest only to the specialist.

The chapter on *The Cell and Cell Division* has been thoroughly revised to incorporate some of the many advances in our understanding of the structure and function of the cell organelles. Irrelevant and confusing material on the chemistry of protoplasm and the structure of chromosomes has been eliminated. The chapter on *Glands and Secretion* was rewritten to present the current concepts of protein synthesis and the release of cell products. More adequate treatment has been given to the cytology of polypeptide and steroid secreting cells; the interrelations among the endocrine glands; and the mechanism of action of hormones on their target organs. The revised chapters on the *Blood* and *Blood Formation* present contemporary views of the function of blood cells and hemopoiesis in the bone marrow and eliminate a number of outmoded concepts concerning the developmental potentialities of lymphoid cells and their relationships to other cells of the blood and connective tissues. The *Urinary System* and *Male Reproductive System* have had extensive revision, while the chapters on *Muscle, Bone, Liver, Pancreas* and *Adipose Tissue,* which were thoroughly rewritten in the previous edition, required only minor modifications. It is a pleasure to acknowledge the helpful suggestions of Dr. George Szabo on *Skin;* Dr. Michael Coppe on *Oral Cavity* and *Teeth;* and Ms. Rosemary Dunn on *The Ear.* Dr. Giuseppina Raviola made important corrections and valuable additions to the chapter on *The Eye.* I am very grateful for their interest and generous assistance.

A complete and authoritative revision of the chapter on *The Nervous System* was undertaken by Dr. Jay Angevine of the University of Arizona School of Medicine. The chapters on *Thymus, Lymph Nodes* and *Spleen* have been written by Dr. Elio Raviola of Harvard Medical School. His new chapter on *The Immune System* should do much to help teachers and students to appreciate the dramatic advances of recent years in our understanding of the biological basis of individuality and the complex mechanisms of immunity.

In a textbook of histology the illustrations are as valuable a learning resource as the text, and it is important that these also be updated to reflect the present state of technical competence in the field and the introduction of new methods. Since the last edition, the scanning electron microscope and the freeze-cleaving technique of specimen preparation for transmission electron microscopy have been added to the research armamentarium of the histologist. Some of the early results of these new methods have been included, and many more will surely appear in future editions. Two hundred fifty-three of the illustrations in the ninth edition, considered substandard or of limited instructional value, have been eliminated. Three hundred thirty new drawings, photomicrographs and electron micrographs have been added, bringing the total number of illustrations to over 900. It is hoped that these will make the text more understandable and will supplement material available to students in the laboratory.

I am indebted to several associates in the Department of Anatomy who have helped in various ways to complete this edition. My secretary, Helen Deacon, has patiently typed and retyped portions of the manuscript. Ms. Sylvia Colard Keene's exceptional talent as an illustrator has contributed much to the beauty and instructional value of the new drawings and diagrams. Mr. Peter Ley has been extraordinarily diligent and helpful in applying his skill to achieve optimal photographic reproduction.

And finally I must express my deep appreciation of the friendship, interest, and encouragement I have received over the years from Mr. John Dusseau. Especially gratifying has been his willingness to see this edition through to completion even after he has put aside many of his duties as Vice President and Editor of the W. B. Saunders Company.

Don W. Fawcett

Contents

1

Methods of Histology and Cytology 1

Methods for Direct Observation of Living Tissues and Cells 2
Isolation of Components of Living Cells by
    Differential Centrifugation 8
Preparation and Examination of Killed Tissue 9
Principles of Microscopic Analysis 21
X-ray Diffraction 31

2

The Cell and Cell Division 35

The Cell 35
    Cytoplasmic Organelles 37
    Cytoplasmic Matrix Components 58
    Cytoplasmic Inclusions 61
    Nuclear Organelles 63
Cell Division 70
    Mitosis 70
    Meiosis 74
    Human Chromosomes 74

3

Epithelium 83

Classification of Epithelia 84
Specializations of Epithelia 90
Specializations of the Free Surface 98

4

Glands and Secretion 108

Exocrine Glands 108
    Synthesis, Storage, and Release of Protein Rich
        Secretory Products 108

Classification of Exocrine Glands 117
Histological Organization of Exocrine Glands 121
Control of Exocrine Secretion 122
Endocrine Glands 123
Cytology of Protein and Polypeptide Secreting
Endocrine Glands 125
Cytology of Steroid Secreting Endocrine Glands 126
Storage and Secretion of Hormones 127
Relation of Endocrine Cells to Blood and Lymph
Vascular Systems 130
Control Mechanisms and Interrelations Within the
Endocrine System 132
Mechanisms of Hormone Action on Target Cells 134

5

Blood 136

Formed Elements of Blood 137
Erythrocytes 137
Blood Platelets 139
Leukocytes 141
Other Components of Blood 153

6

Connective Tissue Proper 158

Loose Connective Tissue 158
Extracellular Components 159
Fixed Cellular Elements 171
Mononuclear Wandering Cells 175
Serous Membranes 186
Dense Connective Tissue 188
Connective Tissue with Special Properties 189
Histophysiology of Connective Tissue 190

7

Adipose Tissue 196

Histological Characteristics of the Adipose Tissues 196
Histogenesis of Adipose Tissue 201
Histophysiology of Adipose Tissue 202

8

Blood Cell Formation 209

Hemopoiesis During Embryonic Development 210
Histological Organization of the Bone Marrow 212

Theories of Hemopoiesis and Cell Lineages 213
Erythropoiesis 216
Thrombopoiesis 221
Granulopoiesis.. 224
Monopoiesis 230
Lymphopoiesis in the Marrow.................................... 231

9

Cartilage 233

Hyaline Cartilage 234
Elastic Cartilage 239
Fibrocartilage 239
Other Varieties of Cartilage and Chondroid Tissue.................. 240
Regeneration of Cartilage.. 241
Regressive Changes in Cartilage 241
Histophysiology of Cartilage 242

10

Bone 244

Macroscopic Structure of Bones 244
Microscopic Structure of Bones.................................. 246
Submicroscopic Structure and Composition of Bone Matrix 253
The Cells of Bone 254
Histogenesis of Bone 262
Histophysiology of Bone 279
Joints and Synovial Membranes.................................. 282

11

Muscular Tissue 288

Smooth Muscle 288
Skeletal Muscle 295
Cardiac Muscle 315
Histogenesis of Muscular Tissue................................. 328
Regeneration of Muscular Tissue 330

12

The Nervous Tissue 333

by Jay B. Angevine

The Structure of the Neuron..................................... 336
Distribution, Forms, and Varieties of Neurons..................... 347
The Nerve Fiber.. 351
Peripheral Nerve Endings 358

Autonomic Nervous System 364
Neuroglia 366
The Synapse and the Relationships of Neurons 369
Development of the Neurons and of the Nervous Tissue 373
Connective Tissue, Choroid Plexus, Ventricles, and the
    Meninges of the Central Nervous System............................ 375
Response of the Neuron to Injury 382

13

Blood and Lymph Vascular Systems 386

Blood Capillaries.. 386
    The Structural Basis of Exchange Across the
        Capillary Wall... 393
Arteries 396
Veins 409
Vascular Specializations and Ancillary Organs 413
The Heart 416
    Impulse Conducting System 418
Histogenesis of the Blood Vessels 420
Lymphatic Vessels.. 420

14

The Immune System 427
by Elio Raviola

Cells of the Immune System 430
    Cytology of the Cells of the Immune System...................... 430
    Histophysiology 434
Lymphoid Tissue 446
Histophysiological Overview of the Immune System 451

15

Thymus 457
by Elio Raviola

Histological Organization 457
Normal, Accidental, and Experimental Involution................... 465
Histophysiology of the Thymus.. 465

16

Lymph Nodes 471
by Elio Raviola

Histological Organization 471
Histophysiology of Lymph Nodes.. 481

17

Spleen 487

by Elio Raviola

Histological Organization 487
Histogenesis and Regeneration of the Spleen 498
Histophysiology of the Spleen 499

18

Hypophysis (Pituitary Gland) 503

Pars Distalis.. 505
    Acidophils (Alpha Cells).. 507
    Basophils (Beta Cells) 509
    Chromophobes (Reserve Cells) 510
    Blood Supply 511
    Histophysiology of the Pars Distalis.......................... 512
    Histophysiological Correlations 515
    Releasing Hormones... 515
Pars Intermedia.. 516
    Histophysiology of the Pars Intermedia........................ 517
Pars Infundibularis or Tuberalis 518
Neurohypophysis.. 518
    Histophysiology of the Neurohypophysis 520

19

The Thyroid Gland... 524

Histological Organization 524
Histophysiology of the Thyroid Gland 528

20

Parathyroid Glands 535

Histophysiology of the Parathyroid.................................. 538

21

Adrenal Glands and Paraganglia 540

The Adrenal Cortex.. 540
The Adrenal Medulla 543
Blood Supply and Lymphatic Drainage of the Adrenal.............. 546
Nerves of the Adrenal 548
Histophysiology of the Adrenal Cortex.............................. 549
Histophysiology of the Adrenal Medulla............................. 551
Histogenesis of the Adrenal Glands 552
The Paraganglia 553

22

The Pineal Gland 556
Histophysiology of the Pineal Gland 560

23

Skin 563
The Epidermis 563
The Melanocyte System 571
Mucocutaneous Junctions 576
The Dermis 577
Hairs 579
Nails 587
Glands 588
Blood and Lymphatic Vessels 592
Nerves 593
Histogenesis of the Skin and Its Accessories 594

24

Oral Cavity and Associated Glands 598
The Oral Cavity 599
The Tongue 601
Glands of the Oral Cavity 605
Tonsils 615
The Pharynx 617

25

The Teeth 621
Histogenesis of the Teeth 631

26

The Esophagus and Stomach 639
Esophagus 639
Glands of the Esophagus 640
Histophysiology of the Esophagus 641
Stomach 643
Gastric Glands 647
Histophysiology of the Stomach 654
Cell Renewal and Regeneration 655

27

Intestines 658
The Small Intestine 658
The Intestinal Mucosa 658

The Appendix.. 673
The Large Intestine 674
The Histophysiology of Intestinal Absorption.......................... 676
Blood Vessels of the Gastrointestinal Tract 680
Lymph Vessels of the Gastrointestinal Tract.......................... 681
Nerves of the Intestinal Tract 682
Histogenesis of Intestines 686

28

The Liver and Gallbladder 688
Liver.. 688
    Histological Organization of the Liver............................ 688
    Regeneration 712
Histophysiology of the Liver... 713
Bile Ducts 717
The Gallbladder and Choledochoduodenal Junction 718

29

Pancreas.. 726
The Exocrine Pancreas 726
The Endocrine Pancreas 729
The Duct System 733
Blood Vessels, Lymphatics, and Nerves 735
Regeneration... 737
Histophysiology of the Exocrine Pancreas.......................... 737
Histophysiology of the Endocrine Pancreas......................... 739

30

Respiratory System 743
The Nose.. 743
The Larynx.. 746
The Trachea 748
The Lungs... 748
    Respiratory Structures of the Lungs............................ 750

31

The Urinary System 766
Kidneys 766
    Uriniferous Tubules 767
    Juxtaglomerular Complex 782
    Blood Supply 784
    Lymphatics 786
    Nerves.. 787
Histophysiology of the Kidneys 787

Passages for the Excretion of Urine 794
Urethra 799

32

Male Reproductive System 805

Testis 805
Seminiferous Tubules 807
The Spermatozoon 811
Spermatogenesis 819
Interstitial Tissue 833
Blood Vessels and Lymphatics of the Testis 835
Histophysiology of the Testis 837
Excretory Ducts of the Testis 841
Ductuli Efferentes 842
Accessory Glands of the Male Reproductive Tract 847
The Penis 851
Semen 855

33

Female Reproductive System 858

Ovary 858
The Oviduct or Fallopian Tube 880
Uterus 883
Endocrine Regulation of the Female Reproductive System 895
Implantation 897
Placenta 898
Vagina 902
External Genitalia 904

34

Mammary Gland 907

Resting Mammary Gland 907
Active Mammary Gland 908
Endocrine Control of Mammary Gland Function 911
Regression of the Mammary Gland 914

35

The Eye 917

Structure of the Eye in General 917
Dimensions, Axes, Planes of Reference 918
Fibrous Tunic 920
The Uvea (The Vascular Tunic) 926
Refractive Media of the Eye 934
The Retina 937
Histophysiology of the Retina 953

Blood Vessels of the Eye 956
Lymph Spaces of the Eye 957
Nerves of the Eye 957
Accessory Organs of the Eye 957
Histogenesis of the Eye 961

36

The Ear 964
   External Ear 964
   Middle Ear 965
      Tympanic Cavity 965
      Tympanic Membrane 966
      Auditory Tube 967
   Internal Ear 968
      The Bone Labyrinth 968
      The Membranous (or Endolymphatic) Labyrinth 970
      The Perilymphatic Labyrinth 981
      Endolymph and Perilymph 983
      Nerves of the Labyrinth 984
      Blood Vessels of the Labyrinth 985
   Embryological Development of the Ear 987
   Functional Considerations 990
Index 993

1
Methods of Histology and Cytology

Anatomy is the branch of science that is concerned with the external form and internal organization of plants and animals. It has as its major aims a thorough understanding of the underlying architectural principles on which living organisms are constructed, the discovery of the structural basis for the functioning of the various parts, and a comprehension of the mechanisms responsible for the development of their complex structure. It is customary to subdivide the broad field of anatomy into several components based upon the method by which the structures are revealed or the size of the subunits studied. Thus *gross anatomy* encompasses all those features accessible to dissection and direct inspection, and *microscopic anatomy* or *histology* includes those minute parts beyond the reach of the naked eye.

The systematic study of the gross structure of the body is the oldest of the sciences basic to medicine, extending back at least to the second century. The investigation of its infinitely small components had to await the development of optical methods and is of relatively recent origin. Significant microscopic observations were recorded by Leeuwenhoek, Hooke, and others in the seventeenth century, but histology did not acquire the status of a separate branch of science until the accumulated observations of the eighteenth and nineteenth centuries led to the enunciation by Schleiden and Schwann of the *cell theory* — the most important general-

ization in the science of morphology. This theory held that cells are potentially independent organisms and that entire plants and animals are aggregations of these living units arranged according to definite laws. To this basic generalization was soon added the concept that all cells originate from pre-existing cells by a process of division in which the nucleus divides into two "daughters" that are precise replicas of the original nucleus. These principles are the foundations upon which much of modern biology and medicine has been built.

The progress of any branch of science is seldom uniform. Introduction of a new instrument or a new technique initiates a period of rapid advance. Then, after a phase of vigorous exploitation, progress slows as the application of existing methods gradually comes to yield diminishing returns of new information. A new period of rapid advance must often await the discovery of a novel approach or the development of a new instrument. Such has been the history of microscopic anatomy. The grinding of improved lenses by Amici in 1827 led directly to the development of the well corrected compound microscopes that made possible the recognition of the cell as the basic unit of living matter. The ensuing classical period of descriptive *histology* and *cytology* established the normal structure of tissues and cells and provided information essential to the development of the allied field of *histopathology*, which had its origins in Virchow's enunciation of the concept that the fundamental changes in human disease can be traced to alterations in cells. Few discoveries have had such a far-reaching influence on the development of scientific medicine, but in time, the pace of new discoveries in both histology and pathology slackened. A little over a hundred years after the perfection of the compound microscope, the first electron microscope was built in 1932 by Knoll and Ruska. The modern instruments, constructed on the same principle, have extended the limits of resolvable tissue structure more than a hundredfold and have opened up for the microscopist a vast area of biological structure that was previously inaccessible. As a consequence, histology is again in a period of rapid advance. The numerous discoveries are leading to entirely new concepts of the structural organization and function of cells and subcellular components.

Important as the microscope is in this branch of science, it is but one of the means by which knowledge is gained. With each major forward step in optical instrumentation, numerous ancillary techniques have been developed that extend the range of its usefulness, sharpen its resolution, and offer the possibility of more accurate and penetrating analysis of biological structure. The student can scarcely hope to acquire a useful knowledge of the substantive content of histology and cytology without an understanding of the principles of microscopic analysis (p. 20) and the other instrumental, observational, and experimental methods by which new information is obtained in this field. This chapter is therefore presented early in the book, so that the student of histology will have some understanding of the principles underlying the various methods that will be referred to again and again throughout the remainder of the book.

METHODS FOR DIRECT OBSERVATION OF LIVING TISSUES AND CELLS

Much of histology is, of necessity, based upon the examination of samples of tissues that have been killed and preserved, but the primary objective of their study is to discover structural relationships that will contribute to an understanding of the vital processes of the *living* organism. It is one of the paradoxes of biology that we often destroy at the outset the very property we most desire to understand. Someone has aptly phrased the problem in a simile: "the quality of being *alive* is like the snowflake on the window pane that vanishes at the warm touch of an inquisitive child."

There is, however, a growing list of methods for the study of living tissues — some relatively crude, others quite refined, but all of them yielding information of a kind that cannot be obtained from dead tissues alone.

Exteriorization and Transillumination of Organs

Some organs have a long vascular pedicle and are sufficiently mobile that they can be brought out of the body cavity of the anesthetized animal and can be maintained in a moist chamber under conditions that permit their transillumination and direct micro-

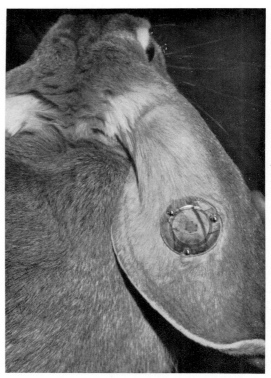

Figure 1-1 Rabbit with a transparent chamber in its ear. This strain of rabbits has unusually large ears that are especially favorable for this purpose. (Courtesy of J. Irwin.)

scopic examination at relatively low power. The smallest laboratory animals have naturally been most useful for this approach because their thinner tissues lend themselves better ,to transillumination. By this simple procedure valuable observations have been made on the dynamics of the circulation of various organs (Knisely). The release of secretory material from the pancreatic cells under the influence of various pharmacological agents has been observed (Covell), and the ovaries of rats have been brought out into a perfusion chamber and the process of ovulation and passage of the ova into the oviduct have been recorded cinematographically (Blandau).

In the applications of this approach, the investigator is 'usually severely limited in the duration of observation and in the magnification that can be employed. There have been numerous efforts, therefore, to create indwelling windows or chambers that will permit prolonged and repeated observations of tissues over a period of days or even months.

Transparent Chamber Methods

One of the most successful means of studying living tissues has involved the installation of chambers of metal and glass in the long flexible ears of rabbits (Figs. 1–1 and 1–2). The tissue to be studied is transplanted between the windows of the thin chamber, where it acquires a blood supply from the neighboring connective tissue and survives for long periods. For periodic examination, the rabbit is trained to rest quietly on the bench beside the microscope with its ear secured to the mechanical stage in such a way that the transparent chamber is centered over the condenser. With such chambers, important observations have been made on the growth of capillaries and nerves (Clark), the emigration of leukocytes from the blood vessels (Florey), the development of adipose cells and many other histophysiological and developmental processes.

The anterior chamber of the eye is a naturally occurring transparent chamber. Small fragments of autologous tissue transplanted into the anterior chamber of the eye acquire a blood supply by ingrowth of capillaries from the corneoiridial angle. They are bathed in a physiological fluid, the aqueous

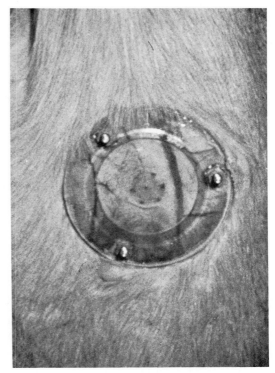

Figure 1–2 A close view of the ear chamber, with the vascular pattern showing through the transparent window. The three threaded studs on the rim are used to hold the chamber onto the stage of the microscope. (Courtesy of J. Irwin.)

humor, and can be observed with a microscope through the transparent cornea. Transplantation of tissue to the anterior chamber of the eye permits the investigator to assess the functional or developmental potentialities of a tissue when removed from its nerve supply and from the influence of neighboring tissues in its normal environment. It has been possible, for example, to transplant fertilized mouse ova to the anterior chamber and to demonstrate their capacity for growth and limited differentiation, independent of the specialized nutritional environment normally provided by the uterus (Fig. 1–4). Similarly, small pieces of the lining of the monkey uterus have been successfully transplanted to the monkey's eye for extended observation of cyclic changes. At the time of the reproductive cycle when the female host was menstruating, the transplants of endometrium in her eye underwent similar changes and bled in the anterior chamber. Thus it was demonstrated by this experi-

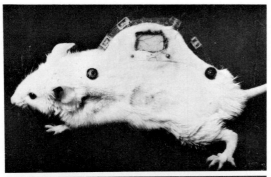

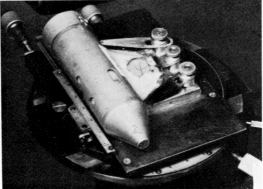

Figure 1–3 An economical transparent chamber for use in mice. A fold of loose dorsal skin and subcutaneous tissue is held in a plastic frame. For observation, the mouse is confined in a brass cylinder on the stage of the microscope *(lower)*. The fin-like chamber projects through a slit in the cylinder and is centered over the condenser of the microscope. (After G. H. Algire and F. Y. Legallais, J. Nat. Cancer Inst., *10*:225, 1949.)

mental device that menstruation is under hormonal rather than nervous control. The transplants also permitted direct microscopic visualization of some of the vascular changes involved (Markee).

Cell and Organ Culture

Tissue culture as an experimental procedure had its inception in the demonstration by Ross Harrison in 1907 that nerve fibers would grow out from fragments of frog spinal cord isolated in clotted lymph. Methods were later developed by Carrel, Warren Lewis, and others for serial propagation of various kinds of cells in vitro. In the classical procedure, an explanted fragment of tissue is embedded in a coagulum of blood plasma containing embryo juice as a growth stimu-

lant. Upon incubation the cells migrate radially from the explant and proliferate in the zone of outgrowth to form a colony, which, in a few days, may be several times the diameter of the original fragment (Fig. 1–5). This may then be subdivided and used to initiate new colonies. The specialized structural features of the original organ are lost in the outgrowth in culture, and there is a simplification of cell form and organization such that the population tends to be reduced to one of three basic patterns of growth: isolated ameboid cells, sheets of flattened polygonal cells, or networks of stellate or fusiform cells. Using these classical methods of tissue culture, Carrel kept a line of cells derived from chick embryo heart in continuous cultivation for long periods. During the early period of experimentation with cultures, much was learned about the characteristics of isolated populations of living cells, but only recently have rapid advances in technical methods made it possible to realize the potential of isolated cell systems for experimental investigations of morphogenesis, malignant transformation, cytogenetic variation, cell-virus relations, cell nutrition, cell interactions, and a host of other interesting problems (Harris).

The classical clot-embedded explant procedures are now of historical interest only. Simplified and chemically defined culture media have now been developed (Parker). Methods have been devised for dissociation of organs to yield cell suspensions for the initiation of cultures in which the cells form a monolayer on the floor of the culture vessel. Some mammalian cells can now be grown in suspension in fluid medium (Gey; Earle). Procedures have been developed for isolation of clones derived from single cells, so that uniform populations of identical cells are available for experiment (Puck and Marcus). Cell populations can be preserved in the frozen state for long periods and retain their viability. These newer methods now make it possible to handle vertebrate somatic cells in much the same way as cultures of microorganisms. The earlier belief that the arrangement of cells in the pattern typical of the tissue of origin is essential for the expression of the specialized physiological capabilities of cells has now been found to be erroneous. Dispersed cultures of cartilage cells continue to elaborate matrix components, and similar cultures of adrenal cells continue to produce their hormones in vitro and respond to stimulation from tropic hormones. The availability of such systems opens the way to correlated structural and biochemical studies of biosynthetic pathways, metabolic control mechanisms, and the mechanism of action of hormones.

The short-term cultures of the white cells of the blood have come into widespread use as the simplest means of studying human chromosomes. Modified chromosomal types or departures from the normal number have been correlated with Down's syndrome (mongolism) and several other congenital disorders.

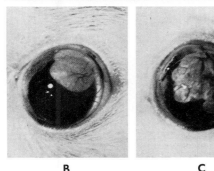

Figure 1-4 A, Photograph of a mouse that had received a fertilized mouse ovum in the eight cell stage in the anterior chamber of the right eye 12 days earlier. The early stages of implantation and development in the corneo-iridial angle could be observed directly through the transparent cornea. (After D. W. Fawcett et al., Am. J. Anat., *81*:413, 1947.) *B,* Photograph of a rat ovary transplanted to the anterior chamber 10 days earlier. No follicles are visible yet. The vascular connections can be seen on the surface of the graft. ×5. *C,* Same animal 21 days after implantation. Many follicles are now present. One, indicated by the dotted line, is hemorrhagic. (After L. Goodman, Anat. Rec., *59*:223, 1934.)

By altering the conditions of cultivation so as to discourage migration and dispersion of the cells, the original organ architecture can be retained. This method is called *organ culture,* and its principal value is that it provides a means of isolating an embryonic organ rudiment for the purpose of assessing its inherent capacity for growth and differentiation in the absence of the external influences that act upon it in the complex environment of the intact organism. An organ primordium from an embryo, when placed upon the surface of a plasma clot in a moist chamber, will often continue to grow for days or even weeks if transferred frequently to a fresh plasma substrate. Among the earliest contributions of this experimental approach was the demonstration that bone rudiments from early embryos would grow in length and undergo calcification outside of the body (Fell and Robison; Maximow). A recent improvement in the procedure involves placement of the primordium on a piece of lens paper floating on a liquid medium. There have been many ingenious applications of this and other modifications of organ culture, which enable the experimenter to control the composition of the environment and thus to influence or even to change the direction of differentiation of embryonic tissues. For example, organ cultures of embryonic chick skin, which normally differentiate feather buds, can be made to develop instead into mucus secreting cells by adding an excess of vitamin A to the culture medium.

Organized populations of neurons and their supporting glial cells from several regions of the brain have been maintained for months in vitro under conditions that permit experimental manipulation and direct visual evaluation of the results on the living cells (Murray). By the use of such simplified model systems it has been shown that blood serum from patients with multiple sclerosis, added to the culture medium, will produce structural and functional changes in vitro that simulate the pathological changes characteristic of the disease in vivo (Bornstein).

Cell (and tissue) culture "affords an ethically acceptable means of experimentation on human tissues and provides an opportunity to isolate living units from the complex environment of the body and to expose them directly to various agents whose effects in vivo might be obscured or confused by irrelevant systemic responses" (Murray).

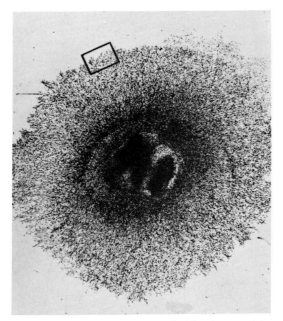

Figure 1-5 A photomicrograph of a tissue culture colony of fibroblasts from mouse subcutaneous tissue. The dense area in the center is the original explant and the broad halo around it represents the zone of outgrowth that has developed in four days of cultivation. ×14. The area indicated in the box is shown at higher magnification in Figure 1-6.

Mechanical Micromanipulation

The exploration of living cells by microsurgery presents a number of intriguing technical problems. Cells are so small that they must be magnified 100 to 1000 times for the relevant structures to be clearly seen, and at the same time they must be maintained in a physiological environment. Cultures provide cells free of connective tissue and spread out on a glass surface, so that they are accessible to microsurgical procedures. By working glass in a microforge, extremely minute instruments are devised—microneedles, micropipettes, and microhooks. These are positioned within an operating chamber on the stage of the compound microscope by highly precise mechanical micromanipulators capable of achieving controlled movements in various planes (Chambers; Kopac).

Micromanipulation has been applied to a variety of fundamental problems in cell biology. Studies have been made of the elasticity and viscosity of protoplasm. The dependence of cell function upon the nucleus has been demonstrated by removal of the nucleus from an ameba. In the absence of the nucleus, synthetic activities were greatly impaired and locomotion ceased, but the anucleate ameba remained viable. Insertion of a nucleus into it restored its motility and other vital activities. This approach has also been used to demonstrate that materials pass from the nucleus into the cytoplasm. The nucleus of an ameba that had incorporated radioactive isotopes into its nucleoplasm was transferred to the cytoplasm of a normal ameba. By autoradiography it was shown that radioactivity introduced in the transplanted nucleus was later found in the surrounding cytoplasm. It is now possible to inject minute amounts of substances directly into the cytoplasm of fertilized mammalian eggs and to assess their effect upon subsequent development (Fig. 1-8). Microinjectors have been developed to handle volumes as small as 1 picoliter (1 $\mu\mu$l or 1/50,000,000 of a drop). Such ingenious and skillfully contrived mechanical devices for microsurgery are no longer the only means available for manipulating cell components.

Use of Radiation Probes

The development of microbeams of protons and beams of ultraviolet light a few micrometers in diameter have made possible the selective irradiation of small areas of living cells. By the use of suitable microapertures, it is possible to get 80 per cent of the protons emitted to fall within a circle 2.5 μm. in diameter (Zirkle and Bloom). With ultraviolet beams (Uretz), the smallest area is about a micrometer in diameter (Fig. 1-9).

A probe of a very few micrometers in diameter is therefore small enough to irradiate parts of individual nuclei or segments of their chromosomes. This method has been used to study the dynamics of cell division. Localized irradiation of a small area of cytoplasm with protons caused no observable abnormality, but a similar irradiation with ultraviolet caused disappearance of spindle elements and disorder of the chromosomes. Segments of chromosomes in the path of the beam become distinctly paler (Figs. 1-10 and 1-11). By irradiating the region of attachment of spindle filaments to a single chromosome, it was shown that this chromosome lost all capacity for directed movements and simply drifted as a micronucleus. Thus, by irradiation it is possible to achieve the selective destruction of specific cell organelles and to assess its effect upon the cell as a whole (see review by Zirkle).

With the recent development of inexpensive lasers, microbeams of extremely intense, focused visible light are now available. By selective supravital staining (see next section) of a cell organelle with a dye, its structure can be photosensitized so that subsequent irradiation with the laser beam will cause destruction of the stained organelle while other parts of the cell, not photosensitized, remain undamaged. Thus the uptake of Janus green by mitochondria makes them vulnerable to subsequent irradiation by ruby laser microbeam (Amy). When acridine orange is introduced into a tissue culture medium for a few minutes, the dye molecules intercalate into the DNA helix, making the chromosomes sensitive to light. Subsequent irradiation of selected chromosomes with intense laser light permits

local destruction of parts of chromosomes (Berns). Improved high power argon lasers now permit microirradiations with more energy than before. This makes it possible to produce discrete lesions in chromosomes or other cell components without previous sensitization with a vital dye.

Vital and Supravital Staining

When certain dyes of relatively low toxicity are injected into living animals (*vital staining*) or applied to surviving cells and tissues removed from the body (*supravital staining*), they are taken up selectively by some cells, subcellular organelles, or extracellular components. The localization of the dye may either aid in identification of the stained component or provide insight into its function.

Alizarin, used as a vital dye, is taken up selectively by the calcifying matrix of bone that is being deposited at the time of administration of the dye. The newly deposited

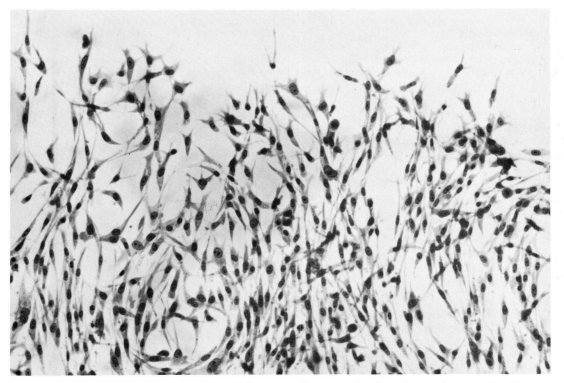

Figure 1-6 Photomicrograph of the edge of the zone of outgrowth of a colony of mouse fibroblasts (see Fig. 1-5). The cells in such a region are free of connective tissue fibers and are favorable for observation in the living state, or in fixed and stained preparations such as this. Harris hematoxylin stain. ×260.

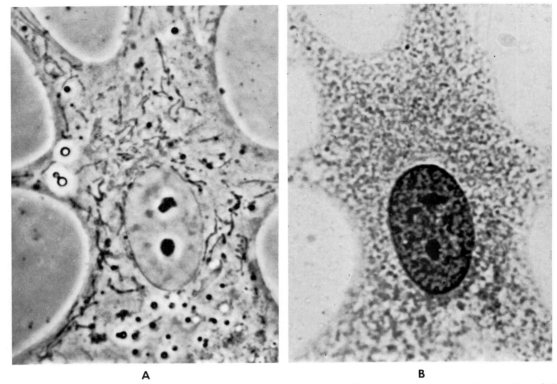

A   **B**

Figure 1–7   *A,* Dark phase contrast photomicrograph of a living fibroblast from a cell culture. Threadlike mitochondria and spherical lipid droplets are clearly visible in the cytoplasm. The cytoplasmic matrix shows little structure and the nucleoplasm is homogeneous except for two prominent nucleoli and a few small karyosomes. *B,* The same cell after fixation in alcohol and staining. The fixation has produced a coarse granular precipitation of the proteins of the cytoplasm and nucleus, and the organelles are no longer visible.

bone is colored red. This classical labeling procedure contributed greatly to our understanding of the mechanism of growth in length and girth of long bones.

Particulate vital dyes, such as trypan blue or lithium carmine, have been widely used to study the phenomenon of *phagocytosis,* a process whereby certain cell types are able to engulf particles from their environment and concentrate them in vacuoles within their cytoplasm. The method is useful for distinguishing certain cell types that are difficult to identify from morphological criteria alone.

The supravital dyes *neutral red* and *Janus green* have been widely used either singly or in combination in studying blood leukocytes. Janus green selectively stains the mitochondria, while neutral red is concentrated in the specific granules of leukocytes, staining the granules of neutrophils light pink, those of eosinophils yellow, and those of basophils

brick red. Janus green has also proved useful in distinguishing mitochondria from other particles isolated from cell homogenates by differential centrifugation. Neutral red is now often used for the identification of lysosomes. Particularly useful in the study of the nervous system has been the ability of methylene blue to stain nerve cells and their processes supravitally under certain conditions.

ISOLATION OF COMPONENTS OF LIVING CELLS BY DIFFERENTIAL CENTRIFUGATION

The function of the various cell organelles can seldom be deduced from morphological observations alone, and their significance was purely conjectural until it became possible to isolate them in bulk and in sufficient purity to permit their biochemical analysis. *Differential centrifugation*, which has become one of the most valuable and widely used methods in biological chemistry, was first developed by the cytologists Bensley and Hoerr in 1934 to separate mitochondria from liver, and in 1937 Bensley made the first chemical analysis of mitochondria. The method was improved some years later by Claude and by Hogeboom, Schneider, and Palade.

In this method, the cells are mechanically disrupted by grinding in glass homogenizers. The resulting homogenate, consisting of a highly heterogeneous suspension of the various cell organelles and inclusions, is layered onto a viscous solution of sucrose and centrifuged at high speed while being maintained at temperatures just above freezing. The heaviest particles are sedimented first, and particles of lower specific densities can be brought down by successive centrifugations at progressively higher speeds (Fig. 1–12). In the case of nuclei and mitochondria, a satisfactory identification and estimate of purity of the fraction can be obtained by examination of the sedimented material with the phase contrast microscope. In the case of microsomes and smaller particles, it is necessary to examine thin sections of the pellets with the electron microscope for morphological identification. Because certain compounds or enzymes have been found to be restricted to a single organelle, these characteristic substances or activities can be used as biochemical markers for identification of centrifugal fractions. Thus deoxyribonucleic acid (DNA) is often used as the identifying marker for a nuclear fraction, succinoxidase or cytochrome oxidase for mitochondria, glucose-6-phosphatase for microsomes, acid phosphatase for lysosomes, and so on.

The newer method of *density gradient centrifugation* is now being widely used because of the improved resolving power of the method and the greater purity of the fractions obtained. The homogenate is layered on top of a stabilized gradient. Prolonged high speed centrifugation causes the particles to sediment only so far as their density permits. They come to rest when they reach a position in the gradient corresponding to their own density.

Centrifugal methods have made it possible to isolate reasonably pure fractions of nuclei, nucleoli, mitochondria, lysosomes, microsomes, ribosomes, pigment granules, and several types of secretory granules (Fig. 1–13). Much of what we know of the chemical composition and enzymatic activities of these cell components is the result of the application of these valuable methods.

PREPARATION AND EXAMINATION OF KILLED TISSUE

Although the histologist seeks to describe and to understand the structure of *living cells* and tissues, the usefulness of direct examination in the living condition is limited by the natural transparency of the tissues, which does not permit easy differentiation of their components, and by their considerable thickness, which interferes with their transillum-

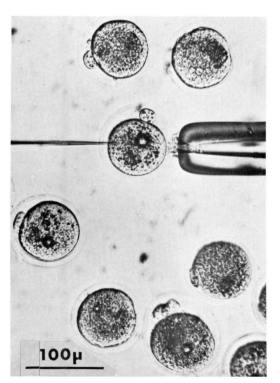

Figure 1–8 Photomicrograph of micromanipulation of mouse ova. The pipette at the right is used to hold the ovum while it is pierced by the micropipette at the left, from which a chemical agent is injected into the cytoplasm. (After T. P. Lin, *Science*, *151*:333, 1966.)

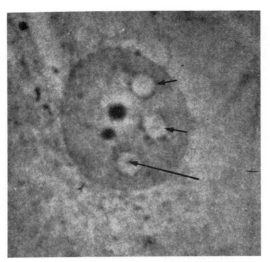

Figure 1–9 Illustration of the potentialities of microbeam irradiation. Living mesothelial cell nucleus of Amblystoma in interphase. It was irradiated three times by the 3 μm. beam of heterochromatic ultraviolet light with a Uretz microbeam. All three areas paled (arrows). In the lowest site of irradiation a bit of chromatin (long arrow) had not paled at the time the cell was photographed. The two dark central bodies are nucleoli.

ination and results in a confusing superimposition of parts. It is usually necessary, therefore, to work with killed, chemically preserved tissues that have been cut into thin slices called *histological sections.* These lend themselves to study by transmitted light and can be stained with various dyes to increase the contrast of the tissue components, so that they can be more easily resolved and recognized with the light microscope. The ideal histological method would be one that resulted in minimum deviation from the condition in the living state and yet permitted maximum resolution of the various components. This goal is difficult to attain, and countless methods of preparing tissues have been developed that claim to approach this ideal more closely in one way or another.

Fixation, Embedding, and Sectioning

The first requirement for preservation of protoplasmic structure is to interrupt the dynamic processes of the cell as promptly as possible and to stabilize the structure with a minimum of change. The essence of the process of *fixation* is to render the structural

components of cells insoluble, and this is accomplished by the use of various chemicals that precipitate the proteins and certain other classes of compounds. It should be borne in mind that in this process structures may be formed that had no precise counterpart in the cell before fixation. Gross distortions that have no basis in the structure of the living cell are referred to as *fixation artifacts.* The best fixatives are those that produce very finely grained precipitates. In general, the more acid the fixative, the more coarsely clumped will be the nuclear material. Because this clumping results in a prominent pattern of chromatin after staining, fixatives producing this result because of their content of picric, acetic, or trichloracetic acid were formerly regarded as "good fixatives." This criterion is no longer accepted. Actually, preparations fixed with solutions containing neutral formalin, osmic acid, and mercuric chloride, singly or in combination, are among the best available for study with the optical microscope. These fixatives produce relatively little clumping of nuclear material and preserve an appearance very close to that of living cells viewed with the phase contrast microscope (Figs. 1–14 and 1–15).

To obtain histological sections that are sufficiently thin for satisfactory examination, it is necessary to infiltrate the tissue after fixation with a solution of gelatin, paraffin, celloidin, or other plastic material, which later solidifies, so that the tissue and the embedding matrix may be sectioned together. The use of paraffin or celloidin requires that the tissue be dehydrated in organic solvents such as ethanol, which remove most of the lipids. Tissues embedded in paraffin may be sectioned rapidly, with a microtome, and may be cut at a thickness of 3 or 4 μm. Embedding with celloidin, which is used at room temperature, disturbs the arrangement of the cells less and causes less shrinkage than does the paraffin method, which requires exposing the tissues to the higher temperatures necessary to keep the wax molten during infiltration. However, infiltration with celloidin is a rather slow process, and sections cannot be cut as thin as those prepared by paraffin embedding.

To avoid the extraction of lipid and other constituents in the process of dehydration, sections of fresh or fixed tissue may also be cut with a freezing microtome after embedding in gelatin or without the use of any embedding medium. The *frozen section* method has the additional advantage of great speed, and it is widely used for surgical biopsies to determine the benign or malignant nature of a lesion while the patient is still on the operating table. In the *freeze-drying method*, the tissue is frozen and then dehydrated at low temperature in a high vacuum. If freezing is carried out with sufficient rapidity to minimize distortions due to ice crystal formation, many structural differences are observable between frozen-dried preparations and those treated with liquid fixatives. This method of dehydration does not render the proteins insoluble, so that additional reagents are required if specimens are to remain "fixed" in aqueous solutions. In the modification of this method, called *freeze-substitution*, the replacement of ice by alcohol or other solvents is carried out at very low temperatures.

Histological Staining

The sections obtained by one of these preparative methods may then be stained by any of a great variety of combinations of dyes that color various tissue constituents more or less selectively. The study of fixed,

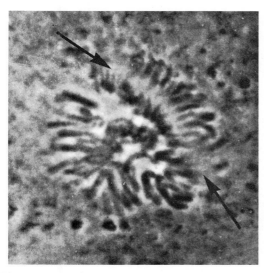

Figure 1–10 Arrows point to "paling" produced in metaphase chromosomes in a living mesothelium cell of Amblystoma by a 3 μm. stripe of ultraviolet light from the Uretz microbeam. Such "paled" areas are Feulgen-negative. Phase contrast photomicrograph of living cell. ×880. (After Bloom and Özarslan, Proc. Nat. Acad. Sci., *53*:1294, 1965.)

sectioned, and stained tissue has long been the principal method of histological investigation, and to it we owe most of what we know now of the microscopic organization of the tissues and organs.

Because living cells are colorless and translucent or transparent, little of their inner structure can be seen without applying one or more biological stains or resorting to phase contrast microscopy (p. 24). The staining methods now in general use were, for the most part, developed empirically, on the basis of their capacity to increase the contrast of the tissue constituents and thus to enable the microscopist to resolve fine structural details. The colors were seldom meaningful as indicators of the chemical nature of the substances stained.

With the most commonly used staining method, *hematoxylin and eosin*, the nuclear structures are stained dark purple or blue, and practically all cytoplasmic structures and intercellular substances are stained varying shades of pink. Actually little else but the character of the nucleus and the extent of the cytoplasm can be seen with this method. To demonstrate other constituents of fixed cells, such as mitochondria, centrioles, and Golgi apparatus, special cytological staining methods must be used. A single staining method does not suffice to reveal all of the functionally significant components of cells that can be preserved by use of appropriate fixatives. Some of the striking differences in the effects of a few of the commonly used fixing and staining agents are shown in Figure 1–14, of cells from the small intestine of the guinea pig. Nuclei appear to have a clearly defined membrane, a prominent body called the nucleolus, and darkly staining granules (chromatin) embedded in a pale ground substance. The cells fixed in neutral formalin and Zenker-formol show much the same structures, although the latter reveals more chromatin material. After treatment with absolute alcohol and two distinctly acid fixatives (Bouin and Zenker-acetic), nuclei have heavily clumped, prominent chromatin. This figure also shows the differences in the effect of these fixatives on mitochondria. These cellular constituents are seen with difficulty in the living cell viewed with bright field microscopy, but are obvious as blue rods and granules after supravital staining with Janus green. They are black in the cells stained with Heidenhain's iron-hematoxylin after fixation

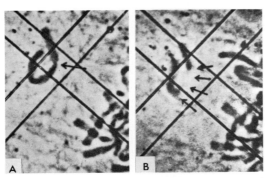

Figure 1–11 Effect of localized ultraviolet irradiation of a portion of a metaphase chromosome of Amblystoma. *A*, Before irradiation, during metaphase (kinetochore at arrow). *B*, Immediately after irradiation, the irradiated segment became "pale," as indicated by the arrows. Phase contrast microscopy. Prints from 16 mm. motion picture film. Each print represents an area 30 × 40 μm. (After Uretz, Bloom, and Zirkle, Science, *120*:197, 1954.)

with hematoxylin-eosin-azure II, one after Zenker-formol fixation and the other a frozen-dried preparation treated with alcohol, should be compared, since the other cells shown in the figure were fixed by the latter method. Toluidine blue is frequently substituted for hematoxylin-eosin-azure II to demonstrate basophilic components. This dye stains both deoxyribo- and ribonucleoprotein. To distinguish staining attributable to one or the other of these, the section can be digested with the enzyme ribonuclease prior to staining. Because the ribonuclease solution may have solvent action other than that due to the enzyme, a better comparison may be made with a section treated with buffer solution. After selective removal of ribonucleoprotein, the areas still stained with toluidine blue can be identified as deoxyribonucleoprotein. Components containing deoxyribonucleoprotein can also be identified

with neutral formalin or Zenker-formol, but are not visible with this stain after Bouin or Zenker-acetic fixation because the mitochondria are destroyed by these highly acid mixtures. Neither are they visible in cells stained with hematoxylin and eosin (H and E) after use of any of these fixatives.

At the extreme right of Figure 1–14 are three cells from the epithelium of guinea pig small intestine, which was dehydrated in the frozen state and sectioned. The sections were then treated with alcohol and stained by the periodate-leukofuchsin method (periodic acid–Schiff or PAS reaction) for insoluble *carbohydrates* and by hematoxylin and eosin to reveal general cell structure. Inasmuch as the cells of the intestine change their shape greatly with the extensive movements of this organ, differences in the size and shape of these cells as shown in Figure 1–14 are not to be ascribed to the influence of the various fixing agents used. However, the impression that the cells and their nuclei are larger when living than after histological preparation is correct.

Some of the features to be seen in unfixed and fixed liver cells with special staining reactions are illustrated in Figure 1–15. Here the usual appearance in hematoxylin and eosin preparations after Zenker-formol fixation is shown. By addition of azure II, additional basophilic regions of nucleus and cytoplasm are revealed. The two cells stained

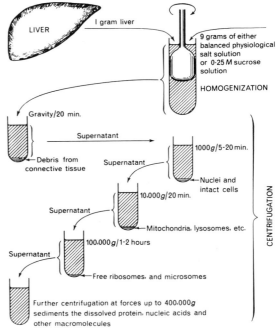

Figure 1–12 A diagram showing the successive stages in fractionation of cell components. The cells are disrupted by the shearing forces created in the homogenizer. Connective tissue fibers and other debris sediment on standing. The supernatant is then centrifuged at a series of increasing speeds and pellets of the various organelles are recovered as indicated. (Modified after K. B. Roberts, *in* G. H. Haggis et al.: Introduction to Molecular Biology. New York, John Wiley & Sons, Inc., 1964.)

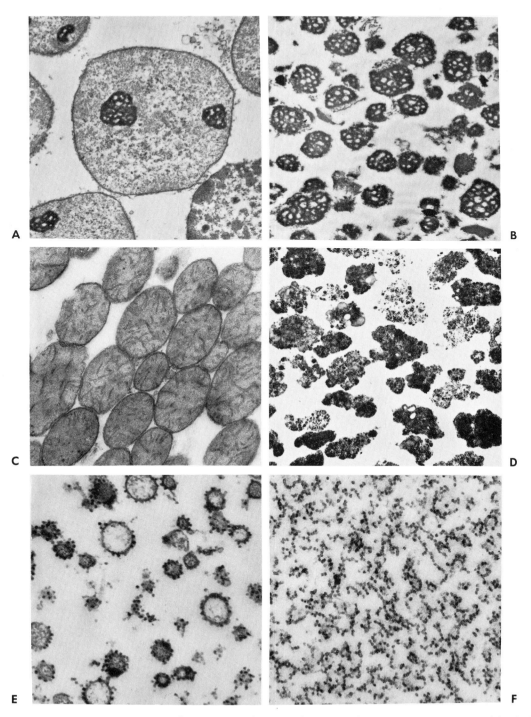

Figure 1–13 Electron micrographs of the pellets of various fractions of cell homogenates isolated by differential centrifugation. *A,* Liver cell nuclei. ×5000. *B,* Liver cell nucleoli. ×16,000. (*A* and *B* after R. Maggio, P. Siekevitz, and G. E. Palade, J. Cell Biol., *18:*267, 293, 1963.) *C,* Liver mitochondria. (Courtesy of S. Malamed.) *D,* Lipofuscin pigment granules from cardiac muscle. (Courtesy of S. Björkerud.) *E,* Microsomes from pancreas. (Courtesy of G. E. Palade.) *F,* Ribosomes from pancreas. (Courtesy of G. E. Palade.)

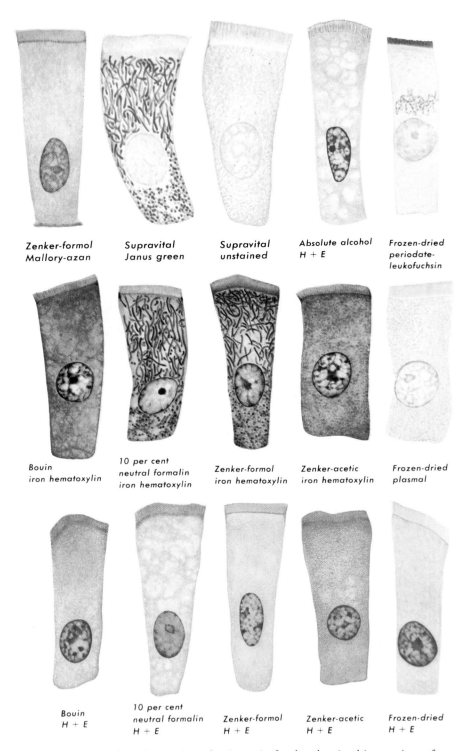

Zenker-formol
Mallory-azan

Supravital
Janus green

Supravital
unstained

Absolute alcohol
H + E

Frozen-dried
periodate-
leukofuchsin

Bouin
iron hematoxylin

10 per cent
neutral formalin
iron hematoxylin

Zenker-formol
iron hematoxylin

Zenker-acetic
iron hematoxylin

Frozen-dried
plasmal

Bouin
H + E

10 per cent
neutral formalin
H + E

Zenker-formol
H + E

Zenker-acetic
H + E

Frozen-dried
H + E

Figure 1–14 Epithelial cells of small intestine of guinea pig fixed and stained in a variety of ways to empha-size the extreme importance of choice of method for the preservation, demonstration, and study of cyto-plasmic and nuclear structures. For explanation, see text. ×1620.

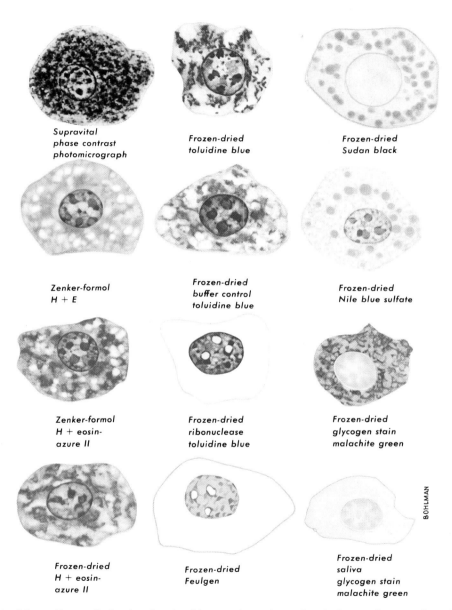

Supravital
phase contrast
photomicrograph

Frozen-dried
toluidine blue

Frozen-dried
Sudan black

Zenker-formol
H + E

Frozen-dried
buffer control
toluidine blue

Frozen-dried
Nile blue sulfate

Zenker-formol
H + eosin-
azure II

Frozen-dried
ribonuclease
toluidine blue

Frozen-dried
glycogen stain
malachite green

Frozen-dried
H + eosin-
azure II

Frozen-dried
Feulgen

Frozen-dried
saliva
glycogen stain
malachite green

Figure 1–15 Mouse liver cells fixed and stained by a variety of cytochemical procedures to show distribution of deoxyribonucleic acid, ribonucleic acid, and lipid droplets. As these tests were all done on material fixed by freezing and drying, some of the sections are compared with similarly stained sections fixed by Zenker-formol. For further orientation, the fixed cell stained by hematoxylin and eosin and the unfixed cell photographed by phase contrast are also shown. ×1500. (Courtesy of I. Gersh.)

by their specific staining with the Feulgen reaction. The glycogen and other carbohydrates in such cells are shown by the periodate-leukofuchsin (PAS) reaction. The effect of prior treatment with saliva on such preparations is also shown. The loss of red staining being due to removal of glycogen by amylase in the saliva, fatty components can be demonstrated if fat solvents are avoided in fixation and dehydration; they are colored with Sudan black and Nile blue. In the cell stained with Nile blue sulfate, the blue component is nonspecific, but the salmon-pink staining occurs in fat droplets.

By use of various methods of fixation and staining, many structures can be demonstrated within the cell. These are artificial to the extent that the structures in fixed material are not the same as those in the living cell, nor are all the structures of the living cell still present in any given preparation. However, with the same fixation and staining methods, the factors of artificiality are constant and the appearance of the cells is reproducible. With improved optical methods for studying living cells, evidence has been found for the presence in the living cell of most of the important structures that had been described on the basis of fixed and stained preparations. The comparison of their form in living and in fixed cells is facilitated by use of phase microscopy and by supravital staining.

THE CHEMICAL BASIS OF HISTOLOGICAL STAINING

In general, the mechanism of the binding of dyes to tissue components is not known, but experiments with model systems (Singer) suggest that it is not too great an oversimplification to assume that in some examples of staining, anionic and cationic dyes form electrostatic (salt) linkages with ionizable radicals of proteins, glycoproteins, and lipoproteins in the tissue section. These constituents of protoplasm are *amphoteric*; that is, they can ionize either as bases or as acids depending upon the pH and certain other conditions in their environment. Whether a protein behaves as an acid or as a base depends upon its net charge—the algebraic sum of its positive and negative charges at the pH at which the staining is carried out. For each kind of protein there

is a pH at which the number of positive charges equals the number of negative charges. This is called its *isoelectric point*. At this pH it stains poorly, but above its isoelectric point, ionization of its anionic groups is favored and it will bind basic (cationic) dyes such as *methylene blue* or *basic fuchsin*. Below its isoelectric point the same protein will have a net positive charge and will combine with acidic (anionic) dyes such as *eosin*, *orange G*, or *light green*.

Proteins of the tissues differ greatly in the relative abundance of their constituent amino acids and therefore have very different isoelectric points. Thus, at the pH ordinarily used for histological staining, some components stain more readily with basic dyes and are said to be *basophilic*, while others, at the same pH, take up acidic dyes and are said to be *acidophilic*. For example, red blood cells, the granules of eosinophilic leukocytes, and the cytoplasm of parietal cells in the stomach all stain with acid dyes at pH 6, while the chromatin of cell nuclei, the ergastoplasm of the cytoplasm in glandular cells and neurons, and the hyaline matrix of cartilage all bind basic dyes. The histologist is therefore able, in a general way, to categorize tissue components on the basis of their affinities for acid or basic dyes under specified staining conditions.

It is important to realize, however, that only a limited number of staining methods involve electrostatic linkages between the dye and the tissue. Hematoxylin, for example, stains chromatin under many conditions and does not behave simply as a basic dye. Some of the most widely used staining methods, such as Mallory's trichrome, Masson's stain, and Heidenhain's azan, combine two or three acid dyes, and the mechanism by which they stain various tissue components differentially is not known. Although these methods provide no insight into the chemical nature of the components stained, they are nevertheless extremely useful to the histologist in providing the contrast necessary for visualization of various components that otherwise would not be distinguishable.

Histochemical and Cytochemical Procedures

Through their desire to get away from the purely empirical use of dyestuffs for improvement of contrast, and to go beyond the description of structure without regard for function, histologists have developed a large number of so-called histochemical methods. *Histochemistry* can be defined as the application to histological preparations of physical and chemical methods of analysis that permit identification of chemical substances in their normal sites in tissues. It differs from biochemistry in its greater emphasis upon the localization of chemical events to particular cellular or subcellular components, and it often provides valuable information that cannot be obtained by the analysis of tissue homogenates. It includes a group of *chemical methods* that permit (1) identification of lipids by their uptake of certain fat soluble dyes; (2) the staining of carbohydrates by means of a reagent that produces a colored compound with the products of their oxidation; (3) the demonstration of deoxyribonucleoprotein by staining of a specific aldehyde group made available by mild hydrolysis; and (4) the localization of numerous enzymes. These latter methods depend upon

incubation of tissue sections with substrates that yield insoluble hydrolytic products that are either already colored or capable of being detected by subsequent conversion to a colored compound.

A group of *physical methods* takes advantage of (1) absorption of ultraviolet light at specific wavelengths to identify and localize nucleoproteins (ultraviolet spectrophotometry); (2) absorption of x-rays of selected wavelengths by calcium and other elements (historadiography); (3) emission of x-rays of specific wavelengths by elements bombarded by an electron beam (electron microprobe analysis); and (4) emission of ionizing particles from unstable isotopes incorporated in tissue components (autoradiography).

Chemical Methods. The requirements for an ideal histochemical procedure that depend upon chemical reactions are the following: (1) the preparation of the tissue section should be carried out without alteration of the position of the chemical constituent being studied; (2) the reaction should

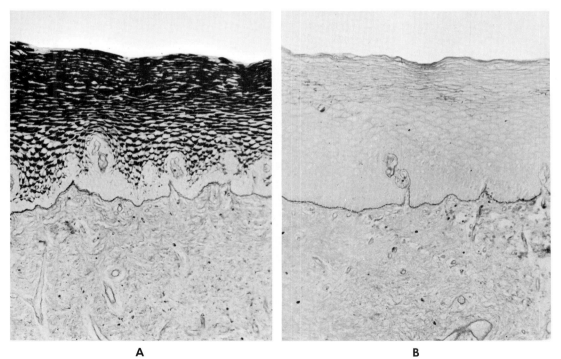

A   B

Figure 1–16   *A,* Photomicrograph of human vaginal epithelium stained with the periodic-acid Schiff (PAS) reaction for carbohydrates. *B,* An adjacent section stained in the same way after digestion with salivary amylase. The abolition of the intense staining of the epithelium by enzymatic digestion demonstrates that the material responsible was glycogen. The faint residual staining is due to protein-polysaccharides of the connective tissue ground substance.

be specific for this substance; and (3) the reaction product should be intensely colored, so that it can be readily visualized with the microscope. In practice, few methods completely satisfy all of these requirements, but many approach them closely enough to be useful. One of the most widely used of this category of staining methods is a group reaction for the identification of carbohydrates, called the periodic acid—Schiff reaction (PAS reaction). In this test the section is exposed to periodic acid, which oxidizes hydroxyl groups on adjacent carbon atoms or adjacent hydroxyl and amino groups to produce aldehydes. The section is then stained with the Schiff reagent, fuchsinsulfurous acid, which forms an addition product with aldehydes to produce a red or magenta reaction product. This widely used method stains glycogen, epithelial mucins, neutral polysaccharides, and glycoproteins. A positive staining reaction in one section that can be abolished by digestion of a parallel section with the enzyme diastase identifies the substance staining as glycogen (Fig. 1–16).

A similar principle is involved in the Feulgen reaction, a highly specific histochemical method for deoxyribonucleoprotein (DNA). The tissue is subjected to mild hydrolysis to remove the purine group of DNA and make available the aldehyde group of deoxyribose. Subsequent treatment with the Schiff reagent results in staining of the DNA of the nuclear chromatin. The Feulgen reaction is perhaps the most specific of the histochemical staining reactions; it owes its specificity to the presence of an aldehyde in deoxyribose and to the fact that no naturally occurring substance other than DNA will yield an aldehyde group under the conditions of gentle hydrolysis employed in this method.

Representative of the methods for enzymes is the classical Gomori-Takamatsu procedure for alkaline phosphatase. A tissue section is incubated in a buffered solution containing the substrate, glycerophosphate, and calcium ions. As hydrolysis of the substrate releases phosphoric acid, it combines with calcium and precipitates as calcium phosphate. This colorless precipitate is converted to brown cobalt sulfide, which is readily visualized with the microscope. It is to be noted that, in methods for enzymes based upon this principle, it is not the enzyme itself that is stained but the product of the enzyme-catalyzed reaction. Diffusion of the reaction product may therefore result in false localization, but methods have been devised for minimizing artifacts of this kind. Methods are now available for localizing a great many enzymes (Figs. 1–17 and 1–18).

Physical Methods. Several useful methods in this category depend upon selective absorption at particular wavelengths in the spectrum of electromagnetic radiation (Fig. 1–25).

ULTRAVIOLET MICROSPECTROPHOTOMETRY. Nucleic acids have the property of absorbing ultraviolet light at a wavelength of 2600 Å. Thus, if intact cells or histological sections being transilluminated with ultraviolet at this wavelength are photographed,

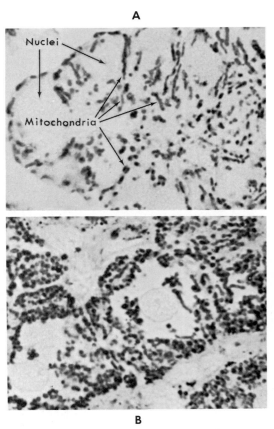

Figure 1-17 Histochemical reaction for an enzyme, showing exceptionally precise localization. *A,* Section of pancreas stained for succinic dehydrogenase. The nuclei and cytoplasm are unstained, but the mitochondria exhibit a strong reaction for the enzyme. *B,* Section of liver, showing a similar localization of the enzyme. (After D. G. Walker and A. Seligman, J. Cell Biol., *16:*455, 1963).

the dark areas in the resulting image will represent the sites of highest concentration of nucleic acids (Fig. 1–19). To ascertain whether nucleic acid absorption in a particular area is due to the presence of ribonucleoprotein or to deoxyribonucleoprotein, the preparation can be photographed before and after digestion with the enzymes ribonuclease or deoxyribonuclease. Areas of absorption removed by a specific enzyme can then be attributed to the corresponding substrate.

HISTORADIOGRAPHY. Absorption of soft x-rays can be related to particular elements in a tissue sample. A thin section of bone, for example, is placed in contact with a fine grained photographic emulsion and exposed to a beam of x-rays at a critical absorption wavelength for calcium. The light areas in the resulting historadiogram represent areas of specific absorption and reflect the distribution of the bone mineral in the section (Fig. 1–20). By densitometric comparison with suitable standards, it is possible to determine the quantity of calcium per unit area with a fairly high degree of accuracy.

It should be pointed out that, as is the case with ultraviolet light, it is the *contrast* afforded by differences in x-ray absorption (in this case, of individual atoms) that is utilized in such techniques as *contact historadiography* and *projection x-ray microscopy*. In these techniques, resolution is not particularly high.

ELECTRON MICROPROBE ANALYSIS. An approach not yet in general use but showing promise of fruitful biological application is the electron probe microanalyzer. In this complex instrument a slender electron beam of low accelerating potential strikes the tissue section, exciting the emission of long wavelength x-rays from a small area of the specimen. An analyzer set for the wavelength characteristic of the element of interest measures the emission in a proportional counter. At the same time, the distribution of the element in the specimen can be recorded in an image in which the pattern of light areas reflects the location and relative abundance of the emitting element (Fig. 1–21). By changing the setting of the analyzer to a new wavelength, the topographical abundance of another element can be recorded from the same specimen. The instrument has the capability of quantitative analysis for

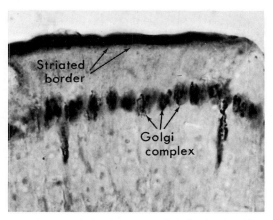

Figure 1–18 A further example of selective histochemical localization of enzymatic activity. A section of epithelium from rat duodenum incubated in the substrate thiamine pyrophosphate for 10 minutes at 37° C., showing localization of phosphatase in the Golgi complex and the striated border. (After A. B. Novikoff et al., *in* R. J. C. Harris, ed.: The Interpretation of Ultrastructure. New York, Academic Press, 1962.)

all elements heavier than fluorine with an error of only a few per cent and a limit of detection as low as fifty parts per million. Its limitations for biological application reside in considerable beam damage to the specimen and in the relatively poor resolution, which at present is probably no better than 5 μm. There appears to be no insuperable technical obstacle, however, to the development of the smaller beams that would provide the resolution needed for regional analysis within cells of ordinary size.

AUTORADIOGRAPHY (RADIOAUTOGRAPHY). A method of extraordinary importance for the tracing of specific substances in the body and for the localization of metabolic events in cells and tissues is autoradiography. When a substance containing a radioactive isotope is injected into an animal, subsequent preparation of autoradiographs makes it possible to detect and establish the location of the labeled compound in the tissues. A histological section containing radioactive material is coated with a photographic emulsion in the dark and put away in a light-tight box to "expose" for a period of days or weeks. The ionizing particles emitted in radioactive decay of the isotope within the tissue strike silver bromide crystals in the overlying emulsion, producing a "latent image" that is sub-

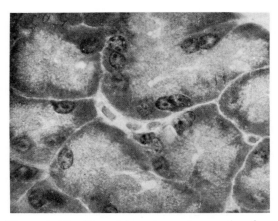

Figure 1-19 Ultraviolet photomicrograph of an unstained section of rabbit pancreas, illustrating the marked absorption by nuclear and cytoplasmic nucleotides that results in an appearance very similar to that found after staining with basic dyes. The absorbing material can be removed by ribo- and deoxyribonuclease. (After T. O. Caspersson, Cell Growth and Cell Function. New York, W. W. Norton Co., 1950.)

sequently "developed" with photographic developer and appears as black dots over the section when the preparation is examined under the microscope. The black spots produced in the emulsion betray the location of the radioactive substance in the underlying tissue section, and it is possible in this way to localize the label with a resolution of 1 to 2 μm. using the light microscope. With the thinner layers of emulsion and the ultrathin sections employed for electron microscopy, the resolution of the method is about 0.2 μm. Autoradiography at the electron microscope level therefore has sufficient precision to make it a valuable technique for localization of substances *within* cells. It can only reveal compounds that are taken up and incorporated into tissue components at sites that are metabolically active during the brief period between injection of the radioactive ("labeled") material and its excretion from the body. This limitation, in a sense, makes the method more valuable than methods for simple identification of stable substances already present in the tissues, because it means that injection of labeled precursors and their subsequent localization in cell products by autoradiography makes it possible to study the dynamics of metabolic processes. This approach has

been employed to study the sequential participation of the various cell organelles in the synthesis and release of various secretions (see Chapter 4).

Another kind of application of autoradiography employs the same principle used in bird banding and enables the investigator to tag the nuclei of cells, so that the marked cells can be traced in the course of their morphogenetic migrations during early development. Tritium labeled thymidine injected into an embryo is incorporated into the deoxyribonucleic acid (DNA) of the nucleus in all of those cells that are preparing for cell division at the time of the injection. The nuclei of these cells and their daughter cells will then be labeled, while those cells that are in other stages of interphase or are not dividing at all will remain unlabeled. Thus such complex problems as the histogenesis of the brain of experimental animals can be approached by preparing autoradiographs of embryos at successive times after administration of labeled thymidine. The path taken by the labeled cells can then be plotted from their site of origin to their ultimate destination in the cerebral cortex. This is proving to be one of the most valuable of the modern morphological methods for studying certain functional and developmental processes.

Immunohistochemical Methods. A highly sensitive method for localization of specific proteins or polysaccharides in tissues is the fluorescent antibody technique. This takes advantage of the fact that the body recognizes foreign protein substances, *antigens*, and makes specific macromolecules called *antibodies* that combine with and inactivate the antigens. The discovery that fluorescent dye molecules could be chemically linked to antibody molecules without interfering with their capacity to react specifically with antigen has opened up a new approach to histochemical localization (Coons). For example, if it is desired to localize the muscle protein, myosin, in mouse tissue, purified myosin from mouse muscle can be injected into a rabbit. In due course the rabbit's blood serum contains antibodies produced against the antigenic mouse myosin. These are precipitated from blood serum, purified, and conjugated in vitro with the fluorescent dye *fluorescein*. This product is then used as a staining reagent. When flooded onto a histological section, the fluorescent antimyosin antibody combines specifically with myosin. When the excess is washed off and the preparation is examined with ultraviolet light under the microscope, the sites of the antigen-antibody complex appear as bright yellow luminescent areas against a dark background (Fig. 1–24). The method has been successfuly used to establish the cell of origin of protein hormones, the intracellular location of various enzymes, and the sites of synthesis of serum albumin (Fig. 1–24C), as well as in many other problems.

Instead of being coupled to the specific antibody, the fluorochrome can be coupled to an antibody against globulins of the species originally reacting to antigen. By this indirect method, the site of antibody production has been localized in the plasma cells (Fig. 6–21).

PRINCIPLES OF MICROSCOPIC ANALYSIS

The principal instrument in histology and cytology is, of course, the *compound microscope*. This basic instrument has been modified in various ways, so that in addition to the common light microscope, we now have available the *phase contrast microscope*, the *interference microscope*, the *polarizing microscope*, the *fluorescence microscope*, and the *ultraviolet microscope*. Each has its own advantages for special purposes and its limitations. These will be considered below after a preliminary discussion of the general principles of microscopic analysis. *Throughout this book, unless otherwise indicated, "microscope" refers to the light microscope using visible light.*

Beams of different wavelengths from different segments of the spectrum of electromagnetic radiation can be thought of as optical probes of varying degrees of coarseness or fineness. The prime considerations in the microscopic analysis of minute structure are that (1) the probe being utilized must not be appreciably larger than the detail to be seen; (2) the probe and the object being investigated must interact; and (3) it must be possible to observe and to interpret this interaction. In no case does the image formed in a microscope ever correspond exactly with the object from which it originates. Certain general rules and considerations governing the relation between object

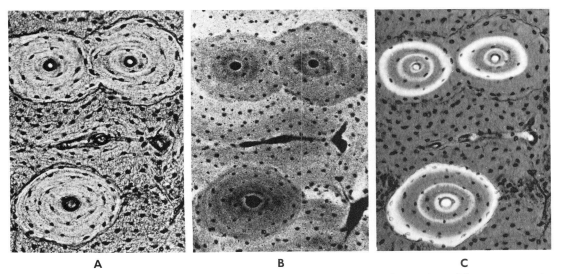

| A | B | C |

Figure 1–20 Photomicrographs of bone, illustrating applications of historadiography and fluorescence microscopy. A ground section of bone from a young dog that had received two courses of treatment with a fluorescent tetracycline compound 19 days apart. *A*, Ordinary microscopy. Three newly formed haversian systems are seen. *B*, In a historadiogram of the same section, the differing shades from black to white reflect the differing concentrations of calcium. In the haversian canals there has been no absorption of the x-rays and the film is therefore black. The areas containing the greatest concentration of calcium are white and regions of intermediate degrees of calcification exhibit shades of gray. *C*, Fluorescence microscopy detects, as two concentric bright rings, the fluorescent tetracycline compound incorporated into the bone during the two periods of treatment. (Courtesy of R. Amprino and R. Marotti.)

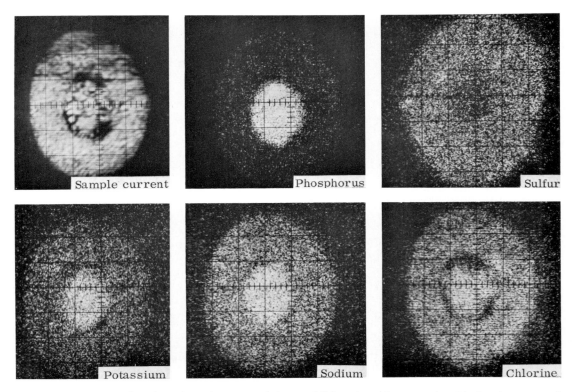

Figure 1–21 Images of nucleated erythrocytes of the amphibian, Amphiuma, made with the electron probe microanalyzer. At the upper left is a sample current image for orientation. The remaining represent analyses for the elements indicated. The light areas represent regions of high concentration of the element. (Courtesy of J. P. Revel and C. A. Anderson.)

and image are applicable to quite diverse, and at first glance unrelated, methods of microscopic analysis.

To begin with, the terms *resolution* and *magnification*, which are used to characterize the performance of a microscope, must be carefully distinguished. Of the two, resolution, or resolving power, is by far the more important criterion. The resolving power of an analytic system is a measure, generally in terms of linear distance, of the smallest degree of separation at which two details can still be distinguished from each other. Magnification, which is the ratio of image size to object size, simply gives us the scale by which we relate object dimensions to image dimensions. Magnification is a useful criterion for ensuring that the image is brought to sufficient size so that all of the resolved detail may be easily viewed. Clearly, any image is capable of indefinite magnification (a photographic transparency may be projected on as large a screen as we care to choose), but once an image is large enough that all of the resolved detail it contains may be viewed comfortably, any further enlargement becomes "empty" rather than "useful" magnification.

The Light Microscope

Historically, the most used and familiar histological probe has been visible light, observed and analyzed in the classical light microscope in its interactions with biological objects. The probe size to be associated with this light is roughly that of its wavelength, or about 0.5 μm. Resolution in the microscope is further determined by the *numerical apertures* of the objective and condenser lenses. Numerical aperture is a measure of the size or angle of the cone of light delivered by the illuminating condenser lens to the object plane and of the cone of light emerging from the object that is collected by the objective lens. Light coming through fine details of the object is diffracted into directions different from that of its original propagation, and the finer the detail involved, the wider the angle over which this light is diffracted. This is analogous to the diffraction and spreading of light coming through small pinholes. Numerical aperture, then, is a measure of the ability of the microscope to collect diffracted light from fine details in the object. The overall resolving power of a well constructed light microscope of high numerical aperture approaches the theoretical limit and is approximately 0.25 μm.

The capacity of the *compound microscope* to reveal structural detail depends upon differences in *absorption* of light by the parts to be differentiated. We commented earlier upon the fact that tissue components are largely transparent. The usefulness of this instrument in biology and medicine depends largely upon the fact that differences in absorption (opacity) can be created by histological staining, and this makes it possible to distinguish components that would otherwise escape detection.

However, even for highly transparent objects, information is available in the image in the form of phase differences, and the methods of *phase* and *interference microscopy* (see pp. 24 and 25) can be used to convert these phase differences into contrasting intensity differences.

Understanding the concept of *index of refraction* and its underlying molecular basis is essential to an understanding of the phase, interference, and polarizing microscopes. Index of refraction is a measure of the rate of propagation of a light wave, or other electromagnetic impulse, through a given medium, and is defined as the ratio of the velocity of light in vacuo to its velocity in the medium. Even for a highly transparent, nonabsorbing medium, there can be a considerable interaction between the medium and a passing light wave or other electromagnetic disturbance. The electrons associated with the atoms and molecules of the medium can oscillate in response to the alternating electric field associated with the passing light. In so doing, these moving electrons act as miniature antennas and radiate secondary energy. This secondary radiation interacts with the primary light coming through. In general, the net result is a retardation in the phase of the oscillating electric field at any point in comparison with what it would have been had

the secondary radiation not been present. This leads to a lowering of the velocity of propagation of the light through the medium. The intensity of this secondary radiation, and, hence, the velocity of propagation through the medium, depends on the freedom of the electrons to respond to the field and will be determined by the wavelength of the light and by the nature of the structure being traversed.

Light coming through an object of higher refractive index will be retarded with respect to light passing through a surrounding medium of lower refractive index; that is, the alternating electromagnetic field of the light wave will be displaced in time relative to the light coming through the sur-

A

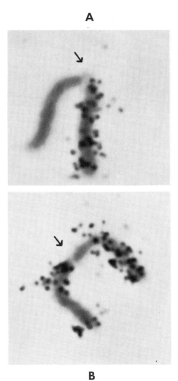

B

Figure 1-22 Autoradiography can be used at the light microscope level to study the distribution of tritium labeled DNA in chromosomes during meiotic division. The dyads shown here are from cells that incorporated labeled thymidine one cell cycle before premeiotic interphase. The arrows indicate the terminal centromeres. In *A,* the silver grains are over one chromatid only and there are no visible exchanges. In *B,* there have been reciprocal exchanges of labeled and unlabeled segments of sister chromatids. (After J. H. Taylor, J. Cell Biol., 25:57, 1965.)

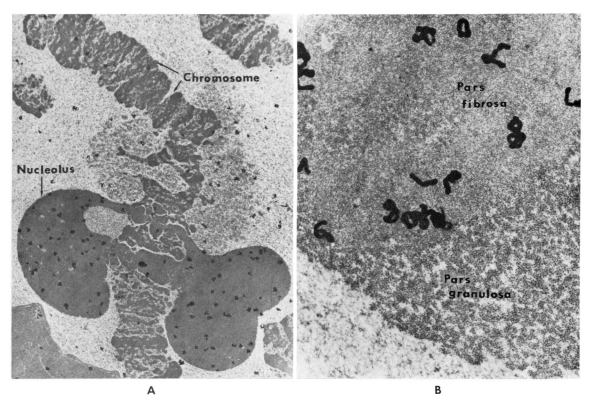

A   B

Figure 1–23 *A*, Electron microscopic autoradiograph of a longitudinal section through chromosome IV of *Chironomus thummi* with its attached nucleolus and an adjacent Balbiani ring. Fingerlike nucleolar processes extend into the chromosome. At this time interval, 27 hours after injection of tritiated uridine, silver grains are distributed over the entire nucleolus and somewhat less abundantly over the Balbiani ring, indicating incorporation into RNA in these sites. (After B. von Gaudecker, Zeitschr. f. Zellforsch., 1967.) *B*, Higher magnification autoradiograph showing silver grains over the pars fibrosa but not the pars granulosa of the nucleolus 13 minutes after injection of ^{3}H-uridine. At 46 hours after the injection (not shown here), most of the label is over the pars granulosa. Thus the resolution of autoradiography at the electron microscope level is good enough to demonstrate that RNA in the fibrous region of the nucleolus subsequently moves into the granular region. (After B. von Gaudecker, Zeitschr. f. Zellforsch., 1967.)

rounding medium. The total retardation of the light wave will be a function of both the index of refraction and the thickness of the object.

The Phase Contrast Microscope

This is essentially an optical device for converting small differences in refractive index that cannot be appreciated by the eye into differences in *intensity* that can be seen. It therefore renders visible certain components of living cells that can ordinarily be seen only in killed stained material (Fig. 1–7). In the image plane of the light microscope, light arriving from areas corresponding to transparent regions of the specimen with an index of refraction different from that of their surroundings will be out of phase with the surrounding light. However, the ordinary light microscope is not sensitive to such phase differences and will therefore show no difference in intensity between these various regions, and hence no contrast. The phase contrast microscope is equipped with special apertures and with absorbing and phase-shifting plates. These serve (1) to partially separate from the background illumination the diffracted light scattered at wide angles from small transparent specimen details, and (2) to shift the phase and intensity of these two components of the light in such a way that they interact in the image plane to produce intensity differences and contrast where only phase differences had been present before.

The phase contrast microscope suffers several major defects: (1) there are halos around the images because of incomplete separation of the background light from the diffracted light; (2) only phase differences from small objects or from border regions of rapidly changing retardation are converted into intensity differences; and (3) in the commonly used phase microscopes, each phase contrast objective is designed to work optimally for only a limited range of retardations.

The Interference Microscope

The interference microscope is designed for observing the same kind of refractile detail in specimens as is the phase microscope, but it utilizes the more straightforward principle of sending two separate beams of light through the specimen. These two beams are then recombined with each other in the image plane. One beam is focused through the detail under observation and the other, a comparison beam, is focused in a neutral area, beside or above or below the observed detail. This instrument allows the direct quantitative measurement of retardation and of the related quantities of index of refraction and thickness, without the presence of halos and with independence of detail size. Such measurements of retardation can be used to measure dry mass per unit area of specimens and to do contour mapping of small objects.

The interference microscope is a more versatile instrument than the phase microscope and the only one of the two to be considered for quantitative measurements. However, it is a more expensive and more cumbersome instrument and, for many types of qualitative observation, the phase microscope is to be preferred. A recent development is differential interference (Nomarski) optics, which are designed to detect localized

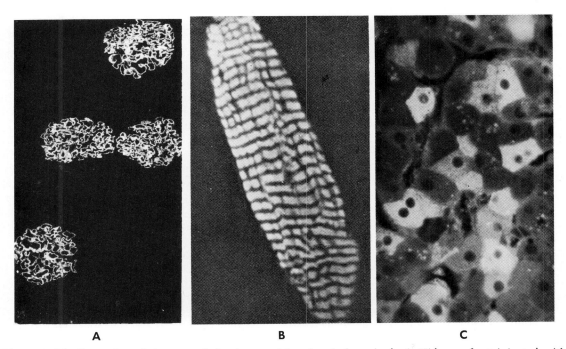

A   B   C

Figure 1-24 Examples of the use of the immunohistochemical method. *A*, Kidney of rat injected with heterologous nephrotoxic α-globulin which binds to the glomerular basement membrane. The antigen is localized by fluorescein-conjugated antibody. (From Hoedmaker et al.: *Lab. Invest.* 26:612, 1972. © 1972, U.S.-Canadian Division of the International Academy of Pathology.) *B*, Chicken muscle stained with antibody against chicken myosin. The fluorescent antibody localizes myosin in the A bands. ×1300. (After H. Finck, H. Holtzer, and J. M. Marshall, J. Biophys. & Biochem. Cytol. [Suppl.], 2:175, 1956.) *C*, Human liver section stained with fluorescent antihuman serum albumin, which localizes serum albumin in certain liver cells and not in others. (After Y. Hamashima, J. G. Harter, and A. J. Coons, J. Cell Biol., 20:271, 1964.)

gradients in refractive index and, in many cases, give most excellent results in the detection of fine transparent detail.

The Polarizing Microscope

Constituents of cells and tissues that are crystalline or fibrous show a high degree of molecular orientation. When a ray of plane polarized light strikes such an object, it acts as if it were split into two rays polarized in planes perpendicular to one another. These two rays have different velocities. Such an object is said to be birefringent. Another way of looking at it is that objects with a high degree of molecular orientation have a different refractive index depending upon the plane of vibration of the ray of polarized light with respect to the orientation of the molecules. This occurs when the cloud of electrons associated with the atoms and molecules of the structure is not free to move equally in all directions under the influence of an external electromagnetic field, or when some other ordering or layering of the structure is present on a scale smaller than the wavelength of the light used. Such ordered structures possessing more than one index of refraction can be studied with the polarizing microscope, which restricts the probing light to preferred directions and orientations and makes it possible to detect the presence of orderly arrangements of fibrous proteins or other arrays of long molecules, even though the molecules are not visible. It is, then, a device that can indirectly provide information about structural arrangement at the molecular level, and it can be applied to the living cell.

The Fluorescence Microscope

Another form of visible light microscopy that is coming into rapidly increasing use is fluorescence microscopy. In this technique light of one wavelength is used to illuminate the specimen. The image seen is the result of emission from molecules that have absorbed the primary exciting light and then re-emitted light of longer wavelength and lower energy. Suitable filters are placed both below the condenser and above the objective to ensure that only the desired secondary emission from the specimen will contribute to the observed image. Under these conditions, the specimen behaves as if it were "self-luminous." The secondary emission may be from naturally occurring "fluorochromes" in the specimens, or from introduced fluorescent dyes bound to certain specific components of the specimen, or from fluorescent dyes coupled to specific antibodies. Owing to the great contrast and specificity inherent in the fluorescent image, this microscopic technique is one with great promise and importance for the future.

The Ultraviolet Microscope

In order to obtain resolution greater than that of the visible light microscope, we must find finer probes. One step in this direction is to use ultraviolet light, with the aid of quartz or reflecting lenses, instead of visible light. Its wavelength of approximately 0.25 μm. allows, in principle, a gain of a factor of two in the smallest spacings that can be resolved. However, in practice the ultraviolet microscope has been used more for the natural contrast it provides, owing to the absorption of nucleic acids and proteins in the ultraviolet region, than for any small increase in resolution.

The Transmission Electron Microscope

A system analogous to that of the visible light microscope, but utilizing very much smaller probes, is that of the electron microscope. In this system, the ordinary light source is replaced by electrons emitted by a tungsten filament, their effective wavelength being determined by the voltage by which they are accelerated; shaped magnetic or electric fields take the place of glass lenses, and a fluorescent screen replaces the human eye for direct viewing. In practice, the requirements of a vacuum-enclosed system, high voltage, and mechanical stability, plus the special treatment and preparation of samples, make for a highly complex and costly microscope system. But it is one well worth the expense and trouble in view of the results obtained to date and those anticipated in the future.

The electron microscope has greatly extended our understanding of the finer structure of cells and tissues. It has been an indispensable instrument for modern morphological research. Many electron micrographs will be found throughout this book.

The problem of resolution with the electron microscope is, in practice, somewhat different from that of the light microscope. At the voltages used, the wavelengths to be associated with the electrons are very short, of the order of 0.05 Å. However, the shaped electric or magnetic lens fields that serve to focus the beam of electrons, being as yet quite crude and imperfect, have numerical apertures of 0.01 to 0.001, rather than the 1.3 to 1.4 associated with a good visible light objective lens. Therefore, the overall limit of resolution of the electron microscope has been about 5 Å, at least until recently. Unlike the ordinary light microscope, the best electron microscope is still far from the theoretical limits for its performance.

One of the serious limitations of the transmission electron microscope is the poor penetrating power of the electron beam. This makes it necessary to cut extremely thin slices (1000 Å) for examination with the standard electron microscope, operating with accelerating voltages of 50 to 100 KV. However, the penetrating power of electrons is known to increase remarkably at higher accelerating voltages. The usefulness of high voltage electron microscopes in biology and medicine is now being explored. The penetrating power of electrons at 800 KV has proved to be sufficient for examination of sections 1 μm. thick. Whereas efforts to understand three dimensional organization in biological fine structure previously required laborious reconstruction from serial ultrathin sections, it is now possible to take stereopairs of micrographs on the high voltage electron microscope and observe, in some depth, the configuration of small components of cells and tissues (Hama; Porter).

The Scanning Electron Microscope

A new type of electron microscope introduced recently is the scanning electron microscope. It is different in principle from light or transmission electron microscopes. In these latter types, the image is formed directly on an image plane. In the scanning microscope, the image is formed indirectly by accumulation of information from the specimen point by point. A sample in the column of the scanning microscope is bombarded with a finely focused beam of electrons 100 Å or less in diameter. The electron beam is scanned over an area of the specimen in a raster pattern. A cathode ray tube on the display panel of the instrument is scanned in synchronization with the electron beam in the column, so that each point on the cathode ray tube corresponds to a point on the specimen. An electron detector placed near the specimen measures the secondary electrons emitted from each point on the specimen as the beam strikes it. Given a biological specimen with an irregularly contoured surface, the intensity of the emission of secondary electrons will vary with the angle at which the electron probe strikes each point on the surface. The intensity of the cathode ray tube is modulated in proportion to the intensity of the secondary electron emission and an image of the specimen is built up point by point on the fluorescent screen of the cathode ray tube. A camera directed at the screen records the varying intensity of the signal along each line of scan, and thus a magnified picture of the specimen is built up.

Because the beam of the scanning microscope does not have to pass through the specimen, there is no need to cut ultrathin sections. Therefore preparation of specimens for examination is relatively simple. Regrettably, the resolution of the scanning electron microscope is only about 100 Å, and thus it does not compare with resolution of 4 to 5 Å achieved by the transmission electron microscope. Its best advantage is its great depth of field (7 to 10 times that of the compound light microscope at comparable magnification), which makes it possible to obtain images with a remarkable three dimensional quality (Fig. 1–25).

Specimen Preparation for Electron Microscopy. Because electrons will form a coherent beam only when traveling in a high vacuum, it is impossible, at least in current conventional electron microscopes, to introduce living cells into the column of the microscope. Therefore, with this instrument, only material that has been killed and dehydrated can be examined. The old and difficult problem of preserving tissue in a lifelike condition has been greatly compounded by the greater resolution of the electron microscope. The majority of the fixatives that are deemed satisfactory for light microscopy produce a precipitation of proteins that is intolerably coarse when viewed with the electron microscope. Of

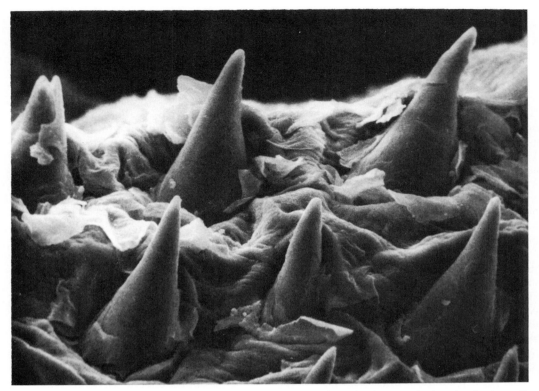

Figure 1–25 Scanning electron micrograph of the epithelium of a rat's glans penis showing in three dimensional effect the spines on the epithelium and squamous cells exfoliating from the surface between spines. (Micrography by Dr. R. Vitale-Calpe.)

the traditional fixatives, only formalin, osmium tetroxide and osmium-dichromate mixtures have been successfully adapted for use in electron microscopy. To these have been added acrolein and glutaraldehyde. With any of these killing agents, it has been found important to maintain the pH of the fixative in the range 7.2 to 7.8 by addition of buffers.

The most widely used fixative is a 1 or 2 per cent buffered solution of osmium tetroxide. This acts not only to preserve the tissue but also stains many of its constituents. "Staining" for the electron microscope does not consist of combination with colored dyes, because registration of color is not possible with an electron optical system. However, reduced osmium from the fixative is bound by the lipoprotein membranes and other components of cells, and because of its high atomic number it increases their electron scattering and therefore enhances the contrast of the electron microscopic

image. Glutaraldehyde as a fixative does not simultaneously stain the tissue, and it is common practice to expose the tissue to osmium afterward for further fixation and, particularly, to take advantage of the osmium staining. The tissues are dehydrated in increasing concentrations of ethanol or acetone and imbedded in acrylic plastic or epoxy resins.

Because an electron beam of the conventional electron microscope has very little penetrating power, the sections of tissue must be extremely thin, 50 to 100 nm. as compared to 5 to 10 μm. for the light microscope. The most challenging part of specimen preparation for electron microscopy, and the most frequent obstacle to success, is the cutting of such exquisitely thin sections, free of compression, scratches and other distortions. This is accomplished on an ultramicrotome, using a knife of fractured plate glass or of cleaved and polished diamond.

To gain additional contrast it is now common practice to restain the tissue by floating the ultrathin sections briefly on a solution of uranyl acetate or lead citrate, or both, in sequence. This additional staining procedure makes it possible to obtain sufficient contrast even in very thin sections (Fig. 1–26).

A relatively new method for preparation of biological materials for electron microscopic study is called *freeze-cleaving* or *freeze-etching*. This method depends upon the fact that high fidelity replicas can be made of the surfaces of frozen aqueous materials at very low temperature in vacuo. One of its principal advantages is the avoidance of chemical fixatives and of dehydrating and embedding agents. The specimens must, however, be protected by binding water to prevent ice crystal distortion during freezing. The tissue is usually impregnated with a 25 per cent glycerol solution prior to rapid

freezing in liquid nitrogen or Freon 12 at −100° C. to −155° C. During the preparative procedure, the frozen tissue is contained in a depression in a cylindrical block of brass. It is cleaved or fractured with a razor blade and then covered with a second brass cylinder, perforated by ports or tunnels through which carbon and platinum can later be deposited to produce a replica of the frozen and fractured surface of the specimen. This second brass cylinder in turn is covered with a lid to prevent contamination of the frozen surface prior to replication. The whole assembly consisting of three nested brass cylinders is transferred to a high vacuum evaporator and the pressure brought down to 10^{-5} mm. of mercury. During this process, the liquid nitrogen boils, freezes and eventually sublimes. The lid of the assembly is then lifted under the vacuum to expose the ports

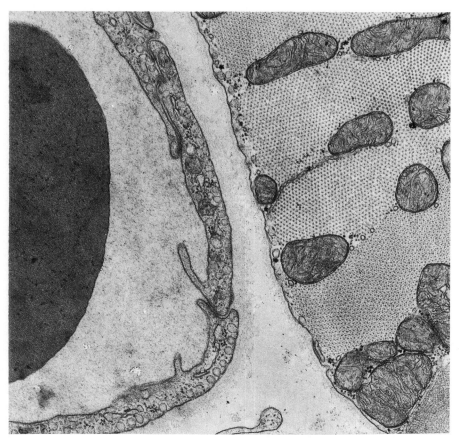

Figure 1–26 Electron micrograph of an ultrathin section of heart muscle. At the left is part of a capillary containing an erythrocyte. At the right is a section of cardiac muscle containing numerous mitochondria and punctate sections of myofilaments. Compare with Figure 1–27.

and carbon is first evaporated vertically onto the surface to produce a carbon replica. Platinum is then deposited at an angle to the surface to produce a "shadowed" effect and bring out its surface features. After warming, the specimen is floated on sodium hypochlorite or strong mineral acid to dissolve the tissue. The replica of the cleaved surface, resisting this digestion, is then picked up on a copper grid and examined with the electron microscope (Fig. 1–27).

The application of this method has clearly demonstrated that the structure of cell organelles in unfixed material corresponds very closely to the interpretations that have been based upon thin sections of chemically fixed cells. This finding has provided reassuring additional evidence

that the routine methods of fixation and embedding for electron microscopy do not produce serious distortions of cell structure. Contrary to the hopes of its developers, the technique of freeze-cleaving of biological materials is not entirely free of artifacts. The distortions produced in freezing are in some respects more difficult to identify than are the artifacts of chemical fixation.

Freeze cleaving has proved to be particularly valuable for the study of membranes and their junctional specializations. It has disclosed within membranes a population of particles 80 to 100 Å in diameter that went undetected with other methods (see Chapter 2). The chemical composition and physiological significance of these particles has yet to be determined. The freeze-cleaving

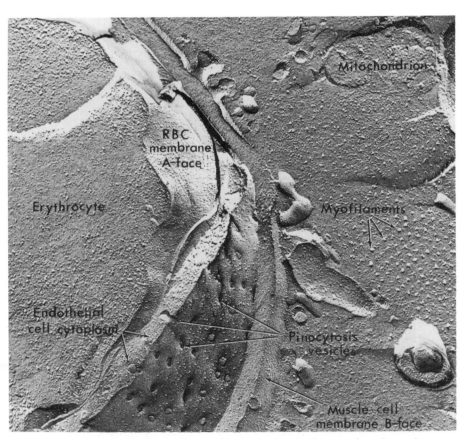

Figure 1–27 Electron micrograph of a replica made on the frozen fractured surface of an area of cardiac muscle similar to that shown in Figure 1–26. The plane of cleavage has passed through the erythrocyte and along its membrane, exposing the outwardly directed inner half membrane (A-Face); then through the endothelium, splitting the abluminal membrane and showing openings of micropinocytosis vesicles. It then cleaves across the muscle fiber in which mitochondria and myofilaments can be identified. (Micrograph courtesy of Dr. Scott McNutt.)

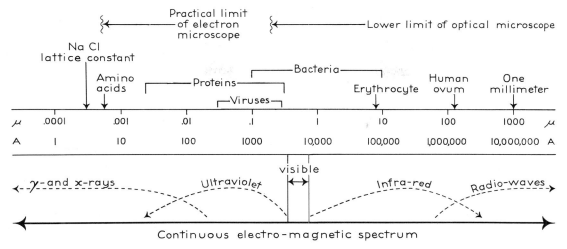

Figure 1-28 Comparison of dimensions of molecules and cells with wavelengths of the electromagnetic spectrum on logarithmic scale. The different names given to overlapping regions of the spectrum do not represent different kinds of radiation. These names were determined historically by the range of sensitivity of the human eye and the varying approaches of investigation and instrumentation centering around different regions of what is actually a single continuous spectrum. (From data supplied by A. B. Hastings, T. F. Young, R. Uretz, and P. Geiduschek.)

method has also proved useful in interpreting the junctional complexes of cells (see Chapter 3).

X-RAY DIFFRACTION

As we proceed farther along the electromagnetic spectrum toward shorter wavelengths and higher energies, we come first to an ultraviolet region known as the vacuum ultraviolet, where radiation is heavily absorbed by almost everything, including the intervening air; and then to the regions of low-energy "soft" x-rays, high-energy "hard" x-rays, and finally gamma rays. It must be emphasized that all of these regions are part of a single continuous electromagnetic spectrum, and that the name associated with a particular wave-length of radiation in a region of overlapping nomenclature usually depends on the source used to produce the radiation in a particular instance (Fig. 1–28).

One would expect that the very short wavelengths associated with x-rays would make them ideal as probes for microscopic analysis, with the ability to resolve interatomic distances accurately. Unfortunately no lenses are available to take full advantage of these short wavelengths by focusing and utilizing them for high resolution studies

with a microscope system analogous to those used with visible light. Alternatively, then, one uses mathematical analysis in lieu of real lenses. In this technique of x-ray diffraction, one allows a narrow beam of x-rays to impinge upon a specimen. Depending upon the fine detail present, these x-rays will be diffracted and scattered by the specimen. In the absence of an objective lens analogous to that used in visible light microscopy, this scattered energy is observed directly, usually by means of a photographic film. Unfortunately, this means that we are restricted to the observation of highly ordered structures, crystalline or semicrystalline in nature, for which x-rays are diffracted in discrete directions and give patterns that are amenable to mathematical analysis. Further, because the diffracted x-ray energy is collected on a photographic film rather than refocused onto an image plane by means of a lens, the information contained in the phase relationships between the secondary x-ray beams diffracted in various directions is lost. This means that the x-ray diffraction pattern obtained is not uniquely and simply related to the object that gave rise to it, but that a series of approximations and trial solutions are necessary in order to decide on the structure that most probably corresponds to the observed pattern. It should

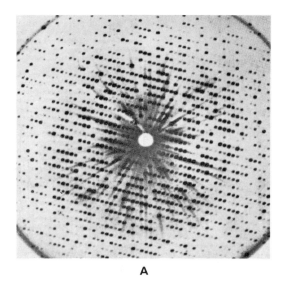

A

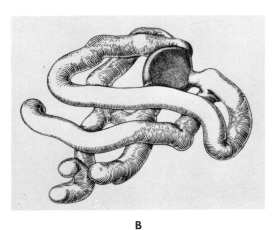

B

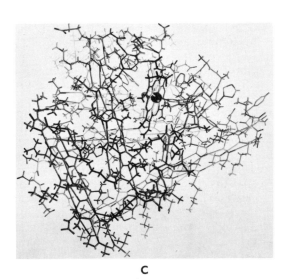

C

be emphasized, also, that in x-ray diffraction, unlike visible light microscopy, we do not see focused individual elements of structure but only the averaged properties of repetitive ordered structures, all elements of which contribute to the observed x-ray diffraction pattern.

For a given wavelength of x-rays, the finer the detail observed, the larger the angle over which the x-rays will be diffracted. This has led to two distinct areas of x-ray diffraction analysis, in which the details of experimental technique are somewhat different: *Large-angle x-ray diffraction*, in which the small distances between individual atoms are studied, and *small-angle x-ray diffraction*, in which more widely spaced repetitions of entire groups of atoms are studied.

In recent years application of x-ray diffraction analysis has led to the determination by Kendrew and Perutz of the secondary and a large part of the primary structure of the molecule of *myoglobin*, a muscle protein involved in oxygen transport (Fig. 1–29), and of *hemoglobin*. It has also made an important contribution to the analysis of the structure of DNA by Wilkins and by Crick and Watson.

In practice a crystal of the protein being analyzed is rotated in the path of a slender beam of monochromatic x-rays. The regularly spaced planes of high electron density within the crystal are thus successively brought to the correct angle to the incident beam. On a photographic plate placed some distance behind the crystal, a pattern of spots is produced, from which the scattering angles and spacing of the scattering centers in the crystal can be calculated. The size and shape of the *unit cell* or repeating group can thus be determined. For a protein, the

---

Figure 1–29 A, X-ray diffraction pattern of myoglobin (Courtesy of J. C. Kendrew. Copyright 1963 by the American Association for the Advancement of Science.) *B,* Drawing of an early model of the myoglobin molecule constructed from an x-ray diffraction analysis with a relatively low resolution (6 Å). (Redrawn after J. C. Kendrew, Nature, *181:* 662, 1958.) *C,* Depiction of the myoglobin molecule as revealed by a higher resolution x-ray diffraction analysis (2 Å). (Painted by I. Geis. From J. C. Kendrew: The three-dimensional structure of a protein molecule. Scientific American, *205:*96, (Dec.) 1961. Reproduced with permission. Copyright © 1961 by Scientific American, Inc. All rights reserved.)

main regions of high electron density are the backbone of the peptide chain and any atoms of high atomic number that may be present. In a relatively low resolution study, these are the only regions localized. In high resolution x-ray diffraction studies, the high density regions are localized more precisely and the less electron dense regions of the unit cell are also studied. Three dimensional contour maps of the electron density within the unit cell of the crystal are produced, and from these, models are constructed showing further detail.

REFERENCES

Transillumination of Exteriorized Organs

Knisely, M. H.: Fused quartz rod technique. *In* Cowdry, E. V., ed.: Microscopic Technique in Biology and Medicine. Baltimore, Williams & Wilkins Co., 1948.

Transparent Chamber Methods

Algire, G. H.: An adaptation of the transparent chamber technique to the mouse. J. Nat. Cancer Inst., *4*:1, 1943.

Algire, G. H., and F. Y. Legallais: Recent developments in the transparent chamber technique as adapted to the mouse. J. Nat. Cancer Inst., *10*:225, 1949.

Fawcett, D. W., G. B. Wislocki, and C. M. Waldo: The development of mouse ova in the anterior chamber of the eye and in the abdominal cavity. Am J. Anat., *81*:413, 1947.

Goodman, L.: Observations on transplanted immature ovaries in the eyes of adult male and female rats. Anat. Rec., *59*:223, 1934.

Lutz, B. R., and G. P. Fulton: The use of the hamster cheek pouch for the study of vascular changes at the microscopic level. Anat. Rec., *120*:293, 1954.

Runner, M.: The development of mouse ova in oculo. Anat. Rec., *98*:1, 1947.

Sandison, J. C.: The transparent chamber of the rabbit's ear, giving a complete description of improved techniques of construction and introduction and general account of growth and behavior of living cells and tissues as seen with the microscope. Am J. Anat., *41*:447, 1928.

Sewell, I. A.: Studies of the microcirculation using transparent tissue observation chambers inserted in the hamster cheek pouch. J. Anat. (Lond.), *100*:839, 1966.

Cell and Organ Culture

Carrel, A.: On the permanent life of tissues outside of the organism. J. Exper. Med., *15*:516, 1912.

Earle, W. R., F. C. Bryant, E. L. Schilling, and V. J. Evans: Growth of cell suspensions in tissue culture. Ann N. Y. Acad. Sci., *63*:666, 1956.

Fell, H. B., and J. Robison: The growth, development and phosphatase activity of embryonic avian femora and limb-buds cultivated *in vitro*. Biochem. J., *23*:767, 1929.

Harris, M.: Cell Culture and Somatic Variation. New York, Holt, Rinehart & Winston, 1964.

Harrison, R. G.: Observations on the living developing nerve fiber. Proc. Soc. Exper. Biol. & Med., *4*:140, 1907.

Maximow, A. A.: Tissue-cultures of young mammalian embryos. Carnegie Contributions to Embryol., *16*:47, 1925.

Moscona, A. A., and H. Moscona: The dissociation and aggregation of cells from organ rudiments of the early chick embryo. J. Anat. (Lond.), *86*:287, 1952.

Parker, R. C.: Methods of Tissue Culture. 3rd ed. New York, Hoeber Medical Division, Harper & Row, 1961.

Puck, T. T., and P. I. Marcus: A rapid method for viable cell titration and clone production with HeLa cells in tissue culture. The use of x-irradiated cells to supply conditioning factors. Proc. Nat. Acad. Sci., *41*:432, 1955.

Puck, T. T., P. I. Marcus, and S. J. Cieciura: Clonal growth of mammalian cells *in vitro*. Growth characteristics of colonies from single HeLa cells with and without a feeder layer. J. Exper. Med., *103*:273, 1956.

Scherer, W. F., and A. C. Hoogasian: Preservation at subzero temperatures of mouse fibroblasts (strain L) and human epithelial cells (strain HeLa). Proc. Soc. Exper. Biol. & Med., *87*:480, 1954.

White, P. R.: The cell as organism, tissue culture, cellular autonomy, and cellular interrelations. *In* Brachet, J., and A. E. Mirsky, eds.: The Cell. Vol. I, New York, Academic Press, 1960.

Micromanipulation

Chambers, R.: Micrurgical studies on protoplasm. Biol. Rev., *24*:246, 1949.

Chambers, R., and M. J. Kopac: Micrurgical technique for the study of cellular phenomena. *In* Jones, R. M., ed.: McClung's Handbook of Microscopical Technique. 3rd ed. New York, Paul B. Hoeber, Inc., 1950.

deFonbrune, P.: Technique de Micromanipulation. Paris, Masson, 1949.

Kopac, M. J.: Cytochemical micrurgy. Int. Rev. Cytol., *4*:1, 1955.

Kopac, M. J.: Micrurgical studies on living cells. *In* Brachet, J., and A. E. Mirsky, eds.: The Cell, Vol. I, New York, Academic Press, 1960.

Radiation Probes

Amy, R. L., and R. Storb: Selective mitochondrial damage by a ruby laser microbeam. An electron microscope study. Science, *150*:757, 1965.

Amy, R. L., R. Storb, B. Fauconnier and R. K. Wertz: Ruby laser microirradiation of single tissue culture cells vitally stained with Janus green G. Exp. Cell Res., *45*:361, 1967.

Berns, M. W., R. S. Olson, and D. E. Rounds: Effects of laser microirradiation on chromosomes. Exp. Cell Res., *56*:292, 1969.

Berns, M. W., W. K. Cheng, A. D. Floyd, and Y. Ohnuki: Chromosome lesions produced with an argon laser microbeam without dye sensitization. Science, *171*:903, 1971.

Bloom, W., and R. V. Leider: Optical and electron microscopic changes in ultraviolet irradiated chromosome segments. J. Cell Biol., *13*:269, 1962.

Bloom, W., and S. Özarslan: Electron microscopy of ultraviolet-irradiated parts of chromosomes. Proc. Nat. Acad. Sci., *53*:1294, 1965.

Bloom, W., R. E. Zirkle, and R. B. Uretz: Irradiation of parts of individual cells. III. Effects of chromosomal and extrachromosomal irradiation on chromosome movements. Ann. N.Y. Acad. Sci., *59*:503, 1955.

Uretz, R. B., W. Bloom, and R. E. Zirkle: Irradiation of parts of living cells. II. Effects of ultraviolet microbeam focused on parts of chromosomes. Science, *120*:197, 1954.

Zirkle, R. E.: Partial cell irradiation. Advances in Biological and Medical Physics. Vol. 5, New York, Academic Press, 1957.

Zirkle, R. E. and W. Bloom: Irradiation of parts of individual cells. Science, *117*:481, 1953.

Isolation of Cell Components by Differential Centrifugation

Allfrey, V.: The isolation of subcellular components. *In* Brachet, J., and A. E. Mirsky, eds.: The Cell. Vol. I. New York, Academic Press, 1960.

Bensley, R. R.: On the fat distribution in mitochondria of the guinea pig liver. Anat. Rec., 69:341, 1937.

Bensley, R. R., and N. L. Hoerr: Studies on cell structure by the freezing-drying method. VI. The preparation and properties of mitochondria. Anat. Rec., 60:449, 1934.

Claude, A.: Fractionation of mammalian liver cells by differential centrifugation. J. Exper. Med., 84:51, 1946.

Hogeboom, G. H., W. C. Schneider, and G. H. Palade: Isolation of intact mitochondria from rat liver; some biochemical properties of mitochondria and submicroscopic particulate material. J. Biol. Chem., *172*:619, 1948.

General Histological Methods

Baker, J. R.: Principles of Biological Microtechnique. New York, John Wiley & Sons, 1958.

Conn, H. J.: Biological Stains. 7th ed. Geneva and New York, Biochemical Publications, 1961.

Jones, R. M., ed.: McClung's Handbook of Microscopical Technique. 3rd ed. New York, Paul B. Hoeber, Inc., 1950.

Histochemical Methods

Barka, T., and P. J. Anderson: Histochemistry—Theory, Practice, and Bibliography. New York, Hoeber Medical Division, Harper & Row, 1963.

Boyd, G. A.: Autoradiography in Biology and Medicine. New York, Academic Press, 1955.

Caro, L. G.: High resolution autoradiography. *In* Prescott, D. M., ed.: Methods in Cell Physiology. Vol. I, p. 327. New York, Academic Press, 1964.

Caspersson, T.: Cell Growth and Cell Function. New York, Morton, 1950.

Coons, A. H.: Histochemistry with labeled antibody. Int. Rev. Cytol., 5:1, 1956.

Coons, A. H.: Fluorescent antibody methods. *In* Danielli, J. F., ed.: General Cytochemical Methods. New York, Academic Press, 1958.

Engstrom, A.: Historadiography. *In* Oster, G., and A. W. Pollister, eds.: Physical Techniques in Biological Research. Vol. I. New York, Academic Press, 1956.

Novikoff, A. B.: The intracellular localization of chemical constituents. *In* Mellors, R. C., ed.: Analytical Cytology. 2nd ed. New York, McGraw-Hill Book Co., 1959.

Pearse, A. G. E.: Histochemistry—Theoretical and Applied. 2nd ed. Boston, Little, Brown & Co., 1960.

Pelc, S. R., T. C. Appleton, and M. E. Wilton: State of light autoradiography. *In* Leblond, C. P., and K. B. Warren, eds.: The Use of Radioautography in Investigating Protein Synthesis. New York, Academic Press, 1965.

Pollister, A. W., and L. Ornstein: The photometric chemical analysis of cells. *In* Mellors, R. C., ed.: Analytical Cytology. 2nd ed. New York, McGraw-Hill Book Co., 1959.

Salpeter, M. M., and L. Bachmann: Assessment of technical steps in electron microscope autoradiography. *In* Leblond, C. P., and K. B. Warren, eds.: The Use of Radioautography in Investigating Protein Synthesis. New York, Academic Press, 1965.

Scarpelli, D. G., and N. M. Kanczak: Ultrastructural cytochemistry: Principles, limitations and applications. Int. Rev. Exp. Path., 4:55, 1965.

Walker, P. M. B.: Ultraviolet absorption techniques. *In* Oster, G., and A. W. Pollister, eds.: Physical Techniques in Biological Research. Vol. I. New York, Academic Press, 1956.

Principles of Microscopic Analysis

Barer, R.: Phase contrast and interference microscopy in cytology. *In* Oster, G., and A. W. Pollister, eds.: Physical Techniques in Biological Research. Vol. I. New York, Academic Press, 1956.

Bennett, H. S.: Microscopical investigation of biological material with polarized light. *In* Jones, R. M., ed.: McClung's Handbook of Microscopical Technique. 3rd ed. New York, Paul B. Hoeber, Inc., 1950.

Hale, A. J.: The Interference Microscope in Biological Research. Edinburgh and London, E. & S. Livingstone Ltd., 1958.

Hale, A. J.: The interference microscope as a cell balance. *In* Walker, P. M. B., ed.: New Approaches in Cell Biology. London, Academic Press, 1960.

Electron Microscopy

Bullivant, S.: Freeze-fracturing of biological materials. Micron *1*:46, 1969.

Everhart, T. E., and T. L. Hayes: The scanning electron microscope. Sci. Amer. *226*:55, 1972.

Fawcett, D. W.: Electron microscopy in histology and cytology. *In* Siegel, B. M., ed.: Modern Developments in Electron Microscopy, New York, Academic Press, 1963.

Goodenough, D. A., and J. P. Revel: A fine structural analysis of intercellular junctions in the mouse liver. J. Cell Biol., *45*:272, 1970.

Hall, C. E.: Introduction to Electron Microscopy. New York, McGraw-Hill Book Co., 1953.

Hama, K., and K. R. Porter: An application of high voltage electron microscopy to the study of biological materials. J. Microsc. 8:149, 1969.

Hama, K., and F. Nagata: A stereoscope observation of tracheal epithelium of mouse by means of the high voltage electron microscope. J. Cell Biol., *45*:654, 1970.

Kimoto, S., and J. C. Russ: The characteristics and applications of the scanning electron microscope. American Scientist, 57:1, 112, 1969.

Koehler, J. K.: The technique and application of freeze-etching in ultrastructure research. Adv. Biol. Med. Physics, *12*:1, 1968.

Pease, D. C.: Histological Techniques for Electron Microscopy. New York, Academic Press, 1960.

Porter, K. R.: Ultramicrotomy. *In* Siegel, B. M., ed.: Modern Developments in Electron Microscopy. New York, Academic Press, 1963.

Staehelin, L. A.: The interpretation of freeze-etched artificial and biological membranes. J. Ultrastr. Res. *22*: 326, 1968.

Weinstein, R. S., and K. Someda: The freeze-cleave approach to the ultrastructure of frozen tissues. Cryobiology, *4*:116, 1967.

2
The Cell and Cell Division

The living substance of plants and animals is described by the general term *protoplasm*. The smallest unit of protoplasm capable of independent existence is the *cell*. The simplest animals consist of a single cell, but the higher animals can be thought of as a colony or complex society of interdependent cells of many kinds, specialized in various ways to carry out the many functions essential to the survival and reproduction of the organism. Cells subserving the same general function are grouped together and united by varying amounts of intercellular substance to form *tissues*, examples of which are bone, cartilage, muscle, nervous tissue, and blood. The several basic tissues function independently in some instances, but more commonly two or more tissues are combined to form larger functional units called *organs*—skin, kidney, blood vessels, glands, and so on. Several organs whose functions are interrelated constitute an *organ system*; examples are the respiratory system (comprising the nose, larynx, trachea, and lungs) and the urinary system (comprising the kidneys, ureters, urinary bladder, and urethra).

Etymologically, *histology* would seem to be the subdivision of anatomy that deals exclusively with the *tissues*, but it is in fact equally concerned with their component cellular and extracellular elements and with the patterns of their interrelation in the formation of the organs. In this broader sense *histology* has come to be synonymous with *microscopic anatomy*. Formerly the boundaries of the field were rigidly limited by the resolving power of the light microscope. The use of the electron microscope by the histologist has greatly extended the scope of his subject, so that it now includes much of the science of cytology and tissue ultrastructure and thus investigates biological structure at all levels of organization from the lower limit of direct visual inspection down to the structure of large molecules. The interests of the modern histologist do not end there, for it is impossible to account for the fine details of the structure of cells and tissues without some understanding of the chemical nature of their submicroscopic components.

THE CELL

In 1665 Robert Hooke observed the microscopic compartmentation of cork and introduced the term *cell* to describe the small chambers demarcated by the inert cellulose walls of that plant tissue. The cellular organization of a number of living plant and animal tissues was subsequently observed by Leeuwenhoek in 1674 and several other early microscopists. The spherical body in the interior of cells which we now know as the *nucleus* was recognized by Brown in 1833. Schleiden in 1838 and Schwann in 1839 assembled persuasive evidence that both plant and animal tissues are made up of aggregations of cellular units. They are therefore generally credited with enunciating the *cell theory*.

Since the 1830's it has been customary to consider the *protoplasm*, the living substance of the cell, as partitioned into two major regions or compartments, the *nucleus*, composed of *nucleoplasm (karyoplasm)*, and the protoplasm surrounding the nucleus, called *cytoplasm*. Both contain a number of structural components of characteristic form and staining properties that permit them to be recognized with the light microscope. On the basis of the generality of their occurrence and assumptions as to their functional significance, these components have traditionally been classified as belonging to one or the other of two categories—*organelles* and *inclusions* (Fig. 2–1). The organelles are structures occurring in nearly all cell types and are regarded as small internal organs of the cell; they are

organized units of living substance having important specific functions in cell metabolism. The inclusions, on the other hand, are considered to be lifeless accumulations of metabolites or cell products, such as stored protein, fat, or carbohydrate, crystals, pigment, secretory droplets, and the like. In contrast to the organelles, these are regarded as dispensable and often temporary constituents of cells.

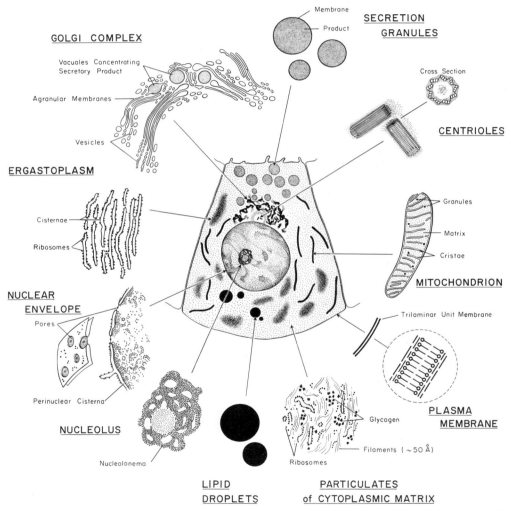

Figure 2–1   In the center of this figure is a diagram of the cell, illustrating the form of its organelles and inclusions as they appear by light microscopy. Around the periphery are representations of the finer structure of these same components as seen in electron micrographs. The ergastoplasm of light microscopy consists of aggregations of submicroscopic membrane-limited elements with granules of ribonucleoprotein adhering to their outer surface. This component is now also called the *granular endoplasmic reticulum*. The illustration of the plasma membrane encircled by an interrupted line is not a structure that has been directly observed but represents one possible interpretation of the arrangement of lipid and protein molecules that may be related to the trilaminar appearance of cell membranes in electron micrographs. See page 69 for comment on "pores" in the nuclear envelope.

Although the distinction between organelles and inclusions is still useful, it should be borne in mind that the assignment of cell components to one category or the other was made at a time when too little was known about their ultrastructure and chemical nature to permit a valid judgment as to whether they were physiologically active or inert, essential or dispensable. Therefore, it is not surprising that as our knowledge of cell biology has increased, the validity of the time honored classification of certain cell structures has become debatable. As a consequence of electron microscopic studies, the list of organelles has been lengthened and a number of new components have been described that are difficult to categorize for lack of precise information as to their chemical nature and function.

CYTOPLASMIC ORGANELLES

Control of the differentiation and function of a cell resides mainly in its nucleus, while most of the responding metabolic and synthetic activities are located in the cytoplasm. The latter, as seen with the light microscope, appears to consist of a structureless medium, the *ground substance* or *cytoplasmic matrix*, and the organelles and inclusions suspended in it. The specialization of cells for different functions is often reflected in their size and shape and in variations in the number and kinds of organelles and inclusions they contain.

The common organelles visible with the light microscope (*mitochondria, Golgi apparatus, ergastoplasm*) were originally described as granules, filaments, lamellae, and so on, implying that they were solid structures. The electron microscope has now shown that these familiar organelles, and several of those newly discovered, are hollow structures bounded by thin lipoprotein membranes and, in some instances, possessing complex internal structure.

Most of the important physiological processes of living organisms take place at surfaces and interfaces. Many of the thousands of enzymes that catalyze specific chemical transformations in the cell are strategically located in the membranes, where they participate in reactions occurring at the interface between the organelles and the cytoplasmic matrix or between the cell and its environment. The internal compartmentation of the cytoplasm achieved by membrane limited organelles no doubt promotes the efficiency of numerous complex chemical reactions by extending the area of the physiologically active interfaces within the cell.

The existence of numerous membrane limited compartments in the cytoplasm may also enable the cell to maintain a separation of enzymes from substrates at some times and at other times to permit their controlled interaction by varying the permeability of a particular membrane or the rate of active transport across it. It is clear that if there were unlimited diffusion and interaction within the cell it would be impossible to maintain the high degree of chemical heterogeneity characteristic of the cytoplasm: enzymes would attack their substrates and all of the potential interactions of the countless chemical constituents of the cell would race out of control. Actually, however, this does not occur. The cell is able to regulate its activities and to hold in reserve a very large repertoire of unexpressed biochemical potentialities. It can call each of these into play at the proper time and at the rate appropriate to the needs of the organism as a whole. That this is possible is probably due in large measure to the prevalence of membrane bounded organelles in the cytoplasm.

Cell Membrane (Plasmalemma)

The cell is enclosed by a thin limiting membrane, called the *plasmalemma* or the *cell membrane*. It is usually too thin to be seen in sections with the light microscope, but its reality as a limiting structure can be demonstrated visually by the outflow of cytoplasm when the membrane is torn by micromanipulation. Numerous physiological experiments on the swelling and shrinking of cells in solutions of different osmolarity also attest to the presence of a limiting membrane and demonstrate its selective permeability. Its low permeability to ions and high permeability to lipid soluble substances early suggested to cell physiologists that the membrane was composed of lipid or a mixture of lipids and protein. Ingenious indirect measurements of its thickness, birefringence, surface tension, and other properties led Danielli and Davson in 1935 to propose that the membrane probably consists of a bimolecular layer of mixed lipids between two layers of adsorbed proteins (Fig. 2–2*A*).

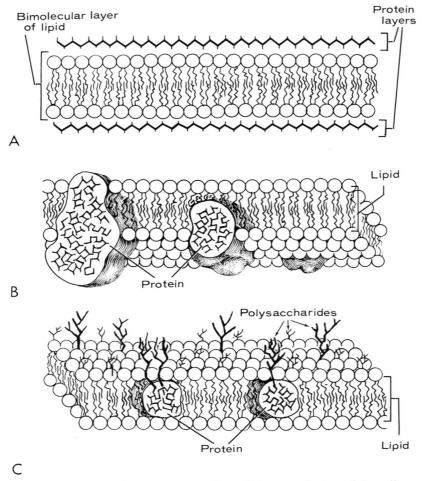

Figure 2–2 Schematic depictions of three interpretations of the organization of the cell membrane. *A*, The classical model of Davson and Danielli: two layers of protein on either side of a bimolecular leaflet of mixed lipid with its hydrophilic ends directed outward and the hydrocarbon chains directed inward. *B*, A lipid-globular protein mosaic model. Globular integral proteins are distributed in a lipid matrix. The protruding parts are presumed to have on their surfaces the ionic residues of the protein. The particles are believed to be free to move laterally within the fluid matrix. (After S. J. Singer and C. K. Nicholson, Science, *175*:720-731, 18 February 1972. Copyright 1972 by the American Association for the Advancement of Science.) *C*, A lipid-globular protein model in which the bulk of the particles is within the thickness of the lipid matrix but polysaccharide chains of glycoprotein and glycolipid constituents project above the surface. Either model *B* or model *C* is more consistent with freeze-cleaving images of membranes than is the traditional Davson-Danielli model.

When it became possible to examine thin sections of cells with the electron microscope, the surface membrane was visualized as a dense linear profile 80 to 100 Å thick. At higher magnification, this line can now be resolved as two dense layers about 25 Å thick separated by a 30 Å light intermediate layer (Fig. 2–3). Some variation in overall thickness is encountered from one cell type to another, and some asymmetry in the relative thickness of the two dense layers occurs, but the same basic trilaminar appearance is found in electron micrographs of all cell membranes. This is now referred to as the *unit membrane* (Robertson). Its three layers have generally been interpreted as corresponding to the two protein layers and the bimolecular leaflet of the Danielli model.

An alternative interpretation of the molecular organization of the membrane, recently proposed, depicts the lipid as forming globular micelles between two layers of protein. A third interpretation considers the membrane to be basically a lipid bilayer with its polar groups directed outward and its hydrocarbon chains directed inward, while the protein or glycoprotein is envisioned as forming intercalated globular units that are either entirely within the lipid bilayer or projecting to varying degrees from the outer surface (Fig. 2–2B). This hypothetical model would account for the asymmetry of the membrane and the random pattern of antigenic sites detected on its outer but not on its inner surface. It is also consonant with the existence of protein lined polar pores that have been postulated to account for certain aspects of membrane permeability.

In its simplest form, the traditional Davson-Danielli model would lead one to expect structural homogeneity within the plane of the membrane. This expectation does not seem to be borne out. Recent applications of the freeze-cleaving technique (p. 29) to frozen cells permits visualization of certain features of the internal structure of their membranes. Electron micrographs of such preparations show "particles" or globular units which vary in their abundance in different cells and in different regions of the limiting membrane of the same cell (Fig. 2–4). This demonstration of heterogeneity within the plane of the membrane does not substantiate the classical Davson-Danielli model but favors a membrane model consisting of globular protein subunits intercalated in a lipid bilayer (Fig. 2–2C). To account for the asymmetry of the membrane and its binding of antibodies and hemagglutinating substances (lectins) it is suggested

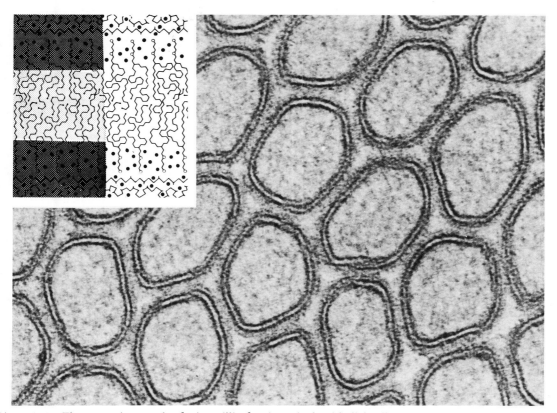

Figure 2–3 Electron micrograph of microvilli of an intestinal epithelial cell in cross section. Each microvillus is enclosed by an extension of the plasma membrane which has a distinct trilaminar appearance—two dense layers on either side of a light intermediate layer. The inset shows the prevailing interpretation of this image as due to deposition of osmium (black dots) in the protein and polar heads of the phospholipid molecules in the traditional Davson-Danielli model. This distribution of osmium would explain the two dark lines of the "unit membrane" while the hydrocarbon chains in the middle would remain light. (Inset modified after W. Stoeckenius.)

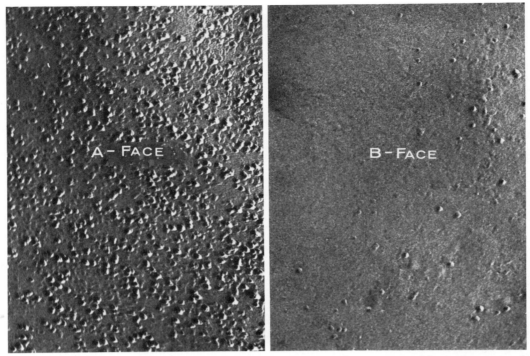

Figure 2-4 Electron micrograph of shadowed replicas of the two faces presented by a plasma membrane when prepared by freeze-cleaving. The outwardly directed inner half membrane (A-Face) bears a large population of particles of rather uniform size. The inwardly directed outer half membrane (B-Face) is relatively free of particles. Why the intramembranous particles adhere more tenaciously to the A-Face is not understood. (Micrograph courtesy of E. Raviola.)

that the polysaccharide chains of glycoprotein and glycolipid components of the membrane extend between the polar heads of the phospholipid molecules and project from the outer surface.

Until more precise information is available a final choice cannot be made from among the three or four hypothetical models of the molecular organization of the cell membrane. The resolution of this problem is of the greatest importance, however, for in the structure and chemical organization of the cell membrane lies the key to its selective permeability, its specific enzymatic activity, its capacity to conduct an impulse, and many other properties upon which life depends.

The outer limit of the cell surface is not always easily defined. On the outer aspect of the unit membrane in plant cells there is an inert layer of cellulose called the *cell wall.* It has recently been found that many animal cells also have a thin external coating of material rich in polysaccharides, some-

times called the *glycocalyx.* This coating is now the subject of intensive research. It is generally regarded as an integral part of the cell membrane rather than an extraneous coating. It may prove to have a very important role in the selective uptake of substances by cells.

Granular Endoplasmic Reticulum (Ergastoplasm)

In stained histological sections, the cytoplasm of many cell types contains a substance that has a strong affinity for basic dyes. This component may be widely dispersed in the cytoplasm and stain diffusely, or it may be concentrated in discrete basophilic masses or clumps of varying size. Classical cytologists referred to this deeply staining material as the *chromidial substance* or the *ergastoplasm.* Later, when reliable histochemical staining reactions and ultraviolet absorption methods were developed for the detection of nucleic acids, the basophilic substance of the cytoplasm was identified as *ribonucleoprotein*.

With the advent of the electron microscope, the cytoplasm of nearly all cells was found to possess a more or less continuous network of membrane bounded cavities. This canalicular system was soon accepted as a new organelle and called the *endoplasmic reticulum*. Its fluid-filled channels facilitate diffusion of metabolites throughout the cytoplasm, and its limiting membranes contain enzyme systems that play an active role in cell metabolism. In its most typical form the endoplasmic reticulum consists of an irregular network of branching and anastomosing tubules that are often continuous with flattened saccular structures commonly referred to as *cisternae*. The latter may occur singly, but more often several become associated to form lamellar systems of parallel flat cavities (Fig. 2–5). In addition to the intercommunicating tubules and cisternae, there may be isolated vesicles that do not form part of the continuous canalicular system but are nevertheless considered to be portions of the endoplasmic reticulum. The degree of development of the reticulum and the relative proportions of its tubular, cisternal, and vesicular elements vary greatly in different cell types and in different phases of the physiological activity of the same cell type.

It is now generally accepted that the ergastoplasmic strands and chromidial bodies of classical cytology correspond to the aggregations of endoplasmic reticulum observed in electron micrographs, but their component tubules and cisternae usually cannot be resolved by the light microscope. The basophilia of these structures resides not in the canalicular elements of the reticulum *per se* but in small particles of ribonucleoprotein, called *ribosomes*, which are found in great numbers adhering to the outer surface of the limiting membrane of the reticulum (Fig. 2–5). The ribosomes are very uniform in size, 120 to 150 Å in diameter. They occur free in the cytoplasmic matrix as well as attached to the membranes. The ribosomes are the sites of synthesis of new protein in the cell. In general, ribosomes found free in the

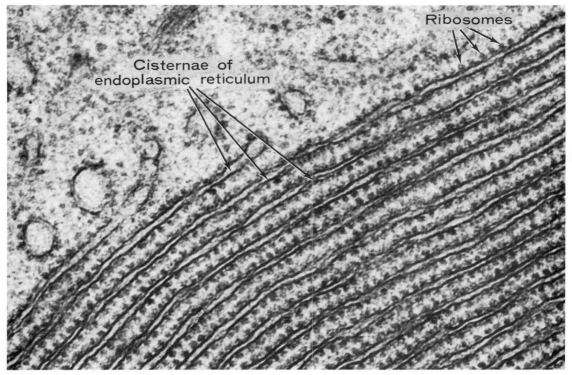

Figure 2–5 Electron micrograph of a basophilic area of cytoplasm from a glandular cell. Many cisternae of the endoplasmic reticulum are arranged in parallel. On the outer surface of their limiting membranes are great numbers of ribosomes (dense particles of ribonucleoprotein about 150 Å in diameter).

cytoplasmic matrix are believed to be sites of synthesis of the protein necessary to sustain cell proliferation and that required for other uses within the cell. Ribosomes attached to membranes are believed to be concerned principally with synthesis of protein that will be secreted by the cell. This generalization cannot be pressed too far, however, for it is clear that ribosomes attached to pre-existing elements of the reticulum are also involved in synthesis of the protein components of new membranes of granular or agranular reticulum arising in the course of physiological adaptation of cells to altered functional demands.

Whether free or attached, ribosomes are usually associated in clusters, called *poly-ribosomes* or *polysomes*, consisting of three to 30 or more ribosomes held together by a slender filament 10 to 15 Å in diameter (see Fig. 4–6). This slender strand is sensitive to ribonuclease digestion and is a single long molecule of a species of ribonucleic acid called *messenger RNA*. This form of nucleic acid arises in the nucleus by transcription of information encoded in the deoxyribonucleic acid (DNA) which comprises the genetic material of the chromosomes. The messenger RNA, formed in close association with the chromosomes, passes out of the nucleus into the cytoplasm carrying the information that determines the sequences of amino acids in the specific proteins that are to be synthesized. In the cytoplasm, ribosomes become attached to the strand of messenger RNA and move stepwise along its length as the appropriate amino acids are added sequentially to the growing polypeptide chain of the nascent protein. When a given ribosome reaches the end of the messenger RNA, the newly synthesized protein is released and the ribosome is detached from the messenger. This fascinating process of assembly of proteins according to information encoded in the structure of the messenger RNA molecule is referred to as *translation* (see Chapter 4).

It is beyond the scope of a morphological text to go into the enzymology and stereochemistry of this process but it is germane to note that the ribosomes consist of two subunits of unequal size. Where polyribosomes are associated with the membranes of the endoplasmic reticulum, it is the larger of the two subunits that is in contact with the membrane. The messenger RNA is thought to be attached in the groove between the ribosomal subunits. There are two attachment sites on the larger subunit, an aminoacyl site and a peptidyl site. The growing peptide is attached to the peptidyl site while the next appropriate amino acid molecule is brought to the aminoacyl site on the ribosome by a third form of nucleic acid called *transfer RNA*. The amino acid is added to the end of the chain, transfer RNA is released, and the messenger moves with respect to the ribosome so that the latter then reads the instruction (codon) for the next amino acid, and so on until the peptide chain is completed. The polypeptide chain associated with a ribosome elongates vectorially so that it penetrates the membrane beneath the larger subunit and is ultimately released into the lumen of the reticulum.

The endoplasmic reticulum is poorly developed in embryonic and other rapidly proliferating cells, but such cells normally contain a large population of free ribosomes, which accounts for their diffuse cytoplasmic basophilia. In glandular cells, on the other hand, in which the basophilia is observed to occur in discrete clumps, this localized staining is attributable to the ribosomes attached to parallel arrays of cisternae of the endoplasmic reticulum.

To investigate the metabolic activities of cell components, biochemists isolate them from tissue homogenates by centrifugation (see Chapter 1, p. 9). In addition to their exploration of the larger organelles—nuclei, nucleoli, and mitochondria—they have devoted much attention in the past 20 years to the properties of a fraction consisting of submicroscopic particles, called *microsomes*, that are rich in nucleic acid. Although it was initially believed that these particles existed as such in the intact cell, it has become evident from electron microscopic examination that the microsomes are small vesicular fragments of the endoplasmic reticulum, fragments produced during homogenization of the cells (Fig. 2–6). They are membrane limited spherical vesicles with an amorphous content and variable numbers of ribosomes on their outer surfaces. By treating the microsome fraction with deoxycholate, the membranes can be solubilized. Further centrifugation at higher speeds then yields a pure fraction of ribosomes.

Most of the ribonucleoprotein of cells can be isolated centrifugally in the form of ribosomes. These are identical to the small dense granules seen in electron micrographs, either free in the cytoplasmic matrix or associated

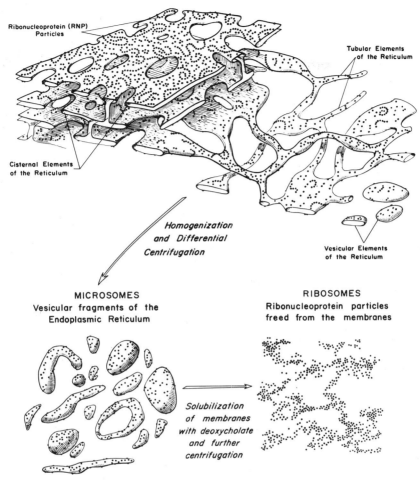

Ribonucleoprotein (RNP) Particles

Tubular Elements of the Reticulum

Cisternal Elements of the Reticulum

Vesicular Elements of the Reticulum

Homogenization and Differential Centrifugation

MICROSOMES
Vesicular fragments of the Endoplasmic Reticulum

RIBOSOMES
Ribonucleoprotein particles freed from the membranes

Solubilization of membranes with deoxycholate and further centrifugation

Figure 2-6 Schematic representation of the relations between the granular endoplasmic reticulum (ergastoplasm) and the *microsome* and *ribosome* fractions isolated by differential centrifugation. The ribosomes are always on the outer surface of the membrane limiting the tubules and cisternae.

with the outer surface of the membranes of the endoplasmic reticulum. They have a sedimentation coefficient of 80S and are composed of two subunits, with sedimentation coefficients of 60S and 40S, held together by hydrogen bonds and magnesium ions. The two units can be taken apart by subjecting ribosomes in vitro to a magnesium free medium. There is no indication as yet that the subunits ever occur separately in cells. The nucleic acid in each of the units is associated with structural protein. Further degradation of the subunits can be achieved by removal of the protein, which leaves two species of RNA, one of 28S and the other of 18S sedimentation coefficient.

Agranular Endoplasmic Reticulum

When it was first discovered that the distribution of parallel arrays of endoplasmic reticulum in electron micrographs was similar to that of the clumps of ergastoplasm seen with the light microscope, it was assumed that areas rich in endoplasmic reticulum were invariably basophilic. As experience was gained with a greater variety of tissues, it soon became apparent that in some cell types the membrane limited tubules comprising the endoplasmic reticulum lack associated ribosomes, and are therefore called *agranular reticulum.* In such cells the cytoplasm is often acidophilic. Possessing no distinctive staining properties at the light microscope level that set it off from the surrounding cytoplasmic matrix, the agranular reticulum went undetected by classical cytologists.

Two categories of endoplasmic reticulum are now distinguished, the granular or rough surfaced form that can be equated with the ergastoplasm or chromidial substance, and the agranular or smooth surfaced reticulum that has no easily identifiable counterpart in stained histological sections. Although the two forms of this organelle are often in continuity with one another, there is reason to believe that the difference between them goes beyond the mere presence or absence of ribosomes. The agranular reticulum is usually a close-meshed tridimensional network of tubules and seldom takes the form of cisternae (Fig. 2–7*A* and *B*). In many cell types either one form of the reticulum or the other greatly predominates. For example, in protein secreting cells such as those of the pancreas, the endoplasmic reticulum is almost exclusively of the granular type, whereas in muscle it is mainly of the smooth surfaced variety. In other cells, such as those of the liver, the two types are represented in nearly equal proportions. It follows that the microsome fraction obtained from homogenates of different tissues will vary in its content of RNA and will contain fragments of both types of reticulum. It has recently become possible to achieve a subfractionation of the microsomes, separating those bearing ribosomes on their surface from smooth surfaced microsomes that are derived mainly from the agranular reticulum.

The biochemical differences between the two kinds of reticulum have not been completely worked out. There is agreement that the granular reticulum is involved in protein synthesis, but it is not yet possible to assign a single function to the agranular reticulum. In striated muscle the agranular form is concerned with the release and recapture of calcium ions in the cycle of contraction

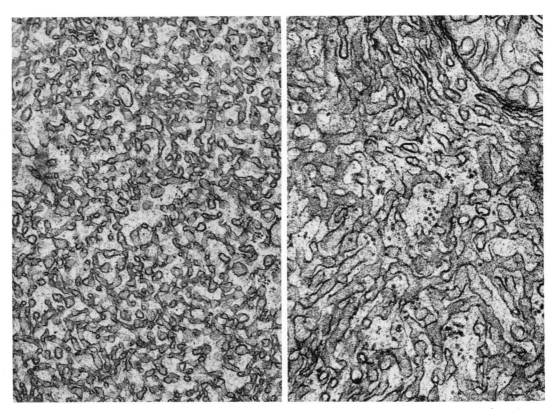

Figure 2–7 Electron micrographs of agranular or smooth-surfaced endoplasmic reticulum. *A* from liver cell of hamster, ×34,000; *B* from the human adrenal cortex, ×50,000. (Courtesy J. Long.)

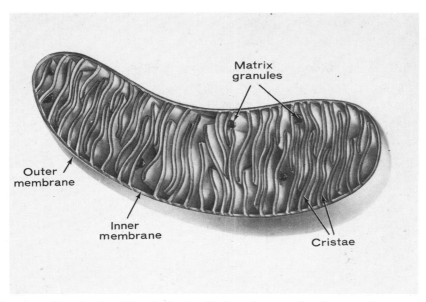

Figure 2–8 Drawing of a mitochondrion in longitudinal section showing the smooth outer membrane and an inner membrane plicated to form the slender folds called cristae that extend into the interior of the organelle.

and relaxation. In a number of endocrine glands it has been implicated in the biosynthesis of steroid hormones, and in the liver it is involved in cholesterol and lipid metabolism and in the hydroxylation of various endogenous and exogenous compounds.

Mitochondria

Mitochondria are the cell organelles concerned principally with the generation of energy to support the various forms of chemical and mechanical work carried out by the cell. They usually appear in living preparations as slender rods or filaments about 0.2 μm. in diameter and 2 to 6 μm. long (Fig. 2–1). They may be randomly distributed, or they may be concentrated at sites of high energy utilization. They can be thought of as mobile "power plants of the cell." Mitochondria are capable of actively changing shape and in living cells are often observed to execute slow, sinuous movements. How their migrations within the cell are directed is not known; nor is it clear whether their movements are a result of flow of the surrounding cytoplasm or of their own intrinsic capacity for changing shape.

When examined in thin sections with the electron microscope, mitochondria have a complex internal structure (Figs. 2–8 and 2–9). They are enclosed by two membranes. The outermost of these, 50 to 60 Å thick, is a smooth-contoured, continuous limiting membrane with the usual trilaminar substructure. The inner membrane is of similar thickness and appearance and generally courses parallel to the outer membrane, but also forms numerous narrow pleats or folds that project into the interior of the organelle. These plications, called the *cristae* of the mitochondrion, are obviously a means of amplifying the surface area of the inner membrane and thus increasing the efficiency of the organelle as an energy generating device. In cells with high energy requirements, the number of cristae per mitochondrion is higher than in those of lower metabolic activity.

The mitochondrial membranes delimit two compartments: a large *intercristal space* comprising all of the area within the inner membrane, and a smaller *membrane space* consisting of the narrow cleft between outer and inner membranes including its inward extensions between the leaves of the cristae (Fig. 2–10). These latter clefts are sometimes designated as the *intracristal spaces*, but it is clear that they are not functionally distinct from the rest of the membrane space. The membrane space is usually only 100 to 200

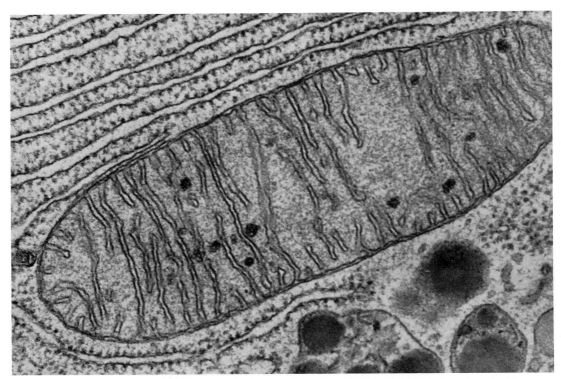

Figure 2–9 Electron micrograph of a typical mitochondrion from the pancreas of a bat, showing the cristae, matrix, and matrix granules. The endoplasmic reticulum is seen at the upper left and some lysosomes at the lower right. ×79,000. (Courtesy of K. R. Porter.)

Å across and evidently contains little or no protein precipitable by chemical fixatives and therefore in electron micrographs it appears empty. The large intercristal space, on the other hand, is occupied by a moderately dense *mitochondrial matrix* which contains a number of morphologically identifiable components.

Although the outer and inner mitochondrial membranes are similar in dimension and appearance after fixation and thin sectioning, both have distinctive morphological features which can be demonstrated only by negative staining of isolated mitochondria. When prepared in this way the outer membrane has a porous appearance, which correlates with studies demonstrating that it is freely permeable to small molecules. The inner membrane, which has the properties of a semipermeable membrane, has no visible porosity. It is distinguishable from the outer membrane because of the presence of great numbers of small particles associated with its inner surface. These *inner membrane*

subunits consist of a globular *head* 90 to 100 Å in diameter, connected by a slender stem or *stalk* (50 Å long and 30 to 40 Å thick) to a *baseplate* (40 by 110 Å) which is incorporated in the inner leaflet of the underlying membrane. The existence of the baseplate has yet to be established to the satisfaction of all investigators, but the head and stem can be detached and isolated. They are found to be the site of the enzymes of oxidative phosphorylation and hydrolysis of adenosine triphosphate (ATP). Mitochondrial membranes stripped of their inner membrane subunits continue to carry out electron transport. The succinoxidase, cytochrome oxidase, and other enzymes concerned with electron transport thus appear to reside in the membrane proper and not in the attached globular subunits.

Mitochondria are self-duplicating organelles that increase their numbers by undergoing division in a manner reminiscent of the binary fission of bacteria. They contain their own supply of the genetic material

DNA. This can occasionally be identified in routine electron micrographs as branching filaments of variable thickness usually located in one or two less dense regions of the mitochondrial matrix (Fig. 2–11). The DNA is studied to better advantage when isolated from mitochondrial fractions and examined in thin spreads, shadowed with metal. In such preparations the mitochondrial DNA is found to consist of double-stranded molecules of circular configuration having a circumference of about 5.5 μm. This DNA differs from that of the cell nucleus in its circular form, its purine and pyrimidine base composition and its much lower molecular weight.

Also present in the matrix of mitochondria is a population of small granules about 120 Å in diameter. These have been shown to consist of ribonucleoprotein and are the counterparts of the ribosomes of the cytoplasmic matrix. Mitochondria thus have all of the chemical components necessary for protein synthesis; namely, their own distinctive DNA, complementary ribosome-like RNA, and a variety of specific transfer RNAs. They seem to be semiautonomous, being able to synthesize some but not all of their constituent proteins. The reduplication of functionally competent mitochondria probably requires cooperative activity of both the genetic systems of the cell and the protein synthesizing machinery of the general cytoplasm, as well as that of the mitochondrial matrix.

The most conspicuous of the matrix components are the *matrix granules*—dense spherical or irregular bodies 300 to 500 Å in diameter occurring anywhere in the inter-

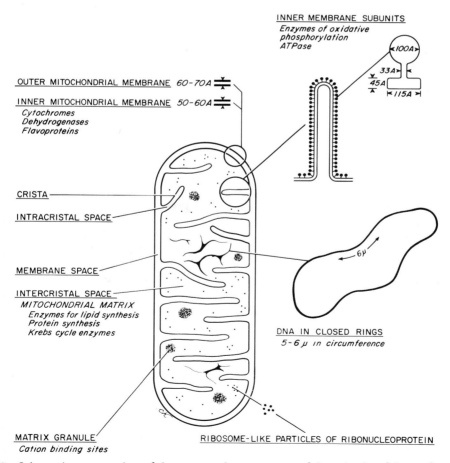

Figure 2–10 Schematic presentation of the structural components of the mitochondrion and some of their functional activities.

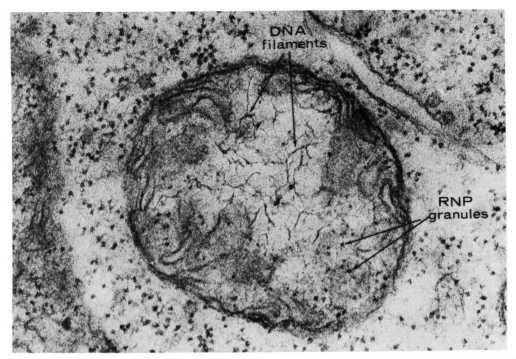

Figure 2–11 Electron micrograph of a mitochondrion from a plant cell showing filaments of DNA and ribosome-like particles of ribonucleoprotein in the matrix. Similar components are demonstrable, but with more difficulty, in mitochondria of animal cells. (Micrograph courtesy of H. Swift.)

cristal space, but often near the bounding inner membrane (Fig. 2–9). They vary in abundance in different cell types. No typical substructure has been defined for these granules, but at high magnification, they sometimes have a loculated appearance. They have not been isolated and analyzed but they are believed to be concerned with the regulation of the internal ionic environment of the mitochondrion. Calcium and other divalent cations accumulate in mitochondria when they are present in high concentration in intact cells or in the fluids bathing isolated mitochondria. Under these conditions large and unusually dense granules are found in the matrix and it seems likely that the accumulated ions are organically bound to the preexisting matrix granules to form larger dense bodies. It has been suggested that the density of matrix granules in electron micrographs of normal cells may be due to their uptake of metal from the fixative rather than their inherent density.

Much is now known about the localization of the enzymes within mitochondria. When isolated mitochondria are disrupted, some of the enzymes residing in the matrix are released into the medium as soluble protein, while others remain bound to the membranes. In general, the respiratory and phosphorylating enzymes are attached to the membranes, while those of the Krebs citric acid cycle and those concerned with protein and lipid synthesis occur in the matrix. Indirect biochemical evidence supports the view that the enzymes and coenzymes associated with the membranes are not randomly distributed but are arranged in a highly ordered repeating pattern that facilitates the sequential catalytic reactions carried out by this organelle.

Lysosomes

The *lysosomes* are newcomers to the ranks of the cell organelles, having first been recognized as a separate category of particles by Christian de Duve in 1955. They are usually dense bodies 0.25 to 0.5 μm. in diameter, limited by a membrane and containing a number of hydrolytic enzymes that are active at acid pH (Fig. 2–13). The enzymes of lysosomes are therefore referred to by the collective term *acid hydrolases*. A partial list of the specific enzymes that have been identified in these particles includes acid phosphatase, acid ribonuclease, acid deoxyribonuclease, cathepsin, β-glucuronidase, β-galactosidase, aryl-sulfatase, and peroxidase.

In normal intact lysosomes these enzymes are bound and are safely contained within an enclosing membrane. A variety of experimental conditions and pharmacological agents may increase the permeability of the lysosomal membrane or cause its complete breakdown, allowing the enzymes to escape and digest or lyse the cell. The term *lysosome* is descriptive of this property.

Such cell digestion is a common occurrence at sites of disease or tissue injury but it is not confined to pathological states. In the programmed cell death that is a normal part of embryonic development; in the regression of the mammary gland after weaning; and in the resorption of the tadpole's tail at metamorphosis the membranes of lysosomes are believed to be altered, permitting escape of acid hydrolases and consequent destruction of the cells.

In certain cell types having a capacity for *phagocytosis* (engulfing extracellular material), lysosomes are an essential part of an intracellular digestive system that enables the cell to break down the ingested material and dispose of the degradation products. For example, two of the types of white blood corpuscles, or leukocytes, contain cytoplasmic granules which are a variety of lysosome. These cells are capable of ingesting bacteria and are therefore in the first line of defense of the organism against invasion by pathogenic microorganisms. When bacteria are engulfed they are taken into the cell in membrane bounded phagocytosis vacuoles or *phagosomes*. Lysosomes of the cell then adhere to the limiting membrane of the phagosome and fuse with it, so that their hydrolytic enzymes are discharged into its cavity, killing and ultimately digesting the bacterium (Fig. 2–14).

Intracellular digestion of material taken into the cell from its environment is referred to as *heterophagy* and the phagosomes which have fused with primary lysosomes are also called *heterophagic vacuoles*. Some of the materials ingested can, in time, be completely broken down. Others may leave indigestible residues which persist in the form of membrane bounded structures called *residual bodies*. These vary greatly in appearance of their contents, containing dense granules of varying sizes and occasionally laminated concentric structures that are interpreted as myelin forms of phospholipid. It has been suggested that cells are capable of divesting themselves of undigestible matter by *exocytosis* —a fusion of the limiting membrane of a residual body with the plasmalemma and discharge of its contents into the extracellular space. However, examples of this process are exceedingly difficult to find in electron micrographs and some cell biologists remain unconvinced of its existence.

The lysosomal digestive system of the cell is also involved in normal turnover of organelles and in the internal remodeling of the structure of the cytoplasm that is associated with marked changes in its physiological activity. Mitochondria, elements of the endoplasmic reticulum, or secretory granules that are damaged or present in

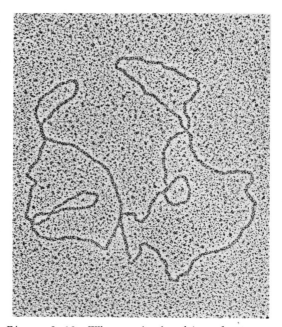

Figure 2–12 When mitochondria of *Xenopus* oocytes are spread on a surface tension film of fluid, the organelle is disrupted and the DNA strands can be collected on a specimen grid and examined with the electron microscope. Mitochondrial DNA is found to be in the form of circles 5.6 to 6 μm. in contour length. (Micrograph courtesy of I. B. Dawid and D. R. Wolstenholme.)

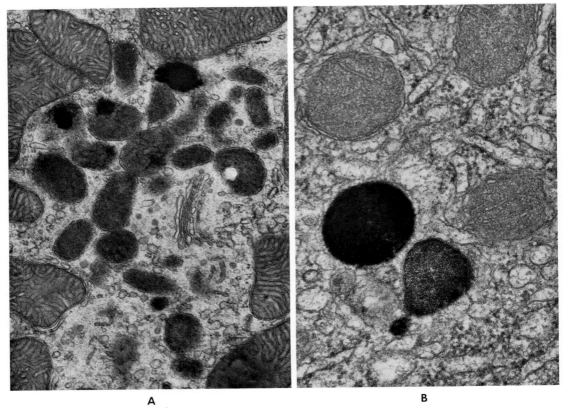

A   B

Figure 2–13 Electron micrographs of lysosomes. *A,* Adrenal cortex lysosomes nonspecifically stained with osmium and lead. ×25,000. *B,* Lysosomes from the rat vas deferens stained for acid phosphatase activity. ×65,000. (Courtesy of D. Friend.)

excess may be segregated and enveloped in a membrane. Lysosomes then fuse with this membrane introducing acid hydrolases into what is now called a *cytolysosome* or *autophagic vacuole.* This process of controlled degradation of organelles in an otherwise healthy, viable cell is called *autophagy,* in contradistinction to *heterophagy,* which is the digestion of substances imported from outside of the cell. The residual bodies resulting from the two processes are not morphologically distinguishable. The indigestible residues of the lysosomal activity, associated with normal wear and tear, accumulate with advancing age in the form of *lipofuscin pigment.*

Lysosomes were discovered by biochemists subfractionating the mitochondrial fraction isolated by differential centrifugation. The presence of a membrane was inferred from the fact that mechanical disruption or treatment with surface active agents was necessary before the enzymes could act upon

their substrates. Lysosomes were defined, therefore, as membrane limited particles containing acid hydrolases. The visual identification of lysosomes in electron micrographs came later, and the appearance of the structures fulfilling these two defining criteria has proved to be surprisingly diverse. Some have a smooth spherical or ovoid shape and a dense, homogeneous interior; others are quite irregular in outline and nonhomogeneous in density; still others are large globular structures with a rather pale matrix; and finally, a few special kinds of lysosomes, such as the specific granules of eosinophilic leukocytes, may contain dense equatorial crystals in a less dense matrix. The diversity of the appearance of this organelle from one cell type to another makes its identification on morphological grounds alone quite uncertain. The uptake by lysosomes of fluorescent vital dyes, such as acridine orange, and their histochemical reactions for acid hydrolases, are valuable additional criteria for their identification (Fig. 2–13).

The functions of lysosomes in the economy of the cell are still being defined. The subject remains somewhat confused, and a complex and cumbersome terminology has developed as an increasing number of morphological types are described. In the current concept the lysosomes and certain other vacuolar structures lacking hydrolytic enzymes are considered to be components of a discontinuous intracellular digestive system for the cell. *Primary lysosomes*, containing enzymes that have not yet been engaged in digestive activities, are distinguished from *secondary lysosomes*, which are vacuolar structures that are the sites of current or past digestive activity. The latter include autophagic and heterophagic vacuoles, residual bodies, and lipochrome pigment deposits.

Lysosomes have been found to participate in the normal secretory activity of some cell types. For example, in the thyroid gland, which stores its secretory product extracellularly in the follicles in the form of thyroglobulin, release of the active hormone thyroxin depends upon uptake of thyroglobulin by pinocytosis and its degradation by lysosomal proteases (see Chapter 4, p. 130).

A variant of the lysosome is the *multivesicular body*. This is a spherical, membrane bounded structure 0.5 to 3.0 μm. in diameter containing variable numbers of small vesicles in a matrix of low density (Fig. 2–15). It is not clear how these organelles relate to the more conventional lysosomes. The matrix of multivesicular bodies exhibits acid phosphatase activity but the included vesicles have no demonstrable enzymatic activity and their origin is obscure.

Interest in lysosomes has been greatly stimulated by the discovery that the storage diseases of man, Gaucher's disease, Tay-Sachs disease. Fabry's disease, and several others, are each traceable to congenital absence of one of the lysosomal enzymes. Absence of an enzyme permits abnormal intracellular accumulation of its corresponding

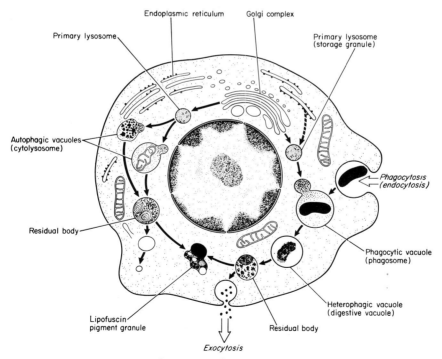

Figure 2–14 Schematic representation of the role of lysosomes in heterophagy (lower right) and in autophagy (upper left). Bacteria or other foreign matter may be taken in by phagocytosis (endocytosis). Primary lysosomes fuse with the heterophagic vacuoles and their enzymes degrade the foreign matter. On the other hand, membranes may be formed around organelles or inclusions and primary lysosomes may fuse with these autophagic vacuoles. End products of either process may be recognized in cells as residual bodies or lipofuscin pigment deposits.

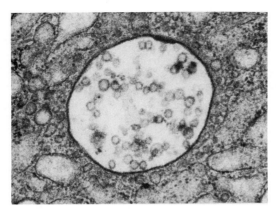

Figure 2-15 An example of a multivesicular body. This is regarded as a variety of lysosome.

substrate, resulting in disturbance of other functions of the cells (Table 2–1).

Peroxisomes (Microbodies)

The term *microbody* was introduced by Rhodin in 1954 to designate spherical cytoplasmic bodies, about 0.5 μm. in diameter, surrounded by a single membrane. They were first observed in the cells of the proximal convoluted tubule of the kidney, and soon thereafter were also reported in the liver.

The microbodies of the kidney have a homogeneous, finely granular matrix of moderate density. Those of the liver show significant species differences. In the rat they contain conspicuous dense *cores* or *nucleoids* that exhibit a highly ordered substructure with the appearance of a crystal. At high magnification, however, this is resolved as a polytubular structure made up of minute tubules of two different sizes: large ones 95 to 115 Å in diameter and smaller ones 45 Å in diameter. In transverse sections, these are arranged in a regular pattern, with each large tubule surrounded by 10 smaller ones, and this unit is repeated throughout the cross section of the core. In longitudinal section this arrangement gives rise to a pattern of parallel lines with alternate narrow and wider spacings. In certain other species, the cores of the microbodies appear to be composed only of the 45 Å tubules in regular hexagonal array. In the hamster the core takes the form of a thin flexuous sheet.

Microbodies isolated from mitochondrial and lysosome fractions by gradient centrifugation are found to contain *urate oxidase, d-amino acid oxidase,* and *catalase.* Because they contain oxidases capable of reducing oxygen to hydrogen peroxide and hydrogen peroxide to water, it has recently been suggested that a more appropriate descriptive name for the microbody would be *peroxisome.*

The matrix is believed to consist mainly of catalase and other soluble proteins. The cores are relatively insoluble and are thought to be the site of the urate oxidase. Consistent with this interpretation is the finding that human liver microbodies, devoid of urate oxidase, also lack cores in electron micrographs.

Although microbodies bear a superficial resemblance to secretory granules, there is no evidence that they are discharged from the cell. It is assumed that they function within the cytoplasm, but their precise role is not understood.

The Golgi Apparatus

This cell organelle, discovered by Camillo Golgi in 1898, was originally called the *internal reticular apparatus* because in silver impregnated preparations viewed with the light microscope it seemed to be a network of intercommunicating channels. It later came to be called the *Golgi apparatus* and since the electron microscope revealed that it is composed of three or four membrane limited structures of different configurations, it is often referred to as the *Golgi complex.* It is not ordinarily visible in living cells and is not stained in routine histological sections. Nevertheless, its location in the cell is sometimes revealed in negative image as an unstained juxtanuclear area (Fig. 2–16*A*). In tissue impregnated with osmium or silver, it is selectively blackened (Fig. 2–16*B*).

In electron micrographs, the Golgi apparatus is seen to be composed of several membrane bounded, flattened saccules or cisternae arranged in parallel array about 300 Å apart. The saccules are disc-like and often slightly curved, so that the stack of saccules presents convex and concave surfaces (Figs. 2–17 and 2–18). The cisternae vary in their structure and dimensions. The outermost cisterna, on the convex surface, is interrupted by numerous fenestrations. Those more deeply situated in the stack are fenestrated near their margins but are continuous in their central portions. Those near the convex surface have a very narrow lumen, while those nearer the concave surface are more dilated. Associated with the normally convex outer surface of each stack of flattened saccules are numerous small vesicles 300 to 800 Å in diameter. The great majority of these have smooth surfaced membranes but a few are limited by a membrane that has a coating of fine radially oriented short filaments or bristles. These are called *coated vesicles* to distinguish them from the larger population of smooth surfaced vesicles. In secretory cell types, a precipitate of the incomplete product may be seen in the lumen of the cisternae at the concave inner aspect of the complex. Also associated with this surface are membrane-limited spherical *condensing vacuoles* containing secretory product in varying degrees of condensation and also mature *secretory granules* with a dense homogeneous content.

The protein constituents of the Golgi membranes are thought to be synthesized on the ribosomes and incorporated into membranes of the granular endoplasmic reticulum. Small *transitional vesicles* are budded off from ribosome-free flat surfaces or from the margins of cisternae of the reticulum. These vesicles are believed to coalesce to form the fenestrated outer saccule of the Golgi complex. This surface is therefore referred to as the *forming face.* At the same time, saccules at the opposite face are expanding to form the limiting membrane of condensing vacuoles and secretory granules. This is called the *maturing face.* Thus at one face of the Golgi complex, new membrane is continually being contributed by the reticulum via the transitional vesicles

while at the same time membrane is continually being lost at the other face. This organelle can therefore be thought of as constantly turning over and maintaining a state of dynamic equilibrium between the rate of accretion of new membrane at the forming face and the rate of membrane loss at the maturing face.

The polarity within the Golgi stacks is also demonstrable by cytochemical staining reactions. The classical method for demonstrating the Golgi apparatus for light microscopy involved prolonged treatment with osmium tetroxide. When tissues treated in this way are examined with the electron microscope, the dense deposits of osmium are found to be confined to one or two saccules at the outer or forming face of the Golgi. On the other hand, when tissues are processed by the histochemical reaction for thiamine pyrophosphatase, the reaction product is found only in the innermost one or two cisternae (Fig. 2–19). Thus there seems to be a functional specialization within the organelle. The functional significance of thiamine pyrophosphatase is not known, but the selectivity of its localization makes it a useful marker for identifying membranes of Golgi origin in centrifugal fractions of tissue homogenates.

The function of the Golgi apparatus is best understood in glandular cells where it has been shown to be a site of accumulation and concentration of the secretory product. In cells secreting protein, the synthesis of the specific protein takes place on the ribosomes. The protein accumulates in the lumen of the endoplasmic reticulum and is transported through it to the Golgi region where transitional vesicles budding off from the

TABLE 2–1 *INBORN LYSOSOMAL DISEASES*

DISEASE	SUBSTANCE ACCUMULATING IN CELLS	ENZYME DEFECT
Glycogen storage disease II (POMPE)	Glycogen	α-Glucosidase
Gaucher's disease	Glucocerebroside	β-Glucosidase
Niemann-Pick disease	Sphingomyelin	Sphingomyelinase
Krabbe's disease	Galactocerebroside	β-Galactosidase
Metachromatic leukodystrophy	Sulfatide	Sulfatidase
Fabry's disease	Ceramide trihexoside	α-Galactosidase
Tay-Sachs disease	Ganglioside GM_2	N-Acetyl-β-glucosaminidase A
Generalized gangliosidoses	Ganglioside GM_1	β-Galactosidase
Fucosidosis	H-isoantigen	α-Fucosidase

A

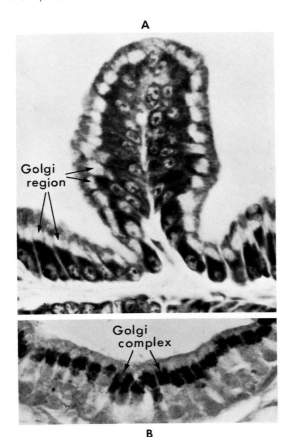

Golgi
region

Golgi
complex

B

Figure 2-16 Photomicrograph of epithelial cells from the prostate. *A*, The Golgi zone in negative image. *B*, The Golgi complex impregnated with osmium in the Da Fano technique. ×500.

reticulum carry small quantities of the product to the Golgi complex. There it is concentrated and inspissated by removal of water, and released from the Golgi complex in the form of secretory granules. In the Golgi apparatus the secretory granules acquire an enveloping membrane with specific properties that permit its fusion with the plasma membrane in releasing the secretory granule from the cell.

In cells that secrete a mucopolysaccharide or glycoprotein, the Golgi complex also has a synthetic role. Isolated Golgi membranes have been shown to contain glucosyl and galactosyl transferases and other enzymes involved in the synthesis of complex carbohydrates and their coupling to protein (Fig. 2–19). Thus, elaboration of glycoproteins is a cooperative venture involving synthesis of polysaccharides in the Golgi complex and their conjugation with protein synthesized on the endoplasmic reticulum. Even in cells that are not usually considered to be glandular, there is reason to believe that carbohydrate components of the cell surface membrane may be made in the Golgi complex and continuously transported to the cell surface.

The Golgi apparatus is also well developed in many cell types that are not secretory, and its function in the economy of these cells remains obscure.

Annulate Lamellae

This is the term that has been applied to a cytoplasmic organelle which consists of parallel arrays of cisternae exhibiting small annuli or circular fenestrae at very regular intervals along their length. The fenestrations are closed by a thin septum or diaphragm and thus very closely resemble the pores of the nuclear envelope (see p. 69). The lamellae or cisternae exhibit a high degree of order, being parallel and very uniformly spaced, with the annuli of the successive cisternae often accurately aligned (Fig. 2–20). Because of the similarity in appearance of the individual lamellae to a segment of the perinuclear cisterna, it has been suggested that they arise by delamination from the nuclear envelope, but this origin has not been firmly established. Annulate lamellae have been described in the germ cells of both invertebrate and vertebrate species, and in a large variety of normal somatic cell types. The functional significance of this organelle is still unknown.

The Centrosome and Centrioles

Centrosome is the term introduced by Boveri in 1888 to describe a specialized zone of cytoplasm containing the *centrioles*, a pair of small granules or short rods. The centrosome, also called the *centrosphere* or *cell center*, is considered to be the center of a number of the activities associated with cell division. It is usually situated adjacent to the nucleus and may occupy a shallow indentation of its surface. The Golgi apparatus often partially surrounds the centrosome on the side away from the nucleus. In some epithelial cell types, however, the centrioles are not associated with the nucleus or the Golgi

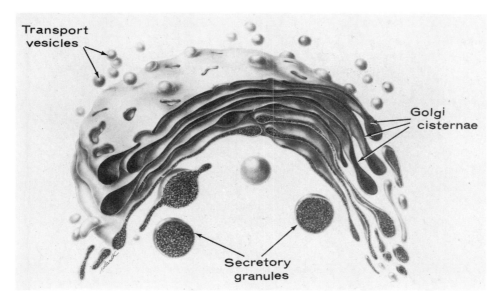

Figure 2-17 A three dimensional representation of the Golgi complex. Small transport vesicles originating from the endoplasmic reticulum are abundant at its convex or forming face. These vesicles fuse with each other and with the outermost flattened saccule or cisterna. In glandular cells secretory granules are associated with the concave or maturing face.

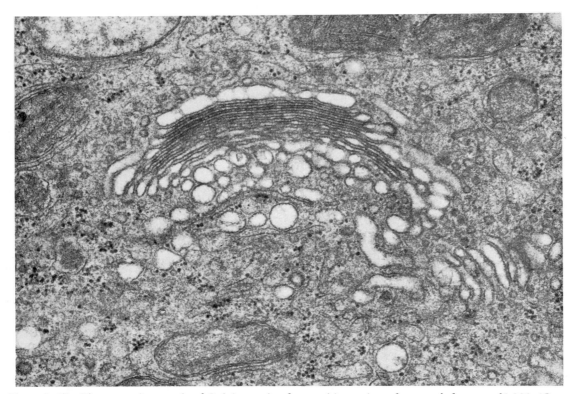

Figure 2-18 Electron micrograph of Golgi complex from a thin section of rat vas deferens. ×65,000. (Courtesy of D. Friend.)

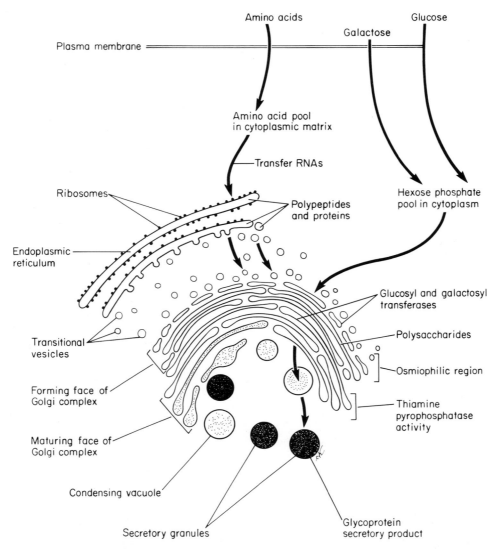

Figure 2–19 Schematic representation of the structure and relations of the Golgi complex to the endoplasmic reticulum. It is involved in concentration of protein secretory products synthesized on the ribosomes of the endoplasmic reticulum. It also has a role in the synthesis of complex carbohydrates and their conjugation with proteins.

apparatus but are located in the apical cytoplasm immediately beneath the free surface of the cell (Fig. 2–21).

In electron micrographs each centriole is found to be a hollow cylinder 150 nm. in diameter and 300 to 500 nm. in length, closed at one end and open at the other. The central cavity is usually occupied by cytoplasm of low density, but it may contain one or more small dense granules. In transverse section, a centriole has a circular outline and its wall is seen to be composed of nine groups of longitudinally oriented parallel subunits. When these were first identified they were considered to be fibers, and this interpretation is still reflected in the terminology. With the resolution now obtained they are clearly seen to be tubular. Each of the nine groups consists of three microtubules aligned and fused together so that in cross section they appear as three circles in a row. The innermost subunit of each triplet is designated subfiber *a* and the others are called subfibers *b* and *c* (Fig. 2–21). The subfibers *a* of the nine triplets are spaced at uniform intervals on the circumference of a circle about 150 nm. in diameter, and subfibers *b* and *c* are aligned so that the axis of each triplet diverges from a tangent to this circle at an angle of about 30 degrees. Subfiber *a* of each triplet is connected to subfiber *c* of the next group by a slender dense line. The arrangement of the triplets in cross section thus resembles a pinwheel or the vanes on a paddle wheel.

As a rule the centrioles occur in pairs, often referred to as a *diplosome*. The long axes of the two centrioles are usually perpendicular. The nature of the forces that maintain this precise orientation is unknown.

Centrioles have traditionally been regarded as self-duplicating organelles that exhibit continuity from one cell generation to the next. They double in number immediately prior to cell division but, contrary to earlier interpretations based upon light microscopy, they do not undergo transverse fission. Instead the new centriole develops in end-to-side relationship to a specific region of each preexisting centriole (Fig. 2–22). The anlage of the new centriole, called a *procentriole*, is a ring-like condensation of fibrogranular material of approximately the same diameter as a mature centriole but initially devoid of microtubular subunits in its wall. The procentriole elongates by accretion to

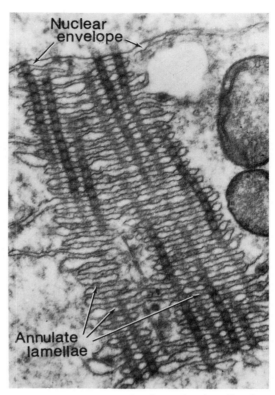

Figure 2–20   An example of annulate lamellae from an oocyte, consisting of parallel arrays of cisternae penetrated by circular pores which are lined by fibrous annuli. These structures are often in register with pores in the nuclear envelope which they closely resemble. (From B. Barton and A. Hertig: Biol. Reprod., 6:98–108, 1972. © The Laboratory for Human Reproduction and Reproductive Biology.)

its distal end and gradually develops microtubules in its wall in the characteristic pinwheel arrangement. After their duplication, the original members of the diplosome separate and each, with its newly formed daughter centriole, moves to opposite poles of the nucleus where they serve as centers for the organization of the microtubules that will form the spindle apparatus of the dividing cell.

Centrioles also serve as the *basal bodies* (*kinetosomes*) and sites of origin of epithelial cilia. Since a ciliated cell may have hundreds of cilia, a large number of centrioles must be formed rapidly as the initial step of ciliogenesis. This rapid proliferation of centrioles was formerly thought to occur by successive replications of the diplosome and its progeny. There is now compelling evidence that, under these conditions, centrioles need not be

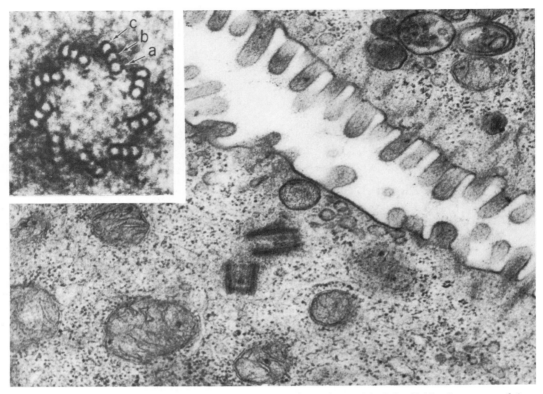

Figure 2–21 Micrograph of a diplosome near the free surface of an epithelial cell. The long axes of the centrioles are usually perpendicular. (Micrograph courtesy of S. Sorokin.) The inset shows a centriole in cross section at higher magnification. The wall is composed of nine triplet microtubules (subunits a, b, c). (Micrograph courtesy of J. André.)

formed one at a time on a preexisting centriole but can also arise de novo by assembly from fibrogranular precursors (see p. 101). The centrioles so formed become arranged in precise linear array immediately beneath the free surface of the epithelial cell. Microtubules then grow out from the distal end of each to form the axoneme of a cilium, which is composed of nine doublet microtubules corresponding to the nine triplets in the wall of the basal body from which it takes origin.

CYTOPLASMIC MATRIX COMPONENTS

Filaments

Some degree of contractility is a fundamental property of protoplasm. The components responsible are filaments. These are most highly developed in cells such as smooth or striated muscle. In striated muscle, there are thin filaments about 70 Å in diameter composed of the protein *actin* and thicker filaments 150 Å in diameter composed of *myosin*. These two classes of filaments are organized in parallel bundles that interdigitate at their ends in such a way that mechanochemical interaction of actin and myosin filaments causes them to slide with respect to one another, producing shortening of the cell (see Chap. 11). In smooth muscle, actin and myosin filaments are also present and interact during contraction, but they are less highly ordered than in skeletal muscle.

In other cell types not specialized for contraction, filamentous components of the cytoplasm are relatively inconspicuous, and 150 Å thick myosin filaments are seldom seen in electron micrographs. There are, however, at least two types of thinner filaments. One type, about 70 Å in diameter, is most abundant in a thin ectoplasmic zone immediately beneath the cell membrane. There the filaments tend to be associated in parallel bundles or are randomly oriented and extensively interwoven. Another type of filament, about 100 Å thick and of indefinite length, may be found in the ectoplasm but it is more often widely distributed throughout the endoplasm. These filaments occur as individual strands or loose fascicles that follow a graceful curving or looping course. The individual filaments cannot be resolved with the light microscope but the bundles formed by their lateral association are easily seen in some cells and were formerly called *tonofibrils* (Fig. 2–23). Tufts of these filaments often converge upon *desmosomes*, dense plaque-like specializations of the cell surface for maintaining cell-to-cell cohesion (see p. 94).

The 70 Å and 100 Å filaments may both be present in the same cell. The rough similarity in their thickness makes it difficult to distinguish them in routine electron micrographs. An ingenious histochemical procedure has been developed for identifying the 70 Å filaments (Ichikawa). Mild tryptic digestion cleaves myosin molecules into two unequal fragments, *light meromyosin* (LMM) and *heavy meromyosin* (HMM). The shorter piece of the myosin molecule (HMM) has the capacity to bind by one end to specific sites on actin filaments (see p. 309), while the remainder of the HMM unit assumes a position oblique to the filament. The binding sites on actin filaments are so distributed that when occupied by HMM subunits, the complex has a highly characteristic "arrow head" configuration. By exposing sections of various cell types to solutions of heavy meromyosin, cytoplasmic filaments composed of actin can be identified by their binding of meromyosin to form "arrow head" complexes. Using this method it has been shown that the smaller 70 Å filaments of cytoplasm are actin. They are presumed to be part of the motility mechanism of the cell.

The 100 Å cytoplasmic filaments do not bind meromyosin. Their chemical nature has not yet been established but they are believed to have a supportive or cytoskeletal function.

Microtubules

In addition to submicroscopic filaments, the cytoplasm contains straight microtubules that can sometimes be followed in electron micrographs for several micrometers before they leave the plane of the section. They have a diameter of 200 to 270 Å and a wall 50 to 70 Å thick. The wall of the microtubule has been shown to be composed of about a dozen filamentous subunits with a center-to-center spacing of 55 to 60 Å. Microtubules occur in small numbers in most cell types during interphase. They may be found in any part of the cytoplasm, but they often converge upon the centrosome and may terminate in small dense *satellites* associated with the centrioles. In mitotic cell division, great numbers of microtubules arise and extend from the chromosomes to the poles and

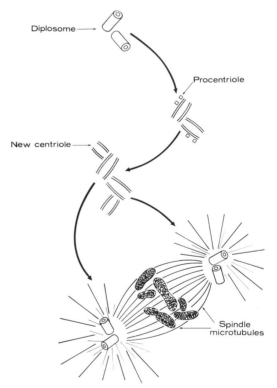

Figure 2–22 In the cell cycle each member of the diplosome becomes a site of nucleation of a new centriole. Its anlage, the procentriole, is a ringlike structure devoid of microtubular substructure. It elongates by accretion to its distal end and acquires triplet microtubules in its wall. Each member of the original diplosome and its newly formed centriole migrates to one pole of the division figure to participate in organization of the spindle. (From D. W. Fawcett, *Genetics of the Spermatozoon.* Amsterdam, Elsevier, 1972.)

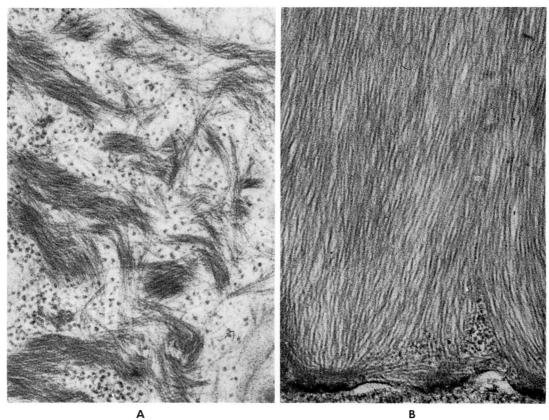

A	B

Figure 2–23 Electron micrographs of filaments in the cytoplasm of epidermal cells. *A*, Bundles of filaments corresponding to tonofibrils of epidermal cells in human skin. ×65,000. (Courtesy of G. Odland.) *B*, Filaments occupy large areas of certain basal cells in the epidermis of the lamprey. Many of these filaments terminate in dense areas of the cell surface called *hemidesmosomes*. ×80,000.

from pole to pole, to constitute what were formerly called the *chromosomal fibers* and the *continuous fibers* of the *spindle apparatus* (Figs. 2–22 and 2–24*A*). After cell division is completed the majority of the microtubules disappear.

In conditions other than mitosis, considerable numbers of microtubules may develop transiently at times of major alterations of cell shape. For example, during the phase of elongation, in the development of spermatozoa, a cylindrical array of microtubules called the manchette is formed around the caudal pole of the nucleus and extends back into the region of the future neck and midpiece (Fig. 2–24*B*). After the period of elongation is over, the manchette disappears. In nucleated erythrocytes of various species, a bundle of microtubules forms the marginal band encircling the cell immediately beneath the plasma membrane. This complex of microtubules is believed to be responsible for maintaining the flattened, discoid shape of the cell.

These observations suggest that the microtubules are cytoskeletal elements influencing cell shape by imparting stiffness to certain regions. Other findings suggest that they may constitute tracks directing flow of cytoplasm or providing for translocation of particles along cell processes.

Microtubules are composed of protein subunits with a sedimentation constant of 65S occurring as a dimer of molecular weight 110,000, separable into two smaller units of 55,000 molecular weight. The naturally occurring alkaloids of plant origin, *colchicine*, *vincristin*, and *vinblastin*, have the property of selectively binding to subunits of microtubule protein and preventing their polymerization to form microtubules. Thus, colchicine blocks cell division by suppressing formation of the mitotic spindle. Several of our inferences as to the physiological significance of microtubules are based upon the functional deficits that result from administration of these compounds. For example, the fact that colchicine prevents the release of the secretory products of certain glands has fostered the speculation that microtubules are required for movement of secretory granules to the cell surface.

It is evident that microtubules are very important components of the cytoplasm, being essential for cell division, involved in maintenance of cell shape, and of importance in the movements of organelles and inclusions. However, how they exert their effects remains an unresolved problem.

CYTOPLASMIC INCLUSIONS

Pigment Granules

In certain tissues scattered throughout the body, particularly in amphibia, there are cells that contain large numbers of dark brown to black granules. These cells are the *melanocytes*, and the granules that contain the pigment *melanin* are called *melanosomes* (Fig. 2–25). In its formative stages the melanosome is limited by a membrane and contains longitudinally oriented lamellae that exhibit a regular periodic structure along their length. As maturation of the granule proceeds, melanin is deposited upon this framework to such an extent that it obscures the internal structure. The melanosome appears as a homogeneous dense granule and its limiting membrane may no longer be evident.

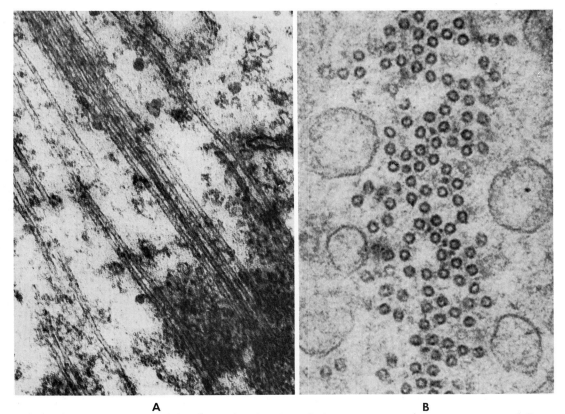

A **B**

Figure 2-24 Electron micrographs of cytoplasmic microtubules. *A*, Microtubules of the mitotic spindle seen here in longitudinal section. The chromosomes are at the lower right. ×70,000. (Courtesy E. Roth.) *B*, The microtubules in transverse section present circular profiles. Those shown here are from the manchette of a mammaliam spermatid. ×140,000.

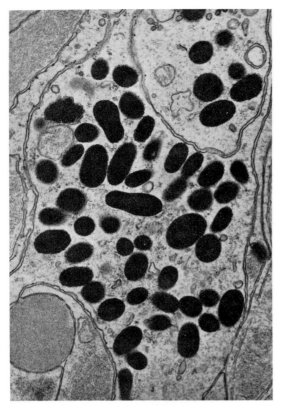

Figure 2–25 Electron micrograph of a portion of a melanocyte from an invertebrate. Numerous exceedingly dense melanosomes are present. ×18,000.

In man, melanosomes are found in the melanocytes in the deep layers of the epidermis, in the basal epidermal cells, in the pigment epithelium of the retina, in the iris, and in certain cells in the brain.

Colored deposits of another pigment called *lipofuscin* are found in many cell types in the body (Fig. 2–26). These deposits are especially abundant in tissues of older animals and humans. They are tan or light brown in unstained preparations and fluoresce as a golden brown in ultraviolet light. They also stain lightly with fat soluble dyes and are insoluble in acid, alkali, and fat solvents. Lipofuscin pigment is now thought to be an end stage of lysosomal activity and is regarded as the indigestible residues of phagocytosed material and degenerated organelles. Because such pigment progressively increases in amount with advancing age, it is sometimes referred to as "wear and tear" pigment.

An additional category of pigment encountered in some tissues is that resulting from the destruction of *hemoglobin*, the iron-containing substance that imparts color to the red blood corpuscles and promotes their efficiency as carriers of oxygen. The red blood cells have a limited life span in the circulation and are then phagocytosed by certain cells in the spleen, liver, and bone marrow. The degradation of hemoglobin within these cells gives rise to a golden brown, iron-containing pigment called *hemosiderin*, which accumulates in irregularly granular masses in the cytoplasm of the phagocytes. There is some hemosiderin in the phagocytes of the normal spleen, liver, and bone marrow, but in diseases that involve an increased rate of destruction of the red blood cells, the amount of this pigment is markedly increased. Hemosiderin may be distinguished from other pigments by staining reactions for iron. In electron micrographs, the masses of pigment include large numbers of 90 Å dense particles of the iron-containing protein *ferritin*.

Glycogen

Animal cells are capable of storing carbohydrate in the form of glycogen, a large polymer of glucose. Glycogen is not apparent in routine histological sections but can be selectively stained by the Best's carmine method or by the periodic acid-Schiff reaction, which colors it a brilliant magenta. Glycogen may appear diffusely distributed in the cytoplasm or in coarse clumps, depending upon the nature of the fixative used. The coarse masses ordinarily observed with the light microscope are composed of submicroscopic particles that can be visualized only with the electron microscope.

The appearance of glycogen in electron micrographs is considerably influenced by the method of specimen preparation, but with the better fixatives it is preserved in the form of dense, roughly isodiametric, 150 to 300 Å particles that are often rather irregular in outline. These are referred to as the *beta particles* of glycogen. In some cell types they occur individually; in others, notably the liver, they form rosette-like aggregates of larger size called *alpha particles* (Fig. 2–27*A* and *B*). The significance of these two forms of glycogen is not understood.

Lipid

Cells often contain stored lipid which, in life, is present in the form of droplets of oil. The simple lipids are neutral fats—triglycerides of fatty acids—and are of such a degree of unsaturation as to be liquid at body temperature. They serve as a local store of energy and also as a source of short carbon chains that can be utilized by the cell in the formation of membranes and other lipid rich structural components. In ordinary histological sections these are likely to appear as round, clear areas in the cytoplasm, because the lipid is extracted by solvents used in the preparation of the specimen. By using sections of frozen tissue, exposure to such solvents can be avoided and the lipid can be colored with a fat soluble dye. Also, by fixation in osmium, lipid can

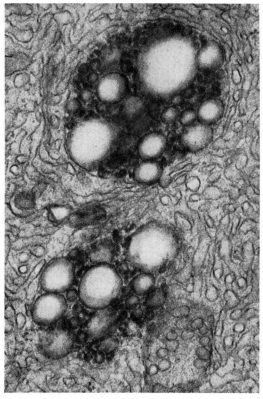

Figure 2–26 Electron micrograph of two lipofuscin pigment deposits in a human adrenal cortical cell. This type of pigment, which accumulates with age, is very heterogeneous in appearance and is thought to represent undigestible residues of lysosomal activity. ×50,000.

be rendered resistant to extraction. It then appears as black spherical droplets of varying size. This is the usual appearance of lipid in electron micrographs (Fig. 2–28), but the degree of blackening depends upon the degree of unsaturation of the lipid and the nature of the fixative used. Some structures other than lipid may blacken with osmium. After preliminary aldehyde fixation, lipid may fail to blacken upon subsequent exposure to osmium, and it then appears pale gray in electron micrographs.

NUCLEAR ORGANELLES

Chromatin and Chromosomes

The nucleus is the archive of the cell, the repository of the genome, and the source of the informational macromolecules (ribosomal RNA; messenger RNA; and transfer RNA) that control the synthetic activities of the cytoplasm. It is an essential organelle present in nearly all cells. Those few cell types that lack a nucleus in the fully differentiated state (erythrocytes, platelets, lens fibers) are incapable of protein synthesis or cell division and are severely limited in their metabolic activities.

The store of the genetic material *deoxyribonucleic acid* (DNA) resides in the chromosomes of the nucleus, but these latter entities are visible as discrete rodlike or threadlike structures only during certain stages of cell division. When the nucleus is reconstituted after division, the filaments of DNA and protein comprising major segments of each chromosome become decondensed or uncoiled. In this dispersed or extended state, the genetic material has ill-defined limits and little or no affinity for histological stains. Other segments of the chromosomes, however, remain condensed and do bind basic dyes. These segments are recognized as irregular clumps of deeply stained material distributed along the nuclear envelope and scattered through the nucleoplasm. This stainable material of the nucleus is called *chromatin* and individual clumps or masses of it are often called *karyosomes*.

The condensed regions of the chromosomes that persist during interphase are described as the *heterochromatin*. Regions of the chromosomes that are dispersed and therefore not readily stainable are referred

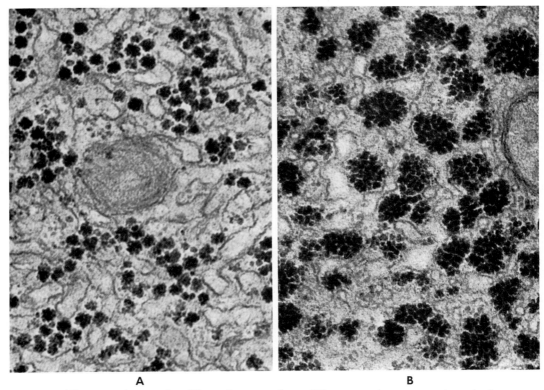

A   **B**

Figure 2–27 Electron micrographs of liver glycogen of two different species at approximately the same magnification. In the salamander liver (*A*), the rosettes or alpha particles are considerably smaller than in the hamster (*B*). In both, the dense glycogen particles are aggregates of smaller subunits. ×60,000.

to as the *euchromatin* (Fig. 2–29). The heterochromatic regions of the chromosomes are thought to be relatively inert, while the euchromatic regions are believed to be those portions that are actively participating in the control of the specific metabolic activities of the cell. Since the cells of the body vary greatly in their functions and in their synthetic activities, they also vary in the proportion of chromatin that remains condensed. Therefore, the depth of staining and the pattern of chromatin in the nucleus differ from cell type to cell type, and may provide useful criteria for their identification.

In addition to the chromatin, the nucleus contains one or more prominent *nucleoli* (Fig. 2–30). These rounded bodies usually stain deeply with basic dyes because of their content of ribonucleic acid (RNA). The faintly stained areas of nucleoplasm not occupied by chromatin or nucleolus have traditionally been described as the *nuclear sap* or *karyo-*

lymph, on the assumption that the stainable elements of the nucleus are suspended in a clear fluid or transparent gel. We now know that much of the area to which these terms were originally applied is occupied by the uncoiled or euchromatic regions of chromosomes and by various submicroscopic granular components of the nucleoplasm. The terms karyolymph and nuclear sap therefore do not describe clearly definable morphological entities and probably should be discarded.

As seen by light microscopy, the condensed chromatin consists of regular clumps of material deeply staining with dyes such as hematoxylin, methylene blue, and methyl green. The affinity of chromatin for these dyes is due principally to its content of deoxyribonucleic acid, but the same dyes are also bound by other acidic substances in the cell and are therefore nonspecific. A widely used specific stain for identification of DNA is the Feulgen reaction. In interphase nuclei with little stainable chromatin, the chromosomes are mainly in the extended or euchromatic condition, in which their DNA presents more synthetically active surface to the nucleoplasm. In cells with abundant coarse blocks of chromatin, on the other hand, a greater proportion of the chromosomal mass is in the condensed or heterochromatic condition, in which its genetic material is believed to be repressed by combination with histones and inaccessible for transcription. The chromatin pattern may thus provide a rough index of a cell's activity.

The finer structural organization of the mitotic chromosomes and of the chromatin in the interphase nucleus is still a matter of dispute. Studies of the physicochemical and optical properties of solutions of purified DNA show that the molecules are long, thin threads, estimated to be about 20 Å in diameter, and formed by the helical intertwining of two DNA chains in such a way that there are alternating deep and shallow helical grooves on its surface. Analysis of the nucleohistones that make up much of the bulk of the chromatin suggests that the histones associated with the DNA molecules lie in the grooves of the double helix.

The DNA double helices, when studied in vitro, undergo profound changes in form with minor changes in pH and salt concentration. Thus it cannot be assumed that they are in the fully extended form when they are in their native state in the nucleus. If they were, one might expect to find in electron micrographs of chromatin, filamentous structures 20 to 30 Å in diameter and of indefinite length. Such is not the case. After the usual fixatives containing osmium the nucleoplasm presents a bewildering array of minute punctate and elongated profiles of varying size and density. The complex texture of chromatin in thin sections permits more than one interpretation. Some investigators consider its characteristic appearance to result from the sectioning of a feltwork of randomly oriented 100 Å filaments. Others visualize it as an interlacing pattern of 30 to 75 Å filaments that branch and anastomose to form a three dimensional lattice with interstices less than 200 Å wide. Still others, particularly those who use glutaraldehyde as the primary fixative, see the areas of chromatin as a mass of 200 Å granules or cross-sectioned filaments. Certainly a fibrillar organization has the appeal that it can most easily be brought into accord with genetic theory and with the biophysical analysis of purified DNA, but the methods of tissue preservation obviously have a profound effect upon the fine structure of the chromatin. Working with thin sectioned nuclei, it is virtually impossible to choose among these conflicting interpretations. Investigators studying whole mounts of condensed chromosomes with the electron microscope (Du Praw) report that they appear to be made up of highly convoluted fibers about 250 Å in diameter. Trypsin digestion of these suggests that each contains a single filament of the dimensions of the Watson-Crick DNA helix arranged in a coiled coil within the chromosomal fiber.

Nucleolus. The nucleolus is visible in the living cell as a conspicuous, rounded refractile body eccentrically placed in the nucleus. In stained sections, it is intensely colored with any of the basic dyes and with some acid dyes as well. The basophilia of the nucleolus is largely due to its content of

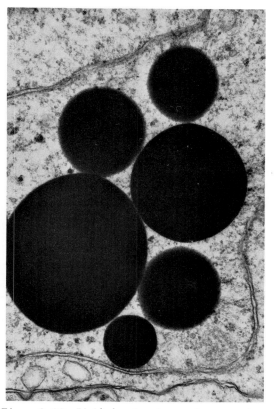

Figure 2-28 Lipid droplets in an electron micrograph of an osmium-fixed Sertoli cell. ×20,000.

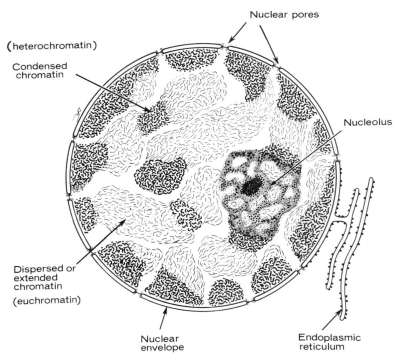

Figure 2–29 Schematic interpretation of the state of the chromatin in the interphase nucleus. The condensed portions of the chromosomes (heterochromatin) are thought to be relatively inactive. The extended or uncoiled segments (euchromatin) are probably the sites of active transcription. The limits of the chromosomes are not identifiable in thin sections. Also shown at the lower right is the continuity of the perinuclear cistern with the granular endoplasmic reticulum.

ribonucleoprotein and therefore it is not colored in preparations stained with the Feulgen reaction for DNA. A rim of Feulgen reactive material often surrounds it, however, and may extend into interstices within it. This is commonly referred to as *nucleolus associated chromatin.*

In electron micrographs, the nucleolus presents a pattern of organization that is more or less characteristic for each cell type. Thus it is difficult to describe a "typical" nucleolus. There are, however, certain common features. There is often one or more rounded masses of closely packed 50 Å filaments. Such areas tend to be in the interior and were formerly described as the *pars amorpha* of the nucleolus. Surrounding this region is a coarse reticulum of anastomosing strands 600 to 800 Å thick that are collectively referred to as the *nucleolonema* (Figs. 2–30, 2–31). This reticular region of the nucleolus is also composed of fine filaments, but interspersed among the filaments are dense granules 120 Å in diameter. The degree of com-

paction of the filaments varies from place to place, so that some regions of the nucleolonema are much denser than others. The distribution of the granular component is also nonuniform. The denser segments of the nucleolonema usually contain few or no granules whereas the latter are abundant in the less dense segments. When the nucleolus is studied by selective cytochemical staining methods for nucleic acids, it is found that both the filamentous and the granular components of the nucleolus are ribonucleoprotein. After their extraction, there remains a protein component that is amorphous at the resolutions attained in such studies.

A generally acceptable descriptive terminology for the nucleolus has been slow to develop. The terms *pars amorpha* and *nucleolonema* were useful regional designations for descriptions of the gross topography of the organelle, but as attention has focused more upon the smaller structural components, many cytologists prefer the terms *pars fibrosa* and *pars granulosa*. However, since

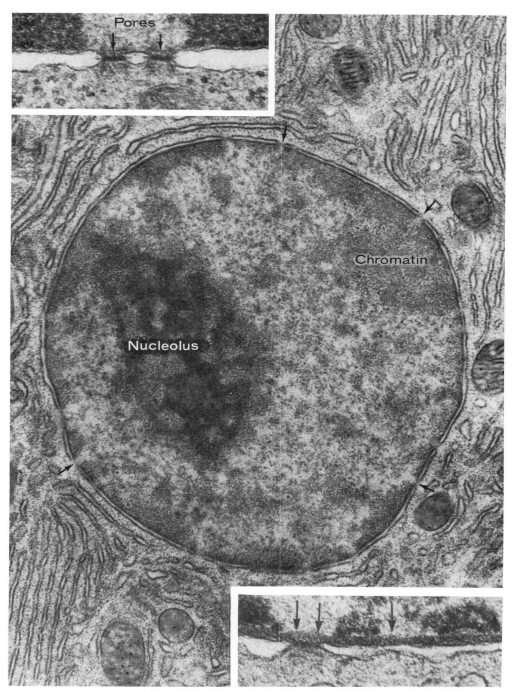

Figure 2-30 Electron micrograph of a typical nucleus with a prominent nucleolus and large clumps of chromatin against a nuclear envelope traversed by numerous pores (arrows). In the inset at the upper left, two nuclear pores are seen at higher magnification to illustrate the septa or pore diaphragms. The inset at the lower right shows a fibrous lamina present on the inner aspect of the nuclear envelope in some cell types.

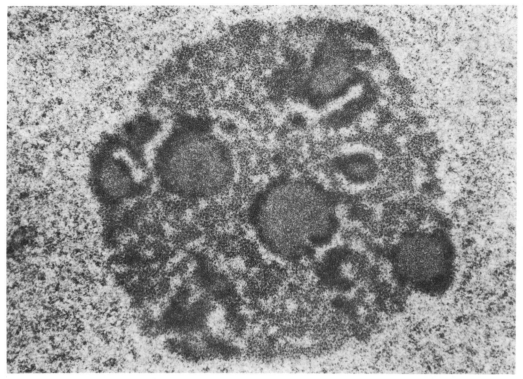

Figure 2-31 Electron micrograph of a nucleolus showing the reticular pattern of the nucleolonema and granular and nongranular portions. (Micrograph courtesy of D. Phillips.)

filaments are present throughout and granules are intercalated among them in certain regions and not in others, pars granulosa and pars fibrosa are not exclusive terms and cannot easily be used in describing the form or pattern of the nucleolus. Until we have a better understanding of the relationship of the filaments and granules and of the physiological significance of the varying patterns of gross topography of the nucleolus, it may not be possible to agree upon a meaningful terminology.

There is now abundant evidence that the principal function of the nucleolus is the production of the ribonucleoprotein of the ribosomes. Labeled precursors of ribonucleic acid are first localized in autoradiographs in the nucleolus and later in the ribosomes of the cytoplasm. Laser beam destruction of the nucleolus results in marked diminution or cessation of incorporation of RNA precursors into ribosomes and in anucleolate mutants of *Xenopus* development is arrested very early because these embryos are unable to synthesize ribosomal RNA. Thus all protein synthesis in the cytoplasm is dependent upon the functional integrity of the nucleolus.

Biochemical studies of isolated nucleoli have shown that there are three major classes of rapidly sedimenting RNA, having sedimentation constants of 45S, 35S, and 28S. Precursors are incorporated most rapidly into 45S RNA and appear somewhat later in the 35S and 28S fractions. In autoradiographic studies using labeled precursors, the grains appear first over the fibrillar regions of the nucleolus and later over the granular areas. It is believed that ribosomal RNAs are first synthesized as long 45S RNA molecules. These subsequently undergo a series of cleavages. Among the products of these cleavages, an 18S fragment is conjugated with protein and passes rapidly out into the cytoplasm, where it appears to be incorporated into the smaller subunit of the ribosome (40S). A 35S fragment acquires protein to form a particle that accumulates in the nucleolus. It is thought that this may correspond to the granular component seen in electron micrographs. The 35S RNA of the nucleolus is ultimately cleaved to a 28S RNA which is incorporated with its associated protein into the larger subunit (60S) of the ribosome.

Although poorly understood, the characteristic structure of the nucleolus is importantly related to its function. The antibiotic actinomycin D binds to DNA and blocks DNA dependent RNA synthesis. When cells are exposed to this substance, there is a loss of normal nucleolar organization and segregation of its fibrillar, granular, and protein components.

The nucleolus varies in size in different cell types, and even within the same cell type it may change in volume in different physiological conditions. As might be expected from its intimate relation to protein synthesis, it is especially large in rapidly growing embryonic or malignant cells and in glandular cells producing large amounts of protein rich secretory products. It is not a permanent organelle but one that disperses when the cell enters mitosis and then is reformed in the daughter cells during reconstitution of their nuclei. The nucleolus forms at particular sites on certain chromosomes. These are called the *nucleolus organizer regions* and are often recognizable as narrowed or poorly stained segments of the chromosomes. These sites are also called *secondary constrictions* to distinguish them from the *primary constriction (kinetochore* or *centromere)* to which the spindle microtubules are attached during anaphase movements of the chromosomes. The number of nucleolus organizer regions in the chromosome set determines the number of nucleoli formed and is theoretically constant for each species. However, the number of nucleoli found may depart somewhat from the basic number characteristic of the species. The number in most somatic cells falls in range from one to four but polyploidy may result in multiples of the basic number. Cinematographic observations of living cells have shown that nucleoli may move about within the nucleus and may fuse with other nucleoli. Coalescence of nucleoli may result in fewer than the expected number. An excess may be produced by their budding or reduplication. This latter phenomenon is rare in somatic cells but occurs regularly in oocytes, in which a thousand or more nucleoli may be formed as a consequence of production of large numbers of extra chromosomal copies of the

cistrons determining ribosomal RNA. This is apparently a unique specialization of the oocyte to provide for the extraordinary needs of the developing early embryo for rapid production of ribosomes.

Nuclear Envelope. The outer limit of the nucleus is clearly demarcated in sections by a thin line that was long interpreted by cytologists as a single thin membrane. It has now been shown by electron microscopy that the *nuclear envelope* is a more complex structure than was previously imagined, consisting of two parallel membranes enclosing a narrow *perinuclear space.* At many points over the surface of the nucleus, the inner and outer membranes are continuous with each other around the circumference of small openings called *nuclear pores* (Figs. 2–29 and 2–30). These openings, which are about 700 Å in diameter, were formerly described as circular, but negatively stained preparations of isolated nuclear envelopes and replicas of nuclei freeze-cleaved *in situ* reveal that they are octagonal in outline. Filamentous material associated with the inner aspect of each pore and extending into it as a lining layer, forms the so-called *annulus* of the pore complex. Although the pores are considered to be potential avenues for exchange of materials between the nucleoplasm and cytoplasm, they clearly do not allow unrestricted diffusion between these two major compartments of the cell. Electrophysiological measurements of resistance have shown that the nuclear envelope constitutes a barrier to diffusion of ions that is several orders of magnitude greater than would be the case if the discontinuities observed were freely communicating passages. Each pore appears to be closed by a delicate septum or diaphragm often somewhat thinner than the usual unit membrane (Fig. 2–30, inset). While very little is known about the molecular organization or permeability properties of this structure, it seems likely that it exercises considerable control over the passage of materials through the pores.

On the inner aspect of the nuclear envelope of some cell types, there is a thin layer of fine filaments comprising the *fibrous lamina* (Fig. 2–30, inset). The significance of this layer is not yet clear. It is possible that it simply provides mechanical support for the nuclear envelope, but it may conceivably have an effect upon its permeability.

Ribosomes are often found on the cytoplasmic surface of the nuclear envelope, and not infrequently its outermost membrane is continuous with the limiting membranes of the system of canaliculi in the cytoplasm known as the endoplasmic reticulum (Fig. 2–29). After mitotic division, the nuclear envelope re-forms by coalescence of flat saccular elements of the reticulum. The cavity of the nuclear envelope is regarded as a *perinuclear cisterna* and is considered to be an integral part of the endoplasmic reticulum.

CELL DIVISION

Growth of nearly all multicellular organisms involves an increase in the number of their cellular units. Many of the specialized cell types of higher organisms have a limited life span and must therefore be continually replaced. The proliferation of cells required for growth and maintenance of the organism takes place by *cell division*. Somatic cells multiply by *mitosis*, a process in which the chromosomes of the nucleus divide and separate with great precision so that two sets exactly alike in number and type pass into each of the two daughter cells and the mass of cytoplasm of the parent cell is constricted to form two cell bodies of equal size. The process of division of the nucleus is called *karyokinesis*, while the partition of the cytoplasm is referred to as *cytokinesis*. Although cytokinesis regularly follows karyokinesis in normal mitosis to produce two separate daughter cells, it is possible to have karyokinesis without cytokinesis, resulting in formation of a binucleate cell.

MITOSIS

The process of cell division extends over a period of 30 to 60 minutes in warm-blooded animals but may take considerably longer in poikilothermic vertebrates. It can now conveniently be studied cinematographically in living cell cultures but most descriptions of mitosis are based upon early light microscopic studies of stained preparations. The resting phase of the cell cycle between episodes of cell division is referred to as *interphase*. Although mitosis is a continuous process, it is arbitrarily divided for convenience of description into four stages—*prophase, metaphase, anaphase* and *telophase* (Figs. 2–32 and 2–33).

During interphase, there is little microscopically resolvable structure to be seen in the living nucleus save for the nucleolus and, in stained preparations, the only additional components that can be made out are a dark rim of peripheral chromatin, a few small karyosomes and the nucleolus associated chromatin. Except for these stainable heterochromatic regions, the chromosomes are too uncoiled and extended to be identifiable as discrete entities. With the approach of cell division, however, the chromosomes are replicated. Their extended segments begin to coil and condense so that they become visible in the living state and stainable in fixed material as continuous threadlike structures.

Prophase of mitosis begins at the moment when the chromosomes first become visible. As they continue to condense during prophase, the chromosomes become thicker and more distinct. Each is double, consisting of two strands called *chromatids*, which are the functional units of the chromosome. They are closely apposed and more or less coiled around one another. As the chromosomes shorten, they undergo further coiling. In addition to the chromosomal changes in prophase, the nucleoli diminish in size and ultimately disappear, the centrioles undergo reduplication and the resulting two pairs of centrioles migrate to opposite poles of the nucleus, and the nuclear envelope breaks down. The disappearance of the nuclear envelope marks the end of prophase.

Metaphase begins with the development of the *mitotic spindle* and the gathering of the chromosomes in the same plane in the middle of the dividing cell, called the *equatorial plate*. The spindle is the organelle responsible for the orderly arrangement and precise separation of the chromosome halves later in division. It arises by polymerization of dispersed protein subunits to form numerous microtubules. These become organized around the centrioles located at opposite poles of the spindle. Some fascicles of microtubules extend from pole to pole as the *continuous fibers* of the spindle while others called *chromosomal fibers* extend only from the poles to the *centromere* or *kinetochore* of each chromosome to which they are attached. The chromosomes may be arranged on the equatorial plate in the axis of a compact spindle or

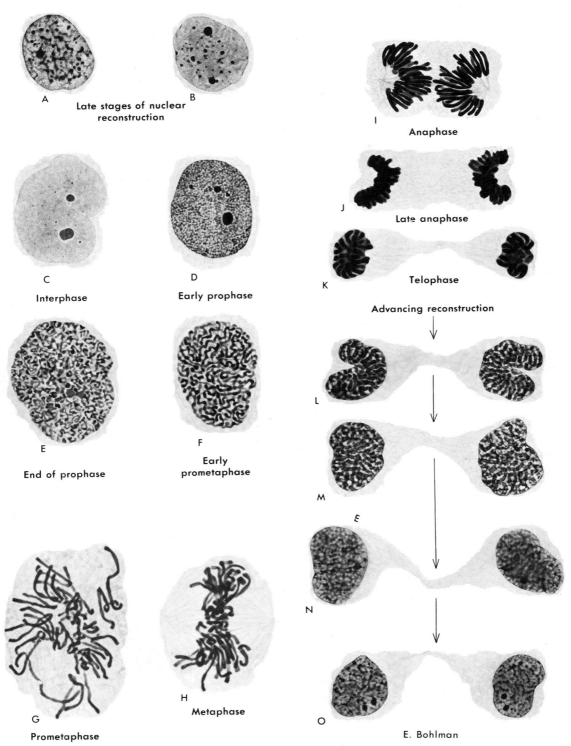

A

B

Late stages of nuclear
reconstruction

C

Interphase

D

Early prophase

E

End of prophase

F

Early
prometaphase

G

Prometaphase

H

Metaphase

I

Anaphase

J

Late anaphase

K

Telophase

Advancing reconstruction

L

M

E

N

O

E. Bohlman

Figure 2-32 Nuclear changes in mitotic mesothelial cells of Amblystoma in culture. (In most of these cells the cytoplasm was much more extensive than is shown.) At the end of prophase the nuclear membrane and the nucleolus are almost gone. In late anaphase, the chromosomes are fusing. With the appearance of the nuclear envelope in telophase the daughter nuclei undergo progressive reconstruction (arrows) until they attain the stage of interphase. Compare with Figure 2–33. Zenker-formol fixed, whole mounts stained with Heidenhain's iron-hematoxylin. ×800.

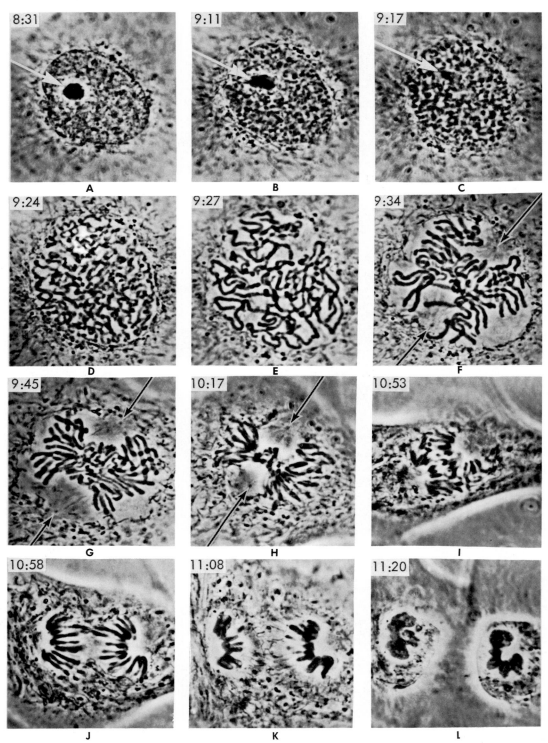

Figure 2–33 Phase contrast micrographs of stages in mitosis of the same living mesothelial cell of Amblystoma in culture. The large white arrows point to the nucleolus; the black arrows indicate centrioles. *A* to *E*, Prophase; *F, G,* and *H*, metaphase; *I, J,* and *K,* anaphase; *L,* telophase. Mitosis proceeds much faster in cells of warm blooded animals.

around the periphery of a hollow spindle with their arms radiating out into the surrounding cytoplasm.

Anaphase is initiated by the doubling of the centromeres or kinetochores of the chromosomes and is marked by the separation of the two chromatids of each chromosome and the beginning of their migration toward opposite poles of the spindle apparatus. During the anaphase movements, the kinetochore regions of the chromosomes usually lead and the arms trail behind. The mechanism of the anaphase movements is still a subject of debate. It is not clear whether the microtubules of the chromosomal fibers shorten actively, or whether elongation of the continuous fibers separates the poles and secondarily draws the chromosomes apart. In any event, at the close of anaphase, the two groups of chromatids, now regarded as daughter chromosomes, are separated and clustered near the spindle poles.

At telophase, discontinuous segments of the nuclear envelope begin to reform around the ends of the chromosomes grouped at the poles. The chromosomes begin to uncoil, become indistinct and lose their stainability except in those regions that remain relatively condensed as the heterochromatin of the interphase nucleus. The normal complement of nucleoli reform and the nuclear envelope, which is at first discontinuous, gradually becomes a complete perinuclear cisterna interrupted only by typical nuclear pores. With these events, karyokinesis is concluded and the two daughter nuclei which are genetically identical have attained the interphase condition.

While the reconstitution of the nuclei is in progress, a constriction of the cytoplasm occurs midway between them. This cleavage furrow advances until it encounters a bundle of microtubules which constitute the remnant of the spindle, particularly its continuous fibers. The cell bodies of the two daughter cells remain connected for a short time in telophase by a slender cytoplasmic bridge filled with spindle microtubules that are held together at their midpoint by dense amorphous material, which is visible at the light microscopic level as a dark dot called the *mid-body*. After a brief delay, the spindle bridge gives way at one side of the mid-body and the two halves retract into their respective daughter cells to complete cytokinesis.

The precise replication of the genetic material DNA prior to cell division, the longitudinal splitting of the chromosome into identical chromatids and the equal distribution of chromatids to the daughter cells insures that the latter are qualitatively and quantitatively of the same genetic make-up as the parent cell from which they were derived.

In cells undergoing rapid growth and division in tissue culture with a constant doubling time, it is possible to identify a repeating sequence of biochemical and morphological events known as the *cell cycle*. The central biochemical event of the cycle consists of the separation of the two helically wound strands of the DNA comprising the chromosomes and the replication of each so that two DNA helices are formed, each of which has one new and one parental strand. This so-called semiconservative replication of DNA characteristic of the somatic cells of mammals occurs during interphase, while the chromosomes are in the extended condition, and is not attended by any visible morphological change in the cell nucleus. It can be detected autoradiographically, however, by following the uptake of radioactive thymidine, a precursor of the newly synthesized DNA. This period of active DNA synthesis lasting 6 to 8 hours is referred to as the *S phase* and occupies 30 to 40 per cent of the cell cycle. It is followed by the G_2 *phase*, during which there is no DNA synthesis but other preparations for division take place. It occupies 10 to 20 per cent of the cycle and is followed by the *M phase*, which consists of the visible morphological events of mitosis described above. Immediately following division is the G_1 *phase*, a period of active RNA and protein synthesis, during which both the nucleus and cytoplasm of the daughter cells enlarge. The G_1 phase extends over 30 to 40 per cent of the cycle. The study of these phases in synchronized cultures has made important contributions to our understanding of the molecular biology of cell proliferation and growth, but it is important to note that these definitions require that the cells of the population are rapidly growing, with a constant doubling time. This type of growth is seldom found in normal adult tissues. Cells may remain for weeks or months in interphase and then undergo one or more division cycles. Some authors refer to these long phases of rest as a G_0 phase, but this is not properly a part of the cell division cycle.

MEIOSIS

All division of somatic cells takes place by mitosis, but the development of the male and female reproductive cells (spermatozoa and ova) involves a special form of cell division called *meiosis*. This consists of two successive nuclear divisions, with only one replication of the chromosomes. It results in separation of the two members of each pair of homologous chromosomes in the first division, thus reducing the chromosomes in each daughter to half the normal number. The second meiotic division involves separation of the two chromatids of each chromosome and results in four nuclei with half the normal number of chromosomes. The gametes that differentiate following meiosis are thus described as *haploid*, and when a male and female gamete unite at *fertilization*, the normal *diploid* number of chromosomes is restored in the fertilized egg, now called the *zygote*.

Meiosis is characterized by a very long prophase, which is divided into six stages. In the earliest of these, called *leptotene*, the chromosomes become visible as long, thin, single strands. In *zygotene*, the homologous chromosomes begin to come together in close lateral apposition with corresponding sites along their length in register. This pairing is also referred to as synapsis. The chromosomes then begin to contract, becoming shorter and thicker in *pachytene*. In this stage, because of the close apposition of homologues, the chromosomes may appear to be present in only the haploid number. The pairs are referred to as *bivalents*.

In *diplotene*, the paired chromosomes separate along their length. Their coiled nature is evident, and it becomes apparent that each is split longitudinally. Each bivalent therefore consists of four *chromatids*. At certain points along their length, the homologous half chromosomes make contact across one another and exchange segments. The sites of crossing are called *chiasmata* and are the morphological expression of the genetic phenomenon of *crossing over*. The shortening and thickening of the chromosomes continues and they tend to clump in the center. The nucleolus, which remained during earlier stages of prophase, begins to fragment in diplotene and may disappear altogether in diakinesis.

In *metaphase*, the nuclear envelope disappears and the spindle forms as it does in mitosis. The bivalents gather on the metaphase plate. In anaphase, the kinetochore or centromere of the bivalents does not divide as it does in mitosis. Consequently in *anaphase* of the first meiotic division, whole chromosomes, not sister chromatids, separate and move to the opposite poles.

The nuclei in mammals are reconstituted in *telophase* for a brief interval, but in other forms the chromosomes may proceed directly into the events of the second division without full reconstitution of the nucleus. In the second meiotic division, the haploid nuclei divide by a mechanism essentially identical to that seen in mitosis. The chromosomes split longitudinally, the kinetochores divide, and sister chromatids move to opposite poles, resulting in formation of four cells with haploid nuclei. The reduction in chromosome number occurs in the first meiotic division. Therefore this is also called the *reductional division* while the second is called the *equational division*. The significance of meiosis is that it provides for constancy of chromosome number from generation to generation by producing haploid gametes. The occurrence of chiasmata provides for variability by insuring that the chromatids emerging from meiosis will be very different genetically than they were before meiosis.

HUMAN CHROMOSOMES

The number of human chromosomes was thought to be 48 until about 20 years ago, when it was clearly demonstrated to be 46 — 22 pairs of homologous autosomes and a pair of sex chromosomes (Tjio and Levan). Soon thereafter it was shown that children born with Down's syndrome (mongolism) have three number 21 chromosomes instead of the two expected in normal human diploid cells (Lejeune et al.). The discovery of a specific chromosomal abnormality in a common congenital disorder aroused great interest in examination of human chromosomes and led to the identification of a number of other examples of disease states associated with visible chromosomal abnormalities. Cytogenetic analysis has now become a routine laboratory procedure in pediatric services of hospitals. It is also possible in some instances to diagnose congenital diseases before birth from a study of chromosomes in cells obtained by amniocentesis (aspiration of fluid from the amnion through a needle). It is necessary therefore for students of medicine to learn something about the basic terminology in this field.

Chromosomes are visible only in dividing cells and the most convenient material for study is a 3- to 4-day tissue culture of leukocytes separated from a sample of blood by centrifugation. The cultures are treated initially with phytohemagglutinin, a substance of plant origin which has the property of stimulating transformation and proliferation of mononuclear leukocytes. After a few days, colchicine is added to the culture medium. This plant alkaloid interferes with formation of the spindle and thus blocks mitotic divisions. This permits an accumulation of cells in metaphase of mitosis. The cells are then exposed to hypotonic solution to cause swelling and thus a better separation of the metaphase chromosomes. Cultures are then fixed and stained, after which they are ready for examination.

The metaphase chromosomes in such preparations appear as double structures, each consisting of two parallel or divergent strands called *chromatids* attached at some point along their length. The region of their attachment is called the *primary constriction* or *centromere*. The chromosomes differ in length and in the location of their centromeres. If the centromere is in the middle and the arms of the chromatids are of about equal length, the chromosome is described as *metacentric*. If the centromere is between the midpoint and one end of the chromosome, it is said to be *submetacentric;* if it is quite near one end, the chromosome is described as *acrocentric*.

To facilitate systematic chromosomal analysis, the chromosomes can be cut out of a photomicrograph. The homologous pairs are identified and arranged in groups on the basis of their differences in length and in position of their centromeres (Fig. 2–34). Such an arrangement of the chromosomes of any given animal species is called the *karyotype*.

The human chromosomal complement is divided into seven groups, within each of which the members are arranged in order of decreasing size: Group 1–3 (Group A) consists of large, approximately metacentric chromosomes; Group 4–5 (Group B) includes four large submetacentric chromosomes; Group 6–12 and the X chromosome (Group C) are medium sized submetacentrics; Group 13–15 (Group D) includes six medium sized acrocentric chromosomes; Group 16–18 (Group E) comprises six short chromosomes, of which number 15 is metacentric and the other two submetacentric; Group 19–20 (Group F) consists of four short metacentrics; and Group 21–22 and the Y chromosome (Group G) are very short acrocentrics. Some cytogeneticists include the X and Y in other groups according to their size, while others prefer to set them apart as a separate group (Fig. 2–34).

Within the seven groups of the human karyotype, it is difficult to recognize individual chromosomes by number. It has recently been found, however, that a characteristic pattern of cross-banding can be revealed by staining the chromosomes with quinacrine mustard and examining them by fluorescence microscopy (Caspersson). Similar patterns can now be demonstrated by a modified Giemsa staining method (Sumner and Evans). These methods provide additional morphological criteria for identification of individual chromosomes.

Chromosomal anomalies of clinical interest may involve changes in number or structure. Cells may have various multiples of the haploid number, and are said to be *polyploid*. More specifically, a *triploid cell* has 69 chromosomes, a *tetraploid* has 92, and so on. Cells with departures from the diploid number that do not involve whole sets of chromosomes are described as *aneuploid*. For example, in Down's syndrome there are 47 instead of 46 chromosomes owing to the presence of an extra chromosome 21 (trisomy 21). Such an abnormality may be the result of nondisjunction, a failure of homologous chromosomes to go to opposite poles during meiosis.

A variety of other accidents of division may occur. One arm of a chromosome may break off and the portion without a centromere may not move to the pole and may be lost. The resulting chromosomal anomaly is called a *deletion*.

During prophase of meiosis, when homologous chromosomes normally cross over, break, and rejoin, an abnormal transfer of a segment of one chromosome to a nonhomologous chromosome may take place. This is called a *translocation* and would result in two chromosomes that would not have the morphology expected in a normal karyotype.

The centromere normally divides longitudinally to permit separation of the chromatids. Rarely it may divide transversely, resulting in metacentric *isochromosomes* consisting of two identical arms of neighboring chromatids joined by a centromere.

Of considerable clinical interest are the examples of aneuploidy involving the sex chromosomes. Loss of one of the X chromosomes (XO) results in Turner's syndrome—producing a phenotypic female whose ovaries are vestigial and usually devoid of germ cells. The presence of an extra X chromosome in a phenotypic male (XXY) results in Klinefelter's syndrome—characterized by underdeveloped testicles, sterility and gynecomastia (enlarged breasts).

About 25 years ago it was discovered

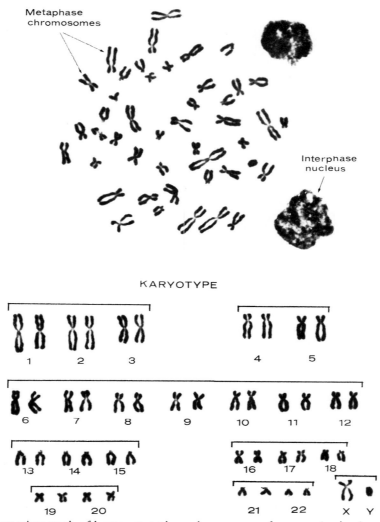

Figure 2-34 Photomicrograph of human metaphase chromosomes from a stained culture of leukocytes. In the lower half of the figure is a human karyotype constructed by cutting out the chromosomes from photographs like that above and arranging them in several groups according to their size and sites of attachment of spindle fibers (primary constrictions). There are 22 pairs of autosomes and an X and Y chromosome. (Photomicrograph courtesy of L. Lisco and H. Lisco.)

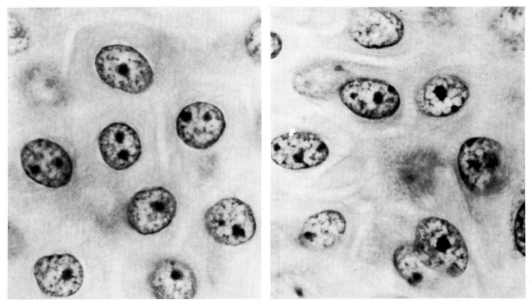

Figure 2-35 Photomicrographs of sections of skin from a male subject on the left and a female subject on the right. In three of the nuclei in the figure at the right a peripherally located mass of sex chromatin can be seen. ×1800. (Courtesy of M. Barr.)

that there is a sexual dimorphism in the interphase nuclei of most mammals, including man (Barr and Bertram). In the female an X chromosome remains condensed during interphase and appears as a small mass of intensely staining chromatin against the inner surface of the nuclear envelope (Fig. 2-35). This *sex chromatin* (or *Barr body*) is not found in the nuclei of normal males. This discovery has made it possible to determine, by simple light microscopic examination of cells, the genetic sex of an individual. This test is also clinically useful in differential diagnosis of abnormalities of sex development.

REFERENCES

General

Brachet, J., and A. E. Mirsky: The Cell: Biochemistry, Physiology, Morphology. Vols I to VI. New York, Academic Press, 1959-1964.

De Robertis, E. D., W. W. Nowinski, and F. A. Saez: Cell Biology. 5th edition. Philadelphia, W. B. Saunders Co., 1970.

Fawcett, D. W.: An Atlas of Fine Structure: The Cell. Philadelphia, W. B. Saunders Co., 1966.

Lima de Faria, A. (ed.): Frontiers of Biology: *Handbook of Molecular Cytology.* Vol. 15. New York, American Elsevier Publishing Co., 1970.

Porter, K. R., and M. Bonneville: An Introduction to the Fine Structure of Cells and Tissues. Philadelphia, Lea and Febiger, 1963.

Wilson, E. B.: The Cell in Development and Heredity. New York, Macmillan Co., 1925.

Cell Membranes

Behnke, O.: Electron microscopic observations on the surface coat of human blood platelets. J. Ultrastruct. Res., *24*:51, 1968.

Bennett, G., and C. P. Leblond: Formation of cell coat material as visualized by radio-autography with L-fucose [3]H. J. Cell Biol., *46*:409, 1970.

Bennett, H. S.: Morphological aspects of extracellular polysaccharides. J. Histochem. Cytochem., *11*:14, 1963.

Branton, D.: Freeze-etching studies of membrane structure. Phil. Trans. Roy. Soc. Lond. *B, 261*:133, 1971.

Ito, S.: The enteric surface coating of cat intestinal microvilli. J. Cell Biol., *27*:475, 1965.

Ponder, E.: The cell membrane and its properties. *In* Brachet, J., and A. E. Mirsky, eds.: The Cell. Vol. II. New York, Academic Press, 1961.

Rambourg, A., and C. P. Leblond: Electron microscopic observations on the carbohydrate-rich cell coat present at the surface of cells in the rat. J. Cell Biol., *32*:27, 1967.

Robertson, J. D.: Unit membranes: A review with recent new studies of experimental alterations and a new subunit in synaptic membranes. *In* Cell Membranes in Development. New York, Ronald Press, 1964.

Shea, S. M.: Lanthanum staining of the surface coat of cells. J. Cell Biol., *51*:611, 1971.

Singer, S. J., and G. L. Nicolson: The fluid mosaic model of the structure of cell membranes. Science, *175*:720, 1972.

Sjostrand, F. S.: A comparison of plasma membrane, cytomembranes, and mitochondrial membrane elements with respect to ultrastructural features. J. Ultrastruct. Res., 9:561, 1963.

Stoeckenius, W.: Some electron microscopic observations on liquid-crystalline phases in lipid-water systems. J. Cell Biol., 12:221, 1962.

Stoeckenius, W., and D. M. Engelman: Current models for the structure of biological membranes. J. Cell Biol., 42:613, 1969.

Yamamoto, T.: On the thickness of the unit membrane. J. Cell. Biol., 17:413, 1963.

Granular Endoplasmic Reticulum

Caro, L. G., and G. E. Palade: Protein synthesis, storage, and discharge in the pancreatic exocrine cell. J. Cell Biol., 20:473, 1964.

Haguenau, F.: The ergastoplasm: Its history, ultrastructure, and biochemistry. Int. Rev. Cytol., 7:425, 1958.

Jamieson, J. D., and G. E. Palade: Intracellular transport of secretory proteins in the pancreatic exocrine cell. I. Role of the peripheral elements of the Golgi complex. J. Cell Biol., 34:577, 1967. II. Transport to condensing vacuoles and zymogen granules. J. Cell Biol., 34:597, 1967. III. Dissociation of intracellular transport from protein synthesis. J. Cell Biol., 39:580, 1968. IV. Metabolic requirements. J. Cell Biol., 39: 589, 1968.

Littlefield, J. W., E. B. Keller, J. Gross, and P. S. Zamecnik: Studies on cytoplasmic ribonucleoprotein particles from the liver of the rat. J. Biol. Chem., 217:111, 1955.

Nonomura, Y., G. Blobel, and D. Sabatini: Structure of liver ribosomes studied by negative staining. J. Mol. Biol., 60:303, 1971.

Palade, G. E.: A small particulate component of the cytoplasm. J. Biophys. Biochem. Cytol., 1:59, 1955.

Palade, G. E.: Studies on the endoplasmic reticulum. II. Simple dispositions in cells *in situ*. J. Biophys. Biochem. Cytol., 1:567, 1955.

Palade, G. E., and K. R. Porter: Studies on the endoplasmic reticulum. I. Its identification in cells *in situ*. J. Exp. Med., 100:641, 1954.

Palade, G. E., and P. Siekevitz: Pancreatic microsomes. An integrated morphological and biochemical study. J. Biophys. Biochem. Cytol., 2:671, 1956.

Porter, K. R.: Observations on a submicroscopic basophilic component of the cytoplasm. J. Exp. Med., 97:727, 1953.

Porter, K. R., A. Claude, and E. F. Fullam: A study of tissue culture cells by electron microscopy. Methods and preliminary observations. J. Exp. Med., 81:233, 1945.

Redman, C. M., and D. D. Sabatini: Vectorial discharge of peptides released by puromycin from attached ribosomes. Proc. Nat. Acad. Sci., 56:608, 1966.

Redman, C. M., P. Siekevitz, and G. E. Palade: Synthesis and transfer of amylase in pigeon pancreatic microsomes. J. Biol. Chem., 241:1150, 1966.

Sabatini, D. D., and G. Blobel: Controlled proteolysis of nascent polypeptides in rat liver cell fractions. II. Location of the polypeptides in rough microsomes. J. Cell Biol., 45:146, 1970.

Sabatini, D. D., Y. Tashiro, and G. E. Palade: On the attachment of ribosomes to microsomal membranes. J. Molec. Biol., 19:503, 1966.

Agranular Endoplasmic Reticulum

Christensen, A. K., and D. W. Fawcett: The fine structure of testicular interstitial cells in the opossum. J. Biophys. Biochem. Cytol., 9:653, 1961.

Christensen, A. K., and S. W. Gillim: The correlation of fine structure and function in steroid secreting cells, with emphasis on those of the gonads. *In* McKerns, K. W., ed.: The Gonads. New York, Appleton-Century-Crofts, 1969.

Conney, A. H.: Pharmacological implications of microsomal enzyme induction. Pharmacol. Rev., 19:317, 1967.

Jones, A. L., and D. W. Fawcett: Hypertrophy of the agranular endoplasmic reticulum in hamster liver induced by phenobarbital. J. Histochem. Cytochem., 14:215, 1966.

Jones, A. L., N. B. Ruderman, and M. G. Herrera: An electron microscopic and biochemical study of lipoprotein production and release by the isolated perfused rat liver. J. Lipid Res., 8:429, 1967.

Long, J. A., and A. L. Jones: Observations on the fine structure of the adrenal cortex of man. Lab. Invest., 17: 355, 1967.

Orrenius, S., J. L. E. Ericsson, and L. Ernster: Phenobarbital induced synthesis of microsomal drug metabolizing enzyme systems and its relationship to the proliferation of endoplasmic membranes. J. Cell Biol., 25:627, 1965.

Palay, S. L., and J. P. Revel: The morphology of fat absorption. *In* Ming, H. C., ed.: Lipid Transport. Springfield, Ill., Charles C Thomas, 1964.

Porter, K. R.: The sarcoplasmic reticulum: its recent history, and present status. J. Biophys. Biochem. Cytol., 10: (Suppl.):219, 1961.

Remmer, H., and H. J. Merker: Drug-induced changes in liver endoplasmic reticulum. Association with drug metabolizing enzymes. Science, 142:1657, 1963.

Remmer, H., and H. J. Merker: Effect of drugs on the formation of smooth endoplasmic reticulum and drug metabolizing enzymes. Ann. N. Y. Acad. Sci., 123:79, 1965.

Strauss, E. W.: Electron microscopic study of intestinal fat absorption in vitro from mixed micelles containing linolenic acid, monoolein and bile salts. J. Lipid Res., 7:307, 1966.

Golgi Complex

Beams, H. W., and R. G. Kessel: The Golgi apparatus: Structure and Function. Int. Rev. Cytol., 23:209, 1968.

Bowen, R. H.: The cytology of glandular secretion. Quart. Rev. Biol., 4:299, 484, 1929.

Dalton, A. J.: Golgi apparatus and secretion granules. *In* Brachet, J., and A. E. Mirsky, eds.: The Cell. Vol. II. New York, Academic Press, 1961.

Fleischer, B., S. Fleischer, and H. Ogawa: Isolation and characterization of Golgi membranes from bovine liver. J. Cell Biol., 43:59, 1969.

Flickinger, C. J.: The development of the Golgi complexes and their dependence upon the nucleus in amoebae. J. Cell Biol., 43:250, 1969.

Friend, D. S., and M. J. Murray: Osmium impregnation of the Golgi apparatus. Am J. Anat., 117:135, 1965.

Golgi, C.: Sur la structure des cellules nerveuses des ganglions spinales. Arch. Ital. Biol., 30:278, 1898.

Hagopian, A., H. B. Bosmann, and E. H. Eylar: Glycoprotein biosynthesis: The localization of polypeptidyl : N —acetylgalactosaminyl, collagen : glucosyl, and galactoprotein : galactosyl transferases in HeLa cell membrane fractions. Arch. Biochem. Biophys., 128:387, 1968.

Jamieson, J. D., and G. E. Palade: Intercellular transport of secretory proteins in the pancreatic cell. I. Role of the peripheral elements of the Golgi complex. J. Cell Biol., *34*:577, 1967.

Morré, D. J., H. H. Mollenhauer, and C. E. Bracker: Origin and continuity of Golgi apparatus. *In* Reinert, J., and H. Ursprung, eds.: Origin and Continuity of Cell Organelles. New York, Springer-Verlag, 1971.

Nassanov, D.: Das Golgische Binnennetz und seine Beziehungen zu der Sekretion. Arch. f. Mikr. Anat., *100*:433, 1924.

Neutra, M., and C. P. Leblond: Radioautographic comparison of the uptake of galactose-H³ and glucose-H³ in the Golgi region of various cells secreting glycoproteins or mucopolysaccharides. J. Cell. Biol., *30*:137, 1966.

Neutra, M., and C. P. Leblond: The Golgi apparatus. Sci. Amer., *220*:100, 1969.

Peterson, M., and C. P. Leblond: Synthesis of complex carbohydrates in the Golgi region as shown by radiography after injection of labeled glucose. J. Cell Biol., *21*:143, 1964.

Rambourg, A., W. Hernandez, and C. P. Leblond: Detection of complex carbohydrates in the Golgi apparatus of rat cells. J. Cell Biol., *40*:395, 1969.

Wagner, R. R., and M. A. Cynkin: Enzymatic transfer of ¹⁴C-glucosamine from UDP-N-acetyl-¹⁴C-glucosamine to endogenous acceptors in a Golgi apparatus rich fraction from liver. Biochem. Biophys. Res. Comm., *35*:139, 1969.

Wagner, R. R., and M. A. Cynkin: The incorporation of ¹⁴C-glucosamine from UDP-N-acetyl-¹⁴C-glucosamine into liver microsomal protein in vitro. Arch. Biochem. Biophys., *129*:242, 1969.

Whaley, W. G., M. Dauwalder, and J. E. Kephart: Golgi apparatus: Influence on cell surfaces. Science, *175*: 596, 1972.

Mitochondria

Altmann, R.: Die Elementärorganismen und ihre Beziehungen zu den Zellen. Leipzig, Veit Co., 1890.

Benda, C.: Weitere Mitteilungen uber die Mitochondrien. Verh. d. Physiol. Ges., *376*, 1899.

Dawid, I. B., and D. R. Wolstenholme: The structure of frog oocyte mitochondrial DNA. *In* Slater E. C., J. M. Tager, S. Papa, and E. Quaglieriello, eds.: Biochemical Aspects of Biogenesis of Mitochondria. Bari, Italy, Adriatica Editrice, 1968.

Gibor, A., and S. Granick: Plastids and mitochondria: Inheritable systems. Science, *145*:890, 1964.

Hackenbrock, C. R.: Ultrastructural bases for metabolically linked mechanical activity in mitochondria. I. Reversible ultrastructural changes with change in metabolic state in isolated liver mitochondria. J. Cell Biol., *30*:269, 1966.

Lehninger, A. L.: The Mitochondrion. New York, W. A. Benjamin, 1964.

Nass, M. M. K., and S. Nass: Intramitochondrial fibers with DNA characteristics. I. Fixation and electron staining reactions. J. Cell Biol., *19*:593, 1963.

Nass, M. M. K., and S. Nass: Intramitochondrial fibers with DNA characteristics. II. Enzymatic and other hydrolytic treatments. J. Cell Biol., *19*:613, 1963.

Novikoff, A. B.: Mitochondria. *In* Brachet, J., and A. E. Mirsky, eds.: The Cell. Vol. II. New York, Academic Press, 1961.

Palade, G.: An electron microscope study of mitochondrial structure. J. Histochem. Cytochem., *1*:188, 1953.

Parsons, D. F.: Mitochondrial structure: Two types of subunits on negatively stained mitochondrial membranes. Science, *140*:985, 1963.

Parsons, D. F.: Recent advances correlating structure and function in mitochondria. Int. Rev. Exp. Path., *4*:1, 1965.

Peachey, L. D.: Electron microscopic observations on the accumulation of divalent cations in intramitochondrial granules. J. Cell Biol., *20*:95, 1964.

Rabinowitz, M., and H. Swift: Mitochondrial nucleic acids and their relation to the biogenesis of mitochondria. Physiol. Rev., *50*:376, 1970.

Sinclair, J. H., and B. V. Stevens: Circular DNA filaments from mouse mitochondria. Proc. Nat. Acad. Sci., *56*: 508, 1966.

Stoeckenius, W.: Some observations on negatively stained mitochondria. J. Cell Biol., *17*:443, 1963.

Swift, H., M. Rabinowitz, and G. Getz: Cytochemical studies on mitochondrial nucleic acids. *In* Slater, E. C., J. M. Tager, S. Papa, and E. Quagliariello, eds.: Biochemical Aspects of Biogenesis of Mitochondria. Bari, Italy, Adriatica Editrice, 1968.

Lysosomes

Axline, S. G., and Z. A. Cohn: In vitro induction of lysosomal enzymes by phagocytosis. J. Exp. Med., *131*: 1239, 1970.

Baudhuin, P., H. Beaufay, and C. DeDuve: Combined biochemical and morphological study of particulate fractions from rat liver. J. Cell Biol., *26*:219, 1965.

Cohn, Z. A., and M. E. Fedorko: The formation and fate of lysosomes. *In* Dingle, J. T., and H. B. Fell, Eds.: Lysosomes in Biology and Pathology. Amsterdam, North-Holland Publishing Company, 1969.

DeDuve, C.: Lysosomes. Sci. Amer. *208*:5, 1963.

DeDuve, C.: Lysosomes. Ciba Foundation Symposium. London, J. & A. Churchill, 1963.

DeDuve, C., and R. Wattiaux: Function of lysosomes. Ann. Rev. Physiol., *28*:435, 1966.

Dingle, J. T., and H. B. Fell, eds.: Lysosomes in Biology and Pathology. Vols. I and II. Amsterdam, North-Holland Publishing Company, 1969.

Essner, E., and A. B. Novikoff: Localization of acid phosphatase activity in hepatic lysosomes by means of electron microscopy. J. Biophys. Biochem. Cytol., *9*:773, 1961.

Friend, D. S., and M. G. Farquhar: Functions of coated vesicles during protein absorption in the rat vas deferens. J. Cell Biol., *35*:357, 1967.

Grove, S. N., C. E. Bracker, and D. J. Marre: Cytomembrane differentiation in the endoplasmic reticulum-Golgi apparatus-vesicle complex. Science, *161*:171, 1968.

Maunsbach, A. B.: Absorption of ferritin by rat kidney proximal tubule cells. Electron microscopic observations of the initial uptake phase in cells of microperfused single proximal tubules. J. Ultrastruct. Res., *16*:1, 1966.

Mego, J. L., and J. D. McQueen: The uptake and degradation of injected labeled proteins by mouse liver particles. Biochim. Biophys. Acta, *100*:136, 1965.

Miller, F., and G. E. Palade: Lytic activities in renal protein absorption droplets: An electron microscopical cytochemical study. J. Cell Biol., *23*:519, 1964.

Nadler, J. J., S. K. Sarkar, and C. P. Leblond: Origin of the intracellular colloid droplets in the rat thyroid. Endocrinology, *71*:120, 1962.

Novikoff, A. B., and W.-Y. Shin: The endoplasmic reticulum in the Golgi zone and its relations to microbodies, Golgi apparatus, and autophagic vacuoles in rat liver cells. J. Microscop., *3*:187, 1964.

Sawant, P. L., I. D. Desai, and A. L. Tappel: Digestive capacity of purified lysosomes. Biochim. Biophys. Acta, *85*:93, 1964.

Smith, R. E., and M. G. Farquhar: Lysosome function in the regulation of the secretory process in the cells of the anterior pituitary gland. J. Cell Biol., *31*:319, 1966.

Strauss, W.: *In* Roodyn, D. B., ed.: Enzyme Cytology. New York, Academic Press, 1967.

Vaes, G.: On the mechanism of bone resorption. The action of parathyroid hormone on the excretion and synthesis of lysosomal enzymes and on the extracellular release of acid by bone cells. J. Cell Biol., *39*:676, 1968.

Wetzel, B. K., S. S. Spicer, and S. H. Wollman: Changes in fine structure and acid phosphatase localization in rat thyroid cells following thyrotropin administration. J. Cell Biol., *25*:593, 1965.

Microbodies (Peroxisomes)

Afzelius, B. A.: The occurrence and structure of microbodies. A comparative study. J. Cell Biol., *26*:835, 1965.

DeDuve, C., and P. Baudhuin: Peroxisomes. Physiol. Rev., *46*:323, 1966.

Hruban, Z., and H. Swift: Uricase: Localization in hepatic microbodies. Science, *146*:1316, 1964.

Centrioles

Andre, J.: Le centriole et la région centrosomienne. J. Microscopie, *3*:23, 1964.

Dalcq, A. M.: Le centrosome. Bull. de l'Acad. Roy. Belgique (Classe de Sciences), *50*:1408, 1964.

DeHarven, E.: The centriole and mitotic spindle. *In* Dalton, A. J., and F. Haguenau, eds.: Ultrastructure in Biological Systems. Vol. 3. New York, Academic Press, 1968.

DeHarven, E. and W. Bernhard: Étude au microscope électronique de l'ultrastructure du centriole chez les vertébres. Zeitschr. f. Zellforsch., *45*:387, 1956.

Dirksen, E. R., and T. T. Crocker: Centriole replication in differentiating ciliated cells of mammalian respiratory epithelium. J. Microscopie, *5*:629, 1965.

Fawcett, D. W.: Observations on cell differentiation and organelle continuity in spermatogenesis. *In* Beatty, R. A., and S. Gluecksohn-Waelsch, eds.: The Genetics of the Spermatozoon. Edinburgh, 1972.

Fulton, C.: Centrioles. *In* Reinert, J., and H. Ursprung, eds.: Origin and Continuity of Cell Organelles. Heidelberg, Springer-Verlag, 1971.

Gall, J. G.: Centriole replication. A study of spermatogenesis in the snail *Viviparus*. J. Biophys. Biochem. Cytol., *10*:163, 1961.

Gall, J., and M. Mizukami: Centriole replication in the water fern *Marsilea*. J. Cell Biol., *19*:26A, 1961.

Henneguy, L. F.: Sur les rapports des cils vibratiles avec les centrosomes. Arch. Anat. Micro., *1*:481, 1897.

Huetter, A. F.: Continuity of the centrioles in *Drosophilia melanogaster*. Zeitschr. f. Zellforsch., *19*:119, 1933.

Renaud, F. L., and H. Swift: The development of basal bodies and flagella in *Allomyces arbusculus*. J. Cell Biol., *23*:339, 1964.

Sorokin, S. P.: Reconstructions of centriole formation and ciliogenesis in mammalian lungs. J. Cell Sci., *3*:207, 1968.

Steinman, R. M.: An electron microscopic study of ciliogenesis in developing epidermis and trachea in the embryo of *Xenopus laevis*. Am. J. Anat. *122*:19, 1968.

Nucleolus

Bernhard, W.: Drug-induced changes in the interphase nucleus. *In* Clementi, F., and B. Ceccarelli eds.: Advances in Cytopharmacology. Vol. 1. New York, Raven Press, 1971.

Bernhard, W., and N. Granboulan: Electron microscopy of the nucleolus in vertebrate cells. *In* Dalton, A. J., and F. Haguenau, eds.: The Nucleus. New York, Academic Press, 1968, p. 81.

Bernhard, W., and N. Granboulan: The fine structure of the cancer cell nucleus. Exper. Cell Res. (Suppl.), *9*:19, 1963.

Birnsteil, M. L., et al.: Properties and composition of isolated ribosomal DNA satellite of *Xenopus laevis*. Nature, *219*, 454, 1968.

Busch, H., and K. Smetana: The Nucleolus. New York, Academic Press, 1970.

Caspersson, T., and J. Schultz: Ribonucleic acids in both nuclei and cytoplasm and the function of the nucleolus. Proc. Nat. Acad. Sci., *26*:507, 1940.

Clyman, M. J.: A new structure observed in the nucleolus of the human endometrial epithelial cell. Am. J. Obstet. Gynec., *86*:430, 1963.

Estable, C., and J. R. Sotelo: Una nueva estructura celular; el nucleolonema. Publ. Inst. Invest. Ciencias Biol., *1*:105, 1951.

Hay, E. D., and J. P. Revel: The DNA component of the nucleolus studied in autoradiographs viewed with the electron microscope. Proceedings V International Congress Electron Microscopy. New York, Academic Press, 1962, Vol. 2, p. O-7.

Hay, E. D.: Structure and function of the nucleolus in developing cells. *In* Dalton, A. J., and F. Haguenau, eds.: The Nucleus. New York, Academic Press, 1968, p. 2.

Hyde, B. B., K. Sankaranarayanan, and M. L. Birnstiel: Observations on the fine structure of pea nucleoli *in situ* and isolated. J. Ultrastruct. Res., *12*:652, 1965.

Jones, K. W.: The role of the nucleolus in the formation of ribosomes. J. Ultrastruct. Res., *13*:257, 1965.

Maggio, R., P. Siekevitz, and G. E. Palade: Studies on isolated nuclei. II. Isolation and chemical characterization of nucleolar and nucleoplasmic subfractions. J. Cell Biol., *18*:293, 1963.

Marinozzi, V., and W. Bernhard: Presence dans la nucleole de deux types de ribonucleoproteines morphologiquement distinctes. Exper. Cell Res., *32*:595, 1963.

Marinozzi, V.: Cytochimie ultrastructurale du nucleole-RNA et proteines intranucleolaires. J. Ultrastruct. Res. *10*:443, 1964.

Monneron, A., and W. Bernhard: Fine structural organization of the interphase nucleus in some mammalian cells. J. Ultrastruc. Res., *27*:266, 1969.

Perry, R. P., and M. Errera: The influence of nucleolar ribonucleic acid metabolism on that of the nucleus and cytoplasm. *In* Mitchell, J. S., ed.: The Cell Nucleus. London, Butterworths, 1958.

Perry, R. P.: The nucleolus and the synthesis of ribosomes. Prog. Nucleic Acid Res. Mol. Biol. *6*:219, 1967.

Phillips, S. G., and D. M. Phillips: Sites of nucleolus production in cultured Chinese hamster cells. J. Cell Biol., *40*:248, 1969.

Schoefl, G.: The effect of actinomycin D on the fine structure of the nucleolus. J. Ultrastruc. Res., *10*:224, 1964.

Tavitian, A., S. C. Uretsky, and G. Acs: Selective inhibition of ribosomal RNA synthesis in mammalian cells. Biochim. Biophys. Acta, *157*:33, 1968.

Terzakis, J. A.: The nucleolar channel system of the human endometrium. J. Cell Biol., *27*:293, 1965.

Uretz, R. B., and R. P. Perry: Improved ultraviolet microbeam apparatus. Rev. Sci. Instr., *28*:861, 1957.

Vincent, W. S.: Structure and chemistry of nucleoli. Int. Rev. Cytol., *4*:269, 1955.

Nuclear Envelope

Barnes, B. G., and J. M. Davis: The structure of nuclear pores in mammalian tissue. J. Ultrastruct. Res., *3*:131, 1959.

Baud, C. A.: Nuclear membrane and permeability. *In* Seno, S., and E. V. Cowdry, eds.: Intracellular Membranous Structure. Okayama, Japan, Chugoku Press, 1965.

Callan, S. G., and S. G. Tomlin: Experimental studies on amphibian oocyte nuclei. I. Investigation of the structure of the nuclear envelope by means of the electron microscope. Proc. Roy. Soc. Lond., *137B*:367, 1950.

Fawcett, D. W.: On the occurrence of a fibrous lamina on the inner aspect of the nuclear envelope in certain cells of vertebrates. Am. J. Anat. *119*:129, 1966.

Feldherr, C. M.: The nuclear annuli as pathways for nucleocytoplasmic exchanges. J. Cell Biol., *14*:65, 1962.

Feldherr, C. M.: A comparative study of nucleocytoplasmic interactions. J. Cell Biol., *42*:841, 1969.

Gall, J. G.: Octagonal nuclear pores. J. Cell Biol., *32*:391, 1967.

Ito, S., and W. R. Lowenstein: Permeability of a nuclear membrane. Changes during normal development and changes induced by growth hormone. Science, *150*:909, 1965.

Kanno, Y., and W. R. Lowenstein: A study of the nucleus and cell membranes of oocytes with an intracellular electrode. Exper. Cell Res., *31*:149, 1963.

Lowenstein, W. R., and Y. Kanno: The electrical conductance and potential across the membrane of some cell nuclei. J. Cell Biol., *16*:421, 1963.

Maul, G. G., J. W. Price, and M. W. Lieberman: Formation and distribution of nuclear pore complexes in interphase. J. Cell Biol., *51*:405, 1971.

Maul, G. G.: On the octagonality of the nuclear pore complex. J. Cell Biol., *51*:558, 1971.

Merriam, R. W.: On the fine structure and composition of the nuclear envelope. J. Biophys. Biochem. Cytol., *11*:559, 1961.

Moses, M.: Breakdown and reformation of the nuclear envelope at cell division. *In* Internat. Cong. Electron Micros., Berlin, 1958. Berlin, Springer, 1958.

Pappas, G. D.: The fine structure of the nuclear envelope of *Amoeba proteus*. J. Biophys. Biochem. Cytol., *2* (Suppl.):431, 1965.

Watson, M.: Further observations on the nuclear envelope of the animal cell. J. Biophys. Biochem. Cytol., *6*:147, 1959.

Watson, M. L.: Pores in the mammalian nuclear membrane. Biochim Biophys. Acta, *15*:475, 1954.

Wiener, J., D. Spiro, and W. R. Lowenstein: Ultrastructure and permeability of nuclear membranes. J. Cell Biol., *27*:107, 1965.

Filaments and Microtubules

Barondes, S. H.: Axoplasmic transport. Neurosciences Res. Prog. Bull, *5*:307, 1967.

Behnke, O.: A preliminary report of "microtubules" in undifferentiated and differentiated vertebrate cells. J. Ultrastruct. Res. *11*:139, 1964.

Brody, I.: The ultrastructure of the tonofilaments in the keratinization process. J. Ultrastruct. Res., *4*:265, 1960.

Burgos, M. H., and D. W. Fawcett: An electron microscope study of spermatid differentiation in the toad, *Bufo arenarum* Hensel. J. Biophys. Biochem. Cytol., *2*:223, 1956.

Byers, B., and K. R. Porter: Oriented microtubules in elongating cells of the developing lens rudiment after induction. Proc. Nat. Acad. Sci., *52*:1090, 1964.

Fawcett, D. W., and F. Witebsky: Observations on the ultrastructure of nucleated erythrocytes and thrombocytes, with particular reference to the structural basis of their discoidal shape. Zeitschr. f. Zellforsch., *62*:785, 1964.

Gray, E. G.: Electron microscopy of neuroglial fibrils of the cerebral cortex. J. Biophys. Biochem. Cytol., *6*:121, 1959.

Hepler, P. K., and E. H. Newcomb: Microtubules and fibrils in the cytoplasm of *Coleus* cells undergoing secondary wall deposition. J. Cell Biol., *20*:529, 1964.

Ledbetter, M. C., and K. R. Porter: A "microtubule" in plant cell fine structure. J. Cell Biol., *19*:239, 1963.

Ledbetter, M. C., and K. R. Porter: Morphology of microtubules of plant cells. Science, *144*:872, 1964.

Robbins, E., and N. K. Gonatas: The ultrastructure of a mammalian cell during the mitotic cycle. J. Cell Biol., *21*:429, 1964.

Roth, L. E., and E. W. Daniels: Electron microscopic studies of mitosis in amebae. II. The giant ameba *Pelomyxa carolinensis*. J. Cell Biol., *12*:57, 1962.

Schmitt, F. O., and F. E. Samson: Neuronal fibrous proteins. Neurosciences Res. Prog. Bull., *6*:113, 1968.

Silveira, M., and K. R. Porter: The spermatozoids of flatworms and their microtubular systems. Protoplasma, *59*:240, 1964.

Smith, D. S., U. Jarlfors, and R. Beranek: The organization of synaptic axoplasm in the lamprey *(Petromyson marinus)* central nervous system. J. Cell Biol., *46*:199, 1970.

Tilney, L. G., and K. R. Porter: Studies on microtubules in Helioza I. Protoplasma, *60*:317, 1965.

Cell Division

Bajer, A.: Chromosome movement and fine structure of the mitotic spindle. Aspects of Cell Motility. Symp. Soc. Exp. Biol. XXII. New York, Academic Press, 1968.

Barnicot, N. A., and H. E. Huxley: Electron microscope observations on mitotic chromosomes Quart. J. Micr. Sci., *106*:197, 1965.

Bloom, W., and S. Ozarslan: Electron microscopy of ultraviolet-irradiated parts of chromosomes. Proc. Nat. Acad. Sci., *53*:1294, 1965.

Bloom, W., R. E. Zirkle, and R. B. Uretz: Irradiation of parts of individual cells. III. Effects of chromosomal and extrachromosomal irradiation on chromosome movements. Ann. N. Y. Acad. Sci., *59*:503, 1955.

Cantor, K. B., and J. E. Hearst: Isolation and partial characterization of metaphase chromosomes of a mouse ascites tumor. Proc. Nat. Acad. Sci., *55*:642, 1966.

Coleman, J. R., and M. J. Moses: DNA and the fine structure of synaptic chromosomes in the domestic rooster (*Gallus domesticus*). J. Cell Biol., *23*:63, 1964.

DeRobertis, E. D. P., W. W. Nowinski, and F. A. Saez: Cell Biology. 5th ed. Philadelphia, W. B. Saunders Co., 1970.

Forer, A.: Local reduction of spindle fiber birefringence in *Nephrotoma suturalis* (Loew) spermatocytes induced by ultraviolet microbeam irradiation. J. Cell Biol., *25*:95, 1965.

Frenster, J. H.: Mechanisms of repression and de-repression within interphase chromatin. *In* Dawe, C. J., ed.: The Chromosome: Structural and Functional Aspects. Tissue Culture Association Symposium. In Vitro, *1*:78, 1965.

Gaulden, M. E., and R. P. Perry: Influence of the nucleolus on mitosis as revealed by ultraviolet microbeam irradiation. Proc. Nat. Acad. Sci., *44*:533, 1958.

Gross, P. R., ed.: Second conference on the mechanisms of cell division. Ann. N. Y. Acad. Sci., *90*:345, 1960.

Harris, M.: Cell Culture and Somatic Variation. New York, Holt, Rinehart and Winston, 1964.

Hughes, A.: The Mitotic Cycle: The Cytoplasm and Nucleus During Interphase and Mitosis. New York, Academic Press, 1952.

Inoué, S.: On the physical properties of the mitotic spindle. *In* Gross, P. R., ed.: Second conference on the mechanisms of cell division. Ann. N. Y. Acad. Sci., *90*:529, 1960.

Lafontaine, J. G.: A light and electron microscope study of small, spherical nuclear bodies in meristematic cells of *Allium cepa, Vicia faba* and *Raphanus sativus.* J. Cell Biol., *26*:1, 1965.

Levine, L., ed.: The Cell in Mitosis. New York, Academic Press, 1963.

Locke, M., ed.: The Role of Chromosomes in Development. New York, Academic Press, 1964.

MacIntosh, J. R., P. K. Hepler, and D. G. Van Wie: Model for mitosis. Nature *224*:659, 1969.

Mazia, D.: Mitosis and the physiology of cell division. *In* Brachet, J., and A. E. Mirsky, eds.: The Cell: Biochemistry, Physiology, Morphology. Vol. III. New York, Academic Press, 1961.

Moses, M. J.: The nucleus and chromosomes: A cytological perspective. *In* Bourne, G. H., ed.: Cytology and Cell Physiology, 3rd ed. New York, Academic Press, 1964.

Nicklas, R. B.: Chromosome micromanipulation. II. Induced reorientation and the experimental control of segregation in mitosis. Chromosoma, *21*:17, 1967.

Perry, R. B.: Changes in ultraviolet absorption spectrum of parts of living cells following irradiation with an ultraviolet microbeam. Exper. Cell Res., *12*:546, 1957.

Perutz, M. F.: Proteins and Nucleic Acids: Structure and Function. New York, Elsevier Publishing Co., 1962.

Porter, K. R., and R. D. Machado: Studies on the endoplasmic reticulum. IV. Its form and distribution during mitosis in cells of onion root tip. J. Biophys. Biochem. Cytol., *7*:167, 1960.

Prescott, D. M.: Comments on cell life cycle. Nat. Cancer Inst. Monogr., *14*:55, 1964.

Revel, J. P., and E. D. Hay: Autoradiographic localization of DNA synthesis in a specific ultrastructural component of the interphase nucleus. Exper. Cell Res., *25*: 474, 1962.

Ris, H.: Ultrastructure and molecular organization of genetic systems. Canad. J. Genet. Cytol., *3*:95, 1961.

Robbins, E., and N. K. Gonatas: The ultrastructure of a mammalian cell during the mitotic cycle. J. Cell Biol., *21*:429, 1964.

Seed, J.: X-irradiation of the nucleolus and its effect on nucleic acid synthesis. *In* Mitchell, J. S., ed. (for the Faraday Society): The Cell Nucleus. New York, Academic Press, 1960.

Serlin, J. L.: The intracellular transfer of genetic information. Int. Rev. Cytol., *15*:35, 1963.

Swift, H. S.: Molecular morphology of the chromosome. In Vitro, *1*:26, 1966.

Taylor, E. W.: Control of DNA synthesis in mammalian cells in culture. Exp. Cell Res., *40*:316, 1965.

Taylor, H. J.: The replication and organization of DNA in chromosomes. *In* Molecular Genetics. Part I. New York: Academic Press, 1963.

Tjio, J. H., and T. T. Puck: Genetics of somatic mammalian cells: chromosomal constitution of cells in tissue culture. J. Exper. Med., *108*:259, 1958.

Watson, J. D.: Molecular Biology of the Gene. New York: W. A. Benjamin, Inc., 1965.

3

Epithelium

In Chapter 2 the microscopic and submicroscopic components of cells were described in some detail. This emphasis upon the cell as the fundamental unit of structure in higher organisms is appropriate, but it is important to realize that isolated cells are seldom encountered in the body. Instead, large numbers of cells usually work together in the performance of a particular function. The cooperating cells are assembled in coherent associations and are bound together by fibrous and amorphous intercellular substances to form *tissues*. The early chapters of this book are devoted to descriptions of the *basic tissues*: epithelium, connective tissue, blood, muscular tissue, and nervous tissue. The later chapters will describe the characteristic patterns in which the various tissues are combined to form the larger functional units known as *organs*.

Epithelium is a tissue composed of closely aggregated cells that are in apposition over a large part of their surface and which have very little intercellular substance. In its simplest form, epithelium consists of a single continuous layer of cells of the same type covering an external or internal surface. Quite commonly, however, multiple layers develop and the cells may differentiate into two or more kinds. To describe the resulting diversity in appearance, several types of epithelium are identified by different terms.

Origin and Distribution of Epithelium

Two of the primary germ layers of the early embryo, the *ectoderm* and *endoderm*, are clearly epithelial in their pattern of growth, and most of the epithelial organs of the body are derived from these germ layers. For example, the epidermis of the skin and the epithelium of the cornea, which together cover the entire external surface of the body, develop from the ectoderm. By invagination and proliferation, this outer covering epithelium gives rise to tubes or solid cords that form the glandular appendages of the skin, such as the sudoriparous, sebaceous, and mammary glands. Similarly, the alimentary tract is lined by epithelium of endodermal origin, and its associated glands—liver, pancreas, gastric glands, and intestinal glands—arise in the embryo by invagination and specialization of epithelial outgrowths from the lining of the primitive gut. Each *exocrine gland* of the adult communicates with an internal cavity or an external surface by way of ducts that open onto the epithelium of the inner or outer surface layer from which it developed during embryonic life. The *endocrine glands*, on the other hand, usually lose their connection with the surface epithelium from which they originally develop.

In addition to the epithelial structures that develop from the ectoderm and endoderm, there are several lining layers and solid organs which are composed of epithelium that arises from mesoderm. Examples are the kidney and the epithelia of the male and female reproductive tracts.

The linings of the peritoneal cavity and of other serous cavities in the adult, and the linings of blood and lymph vessels, which are all derivatives of mesenchyme, were formerly called *false epithelia* to distinguish them from derivatives of the epithelial germ layers. This distinction is no longer considered to be important, and the term has fallen into disuse. From a morphological point of view they are in all respects typical epithelia. Nevertheless, it is convenient and customary to refer to the lining of blood and lymph vessels as *endo-*

thelium and to the lining of serous cavities as *mesothelium.*

Epithelia are specialized for many different functions: *absorption, secretion, transport, excretion, protection* and *sensory reception.* Those that form the outer surface of the body are adapted for *protection* of the organism against mechanical damage and loss of moisture. They also play a role in *sensory reception*, containing nerve endings that provide the warning of pain that make the organism avoid injury. Others contain neural elements, such as taste buds and olfactory cells, specialized to function as chemical receptors. All substances received or given off by the body must traverse an epithelium; thus many of the epithelia lining internal surfaces are modified for *absorption* or *secretion*. Those concerned with secretion may contain only scattered individual cells specialized for secretion, or the whole epithelium may give rise to a gland in which most of the cells are specialized for elaboration of a particular product. Other epithelia, concerned with *excretion,* become modified to increase their efficiency in transport of solutes and water or in elimination of substances from the body.

CLASSIFICATION OF EPITHELIA

Epithelia are classified and named according to the number of cell layers and the shape of the cells. If there is one layer of cells the epithelium is described as *simple;* if there are two or more layers it is said to be *stratified.* The superficial cells can usually be described as *squamous, cuboidal,* or *columnar.* Thus a single layer of flat cells is a *simple squamous epithelium.* A single layer of tall prismatic cells is a *simple columnar epithelium.* The corresponding multilayered epithelia are called *stratified squamous epithelium* and *stratified columnar epithelium.*

Within the same general category of epithelium the cells may or may not have motile cell processes called *cilia* on their free surfaces. In the interest of more precise description it is customary to make note of this surface specialization in naming the epithelium. When such a border is present, the tissue is described as a *ciliated simple columnar epithelium* or a *ciliated stratified columnar epithelium.* Similarly in stratified squamous epithelium,

the superficial cells in some cases accumulate in their cytoplasm a fibrous protein called *keratin* and are reduced to scalelike lifeless residues of cells. To distinguish such epithelia from others in which the superficial cells do not undergo this change, it is customary to describe them as *keratinized stratified squamous epithelium.*

Among the simple columnar epithelia one category is described as *pseudostratified* because the cells are so arranged that the nuclei occur at two or more levels and the epithelium thus appears to be stratified. However, it can be shown by maceration that there is actually only one layer, all of the cells being fixed to the basement membrane but only some of them reaching the free surface. In truly stratified epithelia only the cells of the lowermost layer touch the underlying tissue.

Among the stratified epithelia there are two types that cannot adequately be described by reference to the shape of their surface cells. These are the *transitional epithelium* of the urinary tract and the *germinal epithelium* of the male gonad. Their distinguishing characteristics will be described later.

Simple Squamous Epithelium

Thin platelike cells are arranged in a single layer and adhere closely to one another by their edges (Fig. 3–1). When examined in surface view, especially after the cell limits are stained with silver nitrate, a characteristic mosaic pattern is seen (Fig. 3–2). The individual cells have polygonal or irregular wavy outlines, and each contains a nucleus. In sections perpendicular to the epithelium the cells, in profile, appear as plump spindles or thin rectangles (Fig. 3–6). Because of the large area covered by each flattened cell, a given plane of section will pass through the nucleus of only a fraction of the cells transected.

Epithelia of this variety are found in the human body on the inner surface of the wall of the membranous labyrinth and on the inner surface of the tympanic membrane of the ear; in the parietal layer of Bowman's capsule and in the thin segment of the loop of Henle in the kidney; in the rete testis; and in the smallest excretory ducts of many glands. Also included in this category are the *mesothelium* lining the pleural, peritoneal and other serous cavities (Fig. 3–2) and the *endothelium* lining the walls of the blood and lymph vessels.

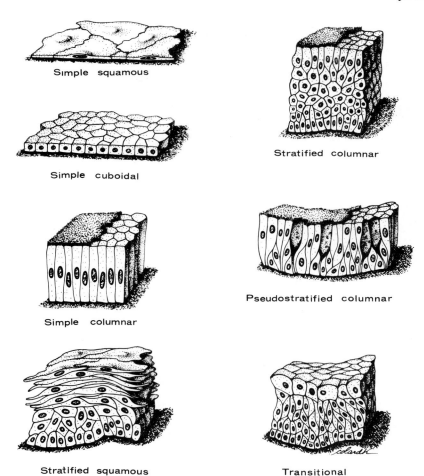

Simple squamous

Simple cuboidal

Stratified columnar

Simple columnar

Pseudostratified columnar

Stratified squamous

Transitional

Figure 3–1 Drawings illustrating the shape and arrangement of cells in the principal types of epithelia.

Simple Cuboidal Epithelium

On surface view this epithelium appears as a mosaic of small, usually hexagonal polygons and in vertical section the sheet of cells appears as a row of square or rectangular profiles.

Epithelium of this kind is found in many glands, as in the thyroid, on the free surface of the ovary, on the choroid plexus, on the inner surface of the capsule of the lens, in the ducts of glands, and as the pigmented epithelium of the retina. Secreting epithelia in the terminal portions of many glands can often be placed in this class, although the cells of acini or in the walls of tubules are usually pyramidal rather than cuboidal.

Simple Columnar Epithelium

In sections parallel to the surface of this type of epithelium one sees a mosaic much like that in other simple epithelia, but one in which the polygonal outlines of the cells are considerably smaller (Fig. 3–1). In sections perpendicular to the surface the rectangular outlines of the cells may be only a little taller than those of cuboidal epithelium (Fig. 3–4A), or they may be very tall and slender, standing upright like columns or fence palings (Fig. 3–4C). In many examples of columnar epithelium, all the oval nuclei are at approximately the same level (Fig. 3–4D). Simple columnar epithelium lines the surface of the digestive tract from the cardia of

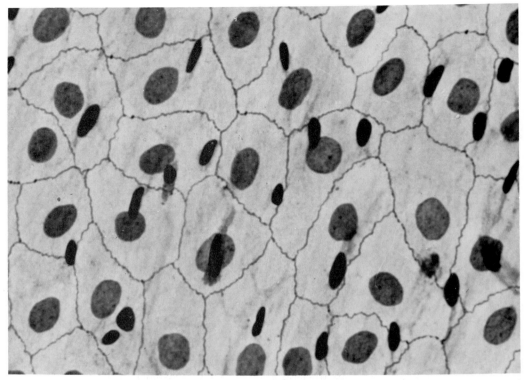

Figure 3–2 A thin spread of guinea pig mesentery treated with silver nitrate and subsequently stained with May-Grünwald and Giemsa stains. The limits of the simple squamous mesothelial cells have been blackened by the silver. The large round or oval nuclei are those of the mesothelial cells. The elongate darker nuclei are those of fibroblasts beneath the layer of mesothelium. ×750.

the stomach to the anus and is also common in the excretory ducts of many glands. Ciliated simple columnar epithelium (Figs. 3–4E and 3–5) is found in the uterus and oviducts, in the small bronchi of the lung, in some of the paranasal sinuses and in the central canal of the spinal cord.

Stratified Squamous Epithelium

The epithelial sheet is thick, and a vertical section of it shows the cells to vary in shape (Figs. 3–4E and 3–6), from base to free surface. The layer next to the basement membrane consists of plump cuboidal or

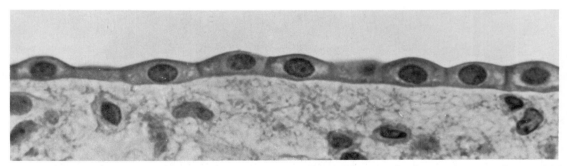

Figure 3–3 The epithelium of the collecting ducts of the dog kidney may be flattened so as to form a thick squamous epithelium such as is shown here, or the cells may be cuboidal. ×960.

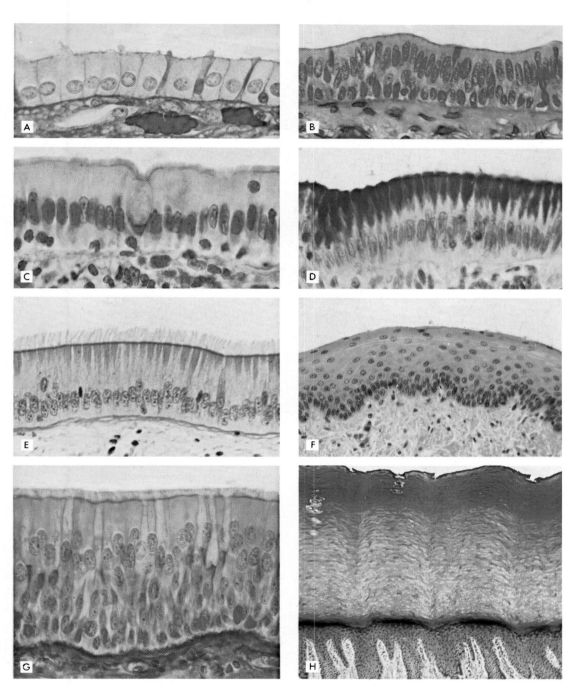

Figure 3–4 Photomicrographs of various types of epithelium: *A*, Simple low columnar epithelium of the pap-
illary duct of the dog kidney. Mallory trichrome stain.
B, Stratified columnar epithelium from a large salivary gland duct. Mallory-azan stain.
C, Simple columnar epithelium from the intestinal mucosa of a cat. The epithelium has a striated border.
Notice the presence of a single goblet cell among the columnar cells. Heidenhain's azan stain.
D, Simple columnar epithelium of mucous cells from the stomach. The mucus is stained a deep magenta.
PAS-hematoxylin stain.
E, Simple ciliate columnar epithelium from the typhlosole of a mollusc. Notice the long cone of rootlets ex-
tending from the basal bodies of the cilia downward into the apical cytoplasm. Chrome alum-hematoxylin-
phloxine stain.
F, Stratified squamous epithelium from the esophagus of a macaque. Hematoxylin and eosin stain.
G, Ciliated pseudostratified columnar epithelium from the human trachea. Mallory-azan stain.
H, Keratinized stratified squamous epithelium of the epidermis of the sole of the foot. Notice the very thick
superficial stratum of fully keratinized devitalized cells.

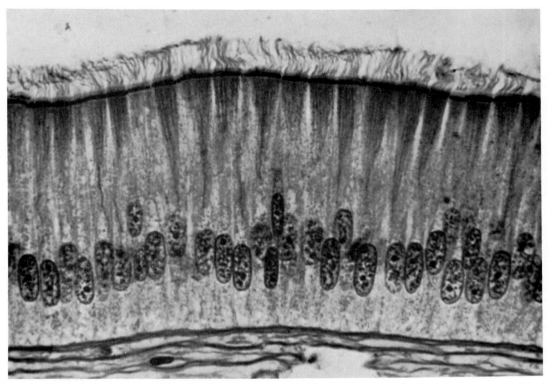

Figure 3–5 Simple columnar ciliated epithelium from the alimentary tract of a fresh water mussel. Notice the dark row of ciliary basal bodies just beneath the free surface of the cells and the cones of fibrous rootlets that extend downward from the basal bodies into the apical cytoplasm. Observe also the distinct "basement membrane" upon which the epithelium rests. Chrome alum-hematoxylin-phloxine stain. ×1200.

even columnar cells with rounded or beveled upper ends. Above this basal layer are additional layers of irregularly polyhedral cells. The nearer to the free surface they occur, the more the cells are flattened (Fig. 3–6). The superficial layers are composed of thin squamous cells.

Epithelium of this kind is found in the epidermis, the mouth, the esophagus, part of the epiglottis, the conjunctiva, the cornea, the vagina and lining a portion of the female urethra. Where stratified squamous epithelium occurs on the exposed outer surface of the body, the superficial cells have lost their nuclei and their cytoplasm has been largely replaced by the scleroprotein *keratin*. The cells are dry, devitalized, scalelike structures. Such epithelium is described as *keratinized stratified squamous epithelium*. On the inner moist surfaces of the body, the superficial cells of this type of epithelium have viable nucleated elements, not unlike the deeper lying cells except for their shape. Under these conditions, the tissue is described as a *nonkeratized stratified squamous epithelium* (Fig. 3–4*F*).

Stratified Columnar Epithelium

The deeper layer or layers consist of small, irregularly polyhedral cells that do not reach the free surface. The superficial cells are prismatic and cuboidal or columnar in form. Stratified columnar epithelium is relatively uncommon. It is found in the fornix of the conjunctiva, in the cavernous urethra, in some small areas of the anal mucous membrane, in the pharynx, on the epiglottis, and in the large excretory ducts of some glands (Figs. 3–1, 3–4*B*, 3–7). Some authors place the epithelium of the enamel organ in this group. On the nasal surface of the soft palate, in the larynx, and transiently in the fetal esophagus one finds *ciliated stratified columnar epithelium.*

Pseudostratified Columnar Epithelium

In pseudostratified columnar epithelium, all the cells are in contact with the basement membrane but not all of them reach the surface (Fig. 3–1). The cells are quite variable in shape: some have fairly broad attachment at the base, narrow rapidly, and extend upward through only a fraction of the thickness of the epithelium. Others extend throughout the thickness of the epithelium but are widest near the free surface and have long slender processes that extend downward between the basally situated cells to attach to the basal lamina. Since the nucleus in both categories is in the widest portion of the

cell, nuclei are found aligned at two or more levels in this class of epithelium, giving a specious appearance of stratification—hence the term pseudostratified.

Pseudostratified epithelium occurs in the large excretory ducts of the parotid and several other glands and in the male urethra. *Ciliated pseudostratified columnar epithelium* lines the greater part of the respiratory passages (Fig. 3–4G), the eustachian tube, a part of the tympanic cavity, and the lacrimal sac.

Transitional Epithelium

This was originally interpreted as an intermediate or transitional form between stratified squamous and columnar epithelium. The term *transitional epithelium* persists, even though its implication of change from one type to another is no longer considered ap-

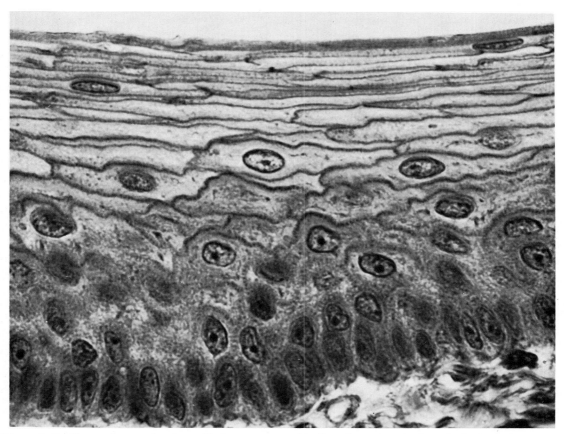

Figure 3–6 Photomicrograph of stratified squamous epithelium from the gingiva of a kitten. Observe the darker-staining cuboidal cells of the basal layer and the progressive flattening of cells in the more superficial layers. ×1500.

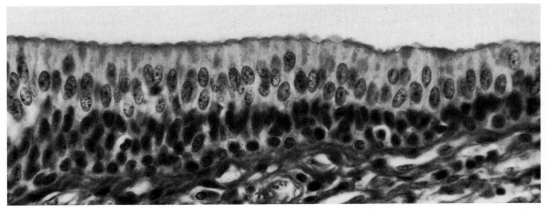

Figure 3-7 Photomicrograph of stratified columnar epithelium from the human male urethra. Notice the columnar form of the superficial layer of cells and the multiple layers of nuclei not attributable to obliquity of section.

propriate. This kind of epithelium varies greatly in appearance depending upon the conditions under which it is fixed. It is found lining hollow organs which are subject to great changes due to contraction and distention. In the contracted condition it consists of many cell layers (Figs. 3–1 and 3–8). The deepest elements have a cuboidal or even a columnar shape; above these are several layers of irregularly polyhedral cells, and the superficial layer consists of large cells with a characteristic rounded free surface. In the stretched condition the interrelations of the cells change to accommodate to the distention of the organ, and usually only two layers can then be distinguished: a superficial layer of large squamous elements over a layer of more or less cuboidal cells. This type of epithelium is characteristic of the mucosa of the excretory passages of the urinary system from the renal calyces to the urethra.

The classification of epithelia that has been presented here applies primarily to the higher vertebrates. Other categories would be necessary to describe adequately the patterns of cell association found in invertebrates and lower vertebrates. In the adult mammal a given type of epithelium is characteristic of the particular organ and under normal conditions it does not change. However, in chronic inflammation or in the development of tumors one type of epithelium may change into another, a process called *metaplasia*. For example, under certain pathological conditions the ciliated pseudostratified epithelium of the bronchi may change to stratified squamous epithelium—a change described as *squamous metaplasia*. A similar transformation can be induced experimentally. If one nostril of a dog is closed surgically, the greater evaporative loss of moisture that accompanies the increased ventilation through the remaining nasal passage causes its pseudostratified ciliated columnar epithelium to transform into stratified squamous epithelium.

SPECIALIZATIONS OF EPITHELIA

A fundamental property of epithelial cells is their inherent tendency to maintain extensive contacts with one another and thus to form coherent sheets covering surfaces and lining cavities. As structural correlates of this property, there are specializations of the plasmalemma on the lateral surfaces of the cells that serve to maintain close cell to cell contact. The free surfaces of the superficial cells may also be modified in various ways to increase the efficiency of the epithelium in carrying out the functions of absorption or transport. Because all substances entering or leaving the body must traverse an epithelium in a direction perpendicular to its surface, the cells are structurally and functionally *polarized*—that is to say, the distal end, toward the free surface, differs from the proximal end, toward the underlying connective tissue. This polarity is evident not only in the specialization of the respective surfaces but also in the arrangement of the organelles in the interior of the cell. The centrosome and Golgi apparatus are usually in an adluminal or supranuclear position. An imaginary line passing through the centrosome and the center of the nucleus defines the *cell axis*, and this is usually vertical or perpendicular to the basement lamina. The long filamentous mitochondria of columnar epithelia tend to be oriented parallel to the cell axis and are often mobilized in greater numbers in the apical cytoplasm (Fig. 3–9).

The evidence of cell polarity is less obvious in stratified squamous epithelia, which are more concerned with protection than with absorption or secretion. In these, the surface specializations for cell attachment are especially well developed, and the cytoplasm contains a conspicuous internal reinforcement or *cytoskeleton* composed of submicroscopic filaments, aggregated in bundles, that comprise *tonofibrils* visible with the light microscope. Such an internal supporting framework is not a prominent feature of columnar epithelia, but in many of these there is

a *terminal web*, consisting of a feltwork of fine filaments immediately beneath the free surface, where it apparently provides for stiffening and mechanical support for the striated or ciliated borders of epithelia.

Specializations for Cell Attachment and Communication

Adjacent epithelial cells cohere so tightly that a relatively strong mechanical force must be applied to separate them. Views as to the basis for their firm adherence have changed greatly since the advent of electron microscopy. According to the traditional interpretation, there was a thin layer of an interstitial substance between cells that acted as an adhesive. This hypothetical substance was referred to as the *intercellular cement*. It was stainable by the periodic acid–Schiff reaction and hence appeared to have a carbohydrate component. It also was a site of selective deposition of metallic silver when tissues immersed in silver nitrate solution were subsequently exposed to sunlight. This method

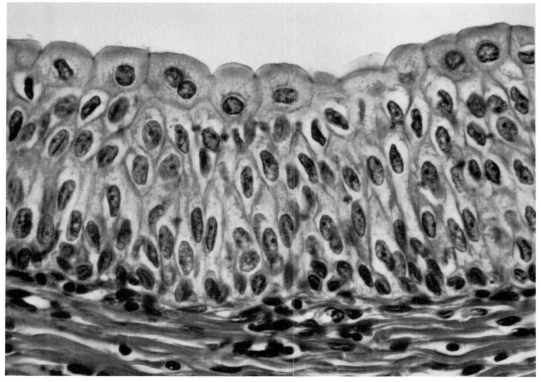

Figure 3–8 Photomicrograph of stratified transitional epithelium from the renal pelvis of a monkey, showing the characteristic superficial layer of large rounded cells, often binucleate. Hematoxylin and eosin. ×700.

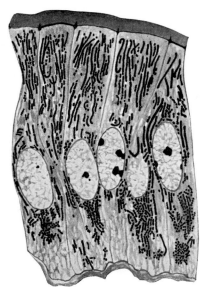

Figure 3–9 Columnar epithelium from rat intestine, showing striated border, terminal bars, and filamentous supranuclear and granular infranuclear mitochondria. Iron-hematoxylin stain. ×1000. (After A. A. Maximow.)

was often used to demonstrate the cell boundaries of epithelia (Fig. 3–2).

Certain epithelial cells, particularly those of stratified squamous epithelium of the epidermis, appeared with the light microscope to adhere to one another by many small processes distributed over the entire surface of the cell. These seemed to extend from cell to cell and were called "intercellular bridges." Between the bridges was a labyrinthine system of expanded intercellular spaces called *interfacial canals*. At the midpoint of each bridge was a densely staining dot called a *desmosome*. Although some histologists insisted that there was protoplasmic continuity from cell to cell through the bridges, others interpreted the desmosomes as special sites of attachment at end to end junctions of short processes on the neighboring cells. With special preparative procedures desmosomes could also be demonstrated on the lateral surfaces of columnar epithelial cells that had no obvious intercellular bridges.

On the boundary between adjacent columnar epithelial cells, immediately subjacent to their free surface, dark dots or dense bars could be seen with the light microscope. These were called *terminal bars*. In horizontal sections at their level, they were seen to form a dense continuous band around the polygonal perimeter of each cell. Traditionally these bars were interpreted as local accumulations of intercellular cement and they were assumed to seal or close the intercellular space at the free surface.

Electron microscopy has now greatly clarified these relationships of epithelial cells and has permitted a more precise definition of their surface specializations.

Zonula Occludens or Tight Junction. Where terminal bars were seen with the light microscope in columnar epithelia, the electron microscope reveals a *junctional complex* often consisting of three distinct components — the *zonula occludens*, the *zonula adherens*, and the *macula adherens* or desmosome (Farquhar and Palade). On the lateral cell boundaries immediately below the free surface of the epithelium, one finds the zonula occludens, a region of surface specialization where the membranes of adjoining cells converge and the outer leaflets of their unit membranes appear to fuse (Fig. 3–10). Within this region, which may occupy 0.1 to 0.3 μm. of the lateral cell boundary, there may be multiple sites of fusion, separated by short regions in which the outer leaflets of the opposing membranes are separated by 100 to 150 Å. This juxtaluminal region of membrane fusion extends in a belt around the perimeter of the cell and serves to close the intercellular space.

When this region is examined in surface replicas of freeze-cleaved preparations, it presents a very distinctive reticular pattern (Fig. 3–11). Each membrane appears to contain straight, rodlike structures that branch and join to form a rectilinear network of ridges on the A-face and a complementary pattern of shallow grooves on the B-face. These intramembranous rods are believed to underlie the lines of membrane fusion seen in this region of the cell membrane in thin sections (Staehelin).

As a consequence of the obliteration of the intercellular space along these circumferential bands around the apex of the cells, substances cannot traverse the epithelium from the lumen entirely via an *intercellular* route. Occluding junctions of this kind seem to be especially important in a transporting epithelium such as that of the gallbladder (see Chapter 28). They make it possible for the cells to pump solute actively through their lateral membranes into the intercellular cleft below the zonula occludens, creating there a standing osmotic gradient that serves to move water across the epithelium, concentrating the luminal contents.

It should be noted that the zonula occludens also has a mechanical role in maintaining the structural integrity of the epithelium. The cells are more firmly attached in this region of membrane fusion than anywhere else on their surface. It is not yet clear whether the membranes in this specialization are sufficiently permeable to ions and small molecules to permit the occluding junctions to participate in cell to cell communication.

The Zonula Adherens. On the epithelial cell boundaries just below the zonula oc-

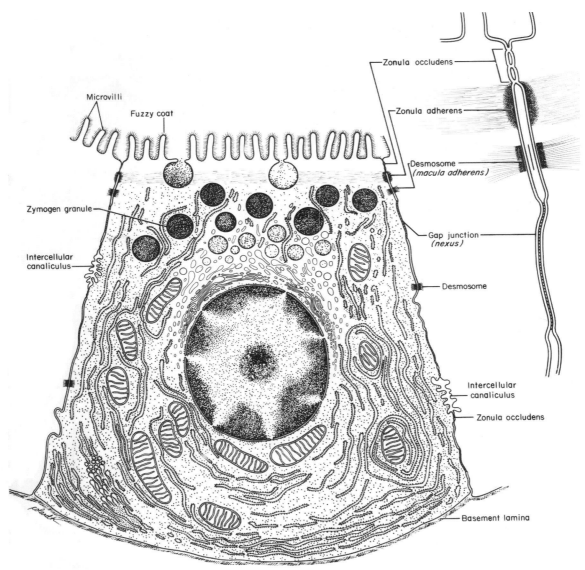

Figure 3–10 Drawing of a typical epithelial cell as seen with the electron microscope, illustrating the basement lamina, microvilli on the free surface, desmosomes on the lateral surfaces and a juxtaluminal junctional complex. This latter consists of a zonula occludens, zonula adherens, and macula adherens. In addition, a nexus or gap junction is depicted near the junctional complex. These specializations for cell-to-cell communication may occur anywhere on the opposed lateral surfaces of epithelial cells. (Drawing from E. Hay, in R. O. Greep: Histology. 2nd ed. New York, McGraw-Hill Book Co., 1965.)

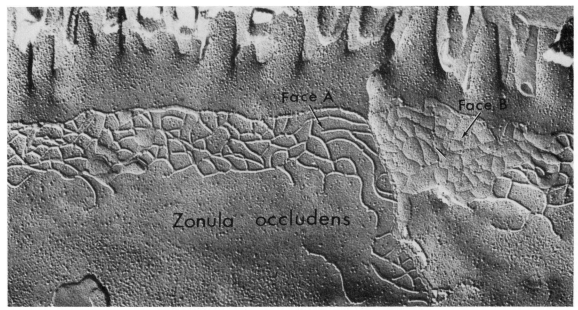

Figure 3–11 Electron micrograph of a replica of a frozen-fractured surface. The membranes were cleaved at a zonula occludens of intestinal epithelium. A reticular pattern of anastomosing rope-like strands is seen on the A-face of the cleaved membrane, and a complementary pattern of grooves on the B-face. (Micrograph courtesty of J. P. Revel.)

cludens, the membranes diverge to a distance of 150 to 200 Å. The opposing unit membranes are unmodified but are reinforced on their cytoplasmic surface by a moderately dense mat of fine filamentous material that forms a continuous band around the cell parallel to the zonula occludens (Fig. 3–10). This junctional element is not identifiable in freeze-cleaved preparations because there seems to be no specialization within the plane of the membrane to distinguish it from other parts of the plasmalemma. The associated condensation of cytoplasmic filaments has ill-defined outer limits and in some epithelia, it blends with the transverse zone of filamentous apical cytoplasm comprising the *terminal web*. No structural elements are seen traversing the intercellular space at the zonula adherens and the nature of the forces that bind the membranes together is not known. Nevertheless, as the name implies, this structure is generally believed to be a band of firm adhesion between neighboring cells.

Owing to the affinity of its filamentous component for stains, it is probable that it was mainly this portion of the epithelial junctional complex that was identified by light microscopists as the terminal bar.

The Macula Adherens or Desmosome. The third component of the typical junctional complex of columnar epithelium is the *macula adherens*, corresponding to the desmosomes of classical histology. These appeared with the light microscope merely as dense dots or fusiform thickenings of the cell boundaries, but they are resolved in electron micrographs as bipartite structures consisting of plaque-like local differentiations of the opposing membranes. The cell surfaces are 150 to 200 Å apart and the unit membranes are of normal dimensions but appear thickened due to the presence of a thin but very dense amorphous layer closely applied to their cytoplasmic surface (Figs. 3–10 and 3–12). Immediately subjacent to this is a thicker layer consisting of a feltwork of fine filaments embedded in a moderately dense matrix. Tonofilaments in the cytoplasm converge upon the desmosomes and appear to terminate in their inner layer. High resolution micrographs studied in stereo pairs suggest that many of the tonofilaments form hairpin loops in the dense layer and turn back into the cytoplasm (Kelly). The desmosomes are thus sites of attachment of the cytoskeleton to the cell surface as well as sites of cell to cell adhesion. As in the case of the zonula adherens, freeze-cleaved preparations show no recognizable internal differentiation of the cell membrane.

In thin sections of desmosomes, a slender intermediate dense line is often seen in the middle of the intercellular space between the two halves of the desmosome (Fig. 3–12). Occasionally, with intense heavy-metal staining, there is also a suggestion of delicate striations traversing the intercellular space. The integrity of desmosomes seems to be dependent upon the presence of calcium. Perfusion of tissue with calcium-free media or immersion in a chelating agent such as ethylenediaminetetraacetic acid (EDTA) results in separation of the two halves.

In simple cuboidal or columnar epithelia, there is often a discontinuous row of desmosomes on the cell boundaries below the zonula adherens forming the third element of the typical junctional complex, but additional desmosomes may be found scattered at random over the cell surface. In stratified squamous epithelia, zonulae occludentes and zonulae adherentes may be absent, but desmosomes are unusually abundant, attaching the ends of the short processes that were erroneously interpreted by light microscopists as "intercellular bridges."

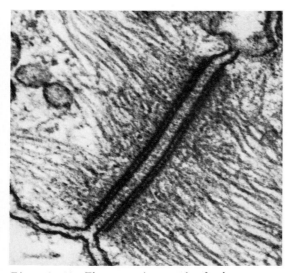

Figure 3–12 Electron micrograph of a desmosome from the epidermis of a larval newt, showing the thickening of the inner leaflet of the cell membrane and the tonofilaments forming "loops" in the condensation of cytoplasm adjacent to the specialized area of the membrane. ×93,000. (Courtesy of Douglas Kelly.)

Half desmosomes are almost never observed along the boundaries between cells; the formation of one half evidently induces the nearly simultaneous formation of the complementary half by the neighboring cell. Half desmosomes are found, however, on the basal surface of stratified squamous epithelia where the cells are exposed to the underlying connective tissue (Fig. 3–13).

The Nexus or Gap Junction. This type of junctional specialization has the form of plaques of variable size where the intercellular space is greatly narrowed but seemingly not obliterated. In thin sections the normal intercellular space is reduced to a narrow slit about 20 Å wide. At low magnifications this junction may be mistaken for a zonula occludens, but the intercellular gap is of constant width throughout and at no point do the opposing membranes appear to be fused. When epithelial tissues are immersed in extracellular electron-opaque tracers, such as lanthanum, these penetrate the intercellular space at the nexus and are visible as a thin dense line about 20 Å wide between the opposing membranes. Where the plane of section passes tangentially to the intercellular gap providing an *en face* view of the nexus, a highly ordered pattern is seen in the specialized portions of the opposing membranes. The lanthanum or other contrast medium outlines hexagonally packed globular subunits with a center to center spacing of 90 Å. When the membrane is cleaved at a nexus with the freeze-fracturing technique, the replica of the outwardly directed inner half-membrane (A-face) shows a high concentration of closely packed particles within the membrane (Figs. 3–14 and 3–15).

It has been found that when cells some distance apart in an epithelial sheet are impaled with microelectrodes, they can be shown to be electrically coupled. The junctional specializations of cells are now the subject of intensive investigation because of the probability that they are sites of low resistance to ion flow that provide for communication between cells and for coordination of their activities. Although the nexus is a site of firm cohesion of cells, it is also believed to be the principal, and possibly the only, type of junction that mediates flow of current between cells. The electrotonic coupling of cells joined by nexuses strongly suggests that these regions of the adjoining membranes are permeable to ions. There is other evidence,

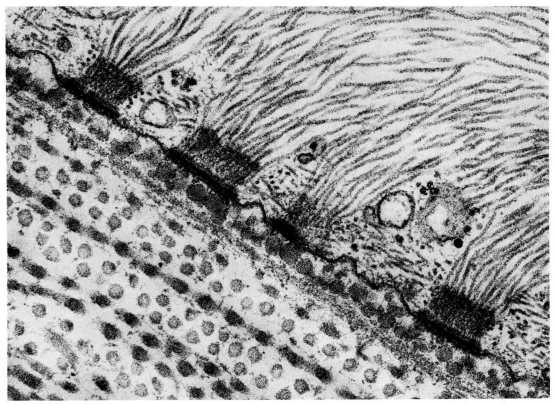

Figure 3–13 Hemidesmosomes along the basal cell membrane in newt epidermal cell. Notice the tonofilaments converging on the dense cytoplasmic component of the hemidesmosomes. At the lower left are cross sections of the collagen fibrils of the basal lamellae. ×80,000. (Courtesy of Douglas Kelly.)

based upon the passage of dye from cell to cell, that these sites also permit passage of substances of molecular weight 300 or more (Lowenstein). Although at present we do not know the nature of the signals that may normally pass between cells, it is speculated that these junctions may have an important role in regulation of growth and differentiation as well as in the coordination of function among groups of cells.

Junctional specializations of this type are not confined to epithelia but are also seen at the so-called electrical synapses in the invertebrate central nervous system (Robertson) and between cellular units of smooth (Dewey) and cardiac muscle (Karrer). There is compelling evidence that in these latter the nexuses or gap junctions are the low resistance pathways through which excitation passes rapidly from cell to cell, permitting the muscle to function as if it were a syncytium (see Chapter 11).

The Basal Surface of Epithelia

Between an epithelium and the underlying connective tissue is an extracellular supporting layer that has long been called the *basement membrane*. It was formerly interpreted as a condensation of the ground substance of the connective tissue at its interface with the epithelium. It is often difficult to see in routine hematoxylin and eosin preparations but can be clearly demonstrated by staining with the periodic acid–Schiff reaction or with silver impregnation methods. It then appears as a thin continuous layer closely applied to the base of the epithelium. It is now apparent that what was formerly identified as the "basement membrane" is not a single structural entity but has two or more distinct components that are not resolved as such with the light microscope. In electron micrographs its most consistent component is a continuous sheet 500 to 800 Å thick and

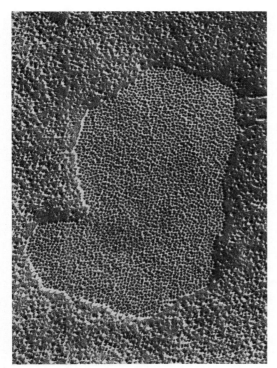

Figure 3-14 Replica of the A-face of an epithelial cell membrane showing a random pattern of intramembranous particles around the periphery of the figure. In the center is a closely packed array of particles comprising a nexus or gap junction.

ly responsible for its impregnation with silver salts, while the periodic acid–Schiff reaction stains principally the polysaccharides of the basal lamina and ground substance. Because the *basal lamina* immediately underlies the epithelium and is the most consistent component of the complex, it is now commonly thought of as synonymous with basement membrane; the latter term is falling into disuse because it leads to confusion with membranes that are parts of cells.

Chemical studies of basal laminae isolated from the kidney indicate that their main structural component is a form of collagen. The collagen does not form cross striated fibrils. It is characterized by a high content of hydroxylysine and hydroxyproline and contains 10 to 20 per cent carbohydrate. Immunochemical studies indicate that the basal lamina possesses at least three antigenic components — collagen, a low molecular weight glycoprotein, and a high molecular weight glycoprotein (Kefalides). There is now strong evidence that this layer is a product of the overlying epithelium and not a condensation of the underlying connective tissue ground substance, as it was formerly thought to be (Hay and Revel). The reticular fibers and their associated polysaccharide matrix, on the other hand, are mainly the products of connective tissue fibroblasts.

composed of a fine feltwork of filaments 30 to 40 Å in diameter embedded in an amorphous matrix. This boundary layer is now called the *basement lamina* or *basal lamina*. It is in contact with the basal plasma membrane of the epithelial cells and conforms closely to their contours. The density of this layer is low immediately adjacent to the cells but increases a short distance away from the membrane. Because this outer condensed zone is more conspicuous in sections, the basal lamina may appear as a linear density running parallel to the cell surface at a distance of 300 to 400 A from the membrane at the base of the epithelium proper.

Outside the basal lamina are small fascicles of unit fibrils of collagen (reticular fibers) embedded in a protein-polysaccharide *ground substance*. All these components — basal lamina, reticular fibers, and ground substance — contribute to the image of the "basement membrane" seen with the light microscope. The reticular fibers are probably large-

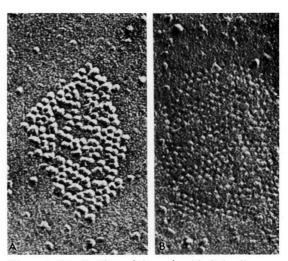

Figure 3-15 Replica of cleaved epithelial cell membrane. *A*, Particles on the A-face of a small nexus. *B*, A pattern of shallow pits on the B-face of a similar but slightly larger nexus. (Micrographs courtesy of A. Yee.)

SPECIALIZATIONS OF THE FREE SURFACE

Striated Border

A number of columnar epithelia possess a refractile border that exhibits delicate vertical striations when examined at high magnification. Such a *striated* or *brush border* (Figs. 3–1 and 3–4C) consists of large numbers of slender cylindrical cell processes 80 to 90 nm. in diameter and 0.5 to 1 μm. long. These are called *microvilli* (Figs. 3–16 and 3–20A). Each is enclosed in an extension of the plasmalemma that has the typical trilaminar structure but which often bears on its outer surface delicate filamentous excrescences 25 to 50 Å in diameter. When present, this surface coating can be shown by histochemical staining reactions to be rich in complex polysaccharides. The cytoplasm in the interior of the microvilli is fine textured and homogeneous except for a bundle of straight parallel filaments that run longitudinally through its core and often extend half a micrometer or more down into the apical cytoplasm. Here the filaments are anchored in the terminal web, which crosses the end of the cell immediately beneath the striated border.

In well developed striated borders such as those of the intestinal absorptive epithelium and proximal convoluted tubule of the kidney, the microvilli are uniform in length and diameter and stand erect in close parallel array. On other epithelia where microvilli are less numerous, their orientation is more variable. In these cells the terminal web and the internal filaments in the microvilli are relatively inconspicuous. These fibrous elements, when present, evidently contribute to the structural stability and to the maintenance of the orderly arrangement of microvilli in the border. It has been shown that the filaments in the interior of the microvilli are actin, but there is as yet no direct evidence that the microvilli are capable of active contraction.

Microvilli occur in limited numbers on the free surface of many epithelia, including some that are secretory. They are present in greatest profusion, however, on cells whose principal function is absorption. Biochemical analysis of striated borders isolated from intestinal epithelium has shown that they contain enzymes that hydrolyze sugar phosphates and split disaccharides to monosaccharides. The enzymes reside in or near the membranes of the microvilli. The brush border thus appears to be an adaptation for greatly increasing the surface area of membrane exposed to substances that are to be absorbed. This amplification of the surface area of an interface, which is a site of important chemical events in digestion and transport, greatly enhances the efficiency of the epithelium in its absorptive function.

Stereocilia

Viewed with the light microscope, the epithelium lining the epididymis is seen to

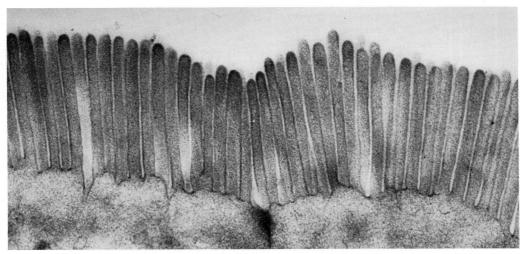

Figure 3–16 Electron micrograph of the microvilli forming the striated border of the intestinal epithelium of a hamster. ×40,000. (Courtesy of S. Ito, after D. W. Fawcett, Circulation, *26*:1105, 1962.)

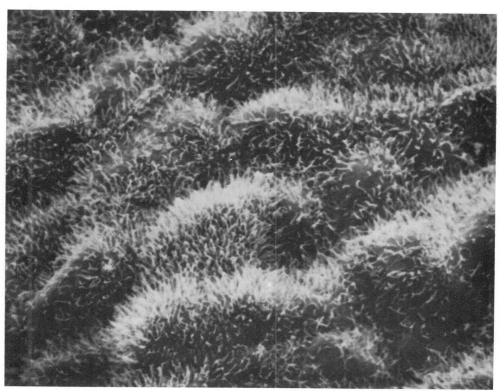

Figure 3–17   Scanning electron micrograph of peritoneal mesothelium showing the numerous microvilli that project from the free surface of the cells. (Micrograph from R. C. Buck, Laboratory Investigation, *26*:604, 1972.)

have an unusual surface specialization in which a long pyriform tuft of slender processes projects into the lumen from each cell (Fig. 3–18). At high magnification, this appears to be composed of thin cilium-like structures that cohere so as to form a tuft that bears a superficial resemblance to the hairs of a watercolor brush. The individual processes are as long as or longer than the vibratile processes called cilia, but they are nonmotile. They were therefore called *stereocilia* in classical histology, and the name persists, although at the submicroscopic level their resemblance to cilia is very slight indeed. In electron micrographs they are found to be very long flexuous microvilli. The filamentous cores that lend a certain degree of stiffness to the shorter microvilli of brush borders seem to be lacking or poorly developed, and although they are parallel at their base, they become increasingly sinuous and entwined toward their tips. Their function is not well established, but the epididymal epithelium is absorptive and it is assumed

that they promote this function by amplifying the cell surface.

Cilia

These are motile processes, larger than microvilli, and with a much more complex internal structure. Their principal function is to propel fluid or mucous films over the surface of the epithelium by active vibratory movements. They are arranged in parallel rows and may number in the hundreds on each epithelial cell. Cilia are 7 to 10 μm. long and about 0.2 μm. in diameter. At the base of each is a dense elongate granule called the *basal body*. Cilia are easily resolved with the light microscope (Figs. 3–4*E*, *G*, and 3–5). Their form and arrangement is seen even more dramatically in a surface view of a ciliated epithelium as recorded by the scanning electron microscope (Fig. 3–19). In living cells cilia can be observed to have a rapid to and fro beat in a consistent direction. When the rate of beat is slowed down in cinemato-

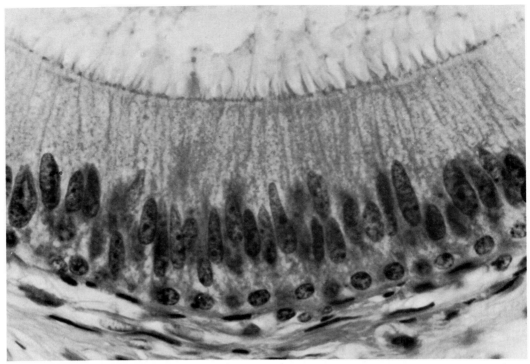

Figure 3–18 Photomicrograph of pseudostratified columnar epithelium of the human epididymis. Notice the tufts of long flexible stereocilia projecting from each cell. ×720.

graphic analysis, each cilium is found to stiffen on the more rapid forward or *effective stroke* and to become flexible on the slower *recovery stroke*. Cilia may have an *isochronal rhythm*, in which all cilia beat together, but more commonly those on epithelia exhibit a *metachronal rhythm*, in which the successive cilia in each row start their beat in sequence so that each is slightly more advanced in its cycle than the preceding one. This sequential activation of the cilia results in the formation of waves that sweep slowly over the surface of the epithelium as a whole. When viewed from above with the microscope, this activity is reminiscent of the waves that run before the wind across a field of grain. The metachronal waves of ciliated epithelia, however, are regular in the periodicity of their occurrence and constant in direction. The effect of this coordinated activity of the cilia is to move a blanket of mucus slowly over the epithelium or to propel fluid and particulate matter through the lumen of a tubular organ.

With the light microscope, no internal structure is discernible in cilia to account for their movement, but under the electron microscope cilia are found to have a core structure called the *axoneme*, consisting of longitudinal microtubules that have a constant number and precise arrangement. In transverse sections, two single microtubules are located in the center of the axoneme, with nine doublet tubules uniformly spaced around them (Figs. 3–20 and 3–21). The structure of the basal body is nearly identical to that of a centriole with nine triplet microtubules in characteristic pinwheel arrangement making up the wall of the hollow cylindrical organelle. The microtubules of the axoneme extend throughout the length of the ciliary shaft. The central pair terminate at the base of the cilium, but the nine peripheral doublets are continuous with the two inner subunits of the nine triplets in the wall of the basal body.

The central pair of microtubules in the axoneme of cilia have much in common with the microtubules in the cytoplasm of many cell types. The doublets are rather different. They are not composed of two similar tubules adherent along one side. Instead, there is one complete tubule with a circular cross section, *subfiber A* and an incomplete tubule, *subfiber B* which has a C-shaped cross section. The latter is fused to subfiber A along its edges so that the resulting doublet has a figure-eight cross section with part of the wall of the complete tubule, A, closing the defect in the incomplete wall of tubule B (Fig. 3–21). Each doublet has two rows of short *arms* that project from subfiber A toward the next doublet in the row. The arms diverge slightly and are directed clockwise from the point of view of an observer looking along the ciliary shaft from base toward tip. Each arm is a molecule of the protein *dynein* which functions as an ATP-splitting enzyme.

The microtubular elements of the axoneme are presumed to be the structures responsible for the active bending of the cilium. How they accomplish this remains unsettled, but two possible mechanisms have been suggested. Either the peripheral doublets must be capable of active shortening, or they must be of constant length and slide with respect to one another in a manner comparable to the sliding filament mechanism for the shortening of striated muscle (see p. 309).

There is no good evidence that microtubules shorten. However, examination of cross sections near the tips of cilia in different phases of their cycle of beating shows that the doublets of the bent cilium terminate at different levels (Fig. 3–22). This suggests that sliding of the doublets is the more likely mechanism (Satir). This interpretation has recently been supported by strong experimental evidence. It has been shown that when ATP is added to isolated flagella whose membranes have been removed with detergent, the sliding mechanism is activated and there is a rapid elongation as the doublets slide past one another and extend from opposite ends of the flagellum (Gibbons).

According to classical cytologists, the formation of cilia was preceded by repeated division of an initial pair of centrioles until the required number of basal bodies was produced. These then became arranged in rows beneath the cell surface, and each gave rise to a cilium. Recent studies of ciliogenesis have shown that the basal bodies arise in two ways: (1) They may originate in the same manner in which centrioles are du-

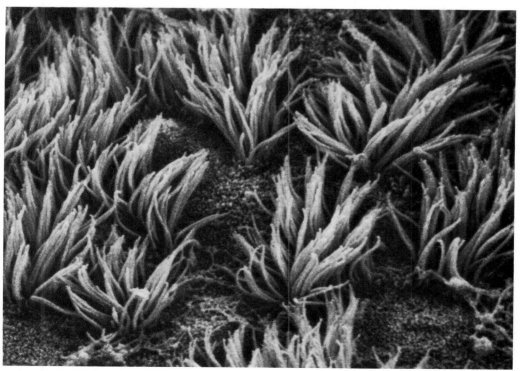

Figure 3–19 Scanning electron micrograph of cilia on pseudostratified ciliated epithelium of the trachea. (Micrograph courtesy of E. R. Dirksen.)

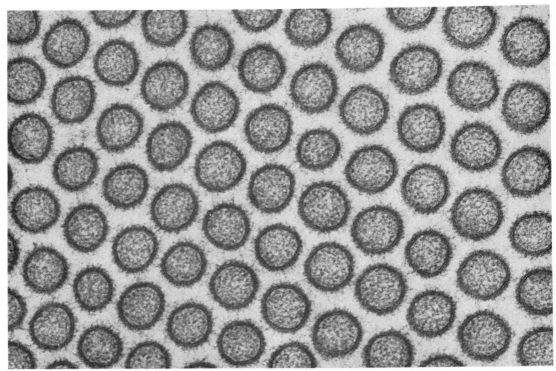

Figure 3--20 A, Electron micrograph of a horizontal section through the striated border of the intestinal epithelium, showing the microvilli in transverse section. They are remarkably uniform in their size and distribution. Compare their lack of internal structure with similar sections of cilia (Fig. 3--20*B*). × 98,000. (Courtesy of S. L. Palay.)

(Illustration continued on opposite page.)

plicated in the mitotic cycle—a dense, ring-like procentriole arising in end-to-side relationship to a preexisting centriole (Fig. 3–23). The centriole seems to act merely as a site of induction or nucleation for a process of self-assembly in which one or several radially arranged new centrioles form from fibrogranular precursor material. (2) Alternatively, multiple basal bodies may arise *de novo* without participation of a preexisting centriole. In this case, they develop around dense spherical bodies variously called *procentriole organizers* or *deuterosomes.* Clusters of small, round, fibrous granules (filosomes) appear to be their precursor material. Multiple *procentrioles* develop around the organizer center and grow by accretion at their ends until they attain the appropriate length. The newly formed centrioles move to the cell surface where they function as basal bodies, initiating polymerization of microtubule protein to form the axonemes of the cilia. Once initiated, the assembly of the ciliary shaft is

rapid and self-perpetuating—the ends of the doublets that polymerize on the ends of the triplets in the wall of the basal body then become sites for deposition of additional subunits until the cilium has attained the normal length (Fig. 3–23).

Flagella

Flagella differ from cilia only in their greater length, the character of their movements, and the number per cell—their internal structure appears to be the same. There is usually a single flagellum per cell, 15 to 30 μm. long, in contrast to hundreds of cilia per cell. Undulatory waves are propagated along the length of the flagellum from base to tip instead of the to and fro lashing strokes characteristic of cilia.

The longest flagella are those of the mammalian spermatozoon which may reach a length of several hundred micrometers. In these an additional row of nine dense lon-

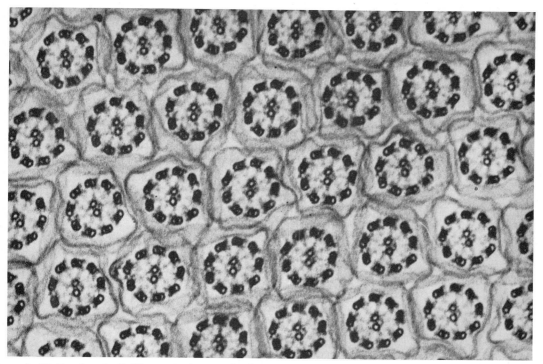

Figure 3–20 Continued B, Electron micrograph of cross sections of cilia from a freshwater mussel. Each contains two central filaments surrounded by nine double ones. This number and arrangement of internal filaments has been found to be of universal occurrence in cilia throughout the plant and animal kingdoms. Notice that one member of each outer doublet appears tubular, whereas the other has a more dense interior and bears, on its outer surface, short arms that project toward the next filament. ×76,000. (From I. R. Gibbons, J. Biophys. & Biochem. Cytol., *11*:179, 1961.)

gitudinal fibers has been added around the periphery of the axoneme (See Chapter 32).

Epithelial flagella are easily overlooked with the light microscope and are only occasionally encountered in electron micrographs of thin sections. They occur, however, in some of the epithelia of nephrons, in the rete testis, and in the ducts of a number of glands. What their function may be is not apparent unless simple agitation of the fluid in the lumen may have some desirable physiological consequences. Still more puzzling is the observation that single short flagella occur on the cells in some epithelial organs that lack a lumen, such as the anterior lobe of the hypophysis and the islets of Langerhans. Here the flagella simply project into the intercellular spaces or into the connective tissue stroma, where their agitation would seem to serve no useful purpose. Similar abortive flagella have been described occasionally on smooth muscle cells, on the stromal cells of the endometrium, and on mesenchymal derivatives in many other organs. Some of these cilia or flagella have a normal appearing axoneme, others lack the central pair of tubules. Because some sensory epithelia employ modified cilia or flagella as receptor organelles, it has been speculated that the nonmotile flagella found sporadically on a wide range of cell types may also have a sensory function, but there is no experimental evidence to support this.

It is an interesting example of the unity of nature that the same basic structural organization is found in cilia and flagella throughout the plant and animal kingdoms. Those that enable the protozoan *Paramecium* to swim about in a drop of pond water have exactly the same cross sectional appearance as those that help to remove dust and bacteria from the sinuses and respiratory passages of man.

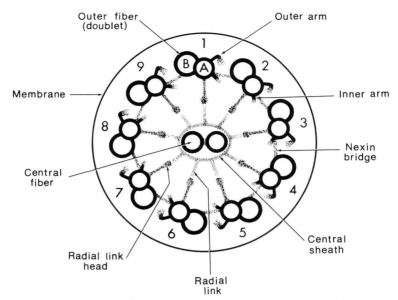

Figure 3–21 Diagram of the cross-sectional appearance of the components in the axoneme of a typical cilium as seen in high resolution electron micrographs. The nexin bridges or links probably extend from one subfiber A to the next, and not from the A to the B subfiber as shown here. (Redrawn after R. Linck.)

Blood Vessels and Nerve Fibers

As a rule, epithelia covering surfaces or lining cavities are not penetrated by blood vessels. The nutritive substances from the blood vessels of the underlying connective tissue reach the epithelial elements after passing through the narrow intercellular spaces between the epithelial cells. If the epithelium is unusually thick, as in the skin, the underlying connective tissue usually forms vascular *papillae*, which project into the deep surface of the epithelium. These facilitate nutrition by shortening the diffusion distance to the cells in the superficial layers. In a few places,

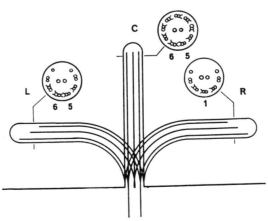

Figure 3–22 An idealized diagram illustrating the sliding filament hypothesis of ciliary binding. At the center, cilium C is straight and the doublets of the axoneme terminate at the same level. A transverse section near the tip would show all peripheral doublets. At the left, cilium L is bent toward peripheral doublets 5 and 6, which project farthest toward the tip. Doublet 1 terminates first and is missing from cross section. Doublets become single near their termination; hence 9 and 2 are shown as single. At the right, cilium R is bent toward doublet 1, which now projects farthest. Doublets on this side of the cilium are present in the transverse section, while doublets 5 and 6 are missing. (Figure after M. A. Sleigh from Endeavour *30*:11, 1971.)

such as the stria vascularis of the cochlea and the maternal layer of certain epitheliochoreal placentae, loops of blood capillaries may actually penetrate among the cells of the epithelium. Such intraepithelial capillaries are rare in other organs.

In the epidermis, olfactory mucosa, and many other epithelia, numerous terminal branches of sensory nerve fibers pierce the basement lamina and run in the interstices among the epithelial cells. The epithelia of the stomach and intestine and the cervix of the uterus, on the other hand, seem to lack sensory nerve endings, and the mucous membranes of these organs can be rubbed or

cauterized in the unanaesthetized patient without discomfort.

Extraneous Cells

Wandering cells normally may enter the epithelium from the connective tissue in some organs. For example, individual lymphocytes are very often found in the epithelium of the intestinal tract. Peyer's patches in the intestinal submucosa are large accumulations of lymphoid cells, and the overlying epithelium is often infiltrated by a multitude of lymphocytes that may push aside and distort the epithelial cells. Similarly, the epithelium

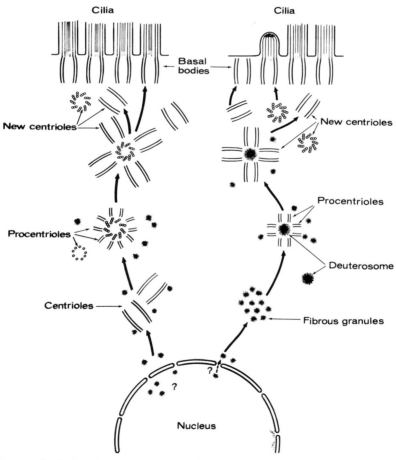

Figure 3-23 Diagram depicting alternative origins of the basal bodies during epithelial ciliogenesis. New basal bodies may form around one or both of the preexisting centrioles as indicated at the left, or they may arise *de novo* from fibrogranular precursors coalescing around centers of organization called procentriole organizers or deuterosomes as shown at the right. The latter mechanism appears to account for the majority of the basal bodies formed. (From D. W. Fawcett: *Genetics of the Spermatozoon.* Eds. R. A. Beatty and S. Glueckson-Waelsch. Edinburgh, 1972.)

overlying the tonsils is extensively infiltrated by lymphocytes. In all of these examples the lymphocytes represent a part of the body's immunological defenses against invasion of microorganisms from the environment. At certain phases of the reproductive cycle of rodents, and to a lesser extent in the human, a great number of leukocytes of various kinds migrate through the vaginal epithelium. It is not surprising that these actively motile cells can insinuate themselves between the sessile epithelial cells, but how they breach the basement lamina and separate the desmosomes and even the so-called "tight junctions" of epithelium, and how these latter are restored to their previous relations after the migratory cell has passed, are problems that remain unsolved.

Renewal and Regeneration of Epithelium

The epithelial layers, especially those that cover the outer surface of the body and the intestinal tract, are subject to constant mechanical and other trauma. Under physiologic conditions, their cells continuously perish and are shed. This is especially manifest in the stratified squamous epithelium of the epidermis, where the superficial cells undergo continuous keratinization, a peculiar kind of differentiation which leads to death and desquamation of the superficial cells. In the gastrointestinal tract, cells are continually exfoliated at the tips of the villi. On the other hand, in the respiratory passages and especially in most of the glands, degeneration of the epithelium is rare, and the cells are correspondingly long lived.

The physiological loss of cells in the epithelium is balanced by a corresponding regeneration. In vertebrates this is always effected through mitotic proliferation of relatively undifferentiated epithelial elements. The keratinized cells lost from stratified squamous epithelium are replaced by new ones which arise through mitotic proliferation of relatively undifferentiated epithelial elements found in the deeper cell layers near the base (stratum germinativum). These cells differentiate and become keratinized during their ascent to the epithelial surface. The simple columnar epithelia of the stomach and the intestine are regenerated from special areas of proliferating undifferentiated epithelial cells in the base of the gastric

foveolae or in the crypts of Lieberkühn. The rate of normal physiological loss and replacement is so great that the epithelial covering of the intestinal villi is entirely replaced every few days (see Chapter 27).

The epithelial cells are nonmotile as a rule. In healing wounds, however, epithelial cells flatten out into a thin sheet that rapidly spreads to cover large denuded areas of connective tissue. In the initial stages of this repair there is no mitotic activity, but proliferation later begins at the margins of the wound, providing the cells necessary to restore the covering epithelium to its normal thickness.

REFERENCES

Specializations of the Free Surface

Andre, J.: Sur quelques details nouvellement comme de l'ultrastructure des organites vibratiles. J. Ultrastruct. Res., 5:86, 1961.

Bennett, H. S.: Morphological aspects of extracellular polysaccharides. J. Histochem. Chyochem., 11:2, 1963.

Fawcett, D. W.: Cilia and flagella. In Brachet, J., and A. E. Mirsky, eds.: The Cell: Biochemistry, Physiology, Morphology. Vol. II. New York, Academic Press, 1961.

Fawcett, D. W.: Surface specializations of absorbing cells. J. Histochem. Cytochem., 13:75, 1965.

Fawcett, D. W., and K. R. Porter: A study of the fine structure of ciliated epithelia. J. Morphol., 94:221, 1954.

Gibbons, I. R.: The relationship between the fine structure and direction of beat in gill cilia of a lamellibranch mollusc. J. Biophys. Biochem. Cytol., 11:179, 1961.

Gibbons, I. R.: Chemical dissection of cilia. Arch. de Biol. (Liege), 76:317, 1965.

Gibbons, I. R., and A. J. Rowe: Dynein: A protein with adenosine triphosphatase activity from cilia. Science, 149:424, 1965.

Ito, S.: The surface coat of enteric microvilli. J. Cell Biol., 27:475, 1965.

Satir, P.: Studies on cilia. III. Further studies on the cilium tip and a "sliding filament" model of ciliary motility. J. Cell Biol., 39:77, 1968.

Sleigh, M. A.: Cilia. Endeavour, 30:11, 1971.

Sleigh, M. A.: The Biology of Cilia and Flagella. Oxford, England, Pergamon Press, 1962.

Junctional Specializations

Barr, L., W. Berger, and M. M. Barr: Electrical transmission at the nexus between smooth muscle cells. J. Gen. Physiol., 51:347, 1968.

Brightman, M. W., and T. S. Reese: Junctions between intimately apposed cell membranes in vertebrate brain. J. Cell Biol., 40:648, 1968.

Farquhar, M. G., and G. E. Palade: Junctional complexes in various epithelia. J. Cell Biol., 17:375, 1963.

Fawcett, D. W.: Intercellular bridges. Exp. Cell Res. 8 (Suppl.):174, 1961.

Furshpan, E. J., and D. D. Potter: Low resistance junctions between cells in embryos and tissue culture. *In* Moscona, A. A., and A. Monroy, eds.: Current topics in Developmental Biology. Vol. 8. New York, Academic Press, 1968.

Gilula, N. B., O. R. Reeves, and A. Steinbach: Metabolic coupling, ionic coupling and cell contacts. Nature, *235*:262, 1972.

Kelly, D.: Fine structure of desmosomes, hemidesmosomes and an adepidermal globular layer in developing newt epidermis. J. Cell Biol., *28*:51, 1966.

Leblond, C. P., H. Puchtler, and Y. Clermont: Structures corresponding to terminal bars and terminal web in many types of cells. Nature, *186*:784, 1960.

Lowenstein, W. R.: Intercellular communication. Sci. Amer., *222*:79, 1970.

Lowenstein, W. R.: Cellular communication through membrane junctions. Arch. Int. Med., *129*:299, 1972.

Revel, J. P., and M. J. Karnovsky: Hexagonal array of subunits in intercellular junctions of the mouse heart and liver. J. Cell Biol., *33*:C7, 1967.

Robertson, J. D.: The occurrence of a subunit pattern in the unit membranes of club endings in Mauthner cell synapses of goldfish brains. J. Cell Biol., *19*:201, 1963.

Basal Lamina

Dodson, J. D., and E. D. Hay: Secretion of collagenous stroma by epithelium grown in vitro. Exp. Cell Res., *65*:215, 1971.

Hay, E. D., and J. P. Revel: Autoradiographic studies of the origin of the basement lamella in Ambystoma. Devel. Biol., *7*:152, 1963.

Kefalides, N. A.: Chemical properties of basement membranes. Internat. Rev. Exp. Path., *10*:1, 1971.

Pierce, G. B., T. F. Beals, J. Sri Ram, and A. R. Midgley: Basement membranes. IV. Epithelial origin and immunological cross reactions. Am. J. Path., *45*:929, 1964.

Pierce, G. B., A. R. Midgley, and J. Sri Ram: Histogenesis of basement membrane. J. Exp. Med., *117*:339, 1963.

Speidel, E., and A. Lazarow: Chemical composition of glomerular basement membrane in diabetes. Diabetes, *12*:355, 1963.

Regeneration and Renewal

Arey, L. B.: Wound healing. Physiol. Rev., *16*:327, 1936.

Bertalanffy, F. D., and K. P. Nagy: Mitotic activity and renewal rate of the epithelial cells of human duodenum. Acta Anat., *45*:362, 1961.

Leblond, C. P., and B. E. Walker: Renewal of cell populations. Physiol. Rev., *36*:255, 1956.

Leblond, C. P., R. C. Greulich, and J. P. M. Pereira: Relationship of cell formation and cell migration in the renewal of stratified squamous epithelia. *In* Montagna, W., and R. E. Billingham, eds.: Advances in Biology of the Skin. Vol. 5. New York, Pergamon Press, 1964.

Lipkin, M., P. Sherlock, and B. Bell: Cell proliferation kinetics in the gastrointestinal tract of man. Gastroenterology, *45*:721, 1963.

Messier, B., and C. P. Leblond: Cell proliferation and migration as revealed by radioautography after injection of thymidine-H3 into male rats and mice. Am. J. Anat., *106*:247, 1960.

Weiss, P.: The biological foundations of wound repair. The Harvey Lectures, *55*:13, 1961:

4
Glands and Secretion

EXOCRINE GLANDS

Secretion is the process by which some cells take up small molecules from the blood and transform them by intracellular biosynthetic mechanisms into a more complex product that is then released from the cell. The chemical transformations involved in secretion are active processes consuming energy in contrast to *excretion* as exemplified by the passive diffusion of carbon dioxide across the epithelium lining the lung, or the filtration of blood in the kidney to form urine.

Cells and associations of cells specialized for secretion are called *glands*. We define two major categories of glands on the basis of how their products are released. Those that deliver their product into a system of ducts opening onto an external or internal surface are called *exocrine glands*. Those that release their product into the blood or lymph for transport to another part of the body are called *endocrine glands*.

Secretion has traditionally been regarded as a function of epithelial cells because it was only in these that accumulation and liberation of the product could be observed directly with the light microscope. However, since indirect, autoradiographic methods have become available for tracing uptake of precursors and discharge of product, it has become obvious that the traditional definition must be extended to include a variety of nonepithelial mesenchymal derivatives such as fibroblasts, chondroblasts, and osteoblasts that release substances into the extracellular space to form the fibrous and amorphous components of the connective tissues.

Much has been learned in recent years about the intracellular sites of synthesis and the mechanisms of secretion by correlating electron microscopic and biochemical observations. These primary events at the subcellular level will be reviewed before we proceed to a discussion of the histological organization and classification of glands.

SYNTHESIS, STORAGE, AND RELEASE OF PROTEIN RICH SECRETORY PRODUCTS

Glandular cells often contain granules or droplets that represent intracellular accumulations of the precursors of their secretory products. Just as all cells are continually performing chemical work in maintaining their structural integrity and internal organization, most glandular cells are synthesizing and secreting their products continually at minimal levels. They can often be stimulated to increase the rate of delivery of their product, and much of the information on secretion gained by traditional histologists depended upon observation of the cytological changes associated with stimulated or exaggerated activity. It was observed, for example, that when glandular cells were stimulated, the number of specific granules in their cytoplasm decreased concomitantly with the increase in outflow of secretion from the ducts. After depletion of the granules, the basophilic substance of the cytoplasm seemed to become more prominent, the

Golgi apparatus hypertrophied, the nucleus increased slightly in volume and the nucleolus became more prominent. Each of these organelles was therefore thought to be involved in some way in the synthetic activities of the cell. As the secretory granules began to reaccumulate, they first appeared in very close association with the Golgi apparatus and this organelle was therefore thought to be the site of concentration of material synthesized elsewhere in the cytoplasm (Bowen).

Progress in electron microscopy and molecular biology has now substantiated these classical observations of light microscopists, and has made it possible to define the respective roles of the various cell organelles in the synthesis and release of protein-rich secretory products. The cell type that has been most thoroughly studied is the pancreatic acinar cell (Fig. 4–1), which secretes several protein enzymes into the digestive juice. The description of the cellular mechanisms of protein synthesis and of the intracellular secretory pathways that follows will be based upon studies of the pancreatic exocrine cells (Palade and Siekevitz), but it applies equally well to a great variety of other secretory cells.

The chemical nature of a cell product is determined by the nucleus. The information or "blueprint" for construction of the structural proteins and the protein products of cells is encoded in the sequence of nucleotides in the DNA molecules of the chromosomes. The substance synthesized by a cell depends upon what regions of its chromosomes are active at the time—in other words, which portions of the DNA molecules are exposed and available for transcription of information. The cell components that are capable of utilizing this information for the synthesis of a particular protein reside in the cytoplasm. There must therefore be intermediaries or messengers to carry the information from the nucleus to the cytoplasm, and there must be avenues of communication between these two compartments of the cell. Three classes of ribonucleic acid molecules have been identified which are essential

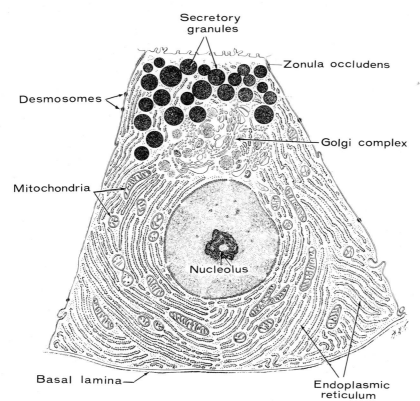

Figure 4–1 Drawing of the fine structure of a pancreatic acinar cell, which can be considered typical of exocrine glandular cells secreting a protein product.

for the transfer of genetic information and its translation during synthesis of proteins: these are *messenger RNA* (mRNA), *transfer RNA* (tRNA), and *ribosomal RNA* (rRNA). All three of these are formed by transcription of specific segments of the chromosomal DNA molecules. A region of one of the chromosomes that is concerned with elaboration of ribosomal RNA is closely associated with the nucleolus. This organelle is believed to be the site of union of ribosomal RNA with protein constituents to form nucleoproteins that then pass into the cytoplasm, where they become subunits of the ribosomes. The morphological pathway which the three types of RNA take to the cytoplasm is thought to be through the pores in the nuclear envelope.

In the cytoplasm, the nucleoprotein subunits from the nucleolus assemble to form microscopically visible ribosomes. These become associated with a site of initiation of protein synthesis at one end of the long mole-cules of mRNA and subsequently move along the length of the molecule, "reading" in each successive set of three nucleotides (codons) the instructions that determine the sequence of assembly of the amino acids in the protein being synthesized. The appropriate amino acid is brought to the site of assembly on the ribosome by a molecule of transfer RNA (Fig. 4–5). There are specific tRNAs for each of the 20 amino acids. A molecule of tRNA carrying its specific amino acid recognizes and attaches itself to the appropriate complementary site on the mRNA. Its amino acid is then inserted into the protein molecule being developed on the ribosome. The ribosome moves along the mRNA to the next codon, and the first tRNA molecule is released. Other ribosomes in turn become attached to the vacated initiator site and follow along after the first, reading the same message and synthesizing the same kind of protein molecule. In this way numerous ribo-

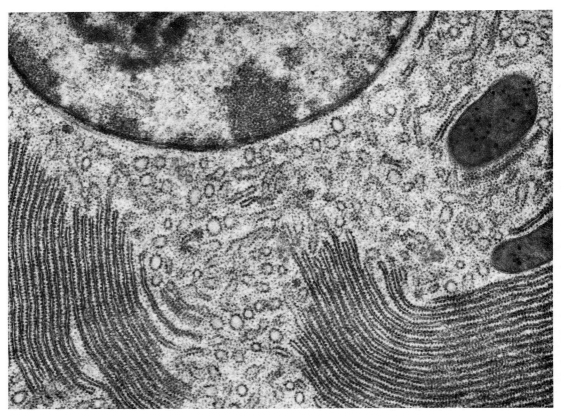

Figure 4–2 Electron micrograph of the basal region of a pancreatic acinar cell. In all protein secreting exocrine glands the granular endoplasmic reticulum (ergastoplasm) is well developed. The associated ribosomes are the sites of synthesis of new protein. ×22,000.

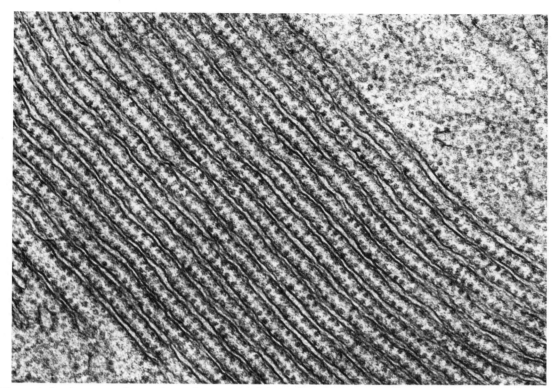

Figure 4-3 An area of cytoplasm from a glandular cell at higher magnification, showing the ribosomes attached to the outer surfaces of several closely spaced cisternae of the endoplasmic reticulum.

somes become associated with the same mRNA molecule to form a chain or rosette of interconnected ribosomes. These assemblages, called *polyribosomes* or *polysomes*, are seen in electron micrographs to occur either free in the cytoplasmic matrix or to be attached to the outer surface of the limiting membrane of the endoplasmic reticulum (Figs. 4–2 and 4–4). In glandular cells producing protein for export from the cell, the vast majority of polysomes are associated with the reticulum. The ribosomes are attached to the membranes by the larger of their two subunits. The elongating polypeptide chain of the new protein molecule forming on each ribosome comes off vectorially, penetrating the underlying membrane (Fig. 4–5). Thus, when the new protein molecules are completed and released from the ribosome, they are found within the lumen of the endoplasmic reticulum. This process, repeated hundreds of thousands of times on polysomes throughout the cytoplasm of the glandular cell, results in rapid accumulation of newly formed protein in the fluid contents of the endoplasmic reticulum. The product is transported through the labyrinthine system of canaliculi comprising this organelle to the supranuclear Golgi region. The lumen of the reticulum is not continuous with the cavities of the Golgi complex, but small evaginations form on smooth surfaced areas of the reticulum and pinch off as free vesicles, each containing a small amount of the newly synthesized protein (Fig. 4–6). These *intermediate* or *transport vesicles* congregate at the forming face of the Golgi where they coalesce with each other and with the outermost flattened saccule of this organelle. The product is thus transferred from the reticulum to the Golgi complex, where it is concentrated in *condensing vacuoles* and ultimately transformed into dense, spherical, secretory droplets or granules, each limited by a smooth contoured membrane. These leave the Golgi complex at its concave or secretory face and accumulate in the apical cytoplasm. When the glandular cell is stimulated to release its product, secretory granules move to the surface and contact the plasmalemma. Their membrane becomes continuous with the cell membrane at the site of contact and the viscous contents of the secretory granule are free to flow out into the lumen (Fig. 4–8). As the granule is evacuated, its membrane is incorporated in the cell surface. Thus, the secretory product leaves the cell without any discontinuity being produced in the plasmalemma. This process of expulsion of material from cells is described by the term *exocytosis*.

In recapitulation, it is the current view that the ribosomes on the endoplasmic reticulum are the sites of synthesis of protein secretory products which are then segregated in the lumen of the reticulum and transported through it to the Golgi region; intermediate vesicles transfer it from the reticulum to the Golgi complex, which functions as a center for concentration and "packaging" of the product. The mitochondria participate in the process only by providing ATP for the energy requiring steps

of protein synthesis and active transport within the cell (Fig. 4–9).

The evidence for the interpretations presented above derives in part from biochemistry and in part from electron microscopy. The degree to which the two approaches have complemented each other has been a gratifying demonstration of the interdependence of the two disciplines. Convincing validation of the sequence and time course of events in the intracellular secretory pathway is provided by autoradiography. Animals given a tritium labeled amino acid intravenously are killed at successive time intervals and the location of the incorporated label is observed in autoradiographs of the pancreas. Within 5 minutes of administration of the tritiated amino acid precursor, reduced silver grains can be found in the photographic emulsion over the endoplasmic reticulum in the basal cytoplasm of the cells where amino acid is being incorporated into newly synthesized protein. In 15 to 20 minutes the label

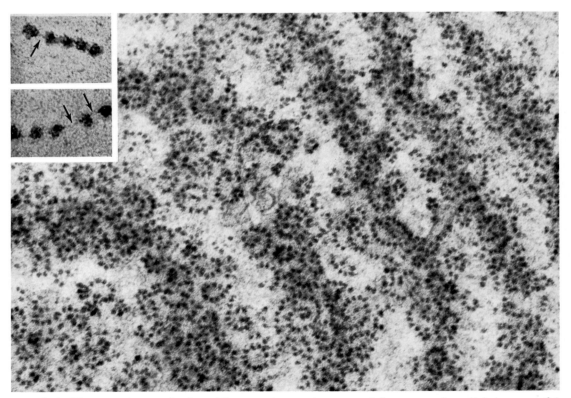

Figure 4–4 Electron micrograph of an oblique section passing tangentially to several parallel cisternae of the endoplasmic reticulum, and showing numerous spiral and rosette configurations of polyribosomes. ×75,000. (Courtesy of E. Yamada.) Insets show positively stained, isolated polyribosomes connected by a thin strand (arrows) representing the messenger RNA. (Courtesy of C. Hall and A. Rich.)

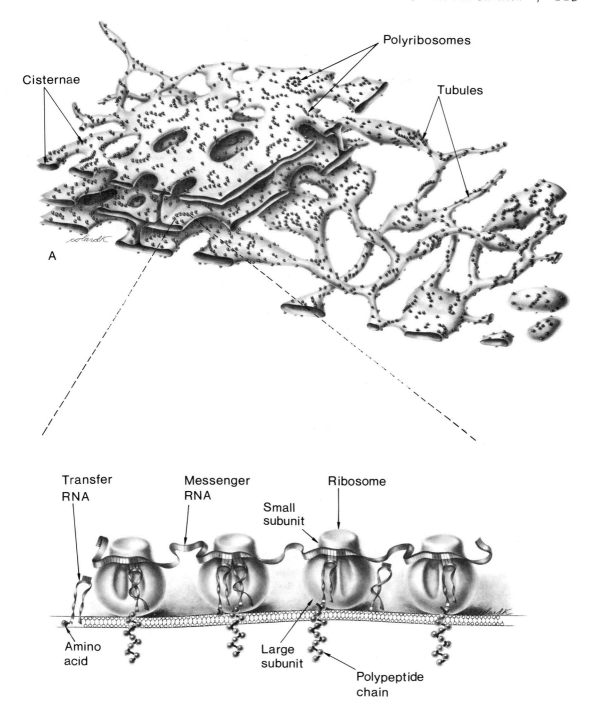

Figure 4-5 *A,* Drawing of the three dimensional configuration of the cisternae and tubules of an area of granular endoplasmic reticulum. Ribosomes occur in rosettes and spirals on the outer surface of the membranes. *B,* A group of four ribosomes is presented at a magnification beyond the reach of the microscope. The drawing is highly schematic and relies upon indirect biochemical and biophysical evidence. For explanation of the mechanism of protein synthesis on the ribosomes, see text.

can be found over the Golgi complex. In 45 minutes the silver grains are over the secretory granules at the cell apex, and after one hour some are already overlying secretion in the lumen of the acinus. These events occur far more rapidly than was previously believed. The mean life span of exportable protein molecules in the pancreatic acinar cell is now estimated to be about 50 minutes (Warshawsky et al.).

Much more is known about the transcription and translation of genetic information and the regulation of protein synthesis than has been indicated here. Some of this will already be familiar to students well prepared in cell and molecular biology. Others may wish to consult a modern textbook of biochemistry for additional details.

In the foregoing account, the Golgi complex was assigned no synthetic role but was considered to be concerned exclusively with the concentration of the secretory product and its enclosure in a membrane capable of coalescing with the plasmalemma. This seems to be true of glandular cells whose product is exclusively protein. However, in cells whose products consist of both protein and carbohydrate there is now compelling evidence that the assembly of the carbohydrate moiety depends upon glycosyltransferases located in the Golgi membranes (Fleischer et al.). In such cells the Golgi apparatus is the principal site of synthesis of polysaccharides and

of their conjugation with protein synthesized on the ribosomes of the endoplasmic reticulum.

Several aspects of the exocrine secretory process remain to be explained. It will have occurred to the reader that during active release of secretion by exocytosis, a large area of membrane is added to the cell surface. Inasmuch as no appreciable redundance of cell membrane is observed under these conditions, it follows that there must be a mechanism for compensatory withdrawal of excess membrane from the cell surface. Some authors have suggested that small, smooth or coated vesicles form at the free surface, pinch off and move back to the Golgi region, providing for bulk interiorization and recycling of membrane. Other investigators, impressed by the paucity of visual evidence of membrane return, have proposed that the surface area is reduced by constituents of the membrane entering the cytoplasm molecule by molecule. The return limb of the cycle would thus be amicroscopic. Clearly much more research will be required to resolve this paradox.

Equally baffling is the basis for the specific properties of the membrane acquired by secretory granules in the Golgi apparatus which permit coalescence with the plasma membrane during release of product, but which seem not to predispose to coalescence with other membranes within the cell. There

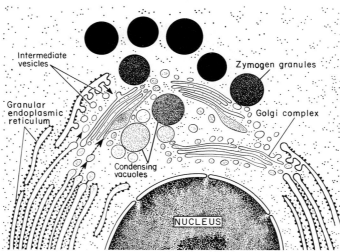

Figure 4-6 Diagram of the Golgi region of a glandular cell, showing smooth surfaced intermediate vesicles budding from the endoplasmic reticulum. The product carried in these vesicles to the forming face of the Golgi complex emerges from its secretory face in condensing vacuoles. These concentrate the product to form zymogen granules.

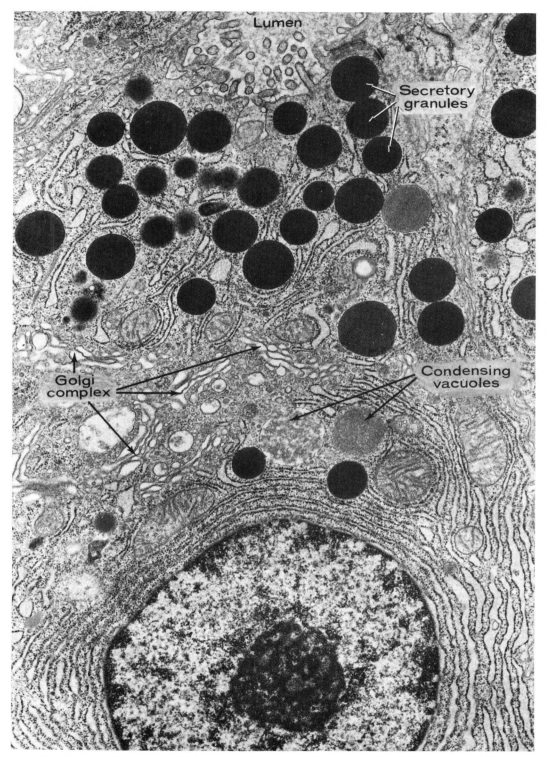

Figure 4-7 Electron micrograph of the supranuclear region of a pancreatic cell illustrating condensing vacuoles in the Golgi region and mature secretory granules at the cell apex. (Micrograph courtesy of S. Ito).

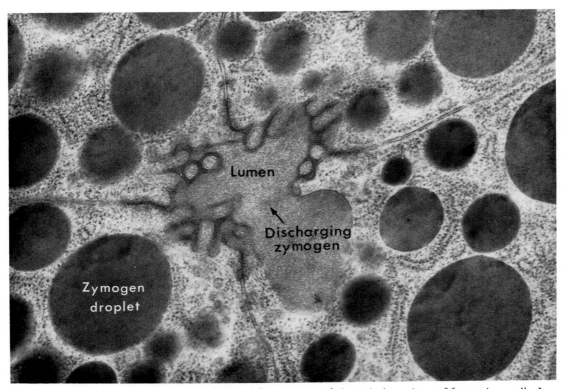

Figure 4-8 Electron micrograph of the lumen of an acinus and the apical portions of four acinar cells. Large dense zymogen droplets or granules are found in the cell apex. The limiting membrane of one of these has fused with the cell membrane and its zymogen is being discharged into the lumen. The free surface of the acinar cells bears short microvilli. ×38,000.

is suggestive evidence that the secretory granules of some cell types have limiting membranes rich in lysolecithin, a substance known to promote membrane fusion. While this might account for their tendency to fuse with the surface membrane it leaves unexplained the fact that secretory granules may be closely packed in the apical cytoplasm but they do not fuse with one another. On the other hand, when one granule has coalesced with the plasma membrane, its properties are immediately changed so that other secretory granules may now fuse with it, producing chains of connected granules communicating at one end with the surface but extending some distance into the apical cytoplasm (Fig. 4–10). The current intense research on biological membranes may soon provide answers to the questions raised by these puzzling morphological observations.

Histologists have traditionally distinguished three mechanisms by which cells discharge their secretory products:

1. *Merocrine secretion* was defined as release through the cell membrane with the cell remaining intact. The limited resolution of the light microscope did not reveal how this was accomplished but it was assumed that the secretory material either diffused through an intact membrane, or, more likely, that whole granules passed out through transient discontinuities in the membrane. Electron microscopic observations have now shown how a product can leave a glandular cell in bulk without the creation of discontinuities in the membrane. Merocrine secretion is now understood to consist of release by the process of exocytosis, which has already been described.

2. *Apocrine secretion* involves loss of part of the apical cytoplasm along with the material secreted. The cell is able to restore continuity of its surface and reaccumulate product. This form of secretion is less common and has been less thoroughly studied. Electron microscopic observations on the mam-

mary gland, which is generally accepted as an apocrine gland, substantiate the belief that some of the cell is lost, but this loss involves only a segment of the membrane and a thin rim of cytoplasm around the lipid component of the secretion—certainly a less drastic loss of cell substance than was envisioned by light microscopists.

3. *Holocrine secretion* consists of release of whole cells into the excretory ducts or total discharge of the contents of cells leading to their complete destruction. In sebaceous glands, the cells break down with an outpouring of their cytoplasm and accumulated lipid. Release of spermatozoa from the seminiferous epithelium of the testis is regarded as a form of holocrine secretion.

Although the terms merocrine, apocrine, and holocrine introduced by light microscopists have required some redefinition, they will continue to be useful until their mechanisms are better understood and a more consistent terminology is developed.

CLASSIFICATION OF EXOCRINE GLANDS

Exocrine glands may be *unicellular* or *multicellular*. The latter are further classified, according to the organization and geometry of their epithelial component, as *tubular*, *alveolar*, *tubuloalveolar*, *saccular*, etc.

Unicellular Glands

In mammals, the most common and indeed virtually the only example of a unicellular gland is the *mucous* or *goblet cell* found scattered among the columnar cells of the epithelium on many mucous membranes. It secretes *mucin*, a protein-polysaccharide, which upon hydration forms a lubricating solution called *mucus*. A fully developed cell of this type has an expanded apical end filled with pale droplets of *mucigen*, and a slender basal end containing a compressed nucleus and a small amount of deeply staining basophilic cytoplasm. The term *goblet cell* is descriptive of the form of the cell, which has an expanded cup-shaped rim of cytoplasm called the *theca* filled with secretory droplets, and a thin base, like the stem of a goblet, extending to the basal lamina of the epithelium (Fig. 4–11).

The mucigen droplets tend to swell and coalesce during specimen preparation and are seldom resolved as separate entities. They are better preserved by freeze-drying and they stain well with the periodic acid–Schiff reaction because of their polysaccharide content.

The finer structure of goblet cells is difficult to study because of the degree to which their organelles are compressed into the basal cytoplasm. The basophilia of the cytoplasm results from the abundance of free and attached ribosomes. The latter are de-

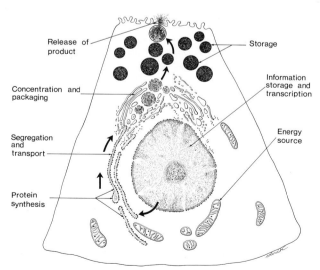

Figure 4–9 Schematic presentation of the role of the various organelles in the secretory process.

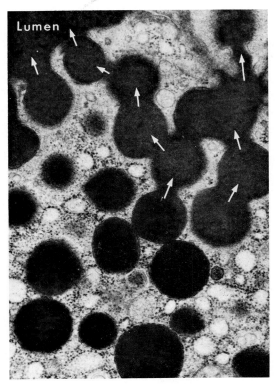

Lumen

Figure 4-10 Electron micrograph of the apical portion of an acinar cell from a dog pancreas. A zymogen granule or droplet opening onto the lumen may be joined to a second and this to a third, so that zymogen may be discharged through several intercommunicating membrane limited vacuoles. ×24,500. (After A. Ichikawa, J. Cell Biol., *24*:369, 1965.)

ployed on the surface of the cisternae arranged roughly parallel to the cell surface in the paranuclear and basal cytoplasm. The Golgi complex is well developed and located between the compressed nucleus and the mucigen droplets in the theca. The individual droplets of mucigen are enveloped by extremely delicate membranes that are usually broken in preparation of the specimen (Moe).

The synthesis of mucigen involves the synthesis of protein in the manner previously described for protein secreting cells in general. However, autoradiography after administration of ^{35}S or ^{3}H-glucose shows that the label goes directly to the supranuclear region, thus establishing that the synthesis and sulfation of the glycoprotein of the mucigen take place in the Golgi complex (Belanger; Florey; Neutra and Leblond).

In the discharging of the secretion, the membrane of individual secretory droplets or of groups of coalesced droplets fuses with and becomes part of the plasma membrane, permitting the mucus to pour out onto the surface (Trier).

The secretion of mucus proceeds more or less continuously and the cell retains its goblet form for most of its life span — which is only two to four days in the intestinal mucosa. Although goblet cells normally pass through only one long secretory cycle, they may be made to expel nearly all of their secretion at once. Under these conditions, they soon resume mucosynthesis and refill their theca.

Multicellular Glands

The simplest form of multicellular gland is a sheet of epithelium consisting of a homogeneous population of secretory cells (Fig. 4–12). The surface epithelium of the gastric mucosa and of the uterine lining at certain stages belong to this category, sometimes described as a *secretory sheet. Intraepithelial glands* are intermediate between a secretory sheet and a simple tubular gland. They are small accumulations of glandular cells (usually mucous) that lie wholly within the thickness of the epithelium but are arranged around a small lumen of their own (Fig. 4–13). In man, examples are found in the pseudostratified columnar epithelium of the nasal mucosa and in the ductuli efferentes and urethra.

All other multicellular glands arise as tubular invaginations of an epithelial sheet and extend into the underlying connective tissue. The glandular cells are usually confined to the *terminal* or *secretory* portions of the tubular invagination. Secretion elaborated by the gland cells reaches the surface directly, or through an *excretory* duct consisting of less specialized, nonsecretory cells.

In many glands, the surface available for release of secretion is further increased by development of many extremely fine canals, the *secretory capillaries* or *canaliculi*, which extend from the lumen between glandular cells. These slender extracellular passages are often branched, and they end blindly before reaching the basal lamina. They have no walls of their own, but are formed by apposition of groove-like excavations in the surface of adjoining cells. They are usually

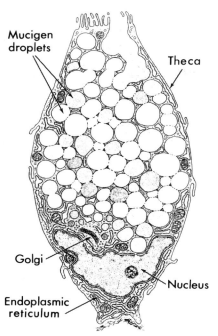

Figure 4–11 Drawing of the fine structure of an intestinal goblet cell. (From T. Lentz, Cell Fine Structure. Philadelphia, W. B. Saunders Company, 1971.)

lined by numerous microvilli. The parietal cells of the gastric glands are exceptional in appearing to have an intracellular system of fine canaliculi. Electron microscopy has shown, however, that these so called *intracellular canaliculi* are not actually within the cytoplasm but are deep invaginations of the cell surface. They are limited by the plasma membrane and their lumen is therefore actually extracellular, like that of the more common *intercellular canaliculi*.

Simple Exocrine Glands. The elaborate scheme of classification of glands may seem to the student unnecessarily complex but it has the advantage of permitting more precise description of the great variety of configurations found in the body. Multicellular glands are designated as *simple* or *compound* depending upon whether or not their communication with the surface is branched. A *simple exocrine gland* is one in which the functional unit is connected directly to the surface epithelium via an unbranched duct (Fig. 4–14). Glands fulfilling this criterion are further categorized on the

basis of the configuration of their terminal or secretory portions. Thus they may be described as *simple tubular, simple coiled tubular, simple branched tubular* and *simple acinar* (or *alveolar*).

In *simple tubular glands*, there is no excretory duct, and the terminal portion is a straight tubule that opens directly onto the epithelial surface. The intestinal glands of Lieberkühn are examples (Fig. 4–14a).

In *simple coiled tubular glands*, the terminal portion is a long coiled tubule, connected to the surface by a long, unbranched excretory duct. The common sweat glands belong to this category. In the large apocrine sweat glands, the terminal portions branch (Fig. 4–14b).

In *simple branched tubular glands*, the tubules of the terminal portion bifurcate into two or more branches, which may be somewhat coiled near their ends. An excretory duct may be absent, as in the glands of the stomach and uterus, or there may be a short

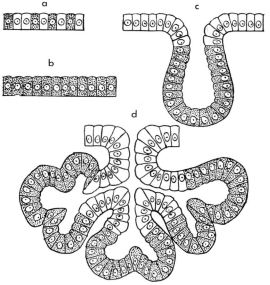

Figure 4–12 Diagram of unicellular and multicellular glands. *a*, Granular; glandular cells are scattered singly among clear, common epithelial cells; *b*, glandular cells arranged in a continuous sheet — secretory epithelial surface; *c*, simplest type of multicellular gland; the area lined with glandular cells forms a saclike invagination into the subjacent tissue; *d*, multicellular gland of greater complexity; the glandular spaces are lined partly with glandular cells (terminal portions), partly with common epithelium (excretory ducts).

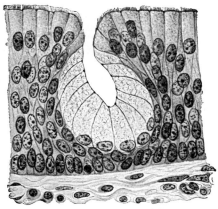

Figure 4–13 Intraepithelial gland from the pseudo-stratified ciliated epithelium of the laryngeal surface of the epiglottis of a woman of 72 years. ×534. (After V. Patzelt, from Schaffer.)

excretory duct, as in some of the small glands of the oral cavity, the tongue, and the esophagus, and in the glands of Brunner in the duodenum (Fig. 4–14*d*).

In the *simple acinar* (or *alveolar*) *glands*, the terminal portion is expanded to form a spherical or elongated sac. If only one acinus is associated with one excretory duct, the gland is a *simple acinar gland* (Fig. 4–14*e*). This type is thought not to occur in mammals. If the acinus is subdivided by partitions into several smaller compartments, or if several acini are arranged along a duct, it is a *simple branched acinar gland* (Fig. 4–14*f*). Examples are the sebaceous glands of the skin and the meibomian glands of the eyelids.

Compound Exocrine Glands. The duct of a compound exocrine gland branches repeatedly. Such a gland can be thought of as consisting of a variable number of simple glands at the ends of an arborescent system of ducts of progressively diminishing caliber (Fig. 4–15). Thus there are *compound tubular, compound acinar, compound saccular glands,* etc.

In *compound tubular glands,* the terminal portions of the smallest lobules are more or less coiled tubules, usually branching. To this category belong the pure mucous glands of the oral cavity, glands of the gastric cardia, some of the glands of Brunner (Fig. 4–16), the bulbourethral glands, and the renal tubules. In special cases, as, for instance, in the testis, the terminal coils anastomose.

In the *compound acinar glands* (also called

compound alveolar glands) the terminal portions were thought to occur in the form of spherical or pear-shaped units with a small lumen (Fig. 4–15*a*). As a rule, however, the form is that of irregularly branched tubules with numerous acinar lateral outgrowths from the wall and on the blind ends. These glands would be more correctly designated *compound tubuloacinar (tubuloalveolar).* To this group belong most of the larger exocrine glands—the salivary glands, glands of the respiratory passages, and the pancreas (Fig. 4–17).

Some authors add another category called *compound saccular glands,* which differ from the compound alveolar type only in their much larger size, and particularly in the larger lumen of their secretory end pieces. The examples commonly cited are the mammary gland and the prostate gland. Other authors, however, include these organs among the compound tubuloacinar glands.

In some cases the excretory ducts do not all join into a single main duct but open independently on a restricted area of a free epithelial surface. Such is the case with the lacrimal, mammary, and prostate glands.

In addition to classification according to histological organization, compound glands are often classified according to the nature of the secretion they produce. Thus they may be designated as *mucous, serous,* or *mixed.* Mucous glands secrete a viscous material with a lubricating or protective function, serous glands have a watery secretion often rich in enzymes (Fig. 4–18).

In mucous glands the major portion of the cell is occupied by mucigen droplets and appears pale and highly vacuolated in histological sections. The nucleus is displaced far to the base and is often greatly flattened by the accumulated mucigen droplets (Fig. 4–18*A*). In serous glands, the cells are generally smaller, their nucleus is spherical and situated in the basal half of the cell surrounded by deeply basophilic cytoplasm. The apex of the cell may be clear, owing to extraction of the secretory material (Fig. 4–18*B*), or, where the secretory product is preserved, it may stain as discrete granules. The ultrastructure of serous cells is similar to that of the pancreatic acinar cell but with somewhat less extensive development of the endoplasmic reticulum.

Mixed glands contain both mucous and serous cells. Mucous cells often make up the

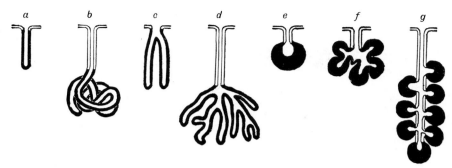

Figure 4–14 Diagrams of simple exocrine glands. *a*, Simple tubular; *b*, simple coiled tubular; *c* and *d*, simple branched tubular; *e*, simple alveolar, *f* and *g*, simple branched acinar. Secretory portions black; ducts double-contoured.

greater part of the gland, with somewhat flattened serous cells forming crescentic caps, called serous *demilunes*, over the ends of the alveoli. These cells are in communication with the lumen via intercellular secretory canaliculi (Figs. 4–19 and 4–20).

HISTOLOGICAL ORGANIZATION OF EXOCRINE GLANDS

There are certain common features in the organization of the larger glands. They are enclosed in a condensation of connective tissue that forms the capsule of the organ. Septa of connective tissue extending inward from the capsule divide the gland into grossly visible subdivisions called *lobes*. These in turn are partitioned by thinner septa into smaller units called *lobules*, still visible with the

naked eye (Fig. 4–21). These are separated to some extent into microscopic *lobules* of glandular units, but as a rule collagenous connective tissue penetrates for only a short distance into the lobule before giving way to a delicate network of reticular fibers surrounding the terminal ducts and secretory acini or tubules.

Blood vessels, lymphatics, and nerves of glands usually show a pattern of distribution similar to that of the connective tissue. They penetrate the capsule and follow the collagenous septa or the thinner partitions between the lobules and from there send branches inward. Within the lobule they are ultimately enclosed by reticular connective tissue. The blood and lymph capillaries form networks around small masses of gland cells and the terminal ducts. The major vascular supply is supplemented in most glands

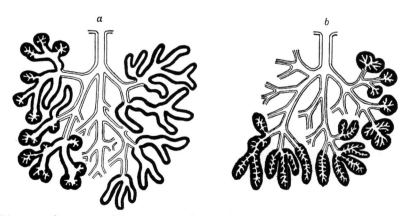

Figure 4–15 Diagram of compound exocrine glands. *a*, Mixed compound tubular and tubuloacinar; *b*, compound acinar. Secretory portions black; ducts double-contoured.

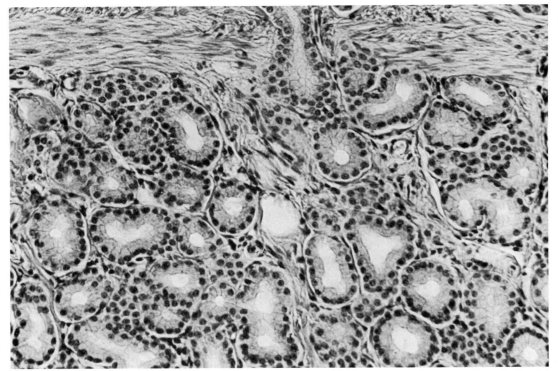

Figure 4–16 Photomicrograph of an intestinal submucosal gland, an example of a simple branched tubular gland. The duct, seen penetrating the muscularis mucosae at the top of the micrograph, is unbranched, but the secretory portion branches repeatedly and presents many cross-sectional profiles when sectioned.

by a collateral circulation mediated through capsular vessels of small caliber. The terminal nerve fibers branch, and their final divisions end in a multitude of small enlargements on the surfaces of gland cells.

The duct system of a complex exocrine gland conducts the product of the gland cells to a free external or internal body surface. The ducts may also modify the secretion during its passage. The *main duct* of the gland divides in the connective tissue to form *lobar ducts*. Their further branchings in the septa between lobules are called *interlobular ducts*, while the ducts of the microscopic lobules are called *intralobular ducts*. The latter are continuous with the *intercalary ducts*, whose branches communicate with the secretory acini either directly, via intercellular canaliculi, or by a combination of these arrangements. The epithelium of the largest ducts may be simple or stratified columnar. As the duct becomes smaller, the epithelium is first simple columnar, then cuboidal, and finally squamous.

CONTROL OF EXOCRINE SECRETION

Many glands secrete more or less continuously at a low level but are stimulated under certain conditions to secrete more abundantly. The mechanisms for physiological control of secretion vary greatly from gland to gland. In a great many, the stimulation is mediated solely via the autonomic nervous system. In other glands, the stimulus is hormonal, and in some there is dual mechanism. It is well known, for example, that the sight or smell of food will increase the secretion of acid, mucus, and digestive enzymes in the stomach. These psychic stimuli are mediated via the vagus nerves and are abolished if these are cut. On the other hand, food placed in the stomach also initiates gastric and pancreatic secretion even if it was not previously seen or tasted. Secretion in this case depends both upon the intrinsic nerves in the organ and upon locally produced hormones. Activation of nerves in the gastric mucosa releases the neurohumor *acetylcholine*, which stimulates release of the hormone *gastrin* from the mucosa, and this in turn activates secretion by the gastric glands.

There are no visible morphological criteria which enable the histologist to determine whether a given gland is under control of hormones, but nervous control can be inferred from the observation of nerve endings in close contact with the secretory cells. In the pancreas, nerve endings can be found inside of the basal lamina of the acini, in close contact with the base of the exocrine cells. These cells are also known to be responsive to the hormone *gastrin*, produced in the stomach, and *pancreozymin*, secreted in the duodenum. Thus, multiple factors are involved in the control of pancreatic secretion.

ENDOCRINE GLANDS

Phylogenetically three main mechanisms have developed in animals to integrate the functions of their different tissues and organs. To some degree these are recapitulated in vertebrate ontogeny. The earliest mechanism to appear involves substances that simply diffuse through the intercellular spaces and influence the behavior or function of other cells at a limited distance from the source. Integration by simple diffusion of chemical messengers is slow, poorly controlled, and of limited usefulness in larger metazoa. This primitive humoral mechanism was later supplemented by development of a nervous system consisting of cells that had acquired the capacity to respond to external stimuli and to rapidly conduct a signal over the surface of their long cell processes to affect other cells. The nervous system increased in complexity and became highly efficient in dealing with elaborate integrated patterns of behavior involving delicate, precise, and rapid motor events. These integrative systems have been supplemented by development of ductless glands whose cells synthesize chemical agents called *hormones* that are carried in the circulating blood to distant parts of the body, where they act

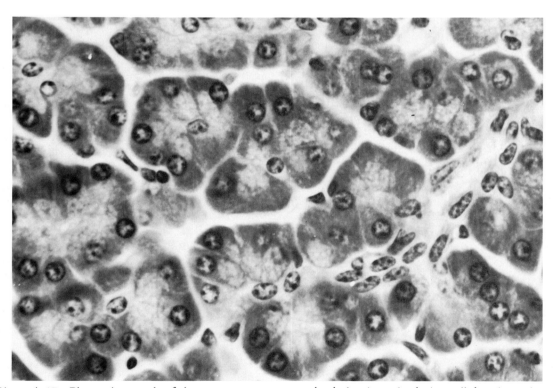

Figure 4-17 Photomicrograph of the pancreas, a compound tubuloacinar gland. A small duct is sectioned longitudinally at the right of the figure. The duct branches to the several acini that are clustered around it.

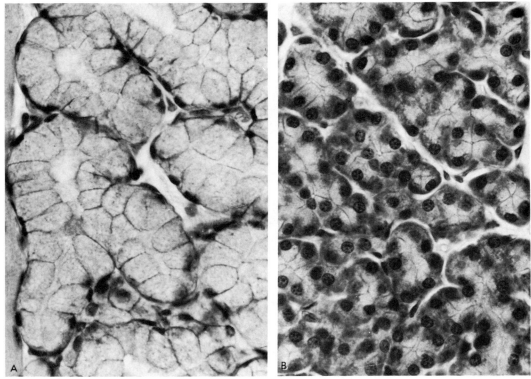

Figure 4-18 Photomicrographs illustrating the contrasting appearance of a mucous gland (*A*) and a serous gland (*B*), both from the tongue.

upon specific *target organs*. These chemical messengers tend to have a longer latent period because they are distributed by the blood, but they produce more sustained effects than the signals carried by nerves.

Endocrine glands arise in the embryo as tubular evaginations or solid outgrowths from lining epithelia, but later in the course of their development their connection with the surface is lost. They are penetrated by blood vessels, which form a very rich capillary plexus in intimate relationship to the cords, follicles, or acini of the endocrine glands. The close proximity of the cells to a dense vascular bed favors release of secretory product into the blood.

The fully developed endocrine gland is usually completely dissociated from exocrine glandular tissue, but in a few instances there is relatively little morphological separation of the endocrine tissue from the exocrine duct system. Thus, the small islets of Langerhans, the endocrine component of the pancreas, are scattered throughout the much greater

bulk of the exocrine portion of the gland (see Chapter 29, Fig. 29–2). Similarly, in the testis, the Leydig cells secreting male sex hormone are located in interstitial tissue between the tubules comprising the exocrine portion of the organ (see Chapter 32, Fig. 32–4). Thus, in these *mixed glands*, one group of cells secretes into the external duct system while another group delivers its internal secretion into the blood. In the rather unique case of the liver, the cells secrete bile into the intercellular terminations of a duct system, but the same cells also release internal secretions into the blood flowing through sinusoids between the sheets of hepatic cells.

The principal endocrine glands are the *hypophysis, thyroid, parathyroid, pancreas, adrenals, pineal, testes,* and *placenta.* These are so diverse in their architecture that they do not lend themselves to classification on the basis of their histological organization. The chemical nature of their hormones is also varied, including modified amino acids, peptides, proteins, glycoproteins, and steroids. It is not surprising, therefore, that one cannot describe cytological features common to all endocrine cells. It is possible, however, to assign them to a few categories related to the chemical nature of their product.

CYTOLOGY OF PROTEIN AND POLYPEPTIDE SECRETING ENDOCRINE GLANDS

As might be expected, endocrine cells secreting peptide, protein, and glycoprotein hormones have many ultrastructural features in common with the protein secreting exocrine cells described previously, but there is a significant difference in the degree of development of the organelles concerned with protein synthesis. The granular endoplasmic reticulum is much less extensive. This is consistent with the great difference in the volume of product produced. The acinar cells of the exocrine pancreas produce over a liter of enzyme rich digestive juice per day, whereas the output of a protein or peptide secreting endocrine gland would be measured in milligram or microgram quantities.

The beta cell of the pancreatic islets, which secretes the hormone *insulin*, can be considered representative of this category of endocrine cells. Electron micrographs of these cells show a few meandering profiles of granular endoplasmic reticulum, and clusters of free ribosomes in a cytoplasmic matrix of low density. There is a small Golgi

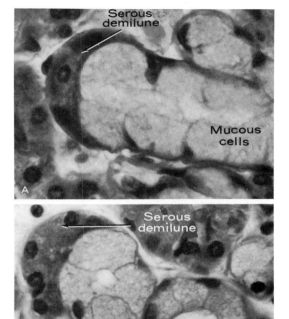

Figure 4-20 Photomicrograph of the terminal portions of the submandibular gland. This is an example of a mixed gland; some of the terminal elements are purely mucous, others have crescentic caps of serous cells called demilunes. The relationship is seen to better advantage in longitudinal section (A) than in transverse section (B).

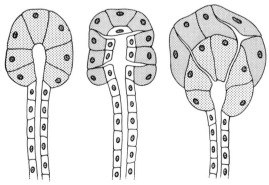

Figure 4-19 Diagram showing relationships of terminal portions of duct system (intercalary duct) and intercellular canaliculi to the secreting cells. Lighter stippled portion generally mucous; darker portion serous. (Modified from Zimmermann.)

apparatus and numerous membrane limited granules 200 to 300 nm. in diameter. As in exocrine glandular cells, the granules appear to be formed in the Golgi complex. They tend to be somewhat more numerous at the vascular pole but occur in considerable numbers throughout the cytoplasm (Fig. 4–22). In man insulin occurs in the form of pleomorphic crystals within membrane limited secretory vesicles, but in common laboratory animals the secretory granules are uniformly dense and homogeneous. With minor differences in cytology and granule size, this same description would apply to the alpha cells of the pancreas, which secrete glucagon (Fig. 4–23), the somatotrophs, thyrotrophs, gonadotrophs and corticotrophs of the hypo-

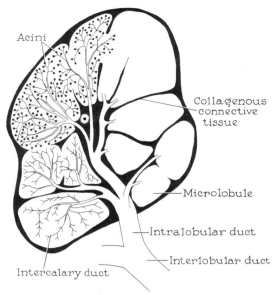

Acini

Collagenous
connective
tissue

Microlobule

Intralobular duct

Interlobular duct

Intercalary duct

Figure 4-21 Diagram showing branches of duct system and relations to secretory portion in a lobule of a compound tubuloacinar gland. Collagenous stroma separates (often incompletely) the microscopic lobules. The main duct shown is a branch of the interlobular duct. The interlobular duct branches into intralobular ducts of several orders. These are continuous with fine terminal intercalary ducts which end in the secretory portion. (Modified from Heidenhain.)

physis (secreting growth hormone, thyroid stimulating hormone, gonadotrophic hormone, and adrenocorticotrophic hormone), and the ultimobranchial cells of the thyroid (secreting calcitonin). In all of these, it is clear that the intracellular secretory pathway involves synthesis on ribosomes, segregation in the reticulum, concentration in the Golgi complex and storage in membrane limited granules. The granules are found throughout the cell instead of being concentrated at a well defined secretory pole.

The thyroid gland belongs to the category of protein secreting endocrine glands, but differs from the others in that its product, *thyroglobulin*, is stored extracellularly. The cells are arranged in a simple cuboidal epithelium bounding spherical follicles with a central cavity. The cells have an extensive endoplasmic reticulum in the form of cisternae distended with the proteinaceous precursor of the secretory product (Fig. 4-24). In the Golgi complex, this material is packaged in membrane limited secretory vesicles

that do not accumulate in the cytoplasm but pass directly to the apical surface and discharge their content into the lumen of the follicle by exocytosis.

CYTOLOGY OF STEROID SECRETING ENDOCRINE CELLS

The steroid secreting endocrine cells of the ovary, testis, and adrenal gland are all quite similar in their ultrastructure, but they are very different from protein and peptide secreting cells. They have little granular endoplasmic reticulum and relatively few free ribosomes. Their most characteristic feature is a remarkably extensive smooth surfaced or agranular endoplasmic reticulum in the form of a close meshed network of branching and anastomosing tubules (Figs. 4-25 and 4-26). The juxtanuclear Golgi complex is very large, but has no associated secretory granules. Lipid droplets are present in the cytoplasm in greater or lesser numbers depending upon the organ and the species. Mitochondria are numerous and of variable size and often have an unusual internal structure, with tubular or vesicular amplifications on the internal membrane instead of the usual lamellar or foliate cristae. These cells also contain lysosomes and peroxisomes and have a tendency to accumulate deposits of lipochrome pigment.

Steroid secreting cells store very little hormone, but they may store a considerable amount of the precursor, cholesterol. The lipid droplets, when present, contain cholesterol esters as well as triglycerides. The steroid secreting cells in some species depend mainly on cholesterol from the blood, while those of other species synthesize much of the cholesterol they utilize for hormone synthesis. The enzymes for synthesis of cholesterol reside mainly in the membranes of the smooth endoplasmic reticulum. The initial step in conversion of cholesterol to steroid hormones is cleavage of its side chain by an enzyme in the mitochondria. Several subsequent steps in steroidogenesis involve enzymes in the reticulum. In the case of the adrenal steroids, there are also additional steps in the synthesis that take place in the mitochondria. Little is known about how cholesterol and the intermediate products in steroidogenesis are moved back and forth between mitochondria and the reticulum to accomplish the successive biosynthetic steps. Since there is no appreciable storage of hormone, these cells must maintain the organelles needed to synthesize steroids on demand. The extensive development of the smooth endoplasmic reticulum thus represents a specialization to insure the presence of the enzymes necessary for rapid synthesis of steroid hormone. The observation that the lipid content of steroid secreting cells diminishes on stimulation is interpreted as a consequence of mobilization and depletion of stored precursors during enhanced hormone production. It is not yet known what role is played by the prominent Golgi complex, but the fact that it increases in size in response to trophic hormone stimulation indicates that it is involved in some way in the secretory process. No consistent morphological changes associated with the release of steroid have been reported, and nothing

can be said at present about the mechanism of release or its regulation.

STORAGE AND SECRETION OF HORMONES

Endocrine glands differ greatly in the amount of hormone stored and in the site of storage. As previously noted, the steroid secreting endocrine glands have no visible secretory granules and they store little or no hormone. They are evidently able to vary their rate of synthesis and release to keep pace with current needs. The thyroid gland, on the other hand, is unique among endocrine glands in that it stores hormone extracellularly in follicles, and ordinarily contains enough to meet normal needs for several weeks. The several endocrine glands that secrete protein, glycoprotein, or polypeptide hormones, as well as those that secrete catecholamines, store their product intracellularly in membrane limited granules in sufficient numbers to represent one to three weeks' supply. This latter category of endocrine glands with intracellular storage have been the most thoroughly studied with respect to the composition of the granules and their mechanism of release.

The neurohypophyseal hormones (*vasopressin* and *oxytocin*) are stored in the neurosecretory granules together with specific soluble proteins called *neurophysins*. These proteins seem to serve as "carriers" for the hormones in the hypothalamo-neurohypophyseal tract. The binding of the hormones to them may prevent diffusion of the biologically active molecules out of the vesicles in which they are stored. Zymogen granules, alpha cell granules of the pancreas, calcitonin containing granules, granules of various pituitary cell types, and the granules of the adrenal medulla all appear dense in electron micrographs and have similar histochemical staining reactions. The presumption is that in all of these, the hormones are bound to or at least associated with a class of proteins comparable to the neurophysins. All of these glands release their secretion by exocytosis entirely comparable to that described for the exocrine pancreas (see p. 112) but less easily observed because the quantities of material

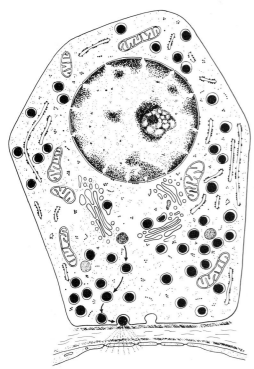

Figure 4-22 Schematic representation of the mechanism of release in endocrine cells producing protein or peptide hormones. Membranes bounding the granules coalesce with the cell membrane. The exteriorized granule disintegrates and the hormone diffuses into the blood through the fenestrated endothelium of an adjacent capillary or sinusoid.

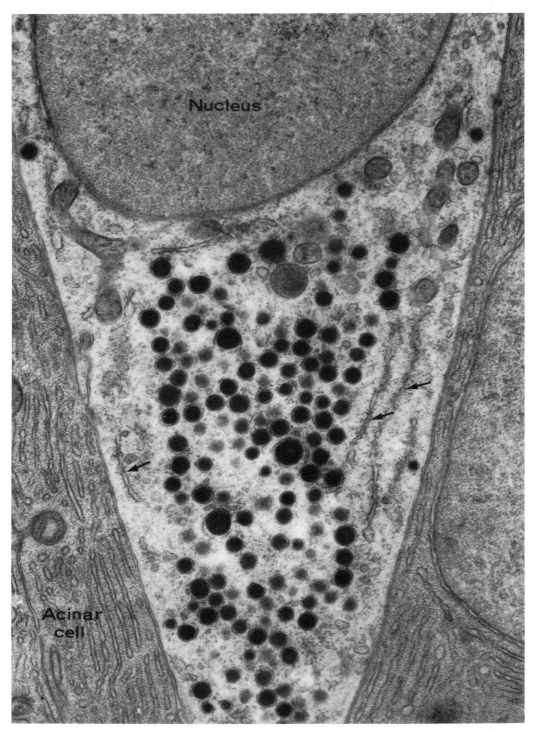

Figure 4-23 Electron micrograph of an alpha cell from pancreas, showing typical dense granules characteristic of many protein and peptide secreting endocrine glands. (From D. W. Fawcett et al., Advances in Hormone Research. Vol. 25. New York, Academic Press, 1969.)

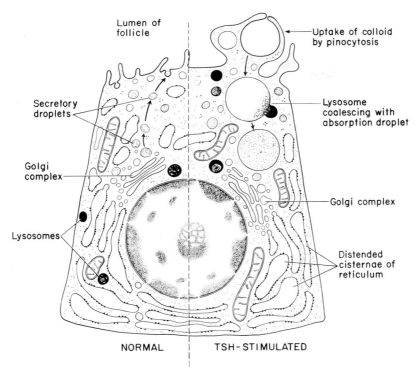

Lumen of
follicle

Uptake of colloid
by pinocytosis

Secretory
droplets

Lysosome
coalescing with
absorption droplet

Golgi
complex

Golgi complex

Lysosomes

Distended
cisternae of
reticulum

NORMAL   TSH-STIMULATED

Figure 4-24 Diagram depicting, at the left, the ultrastructure of the thyroid epithelial cell with secretory droplets of thyroglobulin being formed in the Golgi and discharged at the cell apex for extracellular storage. In the TSH-stimulated cell (at the right), droplets of colloid are taken up by pinocytosis. Lysosomes coalesce with these and their hydrolytic enzymes degrade thyroglobulin to release thyroxin, which diffuses into perifollicular capillaries. (From D. W. Fawcett et al., Advances in Hormone Research. Vol. 25. New York, Academic Press, 1969.)

released are smaller. It follows from this mode of secretion that the soluble protein and other components of the granules are discharged as well as the hormones. Their fate is poorly understood. The biologically active hormones evidently become dissociated from the other constituents extracellularly and are free to diffuse into the blood vessels.

Active hormone secretion requires a mechanism not only for release of the membrane limited granules (exocytosis) but also for transport of the granules to the cell surface. In glands, whether the cells are polarized toward the lumen of an acinus or toward a blood vessel, this transport must be selective and directional. Recent studies indicate that microtubules and possibly the microfilaments of the cytoplasm may be involved in this phase of the secretory process. The evidence for this is more pharmacological than morphological, and rests upon the demonstration that colchicine and other alkaloids

that are known to prevent the aggregation of microtubule subunits also block the release of secretory products. A relation between microtubules and the secretory process was suggested first by the observation that colchicine prevents release of insulin from the pancreatic beta cells (Lacy et al.). Similar observations have since been made for release of catecholamines from the adrenal medulla (Poisner and Bernstein) and for secretion of thyroxin by the thyroid gland (Williams and Dumont).

In the case of the thyroid, there is also evidence for the involvement of the microfilaments of the cytoplasm. The fungal metabolite *cytochalasin B* is known to cause the disappearance of microfilaments and to block a number of cellular processes involving protoplasmic movement. When this substance is added to the medium in which mouse thyroid glands are being maintained in vitro, the normal response to hormonal stimulation is blocked. Both colloid droplet uptake from the follicle

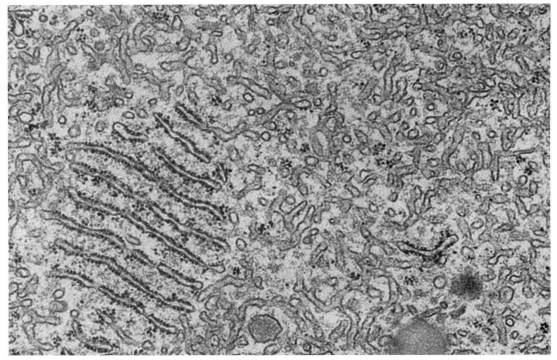

Figure 4-25 Electron micrograph of a small area of cytoplasm from a cell of the human fetal adrenal cortex. A few cisternae of granular endoplasmic reticulum are present, but most of the cytoplasm is occupied by branching tubules of the smooth endoplasmic reticulum. (Micrograph courtesy of N. S. McNutt.)

lumen and release of iodine into the medium are suppressed. The action of cytochalasin B on the secretory process suggests that microfilaments, as well as microtubules, are involved. Since uptake of colloid by macropinocytosis is an initial step in thyroxin release, it may be that the motility of the ectoplasm necessary for formation of the engulfing pseudopods is the process that requires microfilaments. A word of caution may be in order. The conclusions drawn from these observations assume that the action of colchicine and of cytochalasin is specific for microtubules and for microfilaments, respectively. The possibility that either or both may have toxic effects on other components or activities of the cell has not been ruled out.

In the case of the thyroid, which stores its product, *thyroglobulin*, extracellularly, the mechanism for release of hormone into the blood is more complex. Droplets of colloid are taken up by pinocytosis from the lumen of the follicle. Within the cell the droplets fuse with lysosomes, and the thyroglobulin is degraded by hydrolytic enzymes liberating *thyroxin*, which diffuses through the base of the cell into the perifollicular capillaries. Thus, participation of lysosomes is an integral part of the normal secretory process in this particular endocrine gland but occurs in few others (Fig. 4–24).

In a number of endocrine cells, lysosomes do play a role in disposal of unneeded stores of secretion. For example, when the young of a lactating rat are weaned, there is a large excess of secretory granules in the mammotrophic cells of the anterior pituitary. These coalesce with lysosomes and are degraded by autophagy. Endoplasmic reticulum and ribosomes no longer required for minimal rates of hormone secretion suffer a similar fate (Smith and Farquhar).

RELATION OF ENDOCRINE CELLS TO BLOOD AND LYMPH VASCULAR SYSTEMS

Despite their histological and cytological diversity, a common feature of endocrine glands is their great vascularity. Nearly every cell is in close relation to one or more thin-walled vessels of a rich vascular bed. In some glands the vessels are typical capillaries; in others, they are more appropriately described as sinusoids. The latter are generally larger than true capillaries and are more variable in shape—often conforming to the contours of the interstices they occupy among the plates or cords of epithelial cells that constitute the parenchyma of the endocrine gland. In the pituitary and adrenal glands, the endothelium of the sinusoids was formerly believed to be phagocytic to colloidal dyes, and it was traditionally included in the reticuloendothelial system This interpretation has not been substantiated in ultrastructural studies, which show that the phagocytic potential resides in perivascular cells rather than in the endothelium.

Whether the vessels of endocrine glands are true capillaries or sinusoids, the lining endothelium is extremely thin and fenestrated. The only exception is the interstitial tissue of the testis, which has unfenestrated capillaries. In all cases the diffusion distance between the secretory cells and the blood is short, and the intervening structural components to be traversed are: (1) a thin basal lamina around the endocrine cells, (2) a narrow perivascular space, (3) the basal lamina of the capillary endothelium, and (4) the thin diaphragms of the capillary pores. None of these appears to constitute a significant barrier to access of the hormones to the blood.

In addition to the microscopic structure of the vascular bed in relation to release of hormone, a consideration of the pattern of drainage of blood from an endocrine gland, at a somewhat grosser level, may be relevant to an understanding of its function. For example the hypothalamic releasing hormones are liberated into capillaries of the median eminence, which are drained via special hypophyseoportal vessels to responsive target cells immediately downstream in the anterior lobe of the pituitary (see p. 511). Similarly, the mammalian adrenal gland consists of two portions arranged concentrically—an outer *cortex* that secretes steroid hormones and an

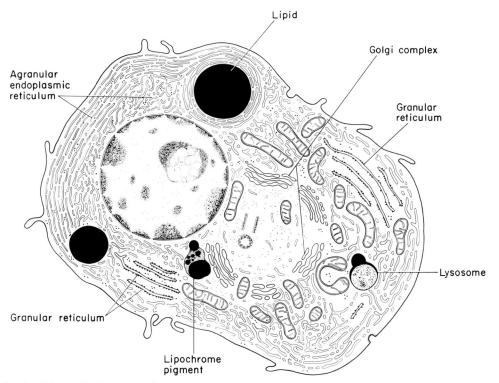

Figure 4-26 Schematic drawing of the characteristic cytological features of a steroid secreting cell. Most notable are the large Golgi complex and extensive smooth surfaced endoplasmic reticulum. (From D. W. Fawcett et al., Advances in Hormone Research. Vol. 25. New York, Academic Press, 1969.)

inner *medulla* composed of cells that synthesize the catecholamines *epinephrine* and *norepinephrine*. No capsule or sharp boundary separates the two zones, and much of the blood supply flows centripetally from the cortex, carrying steroid hormones downstream to the cells of the medulla. It now appears that a relatively high concentration of cortical steroids may be necessary for induction and maintenance of an enzyme in the medulla that is essential for epinephrine synthesis (Wurtman). Thus, the local "downstream" effects of hormones may be as important as their effects exerted at a distance via the general circulation.

In most endocrine organs the hormones are released exclusively into the blood, but recent physiological studies indicate that in a few instances the lymphatics may also be significant pathways for egress of hormones. This is particularly true of the perifollicular lymphatics of the thyroid and the intertubular lymphatics of the rodent testis.

CONTROL MECHANISMS AND INTERRELATIONS WITHIN THE ENDOCRINE SYSTEM

Endocrine glands not only modify the function of specific target organs, but also, in the course of evolution, some have developed the capacity to sense changes in the concentration of metabolites or cell products in the body fluids; others have become specifically responsive to the hormones of other endocrine glands, and still others are stimulated by neurosecretory products of the central nervous system. The activity of the brain and of the endocrine glands has become so closely integrated that changes in one are reflected in alterations in the function of the other. Based upon these interactions, a variety of control mechanisms have evolved which insure the coordinated functioning of organs situated at a distance from one another, and these mechanisms serve to maintain the constancy of the internal environment ("milieu interne") of the organism.

One of the simplest forms of control is the case in which a hormone acts upon a target organ, causing its cells to discharge a substance into the extracellular compartment or to take up a substance from it. The resulting change then acts back upon the endocrine gland to decrease its output of hormone.

This is commonly referred to as a *negative feedback mechanism*. The release of the hormone insulin from the beta cells of the pancreas drives glucose into cells and lowers blood sugar (Fig. 4–27). The lowered concentration of blood sugar, in turn, acts back upon the beta cells to diminish insulin release. Similarly parathyroid hormone acts upon bone cells to mobilize calcium, and the elevated blood calcium, by negative feedback, depresses release of parathyroid hormone.

A somewhat greater degree of complexity is encountered when the endocrine gland is under control of the nervous system. The milk ejection reflex is a good example of a simple neuroendocrine mechanism in which the train of integrated events begins with a peripheral sensory stimulus. In this case, the tactile stimulus to the nipple, evoked by suckling, is conducted over afferent neural pathways via the dorsal nerve root and spinal cord to the brain and thence to cell bodies in the hypothalamic nuclei (Fig. 4–28). Stimulation of these neurosecretory cells causes release of the hormone *oxytocin* from their terminations in the posterior lobe of the pituitary. The hormone carried in the blood back to the breast causes contraction of myoepithelial cells around the glandular acini, resulting in ejection of milk. Feedback control is not an important feature of this reflex.

The neuroendocrine response to stress is

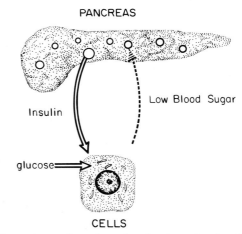

Figure 4–27 Drawing of a simple endocrine feedback mechanism. Insulin, the hormone from the islets of Langerhans in the pancreas, promotes entry of glucose into other cells of the body. The resulting low blood sugar acts back upon the alpha cells in the pancreas to reduce the release of insulin.

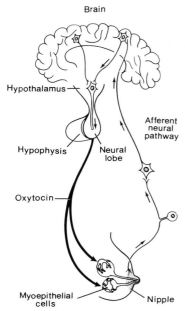

Figure 4-28 Illustration of the neuroendocrine interrelationships involved in the suckling reflex. Stimulation of the nipples generates sensory impulses that pass to the central nervous system via the dorsal root ganglia. In the brain these impulses are relayed to the hypothalamus, where they activate neurosecretory cells whose processes extend into the neural lobe of the hypophysis. Stimulation of these cells results in release of the hormone oxytocin, which is carried in the blood to the breast, where it causes contraction of myoepithelial cells around acini of the mammary gland, expelling milk. No feedback mechanism is involved.

more complex. There are more steps in the sequence of events; it involves a special vascular pathway from hypothalamus to pituitary and it is under negative feedback control. A painful stimulus reaching the hypothalamus over afferent neural pathways stimulates cell bodies whose axons end in close relation to blood vessels in the median eminence (Fig. 4–29). *Adrenocorticotropic hormone releasing factor* (ACTH-RF) is liberated at the nerve ending and carried in the blood via the hypophyseoportal system to the anterior lobe of the pituitary, where it causes specifically responsive cells to release ACTH into the general circulation. When this hormone reaches the adrenal cortex, steroid hormones, called *glucocorticoids*, are released. These reach all of the cells in the body and modify their function in various ways that increase the ability of the organism to tolerate

prolonged muscular activity, trauma, infection, or intoxications. Adrenal steroids carried back to the brain exert a "negative feedback" on the cells of the hypothalamus, diminishing their output of ACTH-RH.

The complex system of neuroendocrine interrelations that control the female reproductive cycle will be discussed in Chapter 33. The few examples cited here may provide sufficient introduction to the mode of operation of the endocrine system to enable the student to appreciate the correlations of structure and function that will appear in this and later chapters.

In the faster acting nervous system, the transmitter substances released at the nerve terminals have a very transient existence, being inactivated in a matter of seconds by

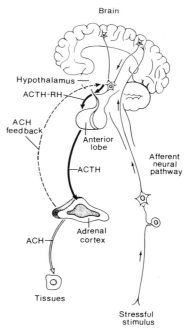

Figure 4-29 More complex neuroendocrine relationships involved in response to stress. A painful peripheral stimulus reaching the brain is relayed to neurosecretory cells in the hypothalamus. These liberate ACTH releasing hormone (ACTH-RH) into the vessels of the hypophysioportal system. Carried downstream to the anterior lobe, this hormone stimulates corticotrophs to release ACTH. The ACTH borne by the blood to the adrenal cortex causes release of corticosteroids (ACH) that are carried to cells throughout the body, inducing protective metabolic responses. Adrenal cortical hormones act back upon the hypothalamus to suppress liberation of ACTH-RH.

specific enzymes at the endings. In the slower acting endocrine integrative system, the hormones are quite variable in their half lives in the circulation, which range from a few minutes to several days. Some hormones are transported in the blood in combination with specific *carrier proteins* (especially steroid hormones and thyroxin). Inactivation or degradation of the hormone may take place at the target organ or in the liver or kidney. Some hormones enter their target cells to exert their effects, others are evidently able to act simply by binding to specific receptor sites on the cell membrane.

MECHANISMS OF HORMONE ACTION ON TARGET CELLS

The biochemical mechanisms by which hormones elicit responses in their target organs have been clarified by the pioneering work of Sutherland. In the course of studies on the effects of norepinephrine and glucagon on liver cells, he found that in binding to receptors on the cell membrane, they activate an associated enzyme called *adenyl cyclase*, which catalyzes the formation of *cyclic AMP* from ATP. Intracellular accumulation of cyclic AMP activates intracellular enzymes called *kinases* which, in turn, activate other enzymes that set in motion a train of events leading to the specific response of the target cell to the hormone.

These findings led to the formulation of the "*second messenger* concept." Briefly stated, a hormone or "first messenger" travels from its cell of origin to the cells of its target tissue, where it activates adenyl cyclase in the surface membrane. This increases the intracellular level of cyclic AMP. This compound acts as a "second messenger," carrying out the work of the hormone within the cell (Fig. 4–30).

We know now that cyclic AMP mediates the action of a great many hormones. It is involved in hormonal stimulation of steroidogenesis, release of insulin from the pancreas, release of the pituitary hormones ACTH, TSH, GH, and LH, and release of calcitonin from the thyroid, among others. It also participates in those examples of exocrine secretion that are initiated by the neurotransmitter, norepinephrine. In all of these examples, the action of the hormone can be duplicated by application of cyclic AMP.

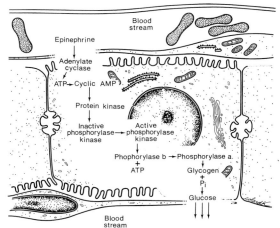

Figure 4–30 Diagram of the mechanism of action of hormones. The hormone epinephrine (first messenger) carried to the liver cell membrane in the blood activates the enzyme adenylate cyclase in the cell membrane, causing it to convert some of the ATP of the cytoplasm into cyclic AMP (second messenger). This then activates a protein kinase, which activates a second kinase. The second kinase initiates a four-step sequence that converts glycogen into glucose, which then passes out into the bloodstream in the hepatic sinusoids.

An explanation for the remarkable diversity of target cell responses to a single second messenger is still being sought, but it appears likely that all of the effects of cyclic AMP are mediated by controlling the activity of protein kinases that catalyze transfer of phosphate from ATP to protein. The diversity of the responses would therefore seem to depend not on the control system but on the specific proteins available for phosphorylation and on the varied biological activities of the resulting phosphorylated proteins.

REFERENCES

Bowen, R. H.: The cytology of glandular secretion. Quart. Rev. Biol., 4:299,484, 1929.

Fawcett, D. W., J. A. Long, and A. L. Jones: The ultrastructure of endocrine glands. Recent Prog. Hormone Res., 25:315, 1969.

Florey, H. W.: The secretion and function of intestinal mucus. Gastroenterology, 43:326, 1962.

Jennings, M. A., and H. W. Florey: Autoradiographic observations on the mucous cells of the stomach and intestine. Quart. J. Exper. Physiol., 41:131, 1956.

Lacey, P. E., S. L. Howell, D. A. Fink, and C. J. Fink: New hypothesis of insulin secretion. Nature (London), 219:1177, 1968.

Liddle, G. W., and J. G. Hardman: Cyclic adenosine monophosphate as a mediator of hormone action. New Eng. J. Med., *285*:560, 1971.

Nassonov, D.: Das Golgische Binnennetz und seine Beziehungun zu der Sekretion. Morphologische und experimentelle Untersuchungen an einigen Saugtierdrüsen. Arch. f. mikr. Anat., *100*:433, 1924.

Neutra, M., and C. P. Leblond: Synthesis of the carbohydrate of mucus in the Golgi complex as shown by electron microscope radioautography of goblet cells from rats injected with glucose-³H. J. Cell Biol., *30*:119–136, 1966.

Palade, G. E.: Functional changes in the structure of cell components. *In* Hayashi, T., ed.: Subcellular Particles. New York, Ronald Press, 1959.

Palade, G. E., P. Siekevitz, and L. G. Caro: Structure, chemistry and function of the pancreatic exocrine cell. *In* de Reuck, A. V. S., and M. P. Cameron, eds: The Exocrine Pancreas. Boston, Little, Brown & Co., 1962.

Palay, S. L.: The morphology of secretion. *In* Frontiers in Cytology. New Haven, Yale University Press, 1958.

Peterson, M., and C. P. Leblond: Synthesis of complex carbohydrates in the Golgi region as shown by radioautography after injection of labeled glucose. J. Cell Biol., *21*:143, 1964.

Poisner, A. M., and J. Bernstein: A possible role of microtubules in catecholamine release from the adrenal medulla: Effect of colchicine, vinca alkaloids, and deuterium oxide. J. Pharmacol. Exp. Therap., *177*:102, 1971.

Rasmussen, H.: Cell communication, calcium ion and cyclic adenosine monophosphate. Science, *170*:404, 1970.

Scharrer, E.: Principles of neuroendocrine integration. *In* Endocrines and the Central Nervous System. Baltimore, Williams and Wilkins Co., 1966.

Scharrer, E., and B. Scharrer: Neurosekretion. *In* von Möllendorff, W., and W. Bargmann, eds.: Handbuch der mikroskopischen Anatomie des Menschen. Vol. 6, part 5. Berlin, Springer-Verlag, 1954.

Smith, A. D.: Storage and secretion of hormones. Scientific Basis of Medicine Annual Reviews, pp. 74–102, 1972.

Sutherland, E. W.: On the biological role of cyclic AMP. J.A.M.A., *214*:1281, 1970.

Trier, J. S.: Studies on small intestinal crypt epithelium. I. The fine structure of the crypt epithelium of the proximal small intestine of fasting humans. J. Cell Biol., *18*:599, 1963.

Turner, C. D. and J. T. Bagnara: General Endocrinology. 5th ed. Philadelphia, W. B. Saunders Co., 1971.

Warshawsky, H., C. P. Leblond, and B. Droz: Synthesis and migration of proteins in the cells of the exocrine pancreas as revealed by specific activity determination from radioautographs. J. Cell Biol., *16*:213, 1963.

Williams, J. A., and J. Wolff: Cytochalasin B inhibits thyroid secretion. Biochem. Biophys. Res. Comm., *44*:422, 1971.

Ziegel, R. F., and A. J. Dalton: Speculations based on the morphology of the Golgi systems in several types of protein-secreting cells. J. Cell Biol., *15*:45, 1962.

5

Blood

The embryonic mesenchyme gives rise to the blood, blood vessels, and various types of connective tissue. The mesenchymal cells are at first irregularly stellate and connected by long slender processes. The wide spaces between their cell bodies are occupied by a soft jelly-like intercellular material. In the earliest stages of development, the endothelial cells of the blood vessels and the blood cells arise simultaneously from the same mesenchymal elements in the so-called blood islands of the yolk sac. The mesenchymal cells differentiate along several lines to give rise to the various cell types of the blood and the connective tissues. The embryonic endothelium for a time also seems to be able to give rise to blood cells but soon becomes more differentiated and independent so that in later stages new vessels originate only by sprouting from preexisting ones. The vessels gradually become confluent to form a continuous circulatory system throughout the embryo. The blood vessels are always accompanied by primitive connective tissue, and some of the cells of this tissue, even in the adult, appear to retain some of the developmental potentialities of mesenchymal cells.

The fibroblasts and other sessile derivatives of mesenchymal cells produce various amorphous and fibrous components of the extracellular matrix in which they reside. All of the connective tissues of the body are composed of cells and varying amounts of intercellular substance. In cartilage, the intercellular substance is a firm gel; in bone it is a highly organized scaffolding of fibers impregnated with calcium salts. Blood has traditionally been classified as a form of connective tissue in which the intercellular substance is fluid. This tissue is obviously not "connective" in the sense of contributing to the structural integrity of the organism, but only in the sense that it maintains communication between the deep lying tissues of the body and atmospheric oxygen in the lungs—a connection that is essential for the continued viability of all of the cells of higher organisms. It also provides for distribution of hormones, those chemical signals produced in one part of the body but influencing the activities of cells at a distance. Thus, blood is essential to the integrative functions of the endocrine system.

The various connective tissues of the body cannot always be sharply separated from one another. The fibers of connective tissue proper extend without interruption into the matrix of cartilage or bone. Similarly, blood cannot be clearly separated from the loose connective tissue through which the blood vessels course, for fluid constituents of the blood are constantly passing through the capillary walls to mingle with the fluid phase of the connective tissue matrix, and at the same time, solutes and metabolites in the tissue fluid are passing in the opposite direction to enter the blood. This continual irrigation with blood and exchange of substances between blood plasma and tissue fluid is of course essential to the survival of nearly all of the tissues and organs of the body.

Similarly, many types of blood cells cannot be separated from those of connective tissue proper. Only the red blood cells and platelets function entirely within the confines of the blood-vascular system. Since methods have become available for tagging cells and following their migrations, it has become evident that the white blood cells are only transients in the blood and that they are constantly migrating through the walls of capillaries and venules to take up residence in the connective tissue. Some may reenter the blood, but most complete their life span and die in the tissues. Thus, the blood simply provides the vehicle by which certain cells, formed in the bone marrow, are disseminated and reach the sites in other tissues and organs where they carry out their appointed tasks.

FORMED ELEMENTS OF THE BLOOD

The blood is a red liquid that circulates in a closed system of blood vessels. In man its volume is about 5 liters, accounting for about 7 per cent of the body weight. The *plasma*, the liquid vehicle of the blood, is a transparent yellow fluid, but it may acquire a milky opalescence after a meal, owing to the suspension in it of minute droplets of absorbed lipid. A clear view of the plasma can only be obtained by centrifuging the blood to sediment the cellular elements normally suspended in it. The cells are of several kinds — erythrocytes (red blood corpuscles), leukocytes (white blood corpuscles), and platelets.

A knowledge of the normal histology of the blood is of great importance to medical and veterinary students, for no tissue is examined more often for diagnostic purposes. Study of stained blood smears not only gives information about a number of diseases that primarily affect the blood and blood forming organs (anemias, leukemias, etc.), but also provides clues to the presence of chemical intoxications (benzene and other solvents) and a variety of viral, bacterial, and parasitic infections (mononucleosis, septicemia, malaria, etc.). Periodic examination of the blood enables the physician to assess the severity of the disease, to follow its course, and to evaluate the effectiveness of his treatment.

ERYTHROCYTES

The minute corpuscles that impart the red color to the blood are called *erythrocytes* or *red blood cells*. Neither term is descriptively accurate, for in mammals they are not true cells — they lack a nucleus, mitochondria and other organelles that are the defining characteristics of cells. The term "erythroplastid" would be more appropriate, but by long usage "erythrocyte" is considered correct. These elements develop in the bone marrow as true cells but extrude their nucleus and lose all capacity for DNA-directed protein synthesis as they become specialized for their primary function — the uptake of oxygen in the lungs, its transport to the tissues, and the return of carbon dioxide to the lungs for exhalation. In fishes, amphibia, reptiles, and birds the erythrocytes retain a nucleus, but it seems to be metabolically inert.

A normal adult has about 35 ml. of erythrocytes per kilogram body weight. The red blood cell count, a measure of their concentration in the blood, is about 5.4 million per cubic millimeter in men and 4.8 million in women. These figures are increased somewhat by residence at high altitudes.

The mammalian erythrocyte has an unusual and highly characteristic shape (Figs. 5–1B, and 5–2). It is a biconcave disc about 7.5 μm. in diameter and 1.9 μm. in thickness at its periphery, and has a surface area of about 140 square micrometers. In the fresh condition it has a faint yellow or tan color due to its content of *hemoglobin*, the respiratory pigment which makes up about 33 per cent of its mass. The biconcave form of the erythrocyte is a shape well adapted to its function. In this form it presents to the plasma a surface 20 to 30 per cent greater in relation to its volume than it would if it were a sphere. This increased surface favors the immediate saturation of its hemoglobin with oxygen as the erythrocyte passes through the pulmonary capillaries. The total surface area of the erythrocytes in an average man is about 3800 square meters or some 2000 times the man's total body surface. These figures indicate that the enormous surface area presented by these cells results in great efficiency in their oxygen and carbon dioxide transport.

Despite the great uniformity in size and shape of erythrocytes as seen in fresh smears, they are in fact extremely soft and elastic and may change their shape to a bell-like or paraboloid form when flowing through capillaries. Their deformation is dependent upon the velocity of flow and seems to be a consequence of hydrodynamic force and viscous drag. It is conceivable, however, that this shape may have some functional significance in gas exchange, since the surface area is further increased in this configuration.

When thick smears of fresh blood are examined under the microscope, the erythrocytes are often observed to associate in stacks called *rouleaux* (Fig. 5–1A). This phenomenon does not occur when blood is circulating but only when it is still or stagnant. It is often considered a surface tension effect but its physical basis is, in fact, poorly understood.

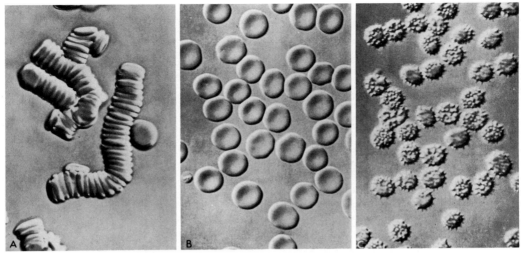

Figure 5–1 Photomicrographs of fresh blood viewed by Nomarski optics. A, In vitro erythrocytes often aggregate like stacked coins. This phenomenon is called rouleau formation. B, Erythrocytes are normally biconcave discs with an obvious central depression and a thicker rim. C, In hypertonic solution, erythrocytes assume a spiny configuration. This change is called crenation, and the crenated cells are sometimes called acanthocytes. (Photomicrographs courtesy of Dr. Marcel Bessis.)

How the biconcave shape of the erythrocyte is maintained is a question still largely unanswered. The membrane is so flexible and deformable that it would seem to have little to contribute to the maintenance of the normal shape. An internal supporting *stroma* has been postulated, and a nonrespiratory protein isolated from packed red cells has been called *stromatin* on the assumption that it subserves a supporting or cytoskeletal function. However, in electron micrographs of thin sections no corresponding internal structural component can be identified.

The shape of the erythrocytes is susceptible to osmotic forces. In hypotonic solution they first swell, becoming spherical, and the membrane stretches so that it becomes leaky or ruptures, allowing hemoglobin to escape and leaving behind an empty membrane, called an *erythrocyte ghost*. This disruptive series of changes is called *hemolysis*. In hypertonic solutions the erythrocytes shrink and take on a curious cockleburr shape (Figs. 5–1C and 5–3). This change is called *crenation*. There is some indication that the biconcave shape depends in part upon a factor present in the plasma called *antisphering substance*, for in the absence of this factor, crenation can occur in isotonic solution and can be reversed by its addition.

The essential biochemical component of the erythrocyte is hemoglobin, a conjugated protein with a molecular weight of about 65,000. It consists of four polypeptide chains, to each of which is bound an iron-containing heme group. Humans are genetically capable of synthesizing and incorporating into hemoglobin four different polypeptide chains designated alpha (α), beta (β), gamma (γ), and delta (δ). Normal human adult hemoglobin, called hemoglobin A (HbA) contains two alpha and two beta chains. This form accounts for 96 per cent of the hemoglobin present, while 2 per cent is of a second type (HbA$_2$), consisting of two alpha and two delta chains, and less than 2 per cent is fetal hemoglobin (HbF) composed of two alpha and two gamma chains. During fetal life HbF greatly predominates over the others but diminishes in amount in the postnatal period. Certain types of anemia (thalassemia) are associated with persistence of abnormally high levels of fetal hemoglobin.

A separate genetic locus determines the structure of each of the four globin chains, and a variety of inherited disorders of hemoglobin synthesis have been discovered which involve relatively minor amino acid substitutions in the beta chain but nevertheless have profound physiological effects. These examples of disease involving defects at the molecular level are now of great interest. A classical example is hemoglobin S (HbS) associated with *sickle cell anemia.* It differs from normal only in the substitution of valine for glutamine at one site on the beta chain, but this substitution is enough to make it less soluble than normal in the reduced condition and results in formation of long tactoids that deform the red cells into bizarre sickle forms, which block capillaries and are prone to hemolysis.

Normally, the erythrocytes in a dry smear of peripheral blood stain deep pink or salmon color with Wright's stain (Fig. 5–6). Some of the young red cells which have lost their nucleus shortly before entering the circulation but are not yet completely mature, may have a bluish or greenish tinge due to the basophilic staining of small numbers of residual ribosomes. These are called *polychromatophilic erythrocytes* or *reticulocytes.* The latter term refers to the fact that when blood smears are stained with brilliant cresyl blue the remaining ribonucleoprotein is precipitated by the dye into a delicate basophilic network in the otherwise acidophilic hemoglobin-rich cy-

toplasm. Within about 24 hours after entering the blood from the bone marrow, the reticulocytes mature into adult erythrocytes. Reticulocyte number in adult man averages about 0.8 per cent of the total erythrocytes of blood. The *reticulocyte count* is used clinically as a rough index of the rate of erythrocyte formation. In patients with anemia, elevation of the count is a valuable sign of response to treatment.

A detailed description of abnormal forms of erythrocytes is more appropriate for textbooks of hematology or pathology, but a few of the descriptive terms may be useful here. Abnormal variation in size of red cells is described as *anisocytosis.* Red cells that are larger than normal are *macrocytes,* and an anemia characterized by such cells is a *macrocytic anemia.* Conversely, where the cells are smaller than normal, the condition is termed a *microcytic anemia.* Deviation from the normal shape is described by the term *poikilocytosis.* The concentration of hemoglobin per cell is less than normal when the rate of red cell formation is relatively greater than the rate of hemoglobin synthesis. Under these circumstances each erythrocyte contains an abnormally small quantity of hemoglobin. It appears paler and is described as *hypochromic,* compared to normal or *normochromic* erythrocytes.

BLOOD PLATELETS

The *platelets* are small, colorless, anucleate corpuscles found in the circulating blood of all mammals. They are round or oval biconvex discs. Seen edge on, they present a fusiform profile (Figs. 5–2 and 5–5*A*). They are 2 to 3 μm. in diameter and they number 250,000 to 300,000 per cu. mm. of blood. It is difficult to number them accurately, for as soon as blood is removed from the circulation, the platelets adhere to one another and to all surfaces with which they come into contact. In a fresh drop of blood spread on a glass slide, the platelets at once aggregate into small and large clusters adhering to the slide. They are the lightest elements of the blood and therefore, when blood is centrifuged, they form the uppermost layer of the so-called buffy coat. They can be preserved for observation by rendering the blood incoagulable through the addition of sodium citrate or heparin.

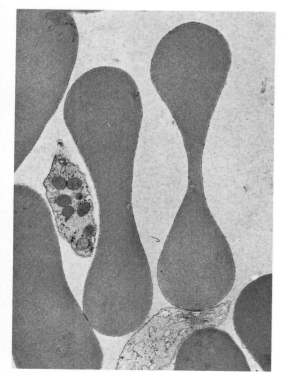

Figure 5–2 Electron micrograph of mature erythrocytes in thin section, showing their biconcave shape and absence of organelles.

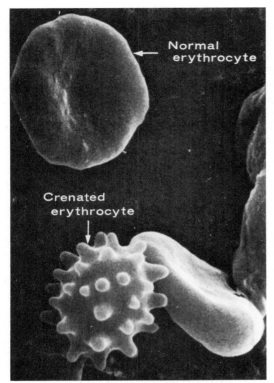

Figure 5–3 Scanning electron micrograph of two normally shaped biconcave erythrocytes and one crenated erythrocyte. (Micrograph courtesy of Dr. Marcel Bessis.)

In dried smears stained with Wright's or some other Romanowsky mixture, and viewed with the light microscope, each platelet is a flattened disc consisting of two concentric zones. The thicker central region is highly refractile and contains small purple-staining granules. This area is called the *granulomere* or *chromomere.* The thin peripheral zone, called the *hyalomere,* is a homogeneous pale blue.

In electron micrographs, the zonation of the platelets is also obvious. The granulomere contains membrane bounded granules that are spherical, about 0.2 μm. in diameter, and have a moderately dense content (Figs. 5–4 and 5–5). Their chemical nature has not been established. These are called *alpha granules* to distinguish them from a second category of very dense granules which are present in some species and are believed to contain serotonin (5-hydroxytryptamine). In addition to the granules, an occasional mitochondrion and variable amounts of glycogen

are observed. The hyalomere is free of granules but at high magnification often exhibits fine filaments. In addition, there is a circumferential bundle of 10 to 15 microtubules which is believed to help maintain the flattened discoid shape of the platelets.

The blood of reptiles, birds, amphibians, and lower vertebrates does not contain platelets but has nucleated cells called *thrombocytes,* which seem to play a similar role in blood clotting.

Blood Clotting

The principal function of platelets is to patch small defects in the endothelial lining of blood vessels and to limit hemorrhage by promoting the coagulation of the blood. Under normal conditions, blood remains a circulating population of free cells and corpuscles suspended in plasma. In a variety of pathological circumstances, the blood clots to a semisolid gel. Local damage to the endothelium results in adherence of platelets and their progressive aggregation to cover the discontinuity in the endothelium with a *platelet thrombus.* Concurrently with platelet aggregation, other complex reactions of blood clotting are set into motion. A substance called *thromboplastin* released from the injured area of the vessel wall initiates a series of reactions in blood plasma that convert *prothrombin* to *thrombin.* Thrombin acts as an enzyme catalyzing the conversion of plasma *fibrinogen* to *fibrin* which polymerizes as a feltwork of cross-striated fibrils that enmesh blood cells and platelets to form a clot. Activation of the enmeshed platelets causes them to extend pseudopodia, release the contents of their granules, and coalesce into a coherent viscous mass. Associated with their degranulation, a phospholipid is released which reacts with other plasma components to produce *platelet thromboplastin.* This in turn acts to promote progression of the clotting process initiated by tissue thromboplastin.

In the process of clotting, the aggregated platelets rapidly change from disc-shaped elements to highly irregular structures with thin, radiating pseudopodia. Concurrently with these changes in shape, filaments appear in abundance in their cytoplasm, and the platelets take on some of the properties of contractile cells. An actomyosin-like complex (*thrombosthenin*) has been reported to constitute 15 per cent of total platelet protein. It has recently been possible to isolate the contractile material of platelets and to identify, in electron micrographs, actin filaments that form "arrow head complexes" with heavy meromyosin prepared from skeletal muscle (Behnke; Pollard). Myosin has also been extracted from human platelets (Pollard et al.). Under appropriate conditions, thick filaments or rods form, which apparently are identical to those formed in extracts of myosin prepared from skeletal muscle. Thus, filaments present in platelets seem to be the counterparts of the thick (myosin) and thin (actin) filaments of muscle (see Chapter 11). It is now believed that the mechanism of platelet contraction has a number of features in common with that of skeletal muscle. In the circulating platelets, the contractile material is present mainly in monomeric form, but platelet activation seems to initiate the polymerization of actin and myosin monomers into their filamentous form. Activation of this mechanism is thought to be the basis of clot retraction.

The clotting process is essential for limitation of hemorrhage but it can also be life-threatening when it is initiated on the walls of diseased coronary arteries—causing *coronary thrombosis.* Similarly, when clots that have formed in injured veins of the extremities break loose, they may be carried to the lungs, resulting in fatal *pulmonary embolism.*

LEUKOCYTES

In addition to the red cells, the blood of all mammals contains a number of types of colorless cells, the *leukocytes* or *white blood corpuscles.* They are true cells with a nucleus and cytoplasm and all are spherical in the blood but more or less ameboid in the tissues or on a solid substrate. There are five kinds of leukocytes in the blood (Fig. 5–6). They are categorized according to the presence or absence of specific cytoplasmic granules (*granular* and *nongranular*) and according to the shape of their nucleus (*mononuclear* or *polymorphonuclear*). The granular leukocytes are further classified according to the staining affinities of their granules (neutrophils, eosinophils, basophils).

The number of circulating leukocytes is normally in the range of 5000 to 9000 per cu. mm. of blood. The number is subject to some variation with age and even at different times of the day. Thus, minor variations are of little clinical significance, but in the presence of acute infections (appendicitis, pneumonia, etc.) the *white blood count* may rise to 20,000 or even 40,000 per cu. mm.

The relative proportions of the various types of leukocytes is normally fairly constant: neutrophils, 55 to 60 per cent; eosinophils, 1 to 3 per cent; basophils, 0 to 0.7 per cent; lymphocytes, 25 to 33 per cent; mono-

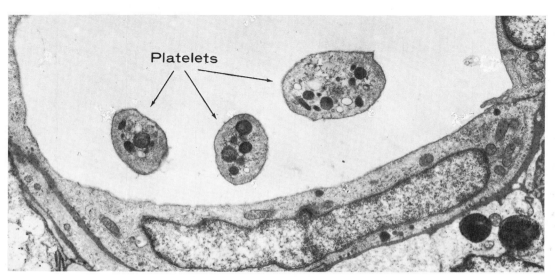

Figure 5–4   Electron micrograph of circulating platelets in the lumen of a capillary.

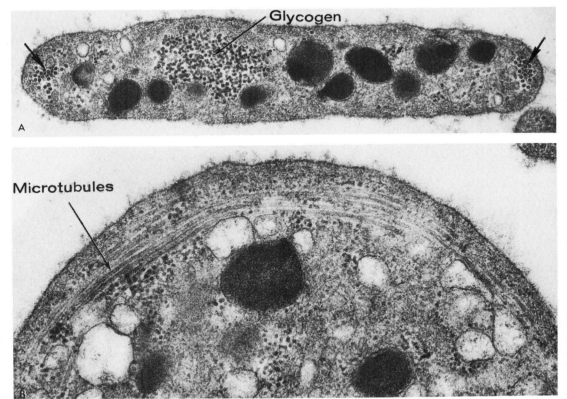

Glycogen

Microtubules

Figure 5–5   A, Electron micrograph of a platelet transected along its narrow surface. The membrane limited dense granules and an aggregation of glycogen particles are shown. At the arrows are seen cross sections of the bundle of microtubules that runs circumferentially around the platelet. ×39,000. B, Platelet sectioned parallel to its flat surface. Here one sees in longitudinal sections the bundles of peripheral microtubules that help to maintain the flattened discoid shape of the platelet. ×57,000. (Micrographs courtesy of Dr. O. Behnke.)

cytes, 3 to 7 per cent. Because different disease processes may affect the numbers of one cell type more than others, the *differential leukocyte count* is diagnostically valuable.

Neutrophilic Leukocytes (Neutrophils)

Neutrophils (*heterophils*) are the most abundant of the leukocytes, constituting 55 to 65 per cent of the total count. In absolute numbers, there are 3000 to 6000 per cu. mm. or 20 to 30 billion in the circulation at any one time. They are 10 to 12 μm. in diameter in dry smears and are easily recognized by their highly characteristic nucleus consisting of two or more lobules connected by narrow strands (Fig. 5–6*A*). The number of nuclear lobes depends in part upon the age of the cell. When these cells are first released into the blood, the nucleus has a simple elongate shape. Such cells are often described as "*band forms*." A constriction subsequently develops, resulting in a bilobed nucleus, and the process of elongation and constriction continues with time until, in older neutrophils, there may be five or more segments or lobes. The proportion of band forms or young cells in the differential count is a useful index of the rate of entry of new neutrophils into the circulation. The variability of nuclear shape is the basis for the other name applied to this cell type— *polymorphonuclear leukocyte*. In clinical parlance this is often abbreviated so that neutrophils are also referred to as "polys."

The nuclear chromatin occurs in deeply staining clumps, and a nucleolus cannot be identified. Since these cells are fully differentiated, with no synthetic capacity, they no longer need a nucleolus as a center of ribosomal assembly. In a small proportion of the

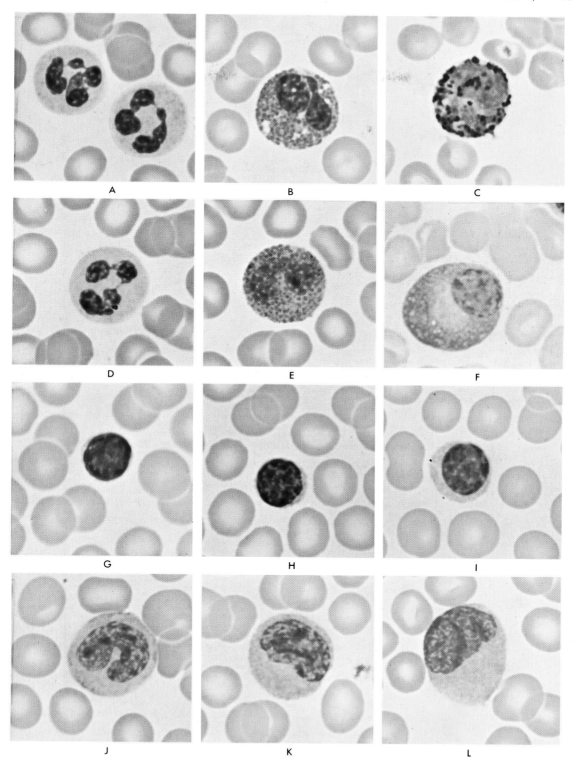

Figure 5--6 Human blood cells from a dry smear stained with Wright's stain. *A* and *D*, Neutrophilic leukocytes. *B* and *E*, Eosinophilic leukocytes. *C*, Basophilic leukocyte. *F*, Plasma cell. This is not a normal constituent of the peripheral blood but is included here for comparison with the mononuclear leukocytes. *G*
and *H*, Small lymphocytes. *I*, Medium lymphocyte. *J*, *K*, and *L*, Monocytes.

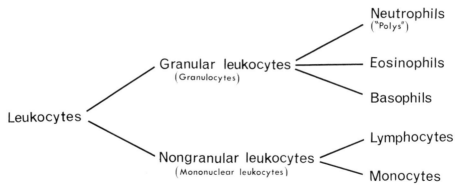

Figure 5-7 Classification of leukocytes. The granular leukocytes, especially the neutrophils, are polymorphonuclear. The term mononuclear leukocytes, widely used for the nongranular leukocytes, is unfortunate in that it implies that other leukocytes may be "polynuclear." The point of contrast is shape, not number of nuclei. Monomorphonuclear would more accurately express the principal morphological distinction between the nongranular leukocytes and the polymorphonuclear granulocytes.

neutrophils of women, the chromatin representing the condensed X chromosomes forms a minute separate lobule—often described as the *"drumstick"* because of its characteristic shape (see Fig. 5-8). Thus, it is possible to determine the genetic sex of the individual by examining, in a blood smear, a large number of neutrophils for the presence of this nuclear appendage.

The cytoplasm of the neutrophil, when properly stained, is stippled with very small granules that have little affinity for the dyes. These are the so-called *specific granules* (Fig. 5-9III). In addition to these there are a few larger, reddish-purple *azurophil granules*. The granules are often quite inconspicuous in routinely stained smears and they are therefore studied to better advantage in living leukocytes viewed by phase contrast microscopy or in electron micrographs of thin sections of the buffy coat from centrifuged blood.

In other mammals, such as the guinea pig and rabbit, the heterophil granules are more conspicuous than in man and are stainable with either acid or basic dyes but show a predilection for eosin (Fig. 5-10). Therefore, in these species they are sometimes called *pseudoeosinophils.*

In electron micrographs the neutrophil granules of man may be found almost anywhere in the cell, but they tend to be absent from a thin peripheral zone of cytoplasm which is rich in fine filaments that seem to be concerned with cell motility (Fig. 5-11). Centrally situated in the cell and more-or-less surrounded by the nucleus is a small Golgi complex and an associated pair of centrioles. The specific granules are round in cross section or elongate like rice grains. In some species the azurophil granules are more spherical and distinctly larger, but in man it is difficult to distinguish the granule types on morphological criteria alone. However, the enzyme myeloperoxidase is localized exclusively in the azurophil granules (Fig. 5-12), and this can be used as a cytochemical marker to identify this granule type (Bainton et al.). In addition to peroxidase, the azurophil granules contain acid phosphatase (Fig. 5-12), and β-glucuronidase and hence are regarded as modified primary lysosomes. The specific granules, which greatly outnumber the azurophils, lack lysosomal enzymes but contain alkaline phosphatase and a variety of poorly characterized basic proteins, called *phagocytins*, which have significant antibacterial activity.

The neutrophils are avidly *phagocytic*, that is, they have the capacity to extend pseudopodia around bacteria and other particulate matter and to take them into the cell in membrane limited vacuoles (Fig. 5-18). Azurophil granules may then coalesce with the vacuoles, discharging into them hydrolytic enzymes that digest their contents (Fig. 5-19). How the specific granules exert their antibacterial effect is less well understood. The neutrophils are clearly a part of the first line of defense of the body against bacterial invasion. At sites of inflammation they adhere to the walls of capillaries and venules, and their ameboid motility enables them to insinuate themselves between the endothelial cells and migrate into the connective tissues to phagocytize and destroy bacteria. In the presence of bacterial infection, some message is transmitted to the bone marrow that stimulates increased production and release of neutrophils. Under these conditions, the number of circulating neutrophils increases and the percentage of young band forms is elevated. The *pus* that accumulates in boils or abscesses consists of millions of dead and dying neutrophil leukocytes. The normal life span of these cells is about eight days, but a major part of this is spent in reserve in the bone marrow.

Eosinophilic Leukocytes (Eosinophils)

Eosinophils constitute 1 to 3 per cent of the leukocyte population of the peripheral blood. They are about the same size as neutrophils—9 μm. in fresh blood and about 12 μm. in diameter when flattened in dried smears. They are easily recognized by their relatively coarse specific granules that stain pink with Wright's blood stain (Figs. 5–6*E* and 5–9*II*).

The nucleus usually has two lobes connected by a narrow isthmus. The chromatin network is fairly dense and no nucleoli are present. In the rat and mouse, the nucleus is not bilobed but is a thick irregular ring. There is a small granule-free cytocentrum with its associated diplosome, and a small Golgi apparatus.

The most conspicuous feature of these cells is their eosinophilic granules. In micrographs of these cells from laboratory rodents, each granule has a single discoid crystal in an equatorial position (Fig. 5–13). In man the crystals within each granule may be single or multiple and are quite variable in form. In the cat the eosiniphil crystals are cylindrical and have a distinctive concentric lamellar substructure. In all species, the crystals are embedded in an amorphous or finely granular matrix of relatively low density and the granule as a whole is enclosed by a membrane. When isolated and analyzed, eosinophil granules are found to contain the common lysosomal enzymes that are present in the azurophil granules of neutrophils but

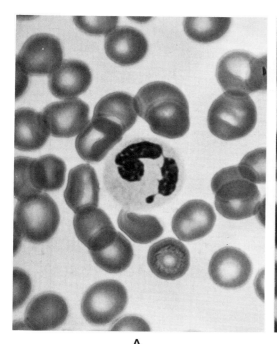
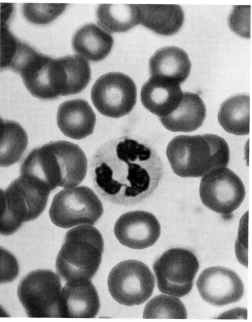

A **B**

Figure 5–8 Erythrocytes and neutrophilic leukocytes from a normal female (*A*) and a normal male (*B*). The female leukocyte shows the "drumstick" appendix of the nucleus that was discovered by Davidson and Smith. From dry smears of human blood. Giemsa stain. ×1800. (Courtesy of Murray Barr.)

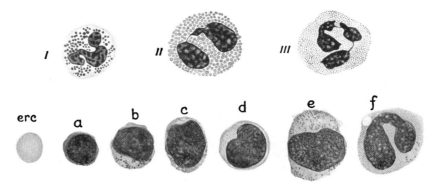

Figure 5–9 *I,* Basophilic leukocyte; *II,* eosinophilic leukocyte; *III,* neutrophilic (heterophilic) leukocyte; *erc,* erythrocyte; *a, b, c,* and *d,* lymphocytes; *e* and *f,* monocytes. From Romanowsky-stained dry smears of human blood, except *I,* which is stained with thionine. (After A. A. Maximow.)

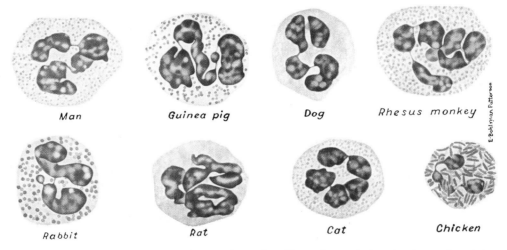

Figure 5–10 Heterophilic leukocytes of several species. Note the variation in size and staining of the granules in those species in which they are present. Wright's stain. (Courtesy of M. Bloch.)

they have a higher concentration of peroxidase. They seem to lack *lysozyme* and the antibacterial protein phagocytin found in neutrophil leukocytes.

Eosinophils are not normally phagocytic for bacteria or foreign red cells, but they will ingest these in the presence of antibacterial or antierythrocyte antibody. They appear to take part in the body's response to foreign protein but their precise role has not yet been defined. There is a marked increase in the numbers of circulating eosinophils in many types of allergic and hypersensitivity states in humans. Repeated injection of any foreign serum or induction of allergic or anaphylactic reactions in experimental animals is attended by local and general increases in eosinophils. Under these conditions, eosinophils are mobilized from large reserves of

these cells in the bone marrow. There are said to be 200 to 300 eosinophils in the marrow for every one in the blood. Therefore, mature or nearly mature eosinophils can be supplied without delay in response to unusual functional demands. While their exact function in the immunological response is still unknown, it is speculated that they may selectively phagocytize and destroy antigen-antibody complexes.

The factors regulating release of eosinophils from the bone marrow are still poorly understood. There is, however, considerable evidence that some eosinotactic substance is formed at sites of antigen-antibody reaction and attendant inflammation in the tissues and that this acts back upon the marrow to cause discharge of eosinophils into the circulation. From the circulation, they emigrate to the tissues. It has long been known that either adrenocorticotropic hormone or hydrocortisone injections cause a fall in the level of circulating eosinophils. These hormones appear to exert this effect by interfering in some way with the mobilization of eosinophil reserves from the marrow.

Basophilic Leukocytes (Basophils)

Basophils are difficult to find in human blood because they make up only about 0.5 per cent of the total number of leukoctyes. Their size is about the same as that of the neutrophilic leukocytes. In a dry smear they measure 10 μm. in diameter. The nucleus is elongated, often bent in the form of a U or an S, and has two or more constrictions (Figs. 5–6 and 5–9I). The chromatin network is looser and paler than in the eosinophilic leukocytes and nucleoli are usually not seen. The granules in the cytoplasm of the living cells have a low refractive index. Their substance, in man, is soluble in water; therefore,

in preparations stained with the usual watery dye solutions, the granules are partly dissolved and distorted. In dry smears or in sections of alcohol fixed material, the cytoplasm contains round granules of different sizes, which stain a metachromatic purple with alcoholic thionine or toluidine blue. Supravital application of neutral red stains the granules a dark red color.

The solubility of the basophilic granules has created confusion, but the use of suitable methods leaves no doubt as to their specific nature. In the guinea pig, the granules are large, oval, and insoluble in water, and they stain but faintly. In the dog, the granules are small and are assembled in a compact group. In the cat, rat, and mouse, the basophilic leukocytes seem to be normally absent from the blood. In the lower vertebrates the variations are still greater.

In electron micrographs, each coarse granule is limited by a membrane and has an internal fine structural pattern that varies from species to species (Fig. 5–14). In the

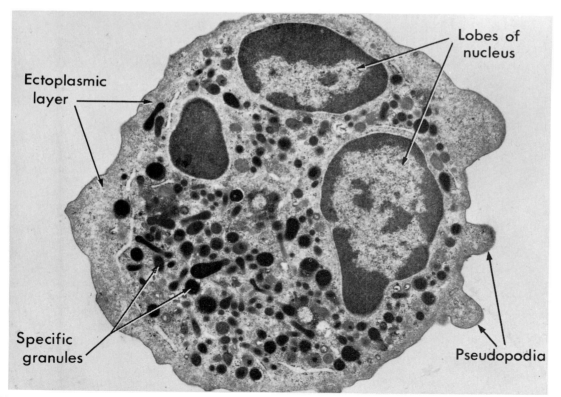

Figure 5–11 Electron micrograph of a heterophilic leukocyte of a guinea pig. The nucleus has several lobes and the cytoplasm is filled with specific granules of varying shape. A thin ectoplasmic layer of cytoplasm that is devoid of granules forms pseudopodia and is probably important in the ameboid locomotion of this cell type. ×12,000.

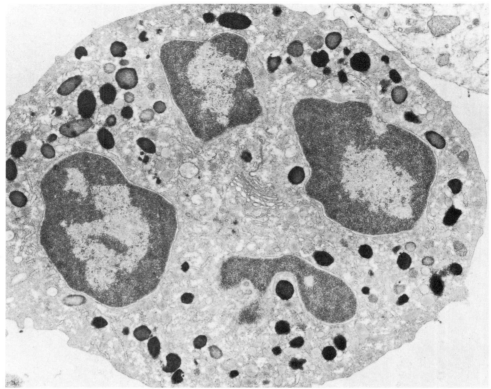

Figure 5-12 Mature neutrophil leukocyte stained by the cytochemical reaction for peroxidase. Clearly, only a fraction of the total complement of granules is positive. Only the persisting azurophil granules can be considered primary lysosomes. (From D. Bainton, J. Ullyot, and M. Farquhar, J. Exp. Med., *134*:907, 1971.)

guinea pig, the granules have a crystalline internal structure; in man, they appear to consist of closely compacted dense granules of uniform size (Fig. 5–15).

The blood basophil resembles in many ways the connective tissue mast cell. Both contain metachromatic granules but those of the basophil are fewer. The basophil is smaller and its nucleus is more polymorphous. The basophil originates in the bone marrow whereas the mast cells arise in the connective tissues. Despite these differences in structure and site of origin, some investigators regard the basophils as a circulating form of mast cell. The granules of both contain histamine and heparin, and both are degranulated by histamine liberating drugs. In sensitized individuals, both discharge their granules when exposed to antigen.

Lymphocytes

Lymphocytes are the second most abundant class of leukocytes in the peripheral blood, constituting 20 to 35 per cent of the circulating white blood cells. They are small cells, with an intensely staining round or slightly indented nucleus and a thin rim of clear blue cytoplasm (Fig. 5–6 *G, H, I*). As a rule, they have no specific granules, but an occasional cell will contain a few small azurophil granules. They are spherical and usually 7 to 8 μm. in diameter. On the average they are only slightly larger than the erythrocytes in blood smears (Fig. 5–9 *a, b, c, d*).

In electron micrographs, they display a tiny Golgi complex, a pair of centrioles, and very few mitochondria. Those circulating in the blood contain small numbers of free ribosomes but essentially no endoplasmic reticulum. Morphologists have traditionally categorized the lymphocytes as large, medium, and small on the basis of their diameter and relative amount of cytoplasm. These were thought to represent progressive stages in their evolution from a larger precursor cell, and the small lymphocytes were long considered to be an end stage capable of surviving only a few hours or days, after which they were presumed to degenerate or to be eliminated from the body. With advances in immunology and introduction of autoradiographic and other means of labeling cells, following their migrations, and measuring their longevity, these earlier concepts of the lymphocyte have been entirely changed. It is now evident that there are at least two distinct categories of small lymphocytes in blood that differ widely in background, life span, and functional potentialities, but these two classes of lymphocytes are not morphologically distinguishable.

The lymphocytes are primarily concerned with the immunological responses of the body. To understand their role, it may be useful to digress briefly in order to describe what those responses are. A variety of foreign substances, usually proteins or polysaccharides, when they are introduced into the body, induce the production of specialized globulins in the blood serum which are capable of combining with and neutralizing the harmful effects of the inducing substance. The animal which has become protected in this way is said to have developed an *immunity*. The foreign substance that induces an immune response is called an *antigen* and the spe-

cific globulin molecules that appear in the blood to counteract it are called *antibodies*. When an antigen is introduced into the body for the first time, there is a conditioning of the antibody producing cells or their precursors which extends over a number of weeks and may result in low levels of circulating antibody. The events taking place in this latent period are described as the *primary response*. If a second exposure to the same antigen occurs weeks or months afterward, there is a dramatic and rapid rise in synthesis of antibody globulin, resulting in a titer of circulating antibody 10 to 100 times the previous level. This is called the *secondary response*, and if a number of injections of antigen are given, the elevated level of circulating antibody may be maintained for years. This component of the bodily defenses, which depends upon blood-borne antibodies, is called the *humoral immune response*. The lymphocytes are the cells that recognize an antigen as foreign to the body and respond to an initial encounter by undergoing certain changes that may have no effect upon their appearance but which endow

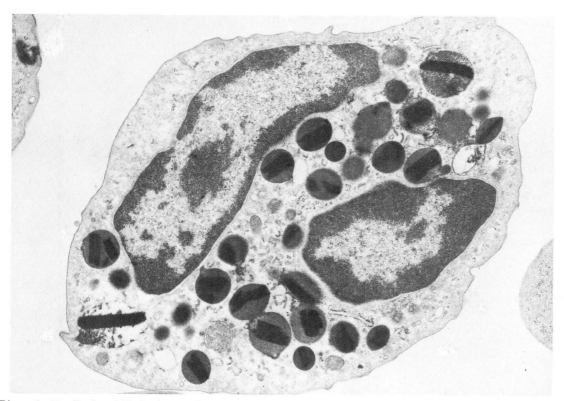

Figure 5–13   Eosinophilic leukocyte from guinea pig. Notice that most of the granules contain one or more dense crystals. ×17,000.

Basophilic granules

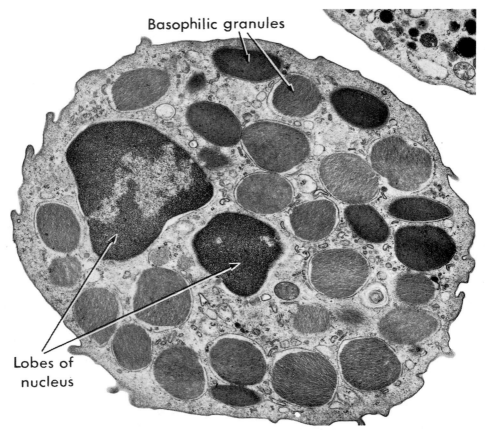

Lobes of
nucleus

Figure 5-14 Electron micrograph of a basophilic granular leukocyte of the guinea pig. The large granules are somewhat irregular in outline and vary in their density. ×16,000.

them with a specific "memory" for that antigen, which conditions their subsequent behavior when exposed at a later time to the same antigen (see Chapter 14).

In contradiction to the traditional view that small lymphocytes are end stages incapable of further development, it has been shown that when lymphocytes of the peripheral blood are placed in tissue culture and stimulated by addition of phytohemagglutinin to the medium, the lymphocytes enlarge progressively, acquire nucleoli and increased numbers of ribosomes, and in 48 hours they have assumed the appearance of very large lymphocytes or lymphoblasts. After the initial period of hypertrophy, they begin to divide (Nowell). The simplicity and reproducibility of this procedure has made it the standard method for obtaining dividing cells for analysis of chromosomes (see p. 75). Of more interest to us here is the subsequent finding that

this unexplained stimulation by phytohemagglutinin duplicates in vitro the normal response of lymphocytes to antigens in vivo. The enlargement and proliferation of lymphoblast-like cells amplifies the antibody response to antigen, since the cells formed then acquire an extensive endoplasmic reticulum, begin to synthesize specific antibody, and take on the cytological characteristics of plasma cells. Their synthesis of antibody can be clearly demonstrated if an enzyme of plant origin, horseradish peroxidase, is used in an experimental animal as an antigen to induce an immune response. Sections of spleen from the hyperimmunized animal are then flooded with antigen, which binds specifically to antibody in the cellular sites of its production. A histochemical reaction for detecting peroxidase then produces a dense reaction product at the sites of the antigen-antibody complex (see Chapter 14, Fig. 14-4). When treated in this way, the plasma cells and their precursors show antibody over the perinuclear cisterna and over the lumen of the cisternae of the endoplasmic reticulum. It is the lymphoblasts and plasma cells developing from stimulated lymphocytes which are mainly responsible for synthesis and release of humoral antibody.

The dependence of the immune mechanisms of the body upon lymphocytes can easily be demonstrated by taking advantage of their sensitivity to x-irradiation. After exposure to an appropriate dose of x-rays, an animal is unable to produce antibodies to new antigens, but if small lymphocytes are later introduced intravenously, the animals again acquire the capacity to produce antibody.

There are a variety of other complex and poorly understood immune mechanisms that

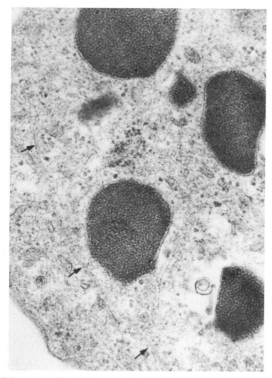

Figure 5-15 Micrograph of a portion of a human basophil, showing that the membrane limited granules consist of closely aggregated small dense granules, in contrast to the highly ordered crystalline structure of these granules in some other species. Arrows indicate microtubules, also present in the cytoplasm. (Micrograph courtesy of Dr. D. Zucker-Franklin.)

depend upon the ability of lymphocytes to "home in" on antigenic foreign cells and to contact and interact with macrophages so as to destroy the antigenic foreign cells by cytotoxic and phagocytic mechanisms. Protective reactions of this kind are distinguished from the *humoral immune response* by the descriptive terms *cell mediated response* or *cellular immunity*. (See Chapter 14.)

The lymphocytes were formerly believed to arise almost exclusively in the lymph nodes and other lymphoid organs, while other leukocytes were formed in the bone marrow. The principal basis for this conclusion was the observation (Yoffey) that if the thoracic duct, which was thought to drain lymph and newly formed lymphocytes from the lymph nodes to the subclavian vein, was severed and exteriorized, the number of lymphocytes in the blood rapidly fell. Since the number entering the blood daily from this source was very large, it seemed to follow that their life span must be very short, for if a comparable number were not leaving the blood daily, the lymphocyte count would rise very rapidly to astronomical numbers. Neither of the conclusions from these observations was entirely correct.

Since it has become possible to label newly formed lymphocytes with tritiated thymidine, our ideas about their movements and life span have changed completely. It was observed (Gowan) that a thoracic duct fistula results not only in a decrease in number of blood lymphocytes, but also in a gradual diminution in the number of lymphocytes emerging from the duct. If this number depended solely upon new formation of lymphocytes in the lymph nodes, the output from the thoracic duct should have been maintained. Thus, it was shown that the lymphocytes entering the blood from the thoracic duct are not all newly formed in the nodes, as was once thought, but a substantial proportion have passed through the nodes from the blood and reentered the lymph. When tritiated thymidine is infused into the afferent lymphatic to a node, it is found that fewer than five per cent of the emerging cells are labeled. The vast majority have migrated through the node from the blood.

It is now universally accepted that lymphocytes are continually migrating between lymph nodes, spleen, and connective tissues, using the blood as a common path. The lymphocytes found in the blood, despite

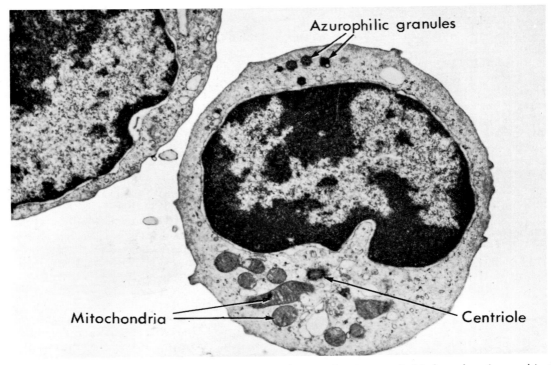

Figure 5–16 Electron micrograph of a guinea pig lymphocyte, showing a typical indented nucleus and in the adjacent cytoplasm a centriole and several mitochondria. Although it is a nongranular leukocyte, the lymphocyte may contain a few azurophilic granules. ×14,000.

their uniform appearance, consist of different populations. The majority are part of the recirculating pool of long-lived (months to years) lymphocytes, capable of participating in cell mediated immunity. A smaller proportion are short-lived (weeks or months) but are capable of being induced to transform into antibody producing cells. (See Chapter 14.)

Monocytes

The typical *monocyte* measures 9 to 12 μm. in diameter, but in blood smears, where they are greatly flattened in the drying process, they may be up to 17 μm. in diameter. They constitute 3 to 8 per cent of the leukocytes of the circulating blood. Their enumeration is subject to some error because they cannot always be sharply differentiated from large lymphocytes. In the typical monocyte, the cytoplasm is more abundant than in lymphocytes, and instead of a clear, pale blue, it tends to have a grayish-blue tint with scattered small azurophil granules (Fig. 5–6 *J, K, L*). In older monocytes, the nucleus

is eccentric in position and oval or reniform. Its chromatin is more finely granular and more uniformly dispersed in the nucleoplasm, so that the nucleus as a whole appears less intensely stained (Fig. 5–9 *e, f*). One or more nucleoli are present, but they are seldom seen in routine blood smears. In preparations stained supravitally with neutral red and Janus green, a group of red staining vacuoles is associated with the juxtanuclear centrosome, and the mitochondria tend to be clustered around the periphery of this rosette of neutral red vacuoles.

In electron micrographs the two or more nucleoli are obvious, and the cytoplasm contains a conspicuous Golgi complex, a few cisternal profiles of granular endoplasmic reticulum, a moderate number of free polysomes, and some glycogen granules. In addition, there are, in each section, 15 to 20 granules about 400 nm. in diameter, with a dense homogeneous content (Fig. 5–17). These correspond to the azurophil granules seen in stained smears. These granules exhibit the cytochemical staining reactions for acid phosphatase, aryl-sulfatase, and peroxidase, and hence are considered to be primary lysosomes (Nichols; Bainton; Farquhar).

The origin of monocytes and their relation to lymphocytes were long obscured by the contradictory theories of blood formation. The development of methods for labeling marrow or lymphoid cells by their incorporation of thymidine or by chromosomal markers and their transfusion into x-irradiated host animals has now resolved much of this controversy. It has now been convincingly demonstrated that monocytes originate from *promonocytes* in the bone marrow, and after a brief developmental period of 1 to 3 days, enter the circulation at random. Those found in the peripheral blood represent a population of cells in transit from the marrow to their ultimate location in the tissues. They spend only about a day and a half in the blood and then migrate into various organs throughout the body, where they differentiate into tissue macrophages. They are capable of mitotic division and of

continued enzyme synthesis in the tissues. They seem to have little function in the blood, but they survive for months in the tissues, where they are a mobile reserve of scavengers that play a valuable defensive role in phagocytosis and intracellular digestion of invading microorganisms. They also seem to be essential for the processing of many antigens prior to the development of antibodies by associated immunocompetent lymphoid cells.

OTHER COMPONENTS OF BLOOD

Since blood is a tissue composed of cells suspended in a fluid extracellular matrix, the *blood plasma*, it may be appropriate to comment briefly upon some of the more important constituents of this matrix. There are three major types of plasma proteins— *albumin, globulin,* and *fibrinogen.*

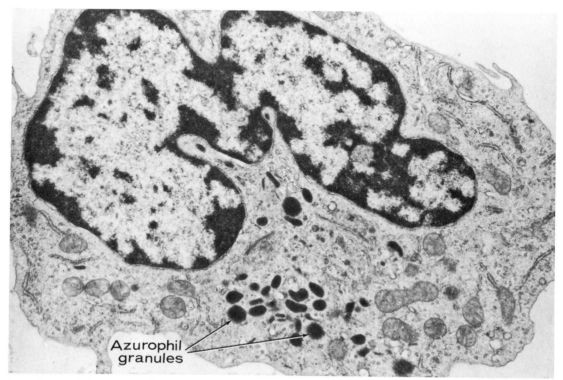

Azurophil granules

Figure 5–17 Micrograph of a typical mature monocyte from rabbit, showing an irregular nucleus with relatively condensed chromatin and a cluster of azurophil granules near the Golgi complex. A few cisternae of endoplasmic reticulum are present near the periphery of the cell. (Micrograph courtesy of Dr. D. Bainton.)

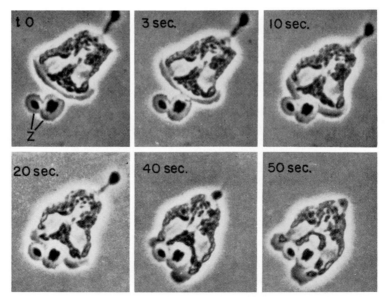

Figure 5–18 Frames from a motion picture of phagocytosis of zymosan particles of yeast cell wall (Z) by a chicken heterophilic leukocyte with its large granules. Note the close apposition of the leukocytic membrane to the zymosan granules. Clear zones seen in the cytoplasm in the 40 and 50 second prints are the result of granule lysis, demonstrated more clearly in Figure 5–19. Note the reduction in content of granules in that part of the cell containing the zymosan particles. Phase contrast microscopy. Approximately ×1000. (Courtesy of J. G. Hirsch, J. Exp. Med., *116*:827, 1962.)

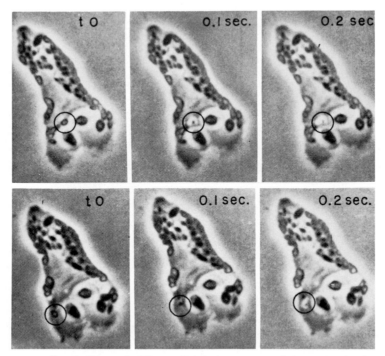

Figure 5–19 The same cell as in Figure 5–18 at a slightly later stage of phagocytosis, showing, in the circled areas, the rapid lysis of two heterophilic granules, one in each of the two rows of micrographs. The area occupied by the circled granule in the upper row appears only as a small vesicle in later micrographs in the lower row. Phase contrast microscopy. Approximately ×2000. (Courtesy of J. G. Hirsch, J. Exp. Med., *116*:827, 1962.)

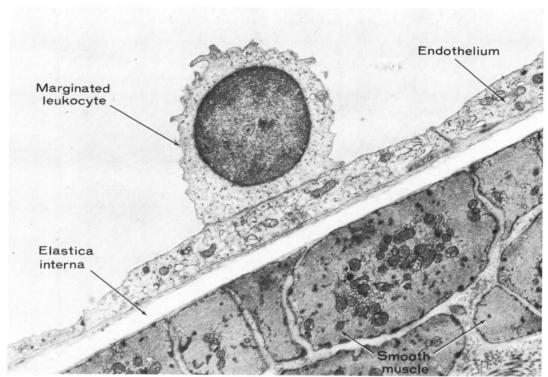

Figure 5-20 A large number of leukocytes in the blood at any one time are not circulating but are temporarily adherent to the endothelium of small blood vessels. These are described as belonging to the "marginated pool" of leukocytes. One example is shown here.

Albumin is the most abundant and smallest of the plasma proteins with a molecular weight of about 59,000. It is synthesized by the liver and its principal function is to maintain the colloid osmotic pressure within the blood capillaries, which prevents excessive loss of fluid to the tissues. In addition, a variety of substances that are relatively insoluble in water dissolve more readily in the presence of blood proteins. Plasma albumin therefore plays an important part in the transport of these metabolic products.

The globulins include proteins of a wide range of molecular weights, 80,000 to several million. They are divided into several fractions. The greatest interest is centered on the *gamma globulins* because this fraction includes the *immune globulins* or *antibodies* that are the basis of the immunological defenses of the body against bacteria, toxins, and other foreign proteins. These important globulins are synthesized in the cells of the lymphoid organs. The *beta globulins* function in the transport of hormones, metal ions, and lipid.

The beta globulin called *transferrin* combines with iron, copper, and zinc. Its principal function is to transport iron. In conditions in which there is increased need for iron for hemoglobin synthesis, as in nutritional deficiency of iron or in pregnancy, there is a compensatory increase in this transport protein. In liver disease or pernicious anemia, the concentration of transferrin is reduced. A protein of rather similar function, *ceruloplasmin*, contains nearly all of the copper of the blood and is believed to regulate utilization of copper by reversibly binding and releasing it at various sites in the body. In the rare inherited disorder of copper metabolism — Wilson's disease — ceruloplasmin is markedly reduced.

Some of the globulins involved in lipid transport attain such a large size that they can be visualized electron microscopically as spherical particulates of varying size. They can therefore be included among the microscopic formed elements of the blood. These serum lipoproteins can be separated from plasma by physical techniques of ultracentrifugal flotation or electrophoresis, and are divided into four major groups on the basis of size. (1) The *chylomicrons*, ranging upward in size from 1000 Å, are the largest and have long been detectable by dark-field light microscopy. (2) The *very low density* lipoproteins (VLDL) generally fall within a size range of 250 to 700 Å and were not visible by light microscopy. (3) The *low density* (LDL) or *beta lipoproteins* are considerably smaller, about 100 Å. In addition to their characteristic sizes, these particles are composed of definite proportions of various classes of lipid associated with specific apoproteins. In the nutrition of mammals, the lipoproteins are the form in which lipids absorbed in the gastrointestinal tract are transported in the blood to and from liver and fat depots. The chylomicrons are transiently increased in the blood after a fat-rich meal. Other classes of lipoproteins are persistently elevated in certain disease conditions. The continued presence of high circulating levels of lipoprotein is thought to predispose to atherosclerosis or hardening of the arteries. The normal lipoproteins are spherical droplets or particles but, interestingly enough, in diseases involving obstruction of the bile duct, abnormal lipoproteins, which have an unusual discoid shape, may appear in the blood. These easily associate in rouleaux under the usual conditions of isolation and negative staining (Hamilton).

The major defense of the body against serious blood loss is the clotting mechanism. An essential protein component of the blood is therefore *fibrinogen*, which is synthesized in the liver and present in the plasma as long asymmetrical molecules of molecular weight 330,000. When *prothrombin*, also present in plasma, is activated by *thromboplastin* of tissue or platelet origin, enzymatically active *thrombin* is produced, resulting in polymerization of fibrin to form the fibrous meshwork of a clot. Various hemorrhagic disorders may result from impaired synthesis of fibrinogen or deficiency of prothrombin.

REFERENCES

Erythrocytes

Bessis, M., and J. P. Thiéry: Les cellules du sang vues au microscope à interferences (système Nomarski). Revue d'Hématologie, *12*:518, 1957.

Bierman, H. R., ed.: Leukopoiesis in health and disease. Ann. N. Y. Acad. Sci., *113*:511, 1964.

Bishop, C., and D. M. Surgenor, eds.: The Red Blood Cells. New York, Academic Press, 1964.

Cowles, J., J. Saikkonen, and B. Thorell: On the presence of hemoglobin in erythroleukemia cells. Blood, *13*:1176, 1958.

Davidson, W. M., and D. H. Smith: A morphological sex difference in the polymorphonuclear leukocytes. Brit. Med. J., *2*:6, 1954.

Davies, H. G.: Structure in nucleated erythrocytes. J. Biophys. Biochem. Cytol., *9*:671, 1961.

Ingram, V.: The Hemoglobins in Genetics and Evolution. New York, Columbia University Press, 1963.

Knisely, M. H.: The settling of sludge during life; first observations, evidences, and significances; a contribution to the biophysics of disease. Acta Anat., *44* (Suppl.):41, 1961.

Macfarlane, R. G., and Robb-Smith, A. H. T., eds.: Functions of the Blood. New York, Academic Press, 1961.

Perutz, M. F.: X-ray analysis of hemoglobin. Science, *140*:863, 1963.

Wintrobe, M.: Clinical Hematology. 5th ed. Philadelphia, Lea & Febiger, 1961.

Granulocytes

Ackerman, G. A.: Cytochemical properties of the blood basophilic granulocyte. Ann. N. Y. Acad. Sci., *103*:376, 1963.

Allen, R. D.: Ameboid movement. In Brachet, J., and A. E. Mirsky, eds.: The Cell: Biochemistry, Physiology, Morphology. Vol II. New York, Academic Press, 1961.

Anderson, D. R.: Ultrastructure of normal and leukemic leukocytes in human peripheral blood. J. Ultrastruct. Res., *9(Suppl.)*:5, 1966.

Archer, R. K.: On the functions of eosinophils in the antigen-antibody reaction Brit. J. Haemat., *11*:123, 1965.

Archer, R. K., and N. Bosworth: Phagocytosis by eosinophils following antigen-antibody reactions in vitro. Austr. J. Exp. Biol. Med. Sci., *39*:157, 1961.

Athens, J. W.: Granulocyte kinetics in health and disease. National Cancer Institute Monograph, No. 30:135, 1969.

Bainton, D. F., and M. G. Farquhar: Differences in enzyme content of azurophil and specific granules of polymorphonuclear leukocytes. II. Cytochemistry and electron microscopy of bone marrow cells. J. Cell Biol., *39*:299, 1968.

Bainton, D. F., J. L. Ullyot, and M. G. Farquhar: The development of neutrophilic leukocytes in human bone marrow: Origin and content of azurophil and specific granules. J. Exp. Med., *134*:907, 1971.

Boggs, D. R.: The kinetics of neutrophilic leukocytes in health and in disease. Sem. Hematol., *4*:359, 1967.

Bond, V. B., T. M. Fliedner, E. P. Cronkite, J. R. Rubini, and J. S. Robertson: Cell-turnover in blood and blood-forming tissues studied with tritiated thymidine. In Stohlman, F., Jr., ed.: The Kinetics of Cellular Proliferation. New York, Grune and Stratton, 1959.

Daems, W. Th.: On the fine structure of human neutrophilic leukocyte granules. J. Ultrastruct. Res., *24*:343, 1968.

Hudson, G.: Eosinophil granuocyte reactions. In Yoffey, J. M., ed.: Bone Marrow Reactions. Baltimore, Williams & Wilkins, 1966.

Hudson, G.: Quantitative study of eosinophil granulocytes. Sem. Hematol., *5*:166, 1968.

Litt, M.: Eosinophils and antigen-antibody reactions. Ann. N. Y. Acad. Sci., *116*:964, 1964.

Speirs, R. S.: Advances in knowledge of the eosinophil in relation to antibody formation. Ann. N. Y. Acad. Sci., 73:283, 1958.

Terry, R. W., D. F. Bainton, and M. G. Farquhar: Formation and structure of specific granules in basophilic leukocytes of the guinea pig. Lab. Invest., 21:65, 1969.

Nongranular Leukocytes

Berman, L., and C. S. Stulberg: Primary cultures of macrophages from normal human peripheral blood. Lab. Invest., 11:1322, 1962.

Caffrey, R. W., W. O. Rieke, and N. B. Everett: Radioautographic studies of small lymphocytes in the thoracic duct of the rat. Acta Haemat., 28:145, 1962.

Cohn, Z. A.: The structure and function of monocytes and macrophages. Adv. Immunol., 9:163, 1968.

Everett, N. B., R. W. Caffrey, and W. O. Rieke: Recirculation of lymphocytes. In Bierman, H. R., ed.: Leukopoiesis in health and disease. Ann. N. Y. Acad. Sci., 113:887, 1964.

Furth, R. V., and Z. A. Cohn: The origin and kinetics of mononuclear phagocytes. J. Exp. Med., 128:415, 1968.

Gowans, J. L.: Life-span, recirculation and transformation of lymphocytes. Int. Rev. Path., 5:1, 1966.

Gowans, J. L., and E. J. Knight: The route of re-circulation of lymphocytes in the rat. Proc. Roy. Soc., B159:745, 1965.

Hirsch. J. G.: Cinemicrophotographic observations on granule lysis in polymorphonuclear leucocytes during phagocytosis. J. Exper. Med., 116:827, 1962.

Maximow, A. A.: The lymphocytes and plasma cells. In Cowdry, E. V., ed.: Special Cytology. 2nd ed. New York, Paul B. Hoeber, Inc., 1932.

Nichols, B. A., D. F. Bainton, and M. G. Farquhar: Differentiation of monocytes. Origin, nature, and fate of their azurophil granules. J. Exp. Med., 50:498, 1971.

Norman, A., M. S. Sasaki, R. E. Ottoman, and A. G. Fingerhut: Lymphocyte lifetime in women. Science, 147:745, 1965.

Nossal, G. J. V., A. Szenberg, G. L. Ada, and C. M. Austin: Single cell studies on 19S antibody production. J. Exper. Med., 119:485, 1964.

Rebuck, J. W., ed.: The Lymphocyte and the Lymphocytic Tissue. New York, Paul B. Hoeber, Inc., 1960.

Reinhardt, W. O.: Some factors influencing the thoracic-duct output of lymphocytes. In Bierman, H. R., ed.: Leukopoiesis in health and disease. Ann. N. Y. Acad. Sci., 113:844, 1964.

Rieke, W. O.: Lymphocytes from thymectomized rats: Immunologic, proliferative and metabolic properties. Science, 152:535, 1966.

Sabesin, S. M.: Lymphocytes of small mammals: Spontaneous transformation in culture to blastoids. Science, 149:1385, 1965.

Shelton, E.: Prolonged survival of rabbit thoracic duct lymphocytes in a diffusion chamber. J. Cell Biol., 12:652, 1962.

Speirs, R. S.: The action of antigen upon hypersensitive cells. In Bierman, H. R., ed.: Leukopoiesis in health and disease. Ann. N. Y. Acad. Sci., 113:819, 1964.

Symposium on differentiation and growth of hemoglobin- and immunoglobin-synthesizing cells. J. Cell Physiol., 67(Suppl.):1, 1966.

Volkman, A.: The function of the monocyte. Bibliotheca Haem., 29:86, 1968.

Volkman, A., and J. L. Gowans: The origin of macrophages from bone marrow in the rat. Brit. J. Pathol., 46:62, 1965.

Weiss, L., and D. W. Fawcett: Cytochemical observations on chicken monocytes, macrophages and giant cells in tissue culture. J. Histochem. Cytochem., 1:47, 1953.

Yoffey, J. M.: The lymphocyte. Ann. Rev. Med., 15:125, 1964.

Yoffey, J. M., G. C. B. Winter, D. G. Osmond, and E. S. Meek: Morphological studies in the culture of human leukocytes with phytohaemagglutinin. Brit. J. Haemat., 11:488, 1965.

Platelets

Biggs, R., and R. G. Macfarlane: Human Blood Coagulation and Its Disorders. 3rd ed. Philadelphia, F. A. Davis Co., 1962.

David-Ferreira, J. F.: Sur la structure et le pouvoir phagocytaire des plaquettes sanguines. Zeitschr. f. Zellforsch, 55:89, 1961.

Davie, E. W., and O. D. Ratnoff: The proteins of blood coagulation. In Neurath, H., ed.: The Proteins. 2nd ed. Vol. III. New York, Academic Press, 1965.

Johnson, S. A., R. W. Monto, J. W. Rebuck, and R. C. Horn, Jr., eds.: Blood Platelets (A Symposium). Boston, Little, Brown and Co., 1961.

Marcus, A. J., and M. B. Zucker: The Physiology of Blood Platelets. New York, Grune and Stratton, 1965.

Porter, K. R., and C. Z. van Hawn: Sequences in the formation of clots from purified bovine fibrinogen and thrombin; a study with the electron microscope. J. Exper. Med., 90:225, 1949.

Seegers, W. H.: Prothombin. Commonwealth Fund. Cambridge, Harvard University Press, 1962.

6

Connective Tissue Proper

Connective tissue proper always consists of *cells* and extracellular *fibers* embedded in an amorphous *ground substance* containing *tissue fluid*. Traditionally the fibers have been considered to be of three kinds, *collagenous*, *reticular*, and *elastic*, but recent evidence indicates that collagenous and reticular fibers may simply be different morphological expressions of a single fibrous protein. There are several types of cells in connective tissue, which can be categorized either as *fixed cells* or as *wandering cells*. The relative abundance of the various kinds of fibers, cells, and ground substance varies greatly from one region of the body to another, depending upon the local structural requirements. For convenience of description an effort is made to classify connective tissues. Classification is difficult and inexact and should not be interpreted too rigidly, for the various types grade into one another through transitional forms, and one type may be transformed into another if the local conditions change.

Descriptive terms are usually assigned according to whether the fibers are loosely woven or densely packed. Thus we distinguish *loose connective tissue* and *dense connective tissue*. Within the second category it is useful to add modifiers to indicate whether the fibers have an ordered or a disordered arrangement. Thus, in *dense irregular connective tissue* the fibers are closely interwoven in a random way, whereas in *dense regular connective tissue* the fibers are arranged in parallel bundles, as in tendons, or in flat sheets, as in aponeuroses. In addition, a number of kinds of connective tissue with special properties are named so as to indicate

the predominating component or the identifying feature: *mucous* connective tissue, *elastic* tissue, *reticular* tissue, *adipose* tissue, *pigment* tissue, etc. These and the cellular *lamina propria* of the intestinal and uterine mucosa are all variants of loose connective tissue, which is a common and simple form that can be taken as the prototype of the connective tissues.

LOOSE CONNECTIVE TISSUE

Loose connective tissue develops from the mesenchyme that remains after the other tissues of the embryo have been formed. An interlacing fabric of fine reticular fibers is deposited in the meshes of the stellate reticulum of mesenchymal cells. As the fibers become more numerous, they associate in coarser bundles and take on the staining properties of collagen. The mesenchymal cells gradually change their character, elongating and stretching out along the surface of the fiber bundles to become *fibroblasts*, the principal cells of the connective tissue. Other cell types, either differentiating from mesenchymal cells or emigrating from the blood, take up residence in the interstices of the fabric of interwoven fibers. Like a collapsed sponge this tissue contains innumerable potential spaces, normally occupied by a small amount of amorphous ground substance but capable of becoming enlarged and distended with fluid. These extracellular interstitial spaces are the minute chambers or compartments seen by the early histologists, who are responsible for the term *areolar tissue* (from *areola*, a small space or area), a common synonym for loose connective tissue.

EXTRACELLULAR COMPONENTS

The functions of connective tissue depend largely upon the properties of its extracellular substance. The fibers are responsible for its tensile strength and resilience, while the aqueous phase of the ground substance is the essential medium through which all nutrients and wastes must pass between the blood and the connective tissue cells. The consistency and degree of hydration of the ground substance can exert an important influence upon this vital exchange.

Collagenous Fibers

Collagenous fibers are present in all types of connective tissue but vary greatly in their abundance. In unstained preparations of loose connective tissue the collagen fibers appear as colorless strands 1 to 10 μm. in thickness and of indefinite length. They run in all directions, and if the connective tissue is not under tension, they tend to have a slightly wavy course (Figs. 6–1 and

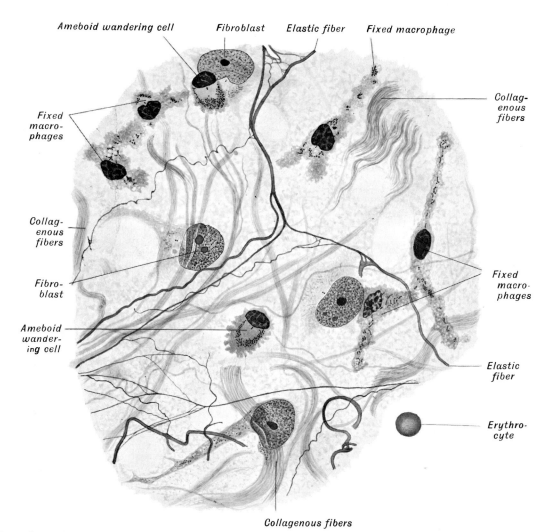

Figure 6–1 Section through slightly edematous, subcutaneous loose connective tissue from the thigh of a man. The figure illustrates various types of cells and fibers found in normal connective tissue. The erythrocyte at the lower right (7 μm.) is for size comparison. ×950. (After A. A. Maximow.)

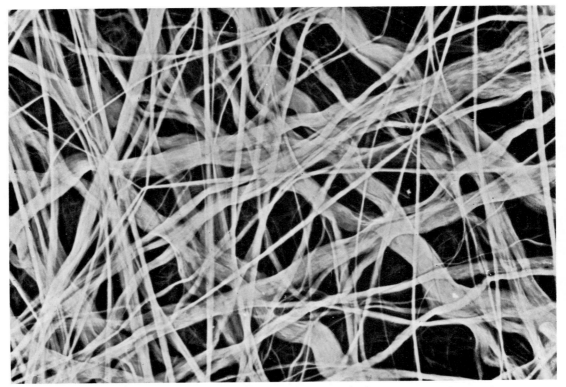

Figure 6–2 Photomicrograph of collagenous fibers in a thin spread of rat mesentery. Notice the variation in size and the wavy course of the larger fibers. The preparation was stained with Paps' silver method and the photograph printed as a negative to simulate more closely their appearance in fresh material. ×550. (After D. W. Fawcett, *in* R. O. Greep, ed.: Histology. Philadelphia, The Blakiston Co., 1953. Reproduced with the permission of the McGraw-Hill Book Co.)

6–2). At high magnification, faint longitudinal striations can be detected in the larger collagenous fibers, suggesting that they consist of bundles of smaller parallel fibrils. With polarization microscopy, even the smallest visible collagen fibrils show form birefringence, indicating the presence of elongated submicroscopic units oriented in the direction of the fiber axis. When the examination is carried down to the electron microscope level, the smallest collagen fibrils detectable with the light microscope are found to be composed of parallel submicroscopic fibrils, 200 to 1000 Å in diameter. These are the oriented subunits responsible for the form birefringence observed when collagen is examined in polarized light. In electron micrographs, the unit fibrils of collagen are seen to be cross striated, with transverse bands repeating every 640 to 700 Å along their length (Fig.

6–3). When collagen fibrils are stained with phosphotungstic acid and viewed at high magnification, several additional bands can be resolved within each 640 Å period (Fig. 6–5A).

The collagenous fibers are flexible but offer great resistance to a pulling force. The breaking point of human collagenous fibers (as in tendon) is reached with a force of several hundred kilograms per square centimeter, and their elongation at this point is only a few percentage points. If collagen is denatured by boiling or by chemical treatment, it yields the familiar substance *gelatin*. With more gentle treatment, some collagen fibrils can be put into solution in vitro without denaturation. When this is done the fundamental units or molecules in solution are called *tropocollagen* and consist of long, slender particles about 2600 Å in length and 15 Å thick. The collagen molecules are made up of three polypeptide chains, each having a molecular weight of about 100,000. These chains, termed α units, have a helical configuration and are coiled around one another in a right-handed direction (Fig. 6–4), and are cross linked. All three are rich in glycine and contain two amino acids, *hydroxyproline* and *hydroxylysine,* which do not occur in significant amounts in other proteins. The content of these amino acids (particularly hydroxyproline) in an organ can therefore be taken as a measure of its collagen content. This fact has proved useful in quantitative chemical studies and autoradiographic localization of sites of collagen synthesis.

Collagen molecules are present in the ground substance of growing connective tissue and can be extracted in cold neutral salt solution. Warming such solutions to body temperature results in spontaneous polymerization of collagen into typical cross-striated fibrils. In this process the long collagen molecules are believed to come together in a parallel arrangement and overlap each other by about a quarter of their

length to produce a staggered array that results in cross striations at 640 Å intervals (Fig. 6–4). The finer lines within each of these periods are presumed to result from alignment of asymmetric areas along the length of the collagen molecules.

Banded patterns that do not occur in nature can be produced by altering the conditions under which the collagen is reconstituted. If a solution of collagen and α-acid glycoprotein of serum is dialyzed against water, the collagen fibers that are formed have a period 2400 Å instead of the 640 Å characteristic of the native fibers. This form is called *fibrous long spacing* (FLS) *collagen* (Fig. 6–6B). Precipitation from acid solution by addition of adenosine triphosphate (ATP) yields segments about 2400 Å long, instead of fibers (Fig. 6–6C). This form is called *segment long spacing* (SLS) *collagen*. Both of these, as well as the native form, can be redissolved and precipitated in either of the other forms, depending upon the physicochemical conditions. In both of the long spacing forms, the collagen molecules are believed to come together side to

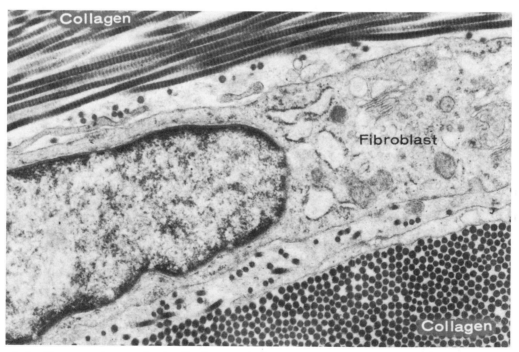

Figure 6–3 Electron micrograph of a fibroblast and adjacent collagen. The collagen fibrils at the upper left have been cut longitudinally and show a regular cross striation. Those at the lower right have been cut transversely. Their uniform size and circular configuration on cross section are apparent.

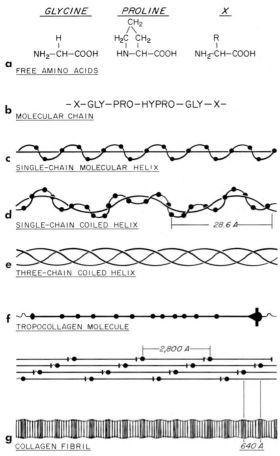

a FREE AMINO ACIDS

b – X–GLY–PRO–HYPRO–GLY–X–
MOLECULAR CHAIN

c SINGLE-CHAIN MOLECULAR HELIX

d SINGLE-CHAIN COILED HELIX ⊢— 28.6 A —⊣

e THREE-CHAIN COILED HELIX

f TROPOCOLLAGEN MOLECULE

⊢—2,800 A—⊣

g COLLAGEN FIBRIL 640 A

Figure 6–4 Diagram depicting the formation of collagen, which can be visualized as taking place in seven steps. The starting materials (*a*) are amino acids, of which only two are shown; the side chain of any of the others is indicated by R in amino acid X. (*b*) The amino acids are linked together to form a molecular chain. (*c*) This then coils into a left handed helix (*d* and *e*). Three such chains then intertwine in a triple stranded helix, which constitutes the tropocollagen molecule (*f*). Many tropocollagen molecules become aligned in staggered fashion, overlapping by a quarter of their length to form a cross striated collagen fibril (*g*). (Redrawn and slightly modified from Collagen by J. Gross. Copyright © May 1961 by Scientific American, Inc. All rights reserved.)

side, in register, so that the length of the period, or of the segment, is approximately the same as the length of the collagen molecules.

Further progress has been made in recent years in understanding the molecular organization of collagen in its different forms. The alpha units of collagen molecules can be separated on cellulose columns into two classes, designated α_1 and α_2. Moreover, several *types* of α_1 polypeptide chains are now known, which differ slightly in their amino acid composition. Thus it is possible for collagens in various locations in the body to differ. Collagen molecules from tendon and skin consist of two α_1, Type I chains linked to an α_2 chain, whereas collagen molecules characteristic of cartilage matrix consist of three α_1, Type II chains. In the extracellular spaces of connective tissue, collagen molecules polymerize in a quarter-staggered, overlapping array that results in formation of cross-striated fibrils with a 640 to 700 Å repeating period. In other sites, such as cartilage that provides a microenvironment for polymerization that is rich in glycosaminoglycans, the molecules may aggregate in fibrils with another pattern. In the lens capsule and other epithelial basal laminae where the collagen molecules are associated with large amounts of neutral polysaccharides, they polymerize to form a feltwork of randomly oriented fine filaments without any obvious cross striation.

Collagen has been identified as a substance capable of inducing the formation of nuclei of hydroxyapatite crystal growth from metastable solutions of calcium and phosphate (Glimcher). These conditions do not prevail in ordinary connective tissue, but this property of collagen appears to be important in the calcification of bone matrix (see Chapter 10).

For the study of histological sections there are no specific staining reactions for collagen, but its recognition usually presents no problem. It stains with eosin in hematoxylin and eosin preparations. It also binds various acid aniline dyes, such as the acid fuchsin of van Gieson's stain and the aniline blue of Mallory's stains. In silver staining methods, such as those of Paps or Bielschowsky, the collagen is tinted tan to brown, in contrast to the blackening of the reticular fibers. Collagen may present physical and possibly chemical differences in different parts of the body and may not always take the form of fibers.

Elastic Fibers

The normal function of some organs requires that their components be able to yield to externally applied force and move with respect to one another. At the same time, the connective tissue that binds them together must have sufficient resilience to restore the original state after deformation. The elastic fibers in the connective tissue stroma of organs provides this property. Elasticity, as strictly defined by physical scientists, means resistance to deformation, but in speaking of elastic fibers of connective tissue, we adhere to the popular usage in which elasticity means the ability to be deformed or stretched by a small force and to recover the original shape and dimen-

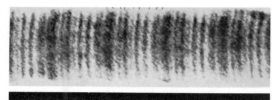

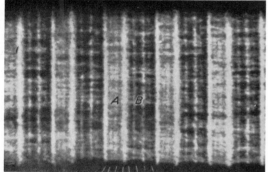

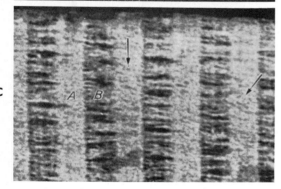

Figure 6–5 Electron micrographs of collagen. *A,* Collagen fibril from rat tail tendon stained with phosphotungstic acid. ×257,000. *B,* Collagen from same source negatively stained with phosphotungstate. ×257,000. *C,* Collagen precipitated from citrate extract of rat skin, negatively stained. Notice that the tropocollagen molecules can be resolved. ×257,000. (After B. R. Olsen, Zeitschr. f. Zellforsch, *59:*184, 1963.)

sions when the force is removed. Elastic fibers stretch easily and when released, they return to their original length rather like rubber bands. Their breaking point occurs when they are stretched to about 150 per cent of their original length. For this degree of stretch, a force of only 20 to 30 kg./cm.² is necessary. When a fiber is broken, the ends retract and spiral or coil up.

In unstained spreads of loose connective tissue, the slender refractile elastic fibers 0.2 to 1.0 µm. in diameter are not plentiful, but they can usually be distinguished from the more abundant collagen fibers by their tendency to branch and anastomose to form networks (Fig. 6–7). They are not ordinarily identifiable in routinely stained histological sections, but can be clearly demonstrated when selectively stained by Verhoeff's stain, Weigert's resorcin fuchsin, or Halmi's aldehyde fuchsin methods. When present in sufficient numbers, elastic fibers impart a yellowish color to the fresh tissue. Certain elastic ligaments, such as the ligamenta flava of the human vertebral column or the ligamentum nuchae of ruminants, are distinctly yellow, and are composed of coarse parallel elastic fibers up to 4 or 5 µm. in diameter. Elastin is not always in the form of fibers. In the walls of arteries for example, it occurs in fenestrated sheets or lamellae, the *elastica interna* and *elastica externa* (see Chapter 13).

Elastic fibers appear homogeneous and are not made up of fibrillar subunits that are visible with the light microscope. Under polarized light, the fibers show a weak birefringence which increases when they are stretched. Examination with the electron microscope at first revealed no characteristic substructure. The fibers or sheets of elastin appeared in electron micrographs as pale, amorphous masses of material that had little or no affinity for lead stain. However, as improvements have been made in methods of specimen preparation, it has become apparent that elastic fibers have two components: *microfibrils*, about 110 Å in diameter, aggregated in bundles that are embedded in a more abundant, amorphous component—*elastin* (Fig. 6–8).

During embryonic life the bundles of microfibrils are laid down first in close apposition to the surface of fibroblasts or other mesenchymal elements. The amorphous material appears later and ultimately con-

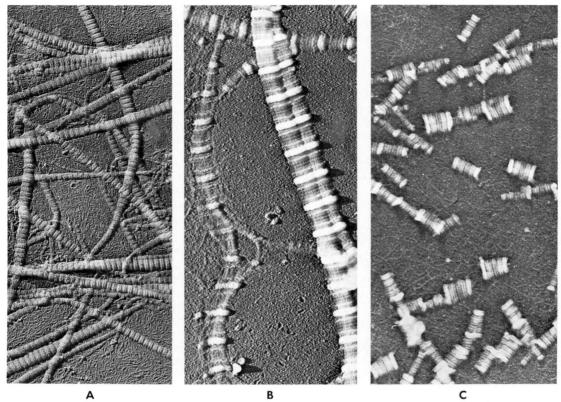

A   B   C

Figure 6–6 Electron micrographs of collagen. *A,* Fibrils with typical collagen period (649 Å), precipitated from collagen solution by dialysis against 1 per cent NaCl. Chromium shadowed. *B,* Fibrous long spacing (FLS), produced by dialysis against water of a mixture of α_1 acid glycoprotein of serum and collagen solution. Stained with phosphotungstic acid hematoxylin. *C,* Segment long spacing (SLS), precipitated from acid solution of collagen by addition of ATP. Chromium shadowed. (Courtesy of J. Gross, F. O. Schmitt, and J. H. Highberger.)

stitutes the bulk of the fiber, with the micro-fibrils forming a layer around its periphery and occurring in small fascicles in its interior.

The amorphous elastin is resistant to digestion by trypsin, but treatment with the enzyme *elastase*, prepared from pancreas, will digest it from sections, leaving cells and collagen intact. Elastin is resistant to boiling and to hydrolysis by dilute acid or alkali. It can be isolated in relatively pure form by taking advantage of its resistance to alkali under conditions that destroy other connective tissue constituents. The microfibrillar component of elastic fibers is rich in cystine, whereas this amino acid is virtually absent from elastin. Thus, contamination of elastin by microfibrillar protein can be eliminated by breaking the disulfide bonds of cystine, thereby solubilizing the microfibrils. (Fig. 6–8*B*).

Upon analysis, the two proteins are found to differ greatly in amino acid composition. Elastin bears some resemblance to collagen in its content of glycine and proline, but differs in its high content of valine. It also contains two unusual amino acids, *desmosine* and *isodesmosine*. These latter are now known to be involved in the cross linking that occurs during polymerization of elastin. The material secreted by the cells lacks desmosines and is called *tropoelastin* by analogy with tropocollagen. Lysine groups on tropoelastin are acted upon extracellularly by the enzyme lysyl oxidase to produce a highly reactive terminal aldehyde. Four of these lysine-derived units join together to form the four-pronged desmosine link tying together four elastin chains.

According to the prevailing interpretation of the genesis of elastic fibers, the elastin precursor, tropoelastin, is synthesized on the ribosomes of fibroblasts, smooth muscle cells, and possibly other mesenchymal derivatives, and is released at the cell surface. It is composed predominantly of hydrophobic or uncharged amino acids, hence the molecule tends to be insoluble in water. At the surface of the developing elastic fiber, the enzyme lysyl oxidase catalyzes the conversion of the lysines of tropoelastin into aldehydes. These condense to form cross links between elastin chains. The role of the microfibrils in the process is not clear, but it is thought that, in some way, they impose a fibrous form on the polymerizing elastin, which does not have filamentous molecular subunits that would predispose to polymerization in the form of fibers.

In the disease osteolathyrism, occurring in animals that eat the plant *Lathyrus odoratus*, or in the comparable condition induced experimentally by administration of β-aminoproprionitrile, the action of lysyl oxidase is inhibited, and both collagen and elastin are incompletely cross linked.

Like collagen, purified elastin has been reported to be capable of inducing the formation of nuclei of hydroxyapatite crystal growth from metastable solutions of calcium and phosphate. It is possible that this process may be involved in pathological calcifications of aorta, skin, etc. (Soble et al.).

Reticular Fibers

These minute fibers tend to form delicate networks rather than coarse bundles, and they are colored more intensely with silver staining methods than are typical collagenous

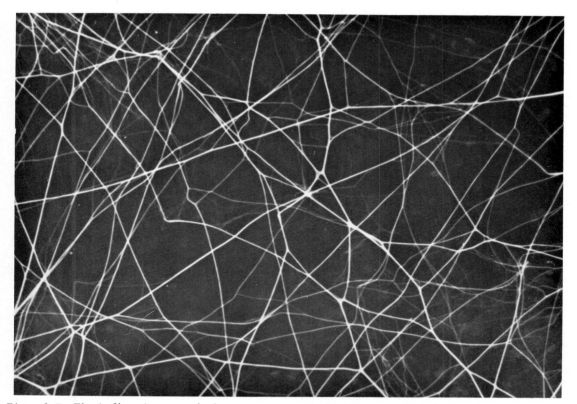

Figure 6–7 Elastic fibers in a spread of rat mesentery stained with resorcin-fuchsin; the photomicrograph is printed as a negative. Notice that the fibers are smaller and less variable in size than collagen bundles and they branch and anastomose to form a network. ×550. (After D. W. Fawcett, *in* Greep, R. O. ed.: Histology. Philadelphia, The Blakiston Co., 1953. Reproduced with the permission of the McGraw-Hill Book Co.)

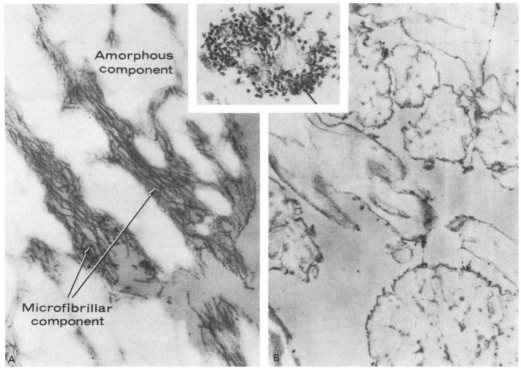

Figure 6-8 Purified preparation of elastic fibers from ligamentum nuchae of a fetal calf. *A*, The stained microfibrils are clearly seen around and between the amorphous appearing unstained elastin. *B*, The microfibrils have been extracted by chemical treatment that breaks disulfide bonds of protein, leaving behind the amorphous component of elastic fibers. The inset shows in cross section an early stage of elastic fiber formation with 110 Å microfibrils around a pale core of newly formed elastin. (Micrographs courtesy of R. Ross and P. Bornstein. Scientific American, June, 1971.)

fibers. The reticular fibers are not apparent in ordinary histological preparations but can be demonstrated by reason of their property of adsorbing metallic silver when treated with alkaline solutions of reducible silver salts (Fig. 6–9). Fibers of this character are the first to appear in the differentiation of mesenchyme into loose connective tissue, but they gradually give way to increasing numbers of collagenous fibers in the loose connective tissue of adults. Reticular fibers persist, however, in delicate networks surrounding adipose cells, supporting the endothelium of capillaries, the sarcolemma of muscle, and the endoneurium of nerves. They are also found in close association with the basal lamina (basement membrane) of epithelia (Fig. 6–12). They constitute the fibrous supporting tissue of lymphoid and blood forming organs and

the stroma of the liver and other epithelial organs.

Because of their arrangement and distinctive staining properties, the *reticular fibers* were formerly considered to be a separate kind of protein fiber, but in electron micrographs they are found to be made up of unit fibrils with the periodic structure typical of collagen. It appears, therefore, that the difference in argyrophilia of reticular and collagenous fibers is not due to a chemical difference but has a physical basis, depending upon the number and arrangement of unit fibrils of collagen and their relation to the protein-polysaccharide matrix that binds them together. Although it now appears that collagen and reticulin are essentially identical, the terms *reticulum* and *reticular fibers* continue to be useful to designate fibrous elements whose size and arrangement are different from those of collagenous fibers.

Ground Substance

The formed elements of connective tissue are embedded in a matrix of *amorphous ground substance* having the properties of a viscous solution or thin gel. It is difficult to characterize this material morphologically because, in the fresh state, it is optically homogeneous and transparent. It is extracted by most of the aqueous fixatives in common use and therefore can seldom be demonstrated in histological sections. The ground substance is preserved to some extent by the method of freeze-drying if the fresh frozen sections are subsequently fixed in ether-formol vapor. In such preparations the ground substance gives a periodic acid–Schiff reaction for carbohydrates and stains metachromatically with toluidine blue. These reactions are attributable to the *mucopolysaccharides* (glycosaminoglycans)* of the ground substance. These are of several kinds, which vary in proportions from one kind of connective tissue

Mucopolysaccharide and *mucoprotein* are terms that have been widely and rather loosely used for a variety of viscous carbohydrate containing secretory products and extracellular matrix components. A concerted effort is now being made to discourage the use of the prefix "muco-" and to secure adoption of the term *glycosaminoglycan* for polysaccharides that contain amino sugars. The terms *glycoprotein* and *glycopeptide* are to be used for proteins and peptides that contain carbohydrates, including those containing amino sugars. Similarly, lipids that contain amino sugars are called *glycosaminolipids.*

In this period of transition we have retained for this edition the more familiar traditional terms, but the student is urged to acquaint himself with this newer and more precise terminology, which is rapidly gaining acceptance.

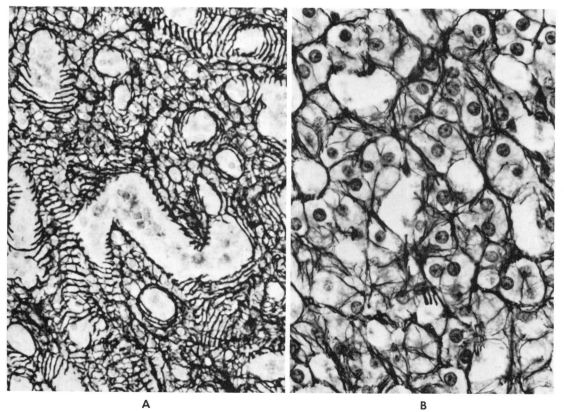

A   **B**

Figure 6-9 Reticular fibers are distinguished from collagenous fibers by their smaller size, their branching pattern, and the fact that they blacken with silver stains. The pattern of reticular fibers is different and characteristic of each organ. *A*, Reticulum of the spleen. ×400. (Preparation by K. Richardson.) *B*, Reticular fibers of the adrenal cortex. ×550.

to another. The most common are *hyaluronic acid, chondroitin-4-sulfate (chondroitin sulfate A)*, and *chondroitin-6-sulfate (chondroitin sulfate C)*, *dermatan sulfate* (chondroitin sulfate B), and *keratan sulfate* (keratosulfate). Each of these polysaccharides is composed of two different saccharide units, which alternate regularly along a long unbranched chain. The saccharides of the *chondroitin sulfates* are galactosamine and glucuronate, and there is one sulfate group in each repeating period of the molecule. Multiple chains of chondroitin sulfate appear to be bound to protein, which accounts for 15 per cent or more of the glycoprotein molecule. The strongly acid sulfate groups are responsible for the basophilia of this component of the extracellular substance. The other polysaccharides, though not sulfated, also carry a very large number of negatively charged groups along their length and are therefore described as polyanions. In the tissues they are always associated with an equivalent number of cations, mostly sodium. The ability of the polyanionic polysaccharides to bind polyvalent cations is the basis for their staining reaction with Hale's iron method or with Alcian blue, which are used for the demonstration of these compounds in tissue sections. These same polyelectrolyte properties are probably also of fundamental importance to the functions of the polysaccharides in the connective tissues.

In hyaluronic acid, the alternating saccharide units are glucosamine and glucuronate. The total molecular weight is 200,000 to 500,000, and if straightened out, the chain would be up to 2.5 μm. in length. The hyaluronic acid is bound to a protein, but this makes up only about 2 per cent of the whole molecule. One of the most important properties of this substance is its very high viscosity in aqueous solutions. This is largely responsible for the physical consistency of the ground substance. If fluid is injected into the connective tissue it does not immediately diffuse away from the site but remains localized for a while in a discrete bleb, as though walled off by the viscous interstitial substance. This property is thought to act as a barrier to the spread of bacteria that may gain access to the tissues. In this connection, it is of interest that some of the most invasive bacteria produce the enzyme *hya-*

luronidase, which enables them to depolymerize the hyaluronic acid of the ground substance. The viscosity of hyaluronic acid in the synovial fluid of joints makes it well suited for its lubricating function, and it is not inconceivable that in dense connective tissues, also, it acts as a plasticizer to diminish friction and wear between collagen fibrils as they move over one another in the flexuous movements of the tissues. The volume of solution occupied by these large diffuse molecules (called their domain) is large (about 4000 Å in diameter), and when these molecules are present in a high enough concentration, they become entangled with each other and with the collagen fibrils that penetrate their domain. The resistance of collagen fibrils to compression in hyaluronic acid solution or in the ground substance appears to be in part a reflection of the resistance of the hyaluronic acid molecule to compression of its domain (Schubert). Though difficult to demonstrate microscopically, the hyaluronic acid of connective tissue is of great importance in determining the structural and physiological properties of the ground substance.

The ground substance also contains variable amounts of *tropocollagen*, which cannot be demonstrated histologically but can be extracted in neutral salt solution and precipitated as cross striated collagen fibers in vitro.

Origin of Connective Tissue Fibers

The sequence of morphological events in formation of collagen is similar whether studied in the embryo, in young scar tissue, or in tissue cultures. Delicate networks of branching and anastomosing argyrophilic fibrils appear among the fibroblasts (Fig. 6–10). The fibrils may follow the outlines of the cells and their processes, but they also extend far into the intercellular substance. When studied in electron micrographs, the finest of the developing fibrils are extracellular and have cross striations (Fig. 6–13). As the fibrils increase in number, they rearrange into parallel wavy bundles of appreciable thickness. These lose their ability to be blackened with silver (Fig. 6–11) and instead accept stains for collagen (Mallory or van Gieson).

The constant association of fibroblasts

with developing collagenous fibers both in vivo and in vitro early suggested that these cells were involved in fibrogenesis, but their exact role has long been a subject of debate. The area of controversy has been considerably narrowed in recent years. It is now widely accepted that reticular and collagenous fibers arise extracellularly by polymerization of molecular collagen secreted into the ground substance by fibroblasts. Consistent with this view is the electron microscopic observation that fibroblasts of growing connective tissue have the extensive endoplasmic reticulum and well developed Golgi complex that we have come to expect of cells actively engaged in protein synthesis. Moreover, if ^{14}C labeled proline is given to animals in which inflammatory new formation of connective tissue has been induced, labeled collagen can be detected in the microsome fraction isolated from connective tissue cells. Incorporation of labeled amino acid in fibroblasts can also be followed autoradiographically in animals with healing wounds. At early time intervals after administration of tritiated proline, the silver grains betraying the location of the labeled precursor are over the endoplasmic reticulum; later they are seen over the Golgi region and still later outside of the cell, over newly formed collagen fibers.

The evidence thus points to a synthetic pathway for collagen, similar to that described for secretion of other proteins (Fig. 6–14). On the ribosomes of the endoplasmic reticulum activated amino acids are assembled into polypeptide alpha chains, each composed of about 1000 amino acids. Hydroxylation of the prolyl and lysyl residues takes place while the nascent alpha chains are still being synthesized. While the alpha chains are still associated with the ribosomes or immediately after their release into the lumen of the endoplasmic reticulum, they associate in helical configuration to form procollagen molecules with a molecular weight of 336,000. The exact location of the other posttranslational events is uncertain, but the procollagen molecules appear to be transported through the lumen of the endoplasmic reticulum, and attachment of carbohydrate (mainly galactose and glycosylgalactose in O-glycosidic linkage to the hydroxyl group of hydroxylysine) is believed to take place in the Golgi complex. Molecular collagen segregated in Golgi vacuoles is released from the fibroblast when these vacuoles move to the cell surface and discharge their contents into the surrounding ground substance.

A recent development in our understanding of collagen synthesis has been the discovery of *procollagen,* an antecedent of the definitive collagen molecule (Church et al.; Bornstein et al.). Procollagen subunits corresponding to α_1 and α_2 chains have been described, which have a molecular weight of 112,000—distinctly larger than the alpha chains of collagen. Their greater length and higher molecular weight is attributed to the presence of an extra peptide on the N-terminal end of the molecule. This is now believed to be the original form in which collagen is synthesized in the cell. The intracellular procollagen molecules are evidently unable to polymerize into collagen fibers. However, an enzyme *procollagen peptidase,* has been identified, which is presumed to be located in the cell or at its surface. This is believed to cleave off the telopeptide converting procollagen to collagen at the time of its release from the cell. The resulting molecules are then free to polymerize extracellularly into cross-striated fibers.

A remaining point of uncertainty concerns the possible role of the cells in determining the arrangement of the fibers. The majority of histologists assume that the cells simply maintain the appropriate physicochemical conditions in the surrounding ground substance to permit collagen fibers to form extracellularly by a process of spontaneous polymerization similar to that occurring in vitro. Such a process could presumably take place at some distance from the fibroblast. The orientation of the fibrils would be in response to mechanical stresses in the tissue and would not be influenced by the cells. A few investigators believe that new fibrils arise only in very close relation to the cell surface, and that the cells exercise a direct control over their formation and their orientation in the connective tissue. It is contended that the orthogonal patterns and other precisely ordered arrangements of collagen fibers in the body are difficult to explain if collagen deposition is a completely independent extracellular phenomenon, whereas, if collagen is deposited on protofibrils that are oriented by fibroblasts, a mechanism is provided for ordering of collagen fibrils by the cells rather than by purely mechanical forces. Further study is needed to resolve this problem.

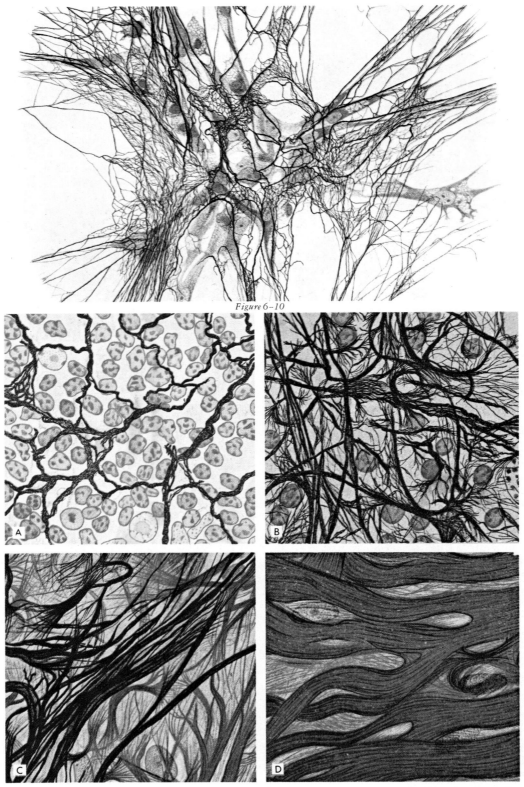

Figure 6–10

Figure 6–11

See legends on opposite page.

FIXED CELLULAR ELEMENTS

It is convenient to think of the cells of loose connective tissue in two categories, a relatively stable population of *fixed cells*— fibroblasts (responsible for production and long term maintenance of the extracellular components) and adipose cells (for storage of reserve fuel), and a population of mobile *wandering cells*, which are mainly concerned with the shorter term events involved in tissue reaction to injury (lymphoid cells, free macrophages, eosinophils, plasma cells, mast cells).

Fibroblasts

These are the common fixed cells of the connective tissue that elaborate the precursors of the extracellular fibrous and amorphous components.* Their shape depends to some extent upon their physical substrate. They are usually deployed along bundles of collagen fibers and appear in sections as fusiform elements with long tapering proc-

---

*The student should be aware of troublesome inconsistency in terminology with respect to this cell type. The suffix *-blast* (Greek *blastos*, germ) is often used in naming the formative stages of various cell types. Thus an *erythroblast* is an early developmental stage of the fully differentiated cell called an *erythrocyte*. Some authors, therefore, use the term *fibroblast* to designate a relatively immature cell actively proliferating and producing components of the extracellular substance, and they apply *fibrocyte* to the relatively quiescent cells of adult connective tissue. This interpretation loses sight of the fact that the term "fibroblast" was originally intended to describe a "fiber forming cell" and not to name an immature form of a cell called a fibrocyte. Moreover, because most histologists recognize *mesenchymal cells*, persisting in postnatal life, as the undifferentiated progenitors of the connective tissue cells, to use "fibroblast" in this sense is to make an unnecessary distinction and to introduce a redundant term. The term *fibroblast*, therefore, is properly used to describe the differentiated cell of adult connective tissue, and it can be considered synonymous with *fibrocyte* (as used by other authors).

esses. In other situations they may be flattened, stellate cells with several slender processes. Their cytoplasm is often eosinophilic like the neighboring collagen. The outlines of the cell bodies are therefore difficult to make out. They are more easily visualized after staining with iron-hematoxylin.

These cells have been extensively studied in tissue culture, where they can be observed free of the interlacing fabric of fibers in which they reside in vivo. In this environment the cells migrate out from the explant into the surrounding medium, with their processes adhering to form a cellular network (Fig. 6–15). It is not unlikely that the fibroblasts in the body also maintain tenuous contacts with one another, but for technical reasons this is difficult to demonstrate.

The elliptical nucleus is usually smoothly contoured but may sometimes be slightly folded. There are one or two nucleoli, and the chromatin is sparse and distributed in very small karyosomes. A pair of centrioles and a small Golgi apparatus are situated near the nucleus. The long, slender mitochondria are found mainly in the cell body, but they may also occur in the processes. Under conditions of stimulation, as in wound healing, when fibroblasts are dividing and actively synthesizing extracellular components, they enlarge and their cytoplasm becomes moderately basophilic. In electron micrographs the quiescent fibroblasts are seen to contain a small Golgi complex and only a few cisternal profiles of granular endoplasmic reticulum, but in growing or repairing connective tissue, the Golgi complex becomes very prominent and the endoplasmic reticulum is much more extensive. The cytoplasm usually contains few inclusions except for occasional small fat droplets. Granules staining with the periodic acid–Schiff reaction become numerous under some conditions and may represent intracellular precursors of the poly-

---

Figure 6–10 Development of reticular fibers in a 20 day culture of adult rabbit thymus. The reticular fibers stain black. Bielschowsky-Foot and Mallory-azan stains. About ×500. (After A. A. Maximow.)

Figure 6–11 Four stages in the development of collagenous fibers in tissue cultures of rabbit lymph node. *A*, Section of lymph node showing cells and blackened reticular fibers. *B*, After four days in vitro the black reticular fibers are branching and more numerous. *C*, After five days in culture the black reticular fibers contrast with the newly developed collagenous fibers stained blue. *D*, After six days in culture only thick bundles of collagenous fibers are present. It is now realized that both types of fiber are composed of collagen, but their staining properties depend upon their size and mode of aggregation. Bielschowsky-Foot and Mallory-azan stains. About ×500. (After R. McKinney.)

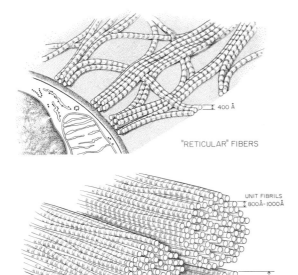

"RETICULAR" FIBERS

UNIT FIBRILS
800Å-1000Å

1-4μ

COLLAGEN FIBERS

Figure 6–12 Diagram showing that the "reticular" fibers" associated with the basal lamina of an epithelial cell (*above*) and the "collagen fibers" of the connective tissue in general (*below*) are both composed of unit fibrils of collagen. Those of reticulum are somewhat smaller and interwoven in loose networks instead of aggregating in large bundles.

saccharides of the ground substance. In electron micrographs, these granules are represented by small vacuoles in the Golgi region and elsewhere, containing a flocculent material that is interpreted as a secretory product.

Fibroblasts normally show no tendency to take up foreign matter, but under intense and prolonged stimulation by injection of a colloidal vital dye, such as trypan blue, they may come to contain a few minute deposits of the dye (Fig. 6–16). Majority opinion holds that fibroblasts are differentiated cells that ordinarily do not give rise to other types of cells in the connective tissue. There is suggestive evidence, however, that in pathological states and under certain experimental conditions, they can develop into bone cells. It is also widely accepted that fibroblasts may accumulate lipid and become typical adipose cells, but in both of these instances, it is difficult to establish with certainty whether it

is actually the fibroblasts or their undifferentiated mesenchymal progenitors that undergo these transformations.

Mesenchymal Cells

It is commonly believed that a population of cells which retain the developmental potentialities of embryonic mesenchymal cells persists in the adult organism. They are somewhat smaller than fibroblasts and less highly differentiated but they have much the same appearance and cannot easily be distinguished from them in ordinary histological sections (Fig. 6–13). In loose connective tissue they are usually deployed along the blood vessels, especially along the capillaries.

The conviction that they are not common fibroblasts but are more primitive, relatively undifferentiated cells is gained from numerous observations which show that under the influence of certain stimuli, such as in inflammation or injection of toxins, or on being explanted to tissue culture, they may develop into other cell types.

Many investigators regard these cells, rather than fibroblasts, as the precursors of adipose cells. When mast cells of connective tissue have been selectively destroyed, they are slowly restored, apparently by differentiation of primitive cells along the blood vessels. When the vessels themselves are obliged to grow and change the character of their walls in response to altered hemodynamic conditions, the smooth muscle cells required seem to be recruited by differentiation of these pluripotential cells in the perivascular connective tissue.

Adipose Cells

Among the fixed cells in loose connective tissue are some that are specialized for the synthesis and storage of lipid. These *adipose cells* or *fat cells* accumulate lipid to such an extent that the nucleus is flattened and displaced to one side, and the cytoplasm becomes so thinned out that it is resolved only as a thin line around the rim of the single large lipid droplet. So inconspicuous are the nucleus and cytoplasm that the fat cells in fresh connective tissue have the appearance of large glistening drops of oil. They may occur singly in the connective tissue but are more often found in groups. There is a marked tendency for them to be located along the course of small blood vessels. When they accumulate in such large numbers that they become the predominant component, crowding out other cell types, the resulting tissue is called *adipose tissue* or *fat* (see Chapter 7). All intermediate grades between loose connective tissue and typical adipose tissue can be found.

In the preparation of the usual histological section the lipid droplets of the adipose cells are dissolved out during dehydration, and there remains only the thin layer of cytoplasm, slightly thickened in one area to accommodate the nucleus. Despite the extreme thinness of the rim of cytoplasm, a juxtanuclear Golgi apparatus can be demonstrated, and filamentous mitochondria are distributed around the entire circumference of the lipid droplet. The individual fat cells are surrounded by a delicate network of reticular fibers.

Adipose cells appear to develop from spindle-shaped cells that resemble fibroblasts, but, as indicated above, these are generally believed to be undifferentiated mesenchymal cells that persist into postnatal life in the adventitia of the small blood vessels of the connective tissue. During their early development they may contain multiple small lipid droplets, but these ultimately coalesce into a single drop (Fig. 6–17). The fully formed fat cell is incapable of mitotic division. Any new areas of adipose cells that develop in adult life must therefore differentiate from fusiform precursors.

Macrophages (Histiocytes)

Stretched out along the bundles of collagen fibers are stellate or fusiform cells that in some regions of the body are almost as abundant as the fibroblasts and are often difficult to distinguish from them (Fig. 6–1). These are the *fixed macrophages* or *histiocytes.*

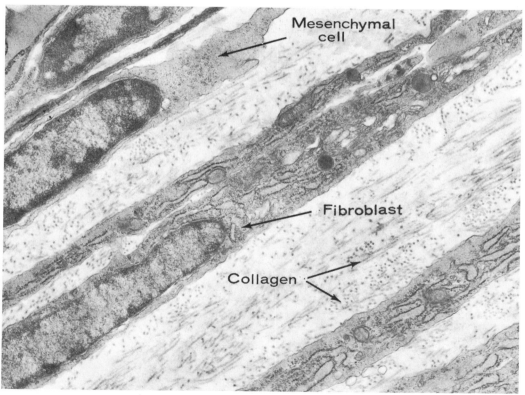

Figure 6–13 Electron micrograph of fibroblasts of developing connective tissue. The active fibroblasts forming collagen have an abundant granular reticulum with distended cisternae. The relatively undifferentiated cell at the upper left has a different chromatin pattern and little differentiation of its cytoplasm. The newly formed collagen fibrils are slender and more or less randomly oriented.

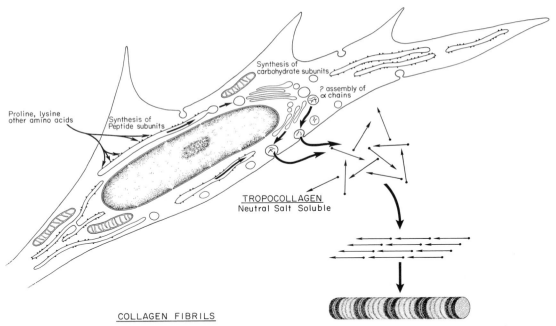

Proline, lysine other amino acids

Synthesis of Peptide subunits

Synthesis of carbohydrate subunits

? assembly of α chains

TROPOCOLLAGEN
Neutral Salt Soluble

COLLAGEN FIBRILS

Figure 6–14   Schematic representation of the intracellular and extracellular events in the elaboration of collagen. Amino acids entering the fibroblast are synthesized into polypeptide subunits at the ribosomes. These are transported to the Golgi complex, where carbohydrate subunits are believed to be synthesized. The α chains of collagen are presumed to be assembled in the Golgi complex into tropocollagen molecules. Tropocollagen molecules released at the cell surface aggregate extracellularly in staggered array to form collagen fibrils. (Redrawn after J. Gross.)

Their nuclei tend to be somewhat smaller and more darkly staining than those of fibroblasts. Near the nucleus is the cytocentrum, containing a diplosome and a closely associated Golgi apparatus. The mitochondria are short rods, usually congregated around the centrosome. The cytoplasm is more heterogeneous than that of fibroblasts, often containing a variety of granules and small vacuoles that stain supravitally with neutral red.

The majority of the macrophages in normal connective tissue are sessile, but when they are stimulated in inflammation they withdraw their processes, detach from the fibers and become actively motile as *free macrophages.* If such macrophages chance to be fixed in different stages of their ameboid migratory movements, they may be highly variable in outline, but as a rule in histological sections they are more or less rounded cells distributed singly or in small clusters in the fibrous meshes of the connective tissue. In electron micrographs they may have many folds and microvillous projections from their

surfaces. The plasma membrane may also be deeply invaginated. The cytoplasm contains many vacuoles, and numerous lysosomes and residual bodies (Fig. 6–19).

These cells have a remarkable capacity for *phagocytosis,* the process wherein blunt pseudopodia or undulating surface folds are extended around foreign particulate matter that is then taken into the cytoplasm in vacuoles. This behavior can be elicited experimentally by injecting into the living animal nontoxic colloidal dyes, such as lithium carmine or trypan blue. The macrophages take up ultramicroscopic particles of the dye by phagocytosis and concentrate them within cytoplasmic vacuoles. Under the same conditions, the fibroblasts and other cell types take up little or none of the dye (Fig. 6–16). The use of such vital dyes is the most certain means of identifying macrophages. They are equally avid in their ingestion of extravasated erythrocytes, debris of dead cells, bacteria, and inert foreign matter. Because of their motility and great phagocytic capacity, the macrophages constitute a mobile reserve of scavenger cells important in the maintenance of the connective tissues and in the local defenses of the body against bacterial invasion. In addition to their phagocytic activity, macrophages are believed to play a significant role in the immunological defenses of the body. They appear to store and process antigens and present them to antibody producing cells in a form with enhanced immunogenicity (see Chapter 14).

The macrophages of the loose connective tissue have also been called *clasmatocytes, rhagiocrine cells, histiocytes, resting wandering cells,* and many other names.

MONONUCLEAR WANDERING CELLS

In addition to the fixed or sessile cell types of connective tissue there are several types of migratory cells that are emigrants from the blood—*lymphocytes, monocytes, eosinophils,* and *neutrophils.* Because of their capacity for ameboid locomotion and their tendency to congregate at sites where their services are needed, their numbers in the connective tissue are highly variable, depending upon the local conditions. They were formerly regarded as blood cells carrying out essential functions in the circulation and only secondarily leaving the blood to take up residence in the connective tissue. The development of ingenious methods of tagging these cells, of determining their life span, and of following their movements in the body has brought about a fundamental change in our interpretation of their mission.

Monocytes

Many of the wandering cells in connective tissue appear to be *monocytes.* The largest of these may be 12 μm. or more in diameter and have an eccentric, kidney-shaped nucleus and a highly heterogeneous cytoplasm containing various vacuoles that stain supravitally with neutral red.

In local inflammatory reactions, additions are made to the resident population of phagocytes in connective tissue by emigration of more monocytes from the blood and their

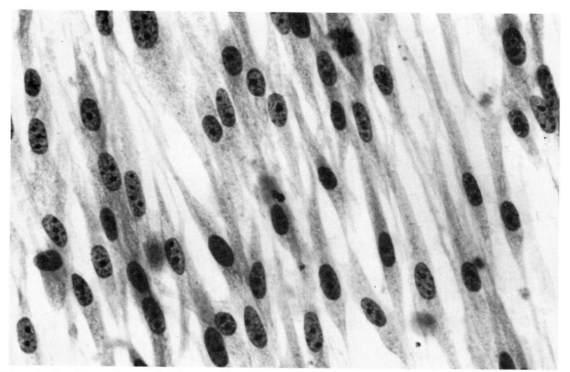

Figure 6-15 Photomicrograph of mouse fibroblasts in tissue culture, illustrating their common spindle shape. Harris hematoxylin stain. ×600.

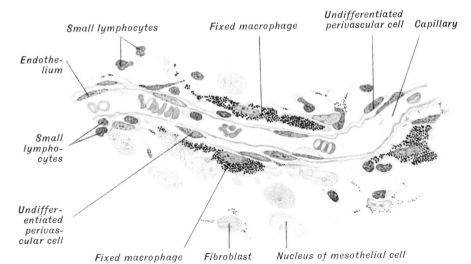

Small lymphocytes   Fixed macrophage   Undifferentiated perivascular cell   Capillary

Endothelium

Small lymphocytes

Undifferentiated perivascular cell

Fixed macrophage   Fibroblast   Nucleus of mesothelial cell

Figure 6–16 Stretch preparation of rabbit omentum vitally stained with lithium carmine, showing undifferentiated perivascular cells, macrophages, and other cellular elements of the connective tissue. Hematoxylin stain. ×500. (After A. A. Maximow.)

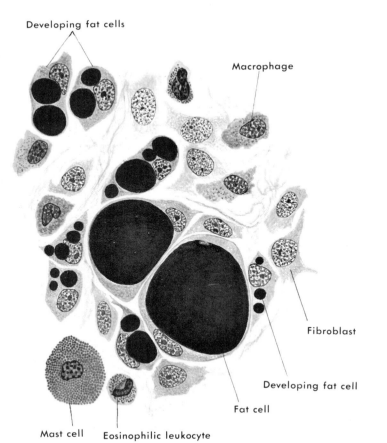

Developing fat cells

Macrophage

Fibroblast

Developing fat cell

Fat cell

Mast cell   Eosinophilic leukocyte

Figure 6–17 Several fat cells from the subcutaneous loose connective tissue of a rat. The fat has been stained black by the osmic acid of the fixation fluid. About ×1000. (After A. A. Maximow.)

transformation into macrophages (Fig. 6–20). In chronic inflammatory reactions the macrophages may become closely packed and may take on the appearance of *epithelioid cells*. Around foreign objects in the tissues that are too large or too resistant to be engulfed and destroyed by intracellular digestion, these phagocytic cells may coalesce to form huge multinucleate masses called *foreign body giant cells.*

The same sequence of transformation of mononuclear wandering cells that occurs in inflamed connective tissue can be observed when mixed leukocytes from blood are cultivated in vitro. Under the conditions prevailing in such cultures the lymphocytes and the monocytes are the only leukocytes capable of prolonged survival. The monocytes are rapidly transformed into macrophages. The effete and dying cellular elements of other kinds are phagocytosed and eliminated. Thus, after a few days, pure cultures of macrophages are obtained (Fig. 6–20). These may later flatten out on the glass substrate and assume an epithelioid appearance. After prolonged cultivation, giant cells are formed. The ability to follow in vitro the same sequence of cellular transformation that occurs in inflamed tissues has made it possible to study in considerable detail the fine structural and cytochemical changes associated with the transition from monocytes to macrophages and to epithelioid and giant cells. Accompanying the acquisition of phagocytic properties, there is an increase in cell volume and a striking enlargement of the Golgi apparatus which becomes the site of active formation of many small lysosomes. During the intracellular digestion of ingested material, the lysosomes discharge their content of hydrolytic enzymes into the phagocytotic vacuoles. Thus the number of lysosomes diminishes during active phagocytosis. They accumulate again in great numbers in the

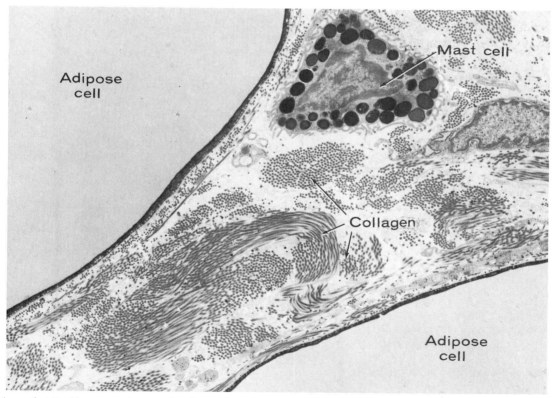

Figure 6–18 Electron micrograph of portions of two adipose cells and the intervening collagenous fibers. Relative to the mast cell and fibroblast at the upper right, the adipose cells are enormous. Only a small portion of each is included in this field, but enough to show the thin peripheral layer of cytoplasm and the homogeneous gray lipid inclusion.

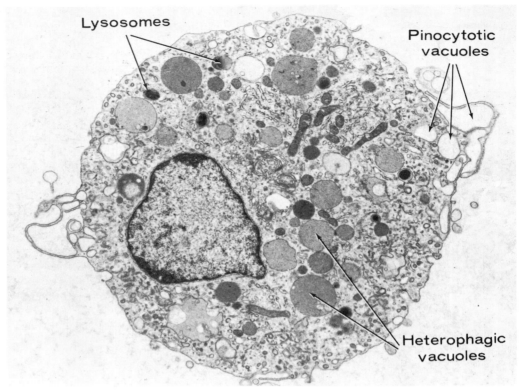

Lysosomes

Pinocytotic vacuoles

Heterophagic vacuoles

Figure 6-19 Electron micrograph of a free macrophage in edematous loose connective tissue, illustrating the heterogeneity of its cytoplasm, which has numerous lysosomes, vesicles and vacuoles. Thin ruffles or folds on its surface were immobilized by the fixative in various phases of their pinocytotic activity.

epithelioid and giant cells that develop after the cellular debris and other material available for phagocytosis has been largely eliminated.

Mononuclear Phagocyte System (Reticuloendothelial System)

The possible portals of entry of infectious microorganisms are many, and the body's defenses need to be widely deployed. The fixed and free macrophages of the connective tissue share the property of phagocytosis and storage of vital dyes with a variety of other cell types broadly distributed in the body. These have been assigned different names in different organs: monocytes of the blood, fixed and free macrophages of the connective tissue, alveolar phagocytes of the lung, the microglia of the brain, reticular cells of bone marrow and lymphoid organs, the Kupffer cells of the liver. Although these cells differ in appearance and in their relation to

the surrounding tissue components, the desirability of grouping them together on the basis of common structural features and their shared property of being avidly phagocytic was generally recognized. They were therefore considered by Metchnikoff (1892) to constitute a diffuse "cell system" which he termed the *macrophage system*. Relying upon the uptake and storage of vital dyes such as trypan blue as a measure of phagocytic capacity, Aschoff (1924) broadened this concept to include the specialized endothelia lining sinusoids in the liver, spleen, and bone marrow, as well as the phagocytic cell types enumerated above, and proposed the term *reticuloendothelial system*, which is still widely used and strongly defended by its proponents (Fig. 6–21).

This more inclusive term is now criticized on several grounds. Trypan blue not only enters highly phagocytic cells but also, when used in high concentrations, may be taken up in small amounts by micropinocytosis in endothelium, reticular cells, fibro-cytes, and even adipose cells—cells with lit-tle phagocytic capacity. As methods have developed for marking cells with radioactive isotopes, or abnormal chromosomes or stable tissue antigens, it has been possible to trace cell lineages and to carry out cytokinetic studies that have substantially changed our concepts of this system. Some specialists in this field now prefer to place all highly phag-ocytic mononuclear cells and their precursors in one system, the *mononuclear phagocyte system* and to exclude such facultative phag-ocytes as fibroblasts, endothelial cells, and the like, which can ingest particles at a very low rate and in the absence of antibodies or complement. Included in the mononuclear phagocyte system are promonocytes of the bone marrow, monocytes of the blood and the free and fixed macrophages of con-nective tissues in many organs. The func-tional criteria for inclusion are avid phago-cytosis, ability to attach firmly to glass in vitro,

and possession on their surface membranes of receptor sites for immunoglobulins and complement, which play an important part in the attachment phase of phagocytosis. In addition to the morphological and functional affinities of these cells, there is increasing evidence that they have a common origin. Mononuclear phagocytes do not appear in embryonic tissues and organs until these have become vascularized. Numerous studies with isotopic or chomosomal markers have shown that mononuclear phagocytes in general orig-inate from precursor cells in the bone mar-row, are transported via the peripheral blood as monocytes, migrate into the tissues, and there become macrophages (Fig. 6–22). The monocytic origin of the Kupffer cells of the liver and the alveolar macrophages of the lung has recently been demonstrated. The promonocyte of the bone marrow is the ear-liest microscopically identifiable cell in this lineage. There must, of course, be a more immature stem cell feeding into the pool of promonocytes, but the morphology of this cell is still unknown. This is part of the more general problem of the nature of the hemo-poietic stem cell of the bone marrow (see Chapter 8).

In the many previous editions of this book, the opinion was expressed that under certain circumstances, lymphocytes can give rise to macrophages. This view, strongly held by Maximow, later derived some sup-port from apparent transformations of this kind in tissue culture. More recently it was reported that in graft-versus-host reactions, macrophages may originate from thoracic duct lymphocytes (Howard), but this has not been confirmed in subsequent studies (Bell and Shand). In short, modern cytokinetic studies have provided no convincing evi-dence of lymphocyte–macrophage transfor-mation and there no longer seems to be any reason to perpetuate this belief. It is now realized that monocytes originate in the bone marrow and are present in the blood as transient elements simply in transit to the connective tissues of various organs, where they carry out their respective functions.

Lymphocytes

The smallest of the wandering cells of connective tissue are the lymphocytes, which are identical to those of the blood and display similar variations in size. The smallest are

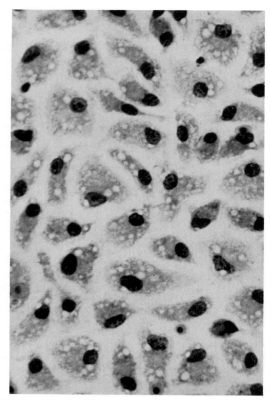

Figure 6–20 Photomicrograph of macrophages which developed from monocytes of chicken blood after a few days in tissue culture. May-Grünwald-Giemsa stain. ×500.

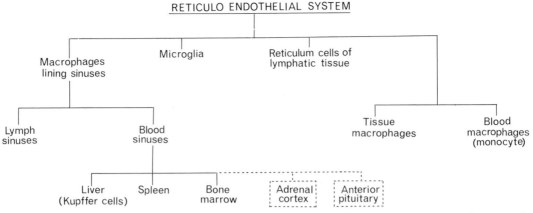

RETICULO ENDOTHELIAL SYSTEM

Figure 6-21 The traditional reticuloendothelial system: a diffuse system of macrophages and special phago-cytic endothelial cells lining blood sinuses in various organs. Though widely separated, they were grouped together because they shared similar phagocytic properties. The sinusoids of the pituitary and adrenal originally included are shown here in interrupted lines because electron microscopy has shown that it is not the endothelial cells in these organs that are phagocytic, but perivascular macrophages. The alleged phagocytic properties of the splenic sinusoids are now also seriously questioned and in the liver these properties reside only in the Kupffer cells and not the endothelium proper. Thus, the endothelial component of the reticulo-endothelial system has been largely eliminated by modern research methods.

7 to 8 μm. in diameter, with a round or slight-ly indented, darkly staining nucleus sur-rounded by a narrow rim of clear, basophilic cytoplasm. In electron micrographs a nucleo-lus can be identified among the clumps of chromatin. A juxtanuclear diplosome, a small Golgi complex, and a few mitochondria are found in the cytoplasm. The endoplasmic reticulum is sparse or absent, but numerous free ribosomes are present. Lymphocytes, as seen in tissue sections, are spheroidal and smooth contoured, showing little evidence of motility. When observed in cell cultures, however, they are actively ameboid and are no doubt migratory in the tissues as well. They are not phagocytic.

The introduction by Ehrlich (1879) of methods for differential staining of blood smears aroused interest in the lymphocytes, but because of their small size and the lack of any means of tagging them, it was difficult for early histologists to carry out meaningful experiments designed to clarify their origin, function, or fate. In the absence of clear evi-dence, there was great diversity of opinion and lively controversy over their function and their capacity to give rise to other cell types. A voluminous and contradictory literature developed, much of which is now only of historical interest. The availability of ³H-thymidine and the development of auto-radiography in the 1950's led to experiments that provided the first solid information about these fascinating cells. It was shown that lymphocytes recirculate from blood to lymph and back to blood (Gowans), and that not all lymphocytes have the same life span (Everett, Caffrey and Rieke). Some are short-lived, persisting for less than a week, while others regularly remain for four or five years in man and some may survive as long as 20 years. It has been clearly established that lym-phocytes are essential agents of the immuno-logical defenses of the body by reason of their ability to generate antibody forming cells and the effectors of cell-mediated immunity. They are not end stages of differentiation, as was once thought, but some are in a pro-longed resting state. When appropriately stimulated by specific antigens, they are capa-ble of transforming into large, immature ap-pearing basophilic cells that proliferate to form additional lymphocytes, and some of these in turn undergo further differentiation into plasma cells that synthesize antibody against the stimulating antigen. The involve-ment of lymphocytes in the immune mechan-isms will be discussed in detail in a later chapter (see Chapter 14). It will suffice here to note that they are present in normal con-nective tissue in small numbers, but they in-crease dramatically in the primary response to foreign protein and in chronic inflamma-tory conditions.

Plasma Cells

Another cell type that has a very impor-tant function in resistance to disease is the *plasma cell*, which is now known to be the prin-

cipal producer of *antibodies,* the immune globulins of the blood that participate in the
body's humoral defenses against bacterial
infection. These cells do not themselves emigrate from the blood, but they differentiate in
the connective tissue from lymphocytes that
have done so. Plasma cells are relatively uncommon in typical loose connective tissue,
but they are plentiful in the highly cellular
connective tissue composing the lamina propria of the gastrointestinal tract. They also
occur in lymphoid tissues throughout the
body. They may be nearly as small as lymphocytes or two or three times that size. They are
ovoid, with a slightly eccentric, round or
oval nucleus and an intensely basophilic cytoplasm. The nuclear chromatin is distributed
in unusually coarse clumps or blocks that
tend to be spaced around the periphery of
the nucleus so as to produce a characteristic
radial pattern that is helpful in identification
of the cell. Adjacent to the nucleus is a conspicuous lightly staining area, which represents the negative image of a prominent
Golgi apparatus (Fig. 6–23). The remainder

MONONUCLEAR PHAGOCYTE SYSTEM

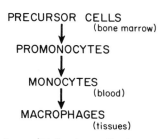

PRECURSOR CELLS
(bone marrow)

PROMONOCYTES

MONOCYTES
(blood)

MACROPHAGES
(tissues)

Connective tissue (histiocytes or fixed macrophages)
Liver (Kupffer cells)
Lung (alveolar macrophages)
Spleen (free and fixed macrophages)
Lymph node (free and fixed macrophages)
Bone marrow (macrophages)
Serous cavity (pleural and peritoneal macrophages)
Nervous system (microglial cells?)

Figure 6–22 The proposed reinterpretation of the
reticuloendothelial system (the mononuclear phagocyte system) which is a group of widely dispersed
cell types that are related not only by their morphology and phagocytic function but also by having
a common origin. It is suggested that the phagocytic
cells in all of the tissues and organs listed are
derived from precursors in the marrow via monocytes of the blood. (Modified slightly from R. Van
Furth, ed., Mononuclear Phagocytes. Oxford, Blackwell Publications, 1970.)

of the cell body has a strong affinity for basic
dyes. The basophilia and pyroninophilia of
the cytoplasm are abolished by digestion with
ribonuclease and hence these properties are
attributed to its high content of ribonucleoprotein. Fully differentiated plasma cells
seldom divide. They exhibit a sluggish motility and have no demonstrable phagocytic
activity. They arise from large lymphoid elements that develop from antigen stimulated
lymphocytes. In the course of this differentiation there is a relative increase in cytoplasm
and an enlargement of the Golgi complex,
while the nucleus becomes smaller and more
chromophilic.

The coarse chromatin pattern seen in
plasma cells with the light microscope is also
evident in electron micrographs (Fig. 6–24).
The juxtanuclear pale zone is the site of a
pair of centrioles and a well developed Golgi
complex. A few membrane bounded spherical bodies associated with the inner face of
the Golgi complex resemble secretory granules but are more likely lysosomal in nature.
The peripheral cytoplasm is occupied by an
extensive system of cisternae of the endoplasmic reticulum. Ribosomes are very numerous, both on the membranes of the reticulum
and in the cytoplasmic matrix. The abundant
ribosomes and highly developed reticulum
are involved in the synthesis of the immune
globulins (antibodies). In some plasma cells
the cisternae are flat and generally parallel
in their arrangement. In others they are
greatly distended with flocculent material of
relatively low density. These different cytological appearances may reflect different degrees of activity or varying degrees of storage
of the product.

Occasionally plasma cells may contain
conspicuous spherical inclusions, called
Russell bodies after the cytologist who first
described them in 1890. These stain with histochemical reactions for both protein and
carbohydrate, but the intensity of their reaction is variable from cell to cell. Their glycoprotein nature suggested that they might
contain immunoglobulin, and their positive
reaction with fluorescein conjugated antibody
against immunoglobulin G seems to bear this
out. In electron micrographs they are found
to be within distended cisternae of the rough
endoplasmic reticulum. Although they contain immunoglobulin, the Russell bodies are
not to be regarded as the normal secretory
product but probably represent an aberrant

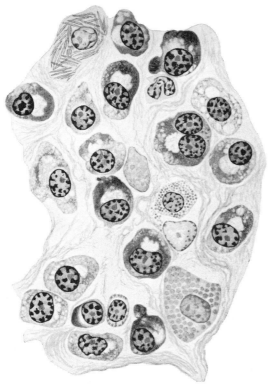

Figure 6-23 Plasma cells from connective tissue near human tonsil. There are transitions from small lymphocytes to plasma cells. Several of the latter contain globular or crystalloid inclusions. Hematoxylin-eosin-azure II stain. (After A. A. Maximow.)

state exhibited by a portion of the population of plasma cells subjected to repeated antigenic stimulation. It is possible that they represent an accumulation of the light chains that are not being used in the biosynthesis of complete globulin molecules. Whether their presence is indicative of a defect in either synthesis or transport remains to be determined.

The normal mechanism of release of immunoglobulin from plasma cells is not understood. There is no evidence of its concentration in the Golgi complex to form secretory granules. Continuity of cisternae of the reticulum with the cell surface has rarely if ever been reported, and images of discharging vesicles or vacuoles are equally rare.

The chain of evidence for the participation of plasma cells in antibody formation extends back over the past 30 years and includes observations and experiments from various disciplines. Human patients with an

excess of circulating antibody (*hyperglobulinemia*) also have a high concentration of plasma cells in their tissues. Persons with congenital *agammaglobulinemia* have a complete failure of antibody synthesis and develop no plasma cells at sites of antigenic stimulation. Intensive immunization of normal animals, on the other hand, is attended by a marked increase in the numbers of these cells in the connective tissues of nearly every organ. Although these correlations strongly supported the inference that plasma cells were the source of antibody, compelling experimental evidence has been obtained only recently. The production of antibody in vitro by individual plasma cells isolated by micromanipulation has now been demonstrated. An ingenious immunohistochemical method adapted for use at the electron microscope level has also made it possible to localize antibody within the cisternae of the endoplasmic reticulum in plasma cells from animals immunized to ferritin (de Petris et al.). Similarly, in animals being immunized against horseradish peroxidase, newly formed antibody can be demonstrated in the cisternae of plasma cells by exposure of sections to the antigen followed by histochemical localization of the enzyme (Leduc, Avrameas, and Bouteille) (Fig. 14–4).

Eosinophils

The eosinophils of connective tissue are identical to the eosinophilic leukocytes of the blood. They emigrate through the walls of the capillaries and venules to settle in the tissues. They are numerous in the loose connective tissue of the rat, mouse, and guinea pig. Eosinophils are less plentiful in the connective tissue of man but are found in the stroma of certain glands, particularly the mammary gland, in the interstitial connective tissue of the lung, and in the omentum. They are abundant in the lamina propria of the small intestine.

In man they usually have a bilobed nucleus, while in the mouse and rat the nucleus is annular (doughnut-shaped). The most distinctive cytological characteristic of the eosinophil is the presence of coarse cytoplasmic granules that stain intensely with eosin and other acid dyes. In electron micrographs the granules are membrane bounded and contain one or more flat crystals embedded in a finely granular matrix. The form of the crystal varies from species to species. In the cat it is cylindrical; in the mouse and rat it is a single flat equatorial disk; in man the crystals tend to be multiple and variable in their shape and orientation.

The eosinophilic granules have been isolated in bulk from horse and rat blood and their chemical properties have been studied. Their eosinophilia appears to reside in their protein matrix, which contains several enzymes, including peroxidase, ribonuclease, aryl-sulfatase, cathepsin, beta glucuronidase, and acid and alkaline phosphatase. Of these enzymes the first four have the highest activity. The range of the hydrolytic enzymes of eosinophilic granules is similar to those of heterophilic leukocytes and rat liver lysosomes. They differ mainly in their higher content of peroxidase and in the absence of lysozyme and phagocytin. The absence of the latter two antibacterial agents is consistent with the fact that eosinophils do not have as one of their major functions the ingestion and destruction of bacteria.

Eosinophils of the connective tissue increase in number in various parasitic infec-tions, in conditions involving allergic hypersensitivity, such as asthma and hay fever, and in the late phases of inflammatory reactions. An accumulation of histamine in the tissues is also associated with these conditions. Studies on experimentally induced inflammatory exudates rich in eosinophils have shown that the total histamine content of the exudate is correlated with the number of eosinophils. Thus there is evidence that these cells contain histamine, but the amount is relatively small compared to the histamine content of mast cells. It is estimated that the mast cell contains 20 to 2000 times as much histamine as the eosinophil.

An accumulation of eosinophils in the tissues can be induced experimentally by repeated injections of foreign protein. The requirement for repeated injections over a considerable period suggests that the appearance of the eosinophils depends in some way upon the development of antibodies against the foreign protein. It has now been shown that intraperitoneal injection of serum from a sensitized guinea pig into a normal guinea

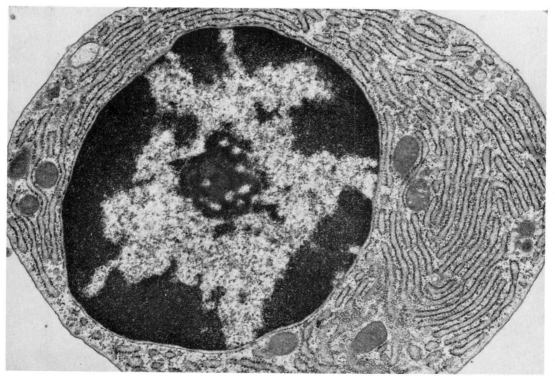

Figure 6-24 Electron micrograph of a guinea pig plasma cell. Notice the coarse pattern of chromatin and extensive granular endoplasmic reticulum. ×16,000.

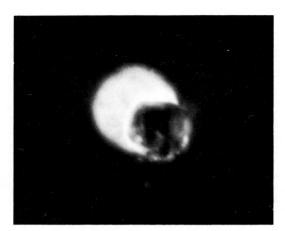

Figure 6–25 Fluorescence photomicrograph of a human plasma cell reacted with fluorescent antibody against γ_2-globulin. The strong fluorescence of the plasma cell cytoplasm identifies this cell type as one of the sites of origin of human immunoglobulins. ×1300. (After R. Mellors and L. Korngold, J. Exper. Med., *118*:387, 1963.)

pig results in an increase in eosinophils in the peritoneal fluid. If the antigenic foreign protein and serum containing antibody are injected together, 15 million or more eosinophils can be recovered by lavage of the peritoneal cavity 24 hours later. These observations have been interpreted as indicating that the presence of antigen-antibody complexes induces eosinophils to emigrate from the bloodstream and accumulate in the connective tissues (Litt).

By ingenious application of immunohistological techniques it has been shown that antigen-antibody complexes not only attract eosinophils but also are phagocytosed by them. A suitable fluorochrome was conjugated with bovine serum albumin to provide a *red* fluorescing *antigen.* Another fluorochrome was used to produce a *green* fluorescing *antibody.* The antigen-antibody complex fluoresced a brilliant yellow. Neither the antigen nor the antibody alone was taken up by eosinophils, but when the doubly labeled complex was injected into the peritoneal cavity of guinea pigs and smears of the exudate were later examined with the fluorescence microscope, numerous eosinophils contained bright yellow intracytoplasmic material. Thus one of the functions of eosinophils may be to phagocytize and destroy immune complexes. Other functions

may well be discovered for these cells in the future.

Mast Cells

Mast cells are found widely distributed in the connective tissues of most vertebrates. They are often especially abundant along small blood vessels. Their cytoplasm is filled with granules that are metachromatic when stained with certain basic aniline dyes. That is to say, the granules, in taking up the dye, change their color. Thus with methylene blue or thionine (also a blue dye), the granules assume a purple hue. Their metachromasia appears to be due to their content of strongly acidic, sulfated mucopolysaccharide. When stained supravitally with neutral red they take on a dark brick-red color (Fig. 6–26).

The size and shape of mast cells vary greatly from species to species. They are large round or ovoid cells in the rat and mouse. They are similar in shape but smaller in man, and in guinea pigs they tend to be slender and fusiform. The round nucleus is small relative to the size of the cell and is often obscured by the large number of intensely stained granules. Binucleate mast cells are not uncommon. The granules are relatively large in murine rodents (0.6 μm.) and smaller in other species. In most species the granules are soluble in aqueous fixatives.

In electron micrographs, mast cells are seen to have numerous small surface folds or villous projections (Fig. 6–27). The Golgi complex is well developed; the endoplasmic reticulum is sparse and the mitochondria are relatively few. The granules are limited by a membrane and display considerable species variability in their fine structure. Their interior is finely granular in rodents, but in man they tend to appear heterogeneous, with coarse subunits made up of lamellar whorls.

The function of mast cells in the connective tissues is poorly understood, and they continue to be a subject of intense investigation. Mast cells have been found to contain at least two compounds of physiological interest, *heparin* and *histamine.* Many years ago it was discovered that a good correlation exists between the number of mast cells in a tissue and the efficacy of extracts of that tissue in preventing coagulation of the blood. It was suggested, therefore, that the mast cells contained the potent anticoagulant heparin. This has since been abundantly verified. In recent years methods have been developed for isolating mast cells from peritoneal fluid in a high degree of purity. When such preparations are analyzed, heparin is the only major mucopolysaccharide found, and it is present in the amount of about 20 picograms (pg.) per cell.

There is a similar correlation between the number of mast cells and the histamine content of tissues. Histamine is a potent substance that increases the permeability of capillaries and venules and also has a marked effect upon the blood pressure. Pharmacological agents that cause a release of histamine in the tissues have been shown to induce mast cells to release their granules, and the amount of histamine released varies directly with the degree of mast cell degranulation. The synthesis and release of histamine thus appears to be another of the activities of mast cells.

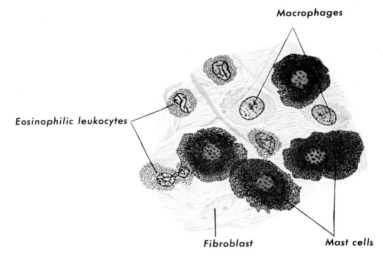

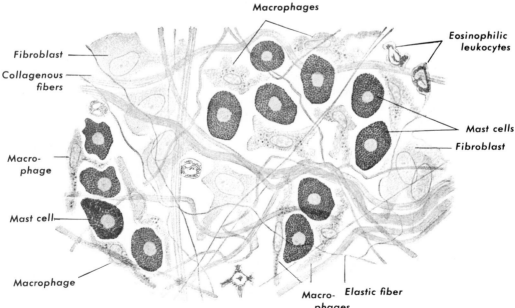

Figure 6–26   Two figures from the loose connective tissue of the rat. *Above*, Fixed and stained with hematoxylin-eosin-azure II. ×600. *Below*, Stained supravitally with neutral red. ×800. (After A. A. Maximow.)

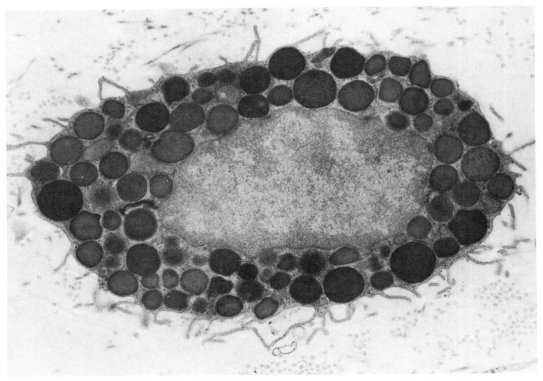

Figure 6–27   Electron micrograph of a mast cell from loose connective tissue of rat.

In the rat and mouse but not in other species, mast cells also contain *serotonin* (5-hydroxytryptamine), a substance that causes constriction of small blood vessels and influences blood pressure.

In mammals the mast cells of the connective tissue and the basophilic leukocytes of the blood are independent cell types, despite similar staining properties of their granules.

SEROUS MEMBRANES

The serous membranes, *peritoneum, pleura,* and *pericardium,* are thin layers of loose connective tissue covered by a layer of mesothelium. When the membranes are folded, forming the omentum or the mesentery, both free surfaces are covered with mesothelium. The cavities lined by serous membranes always contain a small amount of liquid, the *serous exudate.* The cells in this exudate originate from the serous membrane.

All the elements of the loose connective tissue previously described are found in the serous membranes, such as the mesentery. Because they are very thin and require no sectioning the mesenteries have been favorite sites for the microscopic study of loose connective tissue. A mesentery contains a loose network of collagenous and elastic fibers, scattered fibroblasts, macrophages, mast cells, and a varying number of fat cells.

Physiologically the most important and histologically the most interesting of the serous membranes in mammals is the *omentum.* The membrane is pierced by innumerable holes and is thus reduced to a fine lacelike net formed by collagenous bundles covered by mesothelial cells. Such thin, fenestrated areas have few or no vessels. In the thicker areas where the omentum is a continuous sheet, macrophages are numerous. There are also many small lymphocytes and plasma cells and, occasionally, eosinophilic leukocytes and mast cells (Fig. 6–28). The number of lymphocytes and plasma cells varies considerably in different animal species.

In certain areas, the macrophages and

other free cells accumulate in especially dense masses. Such macroscopically visible areas are often arranged along the blood vessels as round or oval patches called *milky spots*. These are sometimes found in the thin netlike part of the omentum. They are especially characteristic of the omentum of the rabbit.

The omentum in man extends downward from the greater curvature of the stomach like a loose curtain or veil over the intestines and is of great clinical importance in the limitation of disease processes in the abdominal cavity. When patients with a recently perforated ulcer are operated upon, it is usually found that the highly mobile omentum has already become locally adherent to the wall of the gut in an effort of nature to close the opening. Similarly, the omentum adheres at sites of inflammation and tends to wall off

the process so that a local abscess will form instead of a generalized and often fatal peritonitis. In addition to the protection afforded by the adhesion of the omentum, the free cells of its connective tissue constitute an important mobile reserve to combat infections in the peritoneal cavity.

Free Cells of the Serous Exudate

Normally, the amount of serous exudate in the body cavities is small, but in pathological conditions it may increase enormously. It contains a variety of freely floating cells, including (1) free macrophages that originate in the milky spots of the omentum and migrate into the cavity; (2) desquamated mesothelial cells that keep their squamous form or round up; (3) small lymphocytes, the vast

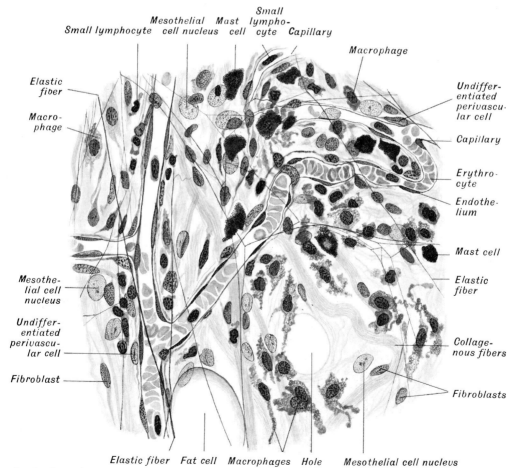

Figure 6-28 Stretch preparation of human omentum. Hematoxylin-eosin-azure II stain. ×450. (After A. A. Maximow.)

majority of which have migrated from the blood vessels of the omentum; (4) eosinophilic leukocytes of hematogenous origin; (5) free mast cells, which are especially abundant in serous exudates of rats and mice; and (6) in pathological inflammatory exudates, enormous numbers of neutrophilic leukocytes from the blood.

DENSE CONNECTIVE TISSUE

Dense connective tissue differs from the loose form mainly in the great preponderance of the fibers over the cellular and amorphous components. Where the fiber bundles are randomly oriented the tissue is described as *dense irregular connective tissue*. Where the fibers are oriented parallel to one another or in some other consistent pattern it is called *dense regular connective tissue*.

Dense Irregular Connective Tissue

This tissue is found in the dermis, the capsules of many organs, sheaths of tendons and nerves, beneath the epithelium in parts of the urinary tract, and in many other sites in the body. Its structure in the dermis of the skin can be taken as typical. The elements are the same as in the loose variety, but the collagenous bundles are thicker and are woven into a compact feltwork. They are accompanied by extensive elastic networks. The fibers from the dermis continue directly into those of the subcutaneous tissue, but there the fiber bundles are thinner and their arrangement is correspondingly looser. There is less amorphous ground substance in the dense connective tissue. Among the densely packed collagenous and elastic fibers are the cells, but these are much more difficult to identify than in the loose tissue. The macrophages are easily recognized only by vital staining. Along the small vessels there are always many inconspicuous nuclei, which probably belong to undifferentiated mesenchymal cells.

Dense Regular Connective Tissue

The collagenous bundles of regular connective tissue are arranged according to a precise plan, and the specific arrangement reflects the mechanical requirements of the particular tissue. In *tendons* the fibers form a

tissue which is flexible but offers great resistance to pulling force. Macroscopically, the tissue has a distinctly fibrous structure and a characteristic shining white appearance.

Its chief constituents are thick, closely packed, parallel collagenous bundles. They show a distinct longitudinal striation. In cross section they appear as finely dotted areas, usually separated from one another by angular lines. Fine elastic networks have been described between the collagenous bundles of tendons.

The fibroblasts, which are the only cells present, are arranged in long, parallel rows in the spaces between the parallel collagenous bundles. The cell bodies are rectangular, triangular, or trapezoidal when seen in surface view and rod-shaped when seen in profile. Their cytoplasm stains darkly with basic dyes and contains a clear centrosome adjacent to the single, flattened nucleus. Although the limits between the successive cells in a row are distinct, the lateral limits of the cells are indistinct. In a stained cross section of a tendon, the cells appear as dark star-shaped figures between the collagenous bundles. A tendon consists of a varying number of small tendon bundles bound by loose connective tissue into larger bundles (Fig. 6–31). The *ligaments* are similar to the tendons, except that the elements are somewhat less regularly arranged.

In other examples of dense regular connective tissue, such as the *fasciae* and *aponeuroses*, the collagenous bundles and fibroblasts are arranged regularly in multiple sheets or lamellae. In each layer the fibers follow a parallel and often slightly wavy course. In the different layers the direction may be the same or it may change. The fibers often pass from one layer into another. Therefore a clear isolation of the sheets is seldom possible. The cells which correspond to the tendon cells adapt their shape to the spaces between the collagenous bundles.

In the fibrous sheets with somewhat less regularly arranged elements, such as the periosteum, sclera, and the like, a section perpendicular to the surface shows successive layers of collagenous bundles cut in the longitudinal, oblique, or transverse direction, and cells which are irregular, flat, or fusiform. In these tissues there are always gradual transitions to neighboring areas, where the elements have a quite irregular, dense arrangement. There is also no sharp distinction between them and the surrounding loose connective tissue.

The cornea is an example of dense regular connective tissue that is made up of successive layers of collagen with the fibrils of one layer oriented at approximately 90 degrees to those in the next layer (Fig. 6–32).

CONNECTIVE TISSUE WITH SPECIAL PROPERTIES

Mucous Connective Tissue

This tissue is found in many parts of the embryo, especially under the skin, and is a form of the loose connective tissue. The classic example of this type of connective tissue is *Wharton's jelly* of the umbilical cord. The cells are large, stellate fibroblasts whose processes often are in contact with those of neighboring cells. A few macrophages and lymphoid wandering cells are also present.

The intercellular substance is very abundant, soft, jelly-like, and homogeneous in the fresh condition. When fixed, much of the ground substance is extracted and the residue contains granules and fibrillar precipitates. It has the staining reactions of mucin and contains thin, collagenous fibers which increase in number with the age of the fetus.

Examples of mucous connective tissue in adult animals are limited to the dermis and hypodermis of the so-called sex skin of monkeys, where the ground substance is extraordinarily abundant, and also the cock's comb. In the latter the ground substance has a very firm consistency.

Elastic Connective Tissue

In the dense connective tissue of a few parts of the body elastic fibers predominate, and the tissue has a yellow color on inspection with the naked eye. It may appear in the form of strands of coarse parallel fibers, as in the ligamenta flava of the vertebral column, in the

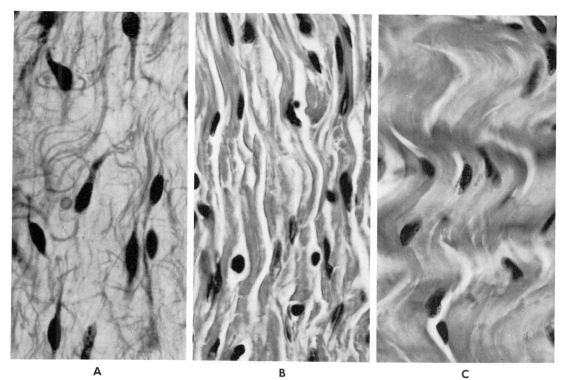

A   B   C

Figure 6–29 Photomicrographs illustrating connective tissue with varying amounts of collagen. *A*, Loose connective tissue from an eight month fetus showing relatively few, slender collagen fibers. ×650. *B*, Moderately dense, irregular connective tissue with coarse, irregularly oriented bundles of collagen. ×500. *C*, Dense connective tissue with very abundant collagen in parallel wavy bundles. ×500.

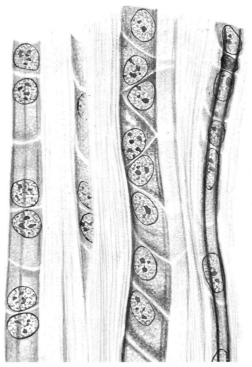

Figure 6–30 Freshly teased tendon of the tail of a rat, stained with methylene blue. The rows of tendon cells run between collagenous bundles. ×380. (After A. A. Maximow.)

vocal cords, in the ligamentum stylohyoideum, and in the ligamentum suspensorium penis. In these situations, the elastic fibers are thick, refringent, and either round or flattened in cross section. They branch frequently and rejoin with one another at acute angles, as in a stretched fishing net. In cross section the angular or round areas representing the fibers form small groups. The spaces between the elastic fibers are filled with a delicate feltwork of collagenous fibers and a few fibroblasts.

An example of *dense regular elastic connective tissue* is found in the massive ligamentum nuchae of grazing animals, which consists of coarse elastic fibers 10 to 15 μm. in diameter, closely associated in parallel bundles.

Scarpa's fascia of the human anterior abdominal wall, which aids in the support of the viscera, consists largely of elastic fibers. The corresponding layer in the large quadrupeds, called the tunica abdominalis, is a thick yellow sheet of dense elastic tissue several millimeters in thickness.

Elastic tissue forms layers in the walls of hollow organs upon which a changing pressure acts from within, as in the largest arteries; in some parts of the heart; and in the trachea and bronchi. In the large elastic arteries, the structural unit of the elastic tissue is a *fenestrated membrane,* a lamella of *elastin* of variable thickness provided with many irregular openings. The fenestrated membranes are arranged in multiple layers concentric with the lumen of the vessel and are connected with one another by oblique ribbon-like branches. The spaces between the lamellae contain a mucoid ground substance and smooth muscle cells of irregular outline. Fibrous elastic networks, as well as fenestrated elastic membranes, exist in the walls of these vessels and it is difficult to distinguish clearly between the two in sections.

Reticular Connective Tissue

Most of the fibrous elements around the sinusoids of the liver and in the stroma of lymphatic tissue, hemopoietic tissue, and the spleen are blackened by silver stains and are thus identified as reticular fibers. The patterns of the fibers in these examples of *reticular connective tissue* are also distinctive. Small bundles of thin collagenous fibrils form complex three dimensional networks, whose interstices are occupied by large numbers of free cells. Stellate cells of mesenchymal origin are also associated with the argyrophilic reticulum in these organs.

HISTOPHYSIOLOGY OF CONNECTIVE TISSUE

Normal Functions

Connective tissue functions in *mechanical support, exchange of metabolites* between blood and the tissues, *storage* of energy reserves in adipose cells, *protection* against infection, and *repair* after injury.

For its mechanical role the fibrous components are most important, and their abundance and distribution are adapted to the local structural requirements. Delicate networks of reticular fibers support the basement lamina of epithelia, surround the capillaries and sinusoids, and envelop individual muscle fibers or the groups of parenchymal cells that form the functional units of organs. The coarser collagenous fibers abound where greater tensile strength is required. They form the tendons and the aponeuroses, the septa and fibrous capsules of organs. Elastic fibers give the tissues their suppleness and their ability to spring back to their normal relations after stretching. They are especially abundant in hollow organs subject to periodic distention. Loose connective tissue, with its abundant, highly hydrated ground substance, is commonly found beneath the integument, between muscles, and in other sites where mobility of the parts is advantageous. On the other hand, where strength is more important than mobility, dense connective tissue is formed, and its bundles of collagen fibers tend to be oriented so as to resist most efficiently the local mechanical stresses.

Connective tissue plays a significant role in the nutrition of the other tissues that it surrounds and permeates. It is evident that all substances reaching the cells of these other tissues from the blood, and all the products of their metabolism that are returned to the blood and lymph, must pass through a layer of connective tissue. These metabolites are believed to diffuse through the aqueous phase of the gelatinous ground substance or along thin films of fluid coating the fibers. The exchange of materials is probably influenced by the viscous properties of the ground substance. The polyelectrolyte properties of its glycosaminoglycans suggest that the connective tissue ground substance may also participate in maintaining water and electrolyte balance. In addition to the storage of energy in adipose cells, it is noteworthy that approximately half of the circulating proteins of the body are in the interstitial spaces and, because the proportions of albumin and globulin there differ from those in plasma, it is speculated that the connective tissue may exercise some selectivity in its depot function.

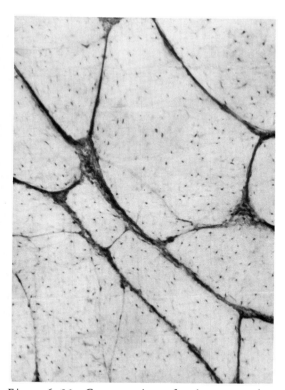

Figure 6-31 Cross section of a human tendon, showing the separation of the tendon bundles by loose connective tissue, which stains darkly. Hematoxylin-eosin-azure II stain. Photomicrograph. About ×120.

Inflammation

Of great importance in the defenses of the organism against disease is the part played by connective tissue in the local reactive process called *inflammation*. Bacteria and other exogenous noxious substances call forth an intense local reaction, in which the cells of the blood and connective tissues are mobilized to bring about the destruction of the foreign substance and the repair of the damage caused. In inflamed connective tissue, leukocytes in great numbers migrate from the capillaries and venules at the very beginning of the process. The majority of these are neutrophils that are capable of phagocytizing bacteria and other foreign matter and digesting it intracellularly through the action of the hydrolytic enzymes in their specific granules (lysosomes). The monocytes from the blood hypertrophy in the first day or two after the onset of inflammation and become transformed into the hematogenous macrophages, which supplement the fixed macrophages already present in the tissue. Stimulated by the noxious material, many of the latter are mobilized at the site as free macrophages (*histogenous macrophages*). Evidence is accumulating that in injured tissue the mast cells may act as migratory unicellular glands, supplying biologically active compounds in the region of local stress.

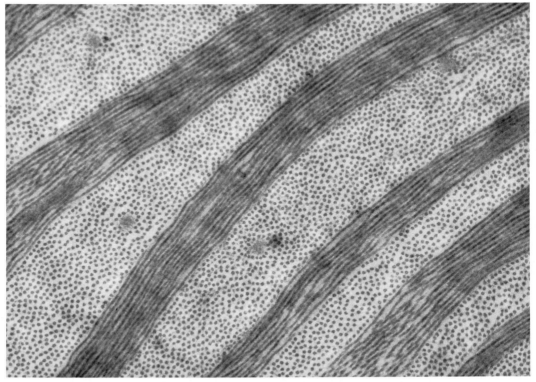

Figure 6–32 An example of dense regular connective tissue in the cornea. The collagen is arranged in lamellae with the fibrils in alternate layers oriented at right angles to those in the intervening layers. Electron micrograph. Osmium fixation. ×35,000. (Courtesy of M. Jakus.)

Their liberation of histamine may serve to increase vascular permeability and may contribute to the local inflammatory edema that dilutes the irritant and promotes its inactivation by antibodies. There is also some indication that release of histamine helps activate phagocytosis of damaged cells and cellular debris.

Repair

The regenerative capacity of fibroblasts and the fact that they respond so readily to injury by proliferation and fibrogenesis make them the principal agents of repair. They are involved in the healing of defects, not only in connective tissue proper, but also in other tissues that have little or no regenerative capacity of their own. For example, the heart muscle that degenerates following a heart attack is replaced by a connective tissue scar.

Although much has been learned about the production of collagen in the histogenesis and repair of connective tissue, it must be realized that there are also mechanisms for the removal of collagen. This is of great importance in the growth and remodeling of bone and other tissues. Systematic study of this process began only recently. It has already been shown that some tissues of tadpoles contain *collagenase*, and that the activity of this enzyme is enhanced by thyroid hormone, which induces metamorphosis and brings about resorption of the tail. Collagenases are now also being detected in mammalian tissues subject to cyclic regression, such as the uterine endometrium.

Hormonal Effects

The adrenocorticotropic hormone of the pituitary and cortisone of the adrenal cortex both tend to lower the glycosaminoglycan content of the ground substance. They also diminish the intensity of the cellular response in inflammation. The response of connective tissues to sex hormones varies greatly with the species, the sex, and the site in the body. The most dramatic effects are on the sex skin of monkeys, where estrogens greatly increase the glycosaminoglycans of the ground substance, and in the cock's comb, where testosterone stimulates accumulation of hyaluronic acid and formation of collagen. Less dramatic hormonal effects are detected in the human female in the periodic increase in hydration of the tissues during certain phases of the menstrual cycle.

Disturbances of Collagen Metabolism

Collagen metabolism is affected by age and nutrition and may be rather specifically disturbed in a number of disease states. In some of these specific disorders, recently acquired knowledge of the mechanisms of fibrogenesis has provided a partial explanation of the defect or has made it possible to identify the step in the process where the normal biosynthetic mechanism fails. It has long been known that *scurvy,* the disease resulting from deficiency of vitamin C (abscorbic acid), is attended by an inability to form collagen fibers in normal abundance. It has now been found that addition of ascorbic acid in vitro to suspensions of fibroblasts from scorbutic animals enhances their conversion of proline to hydroxyproline in collagen. This suggests that the basic defect of collagen metabolism in scorbutic animals may be impaired synthesis of hydroxyproline, one of the amino acids peculiar to collagen.

A disease of domestic animals characterized by bone deformities has been traced to the ingestion of the sweet pea *Lathyrus odoratus.* All of the abnormalities of this disease, called *lathyrism,* can be reproduced by administration of β-aminoproprionitrile, the toxic agent extracted from the sweet pea plant. Tropocollagen appears to be synthesized normally in such animals but is defective in its ability to form stable collagen fibrils. When tropocollagen is extracted at 0° C. from *normal* animals and induced to form fibers by an increase in the temperature to 37° C., the longer it is held at that temperature the less soluble it becomes at 0° C. This time dependent loss of solubility is believed to be due to formation of increased numbers of bonds between the tropocollagen units. In *lathyritic* animals there is a marked increase in the extractability of tropocollagen from connective tissue at 0° C., and although the extracted tropocollagen is capable of forming typical cross-striated fibers on warming, these fibers retain the ability to redissolve upon cooling even after prolonged periods at 37° C. This and other evidence suggest that ingestion of lathyritic agents results in synthesis of abnormal chains that are not able to cross link adequately (Gross).

A rare inherited disease of humans, *Ehlers-Danlos syndrome,* is characterized by short stature, unusually stretchable skin, hypermobility of joints, and a tendency for joint dislocations. There is a related disease of cattle and sheep called *dermatosparaxis* in which the skin is fragile and very easily torn. Recent evidence indicates that the defect may reside in an abnormally low activity of the enzyme *procollagen peptidase,* which normally converts procollagen to collagen by cleaving off a peptide from the aminoterminal ends of the α_1 and α_2 chains of procollagen (Lichtenstein et al.).

REFERENCES

Extracellular Components

Bensley, S. H.: On the presence, properties, and distribution of the intercellular ground substance of loose connective tissue. Anat. Rec., *60*:93, 1934.

Bornstein, P., H. P. Ehrlich, and A. W. Wycke: Procollagen: Conversion of precursor to collagen by a neutral protease. Science, *175*:544, 1972.

Church, R. L., S. E. Pfeiffer, and M. L. Tanzer: Collagen biosynthesis: synthesis and secretion of a high molecular weight collagen precursor (procollagen). Proc. Nat. Acad. Sci., *68*:2638, 1971.

Everett, N. B., R. W. Caffrey, and W. D. Rieke: Recirculation of lymphocytes. Ann. N.Y. Acad. Sci., *113*:887, 1964.

Grant, M. E., and D. J. Prockop: The biosynthesis of collagen. New Eng. J. Med., *286*:194–199 (I), *286*:242–248 (II), *286*:291–300 (III), 1972.

Gross, J., J. H. Highberger, and F. O. Schmitt: Extraction of collagen from connective tissue by neutral salt solutions. Proc. Nat. Acad. Sci., *41*:1, 1955.

Gross, J., and C. I. Levene: Effect of β-aminoproprionitrile on extractibility of collagen from skin of mature guinea pigs. Am. J. Path., *36*:687, 1959.

Hay, E. D.: Origin and role of collagen in the embryo. Amer. Zool. *13*:1085–1107, 1973.

Hodge, A. J., and F. O. Schmitt: The charge profile of the tropocollagen macromolecule and the packing arrangement in native-type collagen fibrils. Proc. Nat. Acad. Sci., *46*:186, 1960.

Hodge, A. J., and F. O. Schmitt: The tropocollagen macromolecule and its properties of ordered interaction. *In* Edds, M. V., ed.: Macromolecular Complexes. New York, Ronald Press, 1961.

Lichtenstein, J. R., G. R. Martin, L. D. Kohn, P. H. Byers, and V. A. McKusick: Defect in conversion of procollagen to collagen in a form of Ehlers-Danlos syndrome. Science, *182*:298, 1973.

Levene, C. I., and J. Gross: Alterations in the state of molecular aggregation of collagen induced in chick embryos by β-aminoproprionitrile. J. Exp. Med., *110*:771, 1959.

Miller, E. G., and V. G. Matukas: Biosynthesis of collagen. Fed. Proc., *33*:1197–1204, 1974.

Olsen, B. R.: Electron microscope studies on collagen. I. Native collagen fibrils. II. Mechanism of linear polymerization of tropocollagen molecules. Zeitschr. f. Zellforsch., *59*:184, 199, 1963.

Petruska, J. A., and A. J. Hodge: A subunit model for the tropocollagen macromolecule. Proc. Nat. Acad. Sci., *51*:871, 1964.

Ramachandran, G. N., ed.: Treatise on Collagen. Vol. 1, Chemistry of Collagen; G. N. Ramachandran, ed. Vols. 2A and 2B, Biology of Collagen; B. S. Gould, ed. Vol. 3, Chemical Pathology of Collagen; R. A. Milch, ed. New York, Academic Press, 1974.

Robertson, W. v.B.: D-Ascorbic acid and synthesis of collagen. Biochem. Biophys. Acta, *74*:137, 1963.

Robertson, W. v.B., and J. Hewitt: Augmentation of collagen synthesis by ascorbic acid *in vitro.* Biochim. Biophys. Acta, *49*:404, 1961.

Ross, R., and P. Bornstein: Elastic fibers in the body. Sci. Am., *224*:44–52, 1971.

Schmitt, F. O., J. Gross, and J. H. Highberger: Tropocollagen and the properties of fibrous collagen. Exper. Cell Res., *3*(Suppl.): 326, 1955.

Schubert, M.: Intercellular macromolecules containing polysaccharides. *In* Connective Tissue: Intercellular Macromolecules. London, J. & A. Churchill Ltd., 1964.

Wolbach, S. B.: Controlled formation of collagen and reticulum; a study of the source of intercellular substance in recovery from experimental scorbutus. Am. J. Path. 9 (Suppl.):689, 1933.

Cellular Elements

Allgöwer, M.: The Cellular Basis of Wound Repair. Springfield, Ill., Charles C Thomas, 1956.

Anderson, H., and M. E. Mattheissen: The histiocyte in human foetal tissues. Its morphology, cytochemistry, origin, functions, and fate. Zeitschr. f. Zellforsch. *72*:193, 1966.

Anderson, P., S. A. Slorach, and B. Uvnas: Sequential exocytosis of storage granules during antigen induced histamine release from sensitized mast cells in vitro. Acta Physiol. Scand., *88*:359–372, 1973.

Aschoff, L.: Das reticulo-endotheliale System. Ergeb. Iun. Med. und Kinderhielk., *26*:1, 1924.

Bell, E. B., and F. L. Shand: A search for macrophages derived from rat thoracic duct lymphocytes during xenogeneic graft-versus-host reaction. Ann. Inst. Pasteur, *120*:356, 1971.

Benditt, E. P., R. L. Wong, M. Arase, and E. Roeper: 5-Hydroxytryptamine in mast cells. Proc. Soc. Exper. Biol. Med., *90*:303, 1955.

Cohn, Z. A.: Structure and function of monocytes and macrophages. Adv. Immunol., *9*:163, 1968.

Cohn, Z. A., M. E. Fedorko, and J. G. Hirsch: The *in vitro* differentiation of mononuclear phagocytes. IV. The ultrastructure of macrophage differentiation in the peritoneal cavity and in culture. V. The formation of macrophage lysosomes. J. Exper. Med., *123*:747, 757, 1966.

Cohn, Z. A., and J. G. Hirsch: The isolation and properties of the specific cytoplasmic granules of rabbit polymor-phonuclear leucocytes. J. Exper. Med., *112*:982, 1960.

Cohn, Z. A., and E. Weiner: The particulate hydrolases of macrophages. I. Comparative enzymology, isolation and properties. II. Biochemical and morphological response to particle ingestion. J. Exper. Med., *118*:991, 1009, 1963.

Deane, H. S.: Some electron microscopic observations on the lamina propria of the gut, with comments on the close association of macrophages, plasma cells and eosinophils. Anat. Rec., *149*:453, 1964.

de Petris, S., G. Karlsbad, and B. Pernis: Localization of antibodies in plasma cells by electron microscopy. J. Exper. Med., *117*:849, 1963.

Downey, H.: The development of histiocytes and macrophages from lymphocytes. J. Lab. Clin. Med., *45*:499, 1955.

DuShane, G. P.: The development of pigment cells in vertebrates. *In* Biology of Melanomas: Results of a Conference held at the New York Academy of Sciences in 1946. New York, New York Academy of Sciences, Special Publication 4, 1948.

Ebert, R. H., and H. W. Florey: The extravascular development of the monocyte observed *in vivo.* Brit. J. Exper. Path. *20*:342, 1939.

Evans, H. M., and K. J. Scott: On the differential reaction to vital dyes exhibited by the two great groups of connective tissue cells. Carnegie Contributions to Embryol., *10*:1, 1921.

Fawcett, D. W.: An experimental study of mast cell degranulation and regeneration. Anat. Rec., *121*:29, 1955.

Gowans, J. L., D. D. McGregor, and D. M. Cowen: Initiation of immune responses by small lymphocytes. Nature, *196*:651, 1962.

Harris, H.: Chemotaxis and phagocytosis. *In* Macfarlane, R. G., and A. H. T. Robb-Smith, eds.: The Functions of the Blood. New York, Academic Press, 1961.

Hirsch, J. G.: Cinematographic observations on granule lysis in polymorphonuclear leucocytes during phagocytosis. J. Exper. Med., *116*:827, 1962.

Hirsch, J. G., and Z. A. Cohn: Degranulation of polymorphonuclear leucocytes following phagocytosis of micro-organisms. J. Exper. Med., *112*:1005, 1960.

Huber, H., and H. H. Fudenberg: The interaction of monocytes and macrophages with immunoglobulins and complement. Series Haemat. *3*:160, 1970.

Lagunoff, D.: Membrane fusion during mast cell secretion. J. Cell Biol., *57*:352–372, 1970.

Leduc, E. H., S. Avrameus, and M. Bouteille: Ultrastructural localization of antibody in differentiating plasma cells. J. Exp. Med., *127*:109, 1968.

Lewis, M. R., and W. H. Lewis: Transformation of mononuclear blood cells into macrophages, epithelioid cells, and giant cells in hanging drop cultures of lower vertebrates. Carnegie Contributions to Embryol., *18*:95, 1926.

Litt, M.: Eosinophils and antigen-antibody reaction. Ann. N. Y. Acad. Sci., *116*:964, 1964.

Maximow, A. A.: Über die Zellformen des lockern Bindgewebes. Arch. f. Mikr. Anat., *67*:680, 1906.

Maximow, A. A.: The morphology of the mesenchymal reactions. Arch. Path. Lab. Med., *4*:557, 1927.

Mellors, R. C., and L. Korngold: The cellular origin of human immunoglobulins. J. Exper. Med., *118*:387, 1963.

Movat, H. Z., and N. V. P. Fernando: The fine structure of connective tissue. I. The fibroblast. II. The plasma cell. Exp. Mol. Pathol., *1*:509, 535, 1962.

Nossal, G. J. V.: Genetic control of lymphopoiesis, plasma

cell formation and antibody production. Int. Rev. Exp. Path., *1*:1, 1962.

Odor, D. L.: Observations of the rat mesothelium with the electron and phase microscopes. Am. J. Anat., *95*: 433, 1954.

Olsen, B. R.: Electron microscope studies on collagen. I. Native collagen fibrils. Zeitschr. f. Zellforsch., *59*:184, 1963.

Ortega, L. G., and R. C. Mellors: Cellular sites of formation of gamma globulin. J. Exp. Med., *106*:627, 1957.

Padawer, J., ed.: Mast cells and basophils. Ann. N. Y. Acad. Sci., *103*:1, 1963.

Padawer, J.: The reaction of mast cells to polylysine. J. Cell Biol., *47*:352–372, 1970.

Porter, K. R.: Cell fine structure and biosynthesis of intercellular macromolecules. *In* New York Heart Association: Connective Tissue: Intercellular Macromolecules. Boston, Little, Brown & Co., 1964.

Rabinovitch, M.: Phagocytosis: the engulfment stage. Sem. Hemat. *5*:134, 1968.

Rawles, M. E.: Origin of pigment cells from neural crest in the mouse embryo. Physiol. Zool., *20*:248, 1948.

Rebuck, J. W., and J. H. Crowley: A method of studying leukocytic functions *in vitro*. Ann. N. Y. Acad. Sci., *59*:757, 1955.

Rifkin, R. A., E. F. Osserman, K. C. Hsu, and C. Morgan: The intracellular distribution of gamma globulin in a mouse plasma cell tumor as revealed by fluorescence and electron microscopy. J. Exper. Med., *116*:324, 1962.

Riley, J. F.: The Mast Cells. Edinburgh and London, E. & S. Livingstone, Ltd., 1959.

Rohlich, P., P. Anderson, and B. Uvnas: Electron microscope observations on compound 48/80 induced degranulation of rat mast cells. J. Cell Biol., *51*:465–483, 1971.

Ross, R.: The fibroblast and wound repair. Biol. Rev. Camb. Phil. Soc., *43*:57, 1968.

Ross, R., and E. P. Benditt: Wound healing and collagen formation. III. A quantitative radioautographic study of the utilization of proline-H³ in wounds from normal and scorbutic guinea pigs. J. Cell Biol., *15*:99, 1962.

Ross, R., and J. W. Lillywhite: The fate of buffy coat cells grown in subcutaneously implanted diffusion chambers. Lab. Invest., *14*:1568, 1965.

Selye, H.: *The Mast Cells*. Washington, Butterworths, 1965.

Sharp, J. A., and R. G. Burwell: Interaction of macrophages and lymphocytes after skin grafting or challenges with soluble antigens. Nature, *188*:474, 1960.

Speirs, R. S., and Y. Osada: Chemotactic activity and phagocytosis of eosinophils. Proc. Soc. Exper. Biol. Med., *109*:929, 1962.

Sutton, J. S., and L. V. Weiss: Transformation of monocytes in tissue cultures into macrophages, epithelioid cells and multinucleated giant cells. An electron microscope study. J. Cell Biol., *28*:303, 1966.

Thiéry, J. P.: Microcinematographic contributions to the study of plasma cells. *In* Ciba Foundation Symposium: Cellular Aspects of Immunity. Boston, Little, Brown & Co., 1960.

Trowell, O. A.: The lymphocyte. Int. Rev. Cytol., *7*:236, 1958.

Unanue, R. R., and Cerotti, J. Ch.: The function of macrophages in the immune response. Sem. Hemat. *7*:225, 1970.

Uvnäs, B.: Release processes in mast cells and their activation by injury. Ann. N. Y. Acad. Sci., *116*:880, 1964.

Van Furth, R.: Origin and kinetics of monocytes and macrophages. Sem. Hemat. *7*:125, 1970.

Van Furth, R., ed.: *Mononuclear Phagocytes*. Oxford, Blackwell Scientific Publications, 1970.

Weiss, L. P., and D. W. Fawcett: Cytochemical observations on chicken monocytes, macrophages, and giant cells in tissue culture. J. Histochem. Cytochem., *1*:47, 1953.

Zagury, D., J. W. Uhr, J. D. Jamieson, and G. E. Palade: Immunoglobulin synthesis and secretion. II. Radioautographic studies of sites of addition of carbohydrate moieties and intracellular transport. J. Cell Biol., *46*: 52, 1970.

7

Adipose Tissue

Twenty-five years ago adipose tissue was considered to be a metabolically inert tissue which passively stored fat, provided insulation against heat loss, and functioned in mechanical support in certain regions of the body. The allocation of a separate chapter to it in recent textbooks of histology is a consequence of its belated recognition as a diffuse organ of primary metabolic importance.

Most animals feed intermittently but consume energy continuously; there must therefore be provision for temporary storage of fuel. Lipid is the most favorable substance for this purpose because it weighs less and occupies less volume per calorie of stored chemical energy than either carbohydrate or protein. Although many tissues contain small amounts of carbohydrate and fat, the adipose tissue serves as the body's most capacious reservoir of energy. About 10 per cent of the total body weight of an average man is fat, representing approximately a 40 day reserve of energy. In obese individuals this may increase to the equivalent of a year or more of normal metabolism. By accumulating lipid in periods of excess food intake and releasing fatty acids in periods of fasting, adipose tissue plays an important role in maintaining a stable supply of fuel. Far from being inert, the cells of this tissue actively synthesize fat from carbohydrate and are highly responsive to hormonal and nervous stimulation.

HISTOLOGICAL CHARACTERISTICS OF THE ADIPOSE TISSUES

In most mammals there are two more or less distinct types of adipose tissue, which differ in their color, distribution, vascularity,

and metabolic activity. One is the familiar yellow or *white adipose tissue*, which comprises the bulk of body fat. The other, called *brown adipose tissue*, is less abundant and occurs only in certain specific areas. There are marked species differences in the relative amounts of the two types of fat. Brown adipose tissue is most abundant in hibernating species. Al-

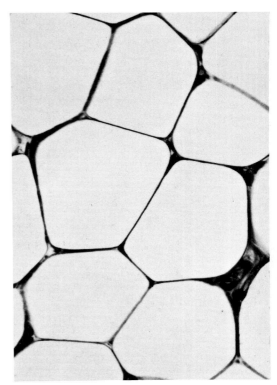

Figure 7-1   Ordinary adipose tissue of a mouse prepared by usual methods of fixation and dehydration. The lipid droplet has been extracted and only a thin rim of cytoplasm of each cell remains. ×400.

though it is present in primates, including man, it is relatively inconspicuous and probably does not assume great importance in the economy of these animals.

The peripheral parts of lobules of brown adipose tissue often have an appearance strongly suggestive of a transition from one form of fat to the other. This has fostered the widespread belief that brown fat is simply an immature or transitional form of ordinary adipose tissue. For this reason it is sometimes referred to in the literature of pathology as *fetal fat*. This term does not seem to be appropriate, however, for in those species in which it is best developed, brown fat persists throughout adult life and is morphologically and metabolically sufficiently different to warrant its designation as a distinct type of adipose tissue. We will return to this point in discussing the histogenesis of the adipose tissues.

Ordinary Adipose Tissue

Fat varies in color from white to deep yellow, depending in part upon the diet. The color resides mainly in the stored lipid. The cells are very large, ranging up to 120 μm. in diameter. They are typically spherical but may assume polyhedral shapes because of mutual deformation (Fig. 7–1). A single droplet of lipid occupies most of the volume of the cell. Therefore, fat cells of this kind are sometimes described as *unilocular* to distinguish them from brown fat cells, which contain multiple small droplets and are termed *multilocular*. The nucleus is displaced to one side by the accumulated lipid and the cytoplasm is reduced to a thin rim comprising only about one fortieth of the total volume of the cell. The lipid is usually dissolved out during preparation of histological sections, so that only the plasmalemma and a thin shell of cytoplasm remain. With silver stains each cell is found to be surrounded by delicate reticular fibers. In the angular spaces between the cells are cross sections of capillaries that form a loose plexus throughout the tissue. If well preserved, adipose tissue appears in section as a delicate network with large polygonal meshes (Figs. 7–1 and 7–2), but the cell rims often collapse to varying degrees during preparation, giving the cells an irregular outline.

Adipose tissue is often subdivided into small lobules by connective tissue septa. This

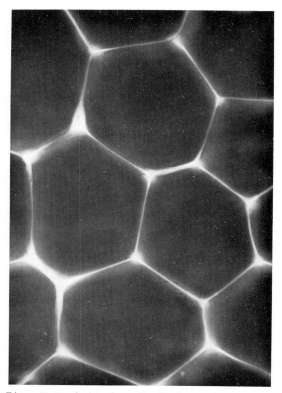

Figure 7–2 A thin formalin fixed spread of adipose tissue in rat mesentery stained with Sudan black without previous dehydration. Here the lipid has been retained and is stained by the fat soluble dye, while the surrounding rim of cytoplasm is essentially unstained. ×400. (After D. W. Fawcett, *in* R. O. Greep, ed.: Histology. Philadelphia, The Blakiston Co., 1953. Reproduced with the permission of the McGraw-Hill Book Co.)

compartmentation, visible with the naked eye, is most obvious in regions where the fat is subjected to pressure and has a cushioning or shock absorbing effect. In other regions, the connective tissue septa are thinner and the lobular organization of the tissue is less apparent.

Examined with the electron microscope, the cytoplasm around the nucleus is found to contain a small Golgi complex, a few filamentous mitochondria, occasional short profiles of endoplasmic reticulum and a moderate number of free ribosomes. Attenuated as it is, the thin layer of cytoplasm around the lipid droplet nevertheless includes a few mitochondria, fine filaments, and minute vesicles, which may represent the agranular reticulum. Not infrequently there are also

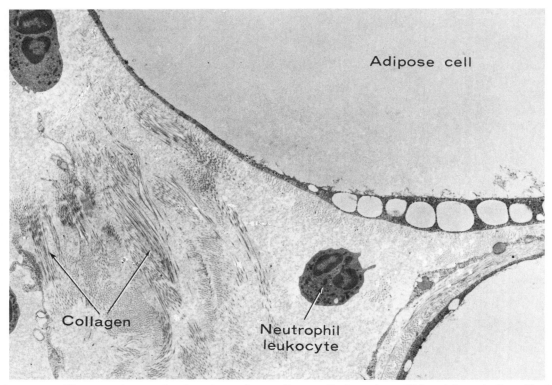

Figure 7-3 Electron micrograph of portions of two adipose cells from the epididymal fat pad of rat. Notice the relative sizes of the neutrophil leukocyte, and the very large adipose cell. The cell at the upper right has a number of small lipid droplets that have not yet coalesced with the large lipid droplet above.

small droplets that represent newly formed lipid which has not yet coalesced with the principal lipid drop (Figs. 7-3 and 7-4). The lipid droplet is not enclosed by a membrane, but it is often set off from the surrounding cytoplasm by 40 to 50 Å filaments in an orthogonal arrangement (Figs. 7-5 and 7-6). Similar filaments occurring singly or in small bundles are found randomly oriented elsewhere in the cytoplasm. The plasma membrane shows numerous minute inpocketings of the kind that are usually interpreted as evidence for a submicroscopic form of pinocytosis. Each adipose cell is invested by a layer of glycoprotein corresponding to the boundary layer or basal lamina of epithelia.

In prolonged fasting or in the emaciation associated with chronic illness, adipose tissue may give up much of its stored lipid and revert to a highly vascular connective tissue containing aggregations of ovoid or polygonal cells with multiple small lipid droplets. The cells seldom or never revert to simple fusiform elements resembling fibroblasts.

Distribution of Ordinary Adipose Tissue

This type of fat is widely distributed in the subcutaneous tissue but exhibits regional differences in amount, which are influenced by age and sex. In infants and young children there is a continuous subcutaneous layer of fat, the *panniculus adiposus*, of rather uniform thickness over the whole body. In adults it thins out in some regions but persists and grows thicker in certain sites of predilection. These sites differ in the two sexes and are largely responsible for the characteristic differences in body form of males and females. In the male, the principal areas are the nape of the neck and the region overlying the seventh cervical vertebra, the subcutaneous area overlying the deltoid and triceps, the lumbrosacral region, and the buttocks. In the female, subcutaneous fat is most abundant in the breasts, the buttocks, the epitrochanteric region, and the anterior aspect of the thigh.

In addition to these superficial fat deposits, there are extensive accumulations in both sexes in the omentum, mesenteries, and retroperitoneal areas. All of these areas readily give up their stored lipid during fasting. There are other areas of fat, however, that do not give up their stored fuel so readily. For example, the adipose tissue in the orbit, in the major joints, and on the palms of the hands and soles of the feet does not seem to be grist for the metabolic mill but instead has the mechanical function of support or protection. These areas diminish in size only after very prolonged starvation.

Brown Adipose Tissue

The color of this form of fat ranges from tan to a rich reddish brown. Its cells are smaller than those of white fat and are polygonal in cross section. The cytoplasm is more abundant, and there are multiple lipid droplets of varying size (Fig. 7–7). The spherical nucleus is somewhat eccentric in position but is seldom displaced to the periphery of the cell. A small Golgi apparatus is present, as well as numerous large spherical mitochondria. In electron micrographs the mitochondria occupy a large part of the cytoplasm and have numerous cristae that may extend across the full width of the organelle (Fig. 7–8). The endoplasmic reticulum is not well developed,

and only a few profiles of the smooth surfaced form can be found. The lipid droplets do not appear to develop within the reticulum but are free in the ground substance of the cytoplasm. Scattered ribosomes and variable amounts of particulate glycogen are also present in the cytoplasmic matrix.

The connective tissue stroma of brown adipose tissue is very sparse and the blood supply exceedingly rich (Fig. 7–9). The cells are therefore in more intimate association with one another and with the capillaries than is the case in ordinary fat. Numerous small unmyelinated nerve fibers can be demonstrated among the brown fat cells by silver staining methods and in electron micrographs. Naked axons are frequently encountered in apposition to the surface of adipose cells.

The histological organization of brown fat is always distinctly lobular, and the pattern of distribution of the blood vessels within lobes and lobules closely resembles that found in glands. In animals subjected to prolonged fasting the brown fat gradually becomes more deeply colored and reverts to a compact, glandlike mass of epithelioid cells bearing no resemblance to connective tissue (Fig. 7–10). The depletion of lipid in brown adipose tissue is more rapid in animals subjected to a cold environment. The brown color of the tissue is in large part attributable

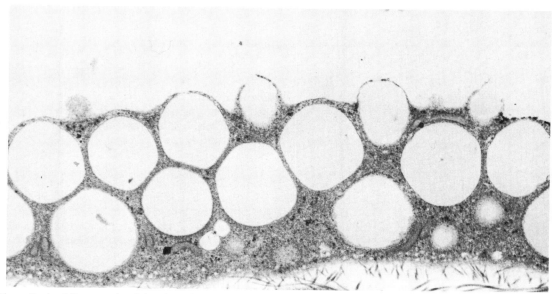

Figure 7–4 Micrograph of the rim of cytoplasm of an adipose cell. Some of the numerous small lipid droplets appear to be discharging their content into the principal lipid drop at the top of the figure.

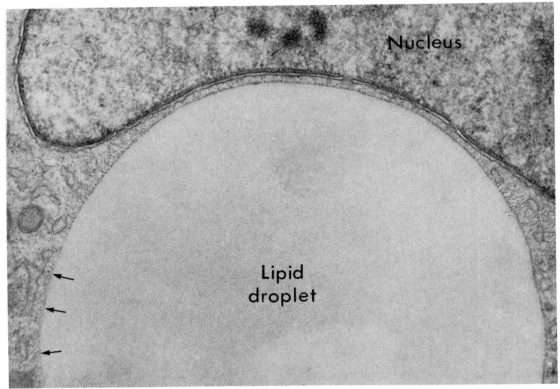

Figure 7-5 Electron micrograph of the nucleus and adjacent lipid droplet of a developing fat cell from chick bone marrow. After glutaraldehyde fixation the lipid shows less staining with osmic acid and the interface between the lipid and the cytoplasm (at arrows) can be seen more clearly. Notice the absence of a membrane around the droplet. ×34,000. (Courtesy of Eunice M. Wood.)

to the high concentration of cytochromes in its mitochondria. The relative oxidative capacity of brown adipose tissue, based on cytochrome oxidase, is said to be greater than that of cardiac muscle.

Distribution of Brown Adipose Tissue

Brown adipose tissue arises in embryonic life in certain specific sites, and no new areas develop after birth. This is in contrast to ordinary fat cells, which may develop in almost any area of loose connective tissue, and new deposits of adipose cells may appear at any time in postnatal life. Brown fat may not occur in all mammals, but its presence has been established in representatives of at least seven of the orders, including primates. It is prominent in the newborn of all the species in which it occurs and it remains a distinct and conspicuous tissue in the adults of hibernating species. In some nonhibernating species, including man, the multilocular condition of the lipid in its cells gradually diminishes postnatally by coalescence of the droplets, so that the cells gradually come to resemble those of ordinary unilocular adipose tissue. For this reason, there has been some debate as to whether or not there are two physiologically distinct types of fat in well nourished human adults. The bulk of the evidence now indicates that two types do exist, even though they may be difficult to distinguish morphologically. Brown fat is well differentiated as early as the twenty-eighth week in the human fetus and in the newborn constitutes about 2 to 5 per cent of total body weight. In adults, all of the fat may seem to be of the unilocular variety, but in the elderly, in persons with chronic wasting diseases, or in starvation, glandlike masses of multilocular fat cells reappear in the same regions where they are found in the newborn. Moreover, two types of fatty tumors, (*lipomas*) occur in man—one resembling ordinary fat and the other resembling brown fat. These observations lend support to the view that both types of adipose tissue are represented in man throughout life.

In the common laboratory rodents, brown fat occurs in two symmetrical interscapular fat bodies, in thin lobules between muscles around the shoulder girdle, and in the axillae. It fills the costovertebral angle and forms long slender lobules on either side of the thoracic aorta. Smaller lobules are also found in the anterior mediastinum, along the great vessels in the neck and in the hilus of the kidney. Brown adipose tissue is less extensive in primates, but in young macaques and in newborn humans, sizable masses can be found in the axillae, as well as at the nape and in the posterior triangles of the neck. Smaller lobules are found near the thyroid, along the carotid sheath, and in the hilus of the kidney.

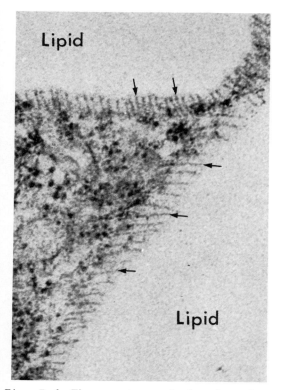

Figure 7-6 Electron micrograph of portions of two lipid droplets and the intervening cytoplasm in a developing adipose cell from the chick. The arrows point to the ordered array of fine filaments at the interface between the lipid and the cytoplasm. ×87,000. (Courtesy of Eunice M. Wood.)

HISTOGENESIS OF ADIPOSE TISSUE

An early view that still has some adherents is that of Flemming (1870), who contended that adipose tissue was merely ordinary connective tissue in which fat had been deposited in the fibroblasts. This view assumes that any and all connective tissue can serve as a repository for fat when dietary intake exceeds energy expenditure. Although connective tissue is ubiquitous, the fact is that in obesity, fat does not become universally and evenly distributed, but instead is deposited in certain sites preferentially, while other areas are spared. For example, the backs of the hands and feet, the eyelids, nose, ears, scrotum, and genitalia seldom accumulate fat. This fact is hard to explain if adipose cells can arise from common fibroblasts wherever they occur. Toldt (1870-1888), on the other hand, maintained that adipose tissue is derived from special formative cells, "lipoblasts," set apart in the embryo in primitive fat forming organs. According to this interpretation the characteristic distribution of fat in the adult would then reflect the distribution and relative abundance of these special fat forming cells. Many would now make no distinction between Toldt's lipoblasts and persisting mesenchymal cells.

Hammar's (1895) interpretation was, in effect, a combination of these two views. He distinguished two processes, the first taking place during embryonic life and called *primary fat formation*. In this process special cells were laid down in lobular, glandlike arrangements of epithelioid cells. These cells first developed multiple small lipid droplets, which later coalesced to form a single large droplet. In addition to this primary fat formation, Hammar believed that fat could form at any time during late fetal or postnatal life directly from relatively undifferentiated connective tissue cells by accumulation of lipid, without these cells becoming arranged in recognizable glandlike lobules. The end products of primary and secondary fat formation in man were said to be indistinguishable in normally nourished individuals.

Certainly two distinct methods of histogenesis of fat are recognizable in human embryos. In postnatal life, however, the cells in those areas that correspond in their anatomical distribution to the brown fat of rodents continue to accumulate lipid. The multiple

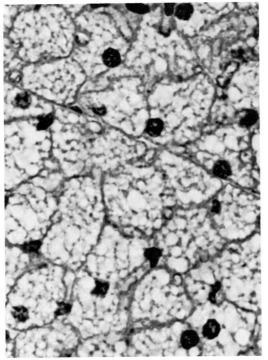

Figure 7-7 Photomicrograph of typical brown adipose tissue. The polygonal cells contain more cytoplasm than those of ordinary fat and have many small lipid droplets. ×650.

cells is replaced each day by new fatty acid. The same kind of continual renewal occurs in man, but the quantities and the time course of these events are not known with the same precision as in the laboratory animals.

The histophysiology of adipose tissue can best be understood by analogy to deposits and withdrawals from a metabolic reserve bank or revolving fund. The "deposits" may be in the form of (1) fatty acids from the chylomicrons formed from dietary lipid, (2) fatty acids synthesized from glucose in the liver and transported to the adipose tissue in the form of serum lipoprotein, or (3) triglyceride synthesized from carbohydrate in the adipose cells themselves. "Withdrawals" are made by enzymatic hydrolysis of triglyceride and release of free fatty acids into the blood. With a continuous supply of glucose, lipolysis and release of free fatty acids are negligible. With alternations of fasting and feeding, which is the usual feeding pattern, lipolysis is increased several fold during periods of fasting. The normal balance is greatly affected by hormones and by the action of the nervous system.

droplets ultimately coalesce into a single droplet, and the cells thus become morphologically indistinguishable from those which develop directly from primitive connective tissue. Thus, in the adult human, there may appear to be only one morphological type of adipose tissue.

HISTOPHYSIOLOGY OF ADIPOSE TISSUE

Since the introduction of isotopic tracers for use in studying metabolism, it has been clearly shown that the lipid in fat depots is not an inert energy reserve drawn upon only in periods of inanition. On the contrary, the lipid is continuously being mobilized and renewed even in an individual in caloric balance. The half life of depot lipid in the rat is about 8 days, which means that almost 10 per cent of the fatty acid stored in adipose

Hormonal Influences

There are marked species differences in the action of the hypophysis on mobilization of depot fat, and the mechanisms involved are still somewhat obscure. Some of the effects of hypophyseal hormones are probably indirect, but it has been suggested that the pituitary secretes an *adipokinetic hormone* which promotes liberation of fatty acids from stored triglyceride. However, the existence of such a hormone has yet to be proved. Administration of adrenocorticotrophic hormone (ACTH) or a synthetic tridecapeptide identical to a terminal portion of the ACTH molecule results in an increase in the plasma level of free fatty acid. This effect is observed in adrenalectomized animals and hence appears to be a direct action of the hormone on adipose cells promoting lipolysis. It may therefore be unnecessary to postulate a separate adipokinetic hormone to account for the observed effects of the hypophysis on adipose tissue.

The characteristic differences in adipose tissue distribution in males and females has already been alluded to. Because hormones circulate freely in the blood and presumably reach all tissues in approximately equal concentrations, these differences in fat distribution imply either that there are genetically determined differences in distribution of cells having the capacity to develop into fat cells, or that there are regional differences in sensitivity of the cells to circulating sex hormones.

This regional difference in sensitivity does not seem to be restricted to the effects of sex hormones, for an excess of *adrenal cortical hormone* results in a characteristic distribution of fat, of which a prominent feature is an accumulation of fat over the lower cervical region, producing a deformity referred to as "buffalo hump."

The hormone *insulin* is the main physiological factor controlling the uptake of glucose by adipose tissue and, secondarily, the synthesis of fat from carbohydrate. Whether given in vivo or added to the medium of adipose tissue incubated in vitro, it appears to stimulate the transport of glucose into the cell and to accelerate its metabolism along all of the paths open to it. It seems to have a specific effect upon the rate at which glucose is converted to glycogen. Oxygen consumption is stimulated because of the accelerated conversion of glucose to fatty acid. These effects of insulin in promoting glycogen deposition can be demonstrated morphologically and are very much more pronounced in brown than in white fat (Figs. 7–12 and 7–13).

In the absence of insulin, as in diabetes, there is a rise in blood glucose, a diminished utilization of glucose, an increase in unesterified fatty acids in the plasma, and an increase in blood lipoproteins. Carbohydrates are normally used preferentially as an energy source, but in the diabetic, in whom carbohydrates cannot be utilized because of the deficiency of insulin, the required energy is derived principally from fat.

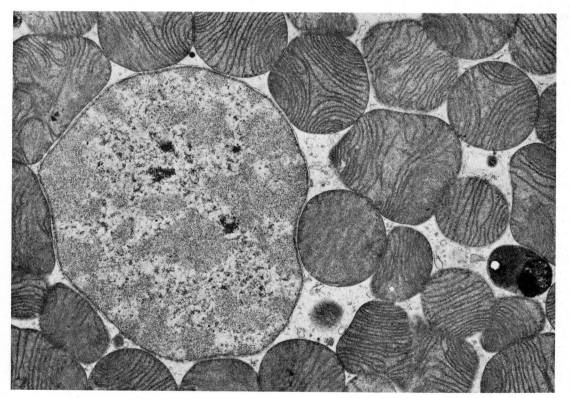

Figure 7–8 Electron micrograph of the nucleus and adjacent cytoplasm of a brown adipose cell from a bat recently aroused from hibernation. Notice the abundance of large spherical mitochondria with numerous long cristae. ×14,000.

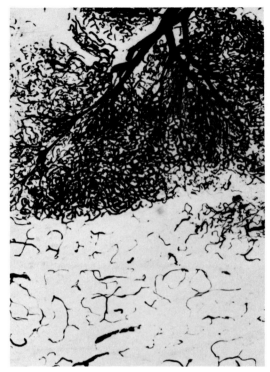

Figure 7-9 A thick section of brown and white adipose tissue in which the blood vessels have been injected with India ink. The vascular bed of the brown fat *(above)* is extraordinarily rich and has a typical glandlike pattern, while that of the white fat *(below)* is relatively sparse. ×70. (After D. W. Fawcett, J. Morphology, 90:363, 1952.)

Influence of the Autonomic Nervous System

Adipose tissue is rather richly innervated, especially the brown fat. The function of the nerves can be demonstrated experimentally by cutting the nerves of the interscapular fat body on one side of the midline, leaving the nerve supply to the other side intact. Within the first few postoperative days it becomes apparent that the fat cells on the denervated side are larger than those on the normal side. The differences in the two sides are more dramatic if the animal is then deprived of food and placed in a cold environment. These environmental conditions ordinarily lead to a rapid mobilization of lipid from the fat depots. In animals unilaterally denervated the fat cells on the side with the nerves intact are rapidly depleted of lipid, while the fat cells on the denervated side retain a nearly normal content of lipid. It is thus demonstrated that the presence of nerves is necessary for normal mobilization of lipid from adipose tissue.

The chemical mediator, norepinephrine, is present in abundance in innervated adipose tissue but is low or absent after denervation. It is apparently through release of norepinephrine from the nerve endings that the nerves control the mobilization of fatty acids from adipose tissue. Injection of small amounts of exogenous norepinephrine inhibits the action of insulin on fat cells and approximately doubles the amount of free fatty acid in the blood plasma. The norepinephrine brings about the activation of adipose tissue lipase, increasing the rate of hydrolysis of triglycerides (Fig. 7–13). In patients who have an adrenal medullary tumor (pheochromocytoma) that secretes excessive amounts of norepinephrine, the plasma con-

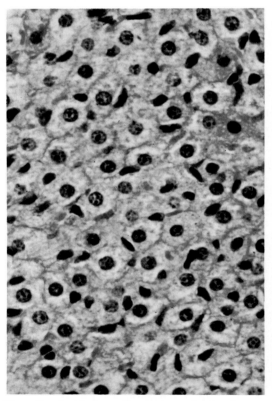

Figure 7-10 Brown adipose tissue that has become depleted of lipid after prolonged fasting, or as a consequence of hypophysectomy, takes on the appearance of a gland. Its cells resemble epithelium rather than fibroblasts. ×750.

centration of fatty acids may be several hundred times the normal level.

Brown Adipose Tissue as a Heat Generator

It has long been noted that brown adipose tissue is more abundant in animal species that hibernate and it was assumed to have a function related to winter dormancy. There is now evidence that one of its functions is to serve as a "chemical furnace" — an oil burner to heat the animal during arousal from hibernation.

When a hibernating animal begins to arouse, there is a marked increase in oxygen consumption and generation of heat. Nerve impulses to the brown adipose tissue release norepinephrine at the nerve endings, which leads to activation of lipase in the fat cells and results in the breakdown of triglyceride to fatty acid and glycerol. Oxidation of fatty acid and re-esterification of some of the fatty acid then occurs, with consumption of oxygen and generation of heat that serves to warm the blood flowing through the fat, secondarily raising the temperature of the animal as a whole.

Correlated with this function are some unusual features of the mitochondria. Oxidative phosphorylation is difficult to demonstrate in mitochondrial fractions from brown

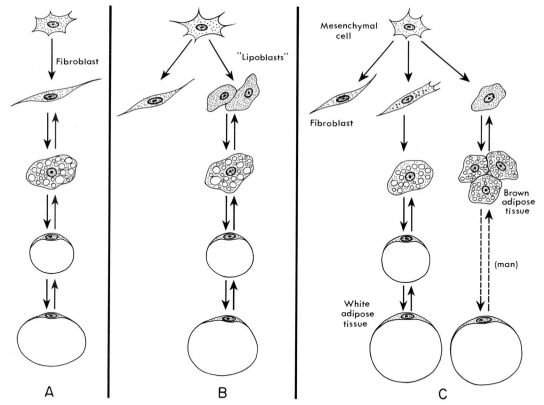

Figure 7-11 Diagrammatic representation of the three principal views concerning the histogenesis of adipose tissue. *A,* This represents the view that adipose cells are merely fibroblasts which have accumulated excess lipid (Flemming). *B,* The view that adipose tissue develops from special formative cells ("lipoblasts") set apart early in embryonic life (Toldt). *C,* The compromise interpretation that recognizes two processes, one leading to the formation of lobular, glandlike masses of epithelioid cells that develop into brown adipose tissue and one in which persisting mesenchymal cells develop directly into ordinary white adipose tissue (Hammar). In rodents that have brown fat in adult life the two types of adipose tissue remain morphologically distinct. In man, the multiple droplets of the brown fat gradually coalesce so that it comes to resemble the white fat except after fasting or prolonged illness.

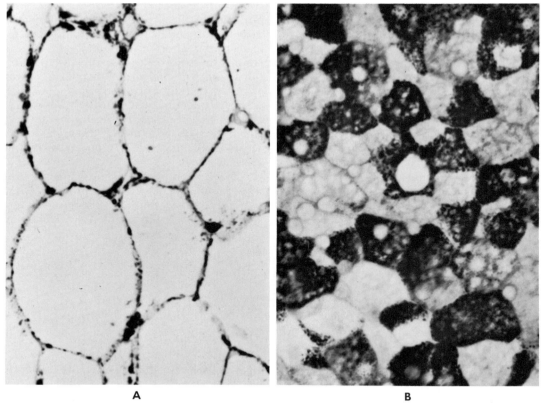

A   **B**

Figure 7-12 *A,* White adipose tissue of a rat re-fed after a period of fasting. The dark granular deposits in the rim of cytoplasm are glycogen. The glycogen subsequently disappears as the carbohydrate is used in the synthesis of fat. ×650. *B,* Under the same conditions, considerably more glycogen is deposited in brown adipose tissue. Not all of the cells respond to the same degree. A similar deposition of glycogen results from administration of the hormone insulin. ×650. (After D. W. Fawcett, J. Morphology, *90*:363, 1952.)

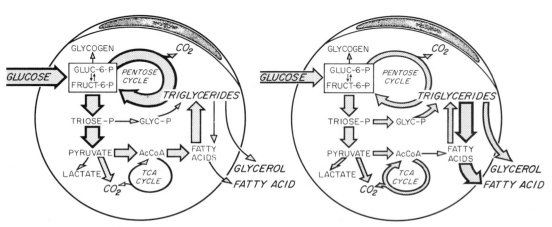

Figure 7-13 Diagram depicting effects of insulin and norepinephrine upon adipose tissue. The widths of the arrows are a rough measure of the quantitative effects on the respective metabolic pathways. (Modified after B. Jeanrenaud, Metabolism, *10*:535, 1961.)

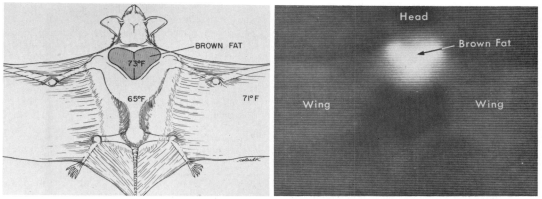

Figure 7-14 Thermograph of a bat made during arousal from hibernation. By scanning for detection of infrared radiation, a "hot spot" is revealed in the area corresponding to the location of the interscapular brown adipose tissue. During arousal this tissue acts as a chemical "furnace" producing heat that helps warm the rest of the body. (Courtesy of J. Hayward.)

adipose tissue. The elementary particles or inner membrane subunits that are usually present on the mitochondrial cristae are thought to be the sites of phosphorylation enzymes. These have not been demonstrated in normal numbers in negatively stained mitochondria from brown adipose tissue. A deficiency of oxidative phosphorylation in mitochondria would be a surprising finding in any other normal tissue, but it is consistent with the needs of a system concerned mainly with heat production (Afzelius). The heat generation by brown fat can be demonstrated visually by the new technique of thermography (Fig. 7–14). The thermograph scans across the body, detecting the infrared radiation from surfaces and registers the temperature dependent intensity of radiation on a photographic plate. When a bat arousing from hibernation is scanned, the thin wing membranes rapidly equilibrate with the ambient temperature, and most of the body is still relatively cool. However, a sharply delineated "hot area" is found on the thermograph, coinciding with the location of the interscapular brown fat. Thus in hibernating species brown adipose tissue performs two important roles during the arousal from dormancy: the oxidation of lipid to produce heat within the brown fat, and the release into the circulation of oxidizable substrates for utilization by other tissues.

When newborns of nonhibernating species such as the rat and rabbit are exposed to the cold or when they are infused with physiological amounts of norepinephrine, there is a substantial increase in oxygen consumption, and thermocouples embedded in their interscapular brown fat register a local production of heat.

It has now been shown that the human infant makes use of the same mechanism for heat generation. When human newborns are removed from an ambient temperature of 35°C. and exposed to 25°C., there is a marked increase in oxygen consumption and a very significant rise in plasma glycerol, indicating increased lipolysis of triglycerides in the brown adipose tissue. Under these conditions, thermography reveals areas of elevated skin temperature over the sites of brown adipose tissue at the nape of the neck and in the axilla. It is possible that this adipose tissue may also have some slight thermogenic function in adults, but this is yet to be demonstrated.

REFERENCES

Afzelius, B. A.: The fine structure of brown fat mitochondria. Proc. 6th Internat. Congr. Electron Microscopy. Tokyo, Maruzen Co., 1966.

Aherne, W. and D. Hull: Brown adipose tissue. Lancet, *1*:765, 1965.

Ball, E. G., and R. L. Jungas: On the action of hormones which accelerate the rate of oxygen consumption and fatty acid release in rat adipose tissue *in vitro*. Proc. Nat. Acad. Sci., *47*:932, 1961.

Dawkins, M. J. R., and J. W. Scopes: Non-shivering thermogenesis and brown adipose tissue in the human newborn infant. Nature, *206*:201, 1965.

Fawcett, D. W.: Histological observations on the relation of insulin to the deposition of glycogen in adipose tissue. Endocrinology, *42*:454, 1948.

Fawcett, D. W.: A comparison of the histological organization and histochemical reactions of brown fat and ordinary adipose tissue. J. Morphol., *90*:363, 1952.

Fawcett, D. W., and I. C. Jones: The effects of hypophysectomy, adrenalectomy, and of thiouracil feeding on the cytology of brown adipose tissue. Endocrinology, *45*:609, 1949.

Hausberger, F. X.: Influence of nutritional state on size and number of fat cells. Zeitschr. f. Zellforsch., *64*:13, 1964.

Hausberger, F. X.: Effect of dietary and endocrine factors on adipose tissue growth. *In* Renold, A. E., and G. F. Cahill, Jr., eds.: Handbook of Physiology, Section 5. Washington, American Physiological Society, 1965.

Havel, R. J.: Autonomic nervous system and adipose tissue. *In* Renold, A. E., and G. F. Cahill, Jr., eds.: Handbook of Physiology, Section 5. Washington, American Physiological Society, 1965.

Hayward, J. S., and E. G. Ball: Quantitative aspects of brown adipose tissue thermogenesis during arousal from hibernation. Biol. Bull., *131*:94, 1966.

Hayward, J. S., C. P. Lyman, and C. R. Taylor: The possible role of brown fat as a source of heat during arousal from hibernation. Ann. N. Y. Acad. Sci., *131*:441, 1965.

Jeanrenaud, B.: Dynamic aspects of adipose tissue metabolism: A review. Metab. Clin. Exp., *10*:535, 1961.

Joel, C. D.: The physiological role of brown adipose tissue. *In* Renold, A. E., and G. F. Cahill, Jr., eds.: Handbook of Physiology, Section 5. Washington, American Physiological Society, 1965.

Joel, C. D., and E. G. Ball: The electron transmitter system of brown adipose tissue. Biochemistry, *1*:281, 1962.

Luckenbill, L. M., and A. S. Cohen: The association of lipid droplets with cytoplasmic filaments in avian subsynovial adipose cells. J. Cell Biol., *31*:195, 1966.

Napolitano, L.: The differentiation of white adipose cells. J. Cell Biol., *18*:663, 1963.

Napolitano, L.: The fine structure of adipose tissues. *In* Renold, A. E., and G. F. Cahill, Jr., eds.: Handbook of Physiology, Section 5. Washington, American Physiological Society, 1965.

Napolitano, L., and D. W. Fawcett: The fine structure of brown adipose tissue in newborn mice and rats. J. Biophys. Biochem. Cytol., *4*:685, 1958.

Napolitano, L., and H. T. Gagne: Lipid depleted white adipose cells. Anat. Rec., *147*:273, 1963.

Rémillard, G. L.: Histochemical and microchemical observations on the lipids of the interscapular brown fat of the female verpertilionid bat, *Myotis lucifugus lucifugus.* Ann. N. Y. Acad. Sci., *72*:1, 1958.

Renold, A. E., A. Marble, and D. W. Fawcett: Action of insulin on deposition of glycogen and storage of fat in adipose tissue. Endocrinology, *46*:55, 1950.

Sidman, R. L.: The direct effect of insulin on organ cultures of brown fat. Anat. Rec., *124*:723, 1956.

Sidman, R. L., and D. W. Fawcett: The effect of peripheral nerve section on some metabolic responses of brown adipose tissue in mice. Anat. Rec., *118*:487, 1954.

Sidman, R. L., M. Perkins, and N. Weiner: Noradrenaline and adrenaline content of adipose tissues. Nature, *193*:36, 1962.

Smith, R. E., and R. J. Hock: Brown fat: Thermogenic effector of arousal in hibernators. Science, *140*:199, 1963.

Smith, R. E., and B. A. Horwitz: Brown fat and thermogenesis. Physiol. Rev., *49*:330, 1969.

Weiner, N., M. Perkins, and R. L. Sidman: Effect of reserpine on noradrenaline content of innervated and denervated brown adipose tissue of the rat. Nature, *193*:137, 1962.

Wells, H. G.: Adipose tissue, a neglected subject. J.A.M.A., *114*:2177, 2284, 1940.

Wertheimer, E., and B. Shapiro: The physiology of adipose tissue. Physiol. Rev., *28*:451, 1948.

8

Blood Cell Formation

The relatively short-lived cells of the blood are maintained in rather constant numbers by continuous replacement from sources outside the circulation. The process of formation of blood cells is called *hemopoiesis,* and the sites where it occurs are referred to as *hemopoietic tissues or organs.* The principal hemopoietic tissue in adult mammals is the *bone marrow,* which produces all of the erythrocytes, platelets, and granular leukocytes. Until recently it was believed that most of the mononuclear leukocytes, particularly the lymphocytes, arose in the lymphoid organs (lymph nodes, thymus, and spleen). Traditionally, therefore, the blood cells have been divided into two categories according to their origin. The mononuclear leukocytes are referred to as the *lymphoid elements* of the blood, and all of the others are referred to as the *myeloid elements.* The formation of the latter in the bone marrow is termed *myelopoiesis,* while the formation of the nongranular leukocytes whether in the lymphoid organs or bone marrow, is described by the term *lymphopoiesis.* Though firmly established in common usage, the usefulness of this distinction in terminology between these two hemopoietic cell lineages has diminished in recent years with the discovery that monocytes arise in the bone marrow and that many of the lymphocytes are also formed there and only secondarily take up residence in the lymphoid organs. Moreover, in embryonic life and in certain pathological conditions in adult life, the liver, spleen, and lymph nodes may become sites of myelopoiesis.

The bone marrow occupies the medullary cavities of long bones throughout the skeleton, the spongiosa of the vertebral bodies, the ribs, sternum, and the flat bones of the pelvis. Because it is so widely dispersed we tend to underestimate its abundance. It has an aggregate volume roughly equal to that of the liver, some 3.5 to 6 per cent of the body weight. Only about half of this volume is active in blood formation in the adult. The marrow varies in its cellular composition in different regions of the skeleton and varies also with the age of the individual. At birth, nearly all of the bones contain deep red, hemopoietically active marrow. Its red color is, in part, attributable to its vascularity but is, in larger measure, a consequence of the enormous numbers of developing red blood cells in its meshes. After birth, the numbers of blood forming cells in some parts of the skeleton decrease and the numbers of adipose cells in the marrow increase. This shift in the relative abundance of these cell types results in a change in the color of the marrow from deep red to yellow. The transformation from highly cellular red marrow to relatively inactive yellow marrow occurs earlier and progresses further in the long bones than it does in the axial skeleton. Thus, in adults the marrow in the bones of the extremities is composed mainly of adipose cells, while hemopoietically active red marrow persists in the vertebrae, ribs, sternum and ilia. The fatty transformation of the marrow in more peripheral elements of the appendicular skeleton is thought to be, in part, a consequence of the slightly lower temperature of these parts (Fig. 8–1). In response to local

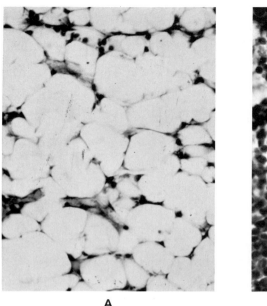
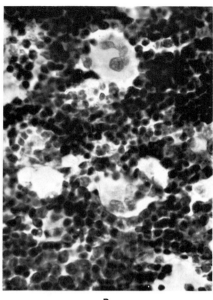

A   B

Figure 8-1 A tail loop was constructed in a 23 day old rat by skinning the distal half of the tail and inserting it surgically in the peritoneal cavity, where it was kept for 125 days. *A*, Section from the cool outside loop, showing fatty bone marrow. *B*, Section from the warm region of the tail in the abdominal cavity, showing hemopoietic marrow. ×500. (Courtesy of C. Huggins.)

change of temperature or to unusual demands for blood cells, fatty marrow can regain its hemopoietic potential.

HEMOPOIESIS DURING EMBRYONIC DEVELOPMENT

In developing embryos three successive phases are recognized in which the principal site of hemopoiesis shifts from one region to another. The formation of blood begins when the embryo is only a few millimeters long, and is first detectable in the mesenchyme of the body stalk and in neighboring areas of the yolk sac. Masses of mesenchymal cells round up and become aggregated to form the so-called *blood islands.* In this early *mesoblastic phase of hemopoiesis,* nearly all of the cells formed are nucleated erythrocytes. The cells of the blood islands differentiate into *primitive erythroblasts* that synthesize hemoglobin and develop into nucleated erythrocytes that are characteristic of the early embryo (Figs. 8–2 and 8–3).

Soon after establishment of blood islands in the yolk sac, accumulations of round basophilic cells appear in the primordium of the liver, initiating the *hepatic phase of hemopoiesis.* These cells are identical in appearance to the erythroblasts found in hemopoietic organs of adults and are called *definitive erythroblasts* to distinguish them from the *primitive erythroblasts* of the yolk sac. In addition to minor differences in the chromatin pattern, the definitive erythroblast ultimately gives rise to anucleate erythrocytes, whereas the erythrocytes arising from primitive erythroblasts never lose their nuclei. Granular leukocytes and megakaryocytes also appear along the sinusoids of the liver in the second month. Somewhat later, the spleen, as well as the liver, becomes a site of hemopoiesis.

During the early stages of development, the embryonic skeleton consists entirely of hyaline cartilage. The *myeloid phase of hemopoiesis* begins with the establishment of ossification centers in the cartilage of the long bones in the fourth and fifth months of intrauterine life (see Chapter 10). As blood vessels penetrate into cavities created by degeneration of chondrocytes in the cartilage model of the bone, they carry mesenchymal cells in with them. Some of these differentiate into bone forming cells, others become primitive reticulum cells that form the stroma of the developing marrow. These in turn may give rise to adipose cells and other connective tissue elements. Hemopoiesis in the liver and spleen declines as the marrow becomes established in the bones and takes over the major part of blood cell formation.

It has been assumed that, in the transition from the mesoblastic to hepatic and myeloid stages of hemopoiesis, mesenchymal

cells in each of these successive sites give rise independently to primitive blood forming cells. The recent demonstrations that stem cells are present in the blood of some species, and that suspensions of marrow cells injected intravenously in adults can repopulate x-irradiated marrow or spleen, now raise the question as to whether the shifts in site of hemopoiesis during embryonic development may depend upon transport of stem cells from the old site to initiate hemopoiesis in the new site.

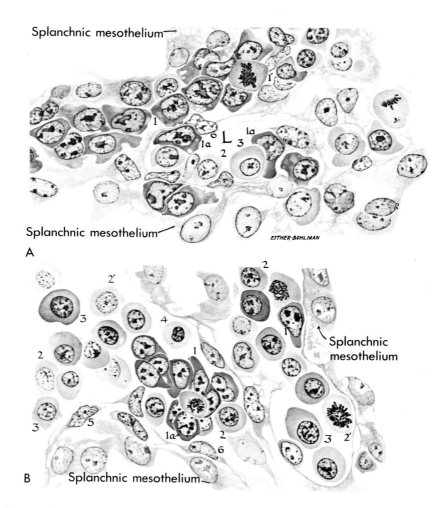

Figure 8–2 Two sections through folds of the wall of the yolk sac of a 24 day human embryo (H1516 Univ. Chicago Emb. Coll.). *A,* Early stage of hemopoiesis, consisting of proliferating extravascular hemocytoblasts (*1, 1′*); *L,* lumen of a small vessel containing a few primitive polychromatophilic erythroblasts. *B,* Later stage of hemopoiesis showing transformation of hemocytoblasts (*1*) into primitive basophilic erythroblasts (*1a*), primitive polychromatophilic erythroblasts (*2, 3*), and primitive erythrocytes (*4*); *5,* mesenchymal cells; *6,* endothelium. Hematoxylin-eosin-azure II stain. ×1100. (From Bloom and Bartelmez, Am. J. Anat., 67:21, 1940.)

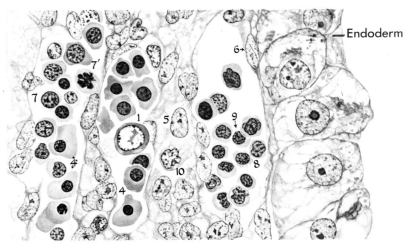

Figure 8–3 Section through yolk sac of a 20 mm. human embryo. In addition to circulating primitive erythrocytes, there are two foci developing polychromatophilic definitive erythroblasts. *1*, Hemocytoblast; *4*, primitive erythrocytes; *5*, mesenchymal cells; *7* and *8*, early and late definitive polychromatophilic erythroblasts with one in mitosis at *7'*; *9*, normoblast; *10*, lymphoid wandering cell. Hematoxylin-eosin-azure II stain. ×1100. (From Bloom and Bartelmez, Am. J. Anat., 67:21, 1940).

HISTOLOGICAL ORGANIZATION OF THE BONE MARROW

The bone marrow consists of blood cells, their precursors, and adipose cells closely packed within the meshes of a loose stroma (Figs. 8–4 and 8–5). The stroma is composed of a framework of reticular fibers supporting *primitive reticular cells* which retain some of the pluripotentiality of embryonic mesenchyme. These cells are not actively phagocytic but can give rise to fixed and free macrophages. They were formerly believed to give rise to the free *stem cells* that are the precursors of the various types of blood cells, but this interpretation is no longer widely accepted (Fig. 8–6).

The vascular supply to the marrow is derived from the nutrient artery to the bone, which not only irrigates the osseous tissue but also ramifies throughout the marrow cavity. The arterioles continue into typical capillaries that are confluent with a complex system of thin-walled sinusoids. Some of these have an open lumen and permit a slow flow of blood, while others are occluded by large numbers of developing cells of the erythrocyte series and newly formed myeloid elements. The channels that are plugged with new blood cells are believed to open from time to time, and their contents are swept into the circulation. Other sinusoids, formerly open, may then become the site of accumulation of new blood cells, with little or no flow through them. The entire system of sinusoidal vessels in the marrow seems never to be open at the same time. The endothelium lining the sinusoids permits the passage through it of large numbers of cells that arise extravascularly, while maintaining its structural integrity. The mechanism of their passage into the lumen, and the factors controlling the relative numbers of each cell type entering the circulation, are poorly understood.

Accounts of the histological organization of the marrow are invariably vague because the close crowding and superimposition of cells in histological sections obscure its basic architecture. Indeed, the description given here depends upon the fact that after x-irradiation nearly all of the free cells disappear. This simplifies the histological picture of the marrow and makes it possible to visualize more clearly the sinusoids and the fibrous and cellular reticulum. There is no assurance, however, that this treatment does not also somewhat alter the basic architecture of the marrow.

THEORIES OF HEMOPOIESIS AND CELL LINEAGES

No subject in histology has given rise to more theories or engendered more controversy than the origin and interrelations of the blood cells. When only morphological criteria were available for identification of cell types, the numerous developmental stages in the marrow could be arranged in a variety of plausible sequences. These were highly subjective, and there were no independent methods for assessing their validity. Only comparatively recently have methods for radiation depletion of the marrow and transfusion of cells labeled with tritiated thymidine or identified by genetic markers made experimental approaches to this problem possible. Application of these methods has eliminated some strongly defended interpretations, but many relationships remain uncertain. It is unneces-

sary to burden the student today with a detailed discussion of this complex subject but some familiarity with the traditional theories will better enable him to understand the current interpretations and to follow the rapidly changing concepts in this field.

The so-called *polyphyletic school of hematologists*, represented by Sabin and coworkers, held that the erythrocytes and leukocytes developed in different sites and from separate stem cells in the marrow. A *stem cell* is defined as a cell capable of self-replication or differentiation or both. In replication, the cell divides mitotically, producing daughter cells indistinguishable from the parent cell. These cells may either remain undifferentiated, perpetuating the *pluripotential stem cell* population (i.e., cells capable of differentiating along a number of alternative lines) or they may differentiate into more mature cells that are *unipotential* (i.e., cells that are committed to develop along only one line). These too can replicate or differentiate. According

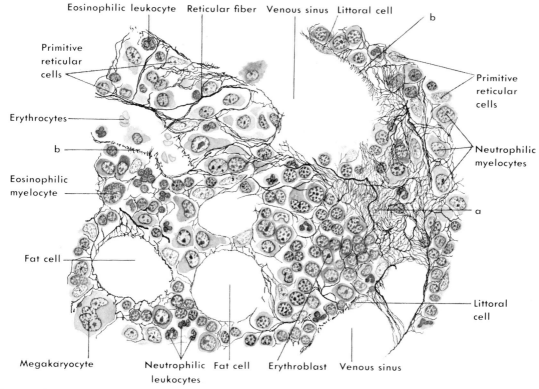

Figure 8–4 Bone marrow from upper epiphysis of a femur of a 6 year old child. The fibrous network of the wall of a vessel is seen from the surface at *a* and in cross section at *b*. Bielschowsky stain. ×500. (After A. A. Maximow.)

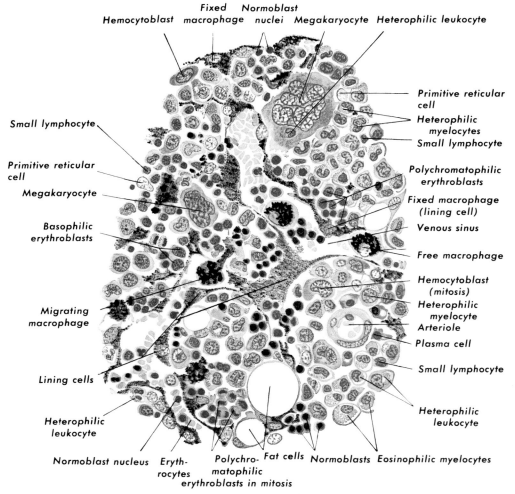

Fixed   Normoblast
Hemocytoblast macrophage nuclei Megakaryocyte Heterophilic leukocyte

Primitive reticular cell
Heterophilic myelocytes
Small lymphocyte

Small lymphocyte
Primitive reticular cell
Megakaryocyte
Basophilic erythroblasts

Polychromatophilic erythroblasts
Fixed macrophage (lining cell)
Venous sinus
Free macrophage
Hemocytoblast (mitosis)
Heterophilic myelocyte
Arteriole
Plasma cell

Migrating macrophage

Small lymphocyte

Lining cells

Heterophilic leukocyte

Heterophilic leukocyte

Normoblast nucleus Eryth-   Polychro- Fat cells Normoblasts Eosinophilic myelocytes
                    rocytes matophilic
              erythroblasts in mitosis

Figure 8–5 Section of bone marrow of rabbit which had injections of lithium carmine and India ink. Hematoxylin-eosin-azure II stain. ×460. (After A. A. Maximow.)

to the polyphyletic school, the erythrocytes developed intravascularly from free stem cells (*erythroblasts*) that originated from the endothelium lining the sinusoids. The granulocytes, on the other hand, were said to arise extravascularly from free stem cells (*myeloblasts*) derived from the primitive reticulum cells in the stroma of the marrow. The mononuclear leukocytes were thought to originate in lymphoid organs or connective tissue, each arising from separate formative cells (*lymphoblasts* or *monoblasts*).

The *monophyletic school*, represented by Maximow, Bloom, Jordan, and others, insisted that the lining of the sinusoids had no hemopoietic potential, but that the primitive reticulum cells in the stroma of both the marrow and the lymphoid organs gave rise to a single type of free stem cell (*hemocytoblast*),

which was capable of differentiating into any of the cell types of the blood. All blood cells were believed to arise extravascularly and to enter the circulation through transient discontinuities in the wall of the sinusoids. According to the followers of this school, the free stem cells of the marrow (hemocytoblasts) normally differentiated into the erythrocytes and granulocytes, while those of the lymphoid organs (lymphoblasts) gave rise to the monocytes and the medium and small lymphocytes of the blood (Fig. 8–6). The hemocytoblast and the lymphoblast or large lymphocyte were considered to be equivalent. The different products of differentiation in the two sites was attributed to different local environmental conditions prevailing in the lymphoid organs and in the bone marrow. This interpretation seemed to be supported by the observation that in certain pathological conditions, involving severe impairment of the hemopoietic function of the marrow, the lymph nodes and spleen may become sites of active granulopoiesis.

The results of modern experimental work have tended to sustain the concept of a single pluripotential stem cell, and it has been clearly established that stem cells can move from organ to organ via the blood—a possibility seldom seriously considered by classical histologists. For example, two rats can be surgically joined in parabiosis (i.e., artificially produced Siamese twins) so that their body walls are continuous and their circulations are confluent. If one is then exposed to x-rays in a dosage sufficient to destroy the proliferative capacity of its hemopoietic cells, its marrow will gradually be colonized and repopulated by proliferation of stem cells that have reached it from the unirradiated partner via the blood. This and other evidence indicate that in rodents, and possibly in man, small numbers of pluripotential cells normally circulate in the blood. Under normal physiological conditions, these may serve to replace wasting populations of unipotential stem cells in lymph nodes, thy-mus, and spleen. These observations have had a profound effect upon current concepts of hemopoiesis. Thus, the occurrence of extramedullary hemopoiesis in pathological conditions may not be due to activation of the latent developmental potencies of extramedullary reticulum cells, as believed by classical monophyletists, but may result from seeding of the spleen and lymph nodes with pluripotential cells carried to them in the blood from the marrow.

It has also been clearly demonstrated in labeling experiments that more mature cells, particularly lymphocytes, move freely from the bone marrow to the lymph nodes, thymus, and spleen. Whereas formerly it was thought that virtually all of the lymphocytes and monocytes of the blood were formed in the lymphoid organs, it is now known that the bone marrow is also an important site of lymphocytopoiesis.

Although hematologists can agree upon a functional definition of a stem cell, they cannot agree upon its cytological characteristics at the light or electron microscope level. Because we lack morphological criteria for their identification, the tendency is to deal with stem cells as a statistical or hypo-

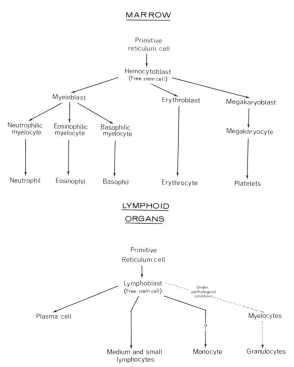

Figure 8–6 Traditional interpretation of the monophyletic school of hematologists. In the marrow, free stem cells were believed to give rise to all of the elements of the blood except the mononuclear leukocytes. The latter were thought to arise in the lymphoid organs from free stem cells (lymphoblasts) that were considered to be essentially the same as the hemocytoblasts of the marrow.

thetical entity rather than a microscopic reality. Kinetic studies indicate that there may be fewer than one stem cell per thousand marrow cells. They are capable of extensive replication but are a *slowly* proliferating population. They differentiate into cells committed to granulopoiesis, erythropoiesis, thrombopoiesis, or lymphopoiesis. These unipotential cells are self-replicating and *rapidly* proliferating. It seems to be these unipotential stem cells that are sensitive to the hormones or *poietins* involved in regulation of the numbers of the various cell types in peripheral blood. Like the pluripotential stem cell, they are poorly defined in morphological terms, but they differentiate into precursors of erythrocytes, granulocytes, and mononuclear leukocytes which are microscopically recognizable (Fig. 8–7). We turn now to a description of those later stages in hemopoiesis for which there are adequate criteria for visual identification of the cell types and where microscopists are on firmer ground

ERYTHROPOIESIS

The red blood corpuscles have a life span of about 120 days. The maintenance of the normal numbers of erythrocytes in the blood depends therefore upon continuing production of these cells. In adult humans, erythropoiesis takes place exclusively in the bone marrow.

The process begins with the slowly replicating pluripotential stem cells. Some of their progeny lose their pluripotentiality and become irreversibly committed to the production of erythrocytes. These constitute a rapidly proliferating population of unipotential stem cells. With further differentiation, these become recognizable in smears as *proerythroblasts*, round cells 14 to 19 μm. in diameter, with a thin rim of basophilic cytoplasm and a large nucleus, which has a rather uniformly dispersed chromatin pattern and two or more nucleoli.

Each proerythroblast undergoes a series of divisions to produce several *basophilic erythroblasts*. Somewhat smaller than their immediate precursors, these have a deeply basophilic cytoplasm, a more coarsely clumped chromatin pattern and no visible nucleoli (Fig. 8–8). The disappearance of nucleoli is associated with cessation of nuclear synthesis of new ribosomal protein. In electron micrographs, the cytoplasm contains a profusion of free polyribosomes but few or

no profiles of endoplasmic reticulum. Synthesis of hemoglobin is already in progress at this stage and the hemoglobin is recognizable in electron micrographs of the cytoplasmic matrix as fine particles of relatively low density. In stained marrow smears observed with the light microscope, its presence is obscured by the intense blue staining of the ribonucleoprotein of the cytoplasm.

The progeny of the division of basophilic erythroblasts are *polychromatophilic erythroblasts*, recognizable by their smaller overall size, smaller nucleus with more condensed chromatin, and a characteristic staining reaction of their cytoplasm, which ranges from bluish-grey through grey-greens of diminishing intensity (Fig. 8–8). Since no new ribosomes are formed after disappearance of the nucleoli, there is a progressive decrease in their concentration as a consequence of the succeeding divisions. At the same time, the hemoglobin synthesized on the polyribosomes steadily accumulates (Fig. 8–9). The range of tinctorial affinities exhibited by the polychromatophilic erythroblasts reflects the progressively changing proportions of ribosomes (which bind the blue components of the Romanovsky dye mixture) and of hemoglobin (which has an affinity for the eosin).

When the cells have acquired nearly their full complement of hemoglobin, their cytoplasm is distinctly eosinophilic with only a slight tinge of residual blue. The nucleus is now small, eccentric and deeply stained. Such cells (7 to 14 μm.) are called *acidophilic* or *orthochromatic erythroblasts* (also called *normoblasts*). In electron micrographs, their heterochromatin is in coarse blocks with little intervening nuclear sap, while the cytoplasm is devoid of organelles except for an occasional mitochondrion (Fig. 8–10). The cytoplasmic matrix presents a rather uniform fine grey granularity, owing to the high concentration of hemoglobin. Widely scattered clusters of ribosomes are still present (Fig. 8–11).

The eccentric nucleus is then extruded, or rather is pinched off, surrounded by a very thin film of cytoplasm and enclosed by a portion of the plasma membrane (Fig. 8–10). The extruded nuclei are ingested and destroyed by phagocytic elements of the marrow, while the anucleate portion is ultimately released into the bloodstream. The newly formed erythrocytes in the peripheral blood contain small amounts of basophilic material dispersed in the hemoglobin and consequently have a slightly greenish tint instead of the clear salmon pink of more mature forms.

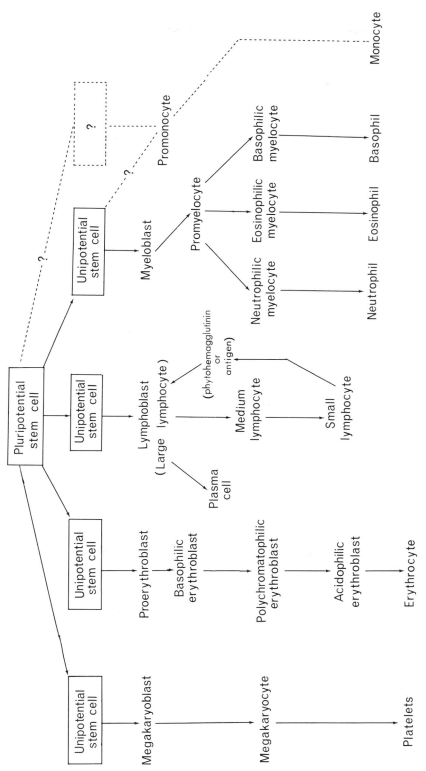

Figure 8-7 Current interpretation of cell lineages in the bone marrow. The hypothetical, pluripotential and unipotential stem cells that are not morphologically identified are shown here in boxes — all others are morphologically distinguishable. It remains undecided as to whether the monocyte comes from the stem cell of the granulocyte series or has a separate unipotential stem cell of its own.

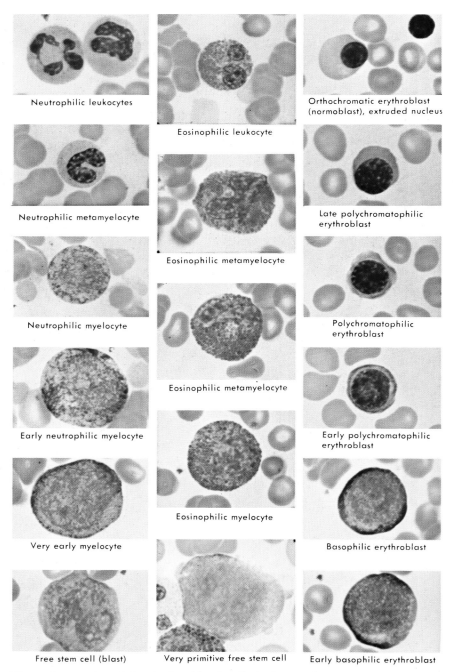

Neutrophilic leukocytes

Eosinophilic leukocyte

Orthochromatic erythroblast (normoblast), extruded nucleus

Neutrophilic metamyelocyte

Eosinophilic metamyelocyte

Late polychromatophilic erythroblast

Neutrophilic myelocyte

Eosinophilic metamyelocyte

Polychromatophilic erythroblast

Early neutrophilic myelocyte

Eosinophilic myelocyte

Early polychromatophilic erythroblast

Very early myelocyte

Basophilic erythroblast

Free stem cell (blast)

Very primitive free stem cell

Early basophilic erythroblast

Figure 8-8 Photomicrographs of developing blood cells in human bone marrow, showing steps in the transformation of stem cells into neutrophilic and eosinophilic leukocytes and into erythrocytes, as seen in dry smears stained with Wright's blood stain.

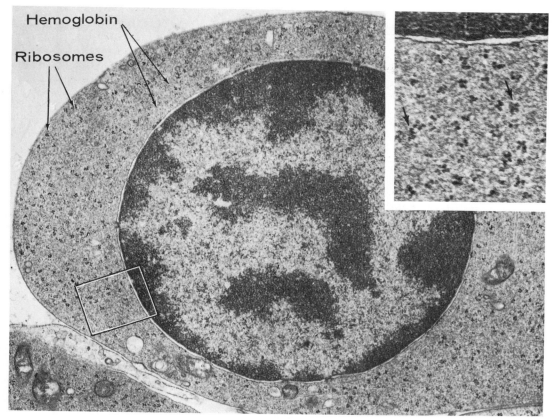

Hemoglobin

Ribosomes

Figure 8–9 Polychromatophilic erythroblast from guinea pig marrow showing coarse blocks of heterochromatin in the nucleus, and cytoplasm consisting mainly of hemoglobin and polyribosomes. In the inset, polyribosomes at the arrows can be distinguished from the smaller, less dense granular background of hemoglobin.

They are called *polychromatophilic erythrocytes* in ordinary blood smears. However, if fresh smears are stained with cresyl blue, the residual ribosomes are clumped and the aggregates formed appear as a bluish skein or network in the otherwise pink cytoplasm. Under these conditions of staining, the recently formed erythrocytes are called *reticulocytes.*

As previously noted (Chapter 7), the percentage of reticulocytes in a blood smear is a dependable index of the rate of formation of new red blood cells and is widely used in following the recovery of patients from blood loss or their response to treatment for anemia. In man, the erythrocyte generation time from stem cell to circulating blood cell is about a week.

Control of Erythropoiesis

The normal numbers of circulating erythrocytes are maintained with remarkable constancy. Transfusion of excess red blood cells is followed by suppression of erythropoiesis, whereas acute blood loss stimulates the marrow to increase its production and release of erythrocytes. An enhanced need for oxygen transport without any change in blood cell volume also stimulates the marrow. For example, in the physiological adaptation to high altitude, the body responds to the hypoxia by increasing the number of circulating erythrocytes (Viault, 1890). This early observation led to the conclusion that the marrow was directly responsive to the oxygen content of the blood. However, it was later shown that when only one member of a pair of parabiotic rats is exposed to hypoxia, both members show enhanced erythropoiesis (Reissman). This and other experiments provided strong evidence that the hypoxic stimulus to the marrow is mediated by a blood borne humoral agent—*erythropoiesis stimulating factor* or *erythropoietin.* This hormone is a glycoprotein with an estimated molecular weight of about 60,000. It appears to act upon unipotential stem cells to promote their differentiation into proerythroblasts. The intracellular site of action of erythropoietin has not been established, but it is speculated that this substance may act as a derepressor, initiating transcription of information for cell differentiation and hemoglobin synthesis.

Erythropoietin can be detected in plasma, lymph, and urine of hypoxic animals and in humans suffering from diseases attended by oxygen deficiency. The site of its synthesis remains uncertain, but indirect evidence implicates the kidney. After nephrectomy experimental animals are unable to respond to hypoxia with enhanced erythropoiesis (Jacobson). Efforts to extract erythropoietin from the kidney have not been successful. Although experimental removal of most other major organs has no effect or erythropoietin levels, there is reason to believe that

other sites of synthesis besides the kidney may exist, and there may be species differences in the site of erythropoietin production.

The maintenance of the normal number of circulating erythrocytes appears to depend upon (1) stimulation of the marrow by erythropoietin, (2) a marrow capable of responding, and (3) an adequate supply of iron to meet the needs of the marrow for synthesis of hemoglobin. A normal marrow not only provides for the necessary basal production to meet the need for daily replacement, but also permits rapid increase in output to four or five times the basal rate. The body contains only limited reserves of iron, associated with a globulin, *transferrin*, in the plasma and occuring in the form of a protein, *ferritin*, in various cells in the marrow and elsewhere. The amount of available iron may therefore limit the response of the marrow to an erythropoietic stimulus.

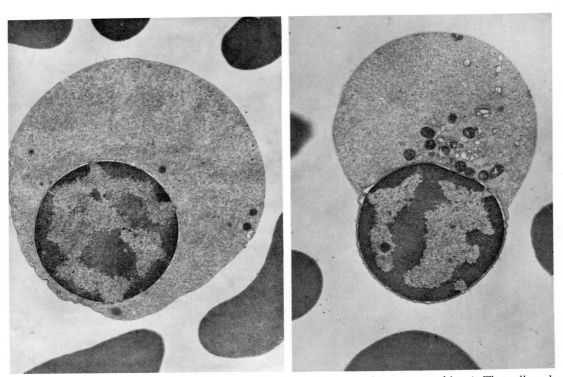

Figure 8–10 Electron micrographs of human orthochromatic erythroblasts (normoblasts). The cell at the right is extruding its nucleus. Notice that the nucleus is pinched off, enclosed in a portion of the cell membrane and a thin layer of cytoplasm, and does not pass through a break in the membrane as was previously believed. ×8000.

THROMBOPOIESIS

The developmental events in hemopoietic organs leading to formation of either the platelets of mammals or the thrombocytes of other vertebrates are called *thromobopoiesis*. Although the platelets were recognized as normal constituents of blood in 1865 (Schultze), their origin from the polymorphonuclear giant cells of the marrow was not described until 1906 (Wright). These huge cells, found in the liver, spleen, and other blood forming organs of the embryo, were called *megakaryocytes* by Howell (1890) to distinguish them from the *polykaryocytes* or *osteoclasts* of normal developing bone (see Chapter 10) and from the multinucleate giant cells found in pathological conditions. The megakaryocytes are distributed among the other hemopoietic elements of the marrow and are conspicuous because of their very large size, some attaining a diameter of 50 to 70 μm. The cell body is roughly spherical in form but often has blunt, irregular pseudopods on its surface. The nucleus is extraordinarily elaborate, with multiple lobes of varying size interconnected by constricted regions. It has a coarse chromatin pattern and numerous indistinct nucleoli. In routine smears the cytoplasm appears rather homogenous, but after appropriate fixation and special staining, a concentric zonation of the cytoplasm can be demonstrated. A relatively narrow perinuclear zone is surrounded by a broad central region stippled with large numbers of fine azurophil granules that are either uniformly distributed or gathered in small, dense clusters, depending upon the stage of development of the megakaryocyte. At the periphery of the cell is a rim of clear cytoplasm of irregular contour and variable thickness, devoid of granules. Groups of centrioles are found among the folds of the nucleus. Mitochondria are numerous and

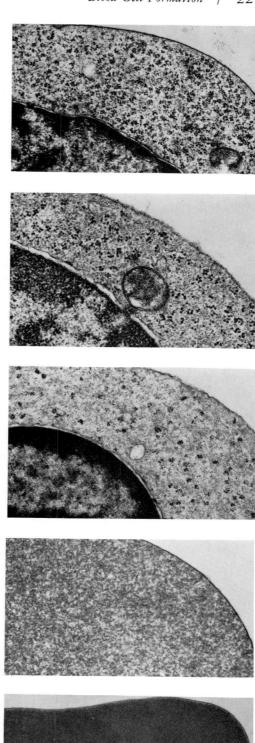

A

B

C

D

E

Figure 8–11 A series of electron micrographs illustrating the decline in number of ribosomes and progressive increase in hemoglobin in the cytoplasm during the differentiation of the guinea pig erythrocyte. *A,* Basophilic erythroblast. *B,* Polychromatophilic erythroblast. *C,* Orthochromatic erythroblast (normoblast). *D,* Reticulocyte. *E,* Erythrocyte. About ×25,000.

small. A compact juxtanuclear Golgi apparatus can be demonstrated in young megakaryocytes, but in more mature forms it tends to be dispersed in multiple small Golgi bodies widely scattered in the cytoplasm.

The youngest recognizable member of the megakaryocytic series is the *megakaryoblast,* a cell 15 to 25 μm. in diameter, usually having two nuclei with a finely stippled chromatin pattern and a thin rim of agranular basophilic cytoplasm. The nuclei subsequently fuse and this $2n$ cell proceeds to undergo a series of peculiar nuclear divisions without accompanying cytokinesis. The centrioles replicate and a complex multipolar spindle arises. The chromosomes become arranged in several equatorial planes at metaphase and give rise, at anaphase, to groups of chromosomes that reconstitute a larger lobulated nucleus without associated constriction of the cytoplasm. After an interval, another episode of division occurs, with daughter groups of chromosomes again fusing in telophase. Thus cells with $4n$, $8n$, and higher degrees of polyploidy are formed. The successive doubling of nuclear chromo-

some content has been verified by microspectrophotometric measurement of megakaryocyte DNA (Odell). The frequencies of $4n$, $8n$, $16n$, $32n$, and $64n$ were 1.6, 10, 71.2, 17.1 and 0.1 per cent, respectively.

A prominent cell center develops in the *promegakaryocyte* stage ($4n$ to $8n$ cells, 30 to 45 μm. in diameter), containing a number of centriole pairs corresponding to the degree of polyploidy. In subsequent differentiation, the volume of cytoplasm increases markedly while its basophilia diminishes and azurophil granules become dispersed throughout the cell. The fully formed megakaryocyte not yet active in platelet formation (sometimes called a *reserve megakaryocyte*) is 50 to 70 μm. in diameter, with a very large, highly lobulated, 16 or $32n$ nucleus and fine azurophil granules widely disseminated in the cytoplasm but generally absent from a narrow rim of pale blue ectoplasm. This rim of clear ectoplasm disappears in the *platelet forming megakaryocyte,* and the azurophil granules become clustered in small groups separated by agranular areas. This is most obvious at the cell periphery, which may be quite

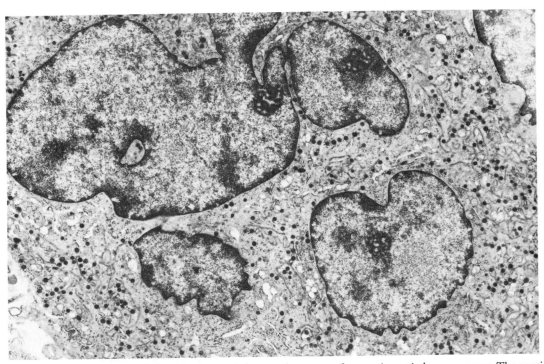

Figure 8–12 Low power electron micrograph of a megakaryocyte from guinea pig bone marrow. The section includes several portions of the highly lobulated single nucleus. Small azurophil granules are scattered throughout the cytoplasm.

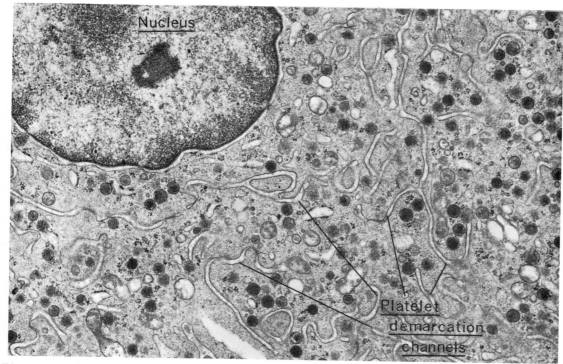

Figure 8–13 Electron micrograph of a small area from a guinea pig megakaryocyte showing the tip of one lobe of the giant nucleus and numerous platelet demarcation channels in the cytoplasm. The granules correspond to the azurophil granules found in the central region of the mature platelet. ×18,000.

irregular and drawn out into pseudopodlike extensions.

Wright accurately described the fragmentation of the megakaryocyte cytoplasm from light microscopic observations, but the actual cellular differentiation that makes this possible had to await electron microscopic examination (Yamada). During their early growth period, the young megakaryocytes are rich in free ribosomes but relatively poor in endoplasmic reticulum. The small, dense azurophil granules initially are randomly dispersed in the cytoplasm (Fig. 8–12). They later become clustered, and there is a concurrent development of small vesicles that become aligned in meandering rows between the groups of granules. If these linear arrays of vesicles could be seen in tridimensional perspective, it would be evident that they actually are in curved planes that intersect to partition the cytoplasm into units 1 to 3 μm. in diameter, each containing a number of granules and representing a future platelet. The initially discontinuous vesicular profiles subsequently elongate and coalesce to form a more or less continuous tridimensional system of paired *platelet demarcation membranes*, which bound the narrow clefts outlining the future platelets (Fig. 8–13). In the activated mature megakaryocyte, the platelet demarcation membranes evidently extend to the cell surface membrane, and masses of platelets are shed, separating along the narrow spaces bounded by membrane pairs, and leaving behind, around the polymorphous nucleus, a thin residual layer of cytoplasm bounded by an intact cell membrane.

It is not known whether the fate of these residual megakaryocytes is disintegration or whether they can reconstitute their cytoplasm and produce another set of platelets. It is generally assumed that they degenerate and are replaced by differentiation of new megakaryocytes from stem cells. About 10 per cent of megakaryocytes observed in the bone marrow appear to be degenerating forms that have lost nearly all of their cytoplasm in the exfoliation of platelets. Degenerate megakaryocytes not infrequently find their

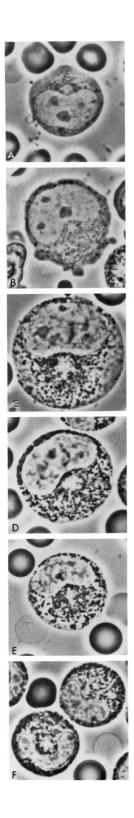

way into the sinusoids of the marrow and are carried with the blood into the capillaries of the lungs, where they remain for a time and then presumably autolyze. Under pathological conditions, embolism of the lung vessels by megakaryocytes may occur on a large scale.

In recent years considerable information has accumulated on the kinetics of thrombopoiesis. The total generation time from stem cell to platelet-producing megakaryocyte is estimated to be about 10 days in man. There appears to be a humoral regulatory mechanism insuring that production is responsive to the need for circulating platelets. Bleeding or performing an exchange transfusion to produce low levels of blood platelets (*thrombocytopenia*) is followed, in several days, by a three- to fourfold increase in megakaryocyte numbers and a rebound in circulating platelets to 150 to 200 per cent of the initial levels. A hypothetical humoral agent, *thrombopoietin*, is believed to be responsible for this positive feedback mechanism. Efforts to isolate this thrombopoiesis stimulating factor from plasma and urine have not been notably successful.

GRANULOPOIESIS

The development of the granular leukocytes begins with further differentiation of unipotential stem cells to form *myeloblasts*, the earliest morphologically recognizable cell of the granulocyte series. The myeloblast is a relatively small cell with a large oval nucleus containing three or more nucleoli. The cytoplasm is basophilic and devoid of granules. In its further development this cell acquires small, metachromatic, purple staining *azurophil granules*. It is then designated a *progranulocyte* or, more commonly, a *promyelocyte*. It has a reniform nucleus, multiple nucleoli, and a dispersed chromatin pattern. In the early promyelocyte, a small number of azurophil granules are clustered near the cell center (Fig. 8–14

Figure 8–14 Phase contrast photomicrographs of promyelocytes (*A, B*), neutrophilic myelocytes (*C, D, E*) and metamyelocytes (*F*) from human bone marrow. (Photographs from A. Ackerman, Zeitschr. f. Zellforsch., *121*:153, 1972.)

A and *B*). In electron micrographs, the granules are dense, 0.1 to 0.25 μm. in diameter, somewhat irregular in outline, and membrane limited. A few cisternal profiles of endoplasmic reticulum are present, as are abundant free ribosomes. The Golgi complex is situated in an indentation of the nucleus and numerous transitional vesicles are observed between the ends of the cisternae of the reticulum and the outer or convex face of the Golgi. In the rabbit, the condensing vacuoles (200 to 150 nm.) contain dense cores (100 to 150 nm.) that are precursors of azurophil granules (Fig. 8–15). These arise from cisternae on the inner or concave surface of the Golgi complex, facing toward the centrioles. The dense-cored vacuoles appear to fuse, forming larger ones containing multiple dense bodies that coalesce to form mature azurophil granules (Bainton and Farquhar). In the human, the condensing vacuoles contain a moderately dense

flocculent precipitate instead of dense cores and morula forms, but otherwise the mechanism of granule formation is not significantly different (Ackerman).

More advanced promyelocytes exhibit a striking increase in size from about 16 to about 24 μm. in diameter (Fig. 8–14 *C* and *D*). There is a concomitant increase in number of azurophil granules which are dispersed throughout the cell. The chromatin becomes more aggregated and is clumped along the nuclear envelope and around the nucleoli. The endoplasmic reticulum is more extensive and often distended during this phase of rapid synthesis of the granule protein.

As a result of one or more mitotic divisions, the late promyelocyte is smaller, the nucleus has a more condensed chromatin pattern, and the nucleoli are inconspicuous. Although azurophil granules still occupy much of the cytoplasm the peak period of

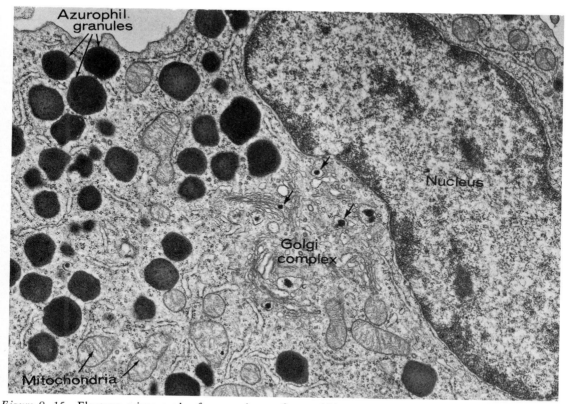

Figure 8–15 Electron micrograph of promyelocyte from rabbit marrow. Dense cored vacuoles associated with the Golgi complex represent formative stages of azurophil granules. Enlargement and coalescence of these gives rise to the large dense mature granules seen elsewhere in the cytoplasm. (Electron micrograph courtesy of D. Bainton and M. Farquhar, J. Cell Biol., 28:277, 1966.)

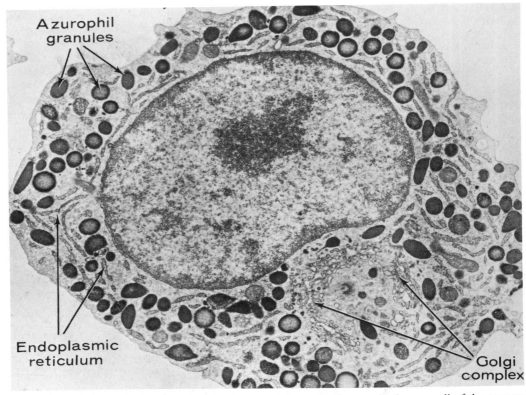

Figure 8-16 Electron micrograph of a polymorphonuclear promyelocyte, the largest cell of the neutrophilic series, treated for peroxidase. The cytoplasm is packed with peroxidase positive azurophil granules, and a positive reaction is seen throughout the reticulum. Specific granules are not yet present. (From D. Bainton, J. Ullyot, and M. Farquhar, J. Exp. Med., *134*:907, 1971.)

their formation has passed, and there is a notable decrease in size of the Golgi complex and the extent of the reticulum. From the stem cell through the late promyelocyte stage the development of all of the granulocytes is essentially the same. The granulocyte lineage diverges along three separate paths of differentiation with the appearance the *secondary* or *specific granules.*

Neutrophilic Myelocyte

This cell is distinguished from the promyelocyte by its smaller size, the more variable shape of its nucleus, the greater condensation of its chromatin, the smaller size of its Golgi complex, and especially by the presence in the cytoplasm of a second type of small granule that has little affinity for stains in routine smears. In electron micrographs, the specific granules are smaller and less dense than the azurophil gran-

ules. The formative stages of the specific granules are said to be associated with the outer or convex surface of the Golgi complex (Bainton and Farquhar). Thus, in the development of neutrophils, two distinct populations of granules develop at different times. The azurophil granules are formed in the promyelocyte stage at the concave face of the Golgi apparatus, and the specific granules form in the myelocyte stage at its convex face. The azurophil granules contain histochemically demonstrable peroxidase, acid phosphatase, aryl-sulfatase, β-galactosidase, β-glucuronidase, esterase, and 5'-nucleotidase and therefore are considered to be primary lysosomes. The specific granules contain alkaline phosphatase and antibacterial proteins.

The metamyelocyte is distinguished from the myelocyte mainly by the shape of its nucleus, which is deeply indented (Fig. 8-17). Two granule types are still present, but their proportions have changed, specific granules now comprising 80 to 90 per cent of the granule population. In the band forms the nucleus is elongated, and in mature neutrophils it becomes constricted into multiple lobules of varying size, connected by extremely attenuated regions. Mitotic divisions stop at the myelocyte stage and, other than the nuclear changes, subsequent differentiation involves some dilatation of the perinuclear cisterna, condensation of the cytoplasm, appearance in it of small amounts of glycogen, and a diminution in number of mitochondria and other organelles.

Eosinophilic Myelocytes

Less numerous than the neutrophil myelocytes are myelocytes with eosinophilic granules (Fig. 8–18). They have a slightly basophilic cytoplasm, and their granules are distinctly larger than those of neutrophil

myelocytes. In electron micrographs, the nuclear chromatin is condensed in conspicuous clumps around the periphery. The cytoplasm contains many cisternal profiles of the endoplasmic reticulum and numerous free ribosomes. Two populations of granules are present—dense azurophil granules and slightly less dense, specific granules. The differences in their sizes and densities are relatively slight.

The specific granules of eosinophils are rich in peroxidase as well as in other lysosomal hydrolytic enzymes. Cytochemical staining reactions are useful for investigating the intracellular pathway for synthesis, segregation, and packaging of the enzymes into specific granules. During the myelocyte stage, peroxidase can be demonstrated in the perinuclear cisterna, in all of the cisternae of the endoplasmic reticulum, and in the Golgi saccules, as well as in immature and mature granules (Fig. 8–19). In later stages, after granule formation has ceased, the

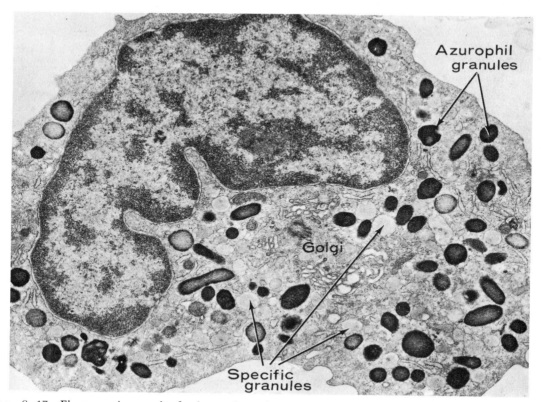

Figure 8–17   Electron micrograph of polymorphonuclear neutrophilic myelocyte stained with the peroxidase reaction. The azurophil granules are strongly reactive but the specific granules are unstained. (Electron micrograph courtesy of D. Bainton, J. Ullyot and M. Farquhar, J. Exp. Med., *134*:907, 1971.)

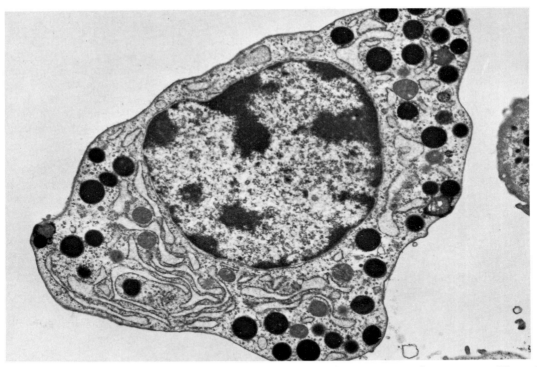

Figure 8-18 Electron micrograph of an eosinophilic myelocyte from guinea pig bone marrow. There is a well developed endoplasmic reticulum and numerous granules that are distinctly larger than those of heterophilic myelocytes. The characteristic equatorial crystal found in the granules of mature eosinophils develops quite late and is not seen at this stage. ×9500.

enzyme is found only in the granules. A similar distribution is reported for acid phosphatase and aryl-sulfatase. Thus, the cells appear to be capable of synthesizing and concentrating several proteins simultaneously.

In eosinophil metamyelocytes the nucleus is indented, and in mature eosinophils it is bilobed. It never acquires the degree of lobulation seen in neutrophils. In late myelocytes and in metamyelocytes, the contents of the specific granules begin to crystalize, so that one finds a heterogeneous population of granules, some remaining dense and homogeneous, others having crystals of varying shape surrounded by a matrix of lower density.

Basophilic Myelocyte

These are much more scarce than the neutrophil myelocytes. They are difficult to study because, in man, their granules are soluble in water and are partially or completely extracted by aqueous fixatives and stains. They are small cells, with a paler staining nucleus than the other myelocytes. The cytoplasm contains varying numbers of metachromatic granules of unequal size. The nucleus of metamyelocytes is deeply indented, and that of mature basophils is S-shaped or constricted into two or three lobules.

Regulation of Granulopoiesis

In normal individuals, the blood granulocyte count shows minor diurnal variations but is, on the whole, maintained at remarkably uniform levels. However, in the presence of bacterial infection or stress, there is a great and rapid increase in the number of circulating neutrophils. How the normal numbers are regulated and what the mechanism is for the response to increased need are still not well understood, but some points are clear. The total population of neutrophils in the blood vascular system can be divided into two categories: (1) those that are flowing with the blood—commonly referred to as the *circulating pool of leukocytes*, and (2) those that are temporarily adherent to the endothelium of vessels in various parts of the peripheral circulatory system—referred to as the *marginated pool of leukocytes*. Cells move randomly back and forth in continual exhange between the two. Normally the neutrophils are about equally divided between these two pools, but in response to violent exercise or epinephrine administration, there may be a massive movement of marginated cells into the bloodstream, doubling the number in the circulating pool without altering proliferative activity in the marrow.

Under normal circumstances maturation through the metamyelocyte stage is necessary before a granulocyte can leave the marrow. Segmented neutrophils enter the blood more readily than band forms or earlier forms.

Eight to 10 days elapse after the last myelocyte division before the progeny complete their maturation and enter the blood (Fig. 8–20). The turnover time of neutrophils in the blood is of the order of 10 hours. Thus, the greater part of the life span of these cells is spent in the marrow, where there are large reserves of band forms and mature neutrophils—approximately 15 times as many as there are in the blood (Boggs). Since these large stores can be mobilized upon demand, very marked increases in the circulating neutrophils can be achieved without a change in production rate. If the unusual demand for neutrophils is continued, there is an increased rate of proliferation of precursors in the marrow. How the information that more neutrophils are needed is transmitted from the periphery back to the marrow is not known. The existence of a humoral agent, *leukopoietin*, comparable to erythropoietin and thrombopoietin, has been postulated.

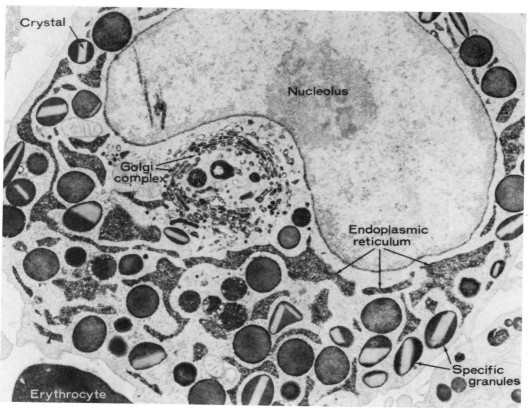

Figure 8–19 Eosinophilic myelocyte of rat, stained by the cytochemical reaction for peroxidase. Reaction product is found in the perinuclear cisterna and throughout the endoplasmic reticulum—also in the Golgi complex and specific granules. (Micrograph from D. Bainton and M. Farquhar, J. Cell Biol., *45*:54, 1970.)

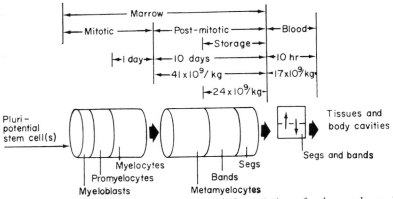

Figure 8-20 Summary diagram of the timing of events in differentiation of polymorphonuclear neutrophils. (From D. Boggs and M. Chernack, J. Reprod. Fertil., Suppl. *10*:32, 1970.)

MONOPOIESIS

The origin of monocytes has long been debated. The classical monophyletic school of hematologists believed that they arose in lymphoid organs, and that they originally were large lymphocytes that had differentiated to become phagocytic. It was argued that in the early phases of an inflammatory reaction they could not be distinguished from lymphocytes, and application of vital staining techniques to animals that developed a monocytosis following infection with *Bacillus monocytogenes* suggested transformation of small lymphocytes into monocytes. Investigators of the polyphyletic school believed that monocytes developed from distinct unipotential stem cells in the marrow called *monoblasts.*

Views on this subject have changed rapidly in recent years. Application of autoradiography (Gowans) and chromosomal marking techniques (Virolainen) have established to the satisfaction of most hematologists that monocytes originate from a rapidly proliferating pool of precursor cells in the bone marrow, and that those found in the blood constitute an early phase in the life cycle of tissue macrophages (see Chapter 6). After a developmental period of a few days in the marrow, they circulate for a day or two and then migrate into the connective tissues and body cavities to carry out their function as macrophages.

Although the origin of monocytes in the marrow has gained wide acceptance, considerable doubt remains as to the identity of their precursors. It has been difficult to settle this matter because monocytes constitute only 1 to 3 per cent of the nucleated cells of the marrow, and immature monocytes are not easily distinguished from early granulocytes. Indeed, some believe that they arise from the same committed stem cells.

Immature monocytes in the marrow have a large oval or round nucleus with two to five nucleoli and an abundant cytoplasm rich in free ribosomes, but with few cisternae of endoplasmic reticulum. The Golgi complex is prominent and numerous small granules associated with it appear to be precursors of azurophil granules.

More nearly mature monocytes are somewhat smaller, have a decreased nuclear-cytoplasmic ratio and fewer polysomes, and their azurophil granules are larger and more numerous. Nucleoli are still present and are also found in monocytes of the blood. In contrast to granulocytes that lose their nucleoli late in development and are no longer able to synthesize new granules, the ultrastructural appearance of the monocytes suggests that they retain considerable synthetic capacity and may continue to form granules in the blood and even in the tissues. The azurophil granules of monocytes are smaller than those of early granulocytes, but like them they contain a variety of hydrolytic enzymes and are regarded as primary lysosomes. Later, in their life in the tissues, the monocytes or macrophages no longer make dense azurophil granules but produce a second type of primary lysosomes consisting of Golgi-derived vesicles distinguishable as lysosomes only by cytochemical techniques (Cohn et al.; Nichols et al.).

LYMPHOPOIESIS IN THE MARROW

Lymphocytes were formerly thought to be produced exclusively in the lymphoid organs, and any found in the marrow were thought to have reached there from the blood. It now appears that there is no large-scale migration of lymphocytes into the marrow, but, on the contrary, the marrow is a major site of proliferation of small lymphocytes (Everett and, Caffrey). The nature of their precursor cells is not entirely clear. Marrow transplantation and chromosome marker studies have shown beyond doubt that lymphocytes originating in the marrow are capable of repopulating thymus, spleen, and lymph nodes. Such migrations are believed to take place normally. There is evidence that the lymphocytes formed in the marrow have a different immunological role than those formed in the thymus. These matters will be discussed in greater detail in relation to the lymphoid organs and the immune system (Chapter 14).

REFERENCES

General References

Downey, H., ed.: Handbook of Hematology. New York, Paul B. Hoeber, Inc., 1938.

McCulloch, E. A., J. E. Till, and L. Siminovitch: Genetic factors affecting the control of hemopoiesis. Proc. 6th Canadian Cancer Res. Conf., 1964, p. 336.

Wintrobe, M.: Clinical Hematology. 5th ed. Philadelphia, Lea & Febiger, 1961.

Yoffey, J. M.: Bone Marrow Reactions. London, Edward Arnold, Ltd., 1966.

Yoffey, J. M., ed.: The Lymphocyte in Immunology and Haemopoiesis. London, Edward Arnold, Ltd., 1967.

Zamboni, L., and D. Pease: The vascular bed of the red bone marrow. J. Ultrastruct. Res., 5:65, 1961.

Erythropoiesis

Ackerman, G. A., J. A. Grasso, and R. A. Knouff: Erythropoiesis in the mammalian embryonic liver as revealed by electron microscopy. Lab. Invest., 10:787, 1961.

Alpen, E. L., and D. Granmore: Observations on regulation of erythropoiesis and on cellular dynamics by Fe⁵⁹ autoradiography. *In* Stohlman, F., Jr., ed.: The Kinetics of Cellular Proliferation. New York, Grune & Stratton, Inc., 1959.

Bessis, M.: Life cycle of the erythrocyte. Sandoz Monographs. Basle, Switzerland, Sandoz Ltd., 1966.

Campbell, F. R.: Nuclear elimination from the normoblast of fetal guinea pig liver as studied with electron microscopy and serial sectioning techniques. Anat. Rec., 160:539, 1968.

Gordon, A. S., and E. D. Zanjani: Some aspects of erythropoietin physiology. In Gordon, A. S., ed.: Regulation of Hematopoiesis. New York, Appleton-Century-Crofts, 1971.

Hillman, R. S., and C. A. Finch: Erythropoiesis: normal and abnormal. Sem. Hematol., 4:327, 1967.

Jacobson, L. O., E. Goldwasser, W. Fried, and L. Plzak: Role of the kidney in erythropoiesis. Nature (London), 179:633, 1957.

Reissmann, K. R.: Studies on the mechanism of erythropoietic stimulation in parabiotic rats during hypoxia. Blood, 5:372, 1950; 16:1411, 1960.

Rifkind, R. A., D. Chui, and H. Epler: An ultrastructural study of early morphogenetic events during the establishment of fetal hepatic erythropoiesis. J. Cell Biol., 40:343, 1969.

Simpson, C. F., and J. M. Kling: The mechanism of denucleation in circulating erythroblasts. J. Cell Biol., 35:237, 1967.

Veault, F.: Sur l'augmentation considérable du nombre des globules rouges dans le sang chez les habitants des hauts plateaux de l'Amérique du Sud. C. R. Acad. Sci., 111:917, 1890.

Yoffee, J. M., ed.: Bone Marrow Reactions, Baltimore, Williams & Wilkins, 1966.

Thrombopoiesis

Abildgaard, C. F., and J. F. Simone: Thrombopoiesis. Sem. Hematol., 4:424, 1967.

Harker, L. A.: Platelet kinetics in man. *In* Greenwalt, T. J., and G. A. Jamieson, eds.: Formation and Destruction of Blood Cells. Philadelphia, J. B. Lippincott Co., 1970.

Wright, J.: Histogenesis of the blood platelets. J. Morphol., 21:263, 1910.

Yamada, E.: The fine structure of the megakaryocyte in the mouse spleen. Acta Anat., 29:267, 1957.

Granulopoiesis

Ackerman, G. A.: Histochemical differentiation during neutrophil development and maturation. Ann. N. Y. Acad. Sci., 113:537, 1964.

Ackerman, G. A.: Ultrastructure and cytochemistry of the developing neutrophil. Lab. Invest., 19:290, 1968.

Ackerman, G. A.: The human neutrophilic promyelocyte. A correlated phase and electron microscopic study. Z. Zellforsch. Mikrosk. Anat., 118:467, 1971.

Ackerman, G. A.: The human neutrophil myelocyte. A correlated phase and electron microscopic study. Z. Zellforsch. Mikrosk. Anat., 121:153, 1971.

Bainton, D. F., and M. G. Farquhar: Origin of granules in polymorphonuclear leukocytes. Two types derived from opposite faces of the Golgi complex in developing granulocytes. J. Cell Biol., 28:277, 1966.

Bainton, D. F., and M. G. Farquhar: Differences in enzyme content of azurophil and specific granules of polymorphonuclear leukocytes. II. Cytochemistry and electron microscopy of bone marrow cells. J. Cell Biol., 39:299, 1968.

Bainton, D. F., and M. G. Farquhar: Segregation and packaging of granule enzymes in eosinophilic leukocytes. J. Cell Biol., 45:54, 1970.

Boggs, D. R.: The kinetics of neurophilic leukocytes in health and disease. Sem. Hematol., 4:359, 1967.

Cartwright, G. E., J. W. Athens, D. R. Boggs, and M. M. Wintrobe: The kinetics of granulopoiesis in man. Series Haemat., 4:1, 1965.

Cronkite, E. P., and T. M. Fliedner: Granulocytopoiesis. New Eng. J. Med., 270:1347, 1964.

Patt, H. M., and M. A. Maloney: A model of granulocyte

kinetics. *In* Bierman, H. R., ed.: Leukopoiesis in health and disease. Ann. N. Y. Acad. Sci., *113*:511, 1964.

Scott, R. E., and R. G. Horn: Ultrastructural aspects of neutrophil granulocyte development in humans. Lab. Invest., *23*:202, 1970.

Development of Monocytes

Howard, J. G., J. L. Boak, and G. H. Christie: Further studies on the transformation of thoracic duct cells into liver macrophages. Ann. N. Y. Acad. Sci., *129*: 327, 1966.

Howard, J. G., J. L. Boak, and G. H. Christie: Macrophage-type cells in the liver derived from thoracic duct cells during graft-vs.-host reactions. *In* The Lymphocyte in Immunology and Haemopoiesis (Symposium). London, Edward Arnold, Ltd., 1967.

Nichols, B. A., D. F. Bainton, and M. G. Farquhar: Differentiation of monocytes: Origin, nature and fate of their azurophil granules. J. Cell Biol., *50*:498, 1971.

van Furth, R., and Z. A. Cohn: The origin and kinetics of mononuclear phagocytes. J. Exper. Med., *128*:415, 1968.

Virolainen, M.: Hematopoietic origin of macrophages as studied by chromosome markers in mice. J. Exper. Med., *127*:943, 1968.

Volkman, A., and J. L. Gowans: The origin of macrophages from bone marrow in the rat. Brit. J. Exper. Pathol., *46*:62, 1965.

Whitelaw, D. M., M. F. Bell, and H. F. Batho: Monocyte kinetics: Observations after pulse labeling. J. Cell. Physiol., *72*:65, 1968.

Lymphopoiesis in the Marrow

Bennett, M., and G. Cudkowicz: Functional and morphological characterization of stem cells: The unipotential role of "lymphocytes" of mouse marrow. *In* The Lymphocyte in Immunology and Haemopoiesis (Symposium). London, Edward Arnold, Ltd., 1967.

Bloom, W.: The hemopoietic potency of the small lymphocyte. Folia Haematol., *33*:122, 1926.

Bruce, W. R., and E. A. McCulloch: The effect of erythropoietic stimulation on the hematopoietic colony-forming cells in mice. Blood, *23*:216, 1964.

Caffrey, R. W., N. B. Everett, and W. O. Rieke: Radioautographic studies of reticular and blast cells in the hemopoietic tissues of the rat. Anat. Rec., *155*:41, 1966.

Craddock, M. D., R. Longmire, and R. McMillan: Lymphocytes and the immune response. New Eng. J. Med., *285*:324, 378, 1971.

Everett, N. B., and R. W. Caffrey: Lymphopoiesis in the thymus and other tissues: functional implications. *In* International Review of Cytology. New York, Academic Press, 1967.

Everett, N. B., W. O. Rieke, and R. W. Caffrey: The kinetics of small lymphocytes in the rat, with special reference to those of thymic origin. *In* Good, R. A., and A. E. Gabrielsen, eds.: The Thymus in Immunology. New York, Hoeber Medical Division, Harper & Row, 1964.

Ford, C. E., H. S. Micklem, E. P. Evans, J. G. Gray, and D. A. Ogden: The inflow of bone marrow cells to the thymus: Studies with part-body irradiated mice injected with chromosome-marked bone marrow and subjected to antigenic stimulation. Proc. 7th Internat. Transplantation Conference. Ann. N. Y. Acad. Sci., *129*:283, 1966.

Ford, W. L. and J. L. Gowans: The traffic in lymphocytes. Sem. Hematol., *6*:67, 1969.

Gowans, J. L.: Life-span, recirculation and transformation of lymphocytes. Int. Rev. Exper. Path., *5*:1, 1966.

Gowans, J. L., and D. D. McGregor: The immunological activities of lymphocytes. Progress in Allergy, *9*:1, 1965.

Micklem, H. S., C. E. Ford, E. P. Evans, and J. G. Gray: Interrelationships of myeloid and lymphoid cells: Studies with chromosome-marked cells transfused into lethally irradiated mice. Proc. Roy. Soc., *B165*: 78, 1966.

Osmond, D. G.: The non-thymic origin of lymphocytes. Anat. Rec., *165*:109, 1969.

Sabesin, S. M.: Lymphocytes of small mammals: Spontaneous transformation in culture to blastoids. Science, *149*:1385, 1965.

Yoffey, J. M., G. Hudson, and D. G. Osmond: The lymphocyte in guinea pig bone marrow. J. Anat., *99*:841, 1965.

9
Cartilage

Cartilage is a specialized form of connective tissue consisting of cells, called *chondrocytes*, and extracellular fibers embedded in an amorphous, gel-like *matrix*. The intercellular components predominate over the cells, which are isolated in small cavities within the matrix. Unlike other connective tissues, cartilage has no nerves or blood vessels of its own. The colloidal properties of its matrix are therefore important to the nutrition of its cells and are in large measure responsible for its firmness and resilience. The capacity of cartilage for rapid growth while maintaining a considerable degree of stiffness makes it a particularly favorable skeletal material for the embryo. Most of the axial and appendicular skeleton is first formed in cartilage models, which are later replaced by bone.

Cartilage is of more restricted occur-

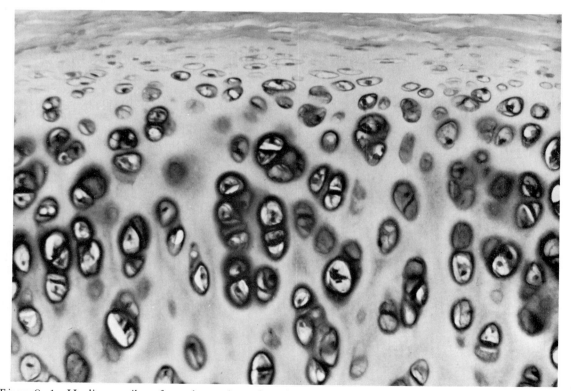

Figure 9-1 Hyaline cartilage from the trachea of a guinea pig. Notice the more intense staining of the capsular or territorial matrix immediately surrounding the groups of isogenous cells. The cells immediately beneath the perichondrium (*top*) recently added in appositional growth are single and elongated. Hematoxylin and eosin stain. ×400.

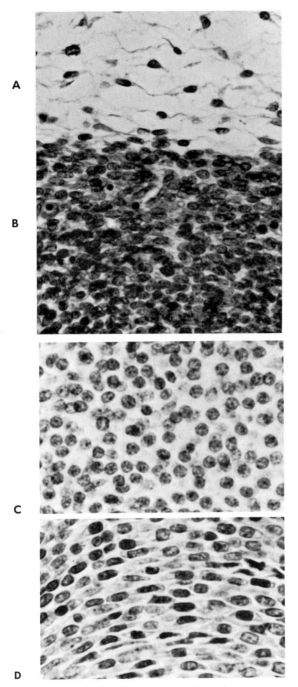

A

B

C

D

Figure 9–2 In the histogenesis of cartilage, mesenchymal cells (A) withdraw their processes and become crowded together to form an area of precartilage (B). In newly formed embryonic cartilage (C), the densely aggregated cells of the precartilaginous stage have been moved apart by deposition of clear hyaline matrix between them. The cells then become angular (D) and isolated in clearly demarcated lacunae. Hematoxylin and eosin stain. ×375.

rence in postnatal life, but it continues to play an indispensable role as the long bones grow in length throughout the growth of the individual, and it persists in the adult on the articular surfaces of the long bones. Except where it is exposed to the synovial fluid in joints, cartilage is invariably enclosed in a dense fibrous connective tissue covering called the *perichondrium*. Three kinds of cartilage, *hyaline, elastic,* and *fibrocartilage,* are distinguished on the basis of the amount of amorphous matrix and the relative abundance of the collagenous and elastic fibers embedded in it. Hyaline cartilage is the most common and most characteristic type, and the others can be regarded as modifications of it (Fig. 9–1).

HYALINE CARTILAGE

In the adult, hyaline cartilage is found on the ventral ends of the ribs, in the tracheal rings and larynx, and on the joint surfaces of bones. It is a somewhat elastic, semitransparent tissue with an opalescent bluish gray tint. Its histological appearance is most easily understood from a consideration of how it develops.

Histogenesis of Cartilage

At sites of future cartilage formation in the embryo, the mesenchymal cells first withdraw their processes and become crowded together in dense aggregations called *protochondral tissue* or *centers of chondrification*. The nuclei of the cells are very close together and the cell boundaries are indistinct (Fig. 9–2A and B). As the cells enlarge and differentiate, they secrete around themselves a metachromatic hyaline matrix (Fig. 9–2C). Tropocollagen is secreted at the same time, but the fibrils that form extracellularly tend to be masked by the hyaline ground substance in which they are embedded. As the amount of interstitial material increases, the cells become isolated in separate compartments or *lacunae* and take on the cytological characteristics of mature cartilage cells or *chondrocytes* (Fig. 9–3).

The continuing growth of cartilage takes place by two different mechanisms. Mitoses are observed among the cells for a rather long period. After the constriction of the cytoplasm in such a division, a new partition

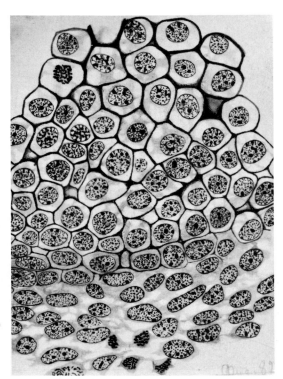

Figure 9–3 Development of cartilage from mesenchyme in a 15 mm. guinea pig embryo. The mesenchyme (*below*) gradually merges into the protochondral tissue with interstitial substance (*above*). Note mitotic figures. ×750. (After A. A. Maximow.)

of interstitial substance quickly develops and separates the two daughter cells. These in turn may divide, giving rise to clusters of four, and so on. The mitotic division of the chondrocytes and the secretion of new matrix between the daughter cells lead to an expansion of the cartilage from within, which is referred to as *interstitial growth*.

The mesenchyme surrounding the cartilage primordium condenses into a special layer, the perichondrium, which merges with the cartilage on one side and the adjacent connective tissue on the other (Fig. 9–4). Throughout embryonic life the cells on the inner or chondrogenic layer of the perichondrium constantly differentiate into chondrocytes, secrete matrix around themselves, and in this way contribute new cells and matrix to the surface of the mass of cartilage. This process is called *appositional growth*. The ability of the perichondrium to form cartilage persists but remains latent in the adult.

The Chondrocytes

In the layers of cartilage immediately beneath the perichondrium or under the free surface of articular cartilage, the lacunae are elliptical in section, with the long axis parallel to the surface, while deeper in the cartilage they are semicircular or angular. The cells in living cartilage usually conform to the shape of the lacunae that they occupy, but fixation and dehydration may result in their retraction from the wall of the lacuna, so that they appear stellate. Actually, mature cartilage cells in higher vertebrates rarely if ever have processes visible with the light microscope, but in electron micrographs their surface is quite irregular. The cells tend to be clustered

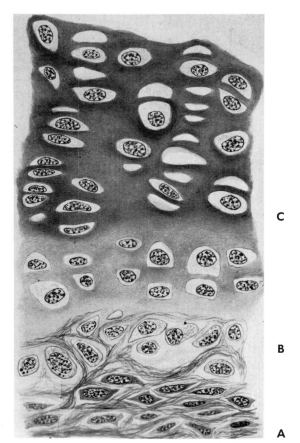

Figure 9–4 Hyaline cartilage from xiphoid process of rat. *A,* Transition layer adjacent to perichondrium. *B,* Continuation of collagenous fibers from perichondrium into interstitial substance of cartilage. *C,* Columns of isogenous groups of cartilage cells, some of which have fallen out of the lacunae in processing. Eosin-azure stain. ×750. (After A. A. Maximow.)

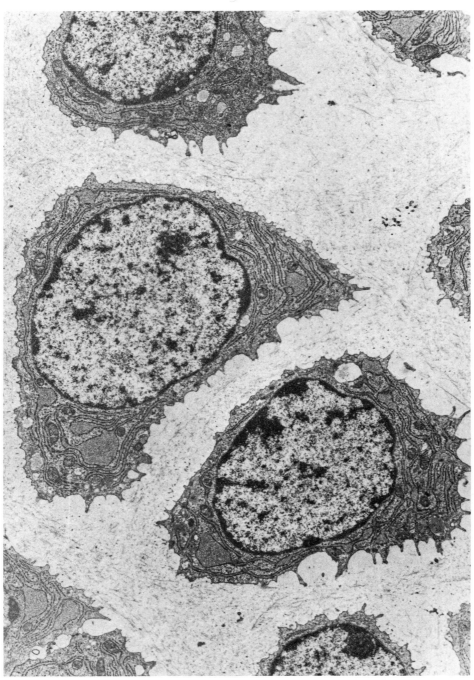

Figure 9-5 An electron micrograph of chondrocytes and matrix of mouse trachea illustrating the irregular outlines of the cells, their well developed granular endoplasmic reticulum, and other organelles. (Micrograph from Seegmiller, R., C. Ferguson, and H. Sheldon, J. Ultrastr. Res., *38*:288, 1972.)

in small groups (Fig. 9–1). Each group is said to be *isogenous* because it represents the progeny of a single chondrocyte that underwent a few mitotic divisions in the course of the interstitial growth of the cartilage. In the cartilage of the epiphyseal plates of long bones, cell division in a consistent plane results in an arrangement of the cartilage cells in long columns that are later invaded by advancing bone (Fig. 9–6).

The nucleus of the chondrocyte is round or oval and contains from one to several nucleoli, depending upon the species. There is a juxtanuclear cell center with a pair of centrioles and a well developed Golgi apparatus. The surrounding cytoplasm contains elongated mitochondria, occasional lipid droplets, and variable amounts of glycogen. When new matrix is being formed in growing or regenerating cartilage, the cytoplasm becomes more basophilic and the Golgi region becomes unusually large. Under these conditions of active growth, electron micrographs show a well developed granular endoplasmic reticulum with moderately distended cisternae. The saccules of the Golgi complex tend to be dilated, and there are numerous associated vacuoles of varying size that sometimes contain a flocculent precipitate. Similar vacuoles are also seen at the cell surface, where they appear to be discharging their contents into the surrounding matrix. In cartilage that is not actively growing, the endoplasmic reticulum is less extensive and the Golgi complex not as prominent.

Cartilage Matrix

In fresh hyaline cartilage the matrix appears homogeneous. This is due in part to the fact that the ground substance and the collagen embedded within it have approximately the same refractive index and in part to the small size of the collagen fibrils. The amorphous ground substance is deeply colored with the periodic acid–Schiff reaction

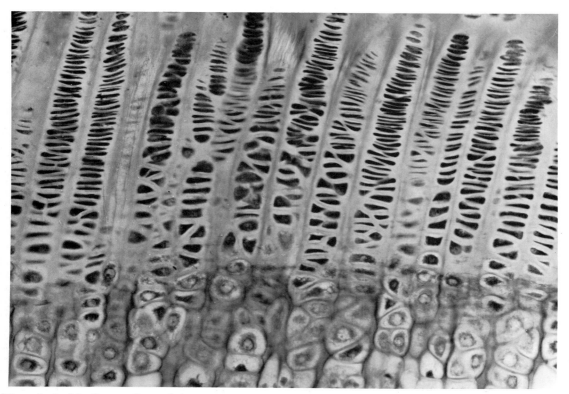

Figure 9–6 Hyaline cartilage of the epiphyseal plate of rabbit tibia. Here the cartilage cells are arranged in long parallel columns. From above downward, zones of cartilage cell proliferation, maturation, hypertrophy, and degeneration can be recognized. Hematoxylin and eosin stain. ×375.

for complex carbohydrates. It also has a marked affinity for basic dyes and stains metachromatically with toluidine blue. The principal constituent of the ground substance is *chondromucoprotein*, a copolymer of a protein and the polysaccharides chondroitin-4-sulfate (chondroitin sulfate A) and chondroitin-6-sulfate (chondroitin sulfate C). It is the strongly acidic sulfate groups of these mucopolysaccharides that are responsible for the basophilia of cartilage matrix.

The matrix immediately surrounding each group of isogenous cells usually stains more deeply than elsewhere (Fig. 9–1). This deeply basophilic rim is called the *capsular* or *territorial matrix*, while the less basophilic matrix between cell groups is called the *interterritorial matrix*. The deeper staining of the territorial matrix suggests that the concentration of the acid mucopolysaccharides is higher in the immediate vicinity of the cells.

Up to 40 per cent of the dry weight of cartilage matrix is collagen in the form of an interlacing fabric of fine fibrils 100 to 200 Å in diameter. Most of these fibrils do not exhibit the 640 Å periodic cross banding characteristic of collagen fibers in connective tissue or bone. They are sparse or absent in the immediate vicinity of the cells but abundant in the intercapsular matrix. Collagen fibrils with 640 Å period do occur in articular cartilage.

Secretion of Matrix Components

The chondrocytes have long been assumed to have some role in the elaboration of the ground substance and fibers of the matrix, but in the absence of obvious precursors in the cytoplasm there was no real evidence that they had a secretory function. With the advent of autoradiography it was shown that injected ^{35}S can be detected at early time intervals in the chondrocytes and later in the matrix (Belanger). Recent adaptations of radioautography for use at the electron microscope level leave no doubt as to the role of the chondrocyte in the production of both collagen and chondromucoprotein. After injection of tritiated proline into animals actively forming cartilage, this precursor of collagen could be localized after 10 to 15 minutes over the endoplasmic reticulum of the chondrocytes. At 30 minutes the label was

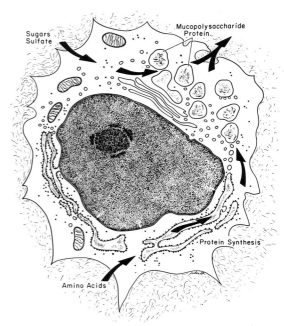

Figure 9–7 Diagram of the intracellular pathway for synthesis of matrix components. Amino acids are incorporated into protein at the ribosomes. Sugar and sulfates are believed to be incorporated into polysaccharide in the Golgi region and combined to form the protein-polysaccharide mucopolysaccharide released into the surrounding matrix. (Courtesy of E. Hay and J. P. Revel.)

over the Golgi region, and at four hours it was over vacuoles at the periphery of the cell and in the adjacent matrix (Revel and Hay). At longer time intervals the cells were cleared and all of the label was over the matrix.

Thus, it has now been demonstrated that the secretion of collagen precursors follows the same intracellular path as the secretion of protein by a glandular cell (Fig. 9–7). Recent studies using tritiated glucose and ^{35}S strongly suggest that the Golgi complex of the chondrocyte is the site of synthesis of the complex carbohydrate constituents of the extracellular matrix. It is probable that sugars and sulfate go directly to the Golgi region, where they are incorporated during the synthesis of sulfated polysaccharide. Labeled amino acid precursors, on the other hand, appear to go to the granular endoplasmic reticulum, where they are incorporated into protein that is later conjugated with polysaccharide in the Golgi apparatus and released from the cell as chondromucoprotein.

ELASTIC CARTILAGE

In mammals this variety of cartilage is found in the external ear, the walls of the external auditory and eustachian tubes, the epiglottis, and in parts of the corniculate and cuneiform cartilages. It differs from hyaline cartilage macroscopically in its yellowish color and its greater opacity, flexibility and elasticity.

Its cells are similar to those of hyaline cartilage; they are of the same rounded shape, are also surrounded by capsules, and are scattered singly or in isogenous groups of two or four cells. The interstitial substance differs from that of hyaline cartilage by being permeated by frequently branching fibers, which are positive in all staining reactions for elastin (Fig. 9–8). They form a network that is often so dense that the ground substance is obscured. In the layers beneath the perichondrium, the feltwork of the elastic fibers is looser. The elastic fibers of the cartilage continue into the perichondrium.

In the histogenesis of elastic cartilage in the embryo, a primitive connective tissue develops, containing fibroblasts and wavy fibrillar bundles that do not give reactions characteristic of either collagen or elastin. These indifferent fibers apparently are transformed later into elastic fibers with typical staining properties. The cells secrete matrix around themselves and become recognizable as chondrocytes. As in hyaline cartilage, a perichondrium is formed and initiates appositional growth.

FIBROCARTILAGE

Fibrocartilage occurs in a few regions of dense connective tissue in the body. In small areas with poorly defined limits typical cartilage cells and a small amount of matrix are

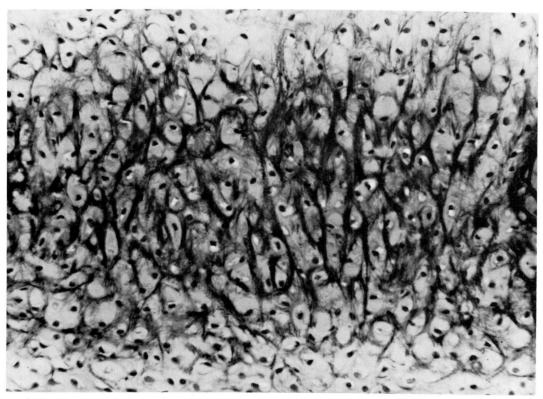

Figure 9–8 Elastic cartilage of the epiglottis of a child. Notice the dark-staining elastic fiber bundles in the matrix between cell groups. Hematoxylin and eosin stain. ×300. (After D. W. Fawcett, *in* R. O. Greep, ed.: Histology. Philadelphia, The Blakiston Co., 1953. Reproduced with the permission of the McGraw-Hill Book Co.)

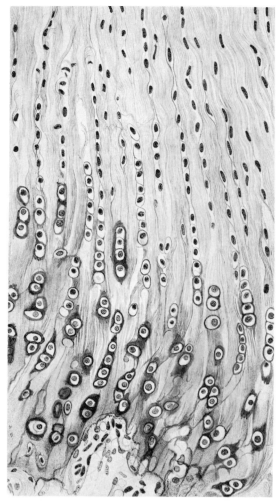

Figure 9–9 Low-power drawing of fibrocartilage at insertion of tendon into the tibia of a rat. Note the direct transformation of rows of tendon cells (*top*) into cartilage cells surrounded by deeply staining matrix. Hematoxylin-eosin-azure II stain. From a preparation of F. C. McLean. (Drawn by Miss A. Nixon.)

found among the abundant fibrous elements. It occurs in the intervertebral disks; in certain articular cartilages; in the symphysis pubis; in the ligamentum teres femoris; and in the sites of attachment of certain tendons to bones. The encapsulated cartilage cells lie singly or in pairs, or are sometimes aligned in rows between bundles of collagen fibers (Fig. 9–9). The ground substance is quite inconspicuous except in the immediate vicinity of the cells,

where its presence can be inferred from the characteristic form of the lacunae.

Fibrocartilage is closely associated with the connective tissue of the capsules and ligaments of joints. It is a transitional form between cartilage and dense connective tissue, and the gradual transformation from one to the other can be observed in the adult, as well as in its histogenesis in the embryo. In the intervertebral disks, for example, the hyaline cartilage connected with the vertebrae shows distinct collagenous fibers in its matrix. These then become associated into thick bundles, which almost entirely displace the homogeneous ground substance while the cartilage cells retain their spherical form and their capsular matrix. Finally this typical fibrocartilage merges into connective tissue, the cells of which are provided with processes and are not enclosed in lacunae.

Fibrocartilage develops in much the same way as ordinary connective tissue. In the beginning there are typical fibroblasts separated by a large amount of fibrillar substance. Then these cells become rounded, are transformed into cartilage cells, and surround themselves with a thin layer of capsular matrix. The abundant fibrous interstitial substance becomes infiltrated only slightly, with amorphous cartilaginous ground substance.

OTHER VARIETIES OF CARTILAGE AND CHONDROID TISSUE

There is a transitory phase in the embryonic development of hyaline cartilage when it is composed of closely adjacent vesicular cells and provided with thin capsules and with collagenous fibers in its interstitial substance. In this undeveloped condition the cartilage may remain throughout life in certain parts of the bodies of higher organisms. It occurs often in lower vertebrates (fishes and amphibians, as in the sesamoid cartilage of the tendon of Achilles in frogs) and is still more common in invertebrates. Such tissue has been called *pseudocartilage, fibrohyaline tissue, vesicular supporting tissue,* and *chondroid tissue.* This tissue serves as a mechanical support for other parts of the body.

The tissue composing the *notochord* of vertebrates has a similar structure. Here there is a shaft of variable thickness which consists of large, closely packed vesicular cells distended with fluid. The notochordal tissue has a different embryological origin from that of the cartilage and of the other connective tissues.

REGENERATION OF CARTILAGE

In amphibians, cartilage is regenerated in a manner resembling histogenesis of cartilage in the embryo, but most workers agree that after a wound or excision of a portion of cartilage in adult mammals, no such independent regeneration takes place. Instead, one sees at first in the injured area only necrotic and atrophic changes. The defect is then filled by newly formed connective tissue, which grows in from the perichondrium or from fascia in the vicinity of the injured area. The fibroblasts of this ingrowing granulation tissue may then round up, produce capsules around themselves and become transformed into new cartilage cells. Thus, if cartilage is replaced in the adult mammal, this takes place mainly by metaplasia of loose connective tissue.

Such a metaplasia sometimes takes place in connective tissue under the influence of simple mechanical forces acting from the outside, such as pressure, particularly when combined with friction. It is claimed that the presence of cartilage on the joint surfaces of bones is related to the constant mechanical influences to which a normal joint is subjected while functioning. When these mechanical conditions disappear, as happens in dislocation of bones, the cartilage often undergoes dedifferentiation. On the other hand, cartilage is laid down in the primordia of the joint surfaces in the embryo at a time when there are probably no mechanical forces acting on the joint.

Although cartilage has only limited regenerative capacity if the cells have been damaged, it has been shown that components of the matrix can be rapidly re-formed if the cells remain intact. Injection of a crude preparation of papain into young rabbits results in a collapse of their ears. This is attended by a loss of basophilia of the cartilage matrix and by a loss of its amorphous and elastic components, demonstrable in electron micrographs. After 48 hours the regeneration of matrix components is already far advanced and the ears are largely restored to their normal erect position.

REGRESSIVE CHANGES IN CARTILAGE

The most important regressive change in cartilage, *calcification*, normally precedes the type of bone formation called *endochondral ossification* (Fig. 9-10). The cartilage cells in a center of ossification undergo a regular sequence of cytological changes accompanied by characteristic changes in the neighboring matrix. In the epiphyseal plate, where the cells become arranged in parallel columns,

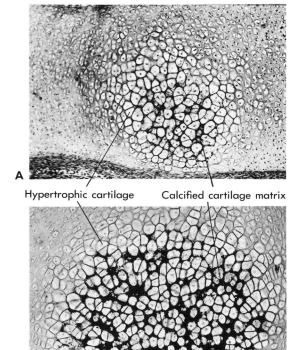

Figure 9-10 Two stages in the calcification of the cartilage model of the calcaneus in rats. *A,* Two days after birth. *B,* Four days after birth. The calcium salts appear black because of the silver nitrate stain. Undecalcified preparations stained with von Kóssa's method and hematoxylin and eosin. ×75. (After W. Bloom and M. A. Bloom.)

these changes are observed in successive zones along the length of the column. Distinct zones of *proliferation, maturation, cartilage cell hypertrophy,* and *cell degeneration* can be recognized (Fig. 9–6). In the zone of hypertrophic cartilage cells, the matrix undergoes calcification.

At sites where cartilage matrix undergoes calcification, small membrane limited structures are found which are called *matrix vesicles* (Anderson). Because they are limited by a typical unit membrane and sometimes contain ribosomes or other recognizable cytoplasmic components, it is assumed that they arise by being budded off from the chondrocytes. The vesicles have been isolated in centrifugal fractions and found to contain acid phosphatase and ATPase activity. They are found at all levels in the epiphyseal plate but are concentrated in the zone of hypertrophic cartilage cells. In the early stages of calcification of the hyaline matrix, minute crystals of hydroxyapatite are seen within and at the surface of the matrix vesicles. It is believed that the vesicles may have the capacity to bind and concentrate calcium, resulting in precipitation of hydroxyapatite in their immediate vicinity. As the nests of apatite crystals enlarge and merge, the cartilage becomes opaque, hard, and brittle. Because of these changes in the matrix, the zone of cartilage cell hypertrophy is also known as the *zone of provisional calcification.* The relation of these events to the process of ossification will be discussed in greater detail in Chapter 10.

In man, ossification of certain cartilages also occurs as a normal age change and may take place in some parts of the larynx as early as 20 years of age.

HISTOPHYSIOLOGY OF CARTILAGE

Cartilage in joints has the remarkable property of sustaining great weight and at the same time allowing the bones, which carry this weight, to move easily and smoothly against one another. In other places, such as the ear and the respiratory passages, cartilage serves as a pliable yet resistant framework that prevents the collapse of the tubular organs. Finally, cartilage in many bones makes possible their growth in length and is important in determining their size and shape.

Far from being an inert tissue, cartilage, through its participation in the growth of bones, is a fairly delicate indicator of certain metabolic disturbances. It reflects *nutritional deficiencies,* especially of protein, minerals, or vitamins. For example, the thickness of the epiphyseal cartilage plate diminishes rapidly when a young rat is placed on a protein deficient diet or on one lacking in vitamin A. When vitamin C is withheld from guinea pigs, producing *scurvy,* cessation of matrix formation may be accompanied by changes in the cells and by distortion of their columnar arrangement. Absence of vitamin D is attended by a deficient absorption of calcium and phosphorus from the diet and leads to *rickets,* in which the epiphyseal cartilages continue to proliferate but fail to calcify, and the growing bones become deformed by weight bearing.

The participation of cartilage in the growth in length of bones is in part under control of several hormones, of which the most important is the pituitary *growth hormone.* Hypophysectomy in young rats leads to a thinning of the epiphyseal plate of long bones, with cessation of mitosis and a decrease in the number and especially in the size of its cells. After a short time the cartilage fails to be eroded, and growth of the bone ceases. When growth hormone is injected into such animals, the cartilage undergoes a striking metamorphosis and within a few days resembles that of a normal, young, growing animal, and the bone resumes its growth. The response of the cartilage varies with the dose level and has been used to assay extracts containing the hormone. Long continued administration of the hormone produces giant rats, this being made possible in part by growth of cartilage after it would normally have ceased growing. Further, the injection of the hormone into older rats, in which cartilage proliferation has stopped, can to some extent reactivate its growth, with subsequent increase in the size of its bones.

When growth of cartilage has been retarded by removal of the thyroid from rats shortly after birth, renewed activity can be stimulated by administering *thyroxin.*

An excess of vitamin A accelerates the normal growth sequences of epiphyseal cartilage cells. It has been shown that these responses are not mediated by the pituitary. Mechanical injury to the cartilage may result in localized disturbance of growth. Lesions produced in the cartilage by x-rays or other high energy radiations frequently result in a marked stunting of growth.

Although much has been learned about the relation of cartilage cells to other mesenchymal derivatives, the interstitial substance is less well understood. Its mode of formation and growth, even its physical state, the organization of its polysaccharides, and the mechanism of calcification, all are fundamental problems that need further study. Perhaps the most difficult problem is the mechanism of interstitial growth in the center of this supporting tissue, with its dense intercellular substance.

REFERENCES

Ali, S. Y., S. W. Sajdera, and H. C. Anderson: Isolation and characterization of calcifying matrix vesicles from epiphyseal cartilage. Proc. Nat. Acad. Sci., 67:1513, 1970.

Amprino, R.: On the incorporation of radiosulfate in the cartilage. Experientia, 11:65, 1955.

Anderson, H. C.: Vesicles associated with calcification of the matrix of epiphyseal cartilage. J. Cell Biol., 41:59, 1969.

Anderson, H. C., T. Matsuzwa, S. W. Sajdera, and S. Y. Ali: Membranous particles in calcifying matrix. Trans. N. Y. Acad. Sci., 32:619, 1970.

Becks, H., C. W. Asling, M. E. Simpson, C. H. Li, and H. M. Evans: The growth of hypophysectomized female rats following chronic treatment with pure pituitary growth hormone. III. Skeletal changes—tibia, metacarpal, costochondral junction and caudal vertebrae. Growth, 13:175, 1949.

Belanger, L. F.: Autoradiographic studies of the formation of the organic matrix of cartilage, bone and the tissues of teeth. *In* Wolstenholme, G. E. W., and O'Connor, C. M., eds.: Bone Structure and Metabolism. London, J. & A. Churchill Ltd., 1956.

Bonucci, E.: Fine structure of early cartilage calcification. J. Ultrastr. Res., 20:33, 1967.

Bonucci, E.: Fine structure and histochemistry of calcifying globules in epiphyseal cartilage. Zeitschr. f. Mikroskop. Anat., 103:192, 1970.

Cameron, D. A., and R. A. Robinson: Electron microscopy of epiphyseal and articular cartilage matrix in the femur of the newborn infant. J. Bone & Joint Surg., 40:163, 1958.

Campo, R. D., and D. D. Dziewiatkowski: A consideration of the permeability of cartilage to inorganic sulfate. J. Biophys. Biochem. Cytol., 9:401, 1961.

Clark, E. R., and E. L. Clark: Microscopic observations on new formation of cartilage and bone in the living mammal. Am. J. Anat., 70:167, 1942.

Dziewiatkowski, D. D., and H. Q. Woodard: Effect of irradiation with x-rays on the uptake of S^{35} sulfate by the epiphyseal cartilage of mice. Lab. Invest., 8:205, 1959.

Fell, H. B., and E. Mellanby: The biological action of thyroxine on embryonic bones grown in tissue culture. J. Physiol., 127:427, 1955.

Glücksmann, A.: Studies on bone mechanics in vitro. II. The role of tension and pressure in chondrogenesis. Anat. Rec., 73:39, 1939.

Godman, G. C., and N. Lane: On the site of sulfation in the chondrocyte. J. Cell Biol., 21:353, 1964.

Godman, G. C., and K. R. Porter: Chondrogenesis, studies with the electron microscope. J. Biophys. Biochem. Cytol., 8:719, 1960.

Leblond, C. P., L. F. Bélanger, and R. C. Greulich: Formation of bones and teeth as visualized by radioautography. Ann. N. Y. Acad. Sci., 60:629, 1955.

McCluskey, R. T., and L. Thomas: The removal of cartilage matrix *in vivo* by papain. J. Exper. Med., 108:371, 1958.

Pelc, S. R., and A. Glücksmann: Sulphate metabolism in the cartilage of the trachea, pinna and xiphoid process of the adult mouse as indicated by autoradiographs. Exper. Cell Res., 8:336, 1955.

Revel, J. P., and E. D. Hay: An autoradiographic and electron microscopic study of collagen synthesis in differentiating cartilage. Zeitschr. f. Zellforsch., 61:110, 1963.

Seegmiller, R., E. C. Fraser, and H. Sheldon: A new chondrodystrophic mutant in mice. Electron microscopy of normal and abnormal chondrogenesis. J. Cell Biol., 48:580, 1971.

Seegmiller, R., C. C. Ferguson, and H. Sheldon: Studies on cartilage. VI. A genetically determined defect in tracheal cartilage. J. Ultrastr. Res., 38:288, 1972.

Sheehan, J. F.: A cytological study of the cartilage cells of developing long bones of the rat, with special reference to the Golgi apparatus, mitochondria, neutral-red bodies and lipid inclusions. J. Morphol., 82:151, 1948.

Sheldon, H., and F. B. Kimball: Studies on cartilage. III. The occurrence of collagen with vacuoles of the Golgi apparatus. J. Cell Biol., 12:599, 1962.

Sheldon, H., and R. A. Robinson: Studies on cartilage. I. Electron microscope observations on normal rabbit ear cartilage. II. Electron microscope observations on rabbit ear cartilage following the administration of papain. J. Biophys. Biochem. Cytol., 4:401, 1958; 8:151, 1960.

Silberberg, R., M. Hasler, and M. Silberberg: Submicroscopic response of articular cartilage of mice treated with estrogenic hormone. Am. J. Path., 46:289, 1965.

Silberberg, R., M. Silberberg, and D. Feir: Life cycle of articular cartilage cells: an electron microscope study of the hip joint of the mouse. Amer. J. Anat., 114:17, 1964.

Streeter, G. L.: Developmental horizons in human embryos (fourth issue); A review of the histogenesis of cartilage and bone. Carnegie Contributions to Embryol., 33:149, 1949.

Thomas, L.: Reversible collapse of rabbit ears after intravenous papain and prevention of recovery by cortisone. J. Exper. Med., 104:245, 1956.

Weiss, P., and A. Moscona: Type-specific morphogenesis of cartilages developed from dissociated limb and scleral mesenchyme in vitro. J. Embryol. Exper. Morphol., 6:238, 1958.

Wolbach, S. B., and C. L. Maddock: Vitamin-A acceleration of bone growth sequences in hypophysectomized rats. Arch. Path., 53:273, 1952.

10
Bone

Bone, in common with other connective tissues, consists of cells, fibers, and ground substance, but unlike the others its extracellular components are calcified, making it a hard, unyielding substance ideally suited for its supportive and protective function in the skeleton. It provides for the internal support of the body and for the attachment of the muscles and tendons essential for locomotion. It protects the vital organs of the cranial and thoracic cavities, and it encloses the blood forming elements of the bone marrow. In addition to these mechanical functions, it plays an important metabolic role as a mobilizable store of calcium, which can be drawn upon as needed in the homeostatic regulation of the concentration of calcium in the blood and other fluids of the body.

Bone has a remarkable combination of physical properties—high tensile and compressive strength while at the same time having some elasticity and being a relatively lightweight material. At all levels of the organization of bones, from their gross form to their submicroscopic structure, their construction ensures the greatest strength with great economy of material and minimal weight. Despite its strength and hardness, bone is a dynamic living material, constantly being renewed and reconstructed throughout the lifetime of the individual. Owing to its continual internal reconstruction and its responsiveness to external mechanical stimuli, it can be modified by the surgical procedures and appliances of the orthopedic surgeon or the orthodontist. It is also surprisingly responsive to metabolic, nutritional, and endocrine influences. Disuse is followed by *atrophy* with loss of substance; increased use is accompanied by *hypertrophy*, with an increase in the mass of bone.

MACROSCOPIC STRUCTURE OF BONES

Upon inspection with the naked eye or hand lens, two forms of bone are distinguish-

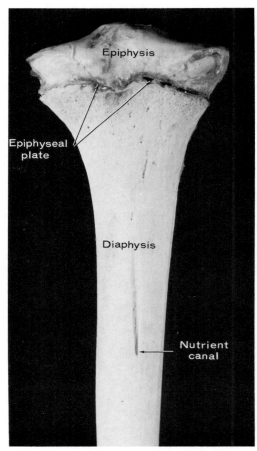

Figure 10-1 Photograph of the upper half of the tibia of young girl, showing the proximal bony epiphysis, the cartilaginous epiphyseal plate, and the shaft or diaphysis.

244

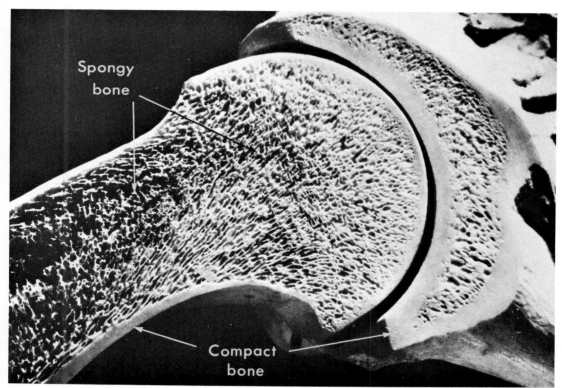

Figure 10-2 Photograph of a sagittal section of the proximal end of the humerus in relation to the glenoid fossa of the scapula at the shoulder joint. These are dry bones, and the cartilaginous articular surfaces of the joint are not present. The figure is presented here to illustrate the appearance and distribution of spongy and compact bone. (After A. Feininger, from *Anatomy of Nature.* Crown Publishers. With permission of Time, Inc.)

able, *cancellous* or *spongy* (substantia spongiosa) and *compact* (substantia compacta). Cancellous bone consists of a three dimensional lattice of branching bony spicules or *trabeculae* delimiting a labyrinthine system of intercommunicating spaces that are occupied by *bone marrow.* Compact bone appears as a solid continuous mass, in which spaces can be seen only with the aid of the microscope. The two forms of bone grade into one another without a sharp boundary (Fig. 10-3).

In typical long bones, such as the femur or the humerus, the *diaphysis* (shaft) consists of a thick walled hollow cylinder of compact bone with a voluminous central *medullary cavity* (marrow cavity) occupied by the bone marrow. The ends of long bones consist mainly of spongy bone covered by a thin peripheral cortex of compact bone (Figs. 10-2 and 10-3). The intercommunicating spaces

among the trabeculae of this spongy bone, in the adult, are directly continuous with the marrow cavity of the shaft. In the growing animal, the ends of long bones, called the *epiphyses,* arise from separate centers of ossification, and are separated from the diaphysis by a cartilaginous *epiphyseal plate* (Fig. 10-1), which is united to the diaphysis by columns of spongy bone in a transitional region called the *metaphysis.* The epiphyseal cartilage and the adjacent spongy bone of the metaphysis constitute a growth zone, in which all increment in length of the bone occurs. On the articular surfaces at the ends of long bones, the thin cortical layer of compact bone is covered by a layer of hyaline cartilage, the *articular cartilage.*

With few exceptions, bones are invested by *periosteum,* a layer of specialized connective tissue, which is endowed with *osteogenic poten-*

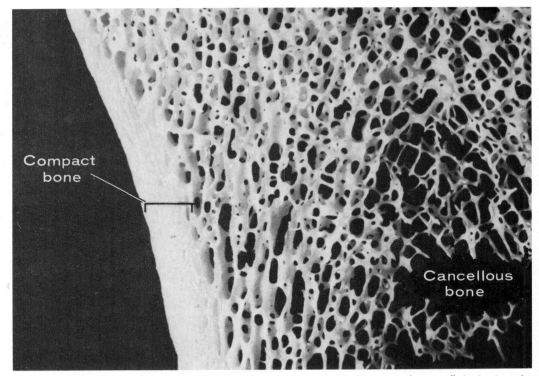

Figure 10-3 A thick ground section of the tibia illustrating the cortical compact bone and the lattice of trabeculae of the cancellous bone.

cy. That is to say, it has the ability to form bone. A covering of periosteum is lacking on those areas at the ends of long bones that are covered with articular cartilage. It is also absent at the sites where tendons and ligaments are inserted and on the surfaces of the patella and other sesamoid bones that are formed within tendons. It is also lacking on the subcapsular areas of the neck of the femur and of the astragalus. Where functional periosteum is absent, the connective tissue in contact with the surfaces of bone lacks osteogenic potency and does not contribute to the healing of fractures. The marrow cavity of the diaphysis and the cavities of spongy bone are lined by the *endosteum*, a thin cellular layer that also possesses osteogenic properties.

In the flat bones of the skull, the substantia compacta forms, on both surfaces, relatively thick layers that are often referred to as the *outer* and *inner tables*. Between them is a layer of spongy bone of varying thickness called the *diploë*. The periosteum on the outer surface of the skull is called the *pericranium*, while the inner surface is lined by the *dura mater*. Although different terms are applied to these connective tissue coverings of the flat bones, they do not differ significantly in their structure or osteogenic potency from the periosteum and endosteum of long bones. However, defects in the calvaria resulting from injury often do not heal completely in adults.

MICROSCOPIC STRUCTURE OF BONES

If a thin ground section of the shaft of a long bone is examined with the microscope, it is apparent that the contribution of the cellular elements of bone to its total mass is small. Compact bone is largely composed of the mineralized interstitial substance, *bone matrix*, deposited in layers or *lamellae* 3 to 7 μm.

thick (Figs. 10–4 and 10–5). Rather uniformly spaced throughout the interstitial substance of bone are lenticular cavities, called *lacunae*, each completely filled by a bone cell or *osteocyte*. Radiating in all directions from each lacuna are exceedingly slender, branching tubular passages, the *canaliculi*, that penetrate the interstitial substance of the lamellae, anastomosing with the canaliculi of neighboring lacunae (Figs. 10–6 and 10–7). Thus, although the lacunae are spaced some distance apart, they form a continuous system of cavities interconnected by an extensive network of minute canals. These slender passages are believed to be essential to the nutrition of the bone cells. Whereas cartilage can be sustained by diffusion through the aqueous phase of the gel-like hyaline matrix, the deposition of calcium salts in the interstitial substance of bone evidently reduces its permeability. However, the maintenance of a system of intercommunicating canaliculi provides avenues for exchange of metabolites between the cells and the nearest perivascular space.

The lamellae of compact bone are disposed in three common patterns. (1) The great majority are arranged concentrically around longitudinal vascular channels within the bone to form cylindrical units of structure called *haversian systems* or *osteons*. These vary in size, being made up of 4 to 20 lamellae. In cross section, the haversian systems appear as concentric rings around a circular opening (Figs. 10–6 and 10–8A). In longitudinal section, they are seen as closely spaced bands parallel to the vascular channels (Figs. 10–5 and 10–9). (2) Between the haversian systems are angular fragments of lamellar bone of varying size and irregular shape. These are the *interstitial systems* (Fig. 10–4). The limits of the haversian systems and interstitial systems are sharply demarcated by refractile lines called *cement lines*. In cross section, the interior of compact bone thus appears as a mosaic of round and angular pieces cemented together (Fig. 10–8A). (3) At the external surface of the cortical bone, immediately beneath the periosteum, and on the internal surface, subjacent to the endosteum, there

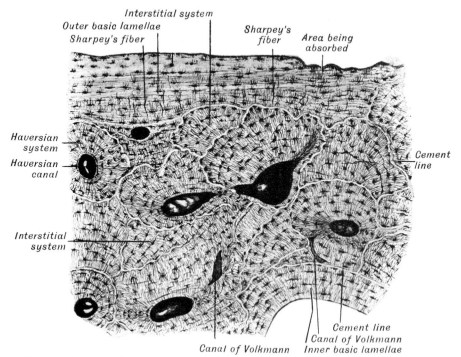

Figure 10–4 Portion of a ground cross section of a human metacarpal bone. Stained with fuchsin, mounted in Canada balsam. ×160. (After Schaffer.)

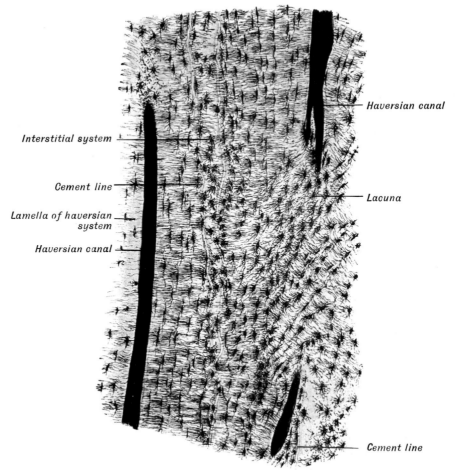

Figure 10-5 Portion of a longitudinal, ground section of the ulna of man; stained with fuchsin. ×160. (After Schaffer.)

may be several lamellae that extend uninterruptedly around much of the circumference of the shaft. These are the *outer* and *inner circumferential lamellae* (Fig. 10–9).

Two categories of vascular channels are distinguished in compact bone on the basis of their orientation and their relation to the lamellar structure of the surrounding bone. The longitudinal channels in the centers of the haversian systems are called *haversian canals*. They are 22 to 110 μm. in diameter and contain one or two blood vessels ensheathed in loose connective tissue. The vessels are, for the most part, capillaries and postcapillary venules, but occasional arterioles may also be found. The haversian canals

are connected with one another and communicate with the free surface and with the marrow cavity via transverse and oblique channels called *Volkmann's canals*. These can be distinguished from the haversian canals in sections by the fact that they are not surrounded by concentrically arranged lamellae but traverse the bone in a direction perpendicular or oblique to the lamellae. The blood vessels from the endosteum and, to a lesser extent, from the periosteum, communicate with those of the haversian systems via Volkmann's canals. The vessels are often larger than those in the osteons.

Although it is basically correct, the traditional description of haversian canals as being longitudinal and Volkmann's canals as being oblique or transverse is an oversimplification. Reconstruction of osteons from serial sections has shown that they are not always simple cylindrical units but may branch and anastomose and have a rather complex three dimensional configuration (Cohen). Thus one may encounter obliquely oriented vascular channels that are surrounded by concentric lamellae. Despite their atypical orientation, these are clearly cross connecting haversian canals.

Cancellous bone is also composed of lamellae, but its trabeculae are relatively thin, and are usually not penetrated by blood vessels. Therefore, there are usually no haversian systems but merely a mosaic of angular pieces of lamellar bone. The bone cells are nourished by diffusion from the endosteal surface via the minute canaliculi

that interconnect lacunae and extend to the surface.

The periosteum is subject to considerable variation in its microscopic appearance, depending upon its functional state. During embryonic and postnatal growth there is an inner layer of bone forming cells, *osteoblasts*, in direct contact with the bone. In the adult, the osteoblasts revert to a resting form (osteoprogenitor cells) and are indistinguishable from other spindle-shaped connective tissue cells. If a bone is injured, however, the bone forming potentiality of these cells is reactivated; they take on the appearance of typical osteoblasts and participate in the formation of new bone. The outer layer of the periosteum is a relatively acellular dense connective tissue containing blood vessels. Branches of these vessels traverse the deeper layer and enter Volkmann's canals, through which they

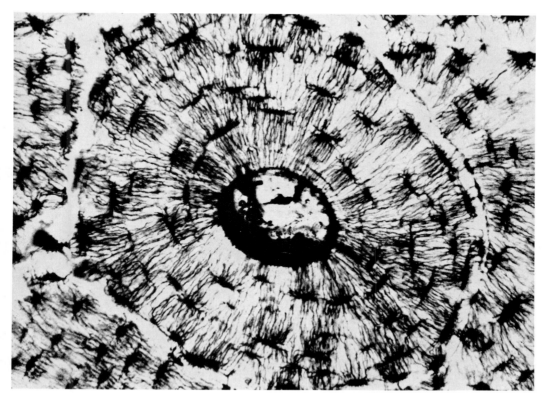

Figure 10-6 Ground section of human femur, showing a typical haversian system and the lacunae and canaliculi. ×300. (After D. W. Fawcett, *in* R. O. Greep, ed.: Histology. Philadelphia, The Blakiston Co., 1953. Reproduced with the permission of the McGraw-Hill Book Co.)

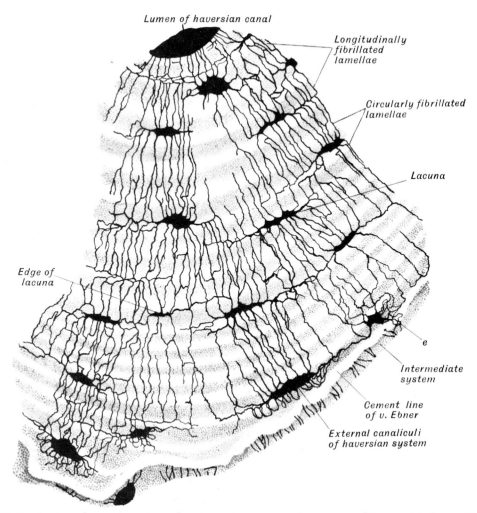

Figure 10-7 Sector of a cross section of an haversian system of a macerated human hip bone. The cavities and canaliculi are filled with a dye: *e*, connection of canaliculi of the haversian system with those of an intermediate system. ×520. (After A. A. Maximow.)

Figure 10-8 Section of bone from the midshaft of the human fibula as revealed by four different optical methods. *A,* Ground section photographed through the ordinary bright field microscope. The lacunae, the haversian systems, and interstitial lamellae are clearly shown. *B,* The same section photographed through the polarizing microscope shows the alternating bright and dark concentric layers in the haversian systems that result from the differing orientation of collagen fibers in the successive lamellae. *C,* In a historadiogram of the same section, the differing shades of grey in the scale from nearly white to nearly black reflect the differing concentrations of calcium. In the haversian canals, there has been no absorption of the x-rays and the film is therefore black. The most recently deposited haversian systems are incompletely calcified and appear dark grey, whereas older ones containing higher concentrations of calcium are lighter. The old interstitial lamellae, being fully calcified, are most highly absorptive and therefore appear white. *D,* The 14 year old girl from whom this specimen was taken had been given a daily dose of the antibiotic Achromycin for 15 consecutive days at one period of her illness. Amputation of the leg was carried out 230 days later. Achromycin is incorporated into the matrix of bone being deposited at the time of its administration and imparts a fluorescence to the newly formed bone. In the section shown here, transilluminated with ultraviolet light in a fluorescence microscope, the white areas represent areas of bone laid down during the 15 day Achromycin treatment. The nonfluorescent central portions of the same haversian systems represent bone deposited after cessation of the treatment. ×125. (Courtesy of R. Amprino.)

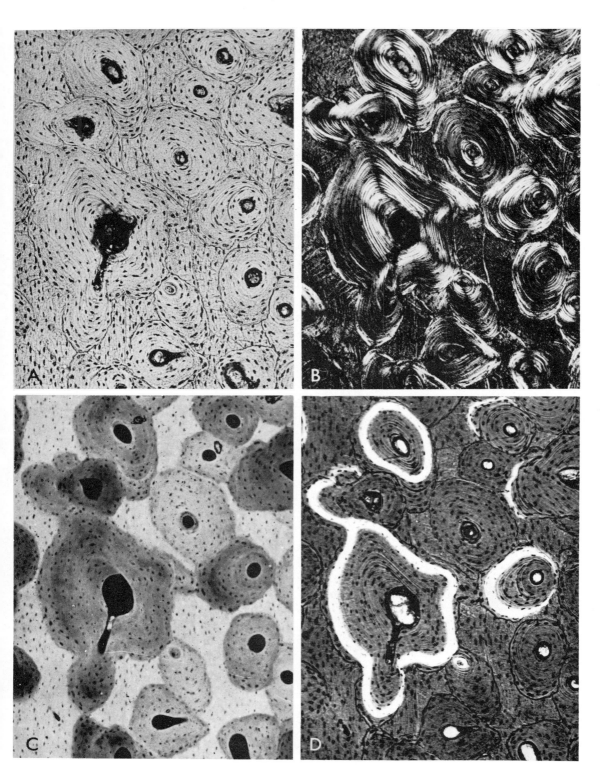

Figure 10–8 See opposite page for legend.

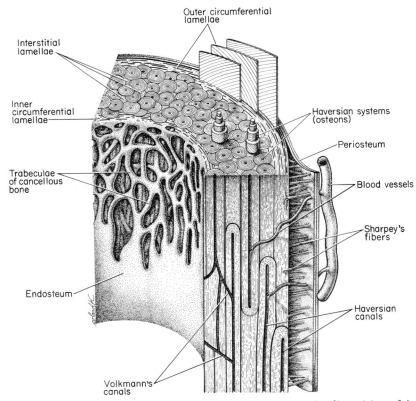

Figure 10–9 Diagram of a sector of the shaft of a long bone illustrating the disposition of the lamellae in the osteons or haversian systems, the interstitial lamellae, and the outer and inner circumferential lamellae. (After A. Benninghoff, Lehrbuch der Anatomie des Menschen. Berlin, Urban und Schwarzenberg, 1949.)

communicate with the vessels of the haversian canals. These numerous small vessels entering Volkmann's canals from the periosteum may contribute to maintaining its attachment to the underlying bone. In addition, coarse bundles of collagenous fibers from the outer layer of the periosteum turn inward, penetrating the outer circumferential lamellae and interstitial systems of the bone. These are called *Sharpey's fibers* or *perforating fibers* (Figs. 10–9 and 10–10). They arise during growth of the bone when thick collagenous bundles become incarcerated in the bone matrix deposited during the subperiosteal formation of new lamellae. When the perforating fibers are uncalcified, they occupy irregular canals penetrating the compact bone from the periosteal surface in a direction perpendicular or oblique to the lamellae. When calcified, they appear as irregular radial streaks in the outer portion of the cortical bone. They serve to anchor the periosteum firmly to the underlying bone. They vary greatly in number in different regions, being particularly numerous in some bones of the skull and at sites of attachment of muscles and tendons to the periosteum of long bones. In addition to Sharpey's fibers, some elastic fibers penetrate the cortical bone from the periosteum, either together with or independent of the collagenous bundles.

The endosteum is a thin layer of squamous cells lining the walls of those cavities in the bone that house the bone marrow. It is the peripheral layer of the stroma of the bone marrow where it is in contact with bone, and it resembles the periosteum in its osteogenic potencies, but is much thinner—usually a single layer of cells without associated connective tissue fibers. All the cavities of bone, including the haversian canals and the marrow spaces within spongy bone, are lined by endosteum which is said to have osteogenic potencies.

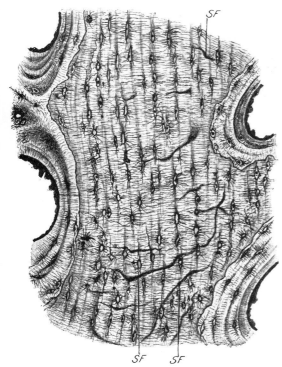

Figure 10-10 Portion of a cross section of a human fibula. *SF*, Sharpey's fibers. ×160. (After Schaffer.)

SUBMICROSCOPIC STRUCTURE AND COMPOSITION OF BONE MATRIX

The interstitial substance of bone is composed of two major components, an organic matrix and inorganic salts. The organic matrix consists of collagenous fibers embedded in an amorphous ground substance. In adult mammals, about 95 per cent of the organic matrix is collagen. The sulfate content of the ground substance is lower than that of hyaline cartilage, and, therefore, bone matrix is usually acidophilic.

Amorphous Ground Substance

The chemical composition of the amorphous extracellular substance of bone has not been studied as thoroughly as that of cartilage, owing in part to the fact that it comprises a relatively small fraction of the organic matrix of bone. The positive periodic

acid–Schiff reaction, the faint metachromasia of some areas of bone matrix, and the autoradiographic demonstration of incorporation of ^{35}S all provide indirect histochemical evidence for the presence of glycosaminoglycans or glycoproteins. Analyses of extracts of whole bones have identified at least three amino-sugar containing macromolecular components—chondroitin sulfate, keratan sulfate, and hyaluronic acid, but since whole bones were used, it is not entirely clear that all of these substances came from the bone proper and not from the small amount of associated cartilage. In either case, it is evident that the concentration of sulfated glycosaminoglycans in the ground substance of bone is much less than in cartilage. Consistent with this is the uniformly eosinophilic staining of bone matrix.

Collagen

The collagen of bone, like that of common connective tissue, occurs in the form of cross-striated fibers 500 to 700 Å in diameter, with a 680 Å repeating period. Collagen of bone differs, however, in some of its physical properties. It fails to swell in dilute acid and is insoluble in solvents used successfully to extract collagens from other tissues. Thus, it seems to have a greater degree of intermolecular bonding.

In mature lamellar bone, the collagen fibers are highly ordered in their arrangement. Those within each lamella of a haversian system are parallel in their orientation, but the direction of the fibers in the successive lamellae changes. This change in orientation of the fibers is responsible for the alternation of bright and dark layers in haversian systems viewed with polarizing optics (Fig. 10-8B). Some disagreement persists as to the precise arrangement of the fibers. In decalcified preparations viewed at high magnification, refractile lamellae with a fine circumferential striation alternate with less refractile layers having a stippled or punctate aspect. This appearance was originally interpreted as indicating a regular alternation of lamellae with circularly and with longitudinally oriented fibrils. This was apparently an oversimplification. Some investigators have insisted that collagen-rich lamellae alternate with collagen-poor lamellae and that this difference is as important as the direction of the fibers in accounting for the microscopic appearance of the haversian systems. Others have suggested that the fibers within a given collagen-rich lamella are not parallel but form two sets of fibers intersecting in a lattice-like pattern (Rouiller). The majority of histologists, however, seem to follow Gebhardt in believing that the fibrils in all of the lamellae run helically with respect to the axis of the haversian canal, but that the pitch of the helix changes sufficiently from one lamella to the next to account for the differences observed under bright-field and polarization microscopes.

Bone Mineral

The inorganic matter of bone consists of submicroscopic deposits of a form of calcium phosphate, very similar, but not identical, to the mineral hydroxyapatite (Ca_{10} [PO_4]$_6$ [OH]$_2$). Bone mineral is probably deposited initially as amorphous calcium phosphate and subsequently reordered to form crystalline hydroxyapatite. In its final phase, the calcium phosphate is present as thin plates or slender rodlike crystals 15 to 30 Å in thickness and a few hundred angstroms long. These are situated on and within the substance of collagen fibers in the matrix. The crystals are not randomly distributed but recur regularly at intervals of 600 to 700 Å along the length of the fibers.

Bone mineral contains significant amounts of the citrate ion, $C_6H_5O_7\equiv$, and the carbonate ion, $CO_3^=$. Citrate is considered to be in a separate phase, located on the surfaces of crystals. The location of carbonate is still a matter of debate; it may be located on the surface of crystals, or it may substitute for $PO_4\equiv$ in the crystal structure, or both. Substitution of the fluoride ion, F^-, for OH^- in the apatite crystal is common; its amount depends mainly on the fluoride content of the drinking water. Magnesium and sodium, which are normal constituents of the body fluids, are also present in the bone mineral, which to some extent serves as a storage depot for these elements. The isotopes, ^{45}Ca and ^{32}P can, of course, substitute for the stable ^{40}Ca and ^{31}P in the hydroxyapatite crystal. Foreign cations, such as Pb^{++}, Sr^{++}, and Ra^{++} (^{226}Ra), if ingested, may also substitute for Ca^{++}. In the fission of uranium in nu-

clear reactors or of uranium or plutonium in the detonation of nuclear weapons, a large number of radioactive elements are liberated. Some of these, on gaining access to the body, are incorporated in bone. The most hazardous of these *bone seeking isotopes* is ^{90}Sr. As a result of their radioactivity, isotopes may cause severe damage to bone and to the blood forming cells in the marrow. A few of these bone seeking isotopes, including ^{239}Pu, do not enter the bone mineral but have instead a special affinity for the organic constituents of bone. Studies of the rate of turnover of the inorganic substances in bone have been greatly aided by the use of bone seeking isotopes.

During development and growth, the amount of organic material per unit volume remains relatively constant, but the amount of water decreases and the proportion of bone mineral increases, attaining a maximum of about 65 per cent of the fat-free dry weight of the tissue in the adults. In the poorly calcified bone of individuals suffering from *rickets* or from *osteomalacia*, the mineral content may be as low as 35 per cent.

If bone is exposed to a weak acid or a chelating agent, the inorganic salts are removed. The bone thus demineralized loses most of its hardness but is still very tough and flexible. It retains its gross form and a nearly normal microscopic appearance. On the other hand, if the organic constituents are extracted from a bone, the remaining inorganic constituents retain the gross form of the bone and, to a certain extent, its microscopic topography, but the bone has lost much of its tensile strength and is as brittle as porcelain. Thus it is clear that the hardness of bone depends upon its inorganic constituents, while its great toughness and resilience reside in its organic matrix, particularly the collagen. Without either one, bone would be a poor skeletal material, but with both, it is a highly ordered, remarkably resistant tissue, superbly adapted, at all levels of its organization, for its chemical and mechanical functions.

THE CELLS OF BONES

In actively growing bones four kinds of bone cells are distinguishable: *osteoprogenitor cells*, *osteoblasts*, *osteocytes*, and *osteoclasts*. Although they are usually described as distinct cell types, there is clear evidence of transformation from one to the other, and it is evidently more reasonable to regard them as different functional states of the same cell type. Such reversible changes in appearance are examples of cell *modulation*, in contrast to *differentiation*, which is the term reserved for progressive and apparently irreversible specialization in structure and function.

Osteoprogenitor Cells

Like other connective tissues, bone develops from embryonic mesenchyme. It retains in postnatal life a population of relatively undifferentiated cells that have the capacity for mitosis and for further structural and functional specialization. These *osteoprogenitor cells* have pale-staining, oval or elongate nuclei and inconspicuous acidophilic or faintly basophilic cytoplasm. They are found on or near all of the free surfaces of bone: in the endosteum; the innermost layer of the periosteum; lining the Haversian canals; and on the trabeculae of cartilage matrix at the epiphyseal plate of growing bones.

The osteoprogenitor cells are active during the normal growth of bones and may be activated in adult life during internal reorganization of bone or in the healing of fractures and repair of other forms of injury. Under any of these conditions, they undergo division and transform into the bone forming cells, osteoblasts, or coalesce to give rise to the bone destroying cells, osteoclasts.

After administration of tritiated thymidine, the osteoprogenitor cells are the only cells found to be labeled in autoradiographs at early time intervals. At later times, silver grains can also be found over the nuclei of osteoblasts or osteoclasts, indicating that some of the osteoprogenitor cells have become transformed into these other cellular elements of bone. It is believed that the more specialized bone cells, osteoblasts and osteoclasts, can also revert to osteoprogenitor cells when osteogenesis subsides.

Many authors refer to these potentially osteogenic cells as mesenchymal cells, but this term implies that they have a broader range of latent developmental potentialities than has been demonstrated. It may yet be shown that these cells can also develop into adipose cells, into fibroblasts and into hemo-poietic cells of the bone marrow. If this should be true, then "mesenchymal cell" would indeed be the more appropriate designation. In the meantime, a majority of contemporary investigators of bone prefer the more limited implications of the term osteoprogenitor cell.

Osteoblasts

The *osteoblasts* are responsible for formation of bone matrix and are invariably found on the advancing surfaces of developing or growing bones. During active deposition of new matrix they are arranged in an epithelioid layer of cuboidal or low columnar cells connected to one another by short slender processes. The nucleus with its single prominent nucleolus is often at the end of the cell farthest from the bony surface. The cells are clearly polarized toward the underlying bone, with a well developed Golgi apparatus situated between the nucleus and the cell base. The mitochondria are elongated and fairly numerous. The cytoplasm is intensely basophilic, owing to its large content of ribonucleoprotein.

The osteoblasts give a strong histochemical reaction for alkaline phosphatase, and the periodic acid–Schiff reaction reveals small pink-staining granules in the cytoplasm that are believed to represent precursors of the bone matrix. When active new formation of bone ceases and the osteoblasts revert to spindle form, these granules disappear from the cytoplasm, and the phosphatase reaction of the cells rapidly declines.

In electron micrographs, osteoblasts are seen to have the structure expected of cells actively engaged in protein synthesis (Fig. 10–11). The endoplasmic reticulum is extensive and its cisternae are often in parallel array. Their membranes are studded with ribosomes, and these are also present in great numbers in the cytoplasmic matrix. The Golgi membranes are well developed and have numerous associated vacuoles. Sizable vesicles containing an amorphous or flocculent material of appreciable density apparently correspond to the PAS staining granules observed with the light microscope. Small lipid droplets and membrane limited dense bodies, interpreted as lysosomes, are also encountered occasionally.

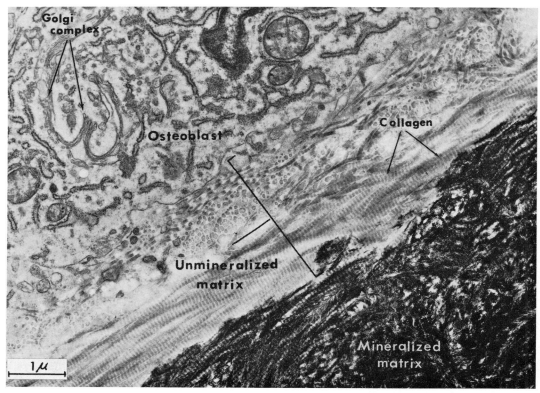

Figure 10-11 Edge of a resorption canal being filled in by lamellar bone. At the upper left is a portion of an osteoblast containing a prominent Golgi zone and abundant granular reticulum. Subjacent to it are the collagen fibrils of two unmineralized lamellae, and at the lower right is the dense mineralized bone. (After R. R. Cooper et al., J. Bone Joint Surg., *48A*:1239, 1966.)

Osteocytes

The principal cells of fully formed bone are the *osteocytes,* which reside in lacunae within the calcified interstitial substance. The cell body is flattened, conforming to the shape of the lenticular cavity that it occupies, but there are numerous slender processes that extend for some distance into canaliculi in the surrounding matrix. How far they penetrate into the canaliculi of adult mammalian bone could not be ascertained by light microscopy. However, recent electron microscopic studies (Holtrop and Weinger) have shown that the processes of neighboring osteocytes are in contact at their ends. Moreover, their apposed membranes are specialized to form gap junctions or nexuses at their sites of contact (Fig. 10-12). Thus the bone cells are not completely isolated in their lacunae but appear to be in communication with one another and ultimately with

the cells at the surface via a series of cell to cell junctions of low electrical resistance permitting flow of ions and possibly of small molecules. This finding may explain how cells deep within the calcified matrix of bone can respond to hormonal stimuli that would seem to have direct access only to cells in the immediate vicinity of blood vessels.

The nuclear and cytoplasmic characteristics of osteocytes at the light microscopic level are similar to those of osteoblasts except that the Golgi region is less conspicuous and the cytoplasm exhibits less affinity for basic dyes. In electron micrographs of osteocytes that have only recently been incorporated into bone, the Golgi apparatus is still rather large and the endoplasmic reticulum is quite extensive (Fig. 10-13). In osteocytes situated deeper in bone matrix, these organelles have undergone some regression (Fig. 10-14). Although these cells appear less active in protein synthesis, they are by no means metabolically inert.

In its development, an osteocyte is essentially an osteoblast that has become surrounded by bone matrix. Isolated within its lacuna, it undergoes some cytological dedifferentiation, but remains active. Considerable indirect evidence has accumulated indicating that the osteocyte exerts an important influence on the surrounding osseous matrix. Bélanger has described the phenomenon of *osteolysis*, an active physiological process whereby the bone matrix immediately surrounding osteocytes is modified and bone salt is resorbed. It is the current belief that the osteocytes play an active role in the release of calcium from bone to blood, and hence participate in the homeostatic regulation of its concentration in the fluids of the body.

Parathyroid hormone is the principal regulator of the blood calcium level. Its administration has a microscopically visible effect on the osteocytes and on the staining reactions of the adjacent bone matrix. Because the response of the blood calcium level to parathyroid hormone is too rapid to be accounted for by osteoclastic erosion of bone, the primary action of the hormone may be to stimulate osteocytic osteolysis.

The osteocyte is believed to be capable of modulation to other cell types. When released from its lacuna during bone resorption, it may revert to a quiescent osteoprogenitor cell, and later undergo modulation to an osteoblast. Some investigators believe that osteocytes liberated from bone matrix may become incorporated into multinucleate osteoclasts; others believe that osteoclasts arise from different progenitor cells (Bingham et al.).

Osteoclasts

Closely associated with areas of bone resorption are the *osteoclasts* — giant cells 20 to 100 μm. in diameter and containing as many as 50 nuclei. They were first described by Kollicker (1873), who believed that they were the active agents in bone resorption. Although this view has been a subject of continuing debate extending over the past century, the great bulk of recent evidence supports this interpretation. Osteoclasts are frequently found in shallow concavities in the surface of bone, called *Howship's lacunae*. It was this relationship that first suggested to early investigators of the histology of bone that these lacunae were formed by an erosive action of osteoclasts. In the turnover and remodeling of bones that occurs in growing animals, osteoclasts are always most abundant in those areas that are known to be undergoing resorption. No one questioned the close topographical relation of these cells to sites of resorption, but some have argued that the osteoclasts arise by coalescence of osteocytes liberated from surrounding matrix in the course of bone resorption, and that they therefore should be regarded as products rather than as agents of bone resorption. This interpretation now has few adherents, as the evidence for an active role of osteoclasts in bone resorption has become more and more compelling. Osteoclasts actively engaged in bone resorption show an obvious polarity. The

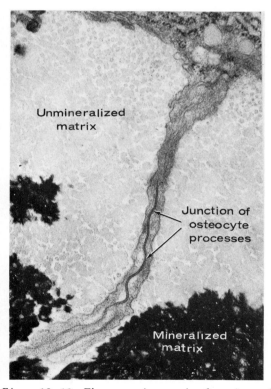

Figure 10–12 Electron micrograph of portions of cell processes from two neighboring osteocytes traversing the zone of unmineralized matrix lining a lacuna. Note the nexus or gap junction where the processes overlap. (From Holtrop, M. E., and M. J. Weinger: Proc. Fourth Parathyroid Conference, Internat. Congress Series No. 243. Amsterdam, Excerpta Medica, 1971.)

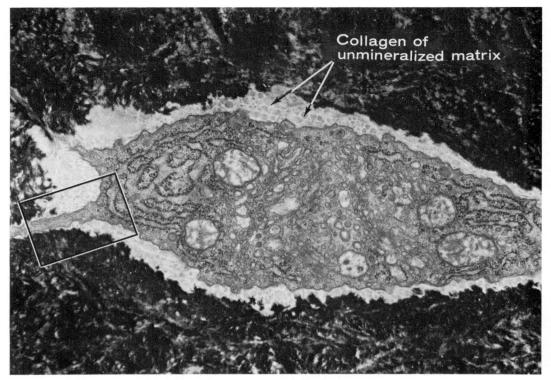

Collagen of unmineralized matrix

Figure 10–13 Electron micrograph of an osteocyte. The plane of section does not include the nucleus. Notice that the Golgi complex is still quite well developed, and numerous cisternal profiles of endoplasmic reticulum are present. At the left, a cell process is seen extending into a canaliculus. An area similar to that in the rectangle is seen at higher magnification in Figure 10–15. (Micrograph courtesy of M. Holtrop.)

nuclei tend to congregate near the outer surface, which is smooth contoured, while the side adjacent to the bone exhibits a radial striation that was long interpreted as a "brush border" but which has now been shown by electron microscopy to have an infolded structure that makes the term "ruffled border" more appropriate. There are deep infoldings of the plasma membrane which delimit a large number of closely packed clavate or foliate processes of highly variable size and shape, separated by narrow extracellular clefts (Fig. 10–16). Small crystals of bone mineral liberated from the bone matrix may be found deep in these clefts.

The plasma membrane itself is specialized in the region of the ruffled border. It bears on its inner or cytoplasmic surface a nap of exceedingly small, bristle-like appendages 150 to 200 Å in length and spaced about 200 Å apart. This bristle coat makes the membrane in this elaborately infolded region appear thicker than the unspecialized unit membrane elsewhere on the cell surface (Kallio et al.). In contrast to a typical brush border, which is a very well ordered and stable differentiation, the ruffled border of the osteoclast seems to be highly active and constantly changing its configuration. Cinematographic studies of these cells in vitro have shown that processes are continually being extended and retracted and changing their position.

The nuclei of osteoclasts resemble those of osteoblasts and are in no way unusual. The cytoplasm is slightly basophilic when stained with basic dyes at controlled pH, but in routine histological sections it is usually eosinophilic and highly vacuolated.

There are multiple Golgi complexes distributed among the nuclei, and a number of centriole pairs corresponding to the number of nuclei. The centrioles may gather together in a centrosome region. The rod-shaped or short filamentous mitochondria of osteoclasts are very numerous and tend to congregate near the ruffled border. In contrast to other bone cells, the cytoplasmic vacuoles of osteoclasts stain supravitally with neutral red—a property that can be used to advantage in locating these multinucleate cells in fresh bone for experimental manipulation (Barnicot). Many of the vacuoles and granules also give a positive histochemical reaction for acid phosphatase, indicative of their lysosomal nature. In electron micrographs, the granules are, for the most part, dense, spherical, 0.2 to 0.5 μm. in diameter, and membrane limited, but larger vesicular structures 0.5 to 3 μm. in diameter may also be a form of lysosome.

Despite the evidence of activity of the osteoclast surface where it is in contact with bone, there is little evidence that these cells are mechanically erosive or even highly phagocytic. The exact mechanisms by which they accomplish the simultaneous degradation of the organic matrix and the dissolution of bone mineral still elude us, but there are rather clear indications that they secrete hydrolytic enzymes, which may be largely responsible for digestion of matrix components.

The experiments upon which this conclusion is based depend upon the fact that maintenance of normal levels of blood calcium in the intact animal depend upon the actions of two hormones that act antagonistically on bone. Administration of *parathyroid hormone* causes mobilization of calcium by promoting bone resorption, while *calcitonin* acts to suppress mobilization of calcium from bone. Both hormones are also effective when applied to isolated bone fragments main-

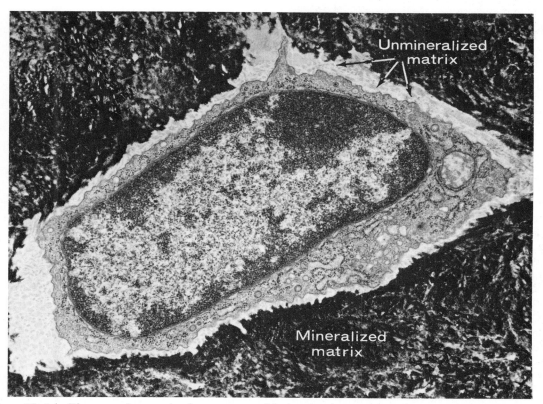

Figure 10-14 Electron micrograph of an osteocyte. Notice that it completely fills its lacuna. The clear area around the cell is in fact occupied by unmineralized matrix in which the collagen fibers are faintly visible. The mineralized matrix is black owing to the electron scattering of the apatite crystals. (Micrograph courtesy of M. Holtrop.)

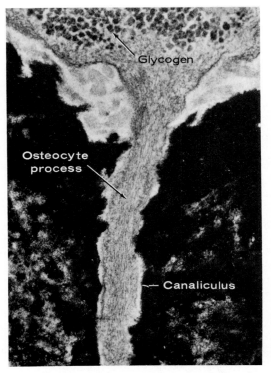

Glycogen

Osteocyte process

Canaliculus

Figure 10-15 Osteocyte process extending from cell body (above) into a canaliculus (below). Notice the high concentration of cytoplasmic filaments in the cell process. (Micrograph courtesy of M. Holtrop.)

tained in vitro. Thus, addition of parathyroid hormone to organ cultures results in appearance of resorption cavities in the bone and markedly accelerates release of calcium and phosphate into the medium as a result of solubilization of bone mineral. There is also an increase in liberation of hydroxyproline from degradation of collagen of the bone matrix. Concomitant with these evidences of bone resorption, appreciable quantities of several lysosomal acid hydrolases are also released into the medium, whereas there is no detectable release of nonlysosomal enzymes from the cells of the culture. It is suggested, therefore, that the lysosomal enzymes are secreted by osteoclasts. Parathyroid hormone also greatly increases the rate of production of lactate and citrate by the bone explants, causing them to acidify their medium much more rapidly than other cells in culture. From consideration of such experiments, it is proposed that lysosomal acid hydrolases of osteoclasts are active in resorption of the organic matrix of bone and that the stimulated local acid production solubilizes bone mineral and at the same time creates a pH favorable to the action of acid hydrolases (Vaes). The surface membrane of osteoclasts around the periphery of the active ruffled border is very smooth and closely applied to the underlying bone. This observation has led to the speculation that the close application of the cell to its substrate in the clear zone around the periphery of the ruffled area might help to seal off the active portion of the cell and enable it to maintain a microenvironment conducive to solubilization of mineral and to optimal activity of hydrolytic enzymes (Schenk et al.).

There is additional physiological evidence for a direct action of hormones on the osteoclast. Administration of parathyroid hormone is reported to cause depolarization of the osteoclast membrane and an increase in the rate of RNA synthesis, while calcitonin polarizes the cell membrane and inhibits the effect of parathyroid hormone on RNA synthesis (Mears). Calcitonin also causes disappearance of the ruffled border, a change in the character of the membrane, and separation of osteoclasts from the bone surface (Zuchner).

Osteoclasts arise by coalescence of mononuclear cells. The identity of the mononuclear cells of origin has been a subject of controversy, but there now is a consensus that fusion of osteoprogenitor cells is the principal source of osteoclasts.

However, recent work on an osteopetrotic strain of mice has provided new evidence for the view that osteoclasts may arise by coalescence of mononuclear cells emigrating from the blood — presumably monocytes. When mutant mice having excessive accumulations of spongiosa in their long bones are joined to normal littermates in parabiosis, the excess spongiosa disappears from their bones within six weeks, and the osteopetrotic animals remain cured even after separation from their normal parabiont. This finding strongly suggests that during parabiosis, progenitors of osteoclasts were recruited from the blood of the normal mouse (Walker). There is reason to believe that these multinucleate cells are not necessarily end stages of differentiation destined to degenerate after a limited life span, but that they may be able to partition their cytoplasm into mononuclear units that revert to progenitor cells (Young).

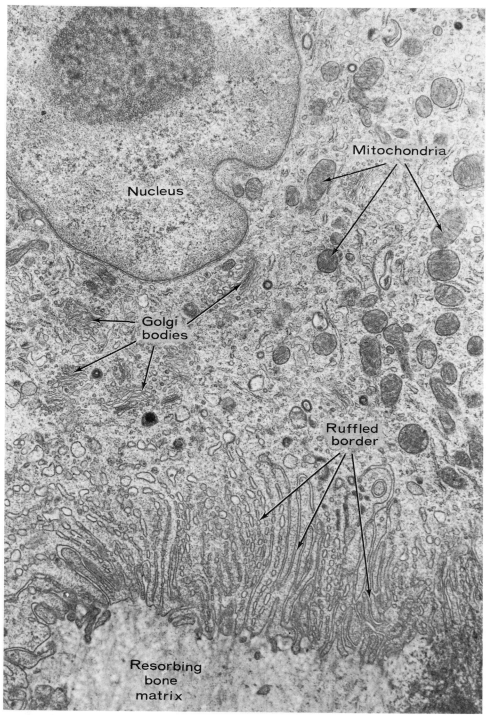

Figure 10–16 Electron micrograph of a portion of an osteoclast, including the nucleus above, several Golgi elements, and the ruffled border closely applied to an area of resorbing bone matrix at the bottom of the figure. (Micrograph courtesy of P. Garrant.)

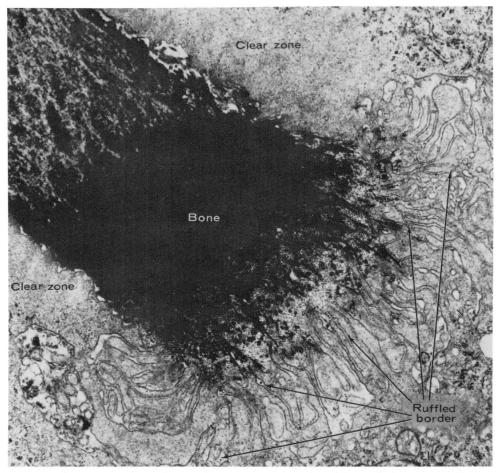

Figure 10-17 Electron micrograph of a portion of an osteoclast around the end of a spicule of bone. Notice the ruffled border at the end of the bone, where it is undergoing resorption. A smooth contoured portion of the osteoclast surface with a subjacent clear zone of ectoplasm is closely applied to the bone around the periphery of the ruffled border. (Micrograph courtesy of M. Holtrop.)

HISTOGENESIS OF BONE

Bone always develops by replacement of a preexisting connective tissue. Two different modes of osteogenesis are recognized in embryos. When bone formation occurs directly in primitive connective tissue, it is called *intramembranous ossification.* When it takes place in preexisting cartilage, it is called intracartilaginous or *endochondral ossification.* In endochondral ossification the bulk of the cartilage must be removed before bone deposition begins, and the distinctive features of this mode of ossification are more concerned with the resorption of cartilage than with deposition of bone. The actual deposition of bony tissue is essentially the same in the

two modes of ossification. Bone is first laid down as a network of trabeculae, the *primary spongiosa,* which is subsequently converted to more compact bone by a filling in of the interstices between trabeculae. Occasionally, under pathological conditions, bone may arise in tissues not belonging to the osseous system, and in connective tissues not ordinarily manifesting osteogenic properties. This is called *ectopic bone formation.*

Intramembranous Ossification

Certain flat bones of the skull—the frontal, parietal, occipital, and temporal bones, and part of the mandible—develop by intramembranous ossification and are referred to as *membrane bones.* The mesenchyme condenses into a richly vascularized layer of connective tissue, in which the cells are in contact with one another by long tapering processes, and the intercellular spaces are occupied by randomly oriented delicate bundles of collagen fibrils embedded in a thin, gel-like ground substance. The first sign of bone formation is the appearance of thin strands or bars of a denser eosinophilic matrix (Fig. 10–18). These strands of bone matrix tend to be deposited approximately equidistantly from neighboring blood vessels, and since the vessels form a network, the earliest trabeculae of bone matrix also develop in a branching and anastomosing pattern (Fig. 10–19). Simultaneously with the appearance of those first strands of eosinophilic extracellular matrix, there are changes in the neighboring primitive connective tissue cells. They enlarge and gather in increasing numbers on the surface of the trabeculae, assuming a cuboidal or columnar form while still remaining adherent to one another via shortened processes. Concurrently with the changes in their size and shape, the cells become intensely basophilic and are thereafter identified as osteoblasts. Through their synthetic and secretory activity, additional bone matrix (osteoid) is deposited, and the trabeculae become longer and thicker.

Collagen macromolecules are secreted together with the amorphous glycoprotein of the matrix, and they polymerize extracellularly to form great numbers of randomly interwoven fibrils of collagen throughout the trabeculae of osseous matrix. This early intramembranous bone in which the collagen fibers run in all directions is often called *woven bone,* to distinguish it from the lamellar bone formed in subsequent remodeling, which contains collagen in highly ordered parallel arrays. Woven bone is permeated by relatively large tortuous channels occupied by blood vessels and connective tissue. The osteocytes are distributed uniformly but oriented at random. In lamellar bone, on the other hand, the osteocytes are arranged in regular concentric order around relatively straight vessels in slender Haversian canals (Fig. 10–20).

At a very early stage in the replacement of the interstitial substances of primitive connective tissue by bone matrix, the latter becomes a site of deposition of calcium phosphate. All of the matrix subsequently se-

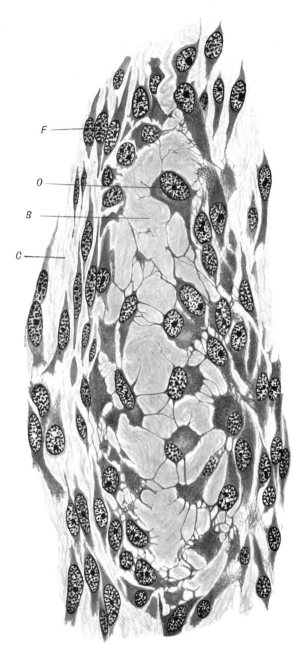

Figure 10–18 Beginning of intramembranous bone formation in the skull of a 5.5 cm. cat embryo. *B,* Homogeneous thickened collagenous fibers, which become the interstitial bone substance; *C,* collagenous interstitial substance; *F,* connective tissue cells; *O,* connective tissue cells, with processes, which become osteoblasts and later bone cells. Eosin-azure stain. ×520. (After A. A. Maximow.)

creted by the osteoblasts calcifies after a very short lag. Thus, in electron micrographs, there is only a narrow zone of osteoid be-

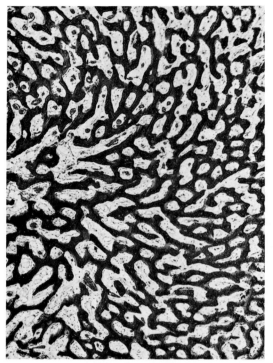

Figure 10-19 Photomicrograph of the pattern of trabeculae in the primary spongiosa of intramembranous bone formation.

tween the bases of the osteoblasts and the heavily mineralized matrix of the underlying trabeculae (Fig. 10–11). As the trabeculae thicken by accretion, some of the osteoblasts at their surface become incarcerated in the newly deposited matrix, and one by one they are buried within its substance to become bone cells—osteocytes. The osteocytes thus sequestered in lacunae within the newly deposited matrix nevertheless remain connected to osteoblasts at the surface by slender processes. The canaliculi of bone are formed by deposition of matrix around these cell processes. As rapidly as the ranks of osteoblasts on the surface of the trabeculae are depleted by their incorporation into the bone, their numbers are restored by differentiation of new osteoblasts from primitive cells of the surrounding connective tissue. Mitotic division is frequent in these progenitor cells but is rarely if ever observed in osteoblasts themselves.

In areas of the primary spongiosa that are destined to become compact bone, the trabeculae continue to thicken at the expense of the intervening connective tissue until the spaces around the blood vessels are largely obliterated. The collagen fibrils in the layers of bone that are deposited on the trabeculae in this progressive encroachment upon the perivascular spaces gradually become more regularly arranged and come to resemble lamellar bone. Although the irregularly concentric layers formed may bear a superficial resemblance to haversian systems, they are not true lamellar bone because their collagen is randomly oriented.

In those areas where spongy bone will persist, the thickening of the trabeculae ceases and the intervening vascular connective tissue is gradually transformed into hemopoietic tissue. The connective tissue surrounding the growing mass of bone persists and condenses to form the periosteum. The osteoblasts that have remained on the surface of the bone during its development revert to the fibroblast-like appearance as growth ceases and persist as the quiescent osteogenic cells of the endosteum or of the periosteum. If they are again called upon to form bone, their osteogenic potentialities are reactivated and they again take on the morphological characteristics of osteoblasts.

Endochondral Ossification

Bones at the base of the skull, in the vertebral column, the pelvis, and the extremities are called *cartilage bones* because they are first formed of hyaline cartilage, which is then replaced with bone in the process called *endochondral ossification*. This can best be studied in one of the long bones of an extremity. The first indication of the establishment of a *center of ossification* is a striking enlargement of the chondrocytes at the middle of the shaft of the hyaline cartilage model (Fig. 10–21). The cells in this region hypertrophy, glycogen accumulates within them, and their cytoplasm becomes highly vacuolated. As the chondrocytes hypertrophy there is an enlargement of their lacunae at the expense of the intervening cartilage matrix, which is gradually reduced to thin fenestrated septa and irregularly shaped spicules. The remaining hyaline matrix in the region of hypertrophic cartilage cells becomes calcifiable, and small granular aggregations and nests of crystals of calcium phosphate are deposited with in it (Fig. 10–25C). Regressive changes in the hypertrophied cartilage cells,

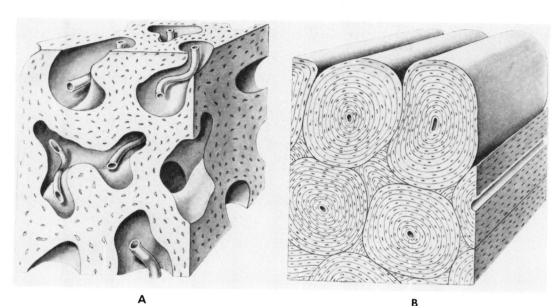

Figure 10–20 A three dimensional diagrammatic representation of the differences in architecture of woven bone (*A*) and lamellar bone (*B*). (From N. M. Hancox: *Biology of Bone.* Cambridge, England, Cambridge University Press, 1972.)

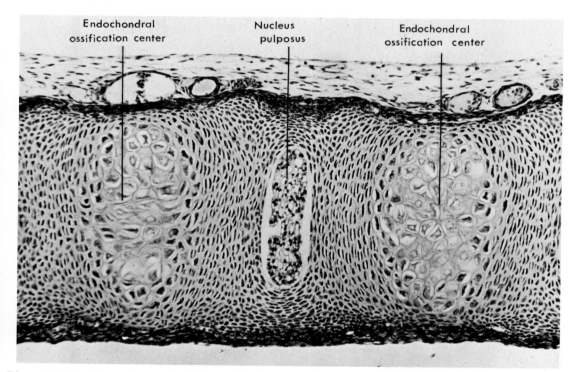

Figure 10–21 Photomicrograph of the cartilaginous vertebral column of a mouse embryo, showing in the center of each vertebra an area of hypertrophied cartilage cells that represents an early stage in the establishment of a center of endochondral ossification.

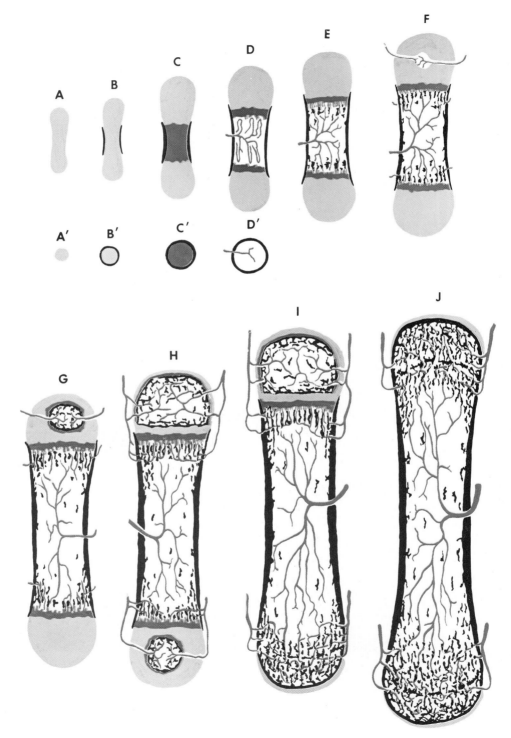

Figure 10–22 See opposite page for legend.

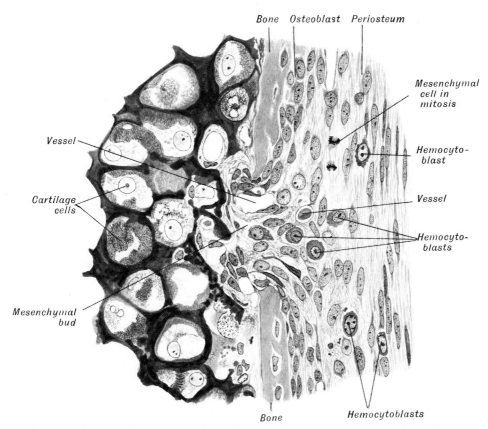

Bone Osteoblast Periosteum

Mesenchymal
cell in
mitosis

Hemocyto-
blast

Vessel

Vessel

Hemocyto-
blasts

Cartilage
cells

Mesenchymal
bud

Bone   Hemocytoblasts

Figure 10-23 Part of longitudinal section through the middle of the diaphysis of the femur of a 25 mm. human embryo. Mesenchyme with vessels entering calcified cartilage through an opening in the periosteal bone collar. Eosin-azure stain. ×560. (After A. A. Maximow.)

including swelling of their nuclei and loss of chromatin, are followed by their death and degeneration.

Concurrently with these hypertrophic and regressive changes in the chondrocytes in the interior of the cartilage model, the osteogenic potencies of cells in the *perichondrium* are activated, and a thin layer of bone, the *periosteal band* or *collar*, is deposited around

the midportion of the shaft (Figs. 10–22*B* and 10–25*A*). At the same time, blood vessels from the investing layer of connective tissue (now called the periosteum) grow into the diaphysis, invading the irregular cavities in the cartilage matrix created by the enlargement of the chondrocytes and confluence of their lacunae (Figs. 10–22*E* and *F*, 10–23, and 10–24). The thin-walled vessels branch and grow toward

Figure 10-22 Diagram of the development of a typical long bone as shown in longitudinal sections (*A* to *J*) and in cross sections *A'*, *B'*, *C'*, and *D'* through the centers of *A, B, C,* and *D*. Pale blue, cartilage; purple, calcified cartilage; black, bone; red, arteries. *A,* Cartilage model; *B,* periosteal bone collar appears before any calcification of cartilage. *C,* Cartilage begins to calcify. *D,* Vascular mesenchyme enters the calcified cartilage matrix and divides it into two zones of ossification (*E*). *F,* Blood vessels and mesenchyme enter upper epiphyseal cartilage and the epiphyseal ossification center develops in it (*G*). A similar ossification center develops in the lower epiphyseal cartilage (*H*). As the bone ceases to grow in length the lower epiphyseal plate disappears first (*I*) and then the upper epiphyseal plate (*J*). The bone marrow cavity then becomes continuous throughout the length of the bone, and the blood vessels of the diaphysis, metaphyses, and epiphyses intercommunicate.

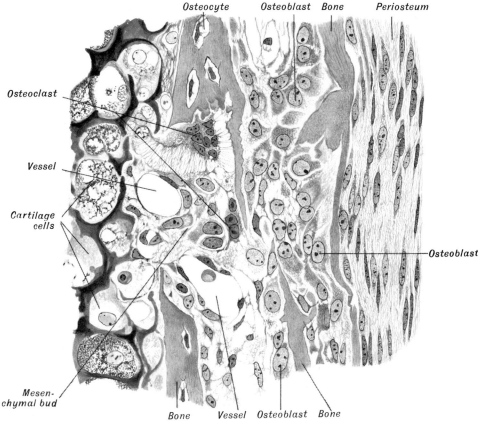

Figure 10-24 Part of longitudinal section through the middle of the diaphysis of the humerus of a human embryo of eight weeks. The process of ossification has advanced slightly farther than in Figure 10-23. Eosin-azure stain. ×560. (After A. A. Maximow.)

either end of the cartilage model, forming capillary loops that extend into the blind ends of the cavities in the calcified cartilage. Primitive pluripotential cells are carried into the interior of the cartilage in the perivascular tissue of the invading blood vessels. Some of these cells differentiate into hemopoietic elements of the bone marrow. Others differentiate into osteoblasts which congregate in an epithelioid layer on the irregular surfaces of spicules of calcified cartilage matrix and begin to deposit bone matrix upon them. The earliest bony trabeculae formed in the interior of the cartilage model thus have a core of calcified cartilage and an outer layer of bone of varying thickness. Owing to the different staining affinities of calcified cartilage and bone, these trabeculae have a mottled heterogeneous appearance and are

easily distinguished from the homogeneous trabeculae of woven bone formed under the periosteum by a form of intramembranous ossification.

It is common practice to include in the term *primary center of ossification* all of the early morphological changes described above whether they occur in the interior of the cartilage model or under the perichondrium. This usage is intended only to distinguish the diaphyseal center, which appears first, from *secondary centers of ossification*, which develop much later in the epiphyses. Some investigators, however, reserve the term primary center of ossification for the subperiosteal collar on the grounds that this is the first true bone formed, even though its formation is heralded by earlier changes in the chondrocytes in the interior of the model.

The Mechanism of Calcification

The mechanism by which mineral is deposited in the organic matrix of cartilage and bone has been a subject of much debate and numerous hypotheses. One of the most widely accepted of these, proposed by Glimcher, holds that the initiation of mineralization in bone is analogous to the familiar induction of crystallization from metastable solutions in vitro by adding a seed crystal or by scratching the wall of the beaker—a proc-

ess called *heterogeneous nucleation*. The foreign matter disturbs the equilibrium in the solution and causes a clustering of molecules that results in formation of small nuclei capable of growing to form crystals. In the case of bone, it is believed to be the highly ordered "crystalline" collagen fibers of the matrix which act as the nucleation catalyst for transformation of calcium and phosphate in solution in the tissue fluids into the solid phase mineral deposits. In support of this theory, it

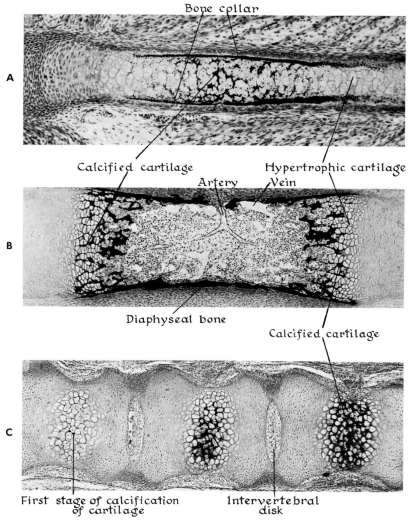

Figure 10–25   Photomicrographs showing several stages of bone formation in developing rats. From formalin-fixed, undecalcified sections stained with silver nitrate to show bone salt (black). *A,* Longitudinal section through second rib of 18 day rat embryo; calcification of the periosteal bone collar is further advanced than that of the cartilage. ×117. *B,* Section of metatarsal of 4 day rat, in which ossification is proceeding toward the epiphyses; the hypertrophic cartilage is not completely calcified. ×63. *C,* Three stages in calcification of vertebrae in 20 day rat embryo. ×57. (W. Bloom and M. A. Bloom.)

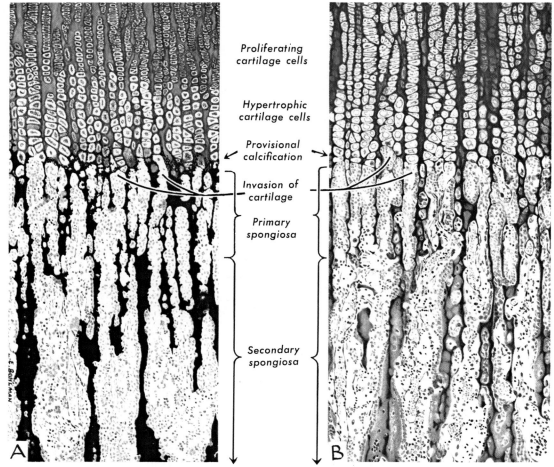

Figure 10–26 Endochondral ossification in longitudinal sections through the zone of epiphyseal growth of the distal end of the radius of a puppy. *A,* Neutral formalin fixation; no decalcification. Von Kóssa and hematoxylin-eosin stain. All deposits of bone salt are stained black; thus, bone and calcified cartilage matrix stain alike. *B,* Zenker-formol fixation; decalcified. Hematoxylin-eosin-azure II stain. Persisting cores of cartilage matrix in trabeculae of bone take a deep blue or purple stain, whereas bone stains red. It is impossible to tell where calcium deposits had been. ×95.

has been shown that reconstituted pure collagen fibers and demineralized bone are able to induce formation of apatite crystals when introduced into metastable solutions of inorganic calcium and phosphate. The fact that fibers of the native type, with 680 to 700 Å periodicity, are the only form of collagen capable of inducing this change led to the speculation that nucleation of bone mineral is dependent upon, or is at least facilitated by, the particular arrangement of molecules in these fibers. This interpretation derives added support from the observation that in electron micrographs of early stages of mineralization, the deposits of calcium phos-phate are localized in specific regions of the cross-banded fibers.

It has been reported that during forma-tion of linear polymers, the collagen mole-cules overlap a short distance (Fig. 10–27). When these linear polymers associate lateral-ly to form fibrils, they pack in such a way that discontinuities or "holes" exist within the fibers between the tails and heads of succes-sive molecules. In negatively stained collagen, the contrast medium penetrates the fiber and fills these holes, producing the broad, dark bands that are characteristic of such prepara-tions (Hodge). The earliest deposits of bone mineral produce a similar pattern of dense bands and therefore are believed to be localized in the holes within the collagen fibers (Fig. 10–27).

Persuasive as the evidence is for this attractive theory, it does not fully explain the localization of the process or the absence of calcification in many other collagen-rich tissues. It is evident too that collagen cannot be the only initiator of calcification. The organic matrix of the developing enamel of teeth, for example, is composed of a very different protein, but it is rapidly and heavily mineralized. A number of investigators insist that collagen does not act alone in vivo but that its interaction with chondroitin sulfate or some other protein-polysaccharide complex in the matrix may result in a particular stereochemical configuration that promotes apatite crystal formation (Miller). Evidence for this hypothesis is fragmentary, but it would seem to be in better accord with morphological observations on early stages of mineralization that show an irregular pattern of crystal deposits on and between collagen fibers. It may also have an advantage over the collagen-centered nucleation theory in helping to explain those instances of mineralization, such as in epiphyseal cartilage, in which the initial deposits are localized without obvious topographical relation to typical 680 Å collagen fibers.

Clearly this chapter in the story of bone development is not closed. Many details of the calcification process and its regulation remain to be worked out.

Growth in Length of Long Bones

In the continuing growth in length of the cartilage model after the appearance of the diaphyseal center of ossification, the chondrocytes in the adjacent regions of the epiphyses become arranged in longitudinal columns instead of in the small groups usually found in hyaline cartilage (Fig. 9–6). The

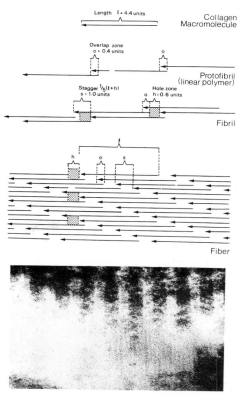

Figure 10-27   Diagram of the overlapping, staggered arrangement of molecules in a collagen fiber, showing the small discontinuities or holes that are thought to be sites of nucleation of apatite crystals in the mineralization of bone. (Modified from M. J. Glimcher and S. M. Krane, *In* Gould, B. S., and G. N. Ramachandran, eds.: A Treatise on Collagen, Vol. II. New York, Academic Press, 1968.)

cells within the columns are separated by thin transverse septa, while adjacent columns are separated by wider longitudinal bars of hyaline matrix. As endochondral ossification progresses from the center of the shaft toward either end of the cartilage model, the chondrocytes undergo the same sequence of changes as described for the establishment of the diaphyseal center, but the process is now more orderly. Along the length of the epiphyseal cell columns are several recognizable zones, corresponding to various stages in the cytomorphosis of the cartilage cells. At some distance from the diaphyseo-epiphyseal junction is a *zone of proliferation*, where frequent division of the small flattened cells provides for the continual elongation of the columns. Next comes a *zone of maturation*, in which the cells that are no longer dividing gradually enlarge. This is followed by a *zone of hypertrophy*, with very large vacuolated cells. Since the matrix in this latter region becomes the site of calcium deposition, this may also be called the *zone of provisional calcification*. And, finally, at the diaphyseal end of the columns is a zone wherein the chondrocytes are degenerating and the open ends of their enlarged lacunae are being invaded by capillary loops and primitive osteogenic cells from the marrow spaces of the diaphysis (Fig. 10–26). As the spaces at the lower ends of the columns are invaded, osteoblasts differentiate and congregate on the surfaces of the irregularly shaped longitudinal bars of calcified cartilage that persist between them. A thin new layer of bone matrix is then deposited on the surface of the cartilage. Under favorable conditions it begins to calcify nearly as rapidly as it is laid down, and thus it becomes bone. Electron microscopy has shown, however, that a superficial layer of uncalcified *preosseous tissue* or *osteoid*, one micrometer or less in thickness, is always present on forming bony surfaces (Fig. 10–11). There may be a further lag in calcification under conditions of local failure in the supply of calcium or phosphate. When such a failure becomes general and osteoid accumulates in excess, the condition is known as *rickets* in growing children or as *osteomalacia* in adults.

The distribution of calcified cartilage and new bone is best demonstrated in undecalcified sections in which the bone mineral has been stained black with silver by the von Kóssa method (Fig. 10–26A). The transitional zone where the cartilage is being replaced by advancing bone is called the *metaphysis*. The primary spongy bone in this zone undergoes extensive reorganization as the growth processes pass it by. As the bone grows longer, the diaphyseal ends of the trabeculae are continually being eroded by osteoclasts at about the same rate that additions are made at the epiphyseal end, with the result that the spongiosa of the metaphysis tends to remain relatively constant in length.

Centers of ossification have appeared in the diaphysis of each of the principal long bones of the skeleton by the third month of fetal life. Much later, usually after birth, the epiphyses show in their interior the characteristic chondrocyte hypertrophy that heralds the onset of endochondral ossification, and they in turn are invaded by blood vessels and osteogenic tissue from the perichondrium to establish *secondary centers of ossification* at either end of the developing long bones (Fig. 10–22G and H). These differ from the diaphyseal center in that there is no associated deposition of subperichondral bone. The expansion of these secondary centers gradually replaces all of the epiphyseal cartilage except that which persists as the *articular cartilage* and a transverse disk between the epiphysis and diaphysis called the *epiphyseal plate* (Fig. 10–22J). The latter contains the cartilage columns whose proliferative zone is responsible for all subsequent growth in length of long bones. Under normal conditions the rate of multiplication of cartilage cells in this zone is in balance with the rate of their degeneration and removal at the diaphyseal end of the columns. The epiphyseal plate therefore retains approximately the same thickness. Growth in length is the result of the cartilage cells continually growing away from the shaft and being replaced by bone as they recede. The net effect is an increase in the length of the shaft.

At the end of the growing period, proliferation of cartilage cells slows and finally ceases. Continued replacement of the cartilage by bone at the diaphyseal end of the columns then results in complete removal of the epiphyseal cartilage, and the bony trabeculae of the metaphysis then become continuous with the spongiosa of the bony epiphysis. This process of elimination of the epiphyseal plate is referred to as *closure of the epiphysis.* When this has taken place, no further longitudinal growth of the bone is possible. The times of closure and the relative contribution of each of the two epiphyses of a long bone to its overall growth may differ markedly. Growth in length of the femur, for example, takes place mainly at the distal epiphysis; growth of the tibia, mainly at the proximal epiphysis. Such information is of clinical value in radiology and orthopedic surgery.

Because all increment in length of a bone is limited to its epiphyseal plates, injury to this region may result in serious impairment of growth. In cases of the retarded growth of one leg attributable to general neurovascular disturbances, such as may occur in the limb of a child who has had poliomyelitis, the orthopedic surgeon can take advantage of existing knowledge of the normal rates of growth at the various epiphyseal plates and of the times of their normal closure to select the appropriate time and site for a surgical obliteration of an epiphysis in the normal leg. Such a procedure, if appropriately timed, may retard growth of the normal leg just enough to permit the slower growing leg to catch up and thus achieve an equalization of leg length by the time growth in stature of the individual ceases.

Growth in Diameter of Long Bones

The long bones of the extremities are first laid down in cartilage models, and, as indicated in the foregoing section, their growth *in length* depends upon endochondral ossification. The growth *in diameter* of the shaft, however, is the result of deposition of new membrane bone beneath the periosteum. The compact bone forming the shaft of a fully developed long bone is almost entirely the product of subperiosteal *intramembranous* ossification.

After establishment of the primary ossification center, the ends of the cartilage model continue to elongate and broaden by proliferation of chondrocytes and elaboration of new matrix, but such interstitial growth is no longer possible in the center of the diaphysis, where the cartilage is regressing and being replaced by bone. The diameter of the endochondral component in the middle of the diaphysis, therefore, cannot be appreciably greater than the diameter of the cartilage model in the early embryo

at the time of establishment of the primary center of ossification. To keep pace with the rapid interstitial growth of the cartilage at the ends, increase in thickness of the shaft is accomplished by a progressive thickening of the *periosteal band* or *collar* formed around the middle of the cartilaginous diaphysis at the onset of ossification. This results in deposition of a lattice of trabeculae of intramembranous woven bone, forming the wall of the diaphysis.

Bone resorption is as important to the growth of bones as is bone deposition, and the deposition of new bone on the outside of the shaft is accompanied by the appearance of osteoclasts that erode the inner aspect of the subperiosteal trabeculae to enlarge the marrow cavity. The rates of external apposition of new bone and internal resorption are so adjusted that the cylindrical shaft expands rapidly while the thickness of its wall increases more slowly.

Because of the continual internal resorption and reorganization of bone during development, the record of the topographical distribution of endochondral and intramembranous ossification in earlier stages of development is continually erased. Therefore, the extent of the contribution of the periosteum to the fully formed long bone is seldom fully appreciated. It is informative in this regard to examine developing long bones of the manatee, an aquatic mammal in which resorption of bone to form the secondary marrow cavity does not take place. In fetal bones of this species (Figs. 10–28 and 10–29), the primary spongiosa of endochondral bone has a characteristic hourglass distribution. The two conical regions, with their apices meeting at the site of the original ossification center, result from uniform growth in length and breadth of the ends of the cartilage model. The area between the diverging sides of the two cones is filled in by a thick collar of trabeculae of periosteal origin. Such bones, lacking the capacity for the resorption that occurs in the histogenesis of long bones in other species, provide an instructive view of the basic topography of the cartilaginous and membranous components of all long bones (Fig. 10–29).

Surface Remodeling of Bones

Although growing bones are constantly changing their internal organization, they retain approximately the same external form

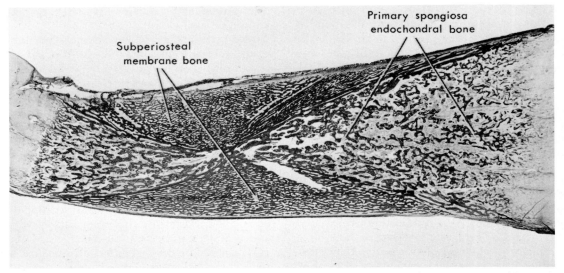

Subperiosteal
membrane bone

Primary spongiosa
endochondral bone

Figure 10-28 Photomicrograph of the humerus in a fetal manatee in longitudinal section. In this species, whose bones lack a secondary marrow cavity, the respective contributions of subperiosteal and endochondral bone to the formation of the shaft of a long bone are more evident than in bones of other species. ×5. (After D. W. Fawcett, Am. J. Anat., 71:271, 1942.)

from an early fetal stage into adult life. It is apparent that this would not be so if new bone were deposited at a uniform rate at all points beneath the periosteum. Instead, the shape of a bone is maintained during growth by a continual remodeling of its surface, which involves bone deposition in some areas of the periosteum and bone absorption in other areas. That this is true was demonstrated in the middle of the eighteenth century by madder feeding experiments. With this method of vital staining, the bone deposited during a period of feeding on madder root was stained red, while areas that were stable or were undergoing resorption remained unstained. It was clearly shown that some areas of the surface of long bones stained while others did not. The general features of these early experiments have now been confirmed and extended by means of newer techniques employing bone seeking isotopes or the antibiotic tetracycline, both of which are deposited preferentially in newly forming bone.

Typical of such experiments are those localizing the sites of osteogenesis in the growing rat tibia (Leblond et al.). This bone supports a large articular surface, and the epiphysis is considerably broader than the shaft. Thus it is possible to distinguish a cylindrical region in the middle of the shaft and a conical region toward the end, where it expands to the width of the epiphysis. If a bone-seeking isotope is given to a growing rat and autoradiographs are then made of longitudinal sections of the tibia, the sites of new bone formation are disclosed by the distribution of silver grains in the overlying emulsion. In the conical region of the bone, the silver grains are aligned immediately subjacent to the endosteum, whereas in the cylindrical portion of the shaft they are found beneath the periosteum (Fig. 10-31). Study of parallel histological sections reveals numerous osteoclasts beneath the periosteum of the conical region and beneath the endosteum of the cylindrical segment. Thus it is clear that in the surface remodeling of this bone, the periosteum plays opposite roles in neighboring regions on the surface of the same bone. Subperiosteal bone deposition is occurring in the cylindrical portion of the shaft while subperiosteal bone absorption is taking place in the conical region. Similarly, bone is being formed at the endosteal surface of the cone and absorbed on the inner aspect of the cylinder. As a consequence of these activities, the midportion of the shaft is expanding radially and its marrow cavity is being enlarged. While the bone as a whole is elongating by growth at the epiphyseal plate, the diverging wall of the conical region of the shaft is being straightened and is contributing, at its lower end, to the lengthening of the cylindrical region of the shaft.

Similarly, in the skull vault, the assumption that growth of the flat bones at the sutures could account for enlargement of the cranial cavity to accommodate the growing brain is not sufficient as an explanation. As the radius of curvature of the growing skull vault increases, the bones become less convex. Therefore, not only must bone resorption take place on the inside of the calvarium concurrently with bone deposition on the outer surface, but also the rates of deposition and absorption must differ from the center to the periphery of each cranial bone in order to account for its flattening as the radius of curvature of the skull vault increases. How these local variations in function of endosteum and periosteum are controlled in space and time to

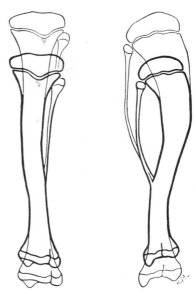

Figure 10–30 Diagram to illustrate remodeling during growth of tibia and fibula of rat, viewed from anterior aspect and in profile. (After Wolbach.)

mold and shape the bone constantly during its growth is a fascinating unsolved problem in morphogenesis.

Internal Reorganization of Bone

The conversion of the primary lattice of trabeculae laid down in intramembranous ossification into compact bone is attributed to thickening of the trabeculae and a progressive encroachment of bone upon the perivascular spaces until these are largely obliterated. As this process advances, bone is deposited in ill-defined layers with randomly oriented collagen fibers but since these are disposed more or less concentrically around vascular channels, they come to bear a superficial resemblance to haversian systems. They are sometimes called *primitive haversian systems*, but they should be clearly distinguished from the more precisely ordered lamellar systems comprising the *definitive haversian systems* of adult bone. The latter arise only in the course of the internal reorganization of primary compact bone that is referred to as *secondary bone formation.*

At scattered points in the compacta, usually in those areas laid down earliest, cavities appear as a result of osteoclastic erosion of primary bone. The formation of such *absorption cavities* was first described by Tomes and

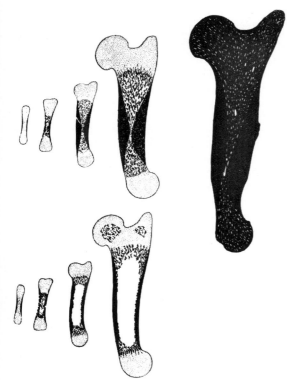

Figure 10–29 Diagrammatic representation of the development of a manatee bone (*above*) compared with that of a typical mammal (*below*). (After D. W. Fawcett, Am. J. Anat., 71:271, 1942.)

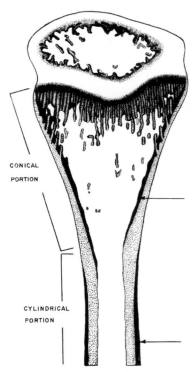

CONICAL
PORTION

CYLINDRICAL
PORTION

Figure 10–31 A diagram based upon an auto-radiograph of the head of the tibia of a growing rat killed a few hours after receiving an injection of ^{32}P. The localization of high concentrations of silver grains in the autoradiograph is depicted here in black. In addition to the new bone in the epiphysis and at the metaphysis, bone is being deposited under the endosteum in the conical portion and beneath the periosteum in the cylindrical portion of the shaft (arrows). (Drawing based upon studies of Leblond et al., Am. J. Anat., 86:289, 1950. After D. W. Fawcett, in R. O. Greep, ed.: Histology. Philadelphia, The Blakiston Co., 1954. Reproduced with the permission of the McGraw-Hill Book Co.)

DeMorgan in 1853. They enlarge to form long cylindrical cavities occupied by blood vessels and embryonic bone marrow. When they reach a considerable length, destruction of bone ceases; the osteoclasts give way to osteoblasts, and concentric lamellae of bone are laid down on the walls of the cavity until it is filled in to form a typical osteon. The lamellae of this and subsequent generations of haversian systems have the ordered arrangement of collagen and the change in its orientation in successive layers that are characteristic of osteons in adult bone. In man from about the age of one year onward,

only lamellar bone of this character is deposited within the shafts of long bones. This secondary bone eventually replaces all of the primitive haversian systems.

The outer limits of secondary haversian systems are defined by distinct *cement lines.* These are layers of bone matrix formed whenever a period of resorption is followed by new bone formation. They are collagen-poor, have staining properties different from other layers of matrix, and are not traversed by canaliculi.

The internal bone destruction and reconstruction do not end with the replacement of primary by secondary bone, but continue actively throughout life. Resorption cavities continue to appear and to be filled in by third, fourth, and higher orders of haversian systems (Fig. 10–32). The interstitial lamellae of adult bone represent persisting fragments of earlier generations of haversian systems largely removed in the continuing internal reorganization. At any one time there may be seen in a cross section: (1) mature osteons, in which all rebuilding activity has come to an end and which form the great mass of structural bone upon which the weight bearing function of the skeleton depends; (2) actively forming new osteons, in which concentric layers of preosseous tissue are being laid down and progressively calcified; and (3) absorption cavities being hollowed out in preparation for formation of new osteons.

The rate of lamellar bone formation can be determined by administration of tetracycline at two different times and measurement of the thickness of bone between the two resulting bands of labeled bone (Fig. 10–33). Such studies show that 1 μm. per day is a fair average for man, and for any given haversian system, the rate of deposition slows as the osteon nears completion. The formation time for an haversian system in the adult is 4 to 5 weeks. Different values are found in young growing bone and in pathological states. The newly deposited lamellar bone continues to calcify over a considerable period of time. A historadiogram therefore reveals a mixture of haversian systems of varying age, displaying all degrees of mineralization (Fig. 10–8C). By this continuous turnover, the organism is assured a continuing supply of new bone to carry out its skeletal and metabolic functions. It also provides the plasticity that enables bone to alter its internal architecture to adapt to new mechanical conditions.

Repair of Bone

After a fracture the usual reactions of any tissue to severe injury are seen, including hemorrhage and organization of the clot by ordinary granulation tissue. The granulation tissue becomes denser connective tissue. Cartilage and fibrocartilage then develop within it, forming a *fibrocartilaginous callus* that fills the gap between the ends of the fragments. The new bone, which will ultimately unite the fragments, begins to form at some distance from the fracture line, by activation of osteoprogenitor cells of the deeper layers of the periosteum and endosteum. A meshwork of subperiosteal trabeculae, the *bony callus*, is formed and a similar formation of new bone of endosteal origin occurs in the medullary cavity around the cartilaginous callus. As healing progresses, the latter is gradually eroded, with only enough cartilage matrix remaining to provide a framework for deposition of new bone in the area. As in endochondral bone formation, ossification of the fibrocartilaginous callus is accomplished by its gradual replacement with bone. *Bony union* of the fracture is complete when the new spongy bone from the two fragments meets and becomes continuous across the fracture line. After this there is compaction and reorganization, with resorption of excess bone and internal reconstruction, resulting finally in a bridging of the gap with compact bone.

In certain locations, where the connective tissue surrounding the bone lacks osteogenic potency, such as the subcapsular areas of the neck of the femur and of the astragalus, and the surfaces of the bones formed within tendons (*sesamoid bones,* e. g., patella, pisiform), healing of fractures occurs without a periosteal reaction and without a fibrocartilaginous callus. If there is good apposition of the fragments, the cancellous bone of the marrow cavity unites, without any callus formation, If apposition is poor or nonexistent, repair may occur only as a relatively weak, fibrous union.

Ectopic Bone Formation

As already stated, intramembranous bone forms from a connective tissue, with the transformation of mesenchymal cells into osteoblasts, osteocytes, and osteoclasts. The return of these cells to fibroblast-like mesenchymal or osteoprogenitor cells has also been described. A common feature in all these transformations, as described heretofore, is that bone has developed only in connection with the osseous system— the skeleton. The influences under which ordinary connective tissue gives rise to bone in the embryo are poorly understood, but it is clear that previously undifferentiated cellular elements of primitive connective tissue are capable of transformation to the cells characteristic of bone.

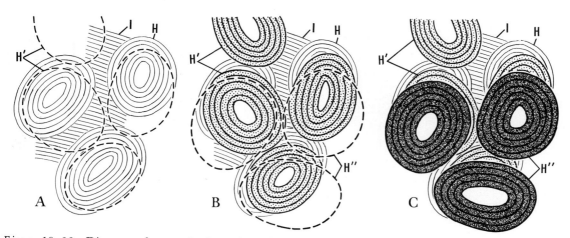

Figure 10–32 Diagram of stages in formation of three generations of haversian system, *H, H',* and *H".* *I,* Interstitial lamellae. (Modified from Prenant.)

It would appear that, once cells have exhibited osteogenic potencies, these can be readily evoked again for an indeterminate period after the cells have returned to an indifferent morphologic state. Thus, in the healing of fractures, cells in the deepest layers of the periosteum and endosteum, under the stimulus of trauma, reassume the form of osteoblasts and once again are actively engaged in osteogenesis. Moreover, cells grown from bone in tissue culture, and having lost the morphologic characteristics of osteoblasts, once again form bone when implanted into the anterior chamber of the eye (Heinen).

Furthermore, under certain conditions, bone may be formed spontaneously from connective tissue that is not in association with the skeleton. This *ectopic ossification* has been described in such diverse locations as the pelvis of the kidney, the walls of arteries, the eyes, muscles, and tendons. In the long tendons of the legs of turkeys, bone formation is a normal event. From these observations it may be inferred that many types of connective tissue have latent osteogenic potencies that are exhibited only rarely. This conclusion is supported by experimental production of bone in connective tissue after ligation of the renal artery and vein and after

a variety of experimental manipulations such as transplantation of bladder epithelium to the fascia of the anterior wall of the abdomen, and after injection of alcoholic extracts of bone into muscle. In fact, alcohol alone may induce osteogenesis in muscle, and it shares this ability with other irritating chemicals.

Many attempts have been made to utilize the osteogenic potencies of periosteum and bone by transplanting these tissues to areas in which it is desired that new bone be formed. The modern "bone bank," which supplies fragments of bone preserved by freezing or by other means, is the fruit of these efforts. Transplants of fresh autogenous bone ordinarily survive and proliferate. Homografts are antigenic and give rise to an immune response characterized by accumulations of lymphocytes and plasma cells forming specific antibodies. This response leads ultimately to death of the transplanted tissue. Heterografts will not survive, but if calf bone is refrigerated and stored, it loses some of its antigenicity and may therefore be suitable for preservation in bone banks and later use. Grafts of such tissue favor induction of new bone formation by the cells of the host.

Primitive connective tissue cells within

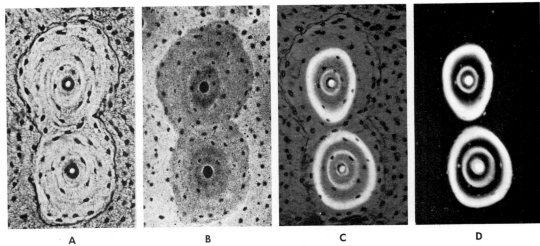

| A | B | C | D |

Figure 10–33 A pair of haversian systems from the midshaft of the tibia of a 9 month old dog given two 5 day courses of treatment with a tetracycline separated by an interval of 19 days. *A*, Ordinary microscopy. *B*, Historadiogram. *C* and *D*, Fluorescence microscopy. The bone deposited during Ledermycin treatment fluoresces, and the design of this experiment permits one to visualize the amount of bone deposited in each 5 day period. Of particular interest is the fact that the inner band, corresponding to the second period of administration, is narrower than the first, demonstrating that in this instance there is slowing down in the rate of concentric bone deposition as the formation of the haversian system progresses. (Courtesy of R. Amprino.)

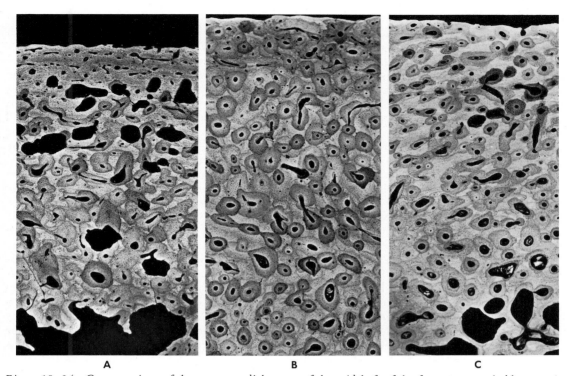

A **B** **C**

Figure 10-34 Cross sections of the anteromedial sector of the midshaft of the femur as revealed by negative historadiography. *A,* At age 7. *B,* At age 20. *C,* At age 65. Notice in the child (*A*) there are large resorption cavities (black) and large, irregularly shaped haversian systems. At the surface of the compacta, the thick zone of periosteal bone is invaded by resorption cavities. Large remnants of periosteal primary bone are found in the interstices between the secondary osteons in the middle zone of the compacta. These remnants are fewer and smaller in the older perimedullary zone at the bottom of the figure. In the 20 year old man (*B*), the compacta is much thicker. Secondary haversian systems and remnants of primary bone persist in the subperiosteal zone. Elsewhere, the osteons are fairly regular in outline and are separated by remnants of preexisting osteons. (Courtesy of R. Amprino.)

the orbit of advancing bone, as in the formation of medullary bone in birds, assume the form of osteoblasts before they actually participate in osteogenesis. This observation, together with those upon the behavior of bone grafts just cited, suggests that the presence of bone itself may be an important factor in activating osteogenic potencies. There is thus histological evidence in favor of *induction* of bone formation, although attempts to isolate a specific *inductor substance* have so far given equivocal results.

HISTOPHYSIOLOGY OF BONE

As the principal tissue making up the skeletal system, bone functions in support of the soft tissues; it carries the articulations and

provides attachment for the muscles involved in locomotion; and it forms a rigid covering for protection of the nervous ststem and of the hemopoietic tissue. In addition to these mechanical functions it plays an important role as a large store of calcium and phosphorus that can be drawn upon to maintain the normal levels of these elements in the blood and to provide for the mineral requirements of other tissues.

Bone as a Store of Mobilizable Calcium

It is impossible to overemphasize the importance of calcium in the vital functions of the body. It is essential for the activity of many enzymes. It is indispensable for maintenance of cell cohesion and of the normal permeability of cell membranes. It is required for contraction of muscles and for coagulation of the blood. It is not surprising, therefore, that the homeostatic mechanisms of the body regulate the concentration of plasma calcium with remarkable constancy, the normal range being between 9 and 11 mg. per 100 ml. Most of the calcium in the body (99 per cent) is, of course, in the bones. There is a constant interchange of calcium between bone and the blood, which results in the maintenance of the relatively constant calcium ion concentration in the plasma. The minute hydroxyapatite crystals present a surface area for exchange with the extracellular fluids that is of the order of 100 to 300 square meters per gram. It has been estimated that during each minute in the life of an adult man, one of every four calcium ions present in the blood exchanges with similar ions in the bones. A dual mechanism for homeostatic regulation of the blood calcium level has been postulated. One part, acting by diffusion and simple equilibrium between blood and the labile fraction of bone mineral, is adequate to maintain a constant but low calcium level of approximately 7 mg. per 100 ml. of blood plasma. Not all of the bone contributes equally to this function. The most labile calcium apparently is located in the younger and incompletely calcified osteons. It is these that are most sensitive to ionic variations in the internal environment. Therefore, the continued remodeling of the adult skeleton has metabolic as well as mechanical significance (Vincent). It provides a pool of young osteons, which can rapidly respond in homeostatic regulation by taking up or releasing calcium. As these osteons mature and become more heavily mineralized, they become progressively less available to the extracellular fluids, and these older osteons probably contribute more to the mechanical function of the skeleton. They are ultimately replaced in their physiologic function by a new generation of osteons. These two categories are sometimes referred to as *metabolic* and *structural bone*. The second part of the dual mechanism required to elevate and maintain the plasma calcium at the normal level of 10 mg. per 100 ml. is mediated by *parathyroid hormone* (Chapter 20), and involves resorption of bone mineral and organic matrix through the action of osteoclasts.

The responsiveness of the skeleton to the metabolic needs of other organ systems is best illustrated in those species in which there are unusual periodic demands for calcium. Perhaps the most striking example is found in birds in the laying cycle, during which considerable amounts of calcium are required in the oviduct for deposition of the egg shell. To meet this need, many trabeculae in the marrow cavities of the long bones are resorbed, only to be restored after the egg is laid and again removed to provide the shell for the next egg in the clutch. Less dramatic examples of mobilization of calcium from the skeleton are also observed in mammals. While the antlers of deer are growing, there is a mild rarefaction of bone throughout the skeleton, and in dairy cows producing large amounts of milk there may be a detectable osteoporosis associated with the considerable calcium loss in the milk. Human reproduction does not involve such unusual demands for calcium. There is no doubt, however, that during pregnancy the maternal skeleton is drawn upon to some extent for calcification of the fetal skeleton, and during prolonged lactation it is the source of some of the calcium lost in the milk. In normal individuals there is no detectable radiological change in the skeleton, but when pregnancy or lactation is superimposed upon severe nutritional deficiency or impaired absorption of calcium, *osteomalacia* results, and may become so severe as to result in pathological fractures.

Endocrine Effects Upon Bone

The skeletal system is affected by several hormones. The most important of these is *parathyroid hormone*. Its participation in maintenance of the normal levels of circulating calcium was referred to earlier. The activity of the parathyroid glands appears to be regulated by a *negative feedback* mechanism, in which the blood Ca^{++} level itself exerts a direct effect upon parathyroid activity. Parathyroid hormone has multiple sites of action. One of the earliest detectable effects after its administration is on the kidney, where it causes a rapid increase in excretion of phosphate in the urine. This in turn affects the plasma calcium levels. The hormone appears to have a dual effect upon bone. Its initial effect is believed to be on osteocytes, stimulating osteocytic osteolysis. A long continued increase in circulating parathyroid hormone results in induction of osteoclast formation and accelerated bone remodeling. Since bone resorption under the influence of parathyroid hormone results in destruction of stable crystals of hydroxy-apatite, as well as of the organic matrix, this mechanism makes available, for homeo-static regulation, an otherwise inaccessible source of calcium.

Grafts of parathyroid to bone in vivo (Barnicot) and confronted cultures in vitro (Gaillard) have demonstrated that the gland causes resorption by direct action on bone. In clinical *hyperparathyroidism*, bone is extensively absorbed and is replaced by fibrous tissue containing large numbers of osteoclasts. This results in the pathological condition described as *osteitis fibrosa* (von Reckling-hausen's disease).

Opposing the action of parathyroid hor-mone is the polypeptide hormone *calcitonin* or *thyrocalcitonin*, which originates from special cells in the thyroid gland (Chapter 19). This hormone inhibits bone resorption and thus tends to lower blood calcium. It is currently hypothesized that parathyroid hormone and calcitonin act together to prevent or counteract any significant pertur-bation of the homeostatic regulation of plas-ma calcium concentration. A fall in plasma calcium below a certain level would pre-sumably result in increased release of para-thyroid hormone and suppression of calci-tonin release. The effect of this would be an increased rate of bone resorption and move-ment of calcium from bone to blood, thereby returning the plasma calcium to normal. Conversely, a supranormal blood calcium concentration would stimulate release of calcitonin and suppress release of parathyroid hormone. These effects would tend to return the elevated plasma calcium to normal.

The effects of the gonadal hormones upon bone vary greatly with the species. In the example of the laying bird cited previous-ly, an entire new system of trabeculae of medullary bone is produced by stimulation of the endosteal lining in the estrogenic phase of the egg laying cycle. These trabeculae serve to accumulate calcium for later use in forma-tion of the egg shell. The same changes can be induced by administration of exogenous *estrogens*. Concurrently with the storage of calcium in medullary bone, the liver forms a phosphoprotein that appears in the blood and is transported to the ovarian follicle, where it is stored in the egg yolk as *phospho-vitellin*, the major source of phosphate for growth and development of the chick embryo.

Mice react to administration of estrogens in a manner qualitatively similar to that of birds. Endosteal bone formation is enhanced, but, in this case, does not seem to serve any physiological function. Endosteal bone for-mation has not been reported in rats. In this species, estrogens inhibit normal resorption of the spongiosa during endochondral ossifi-cation, resulting in a greatly elongated and dense spongiosa in the metaphysis. The osteoporosis occasionally seen in women after the menopause is attributed by some to the decline in ovarian function, but it does not respond favorably to treatment with estrogens.

The gonadal hormones in some way play an important part in determining the rate of skeletal maturation. In normal human devel-opment the time of appearance of the various ossification centers and the time of fusion of the epiphyses with their diaphyses is remark-ably constant. The progress of these events at any given time during development is inti-mately related to the developmental state of the reproductive system. Thus in precocious sexual development, skeletal maturation is accelerated and growth is stunted, owing to premature epiphyseal closure. On the other hand, in testicular hypoplasia or prepubertal castration, epiphyseal union in the long bones is delayed, and the arms and legs become dis-proportionately long.

The growth of bone is also markedly influenced by the *growth hormone* (somatotro-pin) of the anterior hypophysis (Chapter 18). Hypophysectomy results in cessation of growth at the epiphyseal plate; on admini-stration of growth hormone, growth recom-mences. Growth hormone injected into rats that have been both thyroidectomized and hypophysectomized produces skeletal growth, whereas thyroxine produces matura-tion, but only moderate growth. Coordina-tion between growth and maturation may be restored by administration of both hormones.

Nutritional Effects Upon Bone

Growth of the skeleton is quite depen-dent upon nutritional factors. Deficiencies of minerals or of essential vitamins are often detected more easily in bone than in other tissues. A gross dietary deficiency of either calcium or phosphorus leads to rarefaction of bone and increased liability to fractures. Even if the intake of these elements is adequate, a deficiency of *vitamin D* may interfere with their intestinal absorption and lead to *rickets.* In this condition, ossification of the epiphyseal cartilages is disturbed, the regular columnar arrangement of the cartilage cells disappears, and the metaphysis becomes a disordered mixture of uncalcified cartilage and poorly calcified bone matrix. Such bones are easily deformed by weight bearing.

In long-standing deficiency of calcium and of vitamin D, especially when aggravated by pregnancy, the bones of adults come to contain much uncalcified osteoid tissue, a condition known as *adult rickets* or *osteomalacia.* Although the condition is aggravated by the increased demands of pregnancy, the diminution in calcium content in this condition is due mainly to failure of calcification of new bone formed in the turnover of this tissue, rather than to decalcification of previously calcified bone.

Deficiency of *vitamin C* leads to profound changes in tissues of mesenchymal origin, producing the condition known as *scurvy* or *scorbutus,* in which the primary defect is an inability to produce and maintain the intercellular substance of connective tissues. In the case of bone, it results in deficient production of collagen and bone matrix, with consequent retardation of growth and delayed healing of fractures.

Deficiency of *vitamin A* results in a diminution in the rate of growth of the skeleton. The vitamin controls the activity, distribution, and coordination of osteoblasts and osteoclasts during development. Among other things, resorption and remodeling fail to enlarge the cranial cavity and spinal canal at a rate sufficient to accommodate growth of the brain and spinal cord. Serious damage therefore results to the central nervous system. In hypervitaminosis A erosion of the cartilage columns accelerates without a compensating increase in the rate of multiplication of cells in the proliferative zone. The epiphyseal plates may therefore be completely obliterated, and growth may cease prematurely.

JOINTS AND SYNOVIAL MEMBRANES

Bones are joined to one another by connective tissue structures that permit varying degrees of movement between the adjoining bones. Such structures are called joints or articulations. These present extreme variations in character, which depend primarily upon the type of bones which are joined and the varying degrees of motion permitted by the articulation. Thus, in some cases, as in the skull, the joints are immovable, and the connected bones are separated only by a thin connective tissue layer, the sutural ligament. Other joints are slightly movable, such as the intervertebral articulations. Here the succeeding vertebrae are joined by dense fibrous tissue and cartilage. Still other bones are freely movable upon one another, and here the bones are completely separated by cartilage, and the articular surfaces are surrounded by fibrous capsules.

Joints in which there is little or no movement are called *synarthroses.* There are three types of these: if the connection between the bones is of bone, it is a *synostosis;* if it consists of cartilage, a *synchondrosis;* and if of connective tissue, a *syndesmosis.* Joints that permit free movement of the bones are called *diarthroses.*

In the diarthrodial joints there is a cavity. Because this cavity was thought by some to have a continuous lining of flattened, epithelium-like cells, the lining layer was called "mesenchymal epithelium." However, the walls of the joint cavities are in fact composed of a dense connective tissue whose cells are irregularly distributed and seldom suggest epithelium in arrangement. Occasionally, small amounts of cartilage and all transitions between the cartilage cells and the joint or *synovial cells* can be found.

The articular surface of the bones is covered with hyaline cartilage. Where the opposing cartilages touch, they are not covered with dense connective tissue, but at their bases a small area of perichondrium is reflected backward into the membrane of the joint capsule. At this point, there are many cartilage cells extending into the synovial membrane. As is true of much of the cartilage of the body, the articular cartilages contain no blood vessels; it is generally believed that they are nourished by diffusion from the joint fluid and surrounding tissues. The articular cartilages are intimately adherent to a layer of compact bone which lacks haversian systems and has large lacunae, and is said to be free of canaliculi.

Most of the joint capsules are composed

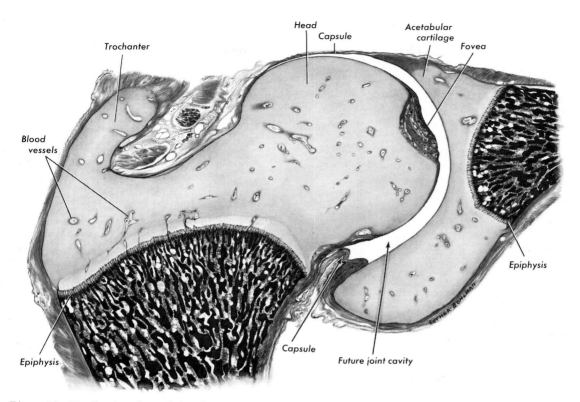

Figure 10--35   Section through head of the femur of a 26 cm. human fetus. ×6. From a preparation of H. Hatcher.

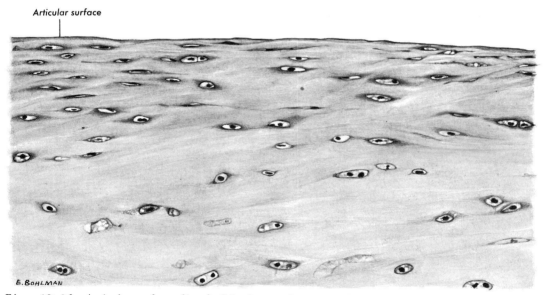

Figure 10--36   Articular surface of head of the femur of a man. ×300. From a preparation of H. Hatcher.

of two fairly distinct layers. The external consists of dense fibrous tissue and is called the *fibrous layer*. The inner is the *synovial layer*, which is more cellular and is thought to secrete the viscid, colorless liquid of the joint cavity. However, the joint membrane exhibits many variations in structure. The synovial layer is sometimes thrown into marked folds, which may project for surprising distances into the cavity. The larger of these folds frequently contain vessels. In other cases the two layers appear fused, or the synovial layer may rest directly on muscle or fatty tissue or periosteum. It has been suggested that the synovia be classified according to the tissues on which they lie: that is, loose connective, dense fibrous, or adipose tissue.

Synovial membranes that rest on loose connective tissue usually cover those parts of the joints not subjected to strain or pressure. As a rule, they have a definite surface layer, separated from the underlying tissue of the joint by loose connective tissue. The surface layer consists of collagenous fibers interspersed with fibroblasts whose processes may extend for long distances, although sometimes the cells are rounded. The collagenous fibers either are irregularly arranged or may be oriented along the main lines of stress. In addition to the fibroblasts, there are a few macrophages, leukocytes, and lymphoid wandering cells. In addition to blood vessels, the loose connective tissue contains many lymphatics.

The fibrous synovial membrane covers the interarticular ligaments and tendons and lines those parts of the joints that are subject to strain. It consists of dense connective tissue; the surface zone is slightly more cellular than the rest. Some of the fibroblasts have capsules. When unusual pressure is applied to the synovial membrane, fibrocartilage develops.

The adipose type of synovial membrane covers the fat pads that project into the joint cavities. The synovial membrane in this case usually consists of a single layer of cells resting on a thin layer of connective tissue.

The fibroblasts of the synovial membrane rarely show mitoses. They may occasionally contain one or two vacuoles. There are no vacuoles within them that stain with neutral red. Mitochondria and a Golgi net have been demonstrated in them.

Folds of the synovial membrane either may be temporary formations, which depend on the position of the joint, or may form permanent villi, which project into the joint cavity. Some of these villi have a broad base and a rather short stalk, while others may be thin and long. The larger folds contain blood vessels, lymphatics, and occasionally lobules of adipose tissue. There is an increase in the size and number of the villi with age. New

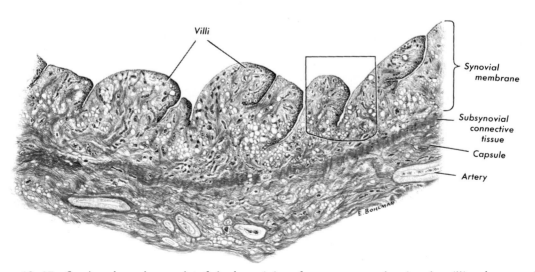

Figure 10-37 Section through capsule of the knee joint of a young man, showing the villi and connective tissue components. The area outlined is shown at higher magnification in Figure 10-38. ×15. From a preparation of H. Hatcher.

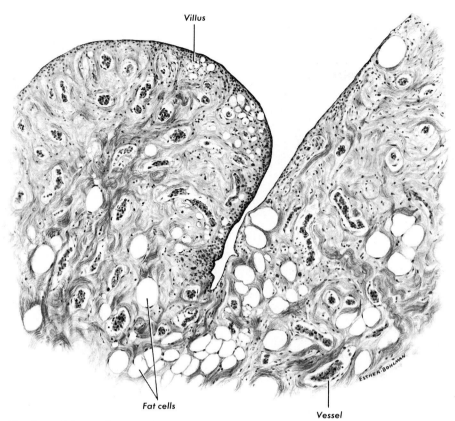

Villus

Fat cells

Vessel

Figure 10-38 Synovial membrane of young adult. (Higher magnification of the area outlined in Figure 10–37.) Note the irregularity in the concentration of cells toward the free surface of the villus and the irregular distribution of fat cells. ×85. From a preparation of H. Hatcher.

islets of cartilage are formed in them, mainly by metaplasia of the synovial fibroblasts.

Blood vessels probably do not lie free on the surface of the synovial membrane. There are two plexuses of lymphatics, as a rule, within the synovial membranes—a superficial and a deep plexus. The nerves which accompany the blood vessels end in the layer beneath the surface in terminal arborizations or end-bulbs or plates. Pacinian corpuscles are always present.

When injured, the synovial membrane reacts, like any other connective tissue, by forming granulation tissue, and after some weeks may be completely regenerated. The synovial fluid is normally small in amount and seems to be a dialysate of blood, to which have been added small amounts of mucin and a very few cells, chiefly lymphocytes, monocytes, and macrophages.

REFERENCES

Current surveys of bone from different points of view range from the relatively brief *Bone: An Introduction to the Physiology of Skeletal Tissue,* by F. C. McLean and M. R. Urist (3rd ed., Chicago, University of Chicago Press, 1967), to the larger and more specialized presentations by many authors in *The Biochemistry and Physiology of Bone,* edited by G. H. Bourne (New York, Academic Press, 1972); *Bone as a Tissue,* edited by K. Rodahl, J. T. Nicholson, and E. M. Brown, Jr. (New York, McGraw-Hill Book Co., 1960); *Bone Biodynamics,* edited by Harold M. Frost (Boston, Little, Brown & Co., 1963); and *The Physiology of Bone,* by J. M. Vaughan (Oxford, Clarendon Press, 1970).

Amprino, R., and A. Engstrom: Studies on x-ray absorption and diffraction of bone tissue. Acta Anat., *15*:1, 1952.
Barnicot, N. A.: Supravital staining of osteoclasts with neutral red; their distribution on parietal bone of normal growing mice, and comparison with mutants grey-lethal and hydrocephalus-3. Proc. Roy. Soc. Lond., *B134*:467, 1947.
Barnicot, N. A.: The local action of the parathyroid and other tissues on bone in intracerebral grafts. J. Anat., *82*:233, 1948.

Bélanger, L. F., J. Robichon, B. B. Migicovscy, D. H. Copp, and J. Vincent: Resorption without osteoclasts (osteolysis.) In Sognnaes, R. F., ed.: Mechanisms of Hard Tissue Destruction. Washington, D. C., American Association for the Advancement of Science, 1963.

Bélanger, L. F.: Osteocytic osteolysis. Calc. Tiss. Res., 4:1, 1969.

Bernard, G. W., and D. C. Pease: An electron microscopic study of initial intramembranous osteogenesis. Am. J. Anat., 125:271, 1969.

Bingham, P., L. Brazell, and M. Owen: The effect of parathyroid extract (PTE) on ribonucleic acid (RNA) and protein synthesis in bone and on the level of calcium in the serum. J. Endocrinol., 45:387, 1969.

Bloom, W., M. A. Bloom, and F. C. McLean: Calcification and ossification: Medullary bone changes in the reproductive cycle of female pigeons. Anat. Rec., 81:443, 1941.

Bonucci, E.: The locus of initial calcification in cartilage and bone. Clin. Orthopaedics, 78:108, 1971.

Cohen, J., and W. H. Harris: The three dimensional anatomy of haversian systems. J. Bone & Joint Surg., 40A:419, 1958.

Cooper, R. R., J. W. Milgram, and R. A. Robinson: Morphology of the osteon. An electron microscopic study. J. Bone & Joint Surg., 48A:1239, 1966.

Doty, S. B., B. H. Schofield, and R. A. Robinson: The electron microscopic identification of acid phosphatase and adenosine triphosphatase in bone cells following parathyroid extract or thyrocalcitonin administration. In Talmage, R. V., and L. F. Bélanger, eds.: Parathyroid Hormone and Thyrocalcitonin (Calcitonin). Excerpta Medica International Congress Series, No. 159, 1968, p. 169.

Dudley, H. R., and D. Spiro: The fine structure of bone cells. J. Biophys. Biochem. Cytol., 11:627, 1961.

Engström, A.: Structure of bone from the anatomical to the molecular level. In Bone Structure and Metabolism. London, J. & A. Churchill, Ltd., 1956.

Fawcett, D. W.: The amedullary bones of the Florida manatee. Am. J. Anat., 71:271, 1942.

Fernández-Moran, H., and A. Engström: Electron microscopy and x-ray diffraction of bone. Biochem. Biophys. Acta, 23:260, 1957.

Fischman, D. A., and E. D. Hay: Origin of osteoclasts from mononuclear leucocytes in regenerating new limbs. Anat. Rec., 143:329, 1962.

Gaillard, P. J.: Parathyroid gland and bone in vitro. VI. Devel. Biol., 1:152, 1959.

Gaillard, P. J.: Parathyroid and bone in tissue culture. In Greep, R. O., and R. V. Talmage, eds.: The Parathyroids. Springfield, Ill., Charles C Thomas Co., 1961.

Glimcher, M. J.: Molecular biology of mineralized tissues with particular reference to bone. In Oncley, J. L., et al., eds.: Biophysical Science—A Study Program. New York, John Wiley & Sons, 1959.

Glimcher, M. J., A. J. Hodge, and F. O. Schmitt: Macromolecular aggregation states in relation to mineralization: the collagen-hydroxyapatite system as studied in vitro. Proc. Nat. Acad. Sci., 43:860, 1957.

Glimcher, M. J., and S. M. Krane: The organization and structure of bone and the mechanism of calcification. In Ramachandran, G. N., and B. S. Gould, eds.: Treatise on Collagen. IIB: Biology of Collagen. London, Academic Press, 1968.

Goldhaber, P.: Oxygen dependent bone resorption in tissue culture. In Greep, R. O., and R. V. Talmage, eds.: The Parathyroids. Springfield, Ill., Charles C Thomas Co., 1961.

Gonzales, F., and M. J. Karnovsky: Electron microscopy of osteoclasts in healing fractures of rat bone. J. Biophys. & Biochem. Cytol., 9:199, 1961.

Hancox, N. M., and B. Boothroyd: The osteoclast in resorption. In Sognnaes, R. F., ed.: Mechanisms of Hard Tissue Destruction. Washington, D. C., American Association for the Advancement of Science, 1963.

Heinen, J. H., G. H. Dabbs, and H. A. Mason: The experimental production of ectopic cartilage and bone in the muscles of rabbits. J. Bone & Joint Surg., 31:765, 1949.

Heller, M.: Bone. In Bloom, W., ed.: Histopathology of Irradiation from External and Internal Sources. National Nuclear Energy Series. New York, McGraw-Hill Book Co., 1948.

Heller, M., F. C. McLean, and W. Bloom: Cellular transformations in mammalian bones induced by parathyroid extract. Am. J. Anat., 87:315, 1950.

Heller-Steinberg, M.: Ground substance, bone salts, and cellular activity in bone formation and destruction. Am. J. Anat., 89:347, 1951.

Holtrop, M. E.: The ultrastructure of osteoclasts during stimulation and inhibition of bone resorption. IV International Congress of Endocrinology, Washington, D. C., 1972.

Holtrop, M. E., and J. M. Weinger: Ultrastructural evidence for a transport system in bone. In Talmage, R. V., and P. L. Munson, eds.: Parathyroid Hormone and the Calcitonins. Amsterdam, Excerpta Medica, 1972.

Jackson, S. F.: The fine structure of developing bone in the embryonic fowl. Proc. Roy. Soc. Lond., B146:370, 1957.

Kallio, D. M., P. R. Garant, and C. Minkin: Evidence of coated membranes in the ruffled border of the osteoclast. J. Ultrastr. Res., 37:169, 1971.

Lacroix, P.: Bone and cartilage. In Brachet, J., and A. E. Mirsky, eds.: The Cell: Biochemistry, Physiology, Morphology. Vol. V. New York, Academic Press, 1961.

Lacroix, P., and A. Budy, eds.: Radioisotopes and bone: A symposium. Oxford, Blackwell Scientific Publications, Ltd., 1962.

Leblond, C. P., et al.: Radioautographic visualization of bone formation in the rat. Am. J. Anat., 86:289, 1950.

McLean, F. C., and W. Bloom: Calcification and ossification; calcification in normal growing bone. Anat Rec., 78:333, 1940.

McLean, F. C., and A. M. Budy: Radiation, Isotopes, and Bone. New York, Academic Press, 1964.

McLean, F. C., and R. E. Rowland: Internal remodeling of compact bone. In Sognnaes, R. F., ed.: Mechanisms of Hard Tissue Destruction. Washington, D. C., American Association for the Advancement of Science, 1963.

Maximow. A. A.: Untersuchungen über Blut und Bindegewebe. III. Die embryonale Histogenese des Knochenmarks der Säugetiere. Arch. f. Mikr. Anat., 76:1, 1910.

Mears, D. C.: Effects of parathyroid hormone and thyrocalcitonin on the membrane potential of osteoclasts. Endocrinology, 88:1021, 1971.

Miller, E. J., and G. R. Martin: The collagen of bone. Clinical Orthopedics, 59:195, 1968.

Neuman, W. F., and M. W. Neuman: The Chemical Dynamics of Bone Mineral. Chicago, University of Chicago Press, 1958.

Robinson, R. A., and D. A. Cameron: Bone. *In* Electron Microscopic Anatomy. New York, Academic Press, 1964.

Schenk, R. K., D. Spiro, and J. Wiener: Cartilage resorption in the tibial epiphyseal plate of growing rats. J. Cell Biol., *34*:275, 1967.

Scott, B. L.: Thymidine-³H electron microscopic radioautography of osteogenic cells in the fetal rat. J. Cell Biol., *35*:115, 1967.

Sledge, C. B.: Some morphologic and experimental aspects of limb development. Clin. Ortho. Rel. Res., *44*:241, 1966.

Sognnaes, R. F., ed.: Calcification in Biological Systems. Washington D. C., American Association for the Advancement of Science, 1960.

Sognnaes, R. F., ed.: Mechanisms of Hard Tissue Destruction. Washington, D. C., American Association for the Advancement of Science, 1963.

Vaes, G.: On the mechanism of bone resorption: The action of parathyroid hormone on the excretion and synthesis of lysosomal enzymes and on the extracellular release of acid by bone cells. J. Cell Biol., *39*:676, 1968.

Vincent, J.: Microscopic aspects of mineral metabolism in bone tissue with special reference to calcium, lead, and zinc. Clin. Orthoped., *26*:161, 1963.

Walker, D. G.: Osteopetrosis cured by temporary parabiosis. Science *180*:875, 1973.

Whitson, S. W.: Tight junction formation in the osteon. Clin. Orthopaed., *86*:206, 1972.

Young, R. W.: Cell proliferation and specialization during endochrondral osteogenesis in young rats. J. Cell Biol., *14*:357, 1962.

Young, R. W.: Specialization of bone cells. *In* Frost, H., ed.: Bone Biodynamics. Boston, Little, Brown, & Co., 1964.

Zichner, D.: The effects of calcitonin on bone cells in young rats: An electron microscope study. Israel J. Med. Sci., *7*:359, 1971.

11
Muscular Tissue

Muscular tissue is responsible for locomotion and for the movements of the various parts of the body with respect to one another. The fundamental protoplasmic property of contractility is highly developed in this tissue, whose cells are elongated in the direction of contraction and organized in long units of structure called *muscle fibers*.

The recognition of two general categories of muscle, *smooth* and *striated*, is based on several distinguishing features. Striated muscle exhibits regularly spaced transverse bands along the length of the fiber. Smooth muscle is composed of individual cellular units and is innervated by the autonomic nervous system and its contraction is not subject to voluntary control. Striated muscle is subdivided into two distinct types, *skeletal* and *cardiac*. Skeletal muscle fibers are syncytial. They are innervated by the cerebrospinal system of nerves, and their contraction is under *voluntary* control. The fibers of cardiac muscle are made up of separate cellular units, and their rhythmical contraction is *involuntary*.

In general, the visceral musculature is composed of *smooth muscle*. The somatic musculature comprising the flesh of the body wall and of the extremities is *striated skeletal muscle*. *Cardiac muscle* makes up the wall of the heart and may extend into the proximal portions of the pulmonary veins.

SMOOTH MUSCLE

Smooth muscle forms the contractile portion of the wall of the digestive tract from the middle of the esophagus to the internal sphincter of the anus. It provides the motive power for mixing the ingested food with digestive juices and for its propulsion through the absorptive and excretory portions of the tract. Smooth muscle is also found in the walls of the ducts in the glands associated with the alimentary tract, in the walls of the respiratory passages from the trachea to the alveolar ducts, and in the urinary and genital ducts. The walls of the arteries, veins, and larger lymphatic trunks contain smooth muscle. In the skin it forms minute muscles called arrectores pilorum, responsible for elevation of hairs. In the areola of the mammary gland it participates in the erection of the nipple, and in the subcutaneous tissue of the scrotum it causes the wrinkling of the skin that accompanies elevation of the testes. In the eye, it forms the musculature of the iris and of the ciliary body, which is concerned with accommodation and with constriction and dilation of the pupil.

The Smooth Muscle Fibers

Smooth muscle fibers are long, spindle-shaped cells. Where they are closely associated in bundles or sheets, their boundaries are difficult to resolve with the light microscope, but by special maceration techniques the fibers can be isolated, and their long fusiform shape is then evident (Fig. 11–1). They vary greatly in length in different organs. In the pregnant human uterus, they may reach a half millimeter in length. Their average length in the musculature of the human intestine is about 0.2 mm. with a thickness of about 5 μm. The smallest smooth muscle cells in the walls of small blood vessels may be only 20 μm. long.

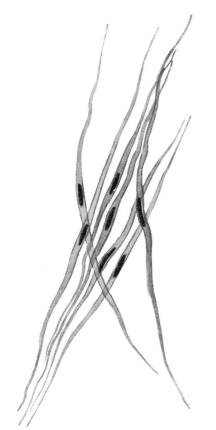

Figure 11–1 Isolated smooth muscle cells from the wall of the stomach of a cat. ×22. (After A. A. Maximow.)

In longitudinal sections, the elongated single nucleus is found to occupy the thickest part of the fiber, about midway along its length. Its long cylindrical profile is rounded at the ends (Fig. 11–2). The chromatin usually forms a delicate pattern uniformly dispersed in the nucleoplasm but in the smooth muscle of some organs it tends to be aggregated along the inner surface of the nuclear envelope. There are two to several nucleoli, depending upon the species. In smooth muscle fixed in contraction, the passively distorted nuclei may be deeply indented along their margins or may take on a helical form.

The cells of smooth muscle are offset with respect to one another, so that the thick middle portion of one is juxtaposed to the thin ends of adjacent cells. In transverse sections, smooth muscle therefore presents a mosaic of rounded or irregularly polygonal profiles varying from less than one micrometer to several micrometers across (Fig. 11–3). Only the largest profiles, those representing sections through the thick middle portion of the fibers, contain a centrally placed cross section of the nucleus. No nucleus is found in the smaller profiles, which represent sections at various levels in the tapering ends of the fusiform cells.

The cytoplasm of muscle cells is called *sarcoplasm.* In smooth muscle it is quite homogeneous in the living state and is almost equally devoid of structure after routine fixation and staining. However, after use of special stains, or after gentle maceration in nitric or trichloracetic acid, fine longitudinal striations can be demonstrated, running the full length of the cell. These are the *myofibrils* and are interpreted as the contractile material of smooth muscle. They are doubly refractile under the polarizing microscope but show no sign of the alternating isotropic and anisotropic transverse bands that are characteristic of the myofibrils of striated muscle.

After appropriate cytological staining methods, mitochondria can be seen throughout the sarcoplasm, but they tend to congregate near the poles of the elongated nucleus. A pair of centrioles and a small Golgi apparatus can also be demonstrated. In some organs the sarcoplasm of smooth muscle may contain considerable glycogen.

In the development of mammary and sweat glands, certain cells of ectodermal origin become specialized for contraction. The cell body of these *myoepithelial cells* has some of the characteristics of epithelial cells but their base is drawn out into several radiating processes that contain myofilaments. In electron micrographs, these portions of the cell have an appearance closely resembling the sarcoplasm of smooth muscle cells (Figs. 23–38 and 34–9).

Mode of Association of Smooth Muscle Fibers

Smooth muscle cells may occur singly or in small groups in ordinary connective tissue, as in the lamina propria of the intestinal villi, where their contraction shortens the villi and helps expel lymph from the lacteals. In the walls of blood vessels, where smooth muscle fibers serve only to change the caliber of the lumen, they are oriented circumferentially,

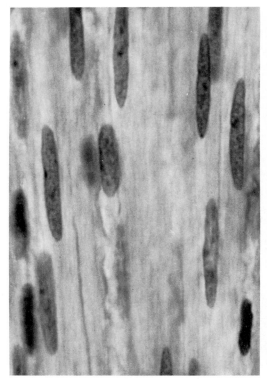 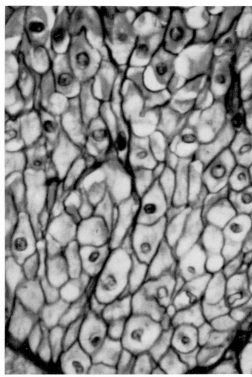

Figure 11–2   *Figure 11–3*

Figure 11–2 Photomicrograph of longitudinal section of smooth muscle from the tunica muscularis of intestine. ×1100.

Figure 11–3 Photomicrograph of transverse section of smooth muscle from the tunica muscularis of human stomach. The section was treated with the periodic acid–Schiff reaction, which stains the glycoprotein coating of the muscle cells, thus accentuating their outline. ×1100.

occurring as isolated fibers in the smallest arterioles and as a continuous layer in vessels of larger size. In the wall of the intestine, smooth muscle is arranged in separate longitudinal and circumferential layers. The coordinated action of these layers forms constrictions that move along the intestine as peristaltic waves, propelling the contents through the lumen. In other hollow organs, such as the bladder or uterus, the smooth muscle forms poorly defined layers of elaborately interlacing coarse bundles oriented in different directions.

The connective tissue fibers outside the muscle layer continue into the spaces between the cells and bind them into bundles. Between the thicker bundles or layers of smooth muscle cells is a small amount of loose connective tissue containing fibroblasts, collagenous and elastic fibers, and a network of capillaries and nerves. Connective tissue cells

are seldom found within smooth muscle bundles, but the clefts between muscle cells are nevertheless penetrated by thin collagenous, elastic, and reticular fibers. The reticular fibers branch irregularly, and their delicate network invests the individual smooth muscle cells. They can be stained with Mallory's aniline blue method and still more distinctly with the Bielschowsky silver impregnation method. The reticular fibers are embedded in an intercellular layer of material that appears in sections stained with the periodic acid–Schiff (PAS) reaction as a continuous pattern of magenta lines outlining every muscle cell (Fig. 11–3).

The pull of each contracting cell in smooth muscle is transmitted to the surrounding sheath of reticular fibers, and these continue into those of the surrounding connective tissue. This arrangement permits the force of contraction of the entire layer of the smooth muscle to be uniformly transmitted to the surrounding parts.

The Fine Structure of Smooth Muscle

In electron micrographs the elongated nucleus of the extended smooth muscle cell is smoothly contoured and rounded at the ends. The juxtanuclear sarcoplasm contains long slender mitochondria, a few tubular elements of granular endoplasmic reticulum, and numerous clusters of free ribosomes. A small Golgi complex is located near one pole of the nucleus. The bulk of the cytoplasm is occupied by exceedingly thin, parallel myofilaments associated in bundles of varying width that correspond to the myofibrils seen with the light microscope. These are oriented, for the most part, parallel to the long axis of the muscle cell. Interspersed among the bundles of myofilaments are mitochondria, occurring singly or in small clusters, and having a prevailing longitudinal orientation. Scattered through the contractile substance of the cell are oval or fusiform dense areas (Figs. 11–4 and 11–5). At high magnification these appear to be traversed by myofilaments embedded in a dense amorphous matrix. Similar dense areas are distributed at intervals along the inner aspect of the plasmalemma. The exact nature of these dense areas in the sarcoplasm is not known. Their fine structural resemblance to the dense regions found at desmosomes, at zonulae adherentes of epithelia, and at the Z bands of striated muscle suggests that the dense component of all of these may be similar and may have a cohesive function. The occurrence of dense bodies in smooth muscle at nodal points where myofilaments seem to be bonded together laterally, and also where they are attached to the cell surface, is consistent with this speculation. The plasmalemma between the specialized sites of myo-

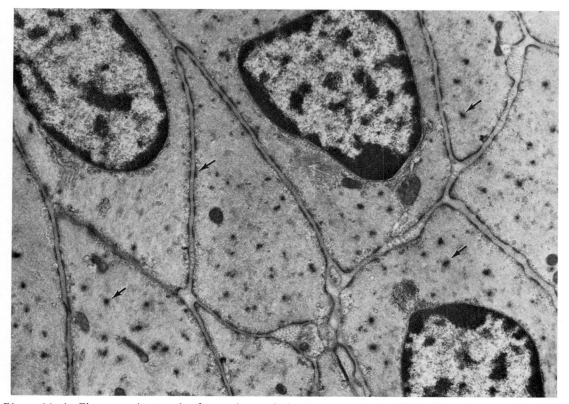

Figure 11–4 Electron micrograph of smooth muscle in transverse section. The cells are separated by rather wide extracellular spaces occupied by glycoprotein and small bundles of collagen fibrils. Scattered through the cytoplasm and around the periphery of the cell (at the arrows) are ill-defined densities that are sites of lateral bonding of myofilaments or sites of insertion of the filaments onto the cell membrane. ×14,000.

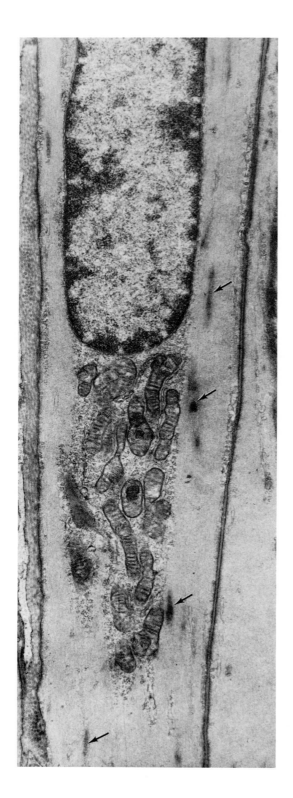

filament attachment is characteristically studded with small vesicular inpocketings or caveoli like those seen in endothelial cells and commonly interpreted as evidence of micropinocytosis.

A number of unstriated invertebrate muscles and all striated muscles of vertebrates have been found with the electron microscope to have two distinct sets of parallel filaments, which are believed to slide past one another during contraction. The widespread occurrence of a two-filament sliding mechanism of muscle contraction (see p. 309) led to the expectation that all muscle cells would be found to have two kinds of filaments. Early electron microscopic studies, however, failed to demonstrate more than one class of myofilament in vertebrate smooth muscle. It has been difficult to determine to what degree this is a technical problem. The myofilaments are very thin, less ordered, and less easily preserved than those of striated muscle. In cross sections at high magnification, it is sometimes possible to distinguish punctate profiles of two sizes, about 30 Å and about 80 Å (Fig. 11–6). These have been interpreted by some investigators as end-on views of two kinds of filaments. The thicker filaments are relatively less numerous, are not distributed as uniformly or in any precise topographical relation to the thin filaments. These two size categories are interpreted as two kinds of myofilaments, comparable to the actin and myosin filaments of skeletal muscle. The thin filaments are always seen in routinely prepared electron micrographs. The thick filaments of smooth muscle are preserved only with difficulty, in contrast to those of striated muscle, which are stable and easily demonstrated. The inconsistency in their preservation has been variously interpreted. Some investigators believe the myosin fila-

Figure 11–5 Electron micrograph of the central portion of a smooth muscle cell in longitudinal section. The uniform grey area at the periphery is occupied by myofilaments, not resolved at this magnification. Conical regions of sarcoplasm extending from the poles of the elongate nucleus contain numerous mitochondria, a few elements of the endoplasmic reticulum, and many free ribosomes. ×20,000.

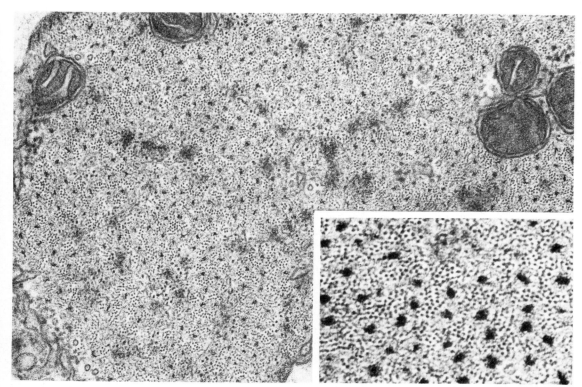

Figure 11–6 Electron micrograph of a vascular smooth muscle cell in cross section, clearly showing thick and thin filaments. ×86,000. The inset shows the same at higher magnification. (×186,000). (Micrograph from A. P. Somlyo, C. E. Devine, and A. V. Somlyo, *In* Vascular Smooth Muscle. Heidelberg, Springer-Verlag, 1972.)

ments are present in vivo but extracted during specimen preparation: others believe that thick filaments are absent in relaxed smooth muscle, but that myosin is organized into thick filaments only at the moment of excitation-contraction coupling. A satisfactory explanation of the variable results is still lacking, but there is growing acceptance of a two filament contractile system in smooth muscle. The ratio of thin to thick filaments is variable, but generally is considerably greater than 12:1, as compared to 5- or 6:1 in skeletal muscle.

In studies of the chemical composition of smooth muscle, two fibrous proteins can be isolated, *actin* and *myosin.* When these are mixed in vitro, they form a complex (actomyosin), which is capable of contracting on addition of adenosine triphosphate. It is reasonable to believe, therefore, that these are the major proteins involved in the contractile mechanism. The localization of actin and myosin to the two microscopically identifiable, filamentous components of the sarcoplasm has been achieved for striated muscle, but their exact relation to the myofilaments in smooth muscle has not been as clearly established.

Cell to Cell Relations in Smooth Muscle

The surface of each smooth muscle cell is invested by a thick extracellular coating that corresponds in its fine structure to the *basal lamina* of epithelia and to the *external lamina* or *boundary layer* of many other cell types. This is clearly the component responsible for the PAS reaction of the intercellular spaces of smooth muscle (Fig. 11–3). Small bundles of collagen fibrils, which correspond to the argyrophilic reticulum, are lodged in clefts between or within the glycoprotein surface coatings of adjacent smooth muscle cells.

Owing to the presence of this thick extracellular layer, adjacent smooth muscle cells are separated by a distance of 400 to 800 Å. Typical desmosomes are not found. However, the specialized dense areas in which the myofilaments terminate at the surface of adjacent cells are too often opposite one another for their distribution to be entirely random. An intermediate dense line may be found in the intercellular material between two such opposing dense regions. Thus, in spite of the considerable distance that separates the cells, there is a complementarity to the specialized areas of their surfaces that suggests cell to cell cohesion at these sites, as at the desmosomes of epithelia. Contraction results in force applied at many points of insertion of myofilaments on the periphery of the cell. The contracted cell becomes ellipsoid and may exhibit numerous invaginations of its surface at points of attachment of myofilament bundles. The force is probably transmitted to neighboring cells, mainly through the reticular connective tissue sheath, but long range forces of attraction acting at multiple dense areas of specialization on the opposing cell surfaces may also be involved.

In certain limited areas of the surface of visceral smooth muscle, the intercellular substance is lacking and the membranes of neighboring cells come into very close association. At these sites, the intercellular space is narrowed to 20 Å or less, and the opposing plasmalemmae are specialized so that in freeze-cleaved preparations they exhibit closely packed 80 to 90 Å particles in hexagonal array within the plane of the membrane. Such junctional specializations are called *gap junctions* or *nexuses*. They are believed to be sites of low electrical resistance, permitting free movement of ions and spread of excitation from one cellular unit to another throughout the muscle mass.

Physiological Properties and Contractile Mechanism of Smooth Muscle

Smooth muscle is distinguished from striated muscle not only by its histological and cytological appearance but by its physiological and pharmacological properties. Its contractions are slower than those of other types of muscle, but it is able to sustain forceful contraction for long periods with relatively little expenditure of energy. Depending upon the site, contraction may be initiated by nerve impulses, hormonal stimulation, or local changes arising within the muscle itself. One of the more important local stimuli initiating contraction is stretching of the muscle fibers, which can change the membrane potential and initiate a wave of contraction. The ability of smooth muscle to respond to stretch is particularly important in the physiology of the bladder, gastrointestinal tract, and other hollow viscera, whose contents are evacuated by contractions.

Although usually treated by morphologists as a single type of muscle, smooth muscle is adapted to a variety of functions and differs markedly in its physiological properties in different organs. *Vascular smooth muscle,* in the blood vessels, behaves rather like skeletal muscle in that its activity is usually initiated by nerve fibers (vasomotor nerves), and there is little evidence of conduction between cellular units. *Visceral smooth muscle,* on the other hand, bears certain functional resemblances to cardiac muscle in that it has a myogenic autorhythmicity; the cells behave like single muscular units and impulses are freely conducted from cell to cell, presumably through the specialized areas of close membrane contact revealed in electron micrographs. Two forms of contraction are recognized in visceral smooth muscle: *rhythmic contraction* and *tonic contraction.* In the former, periodic spontaneous impulses are generated and spread through the muscle, accompanied by a wave of contraction. In addition, smooth muscle maintains a continuous state of partial contraction called *muscle tone* or *tonus.* The cause of the tonic contraction is no better understood than the genesis of the rhythmic contractions. The degree of *tonic contraction* may change greatly, without any change in the frequency of the *rhythmic contraction,* and vice versa. The two forms of contraction thus appear to be independent.

There are several other physiological and pharmacological differences in smooth muscle of different organs. For example, the amounts of *actin* and *myosin* in smooth muscle of the uterus are under endocrine control. Its cells hypertrophy during pregnancy and show a striking increase in the size of the Golgi apparatus and the extent of the granular endoplasmic reticulum. Physiological changes also occur during the normal estrus cycle. Ribonucleic acid synthesis is one of the early responses of the uterus to estrogen stimulation, and the organelles concerned with protein synthesis become more prominent during estrus than at other times. Uterine musculature in the terminal stages of pregnancy is also responsive to the hormone *oxytocin,* elaborated by the posterior lobe of the hypophysis. Smooth muscle in other parts of the body is relatively unresponsive to hormones other than epinephrine.

SKELETAL MUSCLE

Histological Organization

The unit of histological organization of skeletal muscle is the *fiber*, a long cylindrical multinucleate cell visible with the light microscope. Large numbers of parallel muscle fibers are grouped into *fascicles*, which are visible to the naked eye in fresh muscle. The fascicles are associated in various patterns to form the several types of *muscles* recognized by the anatomist—unipennate, bipennate, and so on. The individual muscle fibers, the fascicles, and the muscle as a whole are each invested by connective tissue that forms a continuous stroma, but its different parts are designated by separate terms for convenience of description. The entire muscle is enclosed by a connective tissue layer called the *epimysium* (Fig. 11–7). Thin collagenous septa that extend inward from the epimysium, surrounding all of the fascicles, collectively comprise the *perimysium*, and the exceedingly delicate reticulum that invests the individual

muscle fibers constitutes the *endomysium*. The connective tissue serves to bind together the contractile units and groups of units and to integrate their action; it also allows a certain degree of freedom of motion between them. Thus, although the muscle fibers are very closely packed together, each is somewhat independent of adjacent fibers, and each fascicle can move independently of neighboring fascicles.

The blood vessels supplying skeletal muscle course in the connective tissue septa and ramify to form a rich capillary bed around the individual muscle fibers (Fig. 11–9). The capillaries are sufficiently tortuous to permit their accommodation to changes in length of the fibers, by straightening during elongation and contorting during contraction.

In muscles that do not taper at the ends, such as the sartorius, the fibers apparently continue without interruption through the entire length of the muscle. It is generally believed, however, that in most muscles the fibers are shorter than the muscle as a whole, seldom extending from its origin to its insertion, but being connected at one end to connective tissue septa within the muscle and at the other to the tendon.

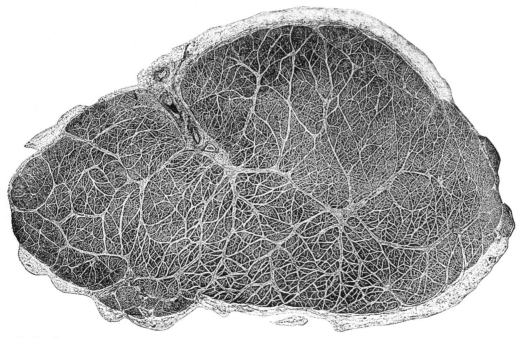

Figure 11–7   Cross section through human sartorius muscle, showing the subdivision into bundles of various sizes by connective tissue. ×4. (Photograph by Müller, from Heidenhain.)

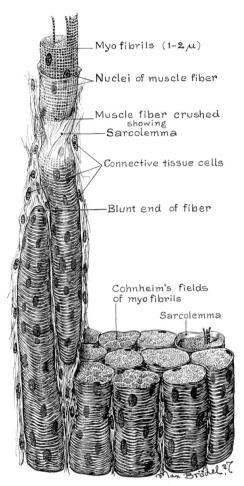

Myo fibrils (1-2 μ)

Nuclei of muscle fiber

Muscle fiber crushed
showing
Sarcolemma

Connective tissue cells

Blunt end of fiber

Cohnheim's fields
of myo fibrils

Sarcolemma

Figure 11–8 Schematic representation of the structure of muscle fibers. (From M. Brödel, Bull. Johns Hopkins Hosp., *61*:295, 1937.)

The thickness of the muscle fibers ranges from 10 to 100 μm. or more, depending upon the species and the particular muscle examined. Fibers within the same muscle may vary considerably in their caliber. During the growth of the organism, the diameter of the fibers increases with age, and in the grown individual it may undergo further increase in response to strenuous muscular activity—a phenomenon referred to as *hypertrophy of use* and exemplified in the bulging biceps of the boxer and the leg muscles of the ballerina. Conversely, the fibers may become thinner in muscle immobilized for long periods as in the treatment of fractures—called *atrophy of disuse*.

Cytology of the Muscle Fiber

The individual fibers can be separated by teasing fresh muscle apart under a dissecting microscope. In addition to the obvious transverse striations that give this type of muscle its name, a more delicate longitudinal striation is also discernible within the muscle fiber. The structural basis of this longitudinal striation becomes apparent when samples of muscle are treated with dilute nitric acid. In such macerated specimens, the limiting membrane of the fiber (the *sarcolemma*) is destroyed, the cytoplasmic matrix (called the *sarcoplasm*) is extracted, and the contractile substance of the muscle fiber separates into a large number of thin, parallel, cross-striated fibrils, the *myofibrils*. The fine longitudinal striation detectable within the fresh muscle fiber is thus attributable to the parallel arrangement of myriad myofibrils within its sarcoplasm. The transverse striation comes about because each myofibril is made up of cylindrical segments or bands of different refractility that alternate regularly along its length. The corresponding segments of the closely packed parallel myofibrils are usually in register, so that the striations appear to extend across the whole width of the fiber (Figs. 11–11 and 11–12).

Each muscle fiber is invested by a delicate membrane just visible with the compound microscope. In teased fresh preparations, where the fiber has been torn or crushed, it appears as a thin, transparent film (Fig. 11–8). This investment has traditionally been called the sarcolemma. It has recently become apparent from electron microscopic studies that this film, visible with the light microscope, is not a single component but a compound structure consisting of the plasmalemma of the muscle fiber, its glycoprotein external coating, and a delicate network of associated reticular fibers. In current usage, the term *sarcolemma* is reserved for the plasmalemma of the muscle fiber, and the other components of the traditional sarcolemma are separately designated. The sarcolemma differs in no essential respect from the limiting membrane of any other cell. It should be realized that this lipoprotein membrane alone is not resolved by the ordinary microscope under the usual conditions of observation, but with the added thickness of its associated amorphous and fibrous investments, a limiting layer is visible.

The nuclei of the striated muscle fiber are numerous. No actual number can be specified, for this depends upon the length of the muscle, but in a fiber several centimeters long, there would be several hundred nuclei. They are elongated in the direction of the fiber. Their position varies according to the type of muscle and the animal species, but in the great majority of skeletal muscles of mammals, the nuclei are located at the periphery of the fiber, immediately beneath the sarcolemma. This is especially apparent in transverse sections (Fig. 11–10). This characteristic position is a helpful criterion for distinguishing skeletal from cardiac muscle, in which the nuclei are centrally located.

The nuclei of the muscle cells usually have one or two nucleoli and moderately abundant chromatin distributed along the inner aspect of the nuclear envelope. A small number of other nuclei, of similar elongated form but with a coarser chromatin pattern, are closely associated with the surface of the muscle fibers. These belong to elongated *satellite cells*, which are flattened against the muscle fiber or occupy shallow depressions in its surface and are enclosed within the same investing layer of glycoprotein and reticular fibers. The cytoplasm of the satellite cell is scanty and its boundary with the muscle fiber usually cannot be resolved with the light microscope. The ontogenetic and functional relationships of these cells to the muscle fibers are not known. It is nevertheless of some importance to be aware that nuclei of slightly different appearance found at the periphery of muscle fibers belong to a separate cell type.

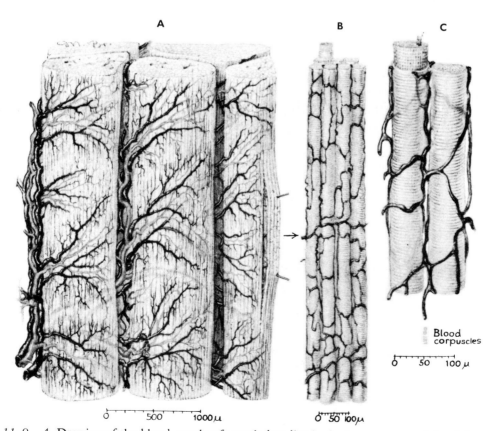

Figure 11–9 *A,* Drawing of the blood supply of muscle bundles in the human rectus abdominis muscle. *B,* The capillary network of muscle fibers; note thick loops crossing the fibers. *C,* The same, at higher magnification, showing red blood cells to establish scale. (From M. Brödel, Bull. Johns Hopkins Hosp., *61*:295, 1937.)

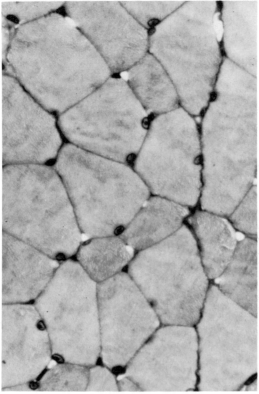

Figure 11-10 Photomicrograph of skeletal muscle fibers in cross section illustrating their polygonal outline and the peripheral position of their nuclei. In well fixed muscle the fibers are quite homogeneous in cross section. It is only where there has been considerable shrinkage that the myofibrils are separated into polygonal areas called Cohnheim's fields. ×450.

The sarcoplasm of a muscle fiber corresponds to the cytoplasm of other types and can be defined as the contents of the sarcolemma exclusive of the nuclei. It consists, therefore, of a typical cytoplasmic matrix and the usual cell organelles and inclusions as well as the myofibrils peculiar to muscle. Though not visible in routine preparations, the Golgi apparatus can be demonstrated by special staining methods. As might be expected in a multinucleate syncytium, there are multiple small Golgi bodies, which are located near one pole of each nucleus throughout the muscle fiber. The mitochondria (formerly called *sarcosomes*) are most abundant near the poles of the nuclei and immediately beneath the sarcolemma, but they also occur in the interior of the fiber, where they are distributed in longitudinal rows between the myofibrils (Fig. 11-12).

Several early cytologists examining preparations of muscle that were impregnated with heavy metals described, in addition to the common organelles, a lacelike network of dark strands in the interfibrillar sarcoplasm. This network appeared to surround all of the myofibrils and was called the *sarcoplasmic reticulum* (Veratti). It was demonstrated with difficulty with the light microscope, and many doubted its reality, but the presence of this organelle has now been verified in electron micrographs (Porter) and will be described later in this chapter.

Lipid droplets are found in varying numbers in the muscles of some species. They may be situated between the myofibrils or among the clusters of mitochondria at the poles of the nuclei and at the periphery of the fiber. In appropriately stained preparations, small amounts of glycogen can be demonstrated throughout the sarcoplasmic matrix. In addition to these microscopically visible inclusions, the sarcoplasm of the living muscle contains the oxygen-binding protein *myoglobin*. In muscle at rest, oxygen probably remains bound to myoglobin, but when demand for oxygen increases, it dissociates from myoglobin and is available for oxidations. In man myoglobin is of relatively little significance in skeletal muscle, but in diving mammals and in birds, it is especially abundant and is probably of great physiological importance.

Most of the interior of the muscle fiber is occupied by myofibrils 1 to 2 μm. in diameter. In transverse sections they are resolved as fine dots either uniformly distributed or grouped in polygonal areas called the *fields of Cohnheim*. Whether this polygonal pattern represents the true distribution of myofibrils or is a consequence of shrinkage was long debated. The weight of evidence now favors its interpretation as a shrinkage artifact, and no functional significance is now attached to Cohnheim's fields.

In longitudinal sections of muscle the feature of greatest interest is the identification of the bands of the cross-striated myofibrils. The cylindrical segments of the myofibrils that are markedly refractile and dark in fresh muscle, stain intensely with iron-hematoxylin in histological sections, while the less refractile, alternate segments remain essentially unstained (Fig. 11-11). When muscle is examined with the polarizing microscope, the contrast of the bands is reversed. The dark-staining bands are now doubly refractile or anisotropic (*A bands*) and therefore appear bright, whereas the *light* staining bands are isotropic (*I bands*) or only very weakly anisotropic and thus appear *dark*. In the most commonly used terminology, the principal bands are named A band and I band, according to their appearance in polarized light. The relative lengths of the bands vary, depending upon whether the muscle is examined at resting length, during contraction, or when passively stretched. The *length of the A band remains constant in all phases of contraction*, but the I band is most prominent in stretched muscle, is shorter at resting length, and is extremely short in contraction. Both in stained preparations and in living muscle viewed with phase contrast, a dark transverse line, the *Z line*, bisects each I band. The re-

peating structural unit, to which all of the morphological events of the contractile cycle are referred, is the *sarcomere*, which is defined as the segment between two successive Z lines and therefore includes an A band and half of the two contiguous I bands. In histological sections of skeletal muscle, the A bands, I bands, and Z lines are usually the only cross striations that are discernible, but in exceptional preparations a paler zone, called the *H band*, may be seen traversing the center of the A band. In its center is a narrow dark line, the *M band* or M line, located precisely in the middle of the A band. Although all of these features of the cross banded pattern of striated muscle can be seen with the light microscope, they can be demonstrated and interpreted more clearly in electron micrographs and will be discussed in greater detail later in this chapter, in the section on the ultrastructure of the sarcoplasm.

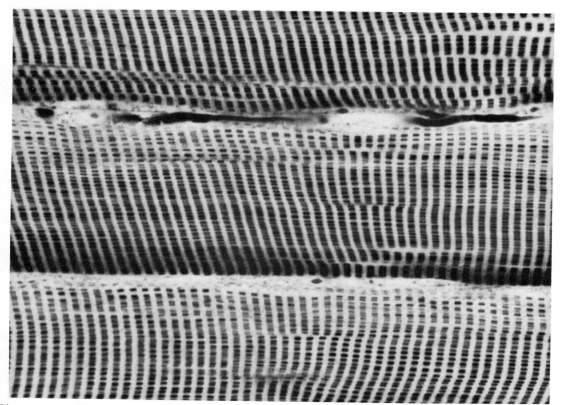

Figure 11–11 Photomicrograph of three muscle fibers from the dog in longitudinal section. The dark transverse A bands and light I bands are clearly differentiated. The dark longitudinal striations visible in the A bands correspond to the myofibrils, the smallest unit of the contractile material visible with the light microscope. Iron-hematoxylin stain. ×1200.

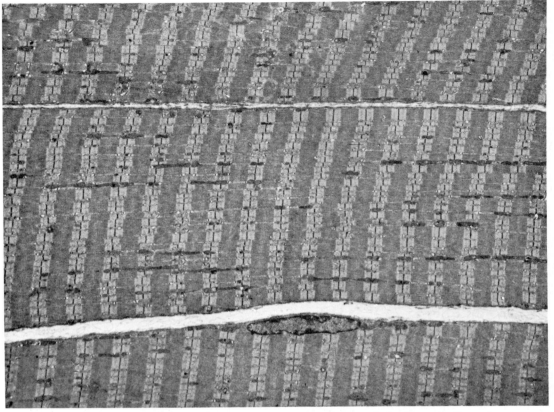

Figure 11–12 Electron micrograph of a longitudinal section of three skeletal muscle fibers from a mouse. Although the magnification is not very much higher than in the photomicrograph of Figure 11–11, the greater resolution of the electron optical image makes it possible to identify the A, I, and Z bands and the mitochondria between the myofibrils. ×3400. (Courtesy of J. Venable.)

Cytological Heterogeneity of Skeletal Muscle Fibers

When muscles are examined in the fresh condition by the naked eye, they differ somewhat in color. It has also been recognized since the late 1800's that the fibers making up a single muscle are not uniform in their size or cytological characteristics. In red muscles, small dark fibers with a granular appearance predominate, whereas in white muscles, paler fibers of larger diameter predominate. Differences among the fibers were not conspicuous in routine histological preparations, but when histochemical methods for localizing enzymatic activity became available, the distinctions between fiber types could be clearly demonstrated and defined more accurately. Staining for the enzyme succinic dehydrogenase clearly identifies the smaller red fibers because of their great abundance of mitochondria. Differences in myoglobin concentration and in myofibrillar adenosine triphosphatase and phosphorylase activity can also be demonstrated.

The multiplicity of fiber types recognizable by these methods has led to some terminological confusion. In the interests of simplicity and continuity with tradition, we adopt here the terms *red, intermediate,* and *white* fibers (Gautier). The red fibers are small, rich in mitochondria and myoglobin (Figs. 11–14, 11–15, and 11–16) and have a richer blood supply. In electron micrographs, the Z lines are thicker, profiles of sarcoplasmic reticulum are more complex in the region of the H band, and the mitochondria located in the periphery of the fibers and in rows between the myofibrils are numerous, large and provided with many cristae. In

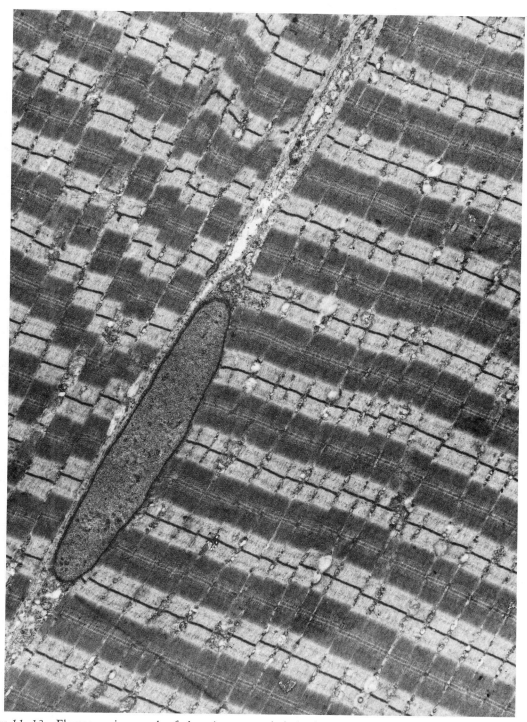

Figure 11–13 Electron micrograph of glycerin extracted skeletal muscle. This treatment improves the con-trast of the myofibrils but damages the mitochondria and sarcoplasmic reticulum. Observe the uniform diam-eter of the myofibrils. The corresponding bands of adjacent myofibrils are usually in register across the mus-cle fiber. Where they are out of register, as at the upper left, this is usually an artifact of specimen preparation.

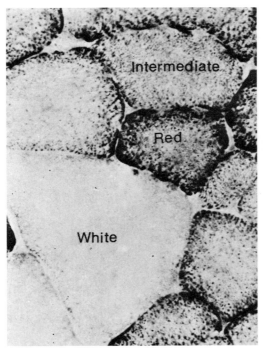

Figure 11–14 Photomicrograph of a transverse section of skeletal muscle stained for the enzyme succinic dehydrogenase, which resides in mitochondria. Three categories of fibers are recognizable: small red fibers rich in mitochondria, especially around the periphery; large white fibers with relatively few mitochondria; and fibers with intermediate characteristics. (Photomicrograph courtesy of G. Gautier.)

The Fine Structure of the Sarcoplasm

The common organelles observed in the sarcoplasm with the light microscope do not depart significantly in fine structure from those in other cell types. The small Golgi complex found near many of the nuclei does not appear especially active. The mitochondria are abundant at the poles of the nuclei and beneath the sarcolemma. In addition, a considerable number are lodged in narrow clefts between the myofibrils. In keeping with the high energy requirements for muscle contraction, the mitochondria have very numerous, closely spaced cristae. Their intimate association with the contractile elements brings the source of chemical energy (ATP) close to the sites of its utilization in the myofibrils.

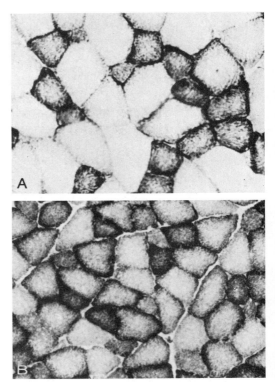

Figure 11–15 Photomicrograph of succinic dehydrogenase reaction. *A,* Plantaris muscle of a normal control guinea pig. *B,* The same muscle of an animal after 8 weeks of running on a treadmill. The fiber population of the exercised muscle is more homogeneous, and nearly all fibers are small and rich in mitochondria. (Photomicrograph courtesy of J. A. Faulkner. *From* Podolsky, R. J., ed.: Contractility of Muscle Cells and Related Processes. Englewood Cliffs, N. J., Prentice-Hall, Inc., 1941.)

larger white fibers, Z lines are relatively narrow, the pattern of sarcoplasmic reticulum is simpler, and the mitochondria are sparse, with subsarcolemmal and interfibrillar accumulations generally absent. The intermediate fibers obviously have intermediate characteristics. There are also differences in the neuromuscular junctions, their overall size and depth of the junctional folds being proportional to the fiber diameter (Gautier and Padykula).

The variations in gross color of different muscles is a reflection of the differing proportion of the three fiber types. The proportions are usually fairly constant for a given muscle, but shifts of population are observed after prolonged forced exercise (Fig. 11–15), thyroxin administration, and denervation. The functional significance of this structural and cytochemical heterogeneity is still poorly understood.

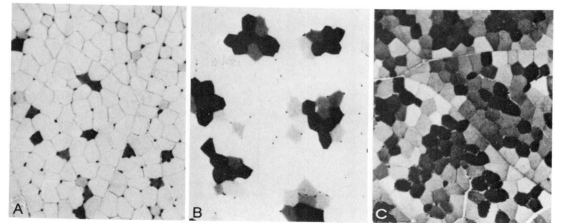

Figure 11–16 Sections of the longissimus muscle of rabbit (*A*), pig (*B*), and ox (*C*), reacted for myoglobin. The species differences in the extent and distribution of myoglobin positive fibers is obvious. (Photomicrographs courtesy of R. G. Cassens, from J. Histochem. Cytochem., *18*:364, 1970.)

An important organelle that cannot profitably be studied with the light microscope is the *sarcoplasmic reticulum*, a continuous system of membrane limited *sarcotubules* that extend throughout the sarcoplasm and form a close-meshed canalicular network around each myofibril (Figs. 11–17 and 11–18). This organelle corresponds to the endoplasmic reticulum of other cell types, but in muscle it is largely devoid of associated ribosomes and exhibits a highly specialized repeating pattern of local differentiations that bear a constant relationship to particular bands of the striated myofibrils. The tubules of the reticulum overlying the A bands have a prevailing longitudinal orientation but anastomose freely in the region of the H band (Fig. 11–18). At regular intervals along the length of the myofibrils the longitudinal *sarcotubules* are confluent with transversely oriented channels of larger caliber called *terminal cisternae*. Pairs of parallel terminal cisternae run transversely across the myofibrils in close apposition to a slender intermediate element, the transverse tubule, commonly called the *T tubule*. These three associated transverse structures constitute the so-called *triads* of skeletal muscle (Figs. 11–17 and 11–18). In amphibian muscle, the triads are found encircling each I band at the level of the Z line (Fig. 11–18). In mammalian muscle there are two triads to each sarcomere, situated at the junctions of each A band with the adjacent I bands. The lumen of the slender T tubule does not open into the adjacent cisternae and, strictly speaking, is not a part of the sarcoplasmic reticulum. Its limiting membrane is continuous with the sarcolemma and its lumen communicates with the extracellular space at the cell surface. It is therefore to be regarded as a slender tubular invagination of the sarcolemma penetrating deep into the interior of the muscle fiber. To emphasize their separate identity and to distinguish the T tubules from elements of the sarcoplasmic reticulum, they are referred to collectively as the *T system* of the muscle fiber.

The Substructure of the Myofibrils. The myofibrils, the smallest units of the contractile material visible with the light microscope (Fig. 11–19*C* and *D*), are found in electron micrographs to be composed of smaller units, the *myofilaments* (Fig. 11–19*E*). These are of two kinds, differing in dimensions and chemical composition. The cross banded pattern of striated muscle reflects the arrangement of these two sets of submicroscopic filaments. The thicker *myosin* filaments, 100 Å in diameter and 1.5 μm. long, are parallel and about 450 Å apart. The parallel arrays of myosin filaments are the principal constituent of the A band and determine its length (Fig. 11–19*E*). The filaments are slightly thicker in the middle and taper toward both ends. They are held in register by

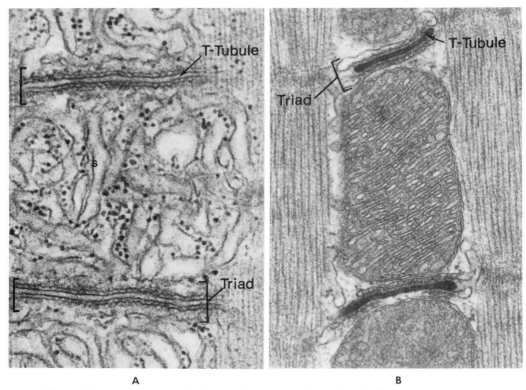

A   **B**

Figure 11–17 A, Electron micrograph of a longitudinal section of skeletal muscle, passing tangential to a myofibril. Observe the longitudinal elements of the sarcoplasmic reticulum and two transversely oriented triads at the level of the A band-I band junction. Glycogen particles are seen among the sarcotubules. B, Longitudinal section of muscle that had been immersed in peroxidase. The peroxidase (revealed here by a dense reaction product) has penetrated into the lumen of the T tubule, thus demonstrating continuity of the T tubule with the extracellular space. (Electron micrograph courtesy of Dr. D. Friend.)

slender cross connections that are aligned at the midpoint of the A band, giving rise to the transverse density recognized as the M line. In cross sections at the level of the H band, the filaments are disposed in an extremely regular array (Fig. 11–19G). The thinner *actin* filaments, 50 Å in diameter, extend about 1 μm. in either direction from the Z line and thus constitute the I band, They are not limited to this band, however, but extend some distance into the adjacent A bands, where they occupy the interstices between the hexagonally packed thick filaments. Thus, in cross sections near the ends of the A band, the punctate profiles of six thin actin filaments are evenly spaced around each myosin filament (Fig. 11–19I). The depth to which the ends of the actin filaments penetrate into the A band varies with the degree of contraction (Fig. 11–21). In the relaxed condition, the thin filaments that extend into the A band

from opposite ends do not meet. The distance between their ends determines the width of the H band, which is defined as the central region of the A band that is not penetrated by the actin filaments. In stretched myofibrils the H band is therefore broad, whereas in the contracted state it is very narrow or entirely absent (Fig. 11–21). In the region of their interdigitation at the ends of the A band, the parallel thick and thin filaments are only 100 to 200 Å apart, and this narrow interval is traversed by regularly spaced cross bridges that extend radially from each myosin filament toward the neighboring actin filaments (Figs. 11–19 and 11–22).

The details of the interrelation of filaments of successive sarcomeres at the Z disc are still a subject of debate, but certain points seem to be adequately established. Each actin filament approaching the Z line appears

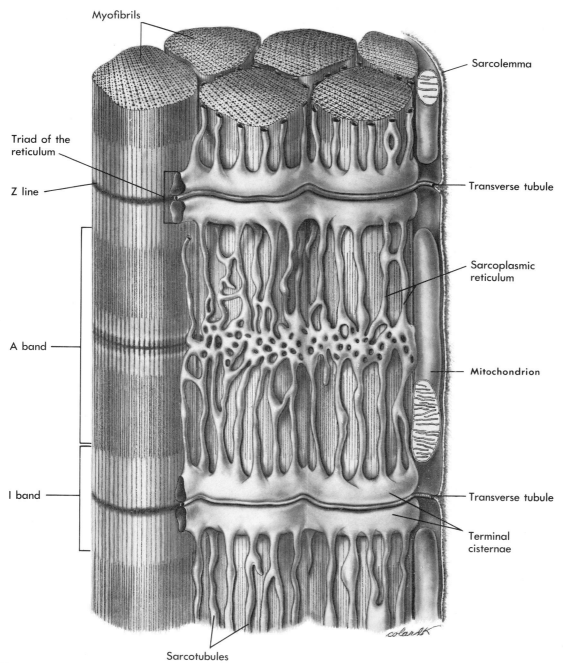

Myofibrils

Sarcolemma

Triad of the reticulum

Z line

Transverse tubule

A band

Sarcoplasmic reticulum

Mitochondrion

I band

Transverse tubule

Terminal cisternae

Sarcotubules

Figure 11–18 Schematic representation of the distribution of the sarcoplasmic reticulum around the myofibrils of amphibian skeletal muscle. The longitudinal sarcotubules are confluent with transverse elements called the terminal cisternae. A slender transverse tubule (T tubule) extending inward from the sarcolemma is flanked by two terminal cisternae to form the so-called triads of the reticulum. The location of these with respect to the cross banded pattern of the myofibrils varies from species to species. In frog muscle, depicted here, the triads are at the Z line. In mammalian muscle, there are two to each sarcomere, located at the A-I junctions. (Modified after L. Peachey: J. Cell Biol., *25*:209, 1965, from D. W. Fawcett and S. McNutt. Drawn by Sylvia Colard Keene.)

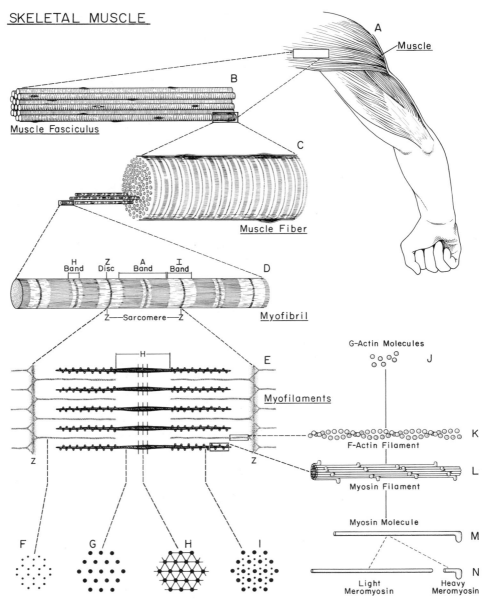

SKELETAL MUSCLE

A
Muscle

B
Muscle Fasciculus

C
Muscle Fiber

H
Band
Z
Disc
A
Band
I
Band
D
Z—Sarcomere—Z
Myofibril

E
Myofilaments
H
Z
Z

G-Actin Molecules
J

K
F-Actin Filament

L
Myosin Filament

Myosin Molecule
M

N
Light
Meromyosin
Heavy
Meromyosin

F   G   H   I

Figure 11–19   Diagram of the organization of skeletal muscle from the gross to the molecular level. *F, G, H,* and *I* are cross sections at the levels indicated. (Drawing by Sylvia Colard Keene.)

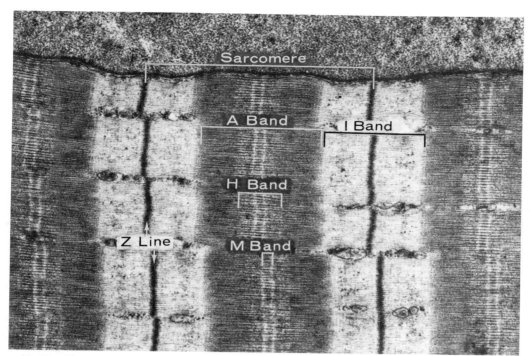

Figure 11–20 Electron micrograph of a juxtanuclear area of sarcoplasm, showing longitudinal sections of five myofibrils labeled to indicate the various bands in the normal pattern of cross striations in relaxed skeletal muscle.

to be continuous with four diverging thin strands called Z filaments (Knappies and Carlsen). Each of these runs obliquely through the Z disc to one of the actin filaments on the other side. The actin filaments approaching the Z line from opposite sides are offset, so that in longitudinal sections the cross-connecting Z filaments produce a characteristic zigzag pattern. In addition to the Z filaments, there appears to be a dense amorphous component simply referred to as "Z disc material" or "Z disc matrix" (Kelly and Cahill). This component varies in abundance in different skeletal muscles and is more easily extractable than the filaments. Its association with the Z disc seems quite selective, for when the matrix material is added to extracted glycerinated muscle, it accumulates around the Z filaments and restores the Z band density (Stromer et al.). The exact chemical nature of the Z filaments is not yet clear.

Although no further detail can be observed in electron micrographs of thin sections of muscle, the analysis of the contractile material has been carried further by mechan-ical disintegration of myofibrils under conditions that permit the release of the individual myofilaments. These have been studied with the electron microscope after metal shadowing and with negative staining procedures. When isolated in this way, the thin filaments are about 1 μm. in length and smooth contoured, and have the chemical properties of *F-actin*. At very high magnification they have a beaded appearance and seem to consist of globular subunits (55 Å) forming two strands entwined in a helix (Figs. 11–19K and 11–24A). Further dissociation of the thin filaments yields globular units with the size, molecular weight, and other properties of *G-actin* (Fig. 11–19J). Each of the two strands making up the thin filaments of muscle is therefore considered to be a polymer of G-actin. Artificial actin filaments formed in vitro from globular actin molecules have an electron microscopic appearance essentially identical to that of naturally occurring thin filaments prepared by dissociation of myofibrils (Fig. 11–24A). An additional muscle protein *tropomyosin* which provides the sensitivity of the actomyo-

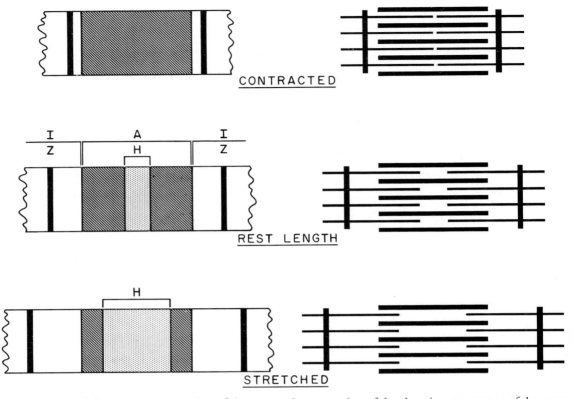

Figure 11–21 Schematic representation of the current interpretation of the changing appearance of the cross striations (*left*) in different phases of contraction, depending upon the degree of interdigitation of the sliding filaments (*right*). The A band is of constant length, but the width of the H band is determined by the depth of penetration of the thin I filaments into the A band. In the contracted state the thin filaments slide more deeply into the A band, obliterating the H band. In stretched muscle the thin filaments are drawn out of the A band and the H band is widened.

sin system to calcium which in turn triggers contraction is believed to be distributed along the entire length of the actin filaments, possibly in the groove between the helically wound strands of actin. Associated with it is another structural protein (50,000 MW) called *troponin* which is distributed along the thin filaments at regular intervals of about 400 Å. Troponin is thought to be attached to the thin filament through the tropomyosin and is responsible for a faint 400 Å periodicity seen in electron micrographs of thin sections of skeletal muscle (Ebashi). It appears that troponin is the calcium receptive protein of the contractile system but it alone cannot sensitize the interaction of actin and myosin but requires the collaboration of tropomyosin.

The isolated thick filaments of muscle are 1.5 μm. long. They have a smooth central segment 0.15 to 0.2 μm. in length, but

toward their ends they are beset with many short projections corresponding to the cross bridges seen between the thick and thin filaments in intact myofibrils. When further dissociation of such fibrils is carried out, myosin molecules are obtained (Figs. 11–19*M* and 11–24*B*). These are rod-shaped and about 1500 Å long, with a globular projection at one end. The thick filaments of muscle are believed to be formed by an antiparallel arrangement of myosin molecules in such a way that the smooth central region of the filament is occupied only by the rodlike parts of the molecules, with the globular heads projecting outward nearer the ends of the fibrils. It has been known for some time that the myosin molecule can be cleaved by brief trypsin digestion into two fragments called *light meromyosin* (LMM) and *heavy meromyosin* (HMM) (Fig. 11–19*N*). It now appears that the light meromyosin makes up the major part of the rodlike backbone of the molecule and the heavy meromyosin comprises a shorter segment bearing the globular lateral projection. The ability to combine with actin, and the adenosine triphosphatase activity, both of which are essential to muscular contraction, reside in the heavy meromyosin fragments, whose lateral projections correspond to the bridges seen between the myosin and actin filaments in micrographs of intact myofibrils.

Sliding Filament Mechanism of Contraction

Though classical cytologists described the changes in the relative lengths of the bands during muscle shortening, these observations suggested no satisfactory explanation of the contractile mechanism. Until fairly recently the commonest speculation envisioned a process of shortening due to reversible folding and cross linking of long molecules. In the past two decades however, the detailed analysis of the submicroscopic organization of muscle by electron microscopy and x-ray diffraction has not only revealed the structural relationships responsible for the cross striations but has also led to an entirely new concept of the mechanism of contraction. Basic to the new theory was the observation that the length of the A band remains constant during contraction, while the lengths of the H band and the I band both decrease. A possible explanation for these changes in the pattern of cross banding became apparent when the electron microscope revealed two interdigitating sets of filaments. According to the *sliding filament hypothesis* (Hanson and Huxley), when a muscle contracts, the thick and thin filaments maintain the same length but slide past each other, so that the ends of the actin filaments extend farther into the A band, narrowing and ultimately obliterating the H band. As a consequence of the deeper penetration of the A band by the I filaments, the Z disc is drawn closer to the ends of the adjacent A bands, and there is an overall shortening of the myofibril (Fig. 11–21).

Because the heads of the myosin molecules forming the cross bridges are the only visible structures by which a force could be developed between the thick and thin filaments, it is assumed that this is their function. However the chemical events responsible for

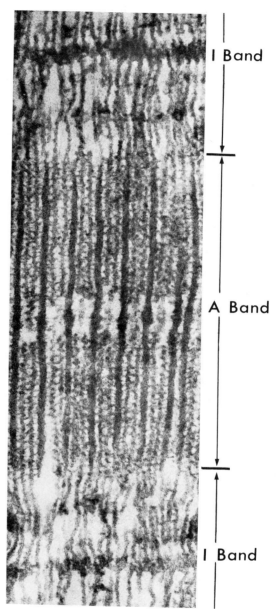

Figure 11–22 Electron micrograph of a thin longitudinal section of rabbit psoas muscle, showing the arrangement of thick and thin filaments. The figure includes one sarcomere length. In the I band at either end, only thin filaments are found. In the A band, occupying the central portion of the figure, the thin filaments of the I band interdigitate with a set of thicker filaments. ×135,000. (Courtesy of H. E. Huxley.)

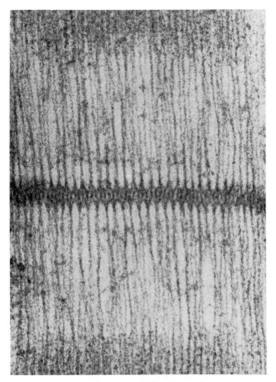

Figure 11-23 High magnification electron micrograph of a Z band from rabbit psoas, showing the offset arrangement of the I filaments approaching the Z band from opposite sides. At the I-Z junction the filaments appear to thicken and to divide into diverging Z filaments. There are varying interpretations of the fine structure of this band. (Courtesy of M. Reedy.)

the longitudinal displacement of one set of fibrils with respect to the other are not yet clear. Since contraction may involve displacements of as much as 3000 Å in each half sarcomere, while displacement of the distal ends of the bridges from the perpendicular is no more than 100 Å, it is inferred that there must be some sort of repetitive interaction of the cross bridges with the actin filaments to produce the observed displacement. A problem with this theory developed when it was observed that the interfibrillar distance in some phases of contraction appeared to be greater than the length of the cross bridges. This paradox has been resolved by the discovery of flexible regions at the base of the globular head and at the junction of the heavy meromyosin subunit with the linear backbone of the myosin molecule. These two flexible couplings permit the HMM heads on the thick filaments to attach

themselves to the actin filaments over a range of different interfilament distances and still preserve the same orientation relative to the actin (Huxley).

A problem remains as to what part of this mechanism is the site of development of the force that results in filament movement. Since it is unlikely that it could reside in the flexible regions of the molecule, current speculation assigns this role to the globular head and postulates an *active* change in effective angle of its attachment to the actin filament. There is little firm evidence for this as yet, and current research is focused upon this problem and upon the mode of attachment of the cross bridge to the actin filament.

The chemical events responsible for the longitudinal displacement of one set of fibrils with respect to the other have yet to be elucidated. The bulk of the evidence to date suggests that the force is produced by a cyclic process occurring at the cross bridges and that each cross bridge on the myosin filament may attach to a succession of sites along the neighboring actin filament, causing the filaments to move past one another. The breakdown of ATP by myosin ATPase localized in the bridges is thought to play a significant role in energizing this process.

Coupling of Excitation to Contraction

The attention of physiologists has long been focused upon the problem of explaining how the myofibrils throughout the muscle fiber are activated simultaneously and almost instantaneously after arrival of an impulse at the sarcolemma. These events take place too rapidly to be explained by inward diffusion of an activating substance liberated from an excitable surface membrane. In a new approach to this problem, Huxley and Taylor applied a microelectrode to the surface of an isolated muscle fiber and showed that a local reduction in membrane potential was not equally effective at all points on the surface. It resulted in inward spread of an impulse, leading to contraction only if the tip of the microelectrode was over certain sensitive spots. In frog muscle, these sensitive points were located only over the I band. There appeared, therefore, to be a structural component at the center of each I band that is responsible for inward conduction.

The discovery of the sarcoplasmic reticulum by Porter and Palade and the finding of transversely oriented triads at the level of each Z line led to the suggestion that these might be the submicroscopic structures involved in the inward spread of activation. The demonstration that the membranes of the T tubules are continuous with the sarcolemma and that their lumen is open to the extracellular space has provided the necessary final link in the evidence for the participation of the T tubules in excitation-contraction coupling. In all of the fast muscle fibers of amphibians so far examined, the T tubules are found at the level of the Z disc, while in the skeletal muscle of mammals they are found near the boundary between the A and I bands. Thus, in mammals there are two T tubules to each sarcomere.

The functions of the longitudinal elements of the sarcoplasmic reticulum are not as well understood, but evidence that they play a part in muscle relaxation is rapidly accumulating. Calcium is required for muscular contraction and it is now known to have an important triggering role in initiating contraction. A "relaxing factor" isolated from muscle homogenates has been shown by electron microscopy to consist of membrane bounded vesicles derived by fragmentation of the sarcoplasmic reticulum. In vitro, these vesicles, in the presence of adenosine triphosphate, rapidly and reversibly bind calcium. It is now speculated that, in the resting state, most of the calcium in muscle is concentrated within the sarcoplasmic reticulum. Excitation of the sarcolemma is conducted inward by the membranes of the T system, somehow causing the sarcoplasmic reticulum to release calcium ions to the myofibrils, triggering their contraction. When contraction is completed, calcium ions are recaptured by the sarcoplasmic reticulum and relaxation ensues. Enzymes splitting ATP and ADP have been demonstrated by histochemical methods at the electron microscope level in the cisternal expansions of the sarcoplasmic reticulum adjacent to the T tubules. The location of a structure containing ATPase in close topographic relation to the T system further suggests that this contact plays a significant role in excitation-contraction coupling by energizing the postulated ATP-driven calcium pump. It is now generally accepted that the contractile material near the center of the muscle fiber is activated as a result of inward spread of an electrical change from the surface membrane along a system of thin, transversely oriented, open mouthed T tubules. There is no doubt that calcium is the immediate activator of contraction, but the mechanism of calcium release from the reticulum is still unknown.

The Myoneural Junction

The specialized junctional region at the termination of a motor nerve on skeletal muscle fibers is called the *motor end plate*. It is recognized with the microscope as a slightly elevated plaque on the muscle fiber marked by a local accumulation of nuclei (Figs. 11–25 and 11–26). The nuclei are of at least two morphologically distinguishable types. The so-called "arborization nuclei" belong to the terminal Schwann cells or sheath cells associated with the motor nerve endings. These are collectively referred to as the *teloglia*. The second category of nuclei, usually larger and less intensely stained, are called "fundamental

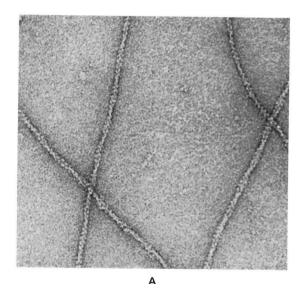

A

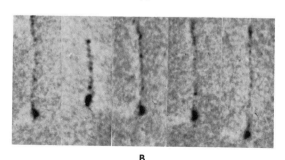

B

Figure 11–24 *A,* A negatively stained preparation of F-actin. The helical structure of the two strands is evident. ×250,000. *B,* Several myosin molecules, demonstrating the knoblike head corresponding to the spines of the intact thick filaments and to the heavy meromyosin fraction. (Micrographs courtesy Dr. H. Huxley.)

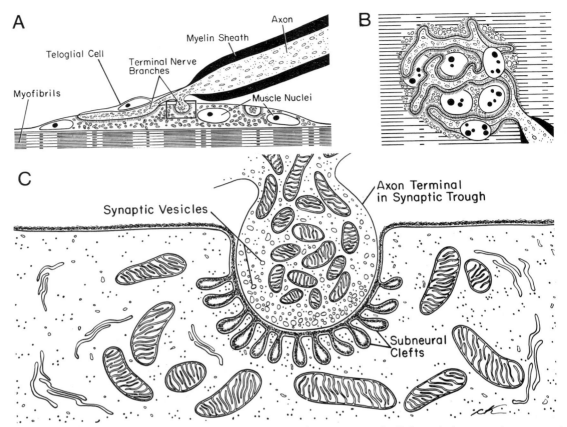

Figure 11–25 Schematic representations of the motor end plate as seen by light and electron microscopy. *A*, End plate as seen in histological sections in the long axis of the muscle fiber. *B*, As seen in surface view with the light microscope. *C*, As seen in an electron micrograph of an area such as that in the rectangle on *A*. (See also Fig. 12–26.) (Modified after R. Couteaux.)

nuclei" or "sole nuclei" in the classical literature. These are simply the nuclei of the underlying muscle fiber that congregate in the region of the myoneural junction. With special methods of metallic impregnation, it can be shown that the axon of the motor nerve, after losing its myelin sheath, forms a terminal arborization among the clustered nuclei of the end plate. The terminal branches of the axons occupy recesses in the surface of the muscle fiber called *synaptic troughs* or *primary synaptic clefts*. When selectively stained, the surface of the underlying muscle fiber is found to be highly differentiated, forming what appear to be evenly spaced, ribbon-like lamellae attached to the sarcolemma by their edges and projecting from the myoneural interface into the underlying sarcoplasm. This specialization of the muscle fiber surface is called the *subneural apparatus.*

Electron microscopy has greatly clarified the relationships at the myoneural junction. The teloglial cells cover the outer surface of the axon terminals but never penetrate into the synaptic clefts. Here the nerve and muscle are directly exposed to one another. The so-called "lamellae" of the subneural apparatus are found to be narrow *secondary synaptic clefts* formed by infolding of the sarcolemma lining the primary synaptic trough (Fig. 11–25). The axolemma and the sarcolemma are separated at all points by a glycoprotein boundary layer similar to that investing the rest of the surface of the muscle fiber. The axoplasm in the nerve terminals contains mitochondria and a very large number of small vesicles (400 to 600 Å), apparently identical to the *synaptic vesicles* seen at axodendritic synapses in the nervous system. These vesicles are generally believed to be the sites of storage of the neurotransmitter substance *acetylcholine.* The subneural sarcoplasm is unremarkable except for the abundance of its mitochondria. Histochemical studies demonstrate cholinesterase activity in the subneural apparatus of the motor end plate (Fig. 11–26). The major part of this activity appears to be due specifically to acetylcholinesterase, which is localized in or near the sarcolemma lining the secondary clefts.

It is the prevailing view that when an action potential reaches the terminal arborization of the nerve at the motor end plate, acetylcholine is released. Diffusing across the synaptic cleft, this activates receptor sites in the postsynaptic membrane, increasing the permeability of the sarcolemma to ions. The resulting increase in ion flow generates an end plate potential, which, upon reaching threshold value, sets off a propagated wave of depolarization that spreads over the muscle fiber and into its interior via the system of T tubules, initiating contraction. The acetylcho-

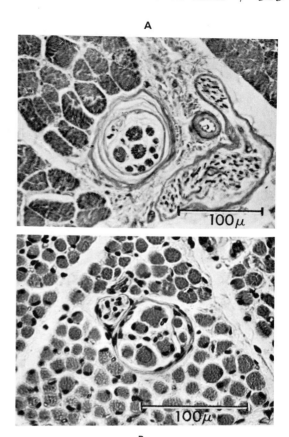

Figure 11–27 A, Photomicrograph of a muscle spindle in the lumbrical muscle of a human hand. The equator of the spindle is seen with its laminated capsule and large periaxial space. There are nine intrafusal muscle fibers; three of these are nuclear bag fibers. The other six small muscle fibers, lying in a group, are nuclear chain fibers. A blood vessel and several nerves are also seen. Transverse section. Holmes' silver method. B, Muscle spindle in human extrinsic eye muscle. Seven of the muscle fibers are surrounded by a thin capsule and there is a small nerve trunk attached. The muscle spindles are usually smaller than those in the limb muscles and have no nuclear bag fibers in man. Transverse section. Hematoxylin and eosin. (Both photomicrographs courtesy of S. Cooper.)

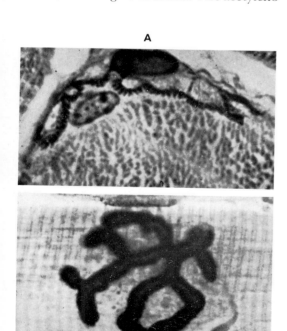

Figure 11–26 Photomicrograph of motor end plates on the intercostal muscle of the hedgehog, stained by the acetylthiocholine method for cholinesterase. A, Cut perpendicular to the long axis of the muscle fiber; the synaptic grooves or gutters of the subneural apparatus are visible. ×3300. B, The branching pattern of the motor end plate in surface view. ×1500. (Courtesy of R. Couteaux.)

line released is rapidly broken down by the acetylcholinesterase in the subneural apparatus, thus limiting the duration of the response.

Neuromuscular Spindles

Skeletal muscle contains complex sensory organs called *muscle spindles.* These fusiform, encapsulated structures consist of several modified striated muscle fibers and their associated nerve endings enclosed in a common sheath. The specialized muscle fibers in the interior of the organ, referred to as *intrafusal fibers*, number from a few to as many as 20, but there are usually about six (Figs. 11–27 and 11–28). The fibers are 1 to 5 mm. long and attached at their ends to tendon or endomysium. For descriptive purposes, they are subdivided into a central or *equatorial segment* and two long tapering *polar segments*. The equatorial segment can be further subdivided on the basis of its structural organization into three regions. The central portion is usually devoid of obvious cross striations and contains an accumulation of 40 to 50 spherical nuclei, which completely fill and often slightly distend the fiber. This region is referred to as the *nuclear bag.* Extending from it toward either pole is a myotube region, in which oval nuclei are aligned in a row in an axial core of sarcoplasm surrounded by a peripheral layer of cross-striated myofibrils. In the slender polar segments the nuclei are scattered at irregular intervals along the axis of the fiber. The capsule closely invests the poles of the intrafusal fiber but diverges from its surface in the equatorial segment to enclose the *periaxial space,* a fluid filled cavity up to 200 μm. in diameter that surrounds the nuclear bag and myotube regions. It has been reported that this space is continuous with the lymphatic system, but this does not seem to have been confirmed, and the space is usually regarded as a closed cavity.

A special kind of nerve ending is associated with each of the three regions of the intrafusal fiber. One or both polar ends are supplied by small efferent myelinated fibers provided with motor end plates similar to those found on ordinary extrafusal muscle fibers. These are referred to as the *fusimotor nerves.* The sensory endings supplied by large myelinated afferent fibers are confined to the equatorial segment. The primary sensory ending is associated mainly with the nuclear

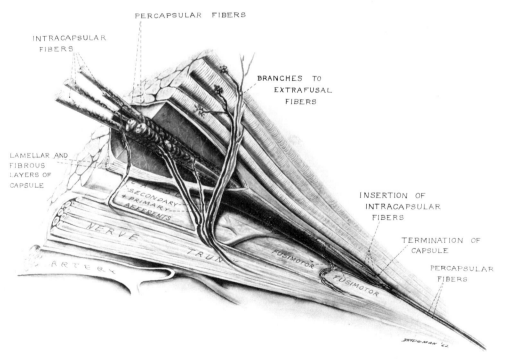

Figure 11–28 Drawing of a muscle spindle and its innervation. The capsule has been cut open to show the periaxial space and the sensory endings of the primary afferent nerves around the central portion of the intrafusal fibers. Near the end of the spindle, fusimotor nerves penetrate, to terminate on the intrafusal fibers in typical motor end plates. (See also Fig. 12–27.) (Drawing courtesy of C. F. Bridgman.)

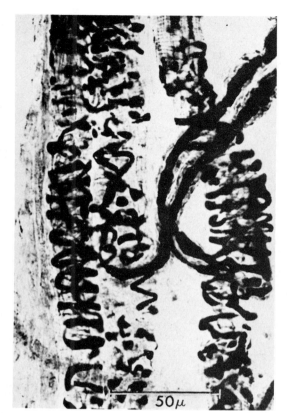

Figure 11–29 Primary nerve ending of a muscle spindle in a cat's plantaris muscle. Two branches of an afferent nerve fiber supply the ending, consisting of two large spirals around the muscle fibers at their nuclear bag regions. Teased gold chloride preparation. (Courtesy of S. Cooper.)

bag region but may extend into the adjacent myotube region. The endings consist of a complex system of half rings and spirals around the fiber (Figs. 11–28 and 11–29). Secondary sensory endings may also be present in the myotube regions. The details of innervation vary greatly from species to species. (See also p. 360 et seq.)

The spindles scattered through skeletal muscles appear to function like miniature strain gauges, sensing the degree of tension in the muscle. The motor innervation of the polar regions of the intrafusal fibers maintains the nuclear bag region under sufficient tension for its stretch receptor endings to be close to their threshold. A further stretch of the equatorial region results in discharge of the spindle afferent fiber, and the frequency of its discharge is proportional to the tension exerted on the intrafusal fiber.

Sensory Nerve Endings in Tendons

There appears to be more than one kind of nerve ending in tendons. In the simplest, unmyelinated nerve fibers ramify over the surface of the collagen bundles. These may possibly give rise to pain sensation on excessive stretch. Of greater interest are the encapsulated *tendon organs*. These are believed to sense tensional stresses produced by muscle pull, and to act as sources of inhibition when muscle contraction becomes excessive. From reconstructions of tendon organs from serial cross sections, it appears that they are composed of specialized, encapsulated fascicles of dense collagen which are subdivisions or branches of the primary tendon of origin or insertion of a muscle. Within this encapsulated region, branches of the entering sensory nerve are entwined among fine bundles of collagen coursing through delicate septa that subdivide the main fascicle of collagen into smaller subunits. Toward the muscle end of the organ, these finer bundles reorganize again into thicker bundles before they interdigitate with the ends of the extrafusal muscle fibers. It is speculated that the spaces between the fine collagen bundles in the relaxed state of the muscle spread open slightly, reducing pressure on the nerve endings lying between them. During muscular contraction, these bundles would straighten and be drawn together, compressing the nerve endings (Bridgman). The compression of the nerve terminals would generate electrochemical events in sensory axons, resulting in transmission of tension information to the central nervous system.

CARDIAC MUSCLE

The vertebrate heart consists of striated muscle fibers that differ in several respects from those of skeletal muscle. (1) The fibers are not syncytial, as was formerly thought, but are made up of separate cellular units joined end to end by special surface specializations, *intercalated discs*, that run transversely across the fiber (Fig. 11–30). (2) The fibers are not simple cylindrical units but they bifurcate and connect with adjacent fibers to form a complex three dimensional network. (3) The elongated nuclei of the cellular units are usually situated deep in the interior of the fiber instead of immediately beneath the sarcolemma (Fig. 11–31 *A* and *B*). The princi-

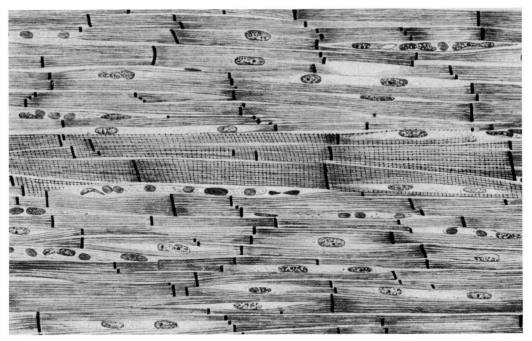

Figure 11–30 Drawing of longitudinal section of human cardiac muscle, stained in thiazin red and toluidine blue to show the intercalated discs. (From H. Heidenhain.)

pal physiological points of difference between cardiac and skeletal muscle are the spontaneous nature of the beat of cardiac muscle and its rhythmical contraction, which ordinarily is not subject to voluntary control.

The Cytology of Cardiac Muscle

The thin sarcolemma of cardiac muscle is similar to that of skeletal muscle, but the sarcoplasm is relatively more abundant and the mitochondria are much more numerous. The longitudinal striation of the fibers is quite obvious with the light microscope, owing to the subdivision of the contractile material into fascicles by rows of mitochondria in the interfibrillar sarcoplasm. The pattern of cross striation of the contractile material and the designation of the A, I, M, H and Z bands is identical to that of skeletal muscle (Figs. 11–30 and 11–32). The myofibrils diverge around the centrally placed nucleus to outline a fusiform axial region of sarcoplasm rich in mitochondria. Near one pole of the nucleus is a small Golgi complex. In the conical regions of sarcoplasm extending in either direction from the poles of the nucleus there are often a few droplets of lipid and, in older animals, deposits of lipofuscin pigment. In aged humans this pigment may come to constitute as much as 20 per cent of the dry weight of the myocardium. In small animal species lipid droplets are plentiful and occur in the interfibrillar sarcoplasm throughout the fiber, often being located between the ends of the mitochondria. The sarcoplasm of cardiac muscle is richer in glycogen than is that of skeletal muscle.

At fairly regular intervals along the length of the fibers, the intercalated discs appear as heavy transverse lines (Figs. 11–30 and 11–38). These are relatively inconspicuous in hematoxylin and eosin stains but are clearly revealed in iron-hematoxylin or phosphotungstic acid–hematoxylin preparations. The disc may extend uninterruptedly across the full width of the fiber, but more often it is divided into segments that are offset longitudinally so as to give the disc a steplike configuration. In the repeating pattern of cross striations, the intercalated discs invariably occur at the level of the I bands. They were formerly interpreted as local contraction bands or specializations for intracellular conduction, but they are now known to be devices for maintaining firm cohesion of the successive cellular units of the myocardium and for transmitting the tension of myofibrils along the axis of the fiber from one cellular unit to the next.

The Submicroscopic Structure of the Sarcoplasm

In electron micrographs, cardiac muscle bears a superficial resemblance to skeletal muscle. Its contractile substance is composed of two sets of myofilaments, thick and thin, in the same interdigitating relationship. In longitudinal section, the tubules of the sarcoplasmic reticulum and rows of mitochondria appear to subdivide the contractile material into myofibrils of variable width (Fig. 11–32). However, upon close examination of transverse sections (Figs. 11–33 and 11–34), it becomes evident that the myofilaments are not organized in discrete myofibrils as they are in skeletal muscle. In cross sections the circular profiles of the sarcotubules are aligned in rows that partially demarcate polygonal or irregular areas of myofilaments, but these are usually confluent, over some fraction of their perimeter, with adjacent areas of myofilaments. Mitochondria often appear completely surrounded by myofilaments (Fig. 11–34). Thus, the contractile substance of cardiac muscle forms a continuum that can be thought of as a large cylindrical mass of parallel myofilaments incompletely subdivided into irregular fascicles by deep incisures and by fusiform or lenticular clefts of sarcoplasm that are occupied by mitochondria and the other organelles essential to the contractile mechanism.

The continuous nature of the contractile mass is not peculiar to cardiac muscle but is also found in certain relatively slow, *tonic* skeletal muscles, particularly in amphibia. The German term *Felderstruktur* has been

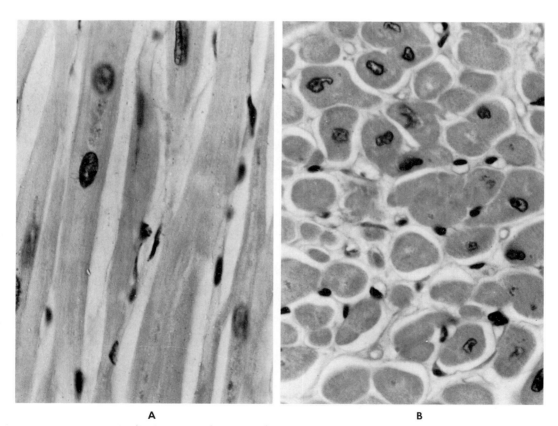

A   **B**

Figure 11–31   *A,* Longitudinal section of human left ventricular muscle, illustrating the variable diameter and branching of the fibers, as well as the central position of the nuclei. In routine hematoxylin and eosin preparations, intercalated discs are not evident. *B,* Cross section of human cardiac muscle. Compare with striated muscle seen in Figure 11–10.

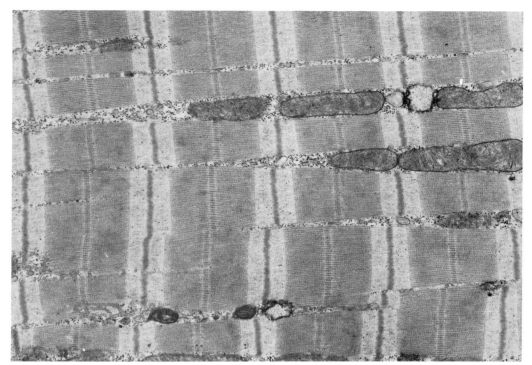

Figure 11–32 Electron micrograph of a portion of a cardiac muscle cell in longitudinal section. The cross banded pattern of the contractile material is similar to that of skeletal muscle. The numerous mitochondria occupy clefts or fusiform spaces that appear in longitudinal section to subdivide the myofilaments in units comparable to the discrete myofibrils of skeletal muscle. They are, however, much more variable in their width.

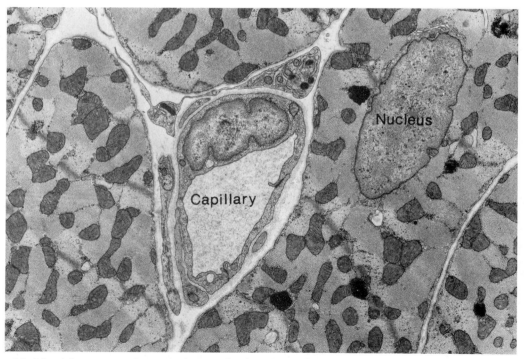

Figure 11–33 A low power electron micrograph of portions of several cardiac muscle fibers in cross section, illustrating the abundance of large mitochondria, the central location of the nucleus, and the intimate relation of the muscle fibers to the capillaries. Cat papillary muscle.

adopted to describe this pattern of organization of the myofilaments, and the term *Fibrillenstruktur* is applied to the pattern of separate myofibrils that is typical of fast, *twitch* muscles.

The large mitochondria of cardiac muscle have very numerous, closely spaced cristae that often exhibit a periodic angulation of their membranes, giving them a zig zag configuration. As a rule, the mitochondria are about the length of one sarcomere (2.5 μm.) but may occasionally be 7 or 8 μm. long. Spherical lipid droplets are often located between the ends of the mitochondria. Glycogen occurs in the form of 300 to 400 Å dense granules crowded into the interstices among the mitochondria. The bulk of the glycogen is located in the interfibrillar sarcoplasm, but particles may also be found aligned in rows between the myofilaments (Fig. 11–36B). They are particularly numerous in the I band and occur more sparsely in the H band. Both the glycogen and the lipid may be used as

energy sources for the contractile activity of the myocardium.

The T System and the Sarcoplasmic Reticulum

The tubular invaginations of the sarcolemma that comprise the T system of cardiac muscle are larger than the corresponding intermediate elements of the triads in skeletal muscle. These tubules, representing inward extensions of the extracellular space, are located at the level of the Z lines instead of at the A-I junction and penetrate to the center of the muscle fiber (compare Figs. 11–18 and 11–35). They are lined by a glycoprotein boundary layer (external lamina) continuous with the layer that coats the sarcolemma (Fig. 11–37). Apparently no point in a cardiac muscle fiber is more than 2 to 3 μm. from the extracellular space, either at the outer surface of the fiber or in one of the transverse tubules. In addition to playing

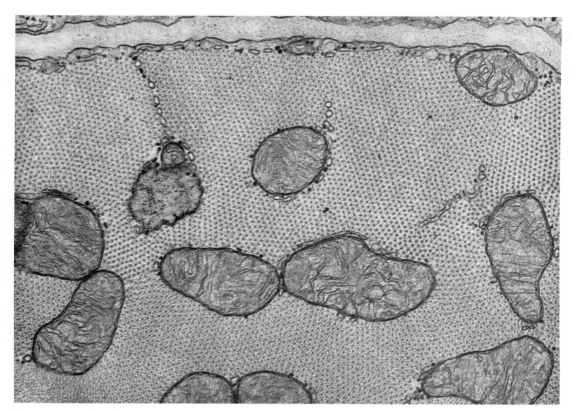

Figure 11–34 Electron micrograph of a small peripheral area of a cardiac muscle fiber in cross section. The cut ends of the myofilaments, seen here, are not associated in discrete myofibrils with clearly defined limits, but instead form a more or less continuous field interrupted by mitochondria. ×44,000.

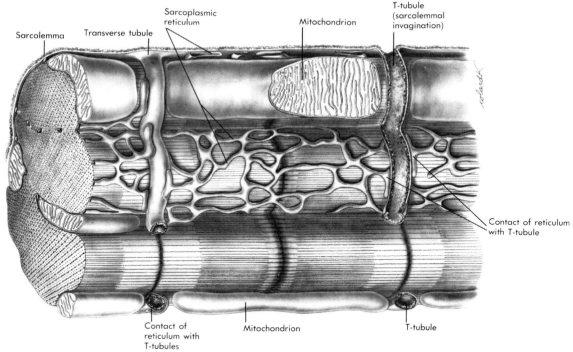

Figure 11–35 Schematic representation of the disposition of the T system and sarcoplasmic reticulum in mammalian cardiac muscle. The transverse tubules are much larger than those of skeletal muscle. The relatively simple sarcoplasmic reticulum has no terminal cisternae and therefore there are no triads. Instead, small expansions of its tubules end in close apposition to the sarcolemma, either at the surface of the fiber or at its inward extension in the T tubules. (After D. W. Fawcett and S. McNutt. J. Cell. Biol., *42*:1, 1969.)

a role in the coupling of excitation to contraction, these channels no doubt provide important additional surface for the exchange of metabolites between cardiac muscle and the extracellular space.

The sarcoplasmic reticulum is not as highly developed as in skeletal muscle. It consists of a simple plexiform arrangement of tubular elements occupying slender clefts within the mass of myofilaments (Fig. 11–36*A*). There are no continuous transverse elements of the reticulum comparable to the terminal cisternae of the triads in skeletal muscle. Instead small terminal expansions of the reticulum here and there are closely applied to the membrane of the T tubes (Fig. 11–37). Similar contacts are made between small flattened expansions of the reticulum and the sarcolemma at the outer surface of the fiber. The total surface area of the many

small sites of apposition of the reticulum to the sarcolemma of cardiac muscle is quite great but would seem to be considerably smaller than the area of contact between the terminal cisternae and intermediate elements of the triads in skeletal muscle. It is noteworthy, too, that the T tubules in cardiac muscle occur only over the Z lines at the ends of the sarcomeres, whereas in mammalian skeletal muscle there are two triads located at the A-I junctions of each sarcomere. The functional significance of this difference in location of the T system is not fully understood.

The Intercalated Disc

On the transverse portions of the intercalated discs, the opposing ends of the cardiac muscle cells have a deeply sculptured surface. A complex pattern of ridges and papillary projections on each cell fit into corresponding grooves and pits in the other cell to form an elaborately interdigitated junction (Fig. 11–39). The entire junctional surface of both cells is specialized in various ways for maintaining cell to cell cohesion, and one can distinguish areas that are similar in their fine structure to the *macula adherens* (desmosome), and the *zonula adherens* of epithelial junctions (see p. 91). However, in the mosaic of different types of surface specialization that constitute the intercalated disc, only the *maculae adherentes* or desmosomes are typical with respect to their shape.

The fine structural counterpart of the zonula adherens actually is not beltlike, as is implied by the term *zonula*. Instead there are multiple, moderately extensive but discontinuous areas having irregular and variable outlines. A descriptive term that has been

suggested for these is *fascia adherens* (pl., *fasciae adherentes*).

In longitudinal sections, the opposing cell membranes at the intercalated disc can be identified as two parallel dense lines that follow a sinuous course separated, for the most part, by a 150 to 200 Å intercellular cleft. Over the greater part of the intercalated disc, the opposing cell surfaces are specialized as fasciae adherentes, with a mat of dense material occurring immediately subjacent to an otherwise unspecialized membrane (Fig. 11–39). The thin filaments of the adjacent I bands terminate in this mat of dense material, which evidently serves to bind the ends of myofilaments to the plasmalemma. At desmosomes or maculae adherentes along the transverse portions of the disc, the inner leaf of each of the opposing unit membranes is thickened and especially dense. A small condensation of sarcoplasm may be associ-

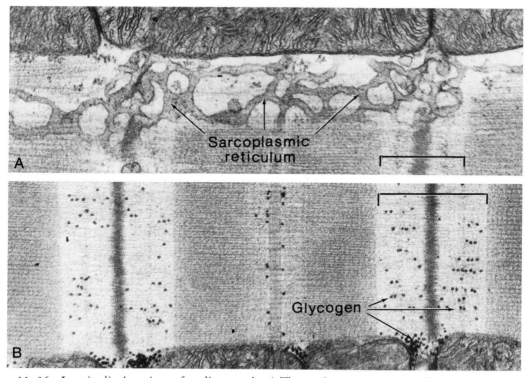

Figure 11–36 Longitudinal sections of cardiac muscle. *A,* The section passes tangentially to an internal surface of the mass of myofilaments and reveals the sarcoplasmic reticulum forming a loose network that continues across the level of the Z lines without any terminal cisternae. *B,* Glycogen particles are seen around mitochondria and between filaments in the I and H bands. The relaxed muscle in these two figures is stretched to different degree. Notice the constancy in length of the I bands, indicated by brackets at the right. (From D. W. Fawcett and N. S. McNutt, J. Cell Biol., 42:1, 1969.)

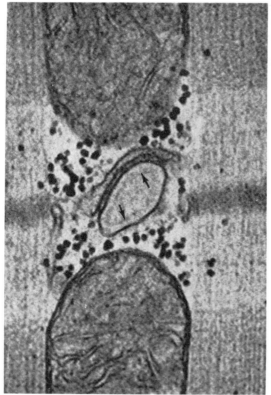

Figure 11–37 Longitudinal section of a small area of a cardiac muscle fiber, illustrating a T tubule cut transversely and a tubule of the reticulum in close apposition to it. The T tubule is lined with a layer of protein-polysaccharide (at arrows) like that coating the sarcolemma at the surface of the fiber. The dense granules in the neighboring sarcoplasm are glycogen. ×70,000.

portions of the intercalated discs, there are more extensive areas of similar close membrane apposition on the longitudinal portions of the steplike cell to cell junctions, where overlapping processes of successive cells are joined side to side. Considerable emphasis is placed upon these junctional specializations, where the intercellular space is narrowed to 20 Å or less, because it is believed that they are areas of low electrical resistance that permit the rapid spread of excitation from cell to cell throughout the heart. Thus they enable the myocardium to behave as though it were a syncytium. The other specializations of the transverse portions of the intercalated discs, where the surfaces do not have hexagonal arrays of intramembranous particles and are not in such close apposition, evidently have a mechanical significance, being mainly concerned with maintaining cell to cell cohesion and transmitting the pull of one contractile unit to the next along the axis of the muscle fibers.

Our understanding of the nature of the forces that bind cells together is still very incomplete, but it is known that calcium ions play an important role. If the beating, isolated heart of an experimental animal is perfused for some time with a calcium free medium, the heart will soon cease beating. If it is then fixed and examined in thin sections, the individual cells of the muscle fibers are found to have come apart at the intercalated discs (Fig. 11–41A and B). At high magnification it can be ascertained that the membranes, for the most part, are intact, and separation has taken place by opening up of the intercellular space. But at the nexus or gap junction where the membranes are apparently in intimate apposition the two elements are unable to separate in calcium-free medium, and one or the other of the cells is denuded of its membrane when the ends of the cells are pulled apart in the agonal contractions of the muscle.

Cytological Differences Between Atrial and Ventricular Cardiac Muscle

The fibers of atrial myocardium are basically similar to those of the ventricle described above, but they have a smaller average diameter and the T tubules are few or absent. When found, they tend to be in the larger fibers. It is possible that the smaller fiber diameter may make unnecessary a well developed system of transverse tubules for

ated with this dense plaque, but the myofilaments usually diverge and do not terminate directly on desmosomes (Fig. 11–39).

At irregular intervals along the disc, the opposing membranes may approach to within 20 Å of one another and run parallel for a short distance. These sites of closer apposition were formerly interpreted as "tight junctions" and were termed *maculae occludentes*. Further study by improved methods of specimen preparation has revealed that these correspond instead to the "nexus" or "gap junctions" of epithelia. There is no fibrous layer or condensation of the adjacent sarcoplasm associated with these regions of close apposition.

In addition to the small gap junctions that occur here and there in the transverse

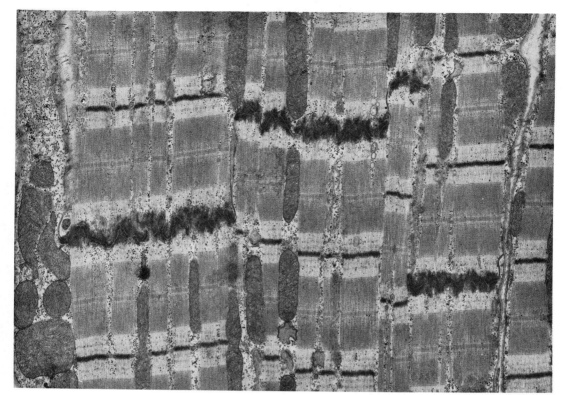

Figure 11–38 Low power electron micrograph of cardiac muscle in longitudinal section, showing a typical steplike intercalated disc. The transverse portions are highly interdigitated and characterized by an abundance of dense material at the insertions of the myofilaments into the end of the cell. The longitudinal portions of the cell boundary are smooth, unspecialized, and difficult to see at this magnification. ×12,000.

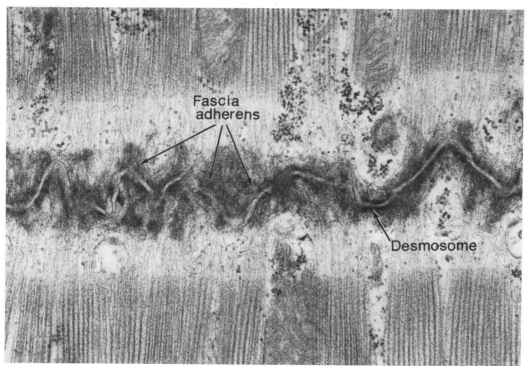

Figure 11–39 Electron micrograph of a transverse segment of an intercalated disc. The portion of the cell junction in which the myofilaments terminate resembles the zonulae adherentes of epithelia, but is here called a fascia adherens. Between sites of myofibril attachment are typical desmosomes. (From D. W. Fawcett and N. S. McNutt, J. Cell Biol., *42*:1, 1969.)

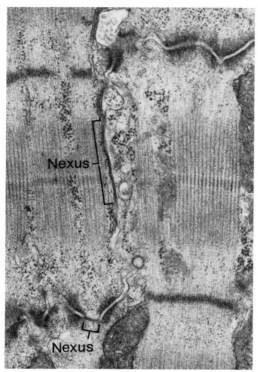

Figure 11–40. Electron micrograph of a longitudinal segment of the junction between successive cellular units of the myocardium. Extensive nexuses are commonly found here.

inward conduction of the impulse to contract. Despite their smaller diameter, conduction of the action potential over the surface of atrial muscle fibers is said to be more rapid than over ventricular fibers.

Another noteworthy difference is the presence of *specific atrial granules* in these cells (Jamieson and Palade). These are membrane bounded spherical granules 0.3 to 0.4 μm. in diameter with a dense homogeneous interior (Fig. 11–42). They are concentrated in the core of sarcoplasm extending in either direction from the poles of the nucleus, usually near the Golgi complex. They may be found in limited numbers in other regions of the cell. Although they have the appearance of secretory granules, their release from the cell has not been demonstrated. They are not stained by the chromaffin reaction and do not incorporate precursors of norepinephrine. Thus, at present there is no evidence that they contain either catecholamines or monoamines. Their functional significance remains unknown.

Specialized Conducting Tissue of the Heart

In addition to those cells of the myocardium whose primary function is contraction, there is a specialized system made up of modified muscle cells whose function is to generate the stimulus for the heart beat and to conduct the impulse to the various parts of the myocardium in such a way as to ensure the contraction of the atria and ventricles in the proper succession, so that the heart acts as an effective pump. This system consists of the *sinoatrial node* (node of Keith and Flack), the *atrioventricular node* (node of Tarawa) and the *atrioventricular bundle* (bundle of His). The sinoatrial node is located beneath the epicardium at the junction of the superior vena cava and the right atrium. The atrioventricular node is found beneath the endocardium in the lower part of the interatrial septum between the attachment of the septal leaf of the tricuspid valve and the opening of the coronary sinus. The atrioventricular bundle originates from the anterior portion of the node and enters the fibrous portion of the interventricular septum, where it soon divides into right and left bundles that are ultimately distributed to the right and left ventricles. Each of these bundles or trunks ramifies beneath the endocardium of its respective chamber to form an extensive plexus, from which fine fibers penetrate the myocardium to come into intimate contact with the ordinary contractile fibers.

The specialized cells of the nodal tissue are distinctly smaller than ordinary cardiac muscle fibers and are arranged in a network embedded in an abundant and rather dense connective tissue. In sections, the slender fusiform nodal cells coursing in various directions among the collagen bundles may be difficult to distinguish from the associated fibroblasts, but careful examination reveals their cross striations. In the mammal no connection between the sinoatrial node and the atrioventricular node via specialized conduction tissue has yet been convincingly demonstrated. The nodal fibers appear to be continuous with ordinary atrial muscle fibers. The node is richly innervated by both the sympathetic and parasympathetic divisions of the autonomic nervous system. Peripheral ganglia of the parasympathetic division are closely associated with the nodal tissue.

In cardiac muscle, which is characterized by the ability to beat rhythmically without nervous or other external stimuli, the cells with the most rapid inherent rhythm establish the rate of beating of the rest of the myocardium. In warm-blooded animals, the fibers of the sinoatrial node have the most rapid rhythm, and this node is therefore referred to as the "pacemaker" of the heart. The evidence for this resides in the fact that the electrical events associated with each beat begin at the sinoatrial node and travel from there over the atria. Warming or cooling the node increases or decreases, respectively, the rate of the heart beat. Although the heart will normally beat at a rate determined by the inherent rhythm of its pacemaker, this rate can be modified by the autonomic nervous system. Parasympathetic (vagal nerve) stimulation brings about a slowing of the heart and sympathetic stimulation accelerates it.

The fibers of the atrioventricular node are small, like those of the sinoatrial node. The fibers of the atrioventricular bundle are similar at their origin, but more distally in the right and left bundle branches they become larger than ordinary cardiac muscle fibers and take on a highly distinctive appearance. These are the so-called *Purkinje fibers* (Figs. 11–43 and 11–44). They have one or two nuclei situated in a clear central mass of sarcoplasm that is rich in mitochondria and glycogen. The myofibrils are relatively sparse and displaced to the periphery, and they are less consistent in their orientation than are those of ordinary muscle fibers.

The Purkinje fibers of ungulates reach very large size, and for this reason these have been more extensively studied than those of other mammals, but they do not seem to differ in any other important respect. Typical intercalated discs are seldom seen in the conducting tissue. At their ends the

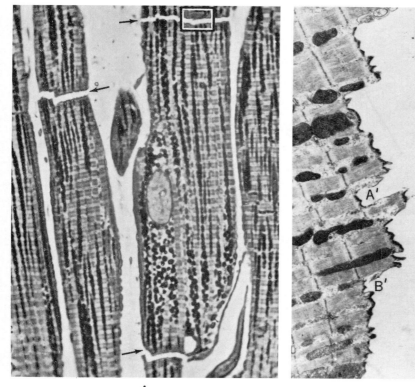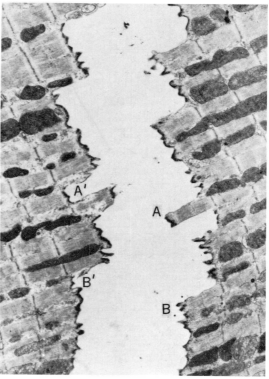

A   **B**

Figure 11–41   *A*, Photomicrograph of cardiac muscle from an isolated heart that had been perfused with calcium free Krebs' solution until it stopped beating. Notice that the muscle cells have come apart at the intercalated discs (arrows). ×1100. *B*, Electron micrograph of an area such as that enclosed in the rectangle at the top of *A*, showing the separated ends of two cardiac muscle cells. Notice the close conformation of the two surfaces: A fits into A', B into B', etc. The separation occurs between the membranes except at the nexus or gap junctions; there, the membrane pulls off one of the cells. ×5000. (Micrographs courtesy of A. Muir.)

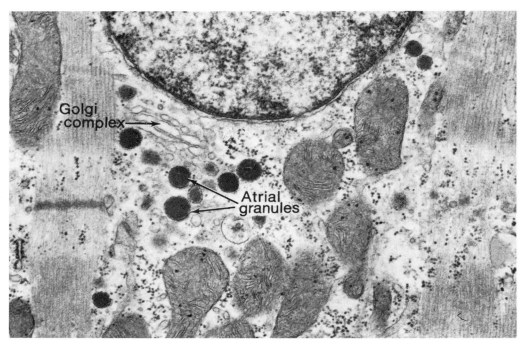

Figure 11–42 Electron micrograph of the juxtanuclear area of a cardiac muscle cell from cat atrium, showing dense spherical atrial granules in the Golgi region. (From N. S. McNutt and D. W. Fawcett, J. Cell Biol., *42:* 45, 1969.)

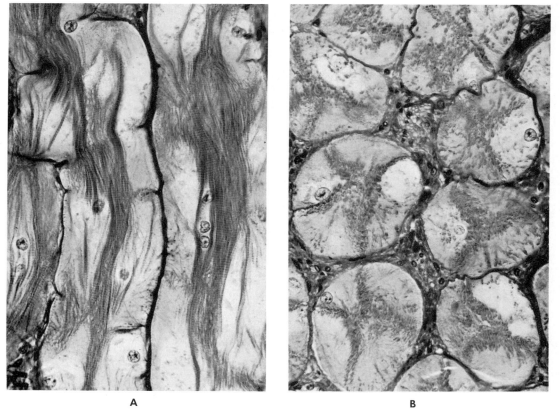

A   B

Figure 11–43 Photomicrographs of the very large Purkinje fibers in the moderator band of the bovine heart. In *A* the fibers are cut longitudinally, and in *B* they are cut transversely. In both, it is evident that the myofibrils occupy only a small part of the sarcoplasm. The large clear areas are rich in glycogen. ×600.

Purkinje fibers are said to lose their specific cytological features and to become continuous with the ordinary muscle fibers of the myocardium.

In electron micrographs, the cytoplasmic matrix of the Purkinje cells is of relatively low density and contains numerous, randomly oriented mitochondria (Figs. 11–45 and 11–46). The myofilaments do not form a continuous contractile mass but are arranged in separate myofibrils that are relatively few in number. Although their prevailing orientation is parallel to the long axis of the cell, they are very poorly ordered compared to those of ordinary cardiac muscle.

The cells have variable and unusual shapes, one often partially surrounding another or sending a large process into a deep recess in the adjoining cell (Fig. 11–46). As a consequence of their irregular shape, the cells are in extensive contact with one another. Although no typical intercalated discs are found, numerous *maculae adherentes (desmosomes)* are distributed at irregular intervals along the cell boundaries. There are also areas of closer apposition corresponding to the nexus or gap junctions of ordinary cardiac muscle. Surprisingly, these do not appear to be as numerous or as extensive as in the unspecialized fibers of the myocardium, and the morphological basis for the more rapid conduction in the atrioventricular bundle is not evident. Disease of the conduction system results in asynchrony in the beating of the ventricles or disorders in the timing of the contraction of the atria and ventricles that result in impaired efficiency of the heart.

Nerves to the Myocardium

Although the initiation of the heartbeat is not dependent upon the nervous system, the heart is richly innervated. The parasympathetic (vagus) and sympathetic divisions of the autonomic nervous system form extensive plexuses at the base of the heart. Ganglion cells and numerous nerve fibers have been described in the wall of the right atrium, particularly in the region of the sinoatrial and atrioventricular nodes. Stimulation of the vagus nerve slows the heart, and release of norepinephrine from sympathetic nerve endings accelerates it. It is commonly assumed that the autonomic nervous system acts indirectly upon the myocardium by modifying the inherent rhythm of the pacemaker. This view is supported by physiological experiment and by light and electron microscopic observations establishing the presence of large numbers of unmyelinated nerve fibers close to the specialized cells of the nodal and conduction systems (Fig. 11–45). In addition, however, a surprising number of unmyelinated fibers are also found in close relation to the ordinary cardiac fibers of the atrium and ventricles. Although it is difficult to determine to which division of the autonomic nervous system these belong, some at least contain granulated vesicles and therefore appear to be sympathetic. Release of catecholamine from these endings apparently exerts a direct effect upon the cardiac muscle.

Neither in ordinary cardiac muscle nor in the conduction tissue do the nerve fibers form specialized endings comparable to the

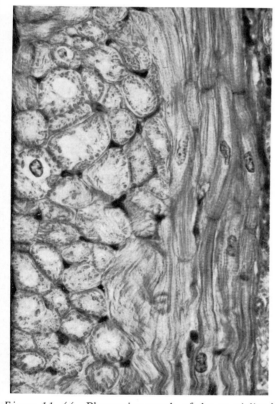

Figure 11–44 Photomicrograph of the specialized conduction tissue of the human atrioventricular bundle. The large Purkinje fibers seen in cross section at the left of the figure can be compared with the smaller unspecialized heart muscle cut longitudinally at the right side of the figure. ×650.

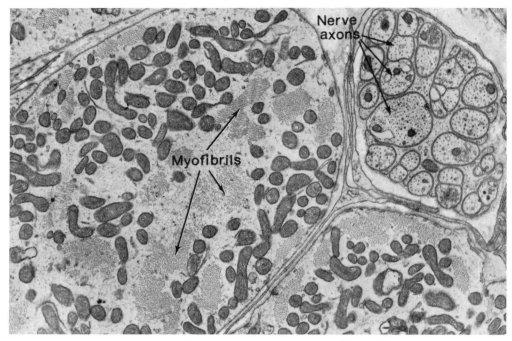

Figure 11-45   Electron micrograph of adjacent areas of two Purkinje fibers and an accompanying nerve in the atrioventricular bundle of the cat heart. The mitochondria are abundant and pleomorphic, and the loosely organized myofilaments occur only in scattered bundles. ×12,000.

myoneural junctions of skeletal muscle. Slender axons merely pass near the surface of the cardiac muscle cells. That these are functional endings and not merely passing axons is inferred from the fact that their axoplasm often contains large numbers of small vesicles identical to those found at other nerve endings and at synapses in the central nervous system.

HISTOGENESIS OF MUSCULAR TISSUE

Smooth Muscular Tissue

Smooth muscle cells arise from the mesenchyme. For example, in blood vessels, which at first consist only of endothelium, mesenchyme cells become arranged at regular intervals along the outside of the tube. They stretch out transversely, multiply by mitosis, and produce myofilaments within their cytoplasm. Then these *myoblasts* come in contact with one another laterally, and a continuous layer of smooth muscle is produced.

The reticular fibers between the muscle cells are probably produced by the same cells —the developing smooth muscle cells have been shown to be capable of elaborating both collagen and elastin.

It is claimed that some of the new smooth muscle cells that develop in the uterus during pregnancy arise from the undifferentiated connective tissue cells in this tissue. In a virgin rabbit, after injection of the female sex hormone, there is mitotic proliferation of the smooth muscle cells of the uterus.

Striated Muscular Tissue

The skeletal muscle fiber is a syncytium resulting from fusion of many separate cells. The mononuclear precursors of muscle, called myoblasts, have large nuclei with prominent nucleoli and a cytoplasm rich in ribosomes. They do not contain myofibrils until after they begin to fuse to form multinucleate muscle fibers. In the continuing differentiation of the contractile material, new filaments are added to the lateral surfaces and ends of the initial myofibrils.

In the later development of the muscular tissue the separate fibers increase in thickness and length, and their number increases through transformation of new myoblasts. The increase in number of fibers in the sartorius muscle stops when the human fetus is 130 to 170 mm. long. The subsequent growth of the muscle depends only on the continued increase in the size of the fibers already present.

Nuclei within syncytial myofibers never synthesize DNA and never divide, but myoblasts persist as *satellite cells* under the basal lamina of the fiber and may continue to proliferate and to fuse with existing fibers even in the young adult (Hay). In mammals, the nuclei at first are in the center and the myofibrils occupy the periphery of the fiber. In later stages, the nuclei move toward the periphery, so that the central parts become occupied by myofibrils.

Contractility begins in the embryonic muscular elements about the time or shortly before the first myofibrils arise in their protoplasm. This contractility, at first slight and slow, gradually increases with the increase in number of myofibrils and their arrangement in bundles. The appearance of voluntary movements is connected with the development of the nervous motor tracts that lead from the spinal cord to the myotomes.

Cardiac Muscular Tissue

Cardiac muscle in the embryo forms from the splanchnopleure adjoining the endothelium of the heart primordium. This part of the splanchnopleure is called the embryonic myocardium and is an epithelium with true desmosomes and special desmosome-like attachments that later develop into intercalated discs. The cells multiply energetically by mitosis, and for the most part they remain mononuclear. The cytoplasm contains many elongated mitochondria, often in groups. Electron micrographic study of embryonic cardiac muscle shows fine bundles of myofilaments developing in the epithelial myocardium. The myocardium is later invaded by blood vessels and mesenchyme that disrupt the epithelium, transforming it into branching cords of mononuclear cells, the definitive cardiac muscle cells. These differentiated muscle cells continue to divide even after birth.

The *Purkinje fibers* soon become distinguishable from the remaining myocardium. A few myofibrils are irregularly distributed at their periphery.

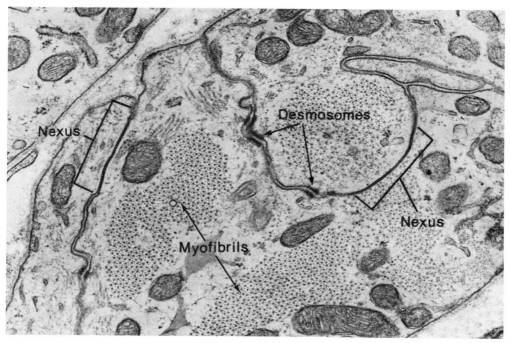

Figure 11–46 Electron micrograph of the cell junctions in the atrioventricular bundle. The cells of the conduction tissue are irregular in shape and have an extensive area of cell to cell apposition, on which are numerous desmosomes and nexuses, ×22,000. (Courtesy of D. Feldman.)

REGENERATION OF MUSCULAR TISSUE

Smooth Muscle

In the vicinity of injured regions in the walls of the intestine or stomach, mitosis has been observed in the smooth muscle cells. But this capacity for regeneration is small, and great defects in smooth muscle heal by scar formation. Whether smooth muscle cells in the adult organism may be formed anew from fibroblasts has not been established; it is practically certain that they can develop from the perivascular mesenchymal cells.

Striated Muscle

During intense activity, the skeletal muscles increase in volume by enlargement of the existing fibers through an increase in the amount of sarcoplasm and not in the number of fibrils.

The regenerative capacity of the striated muscular tissue of higher vertebrates does not always lead to the formation of functioning fibers. After destruction of muscle fibers, regeneration always starts from existing fibers. The most successful regeneration takes place when the nuclei with the surrounding sarcoplasm remain alive. These become separate cells called *myoblasts*, which proliferate and then fuse to form new syncytial muscle fibers in which striated myofibrils develop. In such a regenerative process in vitally stained animals, the myoblasts can easily be distinguished from the macrophages that have penetrated the fiber. A large defect in the muscular tissue is replaced by a connective tissue scar. Connection with motor nerve fibers is necessary for the maintenance of the normal structure of skeletal muscle, as well as for its successful regeneration.

Cardiac Muscle

In various pathological conditions in the adult organism, an increase in volume of the cardiac muscle may take place. This probably depends on the increase in thickness and length of the existing fibers. The regenerative capacity of cardiac muscle tissue has not been studied carefully in mammals. In cardiac diseases such as coronary thrombosis, healing takes place by the formation of scar tissue.

REFERENCES

Smooth Muscle

Bozler, E.: Smooth muscle. *In* Rodahl, K., and S. M. Horvath, eds.: Muscle as a tissue. New York, McGraw-Hill Book Co., 1962.

Burnstock, G.: Structure of smooth muscle and its innervation. *In* Bulbring, E., A. F. Brading, A. W. Jones, and T. Tomita, eds.: Smooth Muscle. London, Edward Arnold Publ., Ltd., 1940.

Choi, J. K.: Fine structure of smooth muscle of chicken gizzard. Proc. 5th Internat. Congr. Electron Microscopy. New York, Academic Press, 1962.

Csapo, A.: Molecular structure and function of smooth muscle. *In* Bourne, G. H., ed.: Structure and Function of Muscle. Vol. I. New York, Academic Press, 1960.

Devine, C. E., and A. P. Somlyo: Thick filaments in vascular smooth muscle. J. Cell Biol., 49:636, 1971.

Dewey, M. M., and L. Barr: Intercellular connection between smooth muscle cells: The nexus. Science 137: 670, 1962.

Hanson, J.: Structure of the smooth muscle fibres in the body wall of the earthworm. J. Biophys. Biochem. Cytol., 3:111, 1957.

Harman, J. W., M. T. O'Hegarty, and C. K. Byrnes: The ultrastructure of human smooth muscle. I. Studies of cell surface and connections in normal and achalasic esophageal smooth muscle. Exp. Mol. Path., 1:204, 1962.

Kelly, R. E., and R. V. Rice: Localization of myosin filaments in smooth muscle. J. Cell Biol., 37:105, 1968.

Lane, B. P.: Alterations in cytological detail of intestinal smooth muscle cells in various stages of contraction. J. Cell Biol., 27:199, 1965.

Lane, B. P., and J. A. G. Rhodin: Cellular interrelationships and electrical activity in two types of smooth muscle. J. Ultrastruct. Res., 10:470, 1964.

Needham, D. M., and C. F. Shoenberg: Proteins of the contractile mechanism of mammalian smooth muscle and their possible location in the cell. Proc. Roy. Soc. Lond., B160:517, 1964.

Prosser, C. L., J. Burnstock, and J. Rahn: Conduction in smooth muscle. Comparative structural properties. Am. J. Physiol., 199:545, 1960.

Rhodin, J. A. G.: Fine structure of vascular walls in mammals with special reference to smooth muscle component. Physiol. Rev., 42:49, 1962.

Ross, R.: The smooth muscle cell. II. Growth of smooth muscle in culture and formation of elastic fibers. J. Cell Biol., 50:172, 1971.

Somylo, A. P., and A. V. Somlyo: Vascular smooth muscle. I. Normal structure, pathology, biochemistry and biophysics. Pharmacol. Rev., 22:249, 1970.

Vihara, Y., G. R. Campbell, and G. Burnstock: Cytoplasmic filaments in developing and adult vertebrate smooth muscle. J. Cell Biol., 50:484, 1971.

Cardiac Muscle

Fawcett, D. W., and N. S. McNutt: The ultrastructure of the cat myocardium. I. Ventricular papillary muscle. J. Cell Biol., 42:1, 1969.

Hirsch, E. F., and A. M. Borghard-Erdle: The innervation of the heart. Arch. Path., 72:100, 1962.

Jamieson, J. D., and G. E. Palade: Specific granules in atrial muscle cells. J. Cell Biol., 23:151, 1964.

Manasek, F. J.: Histogenesis of the embryonic myocardium. Am. J. Cardiol., 25:149, 1970.

McNutt, N. S., and D. W. Fawcett: The ultrastructure of the cat myocardium. II. Atrial muscle. J. Cell Biol., 42:46, 1969.

McNutt, N. S., and D. W. Fawcett: Myocardial ultrastructure. *In*: Mammalian Myocardium. New York, John Wiley and Sons, Inc., 1974.

Muir, A. R.: Electron microscope study of the embryology of the intercalated disc in the heart of the rabbit. J. Biophys. Biochem. Cytol., 3:193, 1957.

Muir, A. R.: Further observations on the cellular structure of cardiac muscle. Journal of Anatomy (London). Proc. Anat. Soc. Gt. Brit. and Ireland, 1963, p. 642.

Nelson, D. A., and E. S. Benson: On the structural continuities of the transverse tubular system of rabbit and human myocardial cells. J. Cell Biol., 16:297, 1963.

Rhodin, J. A., P. Missier, and L. C. Reid: The structure of the specialized impulse-conducting system of the steer heart. Circulation, 24:349, 1961.

Rostgaard, J., and O. Behnke: Fine structural localization of adenine nucleoside phosphatase activity in the sarcoplasmic reticulum and T-system of the rat myocardium. J. Ultrastruct. Res., 12:579, 1965.

Simpson, F. O., and S. J. Oertelis: Relationship of the sarcoplasmic reticulum to the sarcolemma in sheep cardiac muscle. Nature, 189:758, 1961.

Sjostrand, F. S., E. Andersson-Cedergren, and M. M. Dewey: The ultrastructure of the intercalated discs of frog, mouse, and guinea pig cardiac muscle. J. Ultrastruct. Res., 1:271, 1958.

Stenger, R. J., and D. Spiro: The ultrastructure of mammalian cardiac muscle. J. Biophys. Biochem. Cytol., 9:325, 1961.

Truex, R. D.: Comparative anatomy and functional considerations of the cardiac conduction system. *In* de Carvalho, A. P., de Mello, W. C., and Hoffman, B. F., eds.: The Specialized Tissues of the Heart. Amsterdam, Elsevier Publishing Co., 1961.

Truex, R. C., and W. M. Copenhaver: Histology of the moderator band in man and other mammals, with special reference to the conduction system. Am. J. Anat., 80:173, 1947.

Truex, R. C., and M. A. Smythe: Recent observations on the human cardiac conduction system with special considerations of the atrioventricular node and bundle. *In* Electrophysiology of the Heart. New York, Pergamon Press, 1964.

Skeletal Muscle

Andersson-Cedergren, E.: Ultrastructure of motor end plate and sarcoplasmic components of mouse skeletal muscle fiber as revealed by three dimensional reconstructions from serial sections. J. Ultrastruct. Res., Suppl. 1, 1959, p. 1.

Barker, D.: The innervation of the muscle spindle. Quart. J. Micr. Sci., 89:143, 1948.

Bennett, H. S.: The structure of striated muscle as seen by the electron microscope. *In* Bourne, G. H., ed.: Structure and Function of Muscle. Vol. I. New York, Academic press, 1960.

Bourne, G. H., ed.: The Structure and Function of Muscle. 3 Vols. New York, Academic Press, 1960.

Bridgman, C. F.: The structure of tendon organs in the cat: a proposed mechanism for responding to muscle tension. Anat. Rec., 162:209, 1968.

Bridgman, C. F., E. E. Shumpert, and E. Eldred.: Insertions of intrafusal fibers in muscle spindles of the cat and other mammals. Anat. Rec., 164:391, 1969.

Constantin, L. L., C. Franzini-Armstrong, and R. J. Podol-
sky: Localization of calcium accumulating structures in striated muscle. Science, 147:158, 1965.

Cooper, S.: Muscle spindles and other muscle receptors. *In* Bourne, G. H., ed.: Structure and Function of Muscle. Vol. I. New York, Academic Press, 1960.

Couteaux, R.: Motor end plate structure. *In* Bourne, G. H., ed.: Structure and Function of Muscle. Vol. I. New York, Academic Press, 1960.

Davies, R. E.: A molecular theory of muscle contraction: Calcium dependent contractions with H bond formation plus ATP-dependent extensions of part of the myosin-actin cross-bridges. Nature, 199:1068, 1963.

Ebashi, S., and F. Lipmann: Adenosine triphosphate-linked concentration of calcium ions in a particulate fraction of rabbit muscle. J. Cell Biol., 14:502, 1962.

Ebashi, S., A. Kodama, and F. Ebashi: Troponin. I. Preparation and physiological properties. J. Biochem., 64:465, 1968.

Endo, M.: Entry of a dye into the sarcotubular system of muscle. Nature, 202:1115, 1964.

Fischman, D. A.: The synthesis and assembly of myofibrils in embryonic muscle. Current Topics in Developmental Biology, 5:235, 1970.

Franzini-Armstrong, C.: Sarcolemmal invaginations and the T-system in skeletal muscle fibers. J. Cell Biol., 19:24A, 1963.

Gautier, G. F.: The ultrastructure of three fiber types in mammalian skeletal muscle. *In* Briskey, E. J., R. G. Cassens and B. B. Marsh, eds.: The Physiology and Biochemistry of Muscle as a Food. Madison, Wisc., University of Wisconsin Press, 1940.

Gautier, G. F.: The structural and cytochemical heterogeneity of mammalian skeletal muscle fibers. *In* R. J. Podolsky, ed.: Contractility of Muscle Cells and Related Processes. Prentice-Hall, Inc., 1971.

Hanson, J., and L. Lowy: The structure of actin filaments and the origin of the axial periodicity in the I-substance of vertebrate striated muscle. Proc. Roy. Soc. Lond., B160:449, 1964.

Hanson, J., and L. Lowy: Molecular basis of contractility in muscle. Brit. Med. Bull., 21:264, 1965.

Hasselback, W.: Relaxation and the sarcotubular calcium pump. Federation Proc., 23:909, 1964.

Hay, E. D.: The fine structure of differentiating muscle in salamander tail. Zeitschr. f. Zellforsch., 59:6, 1963.

Hay, E. D.: Cellular basis of regeneration. *In* Lash, J. W., and R. Whittaker, eds.: Concepts in Developmental Biology. Stamford, Conn., Sinauer Associates, 1973.

Huxley, A. F.: The activation of striated muscle and its mechanical response. Proc. Roy. Soc. Lond., B178:1, 1971.

Huxley, H. E.: Muscle cells. *In* Brachet, J., and A. E. Mirsky, eds.: The Cell; Biochemistry, Physiology, Morphology. Vol. 4. New York, Academic Press, 1960.

Huxley, H. E.: Electron microscopic studies on the structure of natural and synthetic protein filaments from striated muscle. J. Mol. Biol., 7:281, 1963.

Huxley, H. E.: Evidence for continuity between the central elements of the triads and extracellular space in frog sartorius muscle. Nature, 202:1067, 1964.

Huxley, H. E.: The mechanism of muscular contraction. Science, 164:1356, 1969.

Kelly, D. E., and M. A. Cahill: Filamentous and matrix components of skeletal muscle Z-discs. Anat. Rec., 172:623, 1972.

Lockhart, R. D., and W. Brandt: Notes upon length of striated muscle fiber. J. Anat., 72:470, 1938.

Lowy, J., and J. V. Small: The organization of myosin and

actin in vertebrate smooth muscle. Nature, *227*:46, 1970.

Merrillees, N. C. R.: The fine structure of muscle spindles in the lumbrical muscles of the rat. J. Biophys. Biochem. Cytol., *7*:725, 1960.

Morita, S., R. G. Cassens, and E. J. Briskey: Histochemical localization of myoglobin in skeletal muscle of rabbit, pig and ox. J. Histochem. Cytochem., *18*:364, 1970.

Nonomura, Y., W. Drabikowski, and S. Ebashi: The localization of troponin in tropomyosin paracrystals. J. Biochem., *64*:419, 1968.

Peachey, L. D.: The sarcoplasmic reticulum and transverse tubules of the frog's sartorius. J. Cell Biol., *25*:209, 1965.

Peachey, L. D., and K. R. Porter: Intracellular impulse conduction in muscle cells. Science, *129*:721, 1959.

Pepe, F. A.: Some aspects of the structural organization of the myofibril as revealed by antibody staining. J. Cell Biol., *28*:505, 1966.

Porter, K. R.: The sarcoplasmic reticulum, its recent history and present status. J. Biophys. Biochem. Cytol. *10*(Suppl.):219, 1961.

Porter, K. R., and G. E. Palade: Studies on the endoplasmic reticulum. III. Its form and distribution in striated muscle cells. J. Biophys. Biochem. Cytol., *3*:269, 1957.

Smith, D. S.: The structure of insect fibrillar flight muscle. J. Biophys. Biochem. Cytol., *10*(Suppl.):123, 1961.

Uihara, Y., and K. Hama: Some observations on the fine structure of the frog muscle spindle. I. On the sensory terminals and motor endings of the muscle spindle. J. Electron Microscopy, *14*:34, 1965.

Zacks, S. I.: The Motor Endplate. Philadelphia, W. B. Saunders Co., 1964.

12

The Nervous Tissue

By Jay B. Angevine

The nervous system comprises the entire mass of nervous tissue in the body. The essential function of nervous tissue is *communication,* which depends upon special signaling properties of the nerve cells and their long processes. These properties express two fundamental attributes of protoplasm: the capacity to react to various physical and chemical agents (*irritability*) and the ability to transmit the resulting excitation from one locality to another (*conductivity*).

In signaling the reception of a stimulus from the external or internal environment, various forms of energy are transduced to electrical energy by specialized cellular structures, the receptors. Patterns of electrical messages, or nerve impulses, are transmitted from receptors to nervous centers, where they evoke in other nerve cells additional patterns of signals that result in appropriate sensations or responses. By these means, the organism reacts to the events in the world in which it lives and coordinates the functions of its organs so that the integrity of the body is maintained. In addition, the nervous system provides the structural and chemical basis of conscious experience. It furnishes the mechanism for behavior and the regulation of behavior and for maintenance of the unity of the personality.

The *central nervous system (neuraxis)* consists of the brain and spinal cord and contains the *nerve cells* or *neurons* and a variety of supportive cells, called collectively the *neuroglia.* Nerve impulses conveyed from all parts of the body over the long processes of the nerve cells, called *axons,* come together in the central nervous system. The *peripheral nervous system* comprises all nervous tissue outside of the brain and spinal cord and functions to keep the other tissues of the body in communication with the central nervous system. The functions of all parts of the organism are thus integrated by a central "clearing house" that controls the activity of the individual as a whole.

The sensory, integrative, and motor functions of nerve cells depend mainly upon irritability and conductivity. In addition, however, some nerve cells possess secretory capabilities similar to properties of the endocrine system, which carries out its integrative function by means of blood-borne chemical agents called *hormones.* The secretory products of such nerve cells are released from axon terminals into a perivascular space, transported somehow into the lumen of the vessel, and carried by the blood to the particular target organ. In recent years, a neurosecretory system regulating the activity of the adenohypophysis has been discovered, and subsequently great attention has been devoted to functional interaction between the nervous and endocrine systems.

In the evolution of the nervous systems of higher organisms, certain cells of primitive Metazoa probably developed to a high degree the properties of irritability and conductivity and as a result of their more efficient response and signaling systems gradually evolved into a rudimentary nervous system. By further specialization, some nerve cells developed the capacity to react to special kinds of exogenous stimuli. These cells, with the corresponding accessory structures distributed throughout the body or near its surface, gave rise to three systems of *sensory receptors:* (1) the *exteroceptive system,* receiving stimuli from the body surface; the *interoceptive system,* receiving stimuli from the internal organs; and the *proprioceptive system,* receiving stimuli from the muscles, tendons, and joints.

Other nerve cells became connected with

the peripheral *effector organs*, principally the muscles, forming *neuromotor* systems. Still other nerve cells, collected into a large central mass, assumed the tasks of correlation and integration. These cells receive and modify the impulses arising from the receptors and in turn appropriately influence the effector organs.

The cells of the nervous system primarily involved in its special function are the *neurons*. Each neuron has a cell body consisting of a *nucleus* and the surrounding cytoplasm, which is called the *perikaryon*. Typically the cytoplasm is drawn out into several short radiating processes called *dendrites* and into a single long process called the *axis cylinder* or *axon* (Fig. 12–1). The axon, which may attain great length, often emits branches or *axon collaterals* along its course and at its end may exhibit additional fine ramifications.

The size, shape, and other peculiarities of the nerve cell body and the number and mode of branching of its processes are all subject to variation, which results in many morphologically distinguishable kinds of nerve cells (Fig. 12–2). Functional specializations correlate with this morphological diversity. The neurons are anatomically and functionally related by their processes to other nerve cells, or to epithelial, muscular,

or glandular cells. At *synapses*, points of contact between neurons, influences pass by means of chemical *transmitters* or by electrical coupling, usually in one direction; mixed modes of transmission and reciprocal synapses, however, exist. The countless neurons are morphologically and trophically independent but functionally interrelated at synapses. This fundamental generalization is the *neuron doctrine*, essentially a restatement of the cell theory for the nervous system. The neuron doctrine implies that the nervous system is entirely cellular; that its cells are distinctive in structure and function; and that its cells are not in protoplasmic continuity but are juxtaposed without a significant amount of intervening extracellular substance. Observations with the electron microscope corroborate these tenets of the doctrine and show that the nervous system is a highly specialized epithelium. The nervous system thus reflects its phylogenetic and ontogenetic origin from the ectodermal epithelial layer of the body. Like other epithelia, nervous tissue exhibits characteristic cell-to-cell contacts. These appositional or junctional complexes consist of local specializations of the surfaces of adjacent cells. Their probable function is to maintain the position of the nerve cells and to stabilize

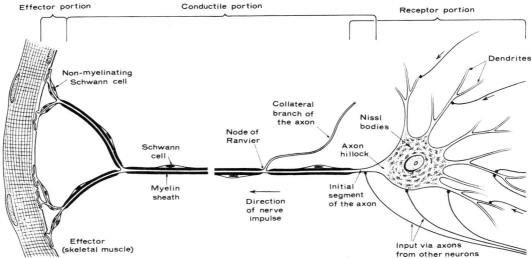

Figure 12–1. Diagrammatic representation of the effector, conductile and receptor portions of a typical large neuron. The effector endings on skeletal muscle identify this as a somatic motor neuron. The effector endings of many neurons may terminate on the receptor portions of a single neuron. The myelin sheath on the conductile portion of the neuron acts as "insulation" and serves to increase its conduction velocity. The discontinuity in the axon indicates that it is much longer than can be illustrated; sometimes a motor neuron to a limb is two or three feet long. (Drawing after Bunge in Bailey's *Textbook of Histology.* 16th Ed.)

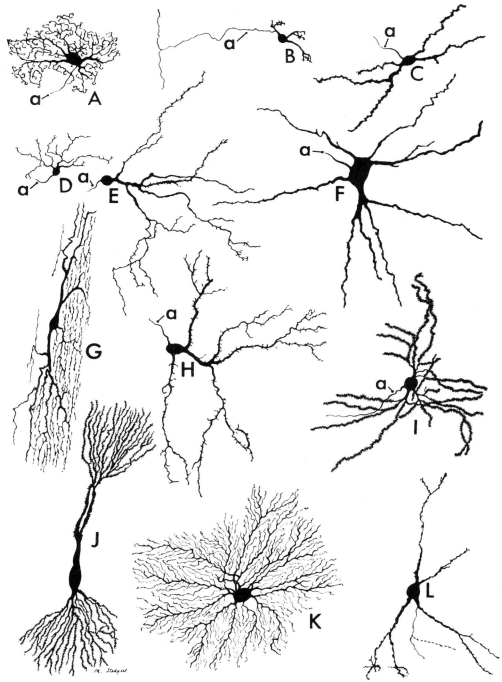

Figure 12–2 Drawing of some characteristic types of neurons whose axons (*a*) and dendrites remain within the central nervous system, illustrating some of the remarkable diversity of cell form exhibited by neurons. *A,* Neuron of inferior olivary nucleus. *B,* Granule cell of cerebellar cortex. *C,* Small cell of the reticular formation. *D,* Small gelatinosa cell of the spinal trigeminal nucleus. *E,* Ovoid cell, nucleus of tractus solitarius. *F,* Large cell of reticular formation. *G,* Spindle-shaped cell, substantia gelatinosa of spinal cord. *H,* Large cell of spinal trigeminal nucleus. *I,* Neuron, putamen of lenticular nucleus. *J,* Double pyramidal cell, Ammon's horn of hippocampal cortex. *K,* Cell from thalamic nucleus. *L,* Cell from globus pallidus of lenticular nucleus. Golgi preparations, monkey brain. (Courtesy of Clement Fox, from R. C. Truex and M. B. Carpenter, Human Neuroanatomy. 6th Ed. Baltimore, Williams and Wilkins, 1969.)

those spatial relations of their processes that are essential to the signaling function of the nervous system.

THE NEURON

The nerve cell, or neuron, is usually large and complex in shape. The volume of cytoplasm in its processes is usually greater — often much greater — than in its perikaryon. The nerve cell body in the central nervous system generally has several processes. The outline of the perikaryon is typically angular or polygonal, with the surfaces between the processes which emerge at the corners of the cell being slightly concave (Figs. 12–3 and 12–4). Motor neurons in general and the pyramidal cells of the cerebral cortex (Fig. 12–5) are two of many examples of angular nerve cell bodies. Cell bodies in the dorsal root ganglia, on the other hand, are rounded,

and only one process projects from the perikaryon (Fig. 12–6). Regardless of shape, the neuron has a number of distinctive cytological characteristics.

Nucleus

The nucleus is large, pale, spherical, or slightly ovoid, and usually centrally placed within the perikaryon. In most cases there is a single conspicuous nucleolus as well as very fine chromatin particles (Fig. 12–4). Because of uniform dispersion of the chromatin, the nuclei of nerve cells, stained with basic dyes, appear empty and pale ("vesicular"). In smaller nerve cells, the concentration of chromatin may be greater and the vesicular character of the nucleus less obvious. In man, but not in all mammals, the sex chromatin of females is prominent and is located either near the nucleolus or at the periphery of the nucleus. Although neurons usually contain only one nucleus, binucleate cells are some-

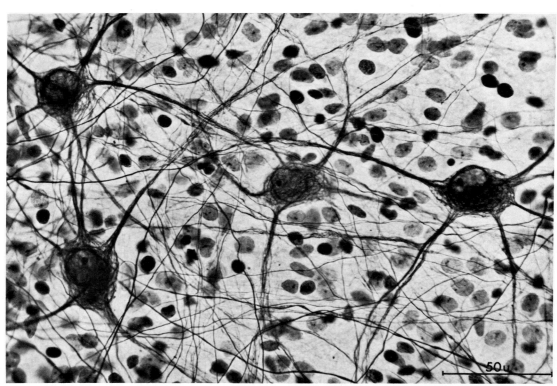

Figure 12–3 In tissue cultures of the nervous system, the three dimensional configuration of the intact neurons can be seen to better advantage than in sections. Shown here are multipolar neurons from the deep nuclei of the rat cerebellum in a 12 day culture. Notice the neurofibrils in the cell bodies. Holmes stain. (From W. Hild, Zeitschr. f. Zellforsch., 69:155, 1966.)

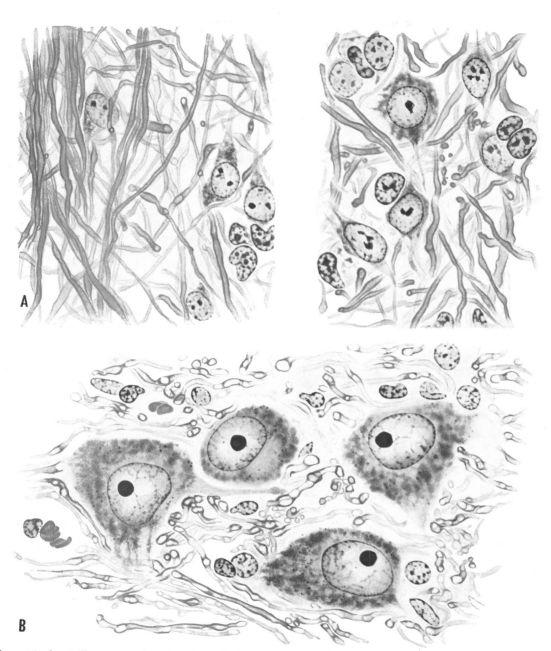

Figure 12–4 *A,* Two areas of section through the optic tectum of a leopard frog, showing blue-stained myelin sheaths and the nerve cell bodies. The small dark nuclei are supporting cells. *B,* Section from pons of man, showing myelin sheaths, nerve cell bodies, and glial cells. *A,* From a frozen section fixed in formalin; *B,* Paraffin section after postmortem formalin fixation. Klüver and Barrera staining methods for cells and myelin sheaths. × 1100. (Drawn by Esther Bohlman.)

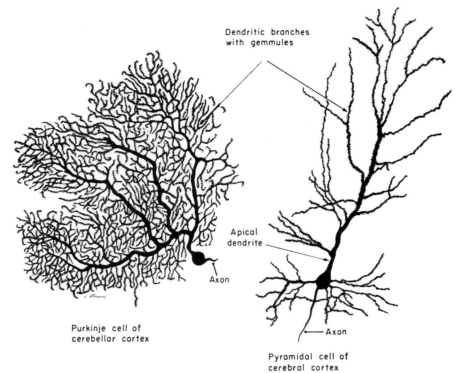

Dendritic branches
with gemmules

Apical
dendrite

Axon

Purkinje cell of
cerebellar cortex

Axon

Pyramidal cell of
cerebral cortex

Figure 12-5 Drawings of two principal cell types in cerebellar and cerebral cortex. Dendritic branches may provide a very extensive area for attachment of synaptic terminals of many other cortical and subcortical neurons. Golgi preparations, monkey brain (Courtesy of Clement Fox, from R. C. Truex and M. B. Carpenter, *Human Neuroanatomy*. 5th Ed. Baltimore, Williams and Wilkins, 1966.)

times encountered in autonomic ganglia. Certain nerve cells—the Purkinje cells of the cerebellar cortex and the hippocampal pyramidal cells—are tetraploid. In electron micrographs, the nuclear envelope and its pores and the fine structure of the nucleolus and karyoplasm (Fig. 12–8) are not significantly different from the corresponding features in other cells. In general, however, little attention has been paid to the fine structure of the nucleus of neurons.

Perikaryon

The cytoplasm of the nerve cell is crowded with filamentous, membranous, and granular organelles arranged more or less concentrically around the nucleus. As identified by light microscopy, these organelles include neurofibrils, chromophilic substance or Nissl bodies, Golgi apparatus, mitochondria, a centrosome, and various inclusions. Although any one of the selective stains for light

microscopic identification of a particular organelle leaves many of the other organelles unstained, electron micrographs show all of the organelles at one time and in the proper relationship to one another, a great advantage for study.

Neurofibrils. The neurofibrils are best developed in large neurons, but they have been demonstrated in almost every variety of nerve cell (Fig. 12–7). When they are impregnated with silver, they appear as slender interlacing threads coursing through the cytoplasm of the perikaryon from one dendrite into another or into the axon. They can be followed into the finest terminal ramifications of all the processes. In electron micrographs, it is evident that neurofibrils seen with the light microscope are formed in part by aggregations of slender *neurofilaments*, about 100 Å in diameter. In the dendrites and axon, these filaments usually lie parallel to the long axis of the process (Fig. 12–7). At high magnification, they appear as minute tubules with a dense wall about 30 Å thick and a clear center. It has been suggested that the neurofilaments may be composed of helically organized protein threads. Similar filaments extracted from the giant axon of the squid have been characterized chemically as a single protein. In addition, *microtubules* (neurotubules) are often abundant, disposed in arcs around the nucleus and passing out into the processes. The neurofilaments and microtubules tend to be arranged in tracts resembling roadways, circumventing the Nissl bodies, and collectively they seem to correspond to the argyrophilic neurofibrils seen with the light microscope (Fig. 12–7).

Chromophilic Substance. The chromophilic or Nissl substance (Figs. 12–4 and 12–7) stands out clearly in the cytoplasm of neurons stained with basic dyes and shows important changes in some pathological conditions. The Nissl bodies are visible in living neurons with phase contrast microscopy, but they are best demonstrated by staining fixed cells with basic aniline dyes—toluidine blue, thionine, or cresyl violet. Thus stained, the bodies appear as deeply basophilic masses or blocks in the perikaryon. The study of Nissl substance in living cells with phase contrast microscopy or by the freeze-drying method establishes the fact that its clumped pattern

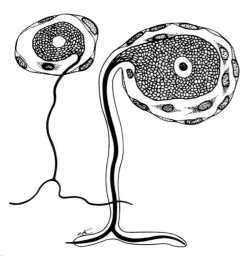

Figure 12–6 Drawing of cells from the nodose ganglion of the vagus nerve. Like neurons in the dorsal root ganglia, their cell bodies are rounded and only one process projects from the perikaryon, which is surrounded by satellite cells. (Redrawn from Ramón y Cajal.)

in histological sections accurately reflects its distribution in life. By use of ultraviolet microscopy and ribonuclease digestion, it has been shown that one of the principal constituents of the Nissl substance is ribonucleoprotein.

In electron micrographs, Nissl bodies are seen to consist of massed cisternae of rough surfaced endoplasmic reticulum in ordered parallel arrays (Figs. 12–8 and 9). Ribosomes, arranged in loops, rows, and spirals, are attached to the outer surface of the membranes, as in the basophilic regions of other cell types. They also occur in clusters or rosettes in the cytoplasm between cisternae. Nissl bodies, like the basophilic substance of pancreatic and hepatic cells, represent sites of protein synthesis.

Nissl substance is abundant throughout the cytoplasm, including the dendrites. In the latter it appears under the electron microscope as anastomosing slender tubules and short cisternae. Sites of dendritic branching are frequently occupied by small Nissl bodies—that is, parallel arrays of cisternae. They are usually absent from the most peripheral region of the perikaryon and from the area of the perikaryon in which the axis cylinder originates (the *axon hillock*), as well as from the axis cylinder itself (Fig. 12–7).

In form, size, and distribution, Nissl bodies vary considerably in different types of neurons. As a rule, they are coarser and more abundant in large neurons, especially motor neurons, and small and scarce in small neurons. Obvious exceptions are encountered, however. The ganglion cells of the dorsal roots of spinal nerves may attain large size yet typically display a uniform distribution of very fine Nissl bodies. Under different physiological conditions, such as rest and fatigue, or in certain pathological states, Nissl bodies change their appearance (this is discussed in more detail later in this chapter).

Golgi Apparatus. The intracellular reticular apparatus, or Golgi complex, is present in all nerve cells and when stained selectively for light microscopy appears as a network of irregular, wavy strands, coarser than the neurofibrillar network. With the electron microscope, the Golgi network appears as clusters of closely apposed, flattened cisternae arranged in stacks and surrounded by multitudes of small vesicles. The ends of

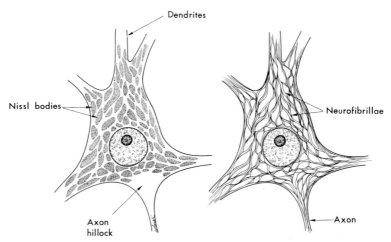

Figure 12–7 Drawings of a motor neuron from the gray matter of the ventral horn of the cat spinal cord stained for Nissl substance (*A*) and stained by a silver method for demonstrating neurofibrillae (*B*). The two images are complementary, the network of neurofibrillae running between the areas occupied by Nissl bodies and continuing into the processes. The Nissl bodies are largely confined to the perikaryon but may extend into the dendrites. They are usually not found in the axon hillock.

the cisternae are frequently dilated; they may be continuous with branching tubules extending into the surrounding cytoplasm. In low power electron micrographs, the distribution of the seemingly isolated arrays of Golgi membranes corresponds to the image obtained with the light microscope. The Golgi complex is arranged in an arc or a complete circle around the nuclear envelope approximately halfway between it and the surface membrane of the perikaryon (Fig. 12–8). A histochemical reaction for the enzyme thiamine pyrophosphatase yields a reaction product concentrated in the cisternae of this organelle and the resulting staining is coextensive with the Golgi apparatus as classically delineated by silver or osmium impregnation methods.

Areas of typical *Golgi membranes* are interconnected by smooth surfaced tubular elements, often interpreted as *agranular endoplasmic reticulum*. These latter in turn are often continuous with tubules or cisternae of the *granular reticulum*. Thus, some workers regard these three types of membrane-limited structures simply as local or regional differentiations of a single organelle.

Mitochondria. Rodlike or filamentous mitochondria are scattered everywhere, intermingling with Nissl bodies and neurofibrils. They are generally smaller than those of non-nervous tissues, varying from 0.1 to

1.0 μm. in diameter, with a preponderance of slender forms that generally measure close to the smaller dimension. They can be demonstrated in fresh nerve cells by supravital staining. Their number varies from cell to cell and in different parts of the same cell; they are especially numerous in axon endings (Fig. 12–36). Their fine structure resembles that of mitochondria in other cells but displays two peculiarities of unknown significance: The cristae are not consistently transversely oriented but often run parallel to the long axis of the mitochondrion, and the dense matrix granules usually present in the inner mitochondrial chamber are either absent or infrequent.

Centrosome. The spherical centrosome contains a pair of centrioles and is characteristic of preneuronal multiplying cells during embryonic development. In adult neurons of vertebrates, a typical centrosome is seldom observed in light microscopic preparations. In electron micrographs, however, a centrosome is occasionally encountered. Since neurons do not proliferate, the role of this organelle in the adult nerve cell is unknown.

Inclusions. In addition to the organelles already described, there are inclusions in nerve cells that are of more restricted occurrence. Pigment granules are frequently encountered. The coarse, dark brown or black granules found in neurons in the sub-

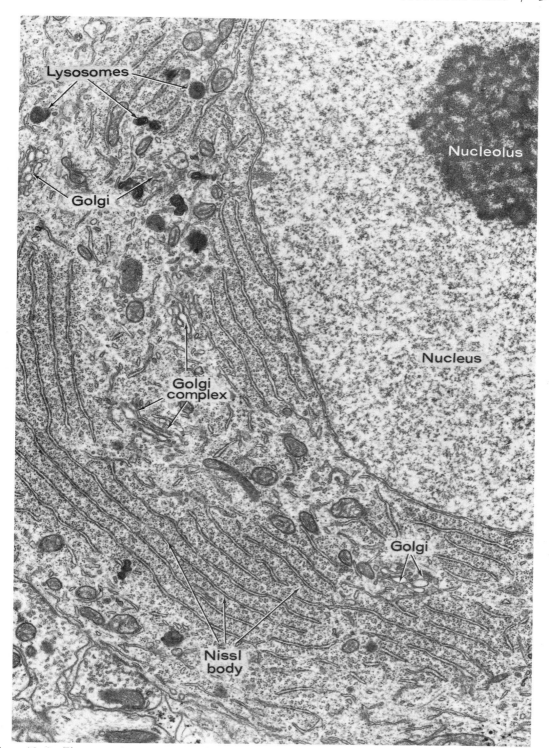

Figure 12–8 Electron micrograph of a portion of the perikaryon of a typical neuron, illustrating the principal organelles. The Golgi complex of the neurons is highly developed and forms a continuous network in the perinuclear cytoplasm; therefore, in a thin section such as this, it is transected at multiple sites. (Micrograph courtesy of Sanford Palay.)

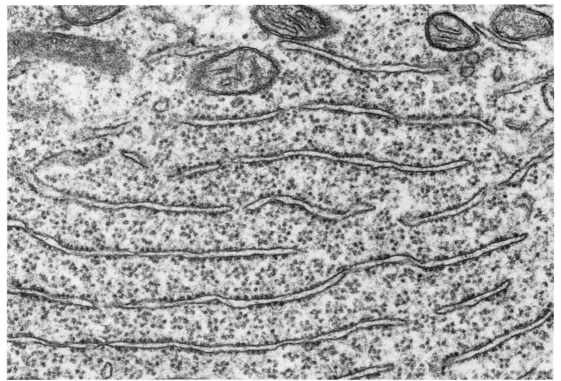

Figure 12-9 Electron micrograph of a Nissl body at higher magnification. It consists of flattened cisternae of the endoplasmic reticulum oriented parallel to each other. In addition to the ribosomes associated with the membranes, there are many clusters of ribosomes in the cytoplasmic matrix between cisternae. (Micrograph courtesy of Sanford Palay.)

stantia nigra of the midbrain, the locus coeruleus near the fourth ventricle, the dorsal motor nucleus of the vagus nerve, and the spinal and sympathetic ganglia are undoubtedly *melanin.* The physiological significance of melanin in these sites is unknown. Of more general occurrence, especially in man, are golden brown pigment granules termed *lipofuscin.* They are probably a harmless by-product of normal lysosomal activity that accumulates within the cytoplasm. Gradual increase in amount of lipofuscin with advancing age may displace the nucleus and organelles far to one side of the neuron. Lipid, encountered as droplets in the cytoplasm, may represent either normal metabolic reserve material or a product of pathological metabolism. Glycogen is found in embryonic neurons, in embryonic neuroglial cells, and in embryonic cells of the ependyma and choroid plexus, but is not present in a histochemically demonstrable quantity in adult nervous tissue. Iron-containing granular deposits are found in neurons of the substantia nigra, the globus pallidus, and elsewhere. Their number increases as the individual grows older.

Processes of Neurons. The cytoplasmic processes of nerve cells are their most remarkable features. In almost all neurons there are two kinds: the dendrites and the axon.

The dendrites provide most of the receptive surface of the neuron, although the cell body, the initial segment of the axon, and axon terminals also may receive afferent fibers (to be discussed in more detail later in this chapter). Dendrites may be direct extensions of the perikaryon or remote arborizations, as in the peripheral branches of a sensory ganglion cell, in which case a length of typical axis cylinder is interposed between perikaryon and dendritic arborization. Dendrites usually contain Nissl bodies and mitochondria. A neuron usually has several main dendrites; rarely there is only one. Where the dendrites emerge from the cell body they are thick, tapering gradually along their length toward the ends. In most neurons the dendrites are relatively short and confined to the immediate vicinity of the cell body. Each dendrite may divide into primary, secondary, tertiary, and higher orders of branches, of variable shapes and sizes, and distributed in diverse ways (Fig. 12–11). The number and length of the dendrites bear little relation to the size of the perikaryon, but their pattern of branching is typical for each variety of neuron. The surface of many dendrites is covered with innumerable minute, thorny *spines* or *gemmules*, which often serve as sites of synaptic contact (Fig. 12–5).

In addition to Nissl bodies and mitochondria, dendrites contain long, straight, parallel microtubules, about 250 Å in diameter. In cross section, the microtubules appear as small circles with a thick wall (60 Å) and a clear center. Neurofilaments are also encountered in small numbers in dendrites (Figs. 12–11 and 12–12). The microtubules and neurofilaments, as well as the larger tubular elements of the endoplasmic reticulum, become progressively more scanty towards the ends of the dendrites. In contrast, mitochondria remain more or less constant in number per unit length and may actually appear relatively increased as they are confined in the finer dendritic ramifications.

Through their synapses with axon terminals, the dendrites receive nerve impulses from other functionally related neurons. The numbers of impulses and of sources from which they are received may be very great. In a Purkinje cell of the cerebellar cortex (Figs. 12–10 and 12–11), the terminals upon the dendritic tree number in the hundreds of thousands. The dendrites play a crucial role in the ability of the neuron to integrate information received from its many inputs. The arriving nerve impulses excite or inhibit electrical activity in localized regions of dendritic membrane and thus continuously shift the neuron toward or away from its threshold for signaling a nerve impulse of its own. Although the impulse carried by the axon behaves in an "all-or nothing" fashion, the integrative capacity of the dendrites depends upon graded changes in electrical potential. Recent studies, however, demonstrate that in certain instances dendrites may transmit as well as receive, exerting influences upon adjacent dendrites through specialized, reciprocal dendrodendritic synapses, or

may exhibit propagated all-or-nothing signaling within long dendritic shafts (see below). Such findings call for flexibility in the functional characterization of dendrites, or for that matter, any part of the nerve cell, whose parts show great adaptability to special requirements in particular situations.

The *axon* or *axis cylinder* differs considerably from the dendrites. Whereas there are usually several dendrites, there is only one axon to each neuron or, in occasional instances (the so-called *amacrine* cells of the retina), no axon at all. This cell process often arises from a small conical elevation on the perikaryon devoid of Nissl bodies, called the *axon hillock.* The axon may arise, however, from the stem of a principal dendrite. The axon carries the response of the neuron in the form of a propagated *action potential;* the axon hillock and initial segment of the axon, from which this potential arises, are sometimes called the "trigger zone." The axon does not contain Nissl bodies and usually is thinner and much longer than the dendrites of the same neuron.* The axoplasm contains longitudinally oriented tubules of the endoplasmic reticulum, long and extremely slender mitochondria, microtubules, and many neurofilaments.

The axons of many nerve cells have a prominent sheath of material called *myelin,* highly refractile in the fresh condition and appearing black in tissue fixed in osmium tetroxide. The *myelin sheath* of the axis cylinder is not part of the neuron but rather a part of an ensheathing cell (see discussion later in this chapter). Its presence or absence exerts an important influence on the physiological properties of the neuron. Because it is associated only with axons, it provides a criterion for recognizing them—except, of course, for those axons that are devoid of a myelin sheath (*unmyelinated axons*). In electron micrographs unmyelinated axons and dendrites of large caliber can usually be distinguished by the fact that there is a much greater number of neurofilaments in the axon. The smaller processes are more difficult to distinguish, because the neurofilaments upon which the identification largely depends are less numerous in small axons.

---

*When the dendritic branches are included in a comparison of axonal and dendritic length, however, the total length of dendritic process usually is much greater.

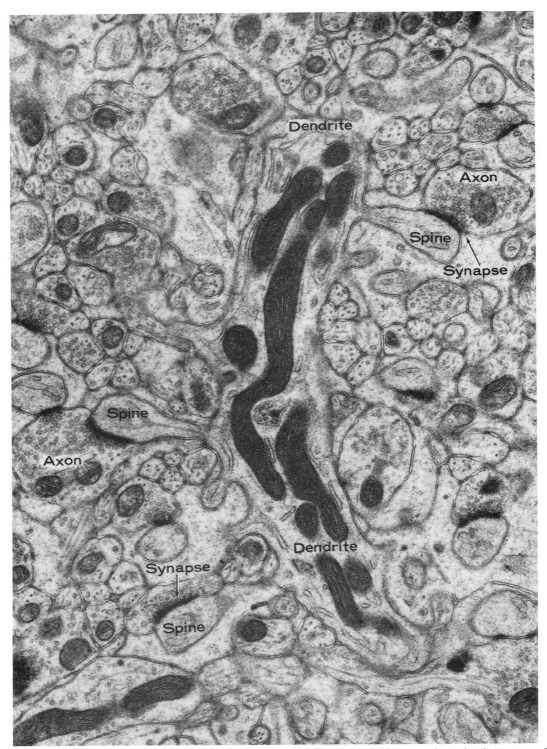

Figure 12-10 Electron micrograph of a small area of cerebellum. A small branch of the dendritic tree of a Purkinje cell running vertically through the field contains several conspicuous mitochondria. Projecting laterally from the dendrite are "spines" or "thorns" with bulbous tips and narrow stalks. Axons of granule cells form synapses with the Purkinje cell dendrite. (From S. L. Palay and V. C. Palay, Cerebellar Cortex. Berlin, Springer-Verlag, 1974.)

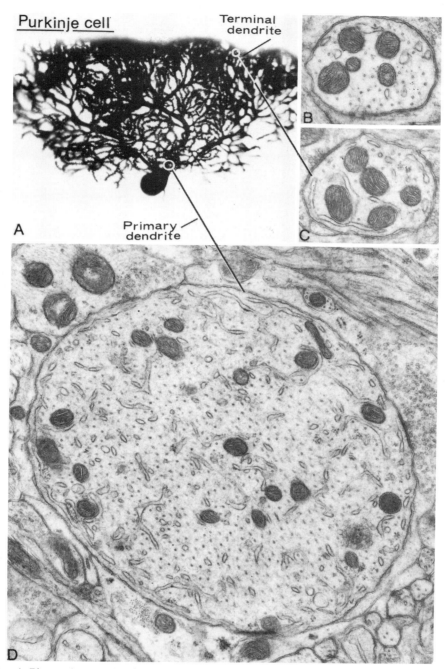

Figure 12–11 *A,* Photomicrograph of a Golgi preparation of a Purkinje cell, showing its highly branched dendritic tree. *B, C,* Electron micrographs of small terminal dendrites of the Purkinje cell located in the molecular layer of the cerebellum. *D,* Cross section of the primary dendrite of a Purkinje cell. Mitochondria, tubular elements of endoplasmic reticulum, and punctate profiles of microtubules are found throughout the dendritic tree, but microtubules are more numerous and more uniformly arranged in the primary dendrite. (Micrograph from Wuerker and Kirkpatrick, International Review of Cytology, eds. G. H. Bourne and J. F. Danielli. Vol. 33. New York, Academic Press, 1972.)

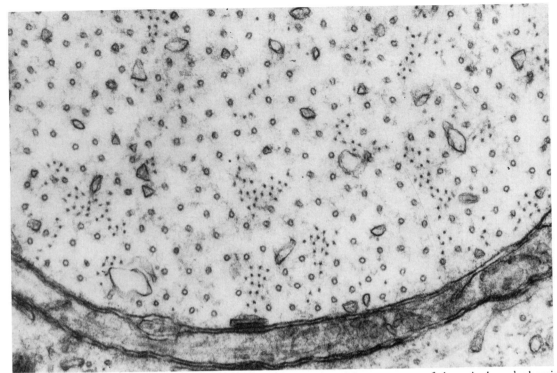

Figure 12-12 Higher magnification of a dendrite from a ventral horn neuron of the spinal cord, showing microtubules and clusters of neurofilaments. (Micrograph courtesy of Raymond Wuerker.)

Along its course, the axon may or may not emit collaterals. Unlike the branches of dendrites, which diverge at an acute angle, axonal branches tend to depart at right angles. In certain instances, a neuron may display an extensive system of axon collaterals, which individually ramify into ever finer branches. In such cases, the total length of axon may approach or even exceed that of the dendrites and can extend the sphere of influence of the neuron to a great number of other neurons. Axon collaterals from many neurons of this kind may combine to form a fibrous plexus of great complexity, enveloping the perikarya of other nerve cells.

The terminal arborization of the axon is composed of primary, secondary, and other branches and buds, varying greatly in number, shape, and distribution. Often its branches assemble into networks that surround the body of the postsynaptic neuron in the form of a basket, or twist around the dendrites like a clinging vine. In simpler cases, the tips of one or two twigs just touch the surface of a dendrite or the body of another neuron.

The perikaryon, like the dendrites, offers electrically excitable membrane upon which excitatory or inhibitory influences from axon terminals of other neurons can be received and integrated. The axon hillock, or subsequent initial segment, may provide a critically placed receptive zone for inhibitory signals. The pseudounipolar neuron of the craniospinal ganglia transmits a nerve impulse directly from the peripheral to the central branch of its long, single, T-shaped process (Fig. 12-6). Its perikaryon has no synaptic contacts from other neurons and is chiefly of trophic significance, even though its membrane may reflect passage of the action potential in the adjacent process.

Through its ending, the axon transmits nerve impulses to other neurons or to muscle fibers and gland cells. The response of the effector cells is always activity, but the response of other neurons may be a varying degree of either excitation or inhibition.

There are many types of axon endings, and the same axon may terminate in several different ways and synapse with several different neurons.

In general, dendrites display local changes in membrane potential in response to impulses received. Certain neurons with very long dendrites, however, exhibit propagated dendritic electrical potentials, similar to the *action potential* characteristic of axons, which appear to summate and convey to the perikaryon weak excitations from remote regions of the dendritic tree.

An important finding is that the nerve cell body is continuously forming new cytoplasm, which flows down the nerve cell processes at a rate of about 1 mm. per day. The perpetual flow of material probably serves to replace catabolized protoplasm, especially proteins, which cannot be synthesized in the axoplasm. Autoradiographic studies with labeled amino acids have demonstrated the synthesis of protein on the Nissl substance of the perikaryon and its progressive transport down the axon. Although substantial transport of axoplasm occurs at this slow rate, recent radioisotope and fluorescence studies demonstrate more rapid rates of translocation of substances along the axon. Certain proteins move two orders of magnitude faster, from a few millimeters to 100 and perhaps up to 500 mm. per day. Catecholamine storage granules (norepinephrine) move from 48 to 240 mm. per day, and glutamate (a suspected nerve-muscle transmitter in the snail) is transported several centimeters per hour (720 mm. per day) when the snail nerve is electrically stimulated. Different materials thus appear to move at different rates, not only in various axons of the same type of neuron but also within a single axon.

DISTRIBUTION, FORMS AND VARIETIES OF NEURONS

The core of the central nervous system, the *gray matter* (Fig. 12–13), contains the cell bodies of the neurons, their dendrites, and proximal portions of the axis cylinders. Clusters of nerve cell bodies in the gray matter are called *nuclei* (not to be confused with cellular nuclei) and represent functional aggregates of neurons. Surrounding the gray matter more or less concentrically is a zone, devoid of nerve cell bodies, which contains axis cylinders of neurons whose cell bodies are located either in the gray matter or in ganglia outside the central nervous system (CNS). This zone is the *white matter*, so called because the axis cylinders here are invested by *myelin*, which is glistening white in the fresh state. Bundles of myelinated fibers in the white matter, which are functional groupings of nerve fibers resembling cables, are called *tracts*. In the cerebral hemispheres and cerebellum, additional gray matter with nerve cell bodies arranged in distinct layers forms the cortex surrounding the white matter (Figs. 12–14 and 12–15).

On the basis of the number, length, thickness, and mode of branching of the processes, and on the shape, size, and position of the cell body, as well as on the synaptic relationships, a very great variety of neurons can be distinguished in the CNS (Fig. 12–2). Neurons may have long axons that leave the gray matter, traverse the white matter, and terminate at some distance in another part of the gray matter. Alternatively, axons may leave the CNS and end in the periphery. Such cells with long axons are termed *Golgi Type I* neurons; this type includes the neurons that contribute to formation of the peripheral nerves and those whose axons form long fiber tracts of the brain and spinal cord. In other neurons, the axon is relatively short and does not leave the region of the gray matter where its cell body lies. These cells with short axons, which are especially numerous in the cerebral and cerebellar cortices and in the retina, are *Golgi Type II* neurons.

The shape of the perikaryon varies; it may be spherical, ovoid, pyriform, fusiform, or polyhedral. The absolute size of the cell body also varies between extreme limits, from dwarf neurons of 4 μm. diameter (smaller than an erythrocyte) to giants approaching 150 μm. The pyramidal cells of Betz in the mammalian cerebral cortex and the paired Mauthner neurons in the medulla oblongata of certain fishes and amphibians are examples of exceptionally large neurons — could they be isolated, they would be visible to the naked eye.

True *unipolar neurons* are rare except in early embryonic stages. In *bipolar neurons*, a process projects from each end of the fusiform cell body. Typical bipolar neurons are found in the retina, in the vestibular and cochlear ganglia, and in the olfactory nasal

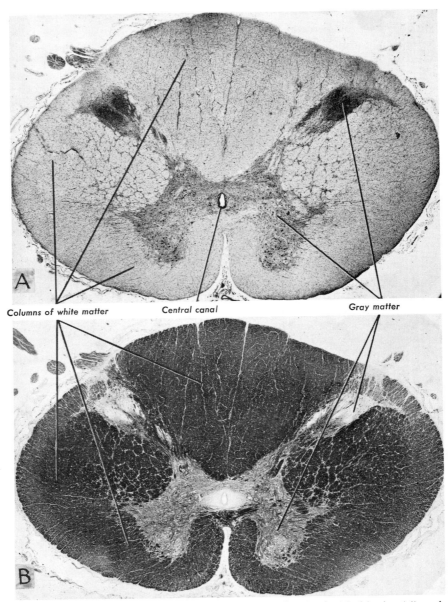

Columns of white matter   Central canal   Gray matter

Figure 12–13 Sections through human upper cervical spinal cord stained with thionine (*A*) to show cells, and with the Weigert-Weil method (*B*) to show myelinated fibers. Note the external arrangement of the fibers (white matter) and the central, cruciate area containing the cell bodies (gray matter). The ventral surface is below. A portion of the dorsal root is seen in the upper left. × 12. (Courtesy of P. Bailey.)

epithelium. In vertebrate embryos, all neurons of the craniospinal ganglia are first bipolar, but during development the opposing processes shift around the perikaryon and combine into a single process. These neurons are thus called *pseudounipolar*. During embryonic stages, the perikaryon of such neurons is progressively set apart from the

region of fusion of the two initial processes. The adult cell body is globular or pear-shaped; a single process arises and divides like the letter T. One branch is directed to the periphery and another traveling in a posterior nerve root to the central nervous system. The single process may be relatively short, as illustrated in Figure 12–6, or may run a considerable distance before bifurcating, sometimes enveloping the cell body of origin in a complex tangle. Except in the smallest examples, the initial single process and the peripheral and central branches are myelinated. The perikaryon of a pseudounipolar neuron is ensheathed by two cellular capsules. The inner is made up of small, flat, epithelium-like *satellite cells* that are continuous with similar *Schwann cells* enveloping the peripheral process. The satellite cells have a relationship to the ganglion cells that is simi-

lar to that of neuroglial cells (oligodendrocytes) to neurons in the CNS. Satellite cells, however, differ in structure and embryonic origin from neuroglial cells. The outer capsule of pseudounipolar neurons is vascular connective tissue, which extends along the cellular process and continues as the endoneurium of the nerve fiber.

In the majority of neurons, shape is determined by the number and arrangement of the dendrites (Fig. 12–2). *Stellate* or *star-shaped neurons* include the motor nerve cells

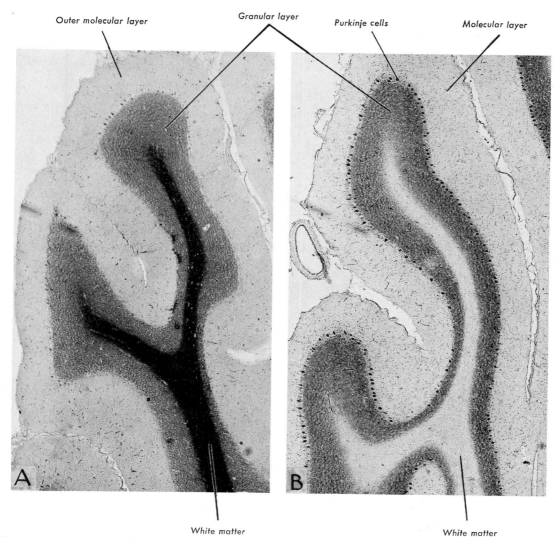

Figure 12–14 Sections of human cerebellar folia stained with the Weigert-Weil method (*A*) for myelinated fibers and with thionine (*B*) for cells. Note the central disposition of the white matter with its myelinated fibers, which stain black with Weigert-Weil and pale with thionine; the outer molecular layer (pale gray), with scattered neurons and the large Purkinje cells; and the intermediate, or granular, layer, composed of cells and fibers. × 32. (Courtesy of P. Bailey.)

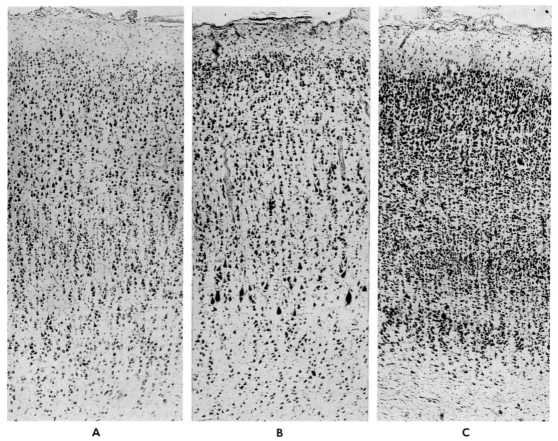

Figure 12-15 Sections from three areas of human cerebral cortex (gray matter), showing distribution of nerve bodies (*A*) in the temporal eulaminate (associational) cortex, (*B*) in the precentral agranular cortex (motor area), and (*C*) in the occipital koniocortex (striate visual cortex). Much stress has been laid on minute differences in lamination of the nerve cells and fibers in these and other areas of the cortex, but there is now a tendency to minimize some of these differences. × 53. (Courtesy of P. Bailey.)

of the ventral gray matter of the spinal cord and of the motor nuclei of the brain stem. Pyramidal neurons are characteristic elements of the cerebral cortex.

Of remarkable shape are the graceful *Purkinje cells* of the cerebellar cortex (Figs. 12–5 and 12–11*A*). One or two thick dendrites covered with innumerable tiny spines arise from the upper end of the cell body. These branch repeatedly to form a large dendritic arborization, oriented in one plane and shaped like a fan turned at right angles to the long axis of the surrounding cerebellar convolution. The axon enters the white matter beneath the cortex; hence the Purkinje cell is a Golgi Type I neuron. Synaptic terminals upon the dendrites and body of the Purkinje cell number several hundred thousand per cell and exhibit, according to

their source, specific places and modes of ending upon the postsynaptic surface.

Many more varieties of neurons are found in the cerebral and cerebellar cortices. In diminutive *granule cells*, a few short dendrites radiate in all directions, while the axon and its collaterals remain either in the immediate neighborhood of the cell or at least within the cortical gray matter. Such neurons qualify as Golgi Type II. Neurons in the reticular formation of the brain stem have large, variously shaped perikarya and extensive but poorly branched dendrites. Great attention has been accorded these neurons in recent years because their morphology and synaptic relationships suggest important integrative functions. The multitude of dendrites frequently overlap in complex fashion and receive an input of axons and axon collaterals derived from many sources. The typically long axon may distribute impulses through ascending and descending branches to a considerable portion of the length of the neuraxis and ramify into rich collateral plexuses at different levels. At first glance, these sprawling neurons convey an impression of disorder in the extreme, yet they are encountered in the core of the brain stem, an area upon which the delicate and exquisite control of homeostatic mechanisms depends.

The few examples described give an incomplete picture of the wealth of different kinds of neurons. Many more have been described by numerous investigators, especially by Ramón y Cajal and his pupils. Recent studies, in which the electron microscope and chrome-silver method of Golgi have played complementary roles, have further refined the knowledge of neuronal types. It is apparent that each ganglion, nucleus, or cortical area is composed of (1) a characteristic variety of neurons in differing proportions, each type of cell designed to meet its special functional requirements, and (2) a complex and highly ordered meshwork of dendritic, axonal, and glial processes whose fine structure and relationships are adapted to provide a framework for a particular form of organized activity. The term used to designate this feltwork of processes is *neuropil*. The details of its dense entanglements cannot be resolved in silver preparations and have only begun to be appreciated with the advent of the electron microscope. The neuropil is of great importance in the communications function of nervous tissue; it provides an enormous area for synaptic contact and functional interaction between the processes of nerve cells. It has been estimated that well over half the cytoplasm of neurons is contained in the neuropil. The great variety of types of neurons and neuropils results in a striking degree of regional heterogeneity in nervous tissue.

The number of nerve cells in the entire nervous system is astronomical, being estimated at 14 billion in man. The tremendous increase in this number in the course of evolution has involved chiefly the integrator cells or *interneurons* of the CNS. The number of *sensory neurons* and associated receptors has also increased, especially in the retina, but to a much lesser extent. The number of *motor neurons* has remained relatively small and in man probably does not exceed two

million. The term *final common pathway* is employed to designate the motor neurons by which nerve impulses from many central sources pass to a muscle or gland in the periphery.

THE NERVE FIBER

The *nerve fiber* is composed of an axon and certain sheaths of ectodermal origin. All peripheral axons are enclosed by a sheath of Schwann cells, which invest the axon almost from its beginning to near its peripheral termination. The larger peripheral axons are also enveloped in a *myelin sheath*, within the *sheath of Schwann*. The smallest axons of peripheral nerves lack a myelin sheath. It is necessary, therefore, to designate axons as *myelinated* or *unmyelinated*. Fresh myelinated fibers appear as homogeneous, glistening tubes. This refractile property of myelin accounts, as noted earlier, for the white color of fiber masses of the brain and spinal cord and of numerous peripheral nerves. In stained preparations, the appearance of various constituents of the nerve fiber differs according to the technique applied. With methylene blue vital staining and with silver methods, the axon is stained blue, brown, or black, the myelin remaining unstained. Unmyelinated fibers, often difficult to observe by routine histological methods, are well demonstrated by these special techniques. Weigert's method and osmium tetroxide darken the myelin, leaving the axon colorless or light gray (Figs. 12–16 and 12–22). Myelin sheaths are stained blue-green by the Klüver-Barrera method (Fig. 12–4).

The Sheath of Schwann

This sheath of flattened cells, sometimes called the *neurilemmal sheath*, forms a thin sleeve around the myelin, which in turn surrounds the axon. The Schwann cells, like the neurons, are of ectodermal origin and represent elements similar to neuroglial cells, but they are derived from neural crest and adapted to the special conditions of the peripheral nervous system. In embryonic life, Schwann cells accompany outgrowing axons and migrate from branch to branch until they form complete neurilemmal sheaths. In the adult their nuclei are flattened; a small Golgi apparatus and a few mitochondria can be

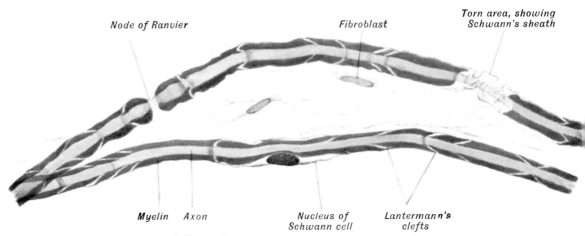

Node of Ranvier   Fibroblast   Torn area, showing Schwann's sheath

Myelin   Axon   Nucleus of Schwann cell   Lantermann's clefts

Figure 12-16 Two myelinated fibers of the sciatic nerve of a frog, treated with osmium tetroxide and picrocarmine and teased. × 330. (After A. A. Maximow.)

demonstrated in their attenuated cytoplasm. The myelin and the Schwann sheaths appear distinct with the light microscope and were formerly considered separate structures. The electron microscope, however, shows that myelin is actually part of the Schwann cell, consisting of spirally wrapped layers of its surface membrane (discussed in more detail later). The outer membrane of the Schwann cell and the glycoprotein boundary layer on its outer aspect were resolved with the light microscope as a single layer, traditionally called the *neurilemma*.* The sheath of Schwann and the myelin sheath are interrupted at regular intervals by *nodes of Ranvier* (Fig. 12-17), which are points of discontinuity between successive Schwann cells along the length of the axon. Here the axon is partially uncovered, being only incompletely enclosed by a complex arrangement of Schwann cell processes (Fig. 12-21). Myelinated axons thus have individual neurilemmal sheaths, divided into segments. Each internodal segment of the sheath between two consecutive nodes of Ranvier is composed of a Schwann cell with its myelin lamellae.

The internodal segments are shorter in the terminal portion of the fiber. The length

varies in different nerve fibers and in different species from about 200 to over 1000 μm. The longer and thicker the fibers, the longer the segments. If an axon gives off collateral branches, this takes place at a node of Ranvier.

In fixed preparations of peripheral nerves, the myelin of each segment appears to be interrupted by oblique cone-shaped discontinuities, the *incisures* or *clefts of Schmidt-Lantermann*, several to each Schwann segment (Figs. 12-16, 12-17 and 12-22). These clefts, seen also in teased fresh or osmicated nerves, represent areas of loosening or local separation of the spirally wrapped myelin lamellae, which are nevertheless continuous across the incisures. The regions between the separated lamellae consist of Schwann cell cytoplasm continuous with that forming the outer sleeve of the nerve fiber on the one hand, and with a thin, inconstant layer of cytoplasm next to the axon on the other.

The exact relationship of the Schwann sheath to unmyelinated axons cannot be visualized with the light microscope, but in electron micrographs it is evident that multiple axons, up to a dozen or more, may occupy deep recesses in the surface of the same Schwann cell (Figs. 12-18 and 12-19). The plasmalemma of the Schwann cell is closely applied to the axon and, as a rule, completely surrounds it. At some point around the periphery of each axon, however, the Schwann cell membrane turns back to form the *mesaxon*, a pair of parallel membranes marking the line of edge-to-edge contact of the encircling sheath cell (Fig. 12-20).

---

*Originally the word *neurilemma*, as employed by European workers early in the twentieth century, meant the connective tissue tunic, continuous with the pia mater, known today as the endoneurium. English-speaking authors, however, used the term to designate the clear layer of Schwann membranes defined above in the text. A related term, *axolemma*, originally referred to the inner membrane of the Schwann cell, but it is now commonly used to signify the plasmalemma of the axon.

Schwann cells are indispensable for the life and function of the axons of peripheral nerve fibers. In regeneration, the new axon grows out of the central stump continuous with the cell body of the neuron and follows the path formed by Schwann cells. In tissue culture, Schwann cells may transform into phagocytes.

The Myelin Sheath

Before the advent of biological electron microscopy, x-ray diffraction analysis suggested that the myelin sheath was composed of concentrically wrapped layers of mixed lipids alternating with thin, possibly unimolecular, layers of neurokeratinogenic protein material. Within the layers, the lipid molecules were thought to be oriented with hydrocarbon chains extending radially and with polar groups aligned at the aqueous interfaces, loosely bonded to the proteins. In general, electron microscopic studies have supported this interpretation of the molecular organization of myelin and have shown that the alternating layers of mixed lipids and proteins are in fact successive layers of the plasma membrane of the Schwann cell wrapped spirally about the axon.

In electron micrographs at high magnifi-

cation, compact myelin presents as a series of light and dark lines in a repeating pattern of about 120 Å (Fig. 12–18). The dark line bounding the repeating unit is called the *major dense line* and is about 30 Å thick; it represents the apposition of the inner (cytoplasmic) surfaces of the unit membrane of the Schwann cell. Between major dense lines is a less dense *intraperiod line*, which represents the union of the outer surfaces of the Schwann cell unit membrane (Fig. 12–20).

Where the laminated myelin sheath is interrupted at each node of Ranvier, the axon is surrounded loosely by a collar of minute finger-like processes of the two adjoining Schwann cells. A distinct gap, however, is found between all the membranes in this unmyelinated part of the node (Fig. 12–22). This gap probably is of significance in relation to current flow between axoplasm and the exterior during propagation of the action potential.

In electron micrographs of myelinating peripheral nerves, successive stages can be found in the development of the sheath from a double-layered infolding of the Schwann cell membrane (Figs. 12–20; 12–21). The mechanism of formation of the spiral, consisting of a few to 50 or more turns around the axon, is still unsettled. It has been sug-

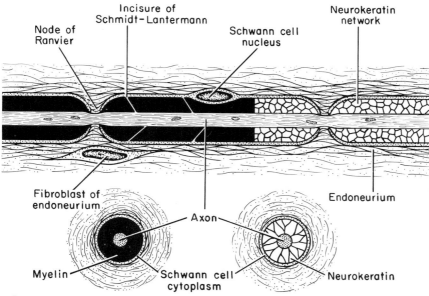

Figure 12-17 Diagrammatic representation of longitudinal sections and cross sections of a single myelinated nerve fiber and its endoneurial sheath. The left half of the drawing represents what would be seen after fixation with osmium tetroxide, which preserves the lipid of myelin. The right half represents the appearance after ordinary methods of histological preparation, which extract the myelin and leave behind an artefactitious network of residual protein described as "neurokeratin." (Redrawn from A. W. Ham, Histology. 5th Ed. Philadelphia, J. B. Lippincott Company, 1965.)

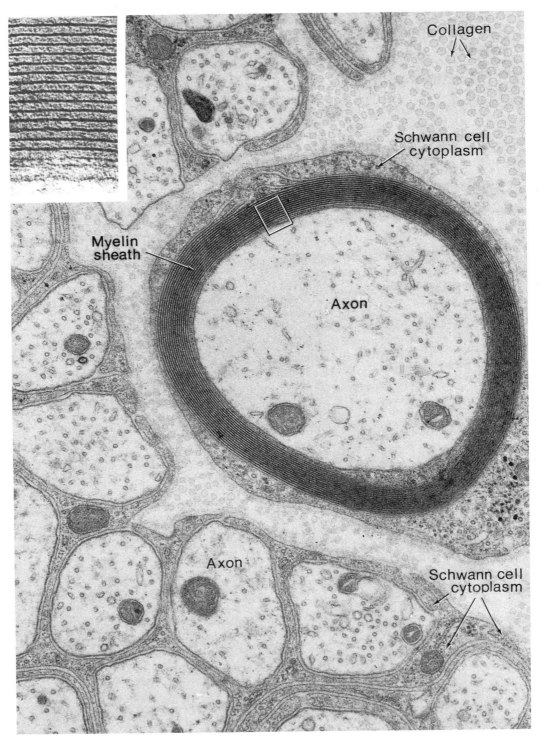

Figure 12-18 Electron micrograph of a small area of rat sciatic nerve in cross section. Included are a large myelinated nerve and several groups of unmyelinated nerve axons occupying deep recesses in the surface of Schwann cells. The area of the myelin sheath enclosed in the box is illustrated at higher magnification in the inset, in which the major dense lines and intraperiod lines of myelin can be seen. (From H. Webster, The Vertebrate Peripheral Nervous System, ed. John Hubbard. New York, Plenum Press, 1974.)

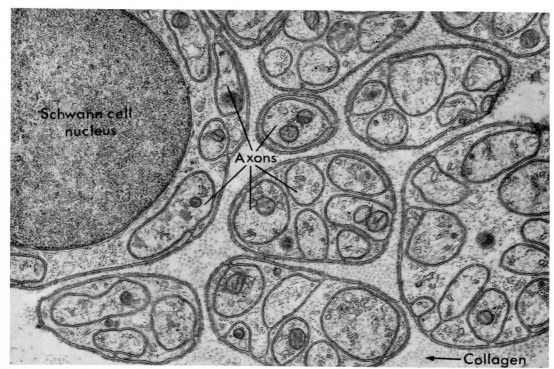

Figure 12-19   Electron micrograph of a small area of an unmyelinated nerve from the rat mesentery, showing multiple axons associated with the cross-sectional profile of each Schwann cell. Between these fascicles of unmyelinated axons are unit fibrils of collagen of the endoneurium. × 25,000.

gested that during myelinization, the spiral disposition of the myelin lamellae is established by rotation of the sheath cells with respect to the axon (Fig. 12–20). It is difficult, however, to imagine how such movements could be initiated or controlled so as to result in formation of the precisely uniform laminated structure observed. Recent studies indicate that the myelin spiral does not develop because of any sort of corkscrew rotation during growth. If this were the mechanism, the direction of spiral for a particular axon would probably be the same in all its myelin segments, and such is not the case.

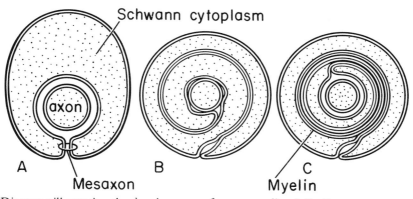

Figure 12-20   Diagrams illustrating the development of nerve myelin. *A,* Earliest stage: axon enveloped by a relatively large Schwann cell. *B,* Intermediate stage: unit membranes of mesaxon and to some extent of axon have come together, line of contact representing future *intraperiod* line of myelin. *C,* Later stage: a few layers of compact myelin have formed by contact of cytoplasmic surfaces of mesaxon loops to make *major dense line* of myelin. (Redrawn from Robertson, Prog. Biophys., *10:*349, 1960.)

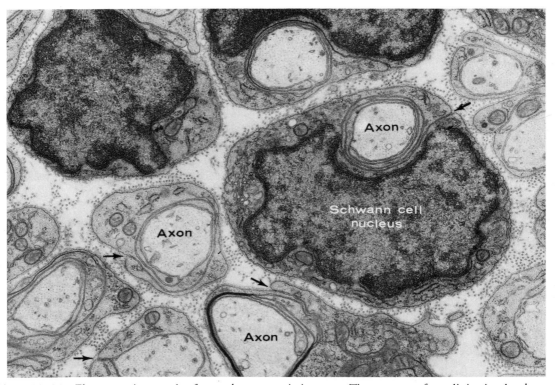

Figure 12–21 Electron micrograph of a newborn rat sciatic nerve. The process of myelinization has begun, and a few loose turns of the spiral of the Schwann cell membrane can be seen around several of the axons. The one at the lower center shows that a few layers of compact myelin have formed on one side of the axon, by contact of the cytoplasmic surfaces of mesaxon loops. The arrows point to the continuity of the two layers of the mesaxons with the Schwann cell surface membrane. (Micrograph courtesy of Henry Webster.)

Apparently the Schwann cell alone actively produces the spiral, and no interaction occurs between individual Schwann cells so far as the direction of spiral is concerned. Formation of new membrane at the free edge of the original infolding of the satellite cell membrane probably extends the fold spirally around the axon without significant change in the relative position of the neuron and its satellite cells. Much remains to be learned concerning the morphogenesis of myelin, but whatever the morphogenetic process, the result is that the axon becomes surrounded by a many-layered sheath. The measurements across lamellae indicate a thickness of about 130 to 180 Å.

In myelinated fibers of the central nervous system, certain neuroglial cells (oligodendroglia) play a role corresponding to that of the Schwann cells in the peripheral nervous system. Nodes of Ranvier occur in the central nervous system, but Schmidt-Lantermann clefts have not been seen.

In ontogenesis, myelin appears relatively late, and the process of myelinization ends some time after birth. Different fiber systems or tracts of the brain and spinal cord become myelinated at different times.

Nerve Fibers as Constituents of Peripheral Nerves, Brain and Spinal Cord

In their course outside the central nervous system, nerve fibers of varying thickness (from 1 or 2 μm. to up to 30 μm.) are associated in fascicles and held together by connective tissue to form nerve trunks. The outer layer of the trunk, the *epineurium*, is made up of connective tissue cells and collagenous fibers, mainly arranged longitudinally (Fig. 12–24). Fat cells may also be found here. Each of the smaller fascicles of a nerve is enclosed in dense, concentric layers of connective tissue, the *perineurium*. Fine longitudinally arranged strands of collagenous fibers, fibroblasts, and fixed macrophages pass into the spaces between the individual nerve fibers to form the *endoneurium.* Where the nerve branches, the connective tissue sheaths become thinner. The smaller branches lack epineurium, and the perineurium cannot be distinguished from the endoneurium, being reduced to a thin, fibrillar layer covered with flat connective tissue cells resembling endothelial cells. Delicate reticular fibrils around each nerve fiber form the tenuous endoneurial sheath. Blood vessels are embedded in the epineurium and perineurium and more rarely in the thicker layers of endoneurium.

It has become customary to classify nerve fibers according to their diameter, because the speed of impulse transmission and the size of the action potential vary with the diameter of the fiber. Diameters cover a wide and continuous range from large myelinated to small unmyelinated fibers. In peripheral nerves the fibers fall into three distinct groups.

The large fibers, group A, conduct at 15 to 100 meters per second and include motor and some sensory fibers. Group B fibers conduct at 3 to 14 meters per second and include mainly visceral sensory fibers. The C group, small unmyelinated fibers conducting at 0.5 to 2 meters per second, carry autonomic and some sensory impulses. Other systems of classification besides this one are used in physiological studies.

Motor nerve fibers of the skeletal muscles are thick and heavily myelinated; those of visceral smooth muscle are thin, lightly myelinated, or without myelin. Tactile fibers are medium-sized and moderately myelinated; pain and taste fibers are thinner, with less myelin or none at all, and olfactory nerve filaments are always unmyelinated. Such histologically defined fiber aggregates therefore constitute functional systems: somatic motor, visceral motor, tactile, gustatory, olfactory, and so forth.

Clear segregation of functionally dif-

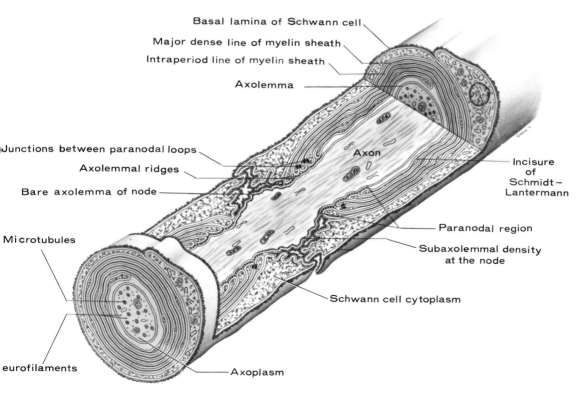

Figure 12-22 Diagrammatic representation of the myelin sheath, node of Ranvier, and incisures of Schmidt-Lantermann in a peripheral nerve. (Courtesy of D. Kent Morest.)

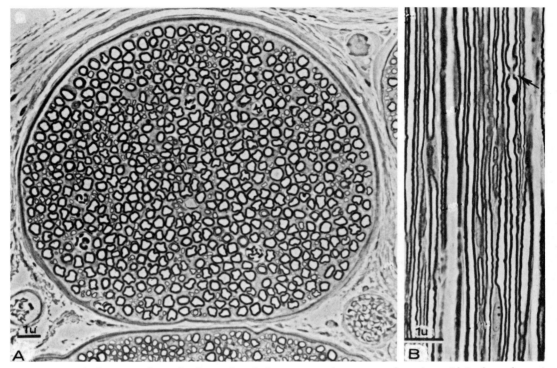

Figure 12–23 A, Cross section of guinea pig sciatic nerve, as it appears after glutaraldehyde and osmium fixation and embedding in eponaraldite. The myelin sheaths have been well preserved and are seen as black rims around the axons. B, Longitudinal section of sciatic nerve similarly prepared. The arrow points to a node of Ranvier. (From H. Webster, The Vertebrate Peripheral Nervous System, ed. John Hubbard. New York, Plenum Press, 1974.)

ferent nerve fibers is found in the *spinal roots.* In the ventral root are motor fibers of several types: (1) coarse and heavily myelinated, innervating ordinary skeletal muscle fibers; (2) small and myelinated, terminating on intrafusal muscle fibers (to be discussed later); and (3) fine and lightly myelinated, belonging to the autonomic nervous system. The dorsal root contains sensory fibers from superficial and deep cutaneous regions, sensory fibers from muscles and tendons, and afferent fibers from viscera. More than half of the dorsal root fibers are very small axons; most of these distribute with the cutaneous rami. The relative numbers of myelinated and unmyelinated fibers vary widely in different spinal segments and in the same segment in different mammalian species. In the mixed trunks peripheral to the spinal ganglia, the fibers of motor and sensory roots mingle, together with sympathetic fibers from the communicating rami. In mixed trunks stained with hematoxylin and eosin or another routine method, the lipid constituents of myelin are dissolved out, leaving a loosely arranged pro-

tein network called *neurokeratin* (Figs. 12–17 and 12–25). A faintly stained axis cylinder can usually be seen in the center of this network. In such preparations, myelinated fibers of various sizes are readily identified by the clear zones of unstained myelin surrounding the darkly stained axons. Unmyelinated fibers tend to assemble in small fascicles: some are sensory fibers from the spinal ganglia; others are postganglionic sympathetic fibers.

In the brain and spinal cord, nerve fibers also segregate into functional systems, the *afferent* (incoming) and *efferent* (outgoing) pathways (spinocerebellar, spinothalamic, corticobulbar, corticospinal, and other fiber tracts whose origins and terminations are indicated by binomial nomenclature). Each has a special function, part of which is well known, but much of which is still obscure.

PERIPHERAL NERVE ENDINGS

Each peripheral nerve fiber, sensory, motor, or secretory, sooner or later ends in some peripheral organ with one or several terminal arborizations. Some nerve fibers ramify as free endings among the non-nervous tissue cells; others attach to tissue cells by means of specialized terminations. The fibers ending in *receptors* are dendrites; those with *motor* or *secretory* endings are axons, their terminations being called *axon endings.* In general, the structure of the ending is adapted to increase the surface of contact between the neuron and its related non-nervous element. The physicochemical changes which mediate the transfer of the various stimuli from, or the nerve impulses to, a peripheral non-nervous structure have been intensively studied. Three groups of nerve terminations can be distinguished: (1) endings in muscle, (2) endings in epithelium, and (3) endings in connective tissue.

Nerve Endings in Smooth and Cardiac Muscle

From complicated plexuses, thin unmyelinated nerve fibers depart and eventually contact or approach the surface of the muscle cells. *Visceral motor endings* terminate by means of one, two, or more terminal swellings. *Visceral sensory fibers* ramify in the connective tissue between smooth muscle bundles or contact the muscle fibers themselves. In cardiac muscle the tissue is permeated by a multitude of thin fibers passing between muscle trabeculae. They appear to end near the surface of the muscle fibers but form no specialized contacts with them.

Terminations of Myelinated Somatic Motor Nerve Fibers on Striated Muscles (Motor End Plates)

These terminations have a more complex structure than those of smooth and cardiac muscle. The motor end plate has already been described in Chapter 11, and need only be reviewed here briefly.

Each motor nerve fiber branches to supply many muscle fibers. The motor neuron together with the muscle fibers it innervates is called a *motor unit.* The myelin sheath ends as a terminal branch of the nerve fiber nears

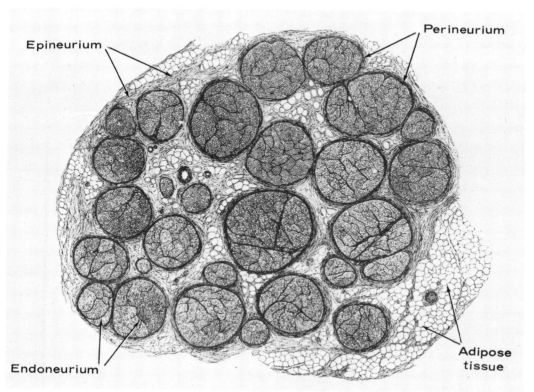

Figure 12-24   Drawing of a histological cross section of a human ulnar nerve at very low magnification, illustrating the perineural adipose tissue, epineurium, perineurium, and endoneurium. (From Bargmann, Histologie und mikroskopische Anatomie des Menschen. Stuttgart, Georg Thieme, 1959.)

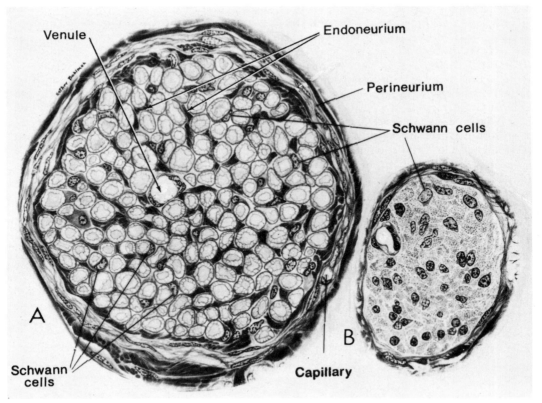

Figure 12-25 Drawing of myelinated (*A*) and unmyelinated nerve (*B*) as they appear in cross section in routine histological preparations.

the muscle fiber. The outer process of Schwann cell cytoplasm continues beyond the termination of the myelin and covers the surfaces of the axonal branch. At the junction of the nerve and muscle fiber is a local accumulation of sarcoplasm rich in mitochondria and muscle nuclei, the *motor end plate* (Fig. 12–26). The terminal branches of the nerve fiber ramify upon it and occupy grooves or troughs in its surface (see Fig. 11–25). Within the expanded axon terminal are numerous mitochondria and *synaptic vesicles*, 200 to 400 Å in diameter. The neurofilaments and microtubules found within the axon do not continue into the terminal. The apposed membranes of the axon and of the muscle fiber do not touch but are separated everywhere by a glycoprotein layer continuous with the boundary layer investing the Schwann cell and the sarcolemma. This layer extends into the trough and the narrow gutters formed by infolding of the sarcolemma of the end plate. The gap

between the surfaces of the axon and muscle fiber varies in width up to 500 Å.

Sensory Nerve Endings in Striated Muscles

These are always present in considerable numbers, some in the muscular tissue, others on tendons or at muscle-tendon junctions. Some terminations are simple, others complex. The *interstitial terminations* are distributed in the connective tissue; the *epilemmal terminations* closely contact the muscle fibers. The interstitial terminations may be simple naked branches of the axons or encapsulated structures. The epilemmal endings likewise may be simple: one or more tortuous axons, after shedding their myelin sheath at approximately the midpoint of a muscle fiber, envelop the sarcolemma in continuous circular and spiral twists. Their varicose twigs terminate with nodular swellings. More complicated *neuromuscular spindles*, found only in higher vertebrates (Fig. 12–27), are long (0.75 to 7 mm. or more), narrow structures arranged parallel to the bundles of ordinary muscle fibers, and situated mainly near the junction of muscles with tendons. Each spindle, enveloped by a connective tissue capsule, consists of one or several long striated muscle fibers, the *intrafusal fibers* (see also Chapter 11). Midway along each fiber, the striations are replaced by a collection of nuclei, the *nuclear bag*. Another type of intrafusal fiber displays a longitudinal array of nuclei, or *nuclear chain*. Each spindle is approached by two types of thick sensory nerve fibers. The larger axons form *annulospiral endings* around the noncontractile nuclear bag. This primary receptor signals both the rate and extent of muscle lengthening. The intrafusal muscle fibers are attached parallel to the other (*extrafusal*) muscle fibers

and are stretched whenever the muscle is stretched. Heightened activity of the primary receptors exerts an excitatory effect upon the motor neurons to the same muscle by a direct reflex connection in the central nervous system. The thinner axons have *flower-spray endings* which innervate the contractile portions of the intrafusal muscle fibers. This receptor signals the extent, more than the rate, of muscle lengthening, but its function is not yet clear.

Neuromuscular spindles are also supplied by thin motor nerves, *gamma fibers*, which emanate from small *gamma motor neurons* in the central nervous system. (The large motor neurons which send axons to the extrafusal muscle fibers are called *alpha motor neurons*). The gamma fibers terminate on the intrafusal muscle fibers with typical motor end plates. These fibers effect shortening of

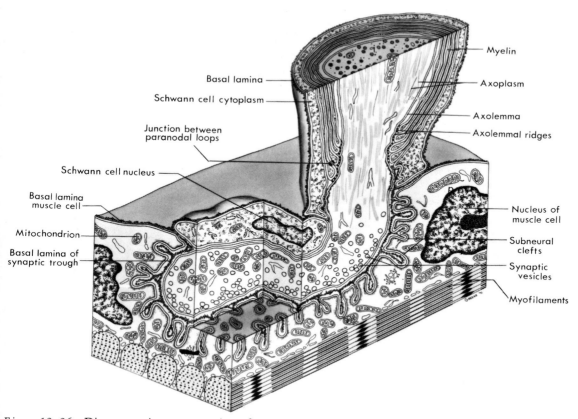

Figure 12–26 Diagrammatic representation of a myoneural junction (motor end plate), illustrating a typical chemical synapse in the peripheral nervous system. Synapses in the central nervous system have some features in common with this, but they occur between neurons, and have no basal lamina or postjunctional folds. (Courtesy of D. Kent Morest.)

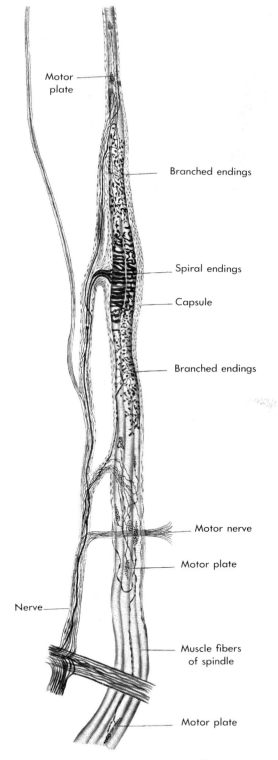

Motor plate

Branched endings

Spiral endings

Capsule

Branched endings

Motor nerve

Motor plate

Nerve

Muscle fibers of spindle

Motor plate

Figure 12-27 Neuromuscular spindle of a cat, showing nerve endings. (Redrawn after Ruffini.)

the striated, contractile portions of the intrafusal fibers. These contractions do not contribute significantly to the tension produced by the muscle but serve instead to stretch the noncontractile nuclear bag where the annulospiral endings are located. Such stretching causes the receptor to discharge more rapidly; hence the function of the gamma fibers is to regulate the sensitivity of the neuromuscular spindle to stretch. The muscle fibers of the spindles are distinguished by their thinness, abundant sarcoplasm, and peripheral nuclei; in this they resemble red muscle fibers (see Chapter 11).

Sensory Nerve Endings in Tendons

These are of several kinds and also may be either simple or encapsulated. In simple forms, the naked nerve fibers and their branches spread over the surface of the tendon fibers in small treelike figures of different types. Such endings in tendons and fasciae probably carry pain sensation. Composite forms, the Golgi tendon organs, which occur at the junction of muscle fibers with intramuscular connective tissue or with tendons, resemble neuromuscular spindles and are sometimes called *neurotendinal spindles.* In contrast to neuromuscular spindles, however, which are placed in parallel with the other muscle fibers, the Golgi tendon organs are in series with the contractile elements. These receptors respond to increase in tension; a heightened activity of the receptors exerts an inhibitory effect, through interneurons of the central nervous system, upon the alpha motor neurons of the same muscle.

The physiological significance of the sensory endings in muscles and tendons has been clarified greatly in recent years, as has their morphology. These receptors participate in postural and phasic adjustments of skeletal musculature. Intimate and complex connections in the central nervous system relate their activity to the alpha and gamma motor neurons. This activity, however, should not be described as "muscle sense" or "position sense"; awareness of the position of the body parts in space appears to be mediated by receptors located in joints.

Nerve Endings in Epithelial Tissue

Histologically, receptors and effectors can be distinguished only in rare instances.

The terminations in the epithelial layers of the skin and mucous membranes are probably only sensory, and those in the epithelial glands partly secretory, partly sensory. Terminations of the cochlear and vestibular nerves of the inner ear are undoubtedly sensory. Endings in glands (lacrimal, salivary, kidneys, and so on) are all unmyelinated sympathetic fibers forming dense nets on the outer surface of the basal lamina; branches penetrate the lamina, often forming a second network on its inner surface, and end between the gland cells.

Free sensory epithelial endings are abundant where sensitivity is highly developed: in the epithelium of the cornea, in the mucous membrane of the respiratory passages and oral cavity, and in the skin. In the epidermis, these branches do not penetrate farther than the granular layer. Free nerve endings in hair follicles are important tactile organs. There are two sets of endings—one circularly arranged in the middle layer of the dermal sheath, the other consisting of fibers running parallel to the hair shaft and terminating in the outer root sheath.

Nerve Endings in Connective Tissue

These are numerous and of many forms, particularly in the dermis, under the epithelium and mesothelium of the mucous and serous membranes, around the joints, in the endocardium, and elsewhere. They are either free or encapsulated endings, or are connected with special tactile cells of epithelial origin. More complex endings are found in skin and hypodermis, mucous and serous membranes, endocardium, cornea, sclera, and periosteum. Nonencapsulated endings are frequent in the papillary layer of the skin, connective tissue of mucous membranes (such as that of the urinary bladder), and pericardium, endocardium, and periosteum; the terminal branches form spherical or elongated structures resembling glomeruli.

Encapsulated Terminal Sensory Endings

In these, a special connective tissue capsule of varying thickness surrounds the actual nerve endings. The capsule attains its greatest thickness in the *corpuscles of Vater-Pacini*

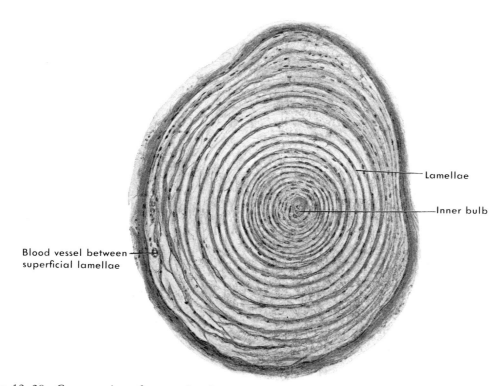

Lamellae

Inner bulb

Blood vessel between superficial lamellae

Figure 12–28 Cross section of corpuscle of Vater-Pacini, from dermis of the sole of a human foot. × 110. (After Schaffer.)

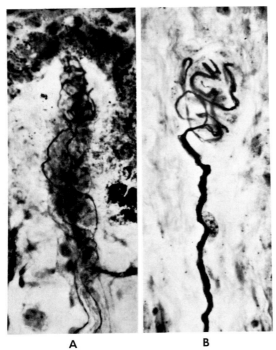

A   B

Figure 12-29 *A,* Genital corpuscle from the glans penis of a 23 year old man. Silver preparation. × 800. (Courtesy of N. Cauna.) *B,* Lingual corpuscle from a filiform papilla on the tongue of a 21 year old woman. Silver stain. × 600. (From N. Cauna, Anat. Rec., *124*:77, 1956.)

(Fig. 12–28), found in the deeper layers of the skin, under mucous membranes, in conjunctiva, cornea, heart, mesentery, and pancreas, and in loose connective tissue. These structures are large (1 to 4 mm. by 2 mm.) and white in color. Each is supplied with one or more thick myelinated fibers, which lose myelin upon entering the corpuscle. Their endoneurial sheaths are continuous with the capsule. *Genital corpuscles,* in the skin of the external genital organs and of the nipple, are similar (Fig. 12–29A). *Meissner's corpuscles* (Figs. 12–30, 12–31 and 12–32), occurring in connective tissue of the skin of the palms, soles, and tips of the fingers and toes, are elongated, pear-shaped, or elliptical formations with rounded ends, located in the cutaneous papillae, with the long axis vertical to the surface. Their size varies (40 to 100 μm. by 30 to 60 μm.). *Corpuscles of Golgi-Mazzoni* and *terminal bulbs of Krause* resemble corpuscles of Vater-Pacini but are smaller and simpler in construction.

AUTONOMIC NERVOUS SYSTEM

Motor neurons of the central and peripheral nervous system concerned with the regulation of visceral activities form the *autonomic nervous system.* This system, as defined long ago, unfortunately excludes the *visceral sensory neurons,* or interoceptive system, which form the afferent side of visceral arcs.

The autonomic nervous system includes numerous small ganglia. The *vertebral ganglia* form a chain, *the sympathetic trunk,* on either side of the spinal column; the sympathetic trunk is connected proximally with the ventral roots of the spinal nerves. Additional ganglia lie at some distance from the central nervous system in certain nerve plexuses *(collateral* or *prevertebral ganglia)* or in the walls of organs *(terminal ganglia).* The autonomic ganglia contain motor nerve cell bodies, which convey impulses originating in the brain and spinal cord to smooth muscle and glands by way of the *visceral* or *splanchnic* nerves (Fig. 12–33). Fibers of some cell bodies in the sympathetic trunk join those in the peripheral nerves and run to the sweat glands and arrector pili muscles. Whatever the destination, the autonomic nervous system mediates activity by *two* motor neurons placed in series; the first lies either in a nucleus of the brain stem or in a special territory of the spinal gray matter, and the second is located in a ganglion. In the peripheral nervous system, only one motor neuron transmits activity to the effector organ. The autonomic system consists of *sympathetic (thoracolumbar)* and *parasympathetic (craniosacral)* divisions: it influences the intrinsic activity of cardiac muscle and supplies nerve fibers to smooth muscle in the viscera, salivary and sweat glands, blood vessels, and other structures. The peripheral nervous system, in contrast, innervates striated skeletal muscle. Despite these distinctions, however, the traditional concept of an autonomic nervous system is justifiable only in terms of convenience; its components and functions are inextricably bound up with the rest of the nervous system and do not possess autonomy.

The sympathetic trunks and their ganglia, as well as the collateral ganglia, are the avenues of communication for the thoracolumbar outflow between the central nervous

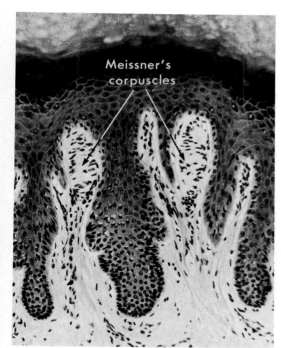

Figure 12–30 Photomicrograph of palmar digital epidermis showing Meissner's corpuscles in two neighboring dermal papillae. Hematoxylin and eosin. × 200.

system and the viscera. Each sympathetic trunk contains ganglia at the level of exit of most of the corresponding spinal nerves. The *communicating branches* (rami communicantes) pass between the trunk and the spinal nerves.

The cell bodies of the sympathetic neurons lie in the *intermediolateral gray column* of the thoracic and upper lumbar spinal cord. The axons pass into the ventral roots of spinal nerves and through the white communicating branches, to end either in a vertebral ganglion of the sympathetic trunk or in a prevertebral ganglion. Most of these axons, the *preganglionic fibers*, with thin myelin sheaths, terminate in a sympathetic ganglion. Here they synapse with secondary visceral motor neurons, whose axons—mostly unmyelinated postganglionic fibers— transmit activity to visceral muscles or glands. Some postganglionic fibers travel to internal viscera over sympathetic nerves, such as the cardiac or splanchnic nerves; others extend from vertebral ganglia through gray communicating branches and spinal nerves to structures of the body wall and extremities: *vasomotor fibers*

chiefly to arteriolar muscles, *pilomotor fibers* to the small muscles of hair follicles, and *sudomotor fibers* to the sweat glands.

The craniosacral division of the autonomic system has preganglionic neurons in the brain and spinal cord. Axons of the cranial component emerge in the oculomotor, facial, glossopharyngeal, and vagus nerves, to synapse with terminal ganglia innervating the head and trunk. From the second, third, and fourth sacral segments of the spinal cord, axons leave via ventral roots and sacral nerves to reach postganglionic neurons in terminal ganglia associated with pelvic viscera.

Postganglionic neurons may exercise a local regulatory control over the viscera to which they are related, secondarily subject to control by components of the central nervous system.

Distributed via both divisions of the autonomic nervous system, the peripheral processes of visceral sensory neurons lead from the viscera through the communicating rami, or through cranial or sacral nerves, to sensory ganglia. Their cell bodies are morphologically indistinguishable from those of the somatic sensory neurons, with which they mingle in the craniospinal ganglia.

Autonomic Nerve Cells

The cell bodies of preganglionic visceral efferent neurons are small, spindle-shaped elements in the intermediolateral gray column. Their perikarya are not studded with innumerable terminal boutons, as are the large nerve cell bodies of somatic motor neurons. Instead, a relatively small number of axodendritic endings is found.

Postganglionic neurons of the craniosacral division lie, as a rule, close to the viscera innervated. The preganglionic fibers, accordingly, are relatively long—as in the vagus nerve—and the postganglionic fibers short. On the other hand, most synapses of the thoracolumbar division are in the sympathetic trunk or collateral ganglia; therefore the postganglionic fibers are longer.

Sympathetic ganglion cells are generally small and have diverse shapes. The cells are generally multipolar, dendrites and axon sometimes being distinguishable but in other cases showing no obvious difference. Preganglionic fibers often synapse with the

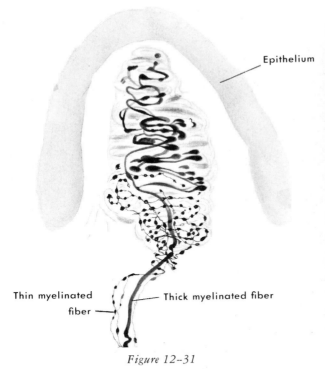

Epithelium

Thin myelinated fiber

Thick myelinated fiber

Figure 12–31

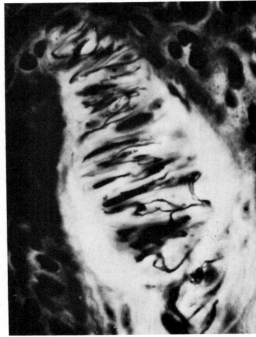

Figure 12–32

Figure 12–31   Meissner's corpuscle of a dermal papilla of a human finger. Methylene blue stain. (Redrawn after Dogiel.)
Figure 12–32   Meissner's corpuscle of an 11 year old girl. Silver stain. (Courtesy of N. Cauna.)

dendrites of the ganglion cell in dense glomeruli. For a typical example, see the description of the postganglionic neurons of the intestine (p. 682).

The cell body may be encapsulated by satellite cells, which, like those of the craniospinal ganglia, are ectodermal elements similar to Schwann cells in the nerve sheaths. In the outlying sympathetic ganglia these capsules may be absent, but Schwann cells accompany the peripheral sympathetic fibers everywhere.

NEUROGLIA

The number of nerve cells within the central nervous system, although enormous, is exceeded, perhaps fivefold, by the number of non-neural supportive cells called the neuroglial cells or neuroglia ("nerve glue"). The term neuroglia is applied to the ependyma, which lines the ventricles of the brain and spinal cord and to *neuroglial cells* and their processes, which mingle with neurons in the central nervous system and retina. The *satellite* or *capsular cells* of periph-

eral ganglia and the *Schwann cells* of peripheral nerves may be considered peripheral neuroglia.

Ependyma

In early embryonic stages the wall of the neural tube is a simple epithelium. Certain thin, non-nervous parts of the brain retain this structure throughout adult life, as for example, the epithelial layer of the choroid plexus (see Figs. 12–40 and 12–41). In most other parts, the wall is greatly thickened by the accumulation of neurons and neuroglial elements. The lining of the inner surface enclosing the ventricular cavities always retains an epithelial character. This membrane, the adult ependyma, is composed of the inner ends of epithelial cells, with their nuclei and some of their cytoplasm.

The embryonic ependyma is ciliated; in some parts of the ventricular lining the cilia may persist into adult life. In the mature brain, the broad bases of ependymal cells taper to long, threadlike processes that branch and are lost among other elements of the brain. In a few places, where the wall is thin, as in the ventral fissure of the spinal cord, some ependymal cells span the entire distance between ventricular and external surfaces, as all do in the early embryonic stages. In these cases, the ependymal cells form a dense *internal limiting membrane* at the ventricular end. The adult ependyma may represent the remaining epithelial cells of the embryonic ventricular zone (see section on development, p. 373) or may be derived from a specialized subventricular zone which appears later in development and persists into adult life.

At the external surface, under the *pia mater*, the ependymal threads and bars expand into pedicles that fuse into a thin, smooth, dense membrane, the *external limiting membrane* of the central nervous system. Similar membranes are formed around the blood vessels.

Neuroglial Cells

In any section of the central nervous system prepared by ordinary histological methods, small nuclei are seen scattered among the nerve cells and their processes. The cytoplasm and long processes of these neuroglial elements are demonstrable by special histological techniques.

Three types of neuroglia are distinguished: *astrocytes, oligodendrocytes,* and *microglia*. The first two, collectively *macroglia*, are ectodermal in origin, as are the nerve cells. The microglia are said to originate from mesodermal cells of the pia mater, which migrate into the central nervous system along the blood vessels.

The astrocytes are of two varieties. The *protoplasmic astrocyte* has a larger nucleus than oligodendrocytes and microglia, abundant

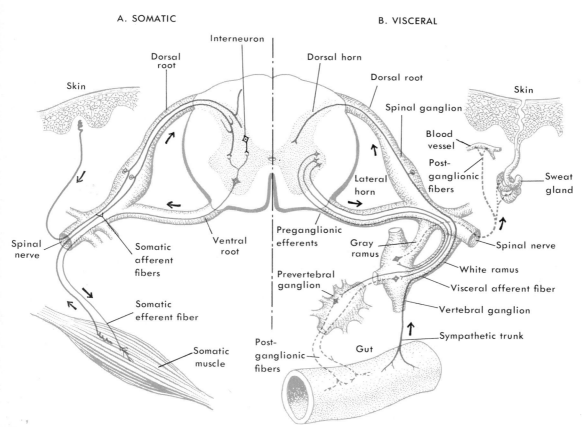

Figure 12-33 A, Somatic nerves. *B,* Visceral nerves. A cross section of spinal cord is shown connected via dorsal and ventral roots to the spinal nerve and to one of the ganglia of the autonomic system. The pattern of afferent (blue) and efferent (red) nerve fibers in both the somatic and visceral system may be directly compared. From Copenhaver and Bunge (eds.), Bailey's Textbook of Histology. 16th Ed. Baltimore, Williams and Wilkins, 1971.

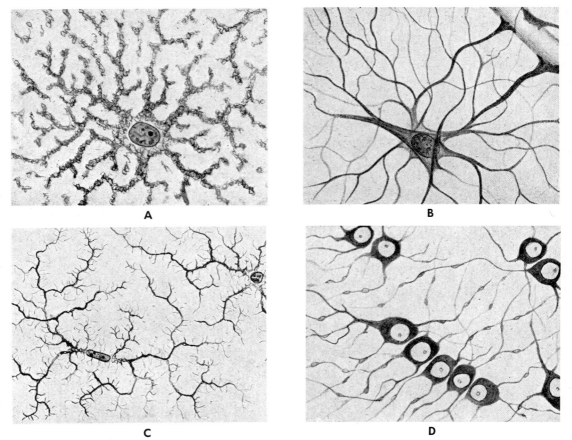

Figure 12-34 Neuroglial cells of the central nervous system. *A*, Protoplasmic astrocyte. *B*, Fibrous astrocyte. *C*, Microglia. *D*, Oligodendroglia. (After del Rio-Hortega.)

granular cytoplasm, and numerous, thick processes (Fig. 12–34*A*). Many processes attach to blood vessels and to the pia mater by means of expanded pedicles. In other cases, the cell body lies directly on the wall of the blood vessel or on the inner surface of the pia mater. Some of the smaller cells of this variety lie close to the bodies of the neurons and represent one type of satellite cell.

The *fibrous astrocyte* (Fig. 12–34*B*) is distinguished by long, relatively thin, smooth, and infrequently branched expansions. Embedded within the cytoplasm are fibrillar structures. Electron micrographs show that the neuroglial fibers of light microscopy result from aggregation of the slender filaments present in profusion in the cytoplasm. These cells also are often attached to blood vessels by means of their processes. Protoplasmic astrocytes are found chiefly in gray matter and fibrous astrocytes in white matter,

insinuated between fascicles of nerve fibers. Mixed or *plasmatofibrous astrocytes* are occasionally encountered at the boundary between gray and white matter; processes that spread into the gray have a protoplasmic character, whereas those that pass into the white are fibrous.

The oligodendrocytes (or oligodendroglia) (Fig. 12–34*D*) are akin to the astrocytes, which they resemble in many respects. They are smaller and have smaller nuclei, although there are many transitional forms. The name signifies that their few and slender processes have few branches. Oligodendrocytes relate intimately to nerve fibers, along which they form rows or columns. Although it is difficult to demonstrate the connection of the oligodendrocyte with the myelin sheath in the adult, studies on the developing nervous system show that this cell forms myelin in the central nervous system. Thus it is the homologue of the neurilemmal cell of Schwann. In gray matter, oligodendrocytes adjoining nerve cells are the principal type of satellite cell. In tissue cultures, oligodendrocytes exhibit rhythmic pulsatile movements. The significance of this behavior in relation to their normal function in the brain is not known. The criteria for identification of the several types of macroglia in electron micrographs have only been partially established.

In the microglia (Fig. 12–34C), the nucleus is small but deeply stained and surrounded by scant protoplasm. The few extensions are short and, unlike the more or less straight extensions of the astrocytes, are twisted in various ways. Also, the processes and the cell body are not smooth, but are covered with numerous tiny pointed twigs or spines. Microglia are scattered everywhere throughout the brain and spinal cord.

In the mature CNS, and also it seems now during development, neuroglia provide an extremely complex framework for the neurons, a scaffolding for migratory young neurocytes and their cell processes. Like the neurons, the supporting neuroglial cells do not form a syncytium, but retain their individuality. In the chambers of a complex labyrinth of glial cells, the nerve cells and their processes are often individually encapsulated and thus insulated from one another. An interesting and probably significant fact revealed by electron microscopy is that wherever nerve cell bodies and their processes are not in synaptic contact with another neuron, they are generally enveloped by the cell bodies or processes of neuroglial cells. The distribution of these neuroglial processes thus appears neither to be random nor merely to fulfill the requirements of mechanical support and nutrition of the neurons. Early in this century, Ramón y Cajal proposed that neuroglial processes are always disposed to prevent contact between processes of nerve cells at sites other than those appropriate to their specific signaling function. On the basis of electron microscopic observations, Palay has revived this hypothesis and has shown that each neuron has a characteristic pattern of neuroglial investment complementary to the specific pattern of its synaptic connections. Only at the synapses are the neuroglial barriers interrupted, and only here is direct contact between the neurons possible. Thus, by isolating and individualizing the many diverse pathways that may converge upon a given neuron, the neuroglial cells may play an essential role in the communications function of the nervous system.

Neuroglial cells seem also to be an important mediator for the normal metabolism of neurons, although little is known in this respect. More is known about the activity of neuroglia in states of injury or disease. Whenever neurons are affected by a local or distant pathological process, the surrounding neuroglial elements always react in some way. They are actively involved in degeneration and regeneration of the nerve fibers, in vascular disorders, and in various infectious diseases. They are the chief source of tumors of the central nervous system. Under certain circumstances, microglia may assume a great variety of forms, with active migration and phagocytosis.

THE SYNAPSE AND THE RELATIONSHIPS OF NEURONS

Essentially, the nervous system consists of complex chains of neurons arranged to permit transmission of activity from one neuron to another in one direction only. The site of transmission is the synapse. Physiologically it is of the utmost importance, for it is here that polarization is established, not along dendrites or the axon, where conduction in either direction is possible.

Anatomically, the synapse was traditionally a place of contact of two neurons *in-series*; it may be from axon to dendrite (axodendritic), from axon to perikaryon (axosomatic), or, frequently, from axon to axon (axoaxonic) (Fig. 12–35). Recently, dendrodendritic synapses and synapses between adjacent perikarya have been found; thus, it appears that any part of a neuron can participate in the formation of a synapse. Indeed, *in-parallel* coupling may be of general evolutionary significance, since it is encountered frequently in the nervous systems of invertebrates. The number of synapses on a neuron varies enormously. Some neurons, such as the granule cell of the cerebellum, have only a few. A motor neuron may possess as many as 1800 synapses. A Purkinje cell of the cerebellum may have several hundred thousand endings upon its dendrites alone. The forms of synaptic end-

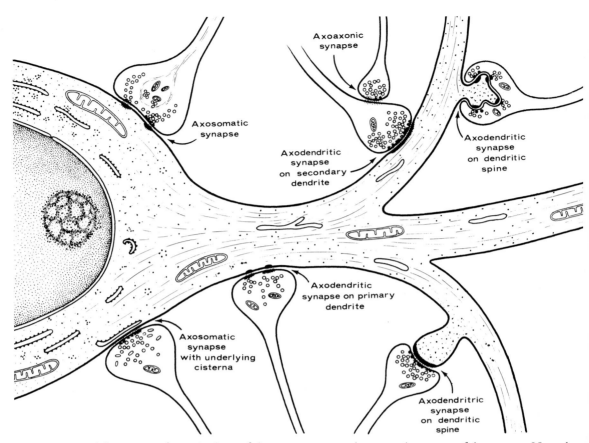

Figure 12–35 The types and terminology of the synapses occurring on various parts of the neuron. Note that the degree of apparent "thickening" of the membrane owing to accumulation of dense material adjacent to it varies in different types of synapses. The material applied to the cytoplasmic side of the presynaptic membrane is often in a regular interrupted pattern rather than a continuous plaque. Redrawn after R. Bunge in Copenhaver and Bunge (eds.), Bailey's Textbook of Histology, 16th Ed. Baltimore, Williams and Wilkins, 1971.

ings also vary in the extreme. Usually they are tiny swellings along the course of axons (synapses *en passant*) or at the tips of axonal branches (*boutons terminaux*), but the terminal twigs may form "bouquets" or loose "baskets," adhering to the body or dendrites of another nerve cell. Each variety of neuron is distinguished by its own form of synaptic terminations, some having endings of several kinds.

In electron micrographs showing synaptic endings in the central nervous system (Figs. 12–36 and 12–37) the axons expand into rounded terminal boutons close to the dendrites or perikarya of other neurons. Neurofilaments may be absent in these endings, which typically contain a cluster of mitochondria and many small organelles (400 to 650 Å), unique to nervous tissue, called *synaptic vesicles*. These are believed to arise by

budding from the ends of the slender tubules of the endoplasmic reticulum present in the axon, and frequently they aggregate near the presynaptic surface. At the synapse, the pre- and postsynaptic membranes are closely apposed, separated only by a narrow extracellular cleft about 200 Å wide, the *synaptic cleft*. Also, at the synapse are local accumulations of filamentous material along the apposing membranes and a subjacent condensation of the cytoplasm (Fig. 12–37). These structures resemble desmosomes and may help to maintain cohesion of the synapsing cells.

The absence of cytoplasmic continuity between neurons forms the basic for the "neuron doctrine"—that each mature nerve cell represents a cellular unit anatomically separate from, and trophically independent of, other neurons. The processes of a neuron depend on the cell body and its nucleus. When cut off from the cell body, the processes die (see p. 382). New processes may, however, grow out from the perikaryon. The body and nucleus of the nerve cell are the trophic center of the entire neuron. If a nerve cell suffers irreparable injury, other nerve cells are not necessarily affected. Nevertheless, certain groups of neurons may atrophy, or degenerate, following interruption of afferent axons or death of other neurons to which they send their efferent output. This phenomenon, *transneuronal degeneration*, for many years has been considered exceptional. It was especially evident in those neuronal subsystems, notably the visual pathway, in which one group of cells along the pathway receives almost all its input from only one other type of cell. Recently, however, it has been found that transneuronal effects are widespread, in both the central and the peripheral nervous systems. Degeneration may be *retrograde* or *anterograde*, depending on the direction, and may involve neurons more than one synapse

removed, hence it may be *primary, secondary, tertiary,* or even *quaternary.* Such findings raise important questions concerning the growth and maintenance of the nervous system and also are crucial facts to consider in interpreting patterns of neuronal atrophy or death after natural or experimental damage to the nervous system.

Transmission of activity from one neuron to another or to an effector is known to involve the passage of a *transmitter substance* across the intervening synaptic cleft. Of particular interest is acetylcholine, found in the central nervous system as well as in peripheral autonomic ganglia and motor end plates. Its hydrolytic (breakdown) enzyme, acetylcholinesterase, has been found in the plexiform layers of the cerebral cortex. Recent fluorescence histochemical methods reveal several central transmitters: norepinephrine, dopamine, and 5-hydroxytryptamine (serotonin); other studies implicate gamma-aminobutyric acid (GABA) as a possible inhibitory transmitter. At certain synapses, the *gap junctions*, in which the apposing cell surfaces

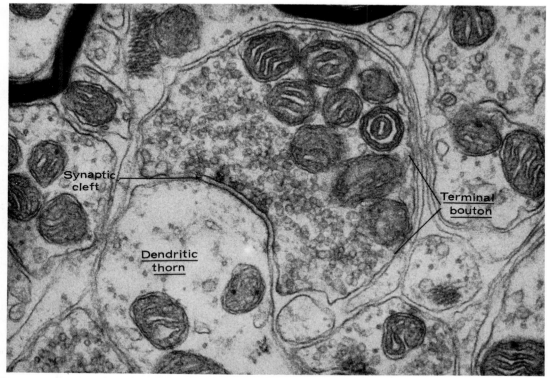

Figure 12-36 Tip of a dendritic thorn, capped by a terminal bouton from the ventral horn of the spinal cord in a rat. The typical features of synapses—mitochondria, clustered vesicles, and the cleft—are well shown. The terminal is enclosed within a thin astrocytic process. × 60,000 (approx.). (Courtesy of S. L. Palay.)

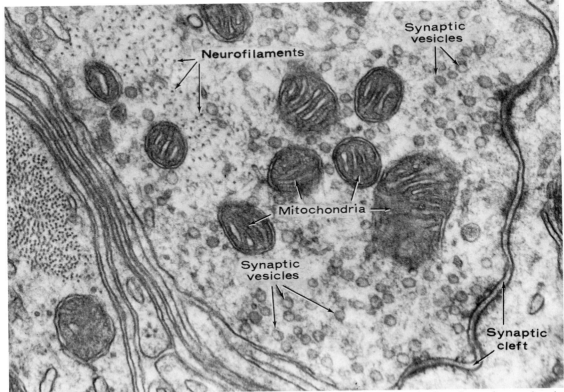

Figure 12–37 Electron micrograph of a typical synapse from the medial trapezoid nucleus of a cat, showing neurofilaments and synaptic vesicles in the nerve ending, a typical synaptic cleft between the pre- and post-synaptic membranes. (Micrograph courtesy M. Jean-Baptiste and D. K. Morest.)

are in especially intimate contact, electrical coupling rather than chemical mediation is the chief mode of transmission (see also Chapter 3).

Examples of Interrelationships of Neurons

Almost every neuron is connected with several or many other neurons. With the aid of the Golgi impregnation and other methods, many types of relationships between neurons have been demonstrated, from complex tangles involving the processes of hundreds of cells to a neuron synapsing upon itself. As an example of the complex type, attached to the body and dendrites of large motor cells in the anterior gray columns of the spinal cord are hundreds of synaptic boutons of axons from neurons in the cerebral cortex, nuclei of the medulla oblongata and elsewhere in the spinal cord. The spinal motor cells serve, accordingly, as the *final common pathway* by

which activity from many sources is transmitted to effector organs. In such arrangements, the response of the postsynaptic cell is determined by the net effect of excitation and inhibition exerted upon it by the many afferent fibers. Thus, in a spinal reflex arc the excitation of peripheral sensory elements is only one of many inputs influencing the response of the motor neurons. The intricate connections between neurons and their enormous numbers (an estimated 9×10^9 neurons in the cerebral cortex alone) indicate the complexity of neural structure and function. Details of the organization of the central nervous system are beyond the scope of this book and must be sought in textbooks of neuroanatomy. It may be instructive, however, to refer back to the photomicrographs of three different parts of the nervous system. Figure 12–13, of the spinal cord, illustrates the white matter, comprising masses of myelinated fibers that surround the relatively small amount of gray matter containing the nerve cell bodies. Figures 12–14 and 12–15 show gray matter located outside the white in the cerebral cortex and cerebellum. White matter, made up of myelinated or unmyelinated axons, serves to transmit patterns of nerve impulses from the body to the central nervous system, or vice versa, and from one part of the brain or cord to another part. There is no evidence that any modification of the nerve impulses occurs in nerves or tracts.

In gray matter, nerve cell bodies mingle with unmyelinated and myelinated fibers. A microscopic preparation shows the bodies of the cells arranged in some order, often in layers. The space between layers, and also between individual cells, is packed with innumerable axons, dendrites, neuroglia, and blood vessels. The axons in these areas usually lack myelin sheaths, which accounts for the gray appearance in fresh condition. Innumerable reciprocal contacts between the various types of neurons permit a variety of mutual influences.

When stained with routine methods, the region between cell bodies has a punctate or stippled appearance and corresponds to the neuropil described above. In the cerebellar and cerebral cortices and in the retina, certain layers consist almost exclusively of naked neuronal or neuroglial processes. Huge numbers of synaptic contacts take place in such synaptic fields.

The pattern of the cells and fibers (*cytoarchitecture*) in gray matter varies from place to place. Every subcortical nucleus, peripheral ganglion, and locality of the cerebral cortex has architectural features of its own. Thus, the cortex in the precentral convolution of the primate brain, the so-called *motor area*, differs noticeably from that of the postcentral convolution, where *somatosensory function* is represented, and from all other parts of the cerebral cortex. One important cortical region having a characteristic cytoarchitecture is the *visual area* along the calcarine fissure of the occipital lobe. Another, in the sylvian fossa, is the *auditory area*. However, careful attempts to correlate cytoarchitectonic and functional findings have largely failed up to the present time.

Anatomical and physiological studies provide compelling evidence that the nervous system is not a random tangle of neurons and neuroglial cells and their processes. Neurons are sometimes considered redundant, but in many regions display remarkable structural and functional individuality. Morphologically the individuality is expressed in the connections between particular cells and in the number, type, and location of synaptic terminals upon different parts of the same cell. Physiologically, particular neurons among the astronomical numbers making up the visual area of the cerebral cortex may respond to highly specific modes of visual stimuli to the retina. Other principles of organization of the nervous system emerge from study of neuroanatomy. Among these are the concepts that the central nervous system is subdivided into a series of interdependent cellular ensembles for analysis and control; that the patterns of connections often permit the reciprocal interactions necessary for modulation of both incoming and outgoing impulses; and finally, that the cells of the central nervous system at all levels from motor neuron to the cell of the cerebral cortex are designed for integrative action.

DEVELOPMENT OF THE NEURONS AND OF THE NERVOUS TISSUE

The neurons of the nervous system develop from embryonic ectoderm. Also of ectodermal origin are the neuroglial cells (except for the mesodermal microglia), the Schwann cells of peripheral nerves and corresponding satellite cells in peripheral ganglia, and certain elements of the meninges.

In early embryonic stages, the future central nervous system separates by folding from the primitive ectoderm to form the *neural tube*. At the time the neural folds meet, some cells leave the junctional region bilaterally to form cellular bands between the neural tube and the prospective epidermis. These bands, the *neural crests*, soon become segmented and are the precursors of the craniospinal and sympathetic ganglia, adrenal medulla, and melanocytes. Schwann cells are also generally regarded as derivatives of the neural crests. Autoradiographic studies with tritiated thymidine, however, show that some Schwann cells originate in the neural tube.

The early neural tube is a type of pseudostratified epithelium in which all cells border on the lumen. Autoradiographic and electron microscopic studies demonstrate a single type of columnar cell, called a *ventricular cell* in a recent revision of terminology. During proliferation, the nuclei of ventricular cells undergo cyclical changes of position in the ventricular zone; nuclei of premitotic cells lie deep, progressively approaching the lumen during prophase. Karyokinesis occurs only at the luminal surface, whereupon the daughter nuclei move again to deeper positions. Even before the closure of the neural tube, the nuclei of *neuroblasts* (immature neurons incapable of further division) derived from ventricular cells migrate peripherally; later such cells will form an *intermediate zone* (future gray matter). A *marginal zone* (future white matter) is already present; it contains the nuclear-free outer processes of the ventricular cells. Neuroglial cells in general originate also from the ventricular zone but, unlike typical neuroblasts, continue to divide after migration to the intermediate and marginal zones. In certain regions of the brain, cells are produced that retain proliferative ability after their origin in the ventricular zone; these give rise to additional neurons and glial cells. One such secondary germinal matrix forms a *subventricular zone* immediately beneath the ventricular cells; it is prominent in the lateral ventricles and persists into adult life. Its cells do not exhibit intermitotic nuclear migrations. Another, similar matrix is found in the development of the cerebellum. A transient layer is formed on the external surface of the embryonic cortex by cells that migrate from the ventricular zone of the underlying brain stem. Proliferation in this external layer produces neuroblasts that descend into the cerebellar cortex. Other cerebellar neurons and most neurons of the cerebral cortex arise directly from the ventricular zone and traverse intermediate and marginal zones to reach their destinations. Autoradiographic studies demonstrate that proliferation of neurons by the ventricular zone is a rigorously timed and highly ordered process, which is followed by active migration and frequent intermingling of neuroblasts as they proceed to their final positions.

The sensory neurons of the craniospinal nerves arise in the neural crests. The peripheral processes grow outward and become axons of the sensory nerve fibers. The dendritic region of these neurons is the receptive zone at the periphery; here, the axon develops a variable pattern of branches, which may or may not be encapsulated. The central processes enter the central nervous system as the axons of dorsal roots and establish connections with interneurons or motor neurons. The cell bodies of the somatic and visceral motor neurons remain within the brain or spinal cord; their axons grow out as ventral roots of the peripheral nerves and terminate in muscles or autonomic ganglia.

The protoplasm of a growing axon shows ameboid movements and insinuates itself between other tissue elements by positive outgrowth. At its advancing tip, a bulbous enlargement, or *growth cone*, thrusts slender, spinelike projections between obstructing cells and fibers. The features of neuronal development seen in fixed and stained material were confirmed by observations on living nerves in tissue culture and by studies of growing nerves in the transparent tail of the living frog tadpole. Axons of neuroblasts grow into the intercellular spaces as slender, protoplasmic strands. In peripheral nerve fibers, all newly formed axons are at first devoid of Schwann and myelin sheaths. The earliest myelin appears near the Schwann cell nucleus, from which locality it spreads proximally and distally.

The forces that direct the course of development of the complex nervous tissue of vertebrates are largely unknown. The importance of an oriented microstructure (micellar orientation and aggregation) as a guide, along whose channels developing axons spread, has been confirmed. There has been no confirmation, however, of the concept of "neurobiotaxis," which assumes that differences in electric potential between dendrites and axons account for migration of nerve cell bodies in the direction of the source from which their stimuli come. No clear-cut effects of electric currents have been seen on either the rate or direction of the growth of nerves. Chemotactic influences upon growing axons have been demonstrated clearly in the optic nerve. Regenerating optic nerve fibers from different parts of the goldfish retina unerringly reach their former terminations in the optic lobes of the midbrain, even after surgical cross-union of medial and lateral optic tracts. There is evidence for refined specificities of growing axons in other regions of the central nervous system, but the role of chemotactic influences on the growth of peripheral nerves remains controversial. There is also evidence to show that the peripheral organs and tissues affect the development of the central nervous system in many ways after contact has been established between the two regions. These effects are both quantitative and qualitative; they act to regulate the number and size of neurons in specific regions of the neuraxis and to influence the pattern of their connections. Another important finding has been the discovery of specific *nerve growth factors*, identified as proteins, which exert powerful effects upon the generation, growth, and maintenance of specific types of nerve cells.

Recent studies with the Golgi method show that many neuroblasts retain for some time the primitive distal process they possessed as ventricular cells. These studies suggest that free ameboid motion of an entire cell may not occur in neurogenesis. Instead, the nucleus may simply shift peripherally from the ventricular zone along this process until reaching its definitive position, perhaps near the external surface of the brain wall, as in the prospective cerebral cortex. Retraction of the attachments of the internal and external processes of the neuroblast takes place from the luminal surface and basal lamina of the neural tube, respectively.

Axon sprouting, growth of dendrites, and other features of neuronal differentiation appear to be independent variables. Such events occur at different times relative to the shift in position of the nucleus and in different sequences, depending on the type of nerve cell and its region of the developing central nervous system.

CONNECTIVE TISSUE, CHOROID PLEXUS, VENTRICLES, AND THE MENINGES OF THE CENTRAL NERVOUS SYSTEM

In addition to the neurons and macroglia, both of which are of ectodermal origin, the brain and the spinal cord contain blood vessels derived from mesenchyme. The three membranes enveloping the brain and cord are likewise composed chiefly of connective tissue. The outermost, the *dura mater* or *pachymeninx*, is dense and firm (Fig. 12–39). The inner membranes, the innermost called the *pia mater* and the intermediate called the *arachnoid membrane* (Fig. 12–38), are composed of looser connective tissue and constitute the *leptomeninges*.

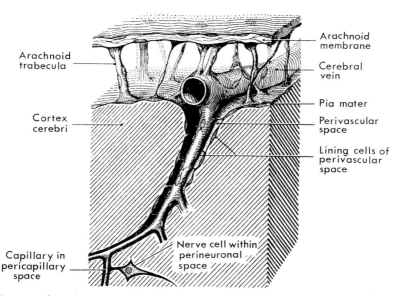

Figure 12–38 Diagram of cerebral pia-arachnoid, showing relations of the subarachnoid space, perivascular channels and nerve cells. (From L. H. Weed, Am. J. Anat., *31*, 1922.)

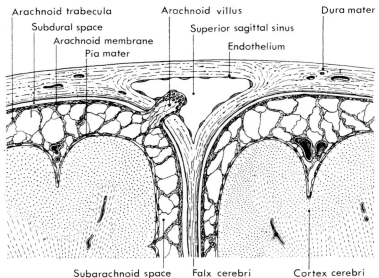

Figure 12-39 Diagram of the organization of the connective tissue sheaths of the brain. Cerebrospinal fluid formed in the choroid plexus circulates in the subarachnoid space and is absorbed by the venous sinuses through the arachnoid villi, one of which is shown here projecting into the sagittal sinus. (From L. H. Weed, Am. J. Anat., *31*, 1922.)

Dura Mater

The dura of the spinal cord and that of the brain differ in their relationships to the surrounding bones. The inner surface of the vertebral canal is lined by its own periosteum; a separate cylindrical dural membrane loosely encloses the cord. The wide epidural space, between periosteum and dura, contains loose connective and fatty tissue and the epidural venous plexus. The dura is firmly connected to the spinal cord on each side by a series of denticulate ligaments. The inner surface of the spinal dura is lined with squamous cells. Its collagenous bundles run for the most part longitudinally. Elastic fibers are less prominent than in the cerebral dura.

The dura mater of the brain in embryonic development also has two layers, but in the adult these are closely joined. Both consist of connective tissue with elongated fibroblasts. The outer layer adheres to the skull loosely except at the sutures and the base of the skull, where it is more firmly adherent. It functions as a periosteum, is richer in cells than the inner layer, and contains many blood vessels; its thick collagenous fibers are arranged in bundles. The inner layer is thinner, with finer fibers forming an almost continuous sheet. Its fibers run from the frontal region backward and upward, oriented opposite to those of the outer layer. The inner surface of the dura is smooth and covered with a layer of squamous mesothelial cells.

Arachnoid

The leptomeninges of the brain and spinal cord are similar in structure. The arachnoid is a thin, netlike membrane devoid of blood vessels, resembling the transparent parts of the omentum. Its outer surface is smooth, but from its inner surface runs a multitude of thin, branching threads and ribbon-like strands, attached to the pia. Microscopically the tissue has a cobweb-like appearance (Figs. 12–38 and 12–39). The arachnoid bridges the sulci and fissures on the surface of the brain and spinal cord, forming subarachnoid spaces of various extent.

Pia Mater

This membrane is a thin connective tissue net closely adherent to the surface of the brain and spinal cord. It contains a large number of blood vessels, from which most of the blood of the underlying nervous tissue is supplied. Attached to the pia are the inner fibrous strands of the arachnoid; these two membranes are so intimately related that their histological structure can best be described together—in fact, these two membranes are often treated as a single entity, the *pia-arachnoid.*

The main elements of the arachnoid and pia are interlacing collagenous bundles surrounded by fine elastic networks. In the pia of the spinal cord an outer longitudinal and an inner circular layer can be distinguished. Among the cells are fibroblasts and fixed macrophages; the latter are especially numerous along the pial blood vessels. They correspond to macrophages of other parts of the body, store vital dyes injected directly into the subarachnoid space, and in inflammation become large, free macrophages or epithelioid cells. In man they often contain considerable amounts of a yellow pigment that sometimes reacts positively to tests for iron.

Along the pial vessels lie scattered single mast cells and small groups of lymphocytes. In certain pathological conditions the latter increase enormously in number and may become plasma cells. The leptomeninges, especially along the pial vessels, also contain many embryonic mesenchymal elements. In the pia, particularly on the ventral surface of the medulla oblongata, a varying number of melanocytes can be found.

The outer and the inner surfaces of the arachnoid, its trabeculae, and the outer surface of the pia are covered with a layer of squamous mesenchymal epithelial cells. Although some investigators describe their rounding off, mobilization, and transformation into free macrophages under the influence of inflammatory stimuli, others trace the origin of macrophages exclusively to fixed macrophages. This question requires further study.

During development of the meninges two zones may be distinguished: an outer zone of condensation of mesenchyme, which gives rise to the periosteum, dura, and membranous arachnoid; and an inner zone, which becomes the pia. Between these two zones the mesenchyme remains loose and later forms spongy tissue permeating the subarachnoid spaces.

Nerves of the Meninges

The dura and pia mater are richly supplied with nerves. All vessels of the pia and of the choroid plexus are surrounded by extensive nerve plexuses in the adventitia. Axons originate in the carotid and vertebral plexuses and in certain cranial nerves and belong to the sympathetic system. Sensory, nonencapsulated nerve terminations, and even single nerve cells, are also present on the adventitia of the blood vessels.

The cerebral dura contains, besides the nerves of the vessels, numerous sensory nerve endings in its connective tissue. The cerebral pia also contains extensive nervous plexuses, especially abundant in the tela choroidea of the third ventricle. The fibers end either in large, pear-shaped or bulbous swellings or in skeins and convolutions similar to those of the corpuscles of Meissner. In the spinal pia the vessels receive their nerves from the plexuses following the larger blood vessels to the cord. Afferent nerve endings are also present, but these are unevenly distributed.

Both myelinated and unmyelinated nerve fibers accompany the blood vessels into the substance of the spinal cord and the brain, ending on the muscle cells of the vessels. These come from similar nerves of the pial vessels, and the two nervous plexuses are continuous.

Meningeal Spaces

Between the dura mater and the arachnoid, the subdural space is a serous cavity containing a minimum of fluid; actually, it is scarcely more than a potential space. Between the outer sheet of arachnoid and pia is the subarachnoid space, traversed by cobwebby connective tissue trabeculae, independent of the subdural space, and containing a large amount of fluid. At the summits of the convolutions it is narrow, but in the sulci it is wide and deep. The subarachnoid space is especially wide throughout the length of the spinal cord. In the brain, it is greatly enlarged in a few places *(cisternae)* where the arachnoid is widely separated from the pia and the trabeculae are rare or absent. The largest cisterna lies above the medulla oblongata and below the posterior border of the cerebellum *(cisterna cerebellomedullaris,* or *cisterna magna).* The fourth ventricle communicates with this cisterna through three openings in the tela choroidea: a medial *foramen of Magendie,* and the two lateral *foramina of Luschka.*

Ventricles

The central nervous system begins development as a neural tube with a wide cavity throughout the length and remains a hollow organ throughout life. The *central canal* or ventricle of the spinal cord in the adult is minute, or it may be obliterated. It does not seem to perform any important function. However, in the normal adult the ventricular cavities of the brain form a continuous channel for flow of cerebrospinal fluid. If part of this channel is occluded by disease so as to prevent free circulation, intracerebral pressure increases, with resulting hydrocephalus or other serious consequences.

The ventricular cavity is dilated in four regions: the two *lateral ventricles* in the cerebral hemispheres, the *third ventricle* in the thalamic region, and the *fourth ventricle* in the medulla oblongata and pons. Choroid plexuses develop in these four regions, and most of the ventricular fluid is derived from the blood vessels of these plexuses.

Choroid Plexus

There are four places where the wall of the brain retains its embryonic character as a thin, non-nervous epithelium. This part of the brain wall is the *lamina epithelialis.* The pia mater which covers it is extremely vascular and is called the *tela choroidea.* Small arteries and capillaries of the pia form glomerular tufts of vessels, covered by the lamina epithelialis and protruding into the ventricle — the *choroid plexus.*

Choroid plexuses are found in the roof of the third and fourth ventricles and in part of the wall of the two lateral ventricles. In each case, the tela choroidea is much folded and invaginated into the ventricle, so that the free surface exposed to the ventricular fluid is large, with tortuous vessels and a rich capillary net (Fig. 12–40).

The epithelium early acquires a peculiar structure, different from that of the cells lining the ventricles elsewhere. In embryonic stages it contains glycogen and carries cilia. In the adult its cells are cuboidal and arranged in a single, regular layer. Each contains a large, round nucleus and a varying number of rod-shaped mitochondria (Fig. 12–41).

On the free surface the cells have a specialized border resembling a brush border. In electron micrographs, however, this border is seen to consist of long microvilli that are irregularly oriented and often somewhat expanded at the tips (Fig. 12–42). Although possibly these terminal expansions are artifacts of fixation, microvilli of other cell types fixed similarly do not have this appearance.

In animals repeatedly injected intravenously with vital dyes, such as trypan blue, the epithelium of the choroid plexus stores large amounts of the dye. Also in the perivas-

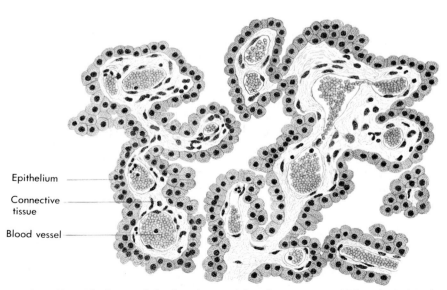

Epithelium
Connective tissue
Blood vessel

Figure 12-40   Choroid plexus of the fourth ventricle of man. × 190. (After A. A. Maximow.)

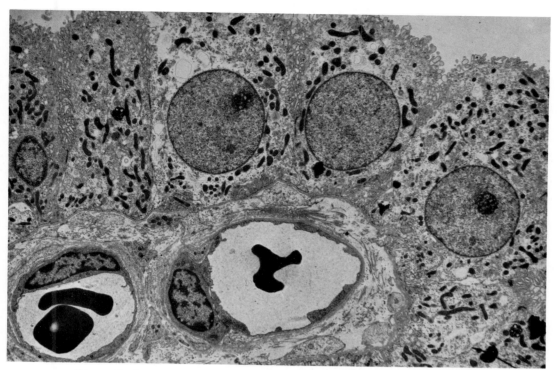

Figure 12-41   Low power electron micrograph of cat choroid plexus. × 4000.

cular connective tissue core of the plexus many fixed macrophages are found, which take up and store great amounts of dye.

On the boundary between adjacent epithelial cells in electron micrographs, a juxtaluminal junctional complex appears to seal the intercellular space. The capillaries beneath the epithelium are unlike those found elsewhere in the brain; they have thin walls and fenestrations or pores closed by thin diaphragms. The junctions between endothelial cells also appear to be more permeable. Following intravenous injection in mice, peroxidase (a protein) can be shown to cross the capillary walls and enter the stromal space. It moves between the epithelial cells but is stopped near the lumen by the junctional complex.

Cerebrospinal Fluid

The central nervous system is bathed and suspended in cerebrospinal fluid as in a water bath. This fluid protects the nervous system from concussions and mechanical injuries and is important for its metabolism.

The subarachnoid spaces freely communicate; cerebrospinal fluid may pass through them from one end to the other of the neuraxis. The amount of the fluid is variable, estimated as 80 to 100 ml., sometimes as much as 150 ml. It is limpid and slightly viscous, has a low specific gravity (1.004 to 1.008), contains traces of proteins, small quantities of inorganic salt and dextrose, and few lymphocytes (about two or three, not more than 10, per milliliter). It resembles the aqueous humor of the eye more closely than it does any other fluid of the body.

Cerebrospinal fluid is constantly renewed. It circulates slowly through the brain ventricles and through the meshes of the subarachnoid space. If the space is opened to the outside by injury, large amounts of fluid steadily drain off—200 ml. or more in a day. The sources of fluid are primarily the blood vessels of the choroid plexus, the pia mater, and the brain substance. From the brain substance the flow is outward into the subarachnoid space; from the choroid plexus it is inward into the ventricles. Fluid may be added to the ventricles in a few other places,

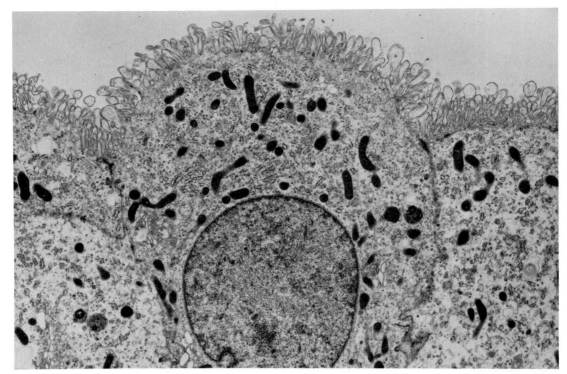

Figure 12-42   Electron micrograph of choroid plexus at higher magnification, illustrating the unusual free border of bulbous or clavate microvilli. × 7200.

notably the area postrema at the caudal margin of the fourth ventricle. The ependymal surfaces in general do not discharge fluid into the ventricles. In contrast, absorption of fluid from the ventricles into nearby veins takes place through the ventricular wall. The plexuses are wholly secretory, not resorptive, and constitute the chief source of fluid. The major channel of ventricular fluid outward into the subarachnoid space is through specially modified places in the membranous roof of the fourth ventricle.

Ventricular fluid normally flows from the lateral ventricles of the cerebral hemispheres, where it derives chiefly from the lateral choroid plexuses, through the foramina of Monro into the third ventricle. Here fluid is added from the choroid plexus of the third ventricle and the augmented flow passes through the aqueduct of Sylvius into the fourth ventricle, where more fluid is added from the choroid plexus there. Fluid then passes into the cisterna magna and diffuses in all directions through the subarachnoid space. Some of the fluid may enter

extracranial lymphatics through perineurial spaces within the cranial nerve roots, part reaching the nasal cavity along sheaths of olfactory nerve filaments. Around the spinal nerve roots, an arrangement of dural veins and sinuses permits passage of cerebrospinal fluid directly into venous blood, rather than into lymphatics. A small amount of fluid enters lymphatics or venous vessels as just described, but most of it passes directly into the large endocranial venous sinuses through the arachnoid villi.

Arachnoid Villi

The large endocranial venous sinuses are surrounded by thick walls of dura mater except in certain places, chiefly in the sagittal sinus of the falx cerebri. Here the dura is perforated by numerous protrusions of the arachnoid, through each of which a finger of arachnoid mesothelium, an *arachnoid villus* (Fig. 12–39), evaginates into the lumen of the sinus. The cavity of the villus, containing a small amount of loose arachnoid tissue, communicates freely with the subarachnoid space, so that at this point fluid of the space is separated from blood in the sinus only by the thin mesothelial membrane.

Arachnoid villi have been found in dogs, cats, monkeys, and humans (infants and adults). In man, with advancing age, they enlarge and become *pacchionian corpuscles* or *granulations.*

The villi provide the main pathway for outflow of cerebrospinal fluid directly into the venous circulation. This flow is rapid. Dyes and other chemicals injected into the subarachnoid space can be detected in the bloodstream in 10 to 30 seconds, and after only 30 minutes they can be found in the lymphatics.

Blood Vessels of the Central Nervous System

The arteries reach the spinal cord with the ventral and dorsal nerve roots (anterior and posterior radicular arteries) and form a dense arterial network in the spinal pia mater. Here several longitudinal arterial pathways can be distinguished (spinal arterial tracts). The most important is the anterior spinal artery; it emits many small branches (central arteries), which enter the ventral median fissure and penetrate to the right and left into the medial part of the anterior gray columns, thus supplying most of the gray matter with blood. Numerous smaller branches of the pial arterial net (peripheral arteries) penetrate the white matter along its circumference. Capillary nets in white matter are loose and have meshes drawn out longitudinally; capillaries in gray matter are much more numerous and dense. The course of the veins does not correspond to that of the arteries. Numerous venous branches emerge from the periphery of the cord and from the ventral median fissure and form a diffuse plexus in the pia, which is especially prominent on the dorsal surface of the cord. From this plexus, blood is drained by veins accompanying the ventral and dorsal roots.

The arterial supply of the brain derives almost entirely from the carotids and the large arteries at its base—the basilar artery and the circle of Willis. Most arteries from these large vessels pass superiorly in the pia mater, from which smaller vessels dip into the brain substance. These vessels are functionally end arteries, since few anastomoses are large enough to be effective in establishing collateral circulation.

As in the spinal cord, the capillary net in cerebral white matter is meager, with elongated meshes; in gray matter the net has a closer mesh. The density of capillaries is a crude indication of the metabolic needs of the tissue supplied. From this, it is clear that gray matter is metabolically much more active; the amount of activity, however, varies from place to place, as reflected in the density of the capillary net.

The linear extent of capillaries per unit volume of brain substance has been measured in a number of representative parts of the central nervous system in various animals. In the rat, parts of both white and gray matter differ in vascularity, but in all cases the gray is more vascular than the white. Motor nuclei are less vascular than sensory nuclei and groups of interneurons.

There are no lymphatics in the central nervous system. Fluid from the capillaries seeps through the tissue but does not collect in lymphatic channels, as in most other parts of the body. The blood vessels that penetrate from the pia are surrounded by perivascular spaces, which open freely at the brain surface into the subarachnoid space. Thus cerebrospinal fluid derived from blood drains from the brain outward toward the meninges.

When certain vital dyes, pigments, or metals are present in circulating blood of adult animals, the central nervous system remains colorless except for the choroid plexuses and certain subependymal areas. In these exceptional regions, dyes and pigments are found within extravascular cells. Thus, a *blood-brain* or *hematoencephalic barrier* exists between the blood and the nervous system. Explanations for this observation include the hypotheses that the capillary endothelium is less permeable than in the rest of the body; that the layer formed by end processes of neuroglial cells on vessel walls excludes certain substances; that the specialized subependymal areas are the barrier; or that a succession of thresholds, including the structures just named, have to be crossed.

In young animals given intravenous dye injections, a distinct but small storage of dye does occur in cells in parts of the brain stem, so that the apparent impermeability of the brain to blood-borne materials develops gradually.

RESPONSE OF THE NEURON TO INJURY

Two important responses of the neuron to injury are the progressive degeneration of an axon severed from its cell body and the morphological changes which occur in the perikaryon of a neuron after axonal transection. These responses, basic to neuropathology, are included here because they exemplify the neuron doctrine and illustrate the trophic influence of the nerve cell body over the axon and its other processes.

When an axon is severed, trauma occurs at both cut edges. Proximally, *primary degeneration* extends only a short distance, depending on the type of injury—one or two internodes in a clean cut, perhaps as much as 2 or 3 cm. from a gunshot wound. Damage is soon repaired and new axonal sprouts appear. Distally, however, the axon, its terminal arborizations, and the myelin sheath completely disintegrate. This *secondary* or *Wallerian degeneration*, first described in peripheral nerves by Waller in 1850, usually proceeds simultaneously along the length of a nerve fiber distal to the point of injury, although a rapid centrifugal sweep of changes may occur. The initial changes in axonal fine structure consist in localized accumulations of mitochondria a few hours after injury; within 12 to 24 hours, neurofilaments and mitochondria vesiculate and disintegrate, and later dense granules aggregate. At about two days, the axis cylinder becomes beaded and shortly begins to fragment and dissolve. Concomitantly, myelin degeneration begins, breaking down into fatty droplets of varying size and concentric lamellar structure, often enclosing an axonal fragment. Macrophages, derived somehow from the endoneurial or Schwann cells, progressively remove the debris. The process of degeneration does not usually spread across the synapse, in accord with the neuron doctrine. Nevertheless, many exceptions are known and additional ones have been suspected (see p. 371). The Schwann cytoplasm remains, and, after axonal and myelin degeneration, forms a tube surrounded by endoneurium and filled with fluid and scattered fragments. The wall of the tube thickens, reducing the original bore until it may be obliterated, and the tube shrinks to perhaps less than half of its original diameter; meanwhile, its constituent Schwann cell nuclei multiply. Ultimately these changes produce a solid, nucleated *band of Büngner*. As myelin disappears, a flexible, ribbon-like peripheral nerve condenses into a dull gray, hardened, and rounded cord. The bands of Büngner may remain for many months, awaiting reinnervation. If regeneration of axons does not occur, the bands gradually become reduced by encroaching endoneurial connective tissue.

Nerve fibers within the central nervous system also undergo Wallerian degeneration. In young animals, degeneration is extremely rapid, but in adult man it proceeds more slowly. Loss of myelin in a heavily myelinated tract, for example, as seen in Weigert stain, may not be evident for two months. Special staining methods for normal and abnormal lipids, however, show myelin catabolism more readily. In the central nervous system, the microglia, equivalent to macrophages elsewhere, break down and remove the myelin and axonal fragments. Whether interfascicular oligodendrocytes undertake similar functions to those of Schwann cells is not known. Wallerian degeneration is widely exploited in neuroanatomical research to trace the course of connections following experimental ablations of nuclei and tracts. Degeneration of terminal boutons, an essential part of Wallerian degeneration, offers a more difficult but higher resolution research method, since it demonstrates the termination of degenerating axons and also serves when brief survival precludes study of the slower reactions of axon or myelin.

The fleeting and restricted traumatic degeneration of the proximal stump of a peripheral nerve is usually soon followed by axonal regeneration, in the form of fine sprouts with protoplasmic *growth cones* or *filopodia* at their advancing tips. Regenerating fibers resemble embryonic ones and grow along the outer edge of a band of Büngner. There they become progressively enfolded by Schwann cells in a fashion similar to the multiple envelopment found in unmyelinated nerves (see p. 352). The rate of growth of the fibers is rapid—three to four millimeters a day in mammals, and perhaps two centimeters per day in the deer antler—but the distance that must be traversed to the terminations may be a meter or more.

Functional recovery depends on reestablishment of appropriate sensory and motor connections at the periphery. The abundance of regenerative sprouts from the original neuron and the capacity of bands of

Büngner to accommodate hundreds of fibers favor successful reinnervation. Although alignment of individual axons is impossible, and regenerating sprouts can negotiate hiatuses of considerable distance, prompt surgical approximation of the two ends of a cut peripheral nerve is nevertheless of cardinal importance. In addition to the abundance of sprouts and their accommodation by the bands of Büngner, peripheral deletion of maladaptive terminations and central remodeling of reflex arcs offer additional possibilities for functional recovery.

Following the regeneration of a peripheral nerve, the axon, myelin, and Schwann cell slowly return to their normal size and condition. During these months, large amounts of axoplasm are resynthesized — possibly 250 times that of the parent cell body.

Retrograde changes in the cell body of origin of a severed axon were first described by Nissl in 1892. Chief among these is *retrograde chromatolysis*, the apparent disappearance of the Nissl substance, obvious and well studied in motor cells, but occurring in varying extent and rate in other types of neurons. With light microscopy, breakup and dissolution of Nissl material is first seen near the axon hillock and in a rim around the nucleus, subsequently spreading to other parts of the cell. In addition, the perikaryon swells, ballooning the normally concave boundaries between dendrites, and the nucleus shifts from its usually central position to a peripheral one away from the axon hillock. Fine structural investigations are few, but have shown dispersion or disappearance of ribosomes and of the cisternal membranes of the granular endoplasmic reticulum, with appearance of numerous coarse neurofilaments. Initially the Golgi apparatus appears normal, but in later stages swarms of small dark vesicles apparently bud from its flattened profiles, suggesting a role in resynthesis of the granular endoplasmic reticulum.

Retrograde chromatolysis begins about one day after axonal injury and is sometimes referred to as *axonal reaction;* it reaches its peak in about two weeks. Similar pathologic changes in the nerve cell body may occur for other reasons. The response, like that of Wallerian degeneration, offers a valuable anatomical method. In this case, the investigator can localize the origin of a tract or nerve, instead of tracing its course; to do this, however, he must be familiar with the normal pattern of Nissl substance for the neurons in the many regions under study. In practice, the neuroanatomist frequently combines anterograde and retrograde degeneration studies.

In general, the more axoplasm that is separated from the cell body, the greater the retrograde chromatolysis. Amputation of a major process close to the perikaryon may lead to the death of the neuron, whereas section of a distal process may produce no detectable response. If the cell body survives and regeneration of the axon takes place, the retrograde changes are slowly reversed. The nucleolus becomes prominent and reconstitution of Nissl substance, often in superabundance, occurs, beginning as a basophilic rim around the nucleus. Return to normal appearance takes several months. The meaning of these changes is not entirely clear, but apparently represents a kind of exhaustion of the nucleoproteins of the perikaryon, stemming from overwork in its attempts to regenerate a severed axon. Very large amounts of axonal cytoplasm may have to be regenerated (see p. 346), entailing an enormous metabolic effort on the part of the cell body and synthesis of immense amounts of cytoplasm relative to the size of the perikaryon, stemming from overwork in its duction and utilization of nucleoprotein, protein, and lipid. Sensory ganglion cells react in a manner similar to motor cells, but show less obvious changes after lesions of the peripheral nerves have occurred and still slighter, perhaps undetectable, changes after section of the dorsal roots. The finely divided Nissl substance in the normal dorsal root ganglion cell and the great length of axon it possesses probably tend to minimize the visible response. In many central neurons, such as Betz cells of the cerebral cortex, retrograde chromatolysis is seldom observed. Unless destruction of the axon and all its branches takes place, intact *sustaining collaterals* are thought to remain functional and to provide enough axoplasm to offset overt retrograde cell change.

REFERENCES

Adams, R. D., and R. L. Sidman: Introduction to Neuropathology. New York, McGraw-Hill, 1968.

Angevine, J. B., Jr.: Time of neuron origin in the diencephalon of the mouse. An autoradiographic study. J. Comp. Neurol., *139*:129, 1970.

Ariëns Kappers, C. U., G. C. Huber, and E. C. Crosby: The Comparative Anatomy of the Nervous System of Vertebrates, Including Man. Vols. I and II. New York, Macmillan, 1936.

Bailey, P., and G. Von Bonin: The Isocortex of Man. Urbana, University of Illinois Press, 1951.

Bodian, D.: Neuron junctions: A revolutionary decade. Anat. Rec., *174*:73, 1972.

Boulder Committee: Embryonic vertebrate central nervous system: Revised terminology. Anat. Rec., *166*:257, 1970.

Boyd, I. A.: The structure and innervation of the nuclear bag muscle fiber system and the nuclear chain muscle fiber system in mammalian muscle spindles. Philos. Trans. Roy. Soc. B, *245*:81, 1962.

Causey, G.: The Cell of Schwann. Edinburgh, E. & S. Livingstone, Ltd., 1960.

Davis, H.: Some principles of sensory receptor action Physiol. Rev., *41*:391, 1961.

Davison, A. N., and A. Peters: Myelination. Springfield, Ill., Charles C Thomas, 1970.

Davison, P. F., and E. W. Taylor: Physical-chemical studies of proteins of squid nerve axoplasm, with special reference to the axon fibrous protein. J. Gen. Physiol., *43*:801, 1960.

Eccles, J. C.: The Physiology of Nerve Cells. Baltimore, Johns Hopkins Press, 1957.

Field, J., H. W. Magoun, and V. E. Hall (eds.): Handbook of Physiology. Section 1: Neurophysiology. 3 Vols. Washington, D.C., American Physiological Society, 1959–1961.

Finean, J. B.: Chemical Ultrastructure in Living Tissues. Springfield, Ill., Charles C Thomas, 1961.

Flexner, L. B.: Events associated with the development of nerve and hepatic cells. Ann. N.Y. Acad. Sci., *60*:986, 1955.

Fox, C. A., and J. W. Barnard: A quantitative study of the Purkinje cell dendritic branchlets and their relations to afferent fibers. J. Anat., *91*:299, 1957.

Fujita, S.: Analysis of neuron differentiation in the central nervous system by tritiated thymidine autoradiography. J. Comp. Neurol., *112*:311, 1964.

Furshpan, E. J.: "Electrical transmission" at an excitatory synapse in a vertebrate brain. Science, *144*:878, 1964.

Gerard, R. W.: Metabolism and Function in the Nervous System. *In* Elliott, K. A. C., I. H. Page, and J. H. Quastel, eds.: Neurochemistry. Springfield, Ill., Charles C Thomas, 1955.

Geren, B. B.: Structural studies of the formation of the myelin sheath in peripheral nerve fibers. *In* Rudnick, D., ed.: Cellular Mechanisms in Differentiation and Growth. Princeton. Princeton University Press, 1956.

Glees, P.: Neuroglia; Morphology and Function. Springfield, Ill., Charles C Thomas, 1955.

Glimstedt, G., and G. Wohlfort: Electron microscope studies on peripheral nerve regeneration. Lunds Universitets Arsskrift, *56*:1, 1960.

Granit, R.: Receptors and Sensory Perception; a Discussion of Aims, Means, and Results of Electrophysiological Research into the Process of Reception. New Haven, Yale University Press, 1955.

Gray, E. G., and R. W. Guillery: Synaptic morphology in the normal and degenerating nervous system. Int. Rev. Cytol., *19*:41, 1962.

Greenfield, J. G.: Neuropathology, Baltimore, Williams & Wilkins, 1967.

Guth, L.: Regeneration in the mammalian peripheral

nervous system. Physiol. Rev., *36*:441, 1956.

Harrison, R. G.: The outgrowth of the nerve fiber as a mode of protoplasmic movement. J. Exper. Zool., *9*:787, 1910.

Hartmann, J. F.: Electron microscopy of motor nerve cells following section of axones. Anat. Rec., *118*:19, 1954.

Herrick, C. J.: An Introduction to Neurology, 5th Ed. Philadelphia, W. B. Saunders Co., 1931.

Herrick, C. J.: The Brain of the Tiger Salamander. Chicago, University of Chicago Press, 1948.

Herrick, C. J.: The Evolution of Human Nature. Austin, University of Texas Press, 1956.

Hild, W.: Das Neuron. *In* von Möllendorff, W., and W. Bargmann, eds.: Handbuch der mikroskopischen Anatomic des Menschen. Vol. 4, part 4, p. 1. Berlin. Springer Verlag, 1959.

Hyden, H.: The Neuron. *In* Brachet, J., and A. E. Mirsky, eds.: The Cell; Biochemistry, Physiology, Morphology. Vol. 4, p. 215. New York, Academic Press, 1960.

Katz, B.: Mechanisms of Synaptic Transmission, and Nature of the Nerve Impulse. *In* Oncley, J. L., et al., eds.: Biophysical Science—A Study Program. New York, John Wiley & Sons, 1959, pp. 254 and 466.

Kuntz, A.: The Autonomic Nervous System. 4th Ed. Philadelphia, Lea & Febiger, 1953.

Lehman, H. J.: Die Nervenfaser. *In* von Möllendorff, W., and W. Bargmann, eds.: Handbuch der mikroskopischen Anatomie des Menschen. Vol. 4, part 4, p. 515. Berlin, Springer Verlag, 1959.

Levi-Montalcini, R.: Events in the developing nervous system. *In* Purpura, D., and J. Schadé, eds.: Progress in Brain Research. Vol. 4, p. 1. Amsterdam, Elsevier Publishing Co., 1964.

Ortiz-Picón, J. M.: The neuroglia of the sensory ganglia. Anat. Rec., *121*:513, 1955.

Palay, S. L.: The structural basis for neural action. *In* Brazier, M. A. B., ed.: Brain Function. Vol. II, p. 69. Berkeley, University of California Press, 1963.

Palay, S. L., and G. E. Palade: The fine structure of neurons. J. Biophys. Biochem. Cytol., *1*:69, 1955.

Penfield, W., ed.: Cytology and Cellular Pathology of the Nervous System. Vols. 1, 2, and 3. New York, Paul B. Hoeber, Inc., 1932.

Peters, A., S. L. Palay, and H. deF. Webster: The Fine Structure of the Nervous System. The Cells and their Processes. New York, Harper & Row, 1970.

Peterson, E. R., and M. R. Murray: Myelin sheath formation in cultures of avian spinal ganglia. Am. J. Anat., *96*:319, 1955.

Polyak, S.: Vertebrate Visual System. Chicago, University of Chicago Press, 1957.

Pomerat, C. M.: Dynamic neurogliology. Texas Rep. Biol. Med., *10*:885, 1952.

Pope, A.: Application of quantitative histochemical methods to the study of the nervous system. J. Neuropath. Exper. Neurol., *14*:39, 1955.

Quarton, G. C., T. Melnechuk, and F. O. Schmitt: The Neurosciences. A Study Program. New York, Rockefeller University Press, 1967.

Ramón y Cajal, S.: Histologie du Systeme nerveux de l'homme et des vertébrés. Paris, A. Maloine, 1909.

Ramón y Cajal, S.: Degeneration and Regeneration of the Nervous System. London, Oxford University Press, 1928.

Reiser, K. A.: Die Nervenzelle. *In* von Möllendorff, W., and W. Bargmann, eds.: Handbuch der mikroskopischen Anatomie des Menschen. Vol. 4, part 4, p. 185. Berlin, Springer Verlag, 1959.

Robertson, J. D.: The ultrastructure of adult vertebrate

peripheral myelinated nerve fibers in relation to myelinogenesis. J. Biophys. Biochem. Cytol., *1*:271, 1955.

Robertson, J. D.: The ultrastructure of Schmidt-Lantermann clefts and related shearing defects of the myelin sheath. J. Biophys. Biochem. Cytol., *4*:39, 1958.

Rodriguez, L. A.: Experiments on the histologic locus of the hematoencephalic barrier. J. Comp. Neurol., *102*:27, 1955.

Rich, T. C., H. D. Patton, J. W. Woodburn, and A. L. Towe: Neurophysiology. 2nd Ed. Philadelphia, W. B. Saunders Co., 1965.

Sauer, F. C.: Mitosis in the neural tube. J. Comp. Neurol., *62*:377, 1935.

Schaltenbrand, G.: Plexus und Meningen. *In* von Möllendorff, W., and W. Bargmann, eds.: Handbuch der mikroskopischen Anatomie des Menschen. Vol. 4, part 2, p. 1. Berlin, Springer Verlag, 1955.

Scharrer, E., and B. Scharrer: Neurosekretion. *In* von Möllendorff, W., and W. Bargmann, eds.: Handbuch der mikroskopischen Anatomie des Menschen. Vol. 6, part 5, p. 953. Berlin, Springer Verlag, 1954.

Schmitt, F. O.: Molecular Organization of the Nerve Fiber. *In* Oncley, J. L., et al., eds.: Biophysical Science — A Study Program. New York, John Wiley & Sons, 1959, p. 455.

Schmitt, F. O.: The Neurosciences. Second Study Program. New York, Rockefeller University Press, 1970.

Schmitt, F. O., et al.: Neurosciences Research Symposium Summaries. Vols. I–V. Cambridge, Massachusetts Institute of Technology Press, 1966–1971.

Sherrington, C. S.: The Integrative Action of the Nervous System. New Haven, Yale University Press, 1906.

Sholl, D. A.: The Organization of the Cerebral Cortex. New York, John Wiley & Sons, 1956.

Speidel, C. C.: Studies of living nerves. VII. Growth adjustments of cutaneous terminal arborizations. J. Comp. Neurol., *76*:57, 1942.

Sperry, R. W.: Chemoaffinity in the orderly growth of nerve fiber patterns and connections. Proc. Nat. Acad. Sci., *50*:703, 1963.

Waelsch, N., ed.: Biochemistry of the Developing Nervous System. New York, Academic Press, 1955.

Watterson, R. L.: Structure and mitotic behavior of the early neural tube. In deHaan, R. L., and H. Ursprung, eds.: Organogenesis. New York, Holt, Rinehart & Winston, 1965.

Weed, L. H.: Certain anatomical and physiological aspects of the meninges and cerebrospinal fluid. Brain, *58*:383, 1935.

Weiss, P., and M. W. Cavanaugh: Further evidence of perpetual growth of nerve fibers; a recovery of fiber diameter after the release of prolonged constrictions. J. Exper. Zool., *142*:461, 1959.

Weiss, P., and H. B. Hiscoe: Experiments on the mechanism of nerve growth. J. Exper. Zool., *107*:315, 1948.

Weston, J. A.: A radioautographic analysis of the migration and localization of trunk neural crest cells in the chick. Develop. Biol., 6:279, 1963.

Windle, W. F.: Regeneration of axons in the vertebrate central nervous system. Physiol. Rev., 36:427, 1956.

Wislocki, G. B., and E. H. Leduc: Vital staining of the hematoencephalic barrier by silver nitrate and trypan blue, and cytological comparisons of neurohypophysis, pineal body, area postrema, intercolumnar tubercle and supraoptic crest. J. Comp. Neurol., 96:371, 1952.

13

Blood and Lymph Vascular Systems

All but the simplest multicellular animals require a mechanism to distribute oxygen, nutritive materials, and hormones to the tissues and to collect from them carbon dioxide and other products of tissue metabolism and to transmit these to the excretory organs. In vertebrates this important function is carried out by the *blood vascular system*, which consists of a muscular pump, the *heart*, and two continuous systems of tubular vessels. One of these, the *pulmonary circulation*, carries blood to and from the lungs; the other, the *systemic circulation*, distributes to and collects from all of the other tissues and organs of the body. In both of these circulations the blood pumped from the heart passes successively through *large elastic arteries, muscular* or *distributing arteries, small arteries, arterioles, capillaries, venules, small veins,* and *large veins,* and back to the heart. The actual exchange between the blood and the inspired air or between the blood and the tissues takes place in the minute thin-walled capillaries and venules. In most organs the network of capillaries of the blood vascular system is paralleled by a plexus of capillaries belonging to the lymphatic system.

BLOOD CAPILLARIES

The endothelium, the main component of the wall of a capillary, is the lining layer common to all parts of the vascular system, including the heart. The endothelial cells, although they differ from fibroblasts in shape, have many similar cytological characteristics. The nucleus is flattened and thus appears elongate or elliptical in section. It contains an inconspicuous nucleolus and fine chromatin particles. The cells are elongated in the direction of the axis of the capillary and have tapering ends. In capillaries of greater diameter they are shorter and broader, and in the lung their outlines are irregularly scalloped. In the smallest capillaries, a single endothelial cell may extend around the entire circumference of the vessel, whereas in capillaries of medium size, two or three curved cells extend around the lumen.

The caliber of the capillaries in various parts of the body varies within relatively narrow limits and is related to the size of the red blood corpuscles. In man it averages about 8 μm. In an organ or tissue that is in a state of minimal functional activity, a considerable number of the capillaries may be narrowed, so that little blood circulates through them. When the organ begins to function actively, these capillaries open up and blood circulates through them. This variability in caliber should be borne in mind, and it should be realized that in tissues fixed by immersion the capillaries appear narrower than in the living animal, while in those fixed by perfusion they may be distended beyond their normal physiological limits.

Intravascular injection of silver nitrate and subsequent exposure to light results in deposition of silver along the cell boundaries. In the majority of capillaries, it is possible by this means to show that the walls consist of separate endothelial cells whose boundaries stand out as sharply stained black lines. This staining reaction was long interpreted as resulting from deposition of metallic silver in an abundant "intercellular cement." Along

386

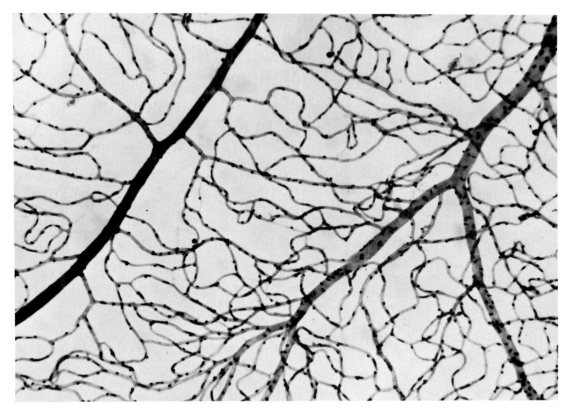

Figure 13–1 Normal human retinal blood vessels. These have been isolated by tryptic digestion of the neural and receptor elements, leaving behind only the vessels. At the left is an arteriole, at the right a venule, and between them is a network of capillaries of very uniform caliber. × 100. (Courtesy of T. Kuwabara.)

the cell boundaries and at the sites of their junction, lenticular or angular blackened regions were seen, and these were thought to be openings in the walls, called *stigmata* or *stomata*. Electron microscopy has shown that there are no such intercellular gaps in normal endothelium. The stomata described earlier were evidently artifacts of the silver nitrate impregnation method. The endothelial cells, like the cells of other simple epithelia, are closely apposed, with an intercellular cleft only 150 to 250 Å wide, which appears empty in electron micrographs. If an intervening layer of intercellular material exists, it is very limited in amount. The concept of an "intercellular cement" has now been largely abandoned.

The capillaries originate from the embryonic connective tissue. They penetrate among the parenchymal elements of various organs and tissues, accompanied along their entire course by thin collagenous or reticular fibers that closely adjoin the endothe-

lium. Whether the capillary endothelium possessed a "basement membrane" was a subject of debate among light microscopists, but this has now been settled by the electron microscopic demonstration of a thin glycoprotein basal lamina similar in all respects to that underlying other epithelia.

Fixed macrophages and undifferentiated mesenchymal cells are associated with the walls of capillaries. The pericapillary mesenchymal cells are clearly demonstrable in whole mounts of thin serous membranes (Fig. 13–2). In certain sites, the pericapillary cells are of quite different nature. For example, scattered along the capillaries in the nictitating membrane of the frog's eye are peculiar cells with long branching processes that surround the capillary wall (Rouget cells). These cells have been seen to contract under electrical stimulation and hence are considered by some to be of the nature of smooth muscle cells. Other cells have been described in very close association

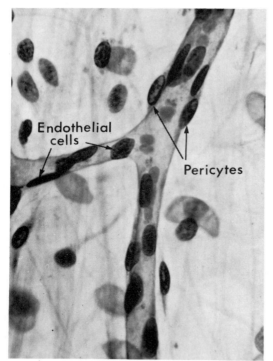

Figure 13-2 Photomicrograph of an intact capillary in a whole mount of rat mesentery. The nuclei of the flattened endothelial cells lining the capillary can be distinguished from those of the pericytes, which bulge outward. May-Grünwald-Giemsa stain. × 475.

with the endothelium but in these contractility has not been demonstrated. Whether or not these are the same as the cells described by Rouget is not clear, and it is now customary to describe all such cells as *pericytes* without attributing to them a special role in regulation of the caliber of the vessel (Fig. 13-3). Microdissection studies have shown that the endothelial cells themselves may contract after direct mechanical stimulation, and therefore it may be unnecessary to ascribe variations in the size of the lumen of a capillary to special cells in its wall.

At the resolution afforded by the light microscope, capillaries in different tissues and organs appear quite similar, but with the electron microscope at least three morphologically distinct types of capillary can be distinguished on the basis of differences in the structure of the endothelium and in its cell to cell junctions. There are indications from physiological studies that there are significant regional differences in permeability among capillaries of the same morphological type.

Continuous Capillaries

This common form of capillary is found in muscles and connective tissues throughout the body and in the central nervous system. The endothelial cells are thickened in the region of their nucleus but may be extremely thin at the periphery (Fig. 13-4). The cytoplasm near the nucleus contains a small Golgi apparatus, a pair of centrioles, and a few profiles of granular endoplasmic reticulum. Most of the cell's complement of mitochondria are near the nucleus, but occasional ones may be found in the thin peripheral parts of the cell. Randomly oriented cytoplasmic filaments and microtubules are present in small numbers.

The adluminal plasma membrane is a typical unit membrane. When stained with ruthenium red or Alcian blue, a fuzzy appearing dense coating can be seen on the outer

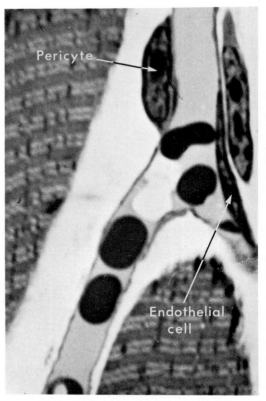

Figure 13-3 Photomicrograph of a capillary in skeletal muscle cut longitudinally. The nuclei of a pericyte, an endothelial cell, and a fibroblast can be distinguished. Several erythrocytes in the lumen give an indication of its dimensions. × 1800. (Courtesy of J. Venable.)

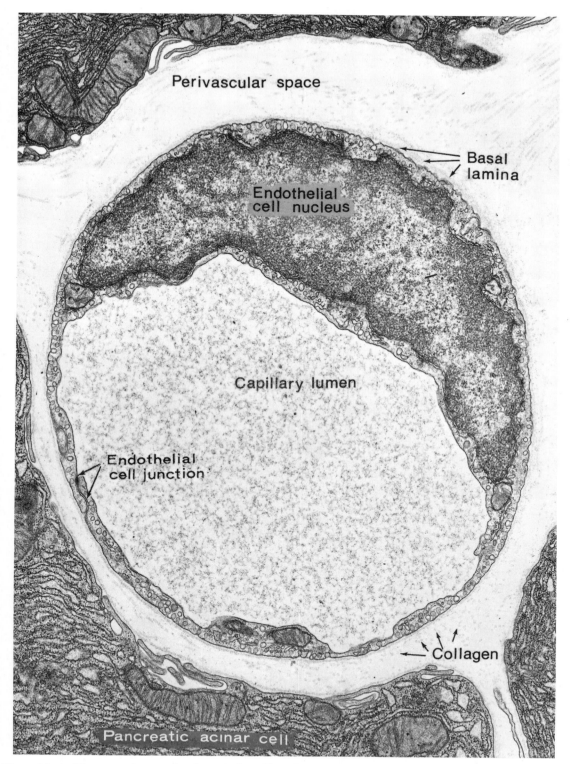

Figure 13-4 Electron micrograph of a typical capillary from guinea pig pancreas. The entire circumference is made up of a single endothelial cell. There is a thin basal lamina and a few associated collagen fibrils. No pericyte is present in this cross section. (Micrograph courtesy of R. Bolender, J. Cell Biol., *61*:269, 1974.)

aspect of the membrane (Luft). This layer, believed to be rich in carbohydrates, may correspond to the "endocapillary layer" described by early investigators of capillary structure, though it would seem to be too thin to be easily resolved with the light microscope.

A conspicuous feature of capillaries of this type is the presence of many small vesicular invaginations (caveolae) of the surface membrane. These are about 800 Å in diameter and are connected to the surface by a narrower neck, giving them a flask-shaped contour in thin sections (Fig. 13–5). The fuzzy coating of the cell membrane extends into the interior of the pits or caveolae. Spherical vesicles of similar dimensions are found within the cytoplasm, suggesting that the surface invaginations pinch off by constriction of their necks and move into the cytoplasm. Similar pits and vesicles are associated with the abluminal membrane of

the endothelial cells, and more rarely they open into the intercellular cleft.

The junction of adjacent endothelial cells may be interdigitated or relatively straight. At the luminal end, the attenuated margin of one cell may be prolonged into a narrow fold or flap (Fig. 13–6). This may lie against the wall of the capillary overlapping the edge of the neighboring cell, or it may project into the lumen. Occasionally both cells have marginal folds. These may have a hydrodynamic effect, retarding flow near the wall of the vessel. It has also been suggested that they may be actively undulatory and under certain conditions may be involved in pinocytosis. Their true significance remains to be discovered.

Along the boundary between endothelial cells, the opposing cell membranes are, for the most part, parallel and 150 to 200 Å apart. At certain points along the interface, however, the membranes come together and

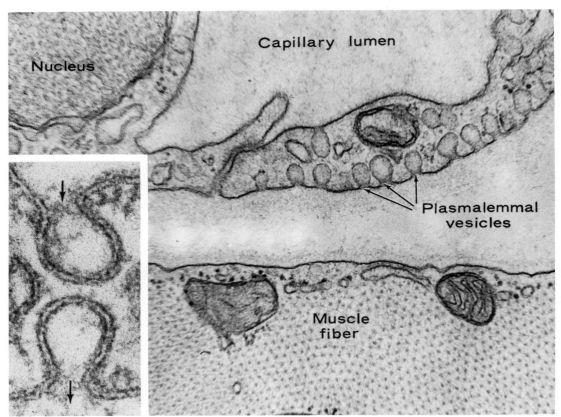

Figure 13–5 Electron micrograph of capillary endothelium, illustrating the small vesicular inpocketings of the luminal and basal surfaces that are characteristic of capillaries in muscle. (From D. W. Fawcett, J. Histochem. and Cytochem., *13*:75, 1965.) The inset shows two such vesicles at high magnification. (From R. Bruns and G. E. Palade, J. Cell Biol., *37*:244, 1968.)

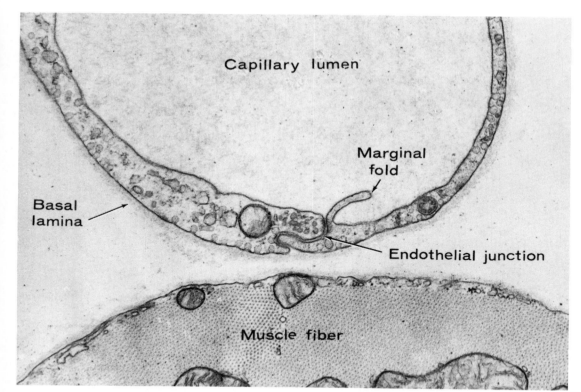

Figure 13-6 Capillary from cardiac muscle, illustrating the interdigitating cell junction and a marginal fold.

the outer layers appear to fuse (Fig. 13–7). These sites are interpreted by some investigators as belt-like occluding junctions (zonulae occludentes) that extend around the entire circumference of the cell, effectively closing the intercellular cleft. Others consider these junctional specializations to be linear sites of fusion of limited extent, interrupted by discontinuities that permit passage of water and small molecules through the intercellular clefts. For technical reasons, it has been difficult to choose between these two interpretations.

The endothelial tube of the capillary is supported on its outside by a thin continuous basal lamina similar in all respects to that of other epithelia. There is good evidence that it is a product of the endothelial cells. Where pericytes or their processes are found this layer splits to enclose them. The principal component of the capillary basal lamina is believed to be collagen in a form not exhibiting cross striations. Typical cross-striated reticular fibers may, however, be closely associated with its outer surface.

Fenestrated Capillaries

Capillaries of the kind just described are found in smooth, skeletal, and cardiac muscle and in various other tissues. Because they have an uninterrupted endothelium and a continuous basal lamina, they may be called *continuous capillaries* to distinguish them from the *fenestrated capillaries*, found in the renal glomeruli, the endocrine glands, the lamina propria of the intestine, and elsewhere (Fig. 13–8). The latter type is characterized by the presence of extremely attenuated areas of endothelium penetrated by circular fenestrae or pores 800 to 1000 Å in diameter (Fig. 13–9). Actually the perforations are only apparent, for they are usually closed by a very thin diaphragm with a slight central thickening. The diaphragm does not seem to be formed by the apposition of the two cell membranes, for it is usually thinner than a single unit membrane. The basal lamina is continuous across the fenestrations on the outside of the capillary. The pores may appear in thin sections to be randomly

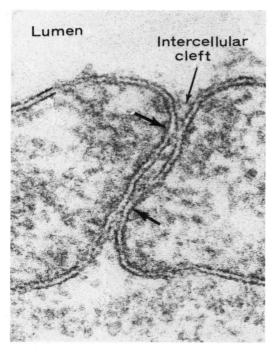

Figure 13-7 High magnification micrograph of an endothelial cell junction. At two points along the intercellular cleft (at arrows), the opposing cell membranes appear to be fused, forming five-layered junctions resembling zonulae occludentes. The linear extent of these junctions is not known. (Micrograph from R. Bruns and G. E. Palade, J. Cell Biol., 37:244, 1968.)

distributed, but in freeze fracture preparations they are often very regularly arranged, with a center to center spacing of about 1300 Å (Fig. 13-10). In any given cross section of a capillary, the areas exhibiting pores make up only a fraction of the circumference of the vessel, the fenestrated areas being separated by slightly thicker, unfenestrated regions. The cell to cell junctions usually occur in the thicker areas of the endothelium and are not significantly different from those of continuous capillaries.

The fenestrated capillaries are not the same everywhere. The fenestrae vary in size, number, and distribution. Although the matter is not entirely settled, it is the consensus that those of the renal glomeruli are exceptional in that they are not closed by diaphragms. The glomerular capillaries also have a basal lamina that is as much as three times thicker than that of other capillaries.

Sinusoids

Sinusoids are very thin-walled vascular channels of relatively large caliber and irregular cross-sectional outline, having a very tenuous connective tissue layer between the vascular wall and the parenchyma of the organ. They often are not cylindrical but conform to the interstices among the epithelial sheets or cords of the organ irrigated. They develop embryologically by ingrowth of the parenchyma (as in the liver) into a large, thin-walled embryonic blood vessel. This mode of development is to be contrasted to that of true capillaries, which branch dichotomously and grow in length by addition of vasoformative cells at the ends of the vessel. Sinusoids are characteristic of the circulation of the liver, spleen, bone marrow, and certain endocrine glands. The cells lining the sinusoids in the liver are phagocytic and thus belong to the reticuloendothelial system.

The anterior lobe of the pituitary gland, the adrenal cortex, and the islets of Langerhans in the pancreas are permeated by *fenestrated sinusoids*. These have a continuous basal lamina and a thin endothelium which has pores that are closed by thin diaphragms, as in fenestrated capillaries.

The liver lobules of many mammalian species have *discontinuous sinusoids*. The endothelial cells lining the sinusoids meet and overlap in typical junctions in some areas, while in other areas there are large gaps between cells (see Chapter 28). A basal lamina is discontinuous or entirely lacking. In certain species, the sinusoids of the liver are said to have a continuous lining and a basal lamina.

The sinusoids of the spleen and bone marrow have peculiarities of their own, which are described elsewhere.

In summary, it may be said that at the light microscopic level few differences were discernible in the smallest blood vessels of the various tissues and organs, and it was commonly assumed that all capillaries were much the same. It has been an important contribution of the electron microscope to have demonstrated that there are a number of different kinds of vessels structurally adapted to the physiological requirements of the particular region in which they are found: (1) capillaries having a continuous endothelium but lacking zonulae occludentes; (2) continuous capillaries with occluding junctions; (3)

fenestrated capillaries; (4) continuous sinusoids; (5) fenestrated sinusoids; and other variants of these major types. We turn now to a consideration of the functional significance of these different structural arrangements.

THE STRUCTURAL BASIS OF EXCHANGE ACROSS THE CAPILLARY WALL

The vascular system carries nutrients, hormones, and gaseous metabolites required by the cells throughout the body, and it takes up the products and by-products of their metabolism for distribution or excretion. One of the most important concerns of physiologists, therefore, is the mechanism of exchange of substances across their walls — *capillary permeability*. The capillaries present an enormous surface area. There is said to be about 2000 capillaries per square millimeter of skeletal muscle, and it is estimated that in a person weighing 150 pounds there would be over 6000 square meters of capillary surface available for exchange of metabolites with the tissues (Bloch).

When large numbers of small vesicles were observed at the luminal and basal surfaces of endothelial cells in electron micrographs, these were interpreted as a submicroscopic form of pinocytosis — "drinking" by cells. It was proposed, therefore, that the endothelial cells are active in capillary exchange, taking into these vesicles small quantities of fluid, transporting it across the cell, and discharging it on the abluminal surface into the perivascular space (Palade). This interpretation met with some resistance among physiologists, for capillary exchange takes place without significant expenditure of energy and to these physiologists the endothelium seemed to exhibit many of the characteristics of an inert, porous membrane, permeable to water and crystalloids but relatively impermeable to large molecules.

Calculations based upon physiological experiments with capillaries of skeletal muscle indicated that the observed rates of exchange could be accounted for by postulating uniform water-filled pores of 45 Å radius and a length of 0.3 μm., corresponding to the average thickness of the endothelium. These need have an aggregate area of only 0.1 to 0.2 per cent of the luminal surface and a frequency of 10 to 20 per μm.^{2} No pores of these dimensions are seen traversing the cytoplasm of the endothelium in electron micrographs of muscle capillaries. Since the intercellular clefts (150 Å wide) would comprise of the order of 0.1 to 0.2 per cent of the surface area, it was assumed that the inter-

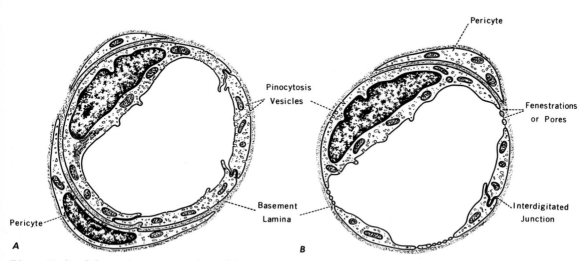

Figure 13–8 Schematic representation of the two commonest types of capillaries. *A*, The continuous or muscle type with an uninterrupted endothelium. *B*, The fenestrated type, in which the endothelium varies in thickness and the thinnest areas have small pores closed by an exceedingly thin membranous diaphragm. (After D. W. Fawcett, in J. L. Orbison and D. Smith, eds.: Peripheral Blood Vessels. Baltimore, Williams and Wilkins, 1962.)

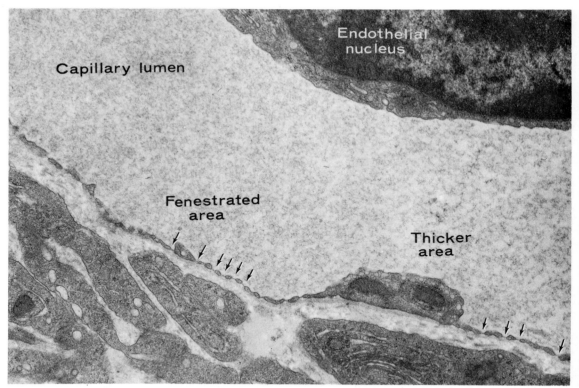

Figure 13-9 Micrograph of a typical fenestrated capillary from the lamina propria of the gastric mucosa. Thin fenestrated areas of endothelium alternate with thicker areas. (Micrograph courtesy of D. Hingson.)

cellular clefts might correspond to the hypothetical "small pore system" (Landis and Pappenheimer). Some of the measurements of permeability to large molecules made it necessary also to postulate the existence of a "large pore system," consisting of openings 400 to 700 Å in diameter. The fractional area occupied by these pores must necessarily be so small that their visual detection would seem to present serious difficulties.

Efforts to establish the morphological counterparts of the "small" and "large" pore systems of the physiologists have led to some disagreement. After intravascular injection, *peroxidase*, a protein tracer of relatively low molecular weight (40,000), could be shown to pass rapidly across the capillary wall through the intercellular clefts of muscle capillaries (Karnovsky). The tracer also entered the caveolae at the luminal surface and the small vesicles within the cytoplasm. A larger particulate tracer, *ferritin* (500,000 mol. wt.), did not pass between cells but did enter the

vesicles. A slow transport of larger molecules across the capillary wall seems to take place via the vesicles (Fig. 13–11). It was concluded from such studies that the endothelial cell junctions having gaps of about 40 Å between the opposing surfaces are the morphological equivalent of the small pore system, and that the vesicular transport may correspond to the "large pore system." The vesicular transport system is considered by many investigators to be too slow and of insufficient magnitude to account for rapid transcapillary exchange of substances of molecular weight below 10,000, but it may play a significant role in transcapillary movement of plasma proteins, hormones, antibodies, and the like.

An opposing school considers a large part of the intercellular pathway to be closed by zonulae occludentes and assigns a much more important role to vesicular transport, believing that it not only corresponds to the large pore system, but also carries out much of the transport of smaller molecules commonly attributed to the small pore system (Bruns and Palade; Simionescu and Palade). Enumeration of the vesicles in representative capillaries yields counts as high as 120 per $\mu m.^2$ of cell surface, and experiments employing myoglobin (17,800 mol. wt.) as a tracer have led to estimates of transit time of less than 1 minute to cross the endothelium. Little is known about the molecular mechanisms involved or energy required for intrusion of the vesicles into the cytoplasm or their transport across the cell. Neither low temperatures nor metabolic poisons seem greatly to affect their numbers, and it has been shown that Brownian motion may be sufficient to account for migration across the cell cytoplasm (Shea and Karnovsky). Clearly much work remains to be done before the relative importance of the intercellular and transcellular pathways is established.

The divergence of opinion concerning the permeability of the intercellular clefts of capillaries may be in part a question of technical differences in specimen preparation, but it is also evident that there are marked differences in the permeability of capillaries in different organs. It has long been known that after intravenous injection, dyes that readily escape from peripheral capillaries and venules are excluded from all but a few areas of the brain. This observation gave rise to the concept of a *blood-brain permeability barrier.* Its morphological basis was formerly thought to reside in special structural relations of the perivascular astrocyte foot-processes to each other and to the capillary wall. Application of tracers and electron microscopy to this problem has shown that the junctions between the endothelial cells of the brain capillaries do not permit the intercellular passage of peroxidase molecules. Although occasional vesicles containing the tracer are found at the luminal surface and in the cytoplasm, there is little evidence of their discharge on the abluminal side of the endothelium. Thus the paucity of transport vesicles in brain capillaries and the presence of occluding junctions between endothelial

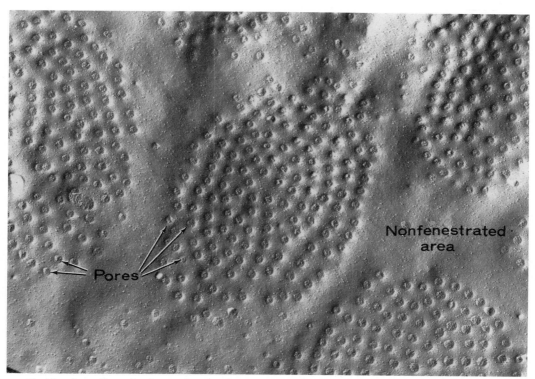

Figure 13–10　A replica of a freeze-fractured preparation of a fenestrated capillary. This extensive surface view of the cleaved membrane of an endothelial cell shows fenestrated areas separated by nonfenestrated areas. Notice the uniform size and spacing of the pores. (Micrograph courtesy of S. McNutt.)

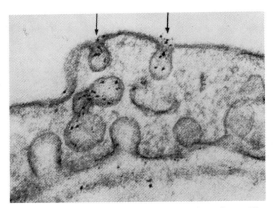

Figure 13-11 Electron micrograph of capillary endothelium, illustrating uptake of particulate matter (saccharated iron oxide) from the lumen by pinocytosis vesicles and its transport across the cell. Although such a mechanism exists, its quantitative importance in capillary exchange is questioned by many. × 100,000. (After M. A. Jennings, V. T. Marchesi, and S. H. Florey, Proc. Roy. Soc. B, *156:* 14, 1962.)

cells seems to account for their lower permeability compared to muscle capillaries (Reese and Karnovsky). A *blood-ocular barrier* has also been described, and a recent study with electron-opaque tracers has established the existence of a *blood-thymus barrier* (Raviola and Karnovsky). Here there is a differential permeability of various segments of the vascular tree within the same organ. The capillary endothelial junctions are impermeable and evidently prevent access of circulating macromolecules to the lymphoid cells of the cortex, while those of the medulla are freely permeable to electron-opaque tracers. The small amount that may be transported by endothelial vesicles in the cortex is immediately sequestered by perivascular macrophages.

In fenestrated capillaries exchange is evidently facilitated by the presence of the fenestrae, even though these are closed by a thin diaphragm. In the glomerular capillaries, where this closure seems to be lacking, fluid passes out of the vessels a hundred times more rapidly than in the continuous muscle capillaries. In discontinuous sinusoids, such as those in the liver, there is of course no barrier to the escape of particles smaller than cells, and the composition of the fluid in the perivascular space is essentially the same as that of plasma.

ARTERIES

Blood is carried from the heart to the capillary networks in the tissues and organs by arteries. These comprise an extensive system of tubular structures beginning with the aorta and pulmonary artery, which emerge from the left and right sides of the heart, respectively. As they course away from the heart, these vessels branch repeatedly and thus give rise to large numbers of arteries of progressively diminishing caliber. Although the diameter of the individual arterial branches steadily decreases as a result of their dichotomous branching, the sum of the cross sectional areas of all the branches gradually increases, and the rate of blood flow diminishes as the capillaries are approached. There is a further rapid expansion of the total cross sectional area of the vascular system at the level of the capillaries. As a consequence, flow through the capillaries is quite slow, thus allowing ample time for efficient exchange with the tissues. It should be borne in mind that it is only at the level of the capillaries and small venules that the vessel walls are thin enough to permit exchange of metabolites with the tissues, which is the essential function of the circulation. At any given moment, less than 10 per cent of the blood volume is in the capillaries and over 90 per cent is on its way to or from them. In all the other vessels of the vascular system, which are concerned with the distribution of the blood, the endothelium is reinforced by networks of elastic fibers, smooth muscle cells, fibroblasts, and collagenous fibers. These several components of the vessel walls vary in their proportions and in their arrangement in different segments of the system.

The basic organization of the wall of all arteries is similar in that three concentric layers or tunics can be distinguished: (1) an inner layer, the *tunica intima*, consisting of an endothelial tube whose cells generally have their long axis oriented longitudinally; (2) an intermediate layer, the *tunica media*, predominantly composed of smooth muscle cells disposed circumferentially, and (3) an outer coat, the *tunica adventitia*, made up of fibroblastic and fibrous elements that are oriented, for the most part, longitudinally. This layer gradually merges with the loose connective tissue that accompanies all blood vessels.

The boundary between the tunica intima and tunica media is marked by the *internal elastic lamina (elastica interna)* which is especially well developed in arteries of medium caliber. Between the tunica media and the tunica adventitia, a thinner *external elastic lamina (elastica externa)* can also be found in many arteries.

There is a continuous gradation in size and in character of the vessel wall from the largest arteries down to the capillaries. Nevertheless, it is customary to designate certain categories of vessels on the basis of their size, their predominant structural component, or their principal function in the arterial system. The large *elastic* or *conducting arteries*, such as the aorta, innominate, subclavian, and common carotid, have walls containing many fenestrated layers of elastin. Their walls may be distinctly yellow in the fresh state because of the abundance of their elastic elements.

These major vessels near the heart are distended during systole, and the subsequent elastic recoil of their walls during diastole serves as a subsidiary pump maintaining continuous flow in the system despite the intermittency of heart beat.

The elastic arteries gradually give way to *muscular* or *distributing arteries*, such as the brachial, femoral, radial, and popliteal. Their tunica media consists primarily of smooth muscle, which can actively alter the diameter of the vessel to adjust the volume of blood to suit the needs of the region irrigated. This category includes the majority of the vessels in the arterial system and spans a wide range of sizes, down to less than half a millimeter in diameter. Beyond the *small arteries* are the *arterioles*. The flow through these is still moderately rapid, but their numbers are so very great that they present an enormous surface area and a correspondingly great fric-

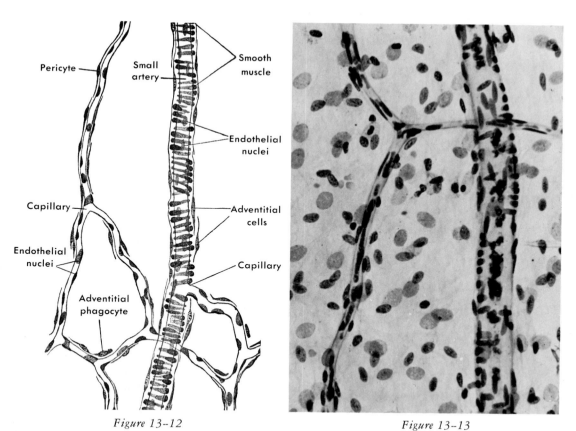

Figure 13–12

Figure 13–13

Figure 13–12 Small artery and capillaries from mesentery of a rabbit. × 187. (After A. A. Maximow.)
Figure 13–13 Photomicrograph of an arteriole and capillary comparable to those drawn in Figure 13–12. Notice in the arteriole the rows of nuclei of the circumferentially oriented smooth muscle cells. Their elongated form is not evident here because they are seen in optical section. × 250.

tional resistance to flow. The peripheral resistance at the level of the arterioles is the principal factor responsible for maintenance of normal blood pressure in the arterial system. Some authors distinguish a transitional category of *precapillary arterioles,* but their limits and morphological characteristics are rather poorly defined.

Arterioles and Small Arteries

The *tunica intima* of the smallest arterioles consists only of endothelium and is surrounded by a media consisting of a single layer of smooth muscle cells (Figs. 13–12, 13–13, and 13–14). In larger arterioles the intima includes an internal elastic lamina, which appears as a thin bright line immediately beneath the endothelium. In cross sections, it usually has a scalloped appearance because the agonal contraction of the muscle in the media throws it into longitudinal folds.

The *tunica media* of small arteries is composed of smooth muscle cells 15 to 20 μm. in length. When seen in surface view they are always oriented transversely to the long axis of the vessel, and in cross sections they are disposed circumferentially. The number of layers of muscle cells depends upon the caliber of the artery (Fig. 13–16).

The *tunica adventitia* approximately equals the tunica media in thickness; it is a layer of loose connective tissue with longitudinally oriented collagenous and elastic fibers and a few fibroblasts. It merges with the surrounding connective tissue. The small arteries lack a definite external elastic lamina.

In electron micrographs of small arterioles, the continuous endothelium is found to be supported by a typical basal lamina and occasional small bundles of collagen fibrils. In vessels having an elastica interna, the endothelium and its basal lamina are closely applied to it (Fig. 13–16). The elastin in vessels of small caliber is in the form of longitudinally oriented bars separated by long slitlike fenestrations. In larger vessels this layer becomes much thicker and is a more nearly continuous sheet but it retains occasional, very narrow fenestrations.

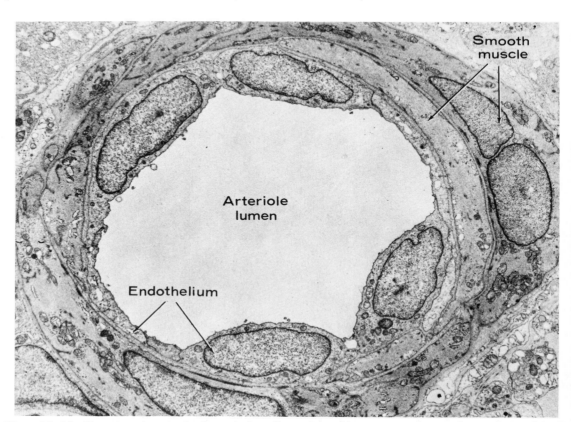

Figure 13-14 Electron micrograph of a typical small arteriole with one or two layers of smooth muscle cells around the endothelium.

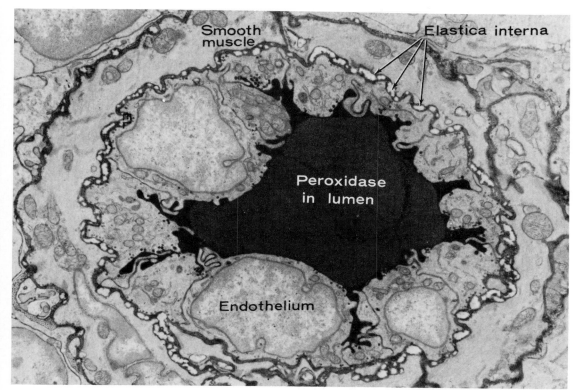

Figure 13-15 Arteriole from the corticomedullary boundary of the mouse thymus, five minutes after intravenous injection of peroxidase. The endothelium is freely permeable to this protein. The dense reaction product is seen in the lumen, between endothelial cells and filling the fenestrations in the elastica interna and the extracellular space around the single layer of smooth muscle cells. (Micrograph from E. Raviola and M. J. Karnovsky, J. Exp. Med., *136*:466, 1972.)

A new cytoplasmic component has been revealed in the endothelial cells of small arteries by electron microscopy. It is a rod-shaped structure 0.1 μm. in diameter and 3 μm. in length and consists of a bundle of fine tubules embedded in a dense matrix and enclosed in a closely fitting membrane. In addition, the endoplasmic reticulum of the endothelial cells often is distended with dense, finely granular material. The significance of these features of arterial endothelium has not been determined (Weibel and Palade).

Muscular or Distributing Arteries

This is the most numerous class of arteries. Beneath the endothelium in the arteries of this group is the elastica interna (Figs. 13–17, 13–18, and 13–19). The basal surfaces of the endothelial cells closely conform to all of the irregularities of contour in the elastica and send slender processes through its fenestrations to establish contact with the underlying smooth muscle cells of the media. It is believed that these discontinuities in the elastica may be essential for the sustenance of the avascular media by permitting diffusion of metabolites from the lumen. The scalloped internal elastic lamina is very well developed, and because of its low affinity for osmium it appears in electron micrographs as a sinuous light layer stippled with cross sectional profiles of fibrils within the substance of the elastin.

The tunica media of muscular arteries consists almost exclusively of smooth muscle cells arranged in concentric layers. The muscle cells are surrounded and separated from one another by a moderately thick layer of glycoprotein analogous to the basal lamina of epithelia. This stains deeply with the periodic acid-Schiff reaction and generally appears amorphous in electron micrographs of low magnification (Fig. 13–16). Embedded within this abundant interstitial material are

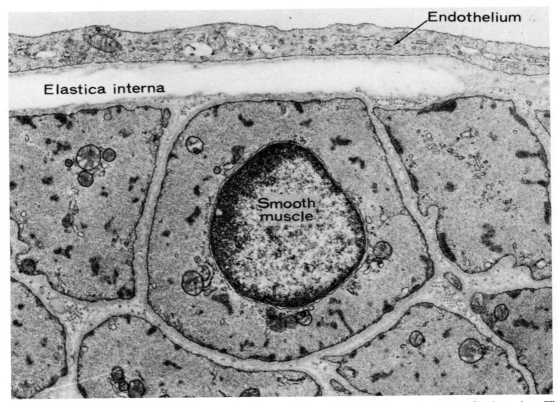

Figure 13-16 Electron micrograph of a portion of the wall of a small artery in longitudinal section. The elastica interna does not stain and therefore appears as a clear area between the endothelium and the smooth muscle of the media.

small bundles of collagen fibrils corresponding to the network of delicate reticular fibers seen surrounding individual muscle fibers in silver stained preparations viewed with the light microscope. Loose networks of thin elastic fibers also course circumferentially in the media and can be recognized as dark wavy lines among the smooth muscle cells in preparations stained with aldehyde-fuchsin or resorcin-fuchsin (Figs. 13–17B and 13–18). In electron micrographs they appear as unstained elongated profiles of irregular outline. The elastica externa may appear in photomicrographs as a continuous layer at the junction of the media and adventitia (Fig. 13–18), but in electron micrographs of cross sections it is an interrupted row of irregular strands of elastin considerably thinner than the elastica interna (Fig. 13–20). In contracted vessels, portions of smooth muscle cells occupy the discontinuities in the elastica externa, sometimes bulging into the adventitia. Closely applied to the elastica on its outer aspect are numerous small fascicles of unmyelinated nerve axons, some containing collections of mitochondria and numerous synaptic vesicles. The nerves ordinarily do not penetrate into the media and ramify among the smooth muscle cells but appear to terminate at the elastica externa (Fig. 13–20). The neural stimulation of the muscle cells may then result from diffusion of the transmitter substance through this layer, and the resulting depolarization of the peripheral muscle cells may be propagated throughout the media via low-resistance cell to cell contacts (nexus) between muscle cells.

The tunica adventitia of distributing arteries is sometimes thicker than the media (Figs. 13–17 and 13–18), and consists of fibroblasts, strands of elastin, and bundles of collagen oriented longitudinally or obliquely. These continue into the surrounding connective tissue without a clearly defined boundary. The loose consistency of the tunica adventitia and predominant longitudinal orientation of its components permits the continual changes in the diameter of the vessel but limits the amount of retraction that takes place when the artery is cut.

Large Elastic Arteries

The resistant elastic wall of a vessel such as the aorta is quite thick, but in proportion to the size of the lumen it is thinner than the wall of muscular arteries.

The tunica intima in the aorta of adult man is about 127 μm. in thickness (Fig. 13–22). Its endothelium differs from that of smaller arteries in that the polygonal cells tend to be less elongated in the axis of the vessel. The thin subjacent layer contains interlacing bundles of collagen fibers and a few fusiform cells. These latter were formerly interpreted as fibroblasts but in electron micrographs they are found to have the cytological characteristics of smooth muscle cells. Occasional wandering cells may be present. The next deeper layer of the intima consists of many branching and anastomosing fibers. Among these elastic fibers are a few collagenous fibers, fibroblasts, and small bundles of smooth muscle cells. Externally these elastic

fibers join a fenestrated elastic lamina corresponding in location to the elastica interna of smaller vessels. In large elastic arteries, however, this does not stand out as a single well defined sheet marking the junction of intima and media but is merely the first of many similar fenestrated elastic laminae found throughout the thickness of the media. Thus in the very large vessels the tunica intima is poorly demarcated from the tunica media.

In the human aorta the tunica media consists largely of elastic tissue, which appears in the form of 50 to 65 concentric fenestrated elastic laminae 2.5 μm. thick and 6 to 18 μm. apart. The successive layers are frequently interconnected by elastic fibers or bands. In the spaces between elastic laminae are thin layers of connective tissue with thin collagenous and elastic fibers, fibroblasts, and smooth muscle cells (Fig. 13–23). The smooth muscle cells, particularly in the inner layers of the tunica media, are flattened, branched elements with irregular outlines and serrated edges; they have characteristic elongated nuclei. Most of them are arranged circumferentially. These smooth muscle cells are closely surrounded by collagenous fibers, which bind them to the elastic laminae. Between these various structures is an appreci-

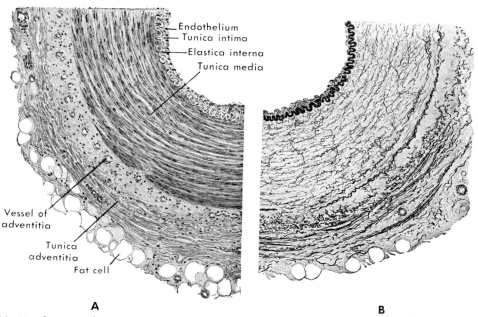

Endothelium
Tunica intima
Elastica interna
Tunica media

Vessel of adventitia

Tunica adventitia

Fat cell

A

B

Figure 13–17 Sectors of two cross sections of the volar digital artery of man. *A*, Stained with hematoxylin and eosin. *B*, Stained with orcein to show elastic tissue. × 80. (Slightly modified from Schaffer.)

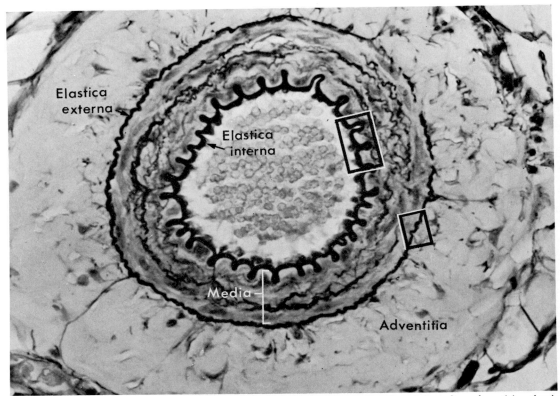

Figure 13–18 Photomicrograph of a muscular artery from the rat, showing the media, adventitia, elastica interna, elastica externa, and scattered elastic fibers in the media. Areas similar to those enlosed in the rectangles are illustrated in Figures 13–19 and 13–20. Aldehyde-fuchsin stain. × 250.

able amount of metachromatic amorphous ground substance. The basophilia and metachromasia of this ground substance is believed to be due to the presence of chondroitin sulfate.

The tunica adventitia in arteries of large caliber is relatively thin. It cannot be sharply distinguished from the surrounding connective tissue. The most external of the fenestrated laminae of the tunica media corresponds to an external elastic lamina. There is a gradual transition from the tunica adventitia into the surrounding loose connective tissue.

The walls of large arteries and veins are too thick to be nourished by diffusion from the lumen. They are provided with small arteries, the *vasa vasorum*, derived either from branches of the main vessel or from neighboring arteries. These break up into a capillary plexus in the deeper layers of the tunica adventitia. As a rule they do not penetrate deeply into the media of arteries, but in large veins they may extend nearly to the intima.

Transitional and Special Types of Arteries

In the gradual transition from one type of artery to another it is sometimes difficult to classify the intermediate region. Some arteries of intermediate caliber (popliteal, tibial) have walls that suggest larger arteries, while some large arteries (external iliac) have walls like those of medium-sized arteries. The transitional regions between elastic and muscular arteries are often designated *arteries of mixed type*. Such are the external carotid, axillary, and common iliac arteries. Their walls contain, in the tunica media, islands of smooth muscle fibers that separate or interrupt the elastic laminae in many places.

Where arteries of mixed or elastic type pass suddenly into arteries of the muscular type, short regions of transition occur; in these regions the vessels are called *arteries of hybrid type*. The visceral arteries that arise from the abdominal aorta are examples of such vessels. In them, for a varying distance, the tunica media may consist of two different layers—the internal being muscular and the external being composed of typical elastic laminae.

In the tunica media of the arteries of the lower limbs, the smooth muscle is more highly developed than it is in arteries of corresponding size in the upper limbs.

The arteries within the skull, which are protected from external pressure or tension, have a relatively thin wall and a well developed elastica interna. Elastic fibers are almost entirely absent in the tunica media.

The umbilical artery has an atypical structure. Its intima consists only of endothelium and an internal elastic layer is lacking. The tunica media contains a small number of elastic fibers and two thick muscular layers, which are sharply separated. The inner layer is composed of longitudinally directed fibers and the outer layer of circumferential fibers. In many places the longitudinal muscle forms longitudinal ridges protruding into both the lumen and the outer circular layer. The extra-abdominal portion of the umbilical artery is provided with numerous oval swellings or varicosities. In these regions the wall becomes thin and consists almost exclusively of circularly arranged muscle.

Physiological Implications of the Structure of the Arterial Walls

The flow of the blood in the arteries is caused by intermittent contraction of the heart, and therefore it is pulsatile. If the walls of the arteries were inflexible, the flow of blood into the capillaries would be intermit-

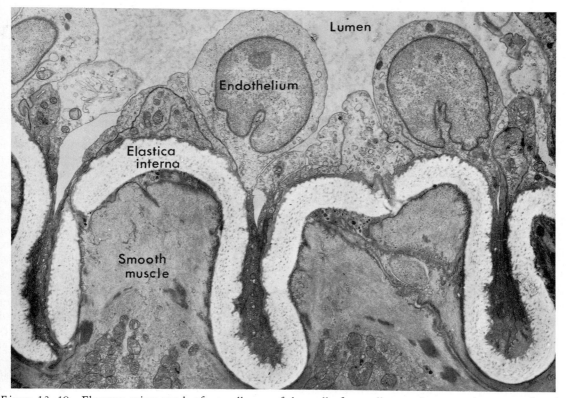

Figure 13–19 Electron micrograph of a small area of the wall of a small muscular artery (see upper box in Figure 13–18). The elastica interna is scalloped because of agonal contraction of the vessel wall. It is penetrated at intervals by slender fenestrations, through which processes extend from the endothelial cells to contact the smooth muscle cells of the media. × 10,000.

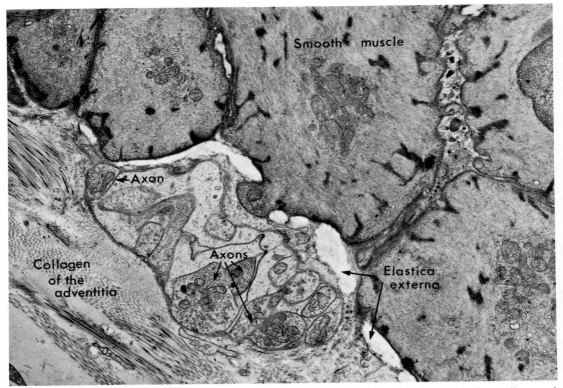

Figure 13-20 Electron micrograph of junctional zone between the media and adventitia of a small muscular artery (see lower box in Figure 13-18). The smooth muscle layer is limited on its outer aspect by a discontinuous elastica externa. Closely applied to this are numerous small nerves, some of whose axons contain many synaptic vesicles. × 10,000.

tent. However, because the large arteries near the heart have expansible elastic walls, only part of the force of cardiac contraction is dissipated in advancing the column of blood in the vessels; the rest of the energy goes to expanding the walls of the large elastic arteries. The potential energy accumulated in the stretching of the walls of these vessels during contraction of the heart (systole) is dissipated in the elastic recoil of the vessel wall during the period when the heart is inactive (diastole). This release of tension in the arterial wall serves as an auxiliary pump, forcing the blood onward during diastole when no forward pressure is exerted by the heart. Thus, although the flow of blood is pulsatile throughout much of the arterial system, the elasticity of the walls of the large elastic vessels insures continuous flow through the capillaries despite the intermittent pumping of the heart.

The musculature in the media of the distributing arteries is normally in a state of partial contraction, referred to as *tone*, but the degree of contraction can be modulated with changes in pressure in the system and variations in activity of various tissues and organs. The *vasoconstriction* and *vasodilation* of arteries is regulated in part by the autonomic nervous system. In the majority of arteries seen in routine histological sections, the smooth muscle of the tunica media has undergone some degree of contraction either after death or in response to the stimulus of immersion in a chemical fixative. One therefore gets a somewhat erroneous impression of the thickness of the arterial wall in relation to the size of the lumen. The remarkable capacity of the arteries to change their caliber is observed best in the living anesthetized animal. If a microdroplet of norepinephrine is placed on an artery, the underlying portion of the vessel wall will undergo marked local vasoconstriction. If the vasculature is then rapidly fixed in this condition and sections are subsequently cut through the open and the adjacent constricted segments of the same vessel, one can clearly observe the great decrease in caliber of the lumen and the striking change in the character of the wall which accompanies vasomotor activity (Figs. 13–24 and 13–25).

Such contractions and relaxations of the muscular walls of arteries obviously influence the distribution of blood to the various organs. They also change the peripheral resistance to flow and therefore affect the blood pressure. Contractility of arteries may be the result of stimulation by sympathetic nerves, or of direct action of local products of injury. This latter effect is important in limiting hemorrhage from torn vessels in sites of tissue injury.

There are other local factors acting at

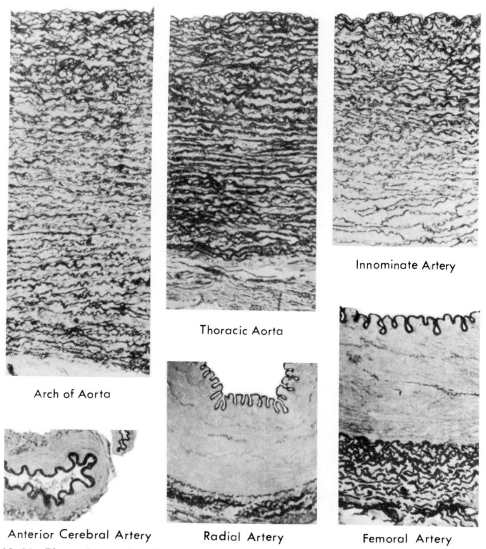

Innominate Artery

Thoracic Aorta

Arch of Aorta

Anterior Cerebral Artery   Radial Artery   Femoral Artery

Figure 13–21 Photomicrographs of the walls of elastic and muscular arteries of a large adult macaque. Elastic tissue has been darkly stained with resorcin fuchsin. In the upper three figures, not all of the adventitia is included. Observe the comparative thickness of the vessel walls and the amount and distribution of elastic tissue. (From E. V. Cowdry, Textbook of Histology. Philadelphia, Lea and Febiger, 1950.)

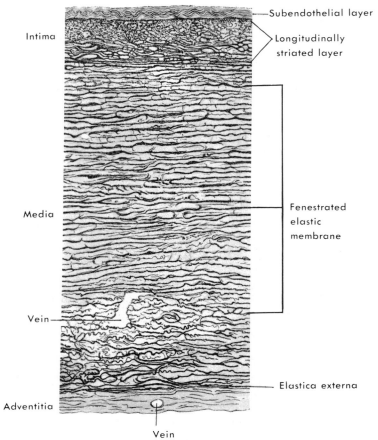

Intima

Subendothelial layer

Longitudinally striated layer

Fenestrated elastic membrane

Media

Vein

Elastica externa

Adventitia

Vein

Figure 13-22 Longitudinal section through posterior wall of human descending aorta. Elastic tissue is black; the other elements are not shown clearly. Elastic fiber stain. × 85. (After Kölliker and von Ebner.)

the level of small arteries and arterioles that tend to regulate blood flow. If blood flow is interrupted briefly, the lack of oxygen and accumulation of carbon dioxide and lactic acid both tend to cause relaxation of smooth muscle and vasodilation, so that when circulation is restored the rate of flow may be two to six times greater than it was before. This important local autoregulation or *reactive hyperemia* correcting metabolic deficits does not depend upon the nervous system.

The maintenance of normal blood pressure depends in large measure upon the peripheral resistance to flow in the system, which in turn is a function of the smooth muscle tone in the walls of arterioles and small arteries. Halving the diameter of arterioles can increase the resistance as much as sixteen-fold and a constriction to one fourth

their original diameter may increase resistance as much as 256 times (Guyton). This is the basis for the powerful effect of catecholamines and vasoactive peptides, such as angiotensin, on blood pressure.

Changes in the Arteries with Age

The arterial blood vessels reach their mature form only in adult life. During the fourth month of embryonic life in man, the arteries acquire their three main layers. From this time the wall of the vessels changes gradually.

In the aorta of a human embryo of four months, the intima consists only of the endothelium and of one rather thick elastic lamina, the elastica interna. The media consists of several layers of circular smooth muscles, between which are flat networks of elastic fibers. The adventitia is thicker than the media and consists of embryonic connective tissue.

At the end of embryonic life, the internal elastic membrane becomes thicker, while the networks of elastic fibers in the media turn into thick elastic laminae. The muscular elements have increased slightly in number but are still inconspicuous. The adventitia by this time has become relatively thinner.

After birth, the number and thickness of the elastic laminae in the media of the aorta gradually increase. By now they are much like the elastica interna. In the intima, between the endothelium and the elastica interna, a musculoelastic layer appears. It arises in part by a splitting of the elastica interna and in part by the new formation of collagenous and elastic fibers, and it gradually increases in thickness. At about the age of 25, the layers are completely differentiated.

The medium-sized muscular arteries, such as the brachial, even in the middle of embryonic life have an intima composed of an endothelium and an elastica interna, a media of circular smooth muscles, and an adventitia. The latter has a pronounced elastica externa surrounded by a connective tissue layer rich in elastic fibers. Toward the end of the embryonic period, the greatly thickened media consists only of circular muscle bounded by the external and internal elastic membranes. After birth, in the arteries of muscular type, in addition to the thickening of the wall as a whole, these arteries gradually develop a connective tissue layer between the endothelium and the elastica interna.

The heart and arteries are always active mechanically and seem more subject to wear and the ravages of age than other systems or organs. Indeed, the final differentiation of the structure of the wall frequently cannot be sharply separated from the regressive changes that develop gradually with age and lead to *arteriosclerosis* or "hardening of the arteries." Some authors view these alterations as physiological, others as pathological. It seems reasonable to regard arteriosclerosis as a pathological process when its degree of development in a given vessel is beyond the norm for this vessel at a particular age. The arteries of elastic type, particularly the aorta, show much greater changes with age than do the arteries of muscular type. Under physiological conditions, the small arteries participate relatively little in this process. The type of pathological change is different in the different types of vessels.

The larger vessels, particularly the aorta and iliac, femoral, coronary, and cerebral arteries, are subject to *atherosclerosis*—a patchy, irregular thickening of the interna with intra-

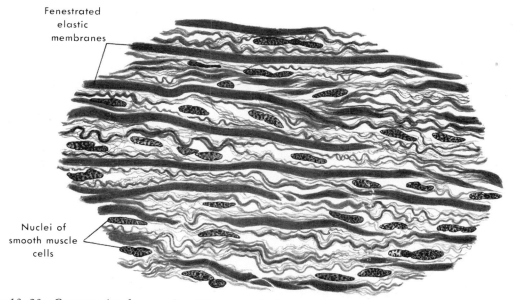

Fenestrated elastic membranes

Nuclei of smooth muscle cells

Figure 13-23 Cross section from media of the aorta of a 5 year old boy. Between the cross sections of fenestrated elastic membranes are wavy bundles of collagenous fibers. Orcein and hematoxylin. × 500. (After A. A. Maximow.)

cellular and extracellular deposition of lipid, followed by degeneration and calcification. Because atherosclerosis can gradually or suddenly interfere with blood flow through the heart or brain, it has serious clinical potentials, such as heart attack and stroke. It is the principal cause of death in the United States.

The pathogenesis of the disease is still poorly understood. This is due, in part, to the fact that a single site in the arterial vasculature cannot be observed more than once, either clinically or in experimentally induced lesions in animals. It is difficult, therefore, to reconstruct accurately the sequence of events in development of the lesions. A currently popular interpretation holds that smooth muscle cells and their products are of central importance. The earliest change appears to be a proliferation of smooth muscle cells in the intima by mitosis and by migration of cells from the

media through the fenestrations in the internal elastic lamina. An accumulation of lipid in these cells and extracellularly results in formation of the early intimal lesions described as "fatty streaks." Deposition of excess collagen, small elastic fibers, and extracellular matrix (glycosaminoglycans) by the smooth muscle cells produces a local thickening of the intima that is recognized grossly as a "fibrous plaque." With the passage of time and progression of the disease process, local hemorrhage, calcification, and necrosis result in what are aptly described as "complicated lesions." These are often the sites of erosion of the luminal surface of the arterial wall and formation of a mural thrombus (clot).

In the medium-sized arteries of muscular type, in addition to the intimal changes and splitting of the elastica interna, there may be degeneration and calcification in the tunica media.

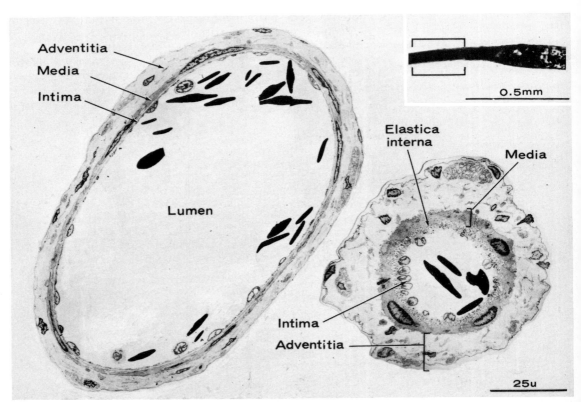

Figure 13–24 Low power micrographs of two cross sections less than a millimeter apart in the same frog arteriole. A microdroplet applied to the living vessel caused local vasoconstriction in the area indicated by the brackets (inset). The vessel was then fixed in situ and sectioned. The two sections offer a dramatic demonstration of the structural correlates of vasoconstriction and vasodilation. (From P. C. Phelps and J. H. Luft, *Am. J. Anat., 125*:399, 1969.)

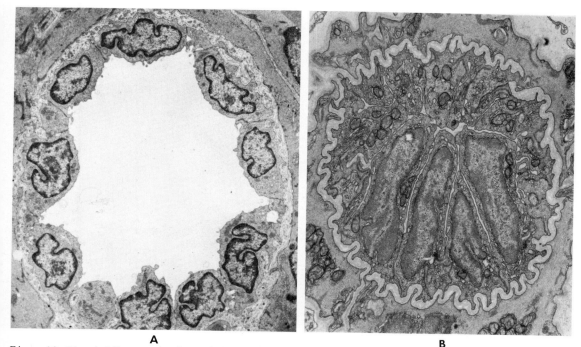

A   **B**

Figure 13-25   *A,* Micrograph of a typical small artery fixed with its lumen open. *B,* Micrograph of an artery of comparable size that has undergone agonal vasoconstriction. The cell bodies of the endothelial cells have increased in height, and they now almost completely occlude the lumen. Such extreme vasoconstriction probably occurs only rarely in normal physiological conditions, but it is evident that at sites of injury, this could effectively reduce hemorrhage. (Micrograph courtesy of R. Bolender.)

VEINS

The blood is carried from the capillary networks toward the heart by the veins. In progressing toward the heart, they gradually increase in caliber, while their walls become thicker. The veins usually accompany their corresponding arteries (Fig. 13-26). The veins are more numerous than the arteries and their caliber is larger, so that the venous system has a much greater capacity than the arterial system. The walls of the veins are always thinner, more supple, and less elastic than those of the arteries. Thus, in sections, the veins are usually collapsed, and their lumen is irregular and slitlike unless a special effort has been made to fix them in distention.

One can frequently distinguish three types: veins of small, medium, and large caliber. This subdivision is often unsatisfactory, for the caliber and structure of the wall cannot always be correlated. Individual veins show much greater variations than do the arteries, and the same vein may show great differences in different parts.

Most authors distinguish three layers in the walls of the veins: tunica intima, tunica media, and tunica adventitia. But the boundaries of these layers are frequently indistinct, and in certain veins these coats, particularly the tunica media, cannot be distinguished. The muscular and elastic tissue is not nearly as well developed in the veins as in the arteries, whereas the connective tissue component is much more prominent.

Venules and Veins of Small Caliber

When several capillaries unite, they form a venule, a cylindrical vessel 15 to 20 μm. in diameter, consisting of a layer of endothelium surrounded by thin, longitudinally oriented reticular fibers with occasional fibroblasts (Fig. 13-27). Although the caliber of the vessel is larger, the structure of its wall is not very different from that of a capillary, but it appears to be more permeable to intravenously injected dyes. Not all of the exchange between the blood and the tissues takes place in the capillaries. The

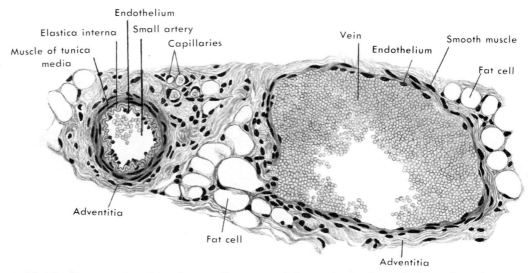

Figure 13-26 Cross section through a small artery and its accompanying vein from the submucosa of a human intestine. × 187. (After A. A. Maximow.)

venules appear to have a significant role in this, and they are particularly important in the changes associated with inflammation.

Early observations on the properties of venules have now been amplified by electron microscopic studies (Majno). When particulate markers are injected intravascularly, the particles are usually found not in the walls of the capillaries but in somewhat larger vessels interpreted as venules. This same category of vessels is also most susceptible to histamine, serotonin, and other substances known to increase vascular permeability (Fig. 13–29). If one of these substances is injected locally into an animal that has previously been injected intravenously with a particulate marker, it induces the appearance of small intercellular gaps in the endothelium. The particles, held back by the basal lamina, accumulate in the gaps, thus marking the vessels and permitting identification of the sites of increased permeability. Although leaks can occasionally be found in capillaries, the vast majority are in small venules. There seems to be a gradient of permeability from the arterial to the venous side, which reaches a maximum in the venules and then diminishes abruptly in vessels of larger size.

When the caliber of venules has increased to about 50 μm., partially differentiated smooth muscle cells appear between the endothelium and the connective tissue. These cells are at first some distance apart. Farther along, in small veins, they become arranged closer and closer together. In small veins with a diameter of 200 μm., these elements form a more or less continuous layer and have a typical long spindle shape.

In still larger veins, thin networks of elastic fibers appear. Their tunica intima consists only of endothelium, and one or several layers of smooth muscle cells form the media. The tunica adventitia consists of fibroblasts and thin elastic and collagenous fibers. Most of these fibrous elements run longitudinally, but some penetrate among the muscle cells of the tunica media.

Veins of Medium Caliber

The veins of medium caliber (2 to 9 mm.) include the cutaneous and deeper veins of the extremities distal to the brachial and the popliteal, and the veins of the viscera and head, with the exception of the main trunks. In the *tunica intima* of these veins, the endothelial cells in surface view are polygons with highly irregular outlines. Sometimes the tunica intima also contains an inconspicuous connective tissue layer with a few cells and thin elastic fibers. Externally, it is sometimes bounded by a network of elastic fibers. Because the tunica intima is often poorly developed, some authors consider the inner and middle coats as forming one layer.

The tunica media is much thinner than in the arteries and consists mainly of circular smooth muscle fibers separated by many longitudinal collagenous fibers and a few fibroblasts (Fig. 13–30). The tunica adventitia is usually much thicker than the media and consists of loose connective tissue with thick longitudinal collagenous bundles and elastic networks. In the layers adjacent to the media, it often contains a number of longitudinal smooth muscle bundles.

Veins of Large Caliber

The tunica intima has the same structure as in the medium-sized veins. In some of the larger trunks its connective tissue layer is of considerable thickness (45 to 68 μm.). The tunica media, in general, is poorly developed and is sometimes absent. Its structure is the same as in the veins of medium caliber. The tunica adventitia makes up the greater part of the venous wall and is usually several times as thick as the tunica media. It consists of loose connective tissue containing thick elastic fibers and longitudinally oriented collagenous fibers. The tunica adventitia contains prominent longitudinal layers of smooth muscle and elastic networks. This is the structure of the inferior vena cava and of the portal, splenic, superior mesenteric, external iliac, renal and azygos veins.

Special Types of Veins

There are longitudinal or circumferential smooth muscle fibers in the subendothelial connective tissue layer of the tunica intima in the iliac, femoral, popliteal, saphenous, cephalic, basilar, umbilical, and other veins. In certain veins the longitudinal orientation is also noticed in the innermost layers of the tunica media.

In a considerable portion of the inferior

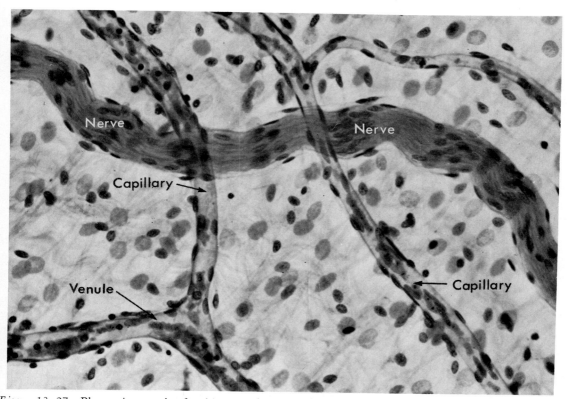

Figure 13-27 Photomicrograph of a thin spread mesentery showing a nerve, venule, and capillaries. May-Grünwald-Giemsa stain. × 300.

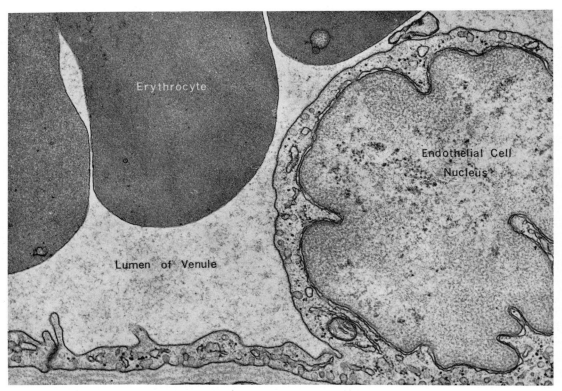

Figure 13-28 Electron micrograph of a portion of the wall of a small venule from the myocardium. The thin continuous endothelium is essentially the same as that of a capillary. The nuclear region of the endothelial cell bulges into the lumen. × 25,000.

vena cava, the tunica media is absent and well developed longitudinal muscle bundles of the tunica adventitia are directly adjacent to the intima. In the pulmonary veins, the media is well developed, with circular smooth muscle, and it is like an artery in this respect. Smooth muscle is particularly prominent in all the layers of the veins in the pregnant uterus.

Certain veins are entirely devoid of smooth muscle tissue and consequently lack a tunica media. In this group belong the veins of the maternal part of the placenta, the spinal pia mater, the retina, and the bones, as well as the sinuses of the dura mater, the majority of the cerebral veins, and the veins of the nailbed and the trabeculae of the spleen. The last two are simply channels lined by endothelium, with a fibrous connective tissue covering.

The adventitia of the vena cava and particularly of the pulmonary vein is provided for a considerable distance with a layer of cardiac muscle fibers arranged in a ring, with a few longitudinal fibers where these vessels enter the heart. In the rat, the pulmonary veins up to their radicles contain a considerable amount of cardiac muscle in the tunica media.

Valves of the Veins

Many veins of medium caliber, especially those of the extremities, are provided with *valves* that prevent the blood from flowing away from the heart. These are semilunar pockets on the internal surface of the wall, with their free edges pointing in the direction of the blood flow (Fig. 13–21). In man the valves are usually arranged in pairs, one opposite the other. Between the valve and the wall of the vein is the *sinus of the valve*, where the wall of the blood vessel is usually thin and somewhat distended.

The valve itself is a thin connective tissue membrane. On the side toward the lumen of the vessel, it contains a network of elastic fibers continuous with those of the tunica intima of the vein. In the thinner region of the wall, comprising the sinus of a valve, the intimal and medial tunics contain only longitudinal smooth muscle fibers. These do not enter into the substance of the valve in man.

Both surfaces of the valve are covered by endothelium. The endothelial cells lining the surface toward the lumen of the vessel are elongated in the axis of the vessel; those that line the surface of the valve facing the sinus are transversely elongated.

VASCULAR SPECIALIZATIONS AND ANCILLARY ORGANS

Portal Systems of Vessels

As a general rule, a capillary network connects the terminal ramifications of the arterial system with those of the venous system, and the transition from arterioles to capillaries to venules is gradual. In a number of regions, however, modifications of this vascular plan are adapted to the special functional requirements of the particular organ.

In one physiologically important modification of the general plan, the flow from one capillary bed passes through a larger vessel or vessels having histological characteristics of veins, to a second capillary network before the blood returns to the heart via the systemic venous circulation. Such a set of vessels interposed between two capillary beds is called a *portal system*. For example, the capillary networks of the intestines and certain other abdominal viscera drain via the *portal vein* to the liver. There the portal vein ramifies into a network of sinusoids throughout the organ. Blood passes from these through a system of converging vessels of gradually increasing caliber to the hepatic vein and thence back to the heart via the inferior vena cava. This arrangement permits nutrient material absorbed in the intestines to be exposed to, and processed by, the liver cells before being distributed throughout the body by the general circulation.

The capillaries in the median eminence of the hypothalamus are continuous with a plexus of small veins, the hypophyseoportal system, which courses along the hypophyseal stalk and then divides into the sinusoids of the anterior lobe of the hypophysis. This arrangement permits releasing factors, which are liberated at the ends of neurosecretory axons in the hypothalamus,

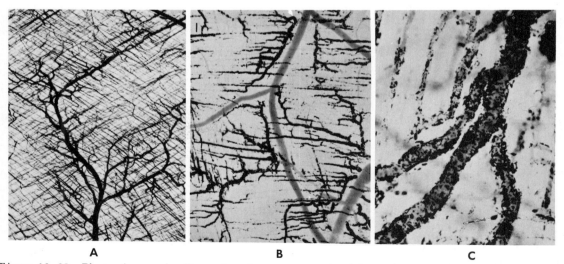

A   B   C

Figure 13-29 Photomicrographs illustrating the greater permeability of venules induced by serotonin. *A*, Cremaster of the normal rat injected with carbon to demonstrate the entire vascular system. *B*, Vascular labeling resulting from leakage of opaque particles from the vessels from local injection of serotonin. The black vessels are venules; the permeability of the many small capillaries visible in *A* has not been enhanced by this treatment. *C*, Higher magnification of a venule after seven days, showing intracellular mass of particulate matter in the vascular wall. (From G. Majno, G. E. Palade, and G. I. Schoefl, J. Biophys. & Biochem. Cytol., *11*:607, 1961.)

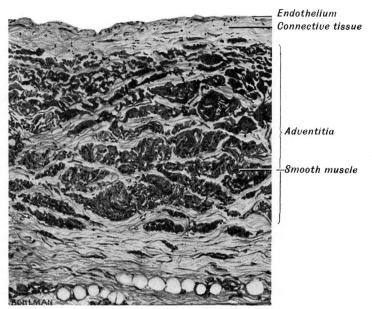

Endothelium
Connective tissue

Adventitia

Smooth muscle

Figure 13-30 Low power view of a cross section of the wall of human vena cava. Note the muscular adventitia. (Drawn by E. Bohlman.)

to be carried downstream to activate endocrine secretory cells in the hypophysis (Chapter 18).

An artery may ramify into a set of capillaries, which are then collected into a larger arterial vessel. An example of this is found in the kidney, in which an afferent arteriole may suddenly break up into a mass of contorted capillaries comprising the glomerulus. These capillaries do not empty into veins but coalesce to form the efferent arteriole, which goes on to break up into another set of capillaries around the kidney tubules. In this case the efferent arteriole is a portal vessel (Chapter 31).

Arteriovenous Anastomoses

In many parts of the body the terminal ramifications of arteries are connected with veins, not only by capillaries, but also by direct arteriovenous anastomoses of larger caliber. They usually arise as side branches from terminal arterioles and run directly to small venules. Their walls are muscular, remarkably thick for the caliber of the vessel, and richly supplied with vasomotor nerves. Observation of living vessels has shown that they contract markedly on stimulation of the sympathetic nerves (Clark). When the arteriovenous anastomosis is contracted, blood passes along the arteriole into the capillary network; when it relaxes, blood can bypass the capillaries and go directly into a thin-walled venule. The arteriovenous anastomoses are therefore considered important structures for regulating the supply of blood to many tissues.

In addition to these simple direct communications, Masson has described highly organized connections between arteries and veins that occur as part of a specific organ, the *glomus*, found in the nailbed, the pads of the fingers and toes, and the ears. The afferent arteriole enters the connective tissue capsule of the glomus, loses its internal elastic lamina, and develops a heavy epithelioid muscle coat and narrow lumen. The arteriovenous anastomoses within the glomus may be branched and convoluted, and they are richly innervated by sympathetic and myelinated nerves. The anastomoses empty into a short, thin-walled vein with a wide lumen, which drains into a periglomic vein and then into the ordinary veins of the skin.

In addition to helping regulate the flow of blood in the extremities, it is claimed that the glomus is concerned with temperature regulation and conservation of heat.

Coccygeal Body

This organ, sometimes erroneously included among the paraganglia, does not contain chromaffin cells. It is situated in front of the tip of the coccyx and measures 2.5 mm. in diameter. It consists of numerous arteriovenous anastomoses embedded in a dense fibrous matrix. The smooth muscle cells have undergone extensive "epithelioid" change. Despite its epithelioid appearance, an internal secretion has not been demonstrated for this organ.

Carotid and Aortic Bodies

The carotid bodies are inconspicuous, flattened structures at the bifurcation of each common carotid artery. Formerly they were erroneously included among the paraganglia (Chapter 21). They are now known to be chemoreceptor organs that sample the arterial blood (deCastro; Heymans). For the control of respiration, the carotid body is virtually the only receptor sensitive to hypoxia. Cutting or cooling its nerve supply abolishes the normal increase in respiratory rate associated with oxygen lack. This body is also sensitive to a rise in carbon dioxide level or a fall in the pH of the blood.

The carotid body is a highly vascular structure, with a high blood flow in relation to its small volume of parenchyma. It is composed of irregular groups of pale-staining epithelioid cells in intimate relation to capillary sinusoids lined with fenestrated endothelium. Two types of parenchymal cells can be distinguished with the light microscope on the basis of differing nuclear characteristics. The validity of this observation has been established by electron micrographs, in which the two cell types are more clearly distinguishable (Ross; Duncan and Yates). The most obvious, the *Type I (glomus cell)*, contains many small, dense-cored vesicles resembling secretory granules. These cells occur in small clusters that are surrounded by *Type II* cells which are devoid of cytoplasmic granules. Many nerves ramify throughout the organ and end on the Type I cells (Biscoe).

It has been the traditional interpretation that the glomus or Type I cells are the chemoreceptors and that they pass information on to associated afferent nerve endings. The Type II cells were believed to be supportive elements. This interpretation has recently been placed in doubt by several observations. The nerve endings on the glomus cells have abundant mitochondria

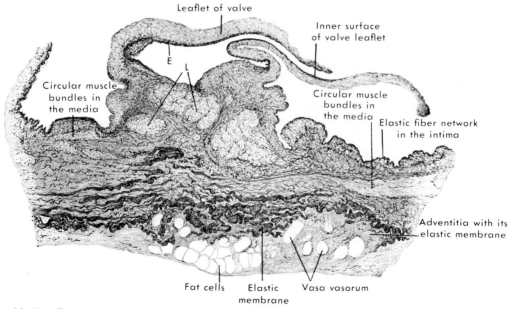

Figure 13–31 From cross section of femoral vein of man. The section passes through the origin of a valve. *E*, Elastic fiber network in the intima on the inner surface of the valve leaflet; *L*, longitudinal muscles of the base of the valve. Acid orcein stain. × 70. (After Schaffer.)

and synaptic vesicles and have all the characteristics ordinarily associated with efferent nerve terminals. After section of the sinus branch of the glossopharyngeal nerve, the endings on the Type I cells degenerate. Thus, it is now suspected that the Type I cell is not the chemoreceptor but part of an efferent system controlling the sensitivity of the sensor. The granules in the glomus cells have been shown to contain catecholamines and 5-hydroxytryptamine. These may serve as secondary transmitters of the efferent system. Which element of the carotid body is the receptor remains to be determined.

On the right side the aortic body lies between the angle of the subclavian and the carotid, while on the left it is found adjacent to the aorta medial to the origin of the subclavian. Although the aortic bodies have been studied less than the carotid bodies, their structure appears to be identical.

THE HEART

The heart is a thick, muscular, rhythmically contracting portion of the vascular system. It lies in the pericardial cavity within the mediastinum. It is about 12 cm. long, 9 cm. wide, and 6 cm. in its anteroposterior diameter, and consists of four chambers: a right and left *atrium* and a right and left *ventricle.* The superior and inferior venae cavae bring the venous blood from the body to the right atrium, from which it passes to the right ventricle. From here the blood is forced through the lungs, where it is aerated, and it is then brought to the left atrium. From there it passes to the left ventricle and is distributed throughout the body by the aorta and its branches. The orifices between the atria and the ventricles are closed by the *tricuspid valve* on the right and the *mitral valve* on the left side. The openings to the pulmonary artery and the aorta, from the right and left ventricles, respectively, are closed by the aortic and pulmonary *semilunar valves.*

The wall of the heart, in both the atria and the ventricles, consists of three main layers: an internal, the *endocardium;* an intermediate, the *myocardium;* and an external, the *epicardium.* The internal layer is directly exposed to the blood; the myocardium is the contractile layer; and the epicardium is the visceral layer of the *pericardium,* a serous membrane that forms the pericardial sac, the serous cavity in which the heart lies.

The endocardium is generally regarded as homologous to the tunica intima of the blood vessels, the myocardium to the tunica media, and the epicardium to the tunica adventitia.

Endocardium

The endocardium is lined with ordinary endothelium, which is continuous with that of the blood vessels entering and leaving the heart. This endothelium consists of polygonal squamous cells. Directly under the endothelium in most places is a thin *subendothelial layer* that contains fibroblasts and collagenous fibers and a few elastic fibers. External to this loose layer is a thick layer of denser connective tissue, which comprises the main mass of the endocardium and contains great numbers of elastic elements (Fig. 13–32). Bundles of smooth muscle fibers are found in varying numbers in this layer, particularly on the interventricular septum.

A *subendocardial layer,* absent from the papillary muscles and from the chordae tendineae, consists of loose connective tissue that binds the endocardium to the myocardium and is directly continuous with the interstitial tissue of the latter. It contains blood vessels, nerves, and branches of the conduction system of the heart. In the spaces between the muscular bundles of the atria, the connective tissue of the endocardium continues into that of the epicardium, and the elastic networks of the two layers intermingle.

Myocardium

The histology and fine structure of the cardiac muscle has been described in Chapter 11. In the embryos of the higher vertebrates, the myocardial fibers form a spongy network. In the adult stage, however, they are bound by connective tissue into a compact mass. This condensation of the myocardium progresses from the epicardium toward the endocardium. Many embryonic muscle fascicles remain in a more or less isolated condition on the internal surface of the walls of the ventricular cavities. These muscle fiber bundles are covered with endocardium and are called *trabeculae carneae.*

Elastic elements are scarce in the myo-

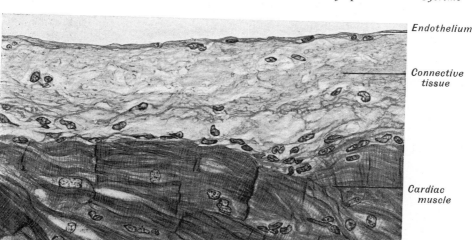

Figure 13-32 Section of the endocardium of the ventricle of man. × 265.

cardium of the ventricles of adult mammals, except in the tunica adventitia of the larger blood vessels in the walls of these chambers. In the myocardium of the atria, however, there are networks of elastic fibers, which run everywhere between the muscle fibers and are directly connected with similar networks in the endocardium and epicardium. They are also continuous with the elastic networks in the walls of the large veins. A large part of the interstitial connective tissue of the cardiac muscle consists of extensive networks of reticular fibrils.

Epicardium

The epicardium is covered on its free surface by a single layer of mesothelial cells. Beneath the mesothelium is a thin layer of connective tissue with networks of elastic fibers, blood vessels, and many nerves. In the loose connective tissue along the coronary blood vessels considerable amounts of adipose tissue are found.

The parietal layer of the pericardium is a serous membrane of the usual type—a flat layer of connective tissue that contains elastic and collagenous fibers, fibroblasts, fixed macrophages, and a covering layer of mesothelial cells. The smooth, moist apposed surfaces of the epicardium and the parietal pericardium permit these layers to glide freely over one another during contraction

and relaxation of the heart. When they become adherent and the potential space between them is obliterated by disease (pericarditis) they may impose considerable restraint upon the action of the heart.

Cardiac Skeleton

The central supporting structure of the heart, to which most of the muscle fibers are attached and with which the valves are connected, is called rather inappropriately the *cardiac skeleton*. It has a complicated form and consists, for the most part, of dense connective tissue. Its main parts are the *septum membranaceum*, the *trigona fibrosa*, and the *annuli fibrosi* encircling the atrioventricular and arterial foramina.

In man the fibrous rings around the atrioventricular foramina contain some fat and elastic fibers but are mainly dense connective tissue. The structure of the septum membranaceum suggests that of an aponeurosis, with its more regular orientation of collagenous bundles in layers. The connective tissue of the trigona fibrosa contains islands of cartilage-like tissue (chondroid) consisting of globular cells resembling chondrocytes. The interstitial substance stains deeply with basic aniline dyes and hematoxylin, and is penetrated by collagenous fibers. In aged persons the tissue of the cardiac skeleton may become calcified in places and sometimes even ossified. In bovine species, bone is normally found in the trigona fibrosa.

Cardiac Valves

Each *atrioventricular valve* consists of a supple sheet of connective tissue, which begins at the annulus fibrosus and is reinforced internally by thin ligamentous strands. It is covered on its atrial and ventricular surfaces by a layer of endocardium. At the free edge of the valve these three layers blend (Fig. 13–33).

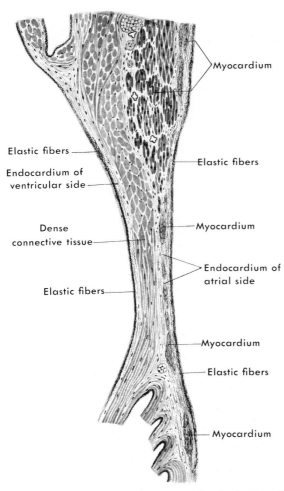

Elastic fibers

Endocardium of ventricular side

Dense connective tissue

Elastic fibers

Myocardium

Elastic fibers

Myocardium

Endocardium of atrial side

Myocardium

Elastic fibers

Myocardium

Figure 13–33 Cross section through mitral valve of man. Atrial surface on the right, ventricular on the left. In the upper left is the attachment of the aortic valve; on the left, below, is the passage of chordae tendineae into the valve. Low magnification. (After Sato.)

The ground plate of connective tissue consists largely of dense chondroid tissue, with small spindle-shaped or rounded cells and a basophilic interstitial substance. The endocardial layer is thicker on the atrial side. Here the subendothelial layer has a small amount of chondroid tissue and rests upon a connective tissue layer, which contains many elastic fiber networks and some smooth muscle fibers. In the vicinity of the annulus fibrosus, the subendocardial layer is quite loose, and the musculature of the atrium penetrates far into it. On the ventricular side, the endocardial layer has a similar structure but is much thinner. In many places the chordae tendineae, which extend from the edge of the valve to the papillary muscles, enter this layer and mingle with the deeper lying connective tissue.

The *aortic* and *pulmonic valves* have the same general structure as the atrioventricular valves. In the middle of the valves are plates of chondroid tissue with collagenous and thin elastic fibers. At the root of the valve these all continue into the annulus fibrosus. At the middle of the free edge they form a thickening called the *nodulus Arantii.*

The aortic and pulmonary valves are normally avascular structures. The mitral and tricuspid valve leaves may be penetrated by small vessels, but only to a distance of a few millimeters from their origin.

IMPULSE CONDUCTING SYSTEM

In the adult mammalian heart, the motor impulse arises in the part of the heart that develops from the embryonic sinus venosus, an area in which the superior vena cava enters the right atrium. There is a specialized mechanism by which the contraction spreads to the atria and then to the ventricles.

An impulse beginning at the *sinoatrial node*, which is the pacemaker of the heart, activates the atrial musculature and is conducted to the *atrioventricular node.* A continuous tract of atypical muscle fibers extends down the interventricular septum from this node to both ventricles, sending branches to the papillary muscles and other portions of the myocardium. This system thus serves to initiate and transmit the contractile impulse. The microscopic and submicroscopic structure of this specialized conduction tissue has been described in Chapter 11. The conduction system, even up to the terminal ramifications in the ventricles, is enclosed within a connective tissue layer that separates it from the working musculature of the myocardium.

At the boundary between the right atrium and the superior vena cava, in the region of the sulcus terminalis, is the sinoatrial node, 1 cm. in length and 3 to 5 mm. in width. Although not sharply outlined, it can be seen with the naked eye. It consists of a dense network of interwoven Purkinje fibers.

The atrioventricular node is a flat, white structure about 6 mm. long and 2 to 3 mm. wide; it is located in the posterior lower part of the interatrial septum below the posterior leaf of the aortic valve. The node consists of Purkinje fibers, which form a tangled dense network whose meshes are filled with connective tissue. These fibers pass into (or between) the usual myocardial fibers, so that the boundary of the node is indistinct. Toward the ventricles the substance of the node converges abruptly into a band about 1 cm. long, the *atrioventricular bundle*. It is located in the dense connective tissue of the trigonum fibrosum dextrum and continues into the septum membranaceum, where it divides into two branches.

The first branch, a cylindrical bundle 1 to 2 mm. thick, runs downward along the periphery of the membranous septum and is located in part directly under the endocardium of the right ventricle. It proceeds along the interventricular septum and splits into many branches, which spread along the entire internal surface of the right ventricle and into the papillary muscles.

The left branch is a wide, flat band that comes forward under the endocardium of the left ventricle in the upper portion of the interventricular septum, under the anterior edge of the posterior cusps of the aortic valve. It divides into two main branches at the border between the upper and middle thirds of the septum; then it separates, as in the right ventricle, into numerous anastomosing thin threads, which are lost to view in the myocardium.

Blood Vessels, Lymphatics and Nerves of the Heart

The blood supply to the heart is carried by the coronary arteries, usually two in number, which arise from the aorta in the sinuses behind two of the valve cusps. They are distributed to the capillaries of the myocardium. The blood from the capillaries is collected by the cardiac veins, most of which empty by way of the coronary sinus into the right atrium. A few small cardiac veins empty directly into the right atrium.

In the coronary arteries of the human heart, the tunica media, which is limited on both sides by the usual internal and external elastic membranes, is divided by a thick fenestrated membrane into an inner and an external layer.

The conduction system and, particularly, both of its nodes are abundantly supplied with blood from special branches of the coronary arteries.

Three groups of lymphatic vessels are described in the heart: (1) large lymphatic vessels, which lie in the grooves of the heart together with the blood vessels. These drain to the lymphatic nodes beneath the loop of the aorta and at the bifurcation of the trachea; (2) lymphatic vessels of the epicardial connective tissue; and (3) lymphatic vessels of the myocardium and the endocardium.

In the subepicardial connective tissue, networks of lymphatic capillaries may easily be demonstrated. Within the subendothelial connective tissue there is an even larger network of typical lymphatic capillaries, the larger vessels being provided with valves. Lymphatic capillaries have also been described in the atrioventricular and semilunar valves, but their presence here in the absence of blood vessels raises some doubts about the validity of these observations.

The lymphatic network in the endocardium used to be confused with the netlike ramifications of the sinoventricular conduction system, for both structures may be demonstrated by the same injection method. However, the conducting system forms much wider meshes, and its cross connections are thicker than those of the lymphatic network.

The myocardium is penetrated by an abundant lymphatic network, which is everywhere connected with the subendocardial plexus and also continues into the pericardial lymphatic network.

The numerous nerves of the heart are in part ramifications of the vagus nerve and in part sympathetic nerves. Some nerve endings in the heart apparently are of effector type, while other endings are of receptor or sensory character.

HISTOGENESIS OF THE BLOOD VESSELS

In mammals the first vessels are laid down in the area vasculosa on the surface of the yolk sac, where they develop from the mesenchymal cells. In the embryo proper, the blood vessels and the heart appear later; at first they are devoid of blood cells and are empty. In the spaces between the germ layers, groups of mesenchymal cells flatten around spaces filled with fluid, which are thus surrounded by a thin endothelial wall. In this way, the primordia of the heart and the main blood vessels, such as the aorta and the cardinal and umbilical veins, are laid down. These originally independent primordia then rapidly unite with one another and with the vessels of the area vasculosa, after which the blood circulation is established. The endothelial cells in these first stages are merely mesenchymal cells adjusted to the new and special function of bounding the blood vessel lumen.

After the closed blood vascular system has developed and the circulation has begun, new blood vessels always arise by "budding" from preexisting blood vessels. The new formation of blood vessels by budding may be studied in sections of young embryos or in the living condition in the margin of the tail in larval amphibians, in the mesentery of newborn mammals, or in the thin layer of inflamed tissue that grows between two coverslips introduced under the skin of an animal. A method has been devised for the continued observation of such chambers in the living rabbit for weeks and even months (Clark and Clark; Sandison).

In the process of budding, a protrusion appears on the wall of the capillary and is directed into the surrounding tissues. From the beginning it often appears to be a simple, hollow expansion of the endothelial wall; in other cases it is at first a solid accumulation of endothelial cytoplasm. This *vascular bud* or sprout enlarges, elongates, and assumes many shapes. Most frequently it appears as a pointed cylinder. It later becomes hollow and thus represents a local outpouching of the blood vessel into which blood cells penetrate.

An endothelial bud may encounter another bud and fuse with its end, or its lateral wall may come into contact with another bud or another capillary. A lumen appears among the fused endothelial cells and unites the two capillaries. In this way a new mesh is formed in the capillary network, and blood begins to circulate through it. Later, new buds may arise from the newly formed vessels. The developing vascular buds are often accompanied by undifferentiated mesenchymal cells and fibroblasts, stretched parallel to the long axis of the buds.

Arteries and veins of all types are always laid down at first as ordinary capillaries. The primary endothelial tube expands and thickens as new elements are added to the outside of the wall. These elements originate from the surrounding mesenchyme in the embryo and play an important part in the formation of new arteries and veins from capillaries, as well as in the formation of large vessels from smaller ones during the development of a "collateral circulation" of the blood. The mesenchymal cells outside the endothelium become young smooth muscle cells, with myofibrils differentiating in their cytoplasm. Soon more layers of smooth muscle fibers join the first layer; these arise in part by the addition of new mesenchymal cells and in part by division of preexisting smooth muscle cells.

The factors that cause the larger arteries and veins to develop in more or less constant patterns in particular places and in definite directions are not completely understood. It is probable that in the earliest embryonic stages the formation of the major vessels is genetically determined, while in the later stages the pattern and growth of the blood vessels are determined by local hemodynamic factors.

LYMPHATIC VESSELS

In most tissues and organs with the exception of the central nervous system, cartilage, bone and bone marrow, thymus, teeth and placenta, the blood capillaries are paralleled by a plexus of *lymph capillaries*. The blood vessels form a closed "circulatory system" with a central pump (the heart), an outflow tract (arteries), and a return system (veins). The lymph vascular system, on the other hand, is a "drainage system" whose smallest vessels, the lymphatic capillaries, end blindly and conduct a clear fluid, called *lymph*, from the extracellular spaces in the periphery back through successively larger *lymphatic vessels* that ultimately converge upon *lymphatic ducts* (thoracic duct and right lymphatic duct) which are confluent with the great veins at the base of the neck. Along the course of the lymphatic vessels are encapsulated accumulations of lymphoid tissue comprising small organs called *lymph nodes* (see Chapter 16). The lymph stream entering the node via *afferent lymphatic vessels* breaks up within it, percolating through a labyrinthine system of minute channels lined with endothelium and phagocytic cells. Lymph then emerges from the node through *efferent lymphatic vessels*. The lymph, exposed to an enormous number of phagocytes, is cleared of foreign matter as it filters through the lymph nodes. Many lymphocytes that enter the lymph nodes from the blood, and others that arise from lymphopoiesis within the node are added to the efferent lymph and are thus carried back to the bloodstream.

Lymph is essentially an ultrafiltrate of the blood plasma formed by continual seepage of fluid constituents of the blood across the capillary walls into the surrounding interstitial spaces. It contains water, electrolytes, and variable amounts of protein (2 to 5 per cent) depending upon the site and conditions of its formation. The walls of blood capillaries are normally freely permeable to water and small molecules. They are less permeable to plasma proteins, which therefore tend to maintain a significant colloid osmotic pressure in the blood. At the arterial end of blood capillaries where the hydrostatic pressure exceeds the colloid osmotic pressure of the blood, water, solutes, and some plasma proteins move across the wall into the tissue. At the venous end, the hydrostatic pressure is lower and the colloid osmotic pressure tends to draw water, electrolytes, and products of tissue catabolism back into the blood. However, some of the fluid and much of the plasma protein that have left the blood do not return directly but are drained off in the lymph and returned to the blood via the lymph-vascular system. A delicate balance is thus maintained, which keeps the volume of extracellular fluid reasonably constant and conserves the small amount of plasma protein that continually escapes through the walls of the blood capillaries.

It follows from this mechanism of lymph formation that the flow of lymph will be increased by (1) an increase in blood capillary permeability, (2) an increase in hydrostatic pressure, or (3) a decrease in colloid osmotic pressure of the blood plasma. Any of these will increase the transudation of fluid. If fluid accumulates in the tissues in excess of the capacity of lymphatic vessels to drain it away, the resulting swelling of the tissues is referred to as *edema*. Thus, increased resistance to venous return in congestive heart failure may raise pressure in the blood capillaries, resulting in edema of the ankles. Similarly, obstruction to the lymphatic vessels of an extremity owing to parasitic disease or radical surgery may result in persistent edema.

The principal function of the lymph vascular system is to return to the blood the fluid and plasma protein that escape from the circulation; to return to the blood the lymphocytes of the recirculating pool; and to add to the blood, immune globulins (antibodies) that are formed in lymph nodes. We are concerned here only with the structure of the vessels; the organization of the associated lymphoid tissue will be discussed in Chapter 16.

Lymphatic Capillaries

Lymphatic capillaries are thin-walled endothelium-lined vessels that differ from blood capillaries in several respects. They branch and anastomose freely and although they are generally cylindrical, they are more variable in shape and caliber than are their counterparts in the blood vascular system. Except in the perinuclear region, the endothelium is usually extremely thin, but it is often rather variable in thickness (Fig. 13–34). Folds or microvilli projecting into the lumen are not uncommon. The thin edges of adjacent endothelial cells often overlap for some distance. There is a distinct intercellular cleft throughout most of this region of overlap, but one or two punctate areas of closer apposition and adherence are usually seen along the boundary. There are no pericytes associated with lymphatic capillaries, and a continuous basal lamina is usually lacking. Extracellular bundles of filaments (50 to 100 Å) have been described terminating on the abluminal plasma membrane of the endothelium and extending outward into the ground substance and between the collagen bundles of the surrounding connective tissue (Leak). These have been called *lymphatic anchoring filaments*, and it is sug-

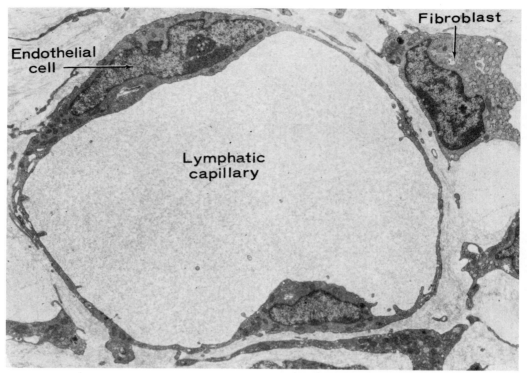

Figure 13-34 Electron micrograph of a subcutaneous lymphatic capillary from guinea pig in cross section. Notice the irregular outline, the thin wall, and the slight variations in thickness of the endothelium. The absence of a basal lamina cannot be verified at this magnification. (Micrograph courtesy of L. V. Leak.)

gested that they have a mechanical role in maintaining the patency of the vessels. The filaments appear to insert in the outer leaflet of the membrane or to terminate in patches of amorphous material on the outer surface of the plasmalemma. These patches bear a superficial resemblance to the material composing the continuous basal lamina of endothelium in blood capillaries. The chemical nature of the anchoring filaments has not been established, but they very closely resemble the filaments associated with elastic fibers and may possibly be identical to them.

The terminal elements of the lymphatic system are quite variable in their form from one organ to another. In the skin and mucous membranes, a plexus of tubular lymphatic capillaries generally occurs parallel to the network of blood capillaries but tends to be more deeply situated. In the lamina propria of the intestine, a single vessel or a simple network of lymphatic capillaries extends from the submucous plexus into the core of each villus and ends blindly near its tip. In the lining of the oviduct, the terminal lymphatics

are not tubular but are narrow, flattened sinusoids extending for considerable distances along the axis of each fold of mucous membrane. In the testis of some rodents, the lymphatics form labyrinthine peritubular sinusoids that have no consistent geometry but conform to the shapes of the intertubular spaces that they occupy and to the contours of the blood vessels and perivascular clusters of Leydig cells which they surround. In man and other large species, the testicular lymphatics are not sinusoidal but occur as one or two tubular vessels in each interstitial space. These are usually much larger than the blood capillaries (Fig. 13–36).

Larger Lymphatic Vessels

These vessels are easily distinguished from blood vessels by the large size of their lumens in relation to the thickness of their walls. The wall is somewhat thicker than that of lymphatic capillaries and is invested by thin collagenous bundles, elastic fibers, and occasional smooth muscle cells. In lymphatics with a diameter greater than 0.2 mm., three layers of wall are recognizable corresponding to interna, media, and adventitia of blood vessels. The boundaries between the layers are often indistinct, so that the division is somewhat artificial. The interna consists of endothelium and a thin layer of interlacing longitudinal elastic fibers. The media is a layer or two of smooth muscle cells, while the adventitia is composed of elastic fibers and collagenous bundles continuous with those of the surrounding connective tissue.

Valves are a conspicuous feature of lymphatics. They occur in pairs with the two members on opposite sides of the vessel and their free edges pointing in the direction of lymph flow. As in veins, the valves are folds of the tunica interna and therefore consist of back-to-back layers of endothelium supported near their base by a thin intervening layer of connective tissue. They occur at much closer intervals along the length of the lymphatic vessel than do the valves of veins. Immediately proximal to a valve, the lymphatic is often slightly expanded. The peri-odic fusiform expansions at the sites of valves give the lymphatic vessels a highly characteristic appearance.

The walls of lymphatic vessels are innervated and there is cinematographic evidence that, in some small mammals, rhythmic contraction of smooth muscle cells in the vessel wall helps to move the lymph along. This does not appear to be true of lymphatics in man and other larger species. Lacking a muscular pump to propel fluid through the system, the flow of lymph in these species is very dependent upon the contraction of skeletal muscles and movements of neighboring structures, which exert pressure on the thin walls of lymphatics, expressing lymph from segments of the vessel, while the presence of valves insures its unidirectional movement. Thus, when an extremity is immobilized, as in an anesthetized animal, there is little or no lymph flow from it, but if passive movements of the extremity are initiated, a slow steady flow of lymph is reestablished comparable to that in the active unanesthetized animal.

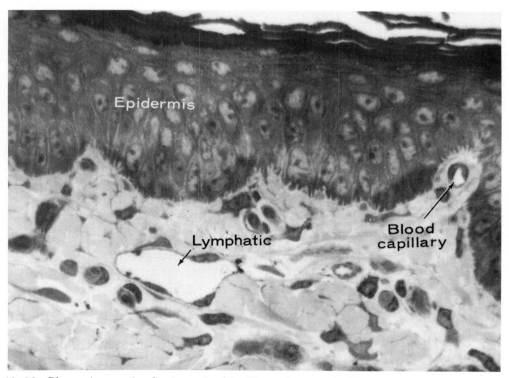

Figure 13-35 Photomicrograph of guinea pig skin, illustrating a typical lymphatic capillary in the dermis. (Photograph courtesy of L. V. Leak.)

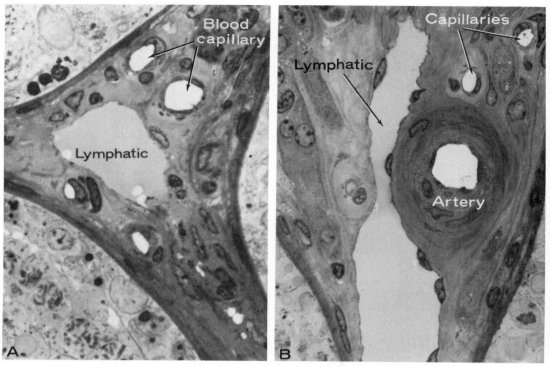

Figure 13-36 *A,* Photomicrograph of a lymphatic in the interstitial tissue of a ram testis. *B,* Lymphatic in interstitium of a bull testis. Both of these preparations have been fixed by vascular perfusion. The blood capillaries are therefore empty, whereas the lymphatics have a light gray content, representing precipitated protein of the lymph. (From D. W. Fawcett, W. B. Neaves, and M. N. Flores, Biol. Reprod., 9:500, 1973.)

Lymphatic Ducts

The lymphatics form progressively larger vessels by their confluence and these latter finally converge to form two main trunks: (1) the *right lymphatic duct,* which is relatively short and carries lymph drainage from the right upper portion of the body; it opens into the right brachiocephalic vein at the junction of the internal jugular and subclavian veins, and (2) the *thoracic duct,* which arises in the abdomen and courses upward along the anterior aspect of the vertebral column through the thorax and into the base of the neck, where it opens into the venous system at the junction of the left jugular and subclavian veins.

The wall of the lymphatic ducts differs from that of the great veins in the greater development of the muscles in the tunica media and by a less distinct division into three layers. The tunica intima consists of the endothelial lining and several thin layers of collagenous and elastic fibers; the latter condense into a layer similar to an internal elastic membrane near the junction with the tunica media. The smooth muscle bundles in the tunica media are penetrated by elastic fibers coming from the elastica interna. The tunica adventitia is composed of longitudinal smooth muscle bundles. The tunica adventitia gradually merges into the surrounding loose connective tissue. The wall of the thoracic duct is provided with small blood vessels that extend into the outer layer of the tunica media. These vessels are similar to the vasa vasorum of the larger blood vessels.

REFERENCES

Capillaries

Bennett, H. S., J. H. Luft, and J. C. Hampton: Morphological classification of vertebrate blood capillaries. Am. J. Physiol., *196*:381, 1959.

Bloch, E. H.: Microscopic observations of the circulating blood in the bulbar conjunctiva in man in health and disease. Ergeb. Anat. Entwickl., *35*:1, 1956.

Brightman, M. W., and T. S. Reese: Junctions between intimately apposed cell membranes in the vertebrate brain. J. Cell Biol., *40*:648, 1969.

Bruns, R. R., and G. E. Palade: Studies on blood capillaries. I. General organization of blood capillaries in muscle. J. Cell Biol., *37*:244, 1968*a*.

Bruns, R. R., and G. E. Palade: Studies on blood capillaries. II. Transport of ferritin molecules across the wall of muscle capillaries. J. Cell Biol., *37*:277, 1968*b*.

Dobbing, J.: The blood-brain barrier. Physiol. Rev., *41*:130, 1961.

Farquhar, M.: Fine structure and function in capillaries of the anterior pituitary gland. Angiology, *12*:270, 1961.

Fawcett, D. W.: Comparative observations on the fine structure of blood capillaries. *In* Peripheral Vessels. Internat. Acad. Pathol., Monograph No. 4. Baltimore, Williams & Wilkins, 1963.

Florey, H.: Exchange of substances between the blood and tissues. Nature, *192*:908, 1961.

Florey, H.: The endothelial cell. Brit. Med. J., *2*:487, 1966.

Guyton, A. C.: *Textbook of Medical Physiology*. 4th Ed. Philadelphia, W. B. Saunders Co., 1971.

Jennings, M. A., V. T. Marchesi, and H. Florey: The transport of particles across the walls of small blood vessels. Proc. Roy. Soc. B., *156*:14, 1962.

Karnovsky, M. J.: Vesicular transport of exogenous peroxidase across capillary endothelium into the T-system of muscle. J. Cell. Biol., *27*:49A, 1965.

Karnovsky, M. J.: The ultrastructural basis of capillary permeability studied with peroxidase as a tracer. J. Cell Biol., *35*:213, 1967.

Karnovsky, M. J.: The ultrastructural basis of transcapillary exchanges. J. Gen. Physiol., *52*:64S, 1968.

Karnovsky, M. J., and R. S. Cotran: The intercellular passage of exogenous peroxidase across endothelium and mesothelium. Anat. Rec., *154*:365, 1966.

Landis, E. M., and J. R. Pappenheimer: Exchange of substances through the capillary walls. *In* Hamilton, W. F., and P. Dow, eds.: Handbook of Physiology. Section 2, Vol. II, p. 961. Washington, American Physiological Society, 1963.

Luft, J. H.: The fine structure of the vascular wall. *In* Jones, R. J., ed.: Evolution of the Atherosclerotic Plaque. Chicago, University of Chicago Press, 1963.

Luft, J. H.: The ultrastructural basis of capillary permeability. *In* Zweifach, B. W., L. Grant, and R. T. McCluskey, eds.: The Inflammatory Process. New York, Academic Press, 1965.

Majno, G.: Ultrastructure of the vascular membrane. *In* Hamilton, W. F., and P. Dow, eds.: Handbook of Physiology. Section 2, Vol. III, p. 2293. Washington, American Physiological Society, 1965.

Majno, G., and G. E. Palade: Studies on inflammation. I. The effect of histamine and serotonin on vascular permeability: An electron microscope study. J. Biophys. Biochem. Cytol., *11*:607, 1961.

Palade, G. E.: Transport in quanta across the endothelium of blood capillaries. Anat. Rec., *136*:254, 1960.

Palade, G. E.: Blood capillaries of the heart and other organs. Circulation, *24*:368, 1961.

Palade, G. E., and R. R. Bruns: Structure and function in normal muscle capillaries. *In* Siperstein, M. D., A. R. Colwell, and K. Meyer, eds.: Small Blood Vessel Involvement in Diabetes Mellitus. Baltimore, Garamond/Pridemark, 1964.

Pappenheimer, J. R.: Passage of molecules through capillary walls. Physiol. Rev., *33*:387, 1953.

Raviola, E., and M. J. Karnovsky: Evidence for a blood-thymus barrier using electron opaque tracers. J. Exp. Med., *136*:466, 1972.

Reese, T. S., and M. J. Karnovsky: Fine structural localization of a blood-brain barrier for exogenous peroxidase. J. Cell Biol., *34*:207, 1967.

Rhodin, J. A. G.: The diaphragm of capillary endothelial fenestrations. J. Ultrastruct. Res., *6*:171, 1962.

Shea, S. M., and M. J. Karnovsky: Brownian motion: A theoretical explanation for the movement of vesicles across endothelium. Nature, *212*:353, 1966.

Speidel, E., and A. Lazarow: Chemical composition of glomerular basement membrane material in diabetes. Diabetes, *12*:355, 1963.

Weinstein, R. S., and N. S. McNutt: Electron microscopy of freeze-cleaved and etched capillaries. *In* Malinin, T. I., et al., eds.: Microcirculation, Perfusion, and Transplantation of Organs. New York, Academic Press, 1970.

Zimmermann, K. W.: Der Feinere Bau der Blutkapillaren. Zeitschr. f. Anat. u. Entwicklungs., *68*:29, 1923.

Blood Vessels in General

Burton, A. D.: Relation of structure to function of the tissues of the wall of the blood vessels. Physiol. Rev., *34*:619, 1954.

Clark, E. R., and E. L. Clark: Microscopic observations on the extraendothelial cells of living mammalian blood vessels. Am. J. Anat., *66*:1, 1940.

Harper, W. F.: The blood supply of human heart valves. Brit. Med. J., *2*:305, 1941.

Heath, D., J. W. DuShana, E. H. Wood, and J. E. Edwards: The structure of the pulmonary trunk at different ages and in cases of pulmonary hypertension and pulmonary stenosis. J. Path. Bact., *77*:443, 1959.

Karrer, H. E., and J. Cox: Electron microscopy study of developing chick embryo aorta. J. Ultrastruct. Res., *4*:420, 1960.

Keech, M. K.: Electron microscope study of the normal rat aorta. J. Biophys. Biochem. Cytol., *7*:533, 1960.

Movat, H. Z., and N. V. P. Pernando: The fine structure of the terminal vascular bed. I. Small arteries with an internal elastic lamina. Exp. Mol. Path., *2*:549, 1963.

Movat, H. Z., and N. V. P. Pernando: The fine structure of the terminal vascular bed. IV. The venules and their perivascular cells. Exp. Mol. Path., *3*:98, 1964.

Pease, D. C., and W. J. Pauli: Electron microscopy of elastic arteries, the thoracic aorta of the rat. J. Ultrastruct. Res., *3*:469, 1960.

Pease, D. C., and S. Molinari: Electron microscopy of muscular arteries: Pial vessels of the cat and monkey. J. Ultrastruct. Res., *3*:447, 1960.

Phelps, P. C., and J. H. Luft: Electron microscopical study of relaxation and constriction in frog arterioles. Am. J. Anat., *125*:399, 1969.

Rhodin, J. A. G.: Fine structure of the vascular wall in mammals. Physiol. Rev., *42*(Suppl 5):48, 1962.

Sabin, F. R.: Studies on the origin of blood vessels and of red blood corpuscles as seen in the living blastoderm of chicks during the second day of incubation. Carnegie Contrib. Embryol., *9*:213, 1920.

Sandison, J. C.: Contraction of blood vessels and observations on the circulation in the transparent chamber in the rabbit's ear. Anat. Rec., *54*:105, 1932.

Simionescu, M., N. Simionescu, and G. E. Palade: Morphometric data on the endothelium of blood capillaries. J. Cell Biol., *60*:128, 1974.

Carotid Body

Adams, W. E.: The Comparative Morphology of the Carotid Body and Carotid Sinus. Springfield, Ill., Charles C Thomas, 1958.

Biscoe, T. J.: Carotid body. Structure and Function. Physiol. Rev., 51:437, 1971.

Boyd, J. D.: The development of the human carotid body. Carnegie Contrib. Embryol., 152:1, 1939.

deCastro, F.: Sur la structure et l'innervation du sinus carotidien de l'homme et des mammifères. Trav. Lab. Recherches. Biol. Univ. Madrid, 25:331, 1927.

Chen, I-Li, and R. Yates: Electron microscopic radioautographic studies of the carotid body following injections of labeled biogenic amine precursors. J. Cell Biol., 42:794, 1969.

Duncan, D., and R. Yates: Ultrastructure of the carotid body of the cat as revealed by various fixatives and the use of reserpine. Anat. Rec., 157:667, 1967.

Edwards, C., D. Heath, P. Harris, et al.: The carotid body in animals at high altitude. J. Path., 104:231, 1971.

Heymans, C.: Action of drugs on carotid body and sinus. Pharmacol. Rev., 7:119, 1955.

Ross, L. L.: Electron microscopic observations of the carotid body of the cat. J. Biophys. Biochem. Cytol., 6:253, 1959.

Yates, R. D., I-Li Chen, and D. Duncan: Effects of sinus nerve stimulation on carotid body glomus cells. J. Cell Biol., 46:544, 1970.

Lymphatic Vessels

Drinker, C. K., and J. M. Yoffey: Lymphatics, Lymph and Lymphoid Tissue. Cambridge, Mass., Harvard University Press, 1941.

Leak, L. V.: Normal anatomy of the lymphatic vascular system. *In* Meessen, H., ed.: Handbuch der algemeine Pathologie. Berlin, Springer Verlag, 1972.

Leak, L. V.: Electron microscopic observations on lymphatic capillaries and structural components of the connective tissue-lymph interface. Microvasc. Res., 2:361, 1970.

Rouvière, H.: Anatomie des lymphatiques de l'homme. Paris, Masson, 1932.

14

The Immune System

By Elio Raviola

Organisms of different species and the various individuals belonging to the same species, with the exception of genetically identical twins, possess a unique chemical identity, because the macromolecular constituents of cells and body fluids have a different composition. The *immune system* protects the individual from exogenous macromolecules, either introduced as such into the body or deployed at the surface of invading viruses, microorganisms or cells; furthermore, it exerts a surveillance function on the appearance in the body of endogenous, abnormal constituents. The immune system encompasses the lymphoid organs (thymus, lymph nodes, spleen, and tonsils), all the aggregates of lymphoid tissue occurring in non-lymphoid organs, the lymphocytes of the blood and lymph, and the whole population of lymphocytes and plasma cells dispersed throughout the connective and epithelial tissues of the body. The various components of the immune system are kept in communication by a continuous traffic of lymphocytes, like a mobile army continuously patrolling the body. The cells of the immune system can be thought of as having "academies," the thymus and the bursa analogue in which they are trained; their "battlefields" are the peripheral lymphoid organs and the connective tissues of the body; their "lines of communication" are the blood and lymph. They dispose of the "invaders" either through attacking them directly or through highly selective weapons, the antibodies, and they are assisted by "mercenary troops" of macrophages.

The science of immunology has developed a rather complex and specialized terminology; therefore, we must present at the outset some concepts and definitions that will be needed to understand the organization and functioning of the immune system.

Lymphocytes have the ability to recognize macromolecules on viruses, on bacteria or on the surfaces of other cells that have chemical patterns different from the normal constituents of the individual they inhabit and are able to set up against them a specific defensive reaction, the *immune response. Antigen* is the term currently used to define any material that bears a surface configuration *(antigenic determinant)* capable of eliciting an immune response upon entry into the internal environment of the body. The *clonal selection theory* holds that during ontogeny of the immune system, and possibly throughout life, lymphocytes arise continuously, each genetically programmed to respond to a limited number of antigens or possibly a single antigen. Thus, the versatility of the immune system in disposing of myriad endogenous or exogenous materials is innate and resides in a population of lymphocytes, all of which are identical from a morphological point of view, but each endowed with the capacity to react to a different antigen. How such a multiplicity of lymphocytes is continuously generated still remains a matter of speculation. Upon first meeting with the appropriate antigen *(primary response)*, the lymphocyte is *stimulated* and undergoes a series of morphological and biochemical changes *(transformation)* which result in *proliferation* and *differentiation*. Proliferation leads to amplification of the population of relevant cells: this is called *clonal expansion*. Differentiation results in the appearance of both *effector cells*

427

and *memory cells*. Effector cells *(activated lymphocytes* and *plasma cells)* are instrumental in causing antigen disposal. Memory lymphocytes revert to the inactive state, but are then capable of setting up an immune response with greater efficiency upon encountering their specific antigen again *(secondary response)*.

As lymphocytes displaying variable degrees of affinity for a given antigen may preexist in the individual, this antigen will represent a better stimulus for those cells which have greater avidity for its surface determinants. Antigen, therefore, exerts a selective pressure upon lymphocyte proliferation, thus simulating on a microscopic scale "natural selection" by which the environment favors the multiplication of genetically fit individuals.

Contact with antigen, however, is not necessarily followed by lymphocyte stimulation and consequent immunization. In special circumstances, lymphocytes may be "paralyzed" and the body may become *tolerant* to the foreign material. The dose of the antigen, its degree of foreignness, and the mode of its presentation (in solution, for example, rather than at the surface of another cell) are among the factors which may result in paralysis rather than stimulation. The mechanism of tolerance is still poorly understood, and the fate of the paralyzed lymphocyte is totally unknown. The importance of this phenomenon, however, is considerable, because self-tolerance rather than innate unresponsiveness is the basis for lymphocyte's inability to attack constituents of the body of which they are a part.

Antigen disposal is based upon two different mechanisms: (1) in the so called *cell-mediated* immunological responses, such as those triggered by transplantation of foreign tissues or application of a chemical sensitizing agent to the skin (delayed hypersensitivity), clones of lymphocytes arise *(cytotoxic* or *killer lymphocytes)* which impair the viability of foreign cells either by attacking them directly or by releasing nonspecific toxic factors; (2) in the *humoral* immunological responses, such as those evoked by most bacterial antigens, lymphocytes and plasma cells synthesize and release proteins called *antibodies*, which specifically combine with the antigen.

Upon binding to the antigen, antibodies may neutralize its harmful effects (if the antigen is a toxin); inhibit its entry into the cells of the body (if the antigen is a virus); enhance the uptake and destruction of bacteria by phagocytic cells such as neutrophils or macrophages (a process called *opsonization);* or induce lysis of bacteria or cells by activating *complement*, a system of proteins that are normally present in the plasma and are necessary for lysis of foreign cells in immunological defenses. Antigen-antibody reactions may also have a detrimental effect upon the host by causing either a severe inflammatory response *(Arthus reaction)* or *anaphylaxis*. This latter is the result of release of pharmacologically active substances by tissue cells which have bound antigen-antibody complexes, the most typical example being the release of histamine by mast cells.

Antibodies are proteins found in the globulin fraction of the plasma. They are also called *immunoglobulins* and are subdivided into several classes. The immunoglobulins G (IgG), represent the bulk of the immunoglobulins of the normal human blood, and their structure is known in great detail. The IgG molecule has a weight of about 150,000 daltons, it consists of about 1400 amino acid residues and contains 2 to 3% carbohydrate. It comprises 4 polypeptide chains; these are paired in such a way that the molecule has identical halves, each consisting of one long or heavy chain (H chain) and one short or light chain (L chain). The four chains are held together by disulfide bonds and noncovalent interactions. In the free IgG molecule, the subunits are folded into a roughly cylindrical unit, about 35×200 Å in dimensions, but the molecule displays a considerable degree of plasticity, and upon combination with antigen, it may acquire a characteristic Y or T shape. Papain splits the antibody molecule into three parts: one, the Fc fragment containing two half H chains, is crystallizable, and does not combine with the antigen. It enables the antibody molecule to bind to complement and to the surface of cells that carry appropriate membrane receptors. Each of the other two parts, the Fab fragments, contains a combining site for antigen and consist of the whole L chain and the remaining portion of the H chain; both chains contribute to the combining site for the antigen. Therefore, the IgG molecule as a whole is bivalent (i.e., it is capable of combining with two entities), and this property permits formation of polymeric aggregates of antigen and antibody, which facilitate the attachment of complement and the uptake of the complex by phagocytes. The IgG antibodies have high affinity for the antigenic determinant; thus they are very effective in neutralizing bacterial toxins or in protecting the body against virus infections; they exchange readily between blood and extravascular space. However, they are produced late during the primary immune response and are rather ineffective in activating complement.

The immunoglobulins M (IgM) are large, complex molecules with a weight of about 900,000 daltons and a 10% content of carbohydrate. They consist of 20 polypeptide chains, joined by disulfide bonds. They probably represent a pentamer of subunits, each resembling IgG in its general organization. The IgM molecules are not as specific as IgG for the antigenic determinant and therefore are not very effective in neutralizing the harmful effects of toxic antigens. However, even a single IgM molecule is capable of activating complement; thus, IgM readily induces lysis of foreign cells. Furthermore, it is much more effective in antigen agglutination and opsonization. Both IgG and IgM can also represent an integral component of the plasma membrane of some lymphocytes (see page 435).

The immunoglobulins A (IgA), when present in the plasma, are 170,000 daltons in molecular weight and, like IgG, they consist of four polypeptide chains, but these may be linked to each other in a polymeric form. IgA is also contained in a variety of secretory products, such as colostrum, saliva, tears, and nasal and tracheobronchial mucus, and it is released into the intestinal lumen. The secretory form of IgA has a molecular weight of 390,000 daltons because two antibody molecules become united to each other by an additional polypeptide chain called the T chain and the resulting complex is bound to a glycoprotein with a high carbohydrate content, called the *secretory piece*, which is produced by the epithelial cells. Secretory IgA is very resistant to proteolytic enzymes; therefore, it has been speculated that the secretory piece confers stability to the immunoglobulin molecule and prevents its catabolism in the intestinal lumen. IgA probably plays a protective role at the surface of mucous membranes.

Two additional types of immunoglobulins have been described: the IgE, which induce release of histamine by mast cells and are responsible for certain allergic reactions, and the IgD, whose function is still poorly understood. IgD is found normally on the surface of about one-fourth of normal human blood lymphocytes together with IgM. It is the main immunoglobulin on the surface of lymphocytes in the newborn and is present with IgM in most cases of chronic lymphatic leukemia. It seems, therefore, to be an embryonal kind of immunoglobulin.

Although a cell-mediated immune response and secretion of antibody may both occur upon introduction of a single antigen, they represent the activity of two morphologically similar, but functionally distinct, classes of lymphocytes, commonly referred to as *thymus-dependent* or *T lymphocytes* and *bursa-dependent* or *B lymphocytes*. T lymphocytes have been preconditioned under the influence of the thymus to respond to antigen by differentiating into cytotoxic lymphocytes; B lymphocytes, on the other hand, have acquired (under the influence of an organ, which is still unknown in mammals) the ability to respond to antigen by differentiation into antibody secreting lymphocytes and plasma cells. In birds, the site of production or preconditioning of B lymphocytes is the *bursa of Fabricius*, an appendix-like diverticulum of the cloaca.

Both T and B lymphocytes manifest immunological specificity, that is, both are genetically programmed to respond to a specific antigen, both carry "memory," and can become "tolerant." The functions of T and B lymphocytes are not independent of each other, however, but are intimately interrelated. Only certain antigens directly stimulate B cells and lead to antibody secretion without participation of T cells. With most antigens which elicit a humoral response, T lymphocytes cooperate with B cells, helping them to become stimulated and regulating their differentiation. Although lymphocytes are the only cells that confer specificity on the immunological response, they are assisted by macrophages in the process of antigen recognition. Phagocytic cells are also involved in antigen disposal, and eosinophils seem to destroy the complexes of antibody with soluble antigens.

Lymphocytes originate from stem cell precursors which, in the embryo, arise from the mesenchyme intervening between the endoderm of the yolk sac and the splanchnopleuric mesoderm. During postnatal life, the source of the stem cells becomes the bone marrow. The differentiation of the stem cells into T lymphocytes takes place in the thymus, a *central* or *primary lymphoid organ*, made up of a special variety of *lymphoid tissue*. In birds, the differentiation of stem cells into B lymphocytes occurs in the bursa of Fabricius, whereas in mammals, the analogue of the bursa has not yet been identified, and it may not exist as an anatomically discrete entity. In both the thymus and the avian bursa (or its unknown mammalian equivalent), the stem cell precursors undergo *antigen-independent* proliferation and differentiation into lymphocytes that are genetically programmed to set up a specific type of immune response upon meeting their appropriate antigen. They subsequently populate the blood and lymph, are disseminated throughout the connective tissues of the body, and infiltrate most epithelia. Together with macrophages and plasma cells, which arise from differentiation of B lymphocytes, they become associated with reticular cells and reticular fibers, thus giving rise to a second variety of lymphoid tissue, which represents the bulk of the *peripheral* or *secondary lymphoid organs* such as the lymph nodes, the spleen and tonsils. In the secondary lymphoid organs, T and B lymphocytes undergo *antigen-dependent* proliferation and differentiation into effector and "memory" cells.

CELLS OF THE IMMUNE SYSTEM

CYTOLOGY OF THE CELLS OF THE IMMUNE SYSTEM

Lymphocytes

This cell type has already been considered as a component of the blood (Chapter 5) and connective tissue (Chapter 6), but the foregoing descriptions need review and amplification in the context of the immune system. The term "lymphocyte" actually refers to a family of cells characterized by lack of specific granules, a round, centrally located nucleus, and a cytoplasm displaying various degrees of basophilia, due to the presence of free ribosomes (Figs. 14–1, 14–2, and 14–3). As previously stated, although they are morphologically similar, lymphocytes are physiologically heterogeneous; not only does this cell type include two major classes of cells, the T and B lymphocytes, but also within these two classes, individual

lymphocytes have the ability to recognize different antigens and may vary in their life span, functional competence, and sensitivity to ionizing radiations and hormones. Lymphocytes circulate with blood and lymph and infiltrate connective tissues and epithelia; they are present in the bone marrow and compose the bulk of the thymus, lymph nodes, white pulp of the spleen, and lymphoid masses associated with the digestive, respiratory, and urinary passages.

When suspended in a fluid medium nonmotile lymphocytes are round. When crowded together in tissues, they mutually deform one another into polyhedral shapes. Motile lymphocytes display a slow, ameboid progression and conform to the shape of the interstices through which they are advancing. When moving on a solid, flat substrate, they acquire a characteristic hand-mirror shape, with the nucleus ahead, followed by a tail of cytoplasm in which most organelles are concentrated.

The size of the lymphocytes varies in different organs and in various functional situations. Lymphocytes circulating in the blood have a diameter of 4 to 8 μm. but upon flattening, as when they are smeared and dried on a slide, this increases to 7 to 10 μm. (Fig. 14–1A). In lymphoid organs and tissues not involved in an acute immunological response, lymphocytes range between 4 and 15 μm. in diameter, the larger forms being rather uncommon. It is customary to subdivide them into small (4 to 7 μm.), medium-sized (7 to 11 μm.) and large lymphocytes (11 to 15 μm.) on the basis of cell size, nuclear morphology, and intensity of the cytoplasmic basophilia (Fig. 14–2); such a subdivision, however, is useful for descriptive purposes, but is rather arbitrary, because lymphocyte diameter and organization vary in a continuous fashion. According to this classification, blood lymphocytes are represented exclusively by small and medium-sized cells; lymphocytes of the lymph include a variable proportion of large cells, whereas lymphoid organs and tissues contain the whole spectrum of cell dimensions. As a consequence of stimulation by antigen or mitogens, mononuclear cells arise which are up to 30 μm. in diameter (Figs. 14–1C and F). These were variously termed *blast cells, immunoblasts, large pyroninophilic cells, hemocytoblasts, lymphoblasts*. There is now good evidence that these large elements result from transformation of small lymphocytes and that

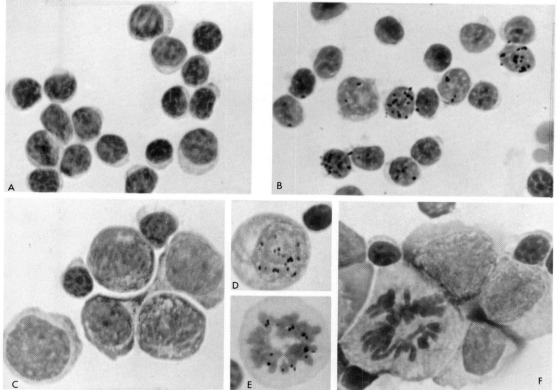

Figure 14–1 *A,* Smear preparation of small lymphocytes from the thoracic duct lymph of the rat stained with the May-Grünwald and Giemsa mixtures. × 1200. *B,* Autoradiograph of rat thoracic duct lymphocytes obtained two weeks after ^{3}H-thymidine administration. Only long-lived small lymphocytes are labeled. ×1200. *C* and *F,* When the lymphocytes from the rat thoracic duct lymph are cultured three days on a monolayer of mouse embryo cells, the contact with the foreign cells stimulates a proportion of the small lymphocytes to transform into lymphoblasts and large lymphocytes. Transformation is followed by proliferation, as shown by the dividing cell in *F.* ×1200. *D* and *E,* Autoradiograph of the transformed lymphocytes which arose from the labeled long-lived small lymphocytes of the rat after two days' culture on monolayer of mouse embryo cells. Note that the grain count is essentially the same as that of the labeled small lymphocytes in *B*; this shows that transformation by antigen precedes cell division. ×1200. (Courtesy of N. B. Everett.)

they may in turn generate small lymphocytes. Therefore, these cells will be referred to as lymphoblasts.

Small lymphocytes have a dense nucleus surrounded by a thin rim of cytoplasm (Fig. 14–3). The nucleus is central, round, or slightly indented, very rich in randomly dispersed, heterochromatic masses; the nucleolus is small and scarcely identifiable in smear preparations. The cytoplasm is slightly basophilic and contains a variable number of azurophilic granules when stained with the Giemsa mixture. The electron microscope shows a diplosome located at the nuclear indentation, surrounded by a small Golgi apparatus and by a few mitochondria. Free ribosomes in moderate numbers are scattered as single units throughout the cytoplasm;

cisternae of the granular endoplasmic reticulum are found only exceptionally. Small numbers of lysosomes, which represent the ultrastructural counterpart of the azurophilic granules, complete the list of cytoplasmic organelles. An occasional small lipid droplet may also be observed.

Medium-sized lymphocytes have a nucleus with a larger nucleolus and more abundant euchromatin; the cytoplasm displays more basophilia, due to a greater abundance of free ribosomes. In large lymphocytes and lymphoblasts (Fig. 15–4), the nucleus is largely euchromatic and contains one or two prominent nucleoli. The cytoplasm is abundant and intensely basophilic, owing to the presence of large numbers of free polyribosomes. Cisternae of the

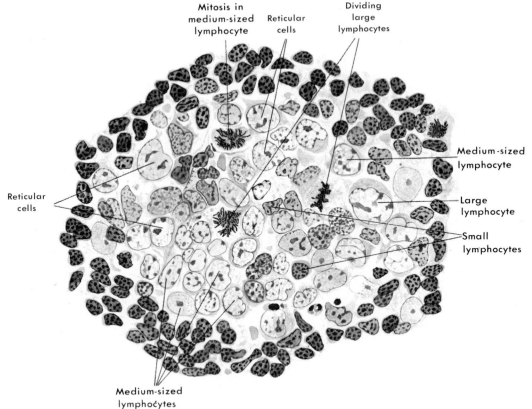

Figure 14–2 Various types of lymphocytes in a section of a human lymph node. Hematoxylin-eosin-azure II. ×750. (After A. A. Maximow.)

granular endoplasmic reticulum are, however, scarce. The Golgi apparatus is moderately enlarged and mitochondria and lysosomes are slightly increased in number.

Plasma Cells (Plasmacytes)

The term "plasma cell" includes a range of immature and mature elements, characterized by presence of considerable but varying numbers of cisternae of the granular endoplasmic reticulum. Their function is the synthesis and release (secretion) of antibody. They probably represent the late stages of differentiation of the B lymphocytes. Plasma cells are found in the medullary cords of resting lymph nodes, the marginal zone and cords of the resting spleen, and scattered throughout the connective tissues of the body. They are especially numerous in the lamina propria of the intestinal mucosa, where most of them have been shown by immunofluorescent methods to produce immunoglobulins A. During the acute phase of a humoral immune response, large numbers of immature plasma cells appear in the deep portion of the cortex of lymph nodes and at the boundary between white and red pulp of the spleen. Mature plasma cells are sessile elements and apparently never enter blood and lymph. After an antigenic challenge, however, immature forms appear in the lymph; furthermore, a limited number of elements appear in the blood which at the light microscope level resemble small lymphocytes in size and have a centrally located, darkly stained nucleus, but which in electron micrographs display the abundant granular endoplasmic reticulum typical of the plasma cell line.

Plasma cells are 6 to 20 μm. in diameter and have a rounded, elongated or polyhedral form, depending upon their location (Fig. 6–23). Seen with the light microscope, mature elements are small; they possess an eccentric, rounded nucleus with a small nucleolus and radially arranged coarse heterochromatic masses adjacent to the nuclear envelope, resulting in a cartwheel configuration. The cytoplasm is strongly basophilic, except for a conspicuous juxtanuclear, pale area, which contains the diplosome and surrounding Golgi apparatus.

It is evident in electron micrographs that the cytoplasmic basophilia of plasma cells is due to their highly developed granular endoplasmic reticulum, often distended with flocculent material (Figs. 6–24 and 14–4A). Experiments involving immunolabeling with

ferritin or horseradish peroxidase (Fig. 14–4B) have shown that the content of the cisternae of the granular reticulum consists largely of antibody. The Golgi apparatus of mature plasma cells is large; the mitochondria are few and unremarkable in their internal structure. In a small percentage of plasma cells, one or more cisternae of the granular reticulum are greatly distended with a mass of dense material. These inclusions (Russell bodies) are readily seen with the light microscope and consist of incomplete immunoglobulin molecules. It has been suggested that Russell bodies are indicative of an aberrant synthesis or faulty intracellular

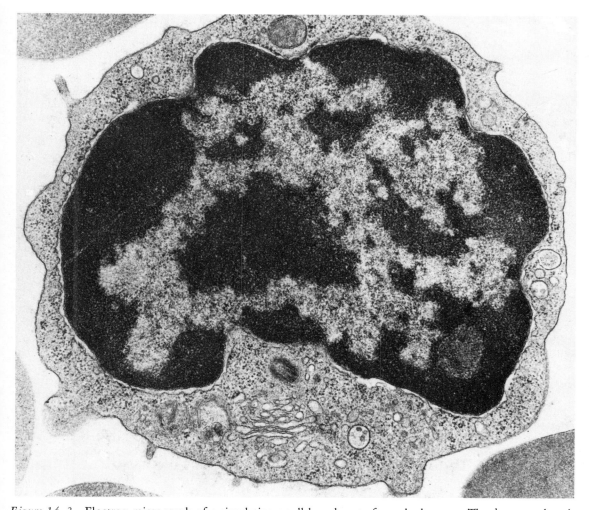

Figure 14–3 Electron micrograph of a circulating small lymphocyte from the hamster. The dense nucleus is surrounded by a thin rim of cytoplasm. A centriole and a small Golgi apparatus are located at a nuclear indentation. Free ribosomes in moderate numbers are scattered as single units throughout the cytoplasm. One mitochondrion (top) and multivesicular bodies complete the list of cytoplasmic organelles. Notice the absence of cisternae of the granular endoplasmic reticulum. ×23,000. (Micrograph by David Phillips.)

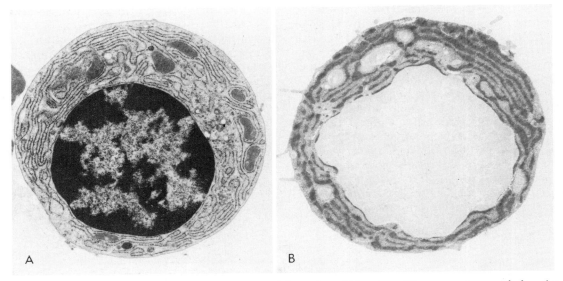

Figure 14–4   A, Electron micrograph of a plasma cell from the rabbit spleen. The eccentric, rounded nucleus contains masses of heterochromatin adjacent to the nuclear envelope. The cytoplasm displays a highly developed granular endoplasmic reticulum. *B,* Plasma cell from the spleen of a rabbit, which was injected with the enzyme horseradish peroxidase as an antigen. The antibody-containing spleen cells were subsequently treated with the antigen and stained with the histochemical method for demonstration of peroxidase activity. Dense reaction product is seen in the lumen of the cisternae of the granular endoplasmic reticulum, indicating the presence of anti-horseradish peroxidase antibody. ×6500. (Courtesy of E. H. Leduc and S. Avrameas.)

transport of antibody, but this speculation lacks conclusive evidence.

Very immature precursors of the plasma cell line *(plasmablasts)* are difficult to distinguish from lymphoblasts or large lymphocytes. The nucleus is rich in euchromatin and provided with a large nucleolus; the cytoplasm contains many free polyribosomes as well as narrow cisternae of the granular endoplasmic reticulum. The transition from plasmablasts to plasmacyte involves progressive condensation of the chromatin, reduction in size and complexity of the nucleolus, disappearance of the free polyribosomes, enlargement of the Golgi apparatus and appearance of a highy organized granular endoplasmic reticulum. The cisternae of the reticulum may form parallel, concentric arrays or become distended with accumulated antibody. The intermediate stages in the course of this differentiation are often referred to as *proplasmacytes.*

Macrophages

The structure of macrophages was discussed in Chapter 6 and will not be repeated here.

HISTOPHYSIOLOGY

Surface Properties of T and B Lymphocytes

The terms "T" and "B lymphocyte" describe two functionally distinct types of lymphocytes which circulate with blood and lymph and inhabit the peripheral lymphoid tissues. The lymphocytes of the thymus have different properties than those of T lymphocytes, but they probably represent the precursors of the T cells (see page 468). T lymphocytes cannot be distinguished from B lymphocytes by light or transmission electron microscopy. With the scanning microscope it has been shown that in the human blood T cells are smaller and possess a smooth surface, whereas B cells are larger and covered with microvilli (Figs. 14–5 and 14–6). This difference, however, reflects a transient functional state of the cell surface and it cannot always be relied upon as a criterion for identification in other tissues or functional states. T and B lymphocytes also have distinct surface properties demonstrable by indirect methods. If antibody is produced against immunoglobulins by injecting the antibody of one species into an animal of a different species, the anti-immunoglobulin antibody produced by the recipient can be isolated, purified, and conjugated to a visible marker. For example, the anti-immunoglobulin antibody can be conjugated with a fluorescent dye and then after interaction with lymphocyte surface, it can be localized with the fluorescence microscope (Fig. 14–7 *A, B, C*). Alternatively, the antibody can be labeled with radioiodine and its localization studied with light or electron microscopic autoradiography (Fig. 14–8); finally, in a third method, the antibody can be conjugated to the electron opaque particulate ferritin or hemocyanin (Figs. 14–9 and 14–10) or to the enzyme horseradish peroxidase and visualized with the electron microscope either directly or after appropriate histochemical reaction. With these techniques, it has been shown that B lymphocytes incubated at 0° C. with labeled anti-immunoglobulin bind the antibody over their entire surface (Figs. 14–7*A* and 14–8*A*). This property is attributable to the presence of immunoglobulins, predominantly of the IgM type, bound to

the cell membrane. There is evidence that this antibody at the cell surface represents the receptor which combines with antigen. On the other hand, the plasma membrane of T lymphocytes has little affinity for anti-immunoglobulins; thus, definitive evidence for the antibody nature of their antigen receptors is still lacking. The plasma membrane of B cells is also able to bind antibody by means of the Fc fragment of their molecule and the C′3 component of the complement system. T cells lack both of these kinds of surface receptors.

In man, a large proportion of T lymphocytes, and possibly all of them, bind sheep erythrocytes, and to a lesser extent pig erythrocytes, forming characteristic clusters or rosettes. The significance of this phenomenon, which lacks immunological specificity, is poorly understood. Nevertheless, spontaneous rosette formation seems to provide a reliable clinical test for evaluation of the size of the T cell population in human patients.

When T lymphocytes are transferred from a donor mouse into a recipient of the

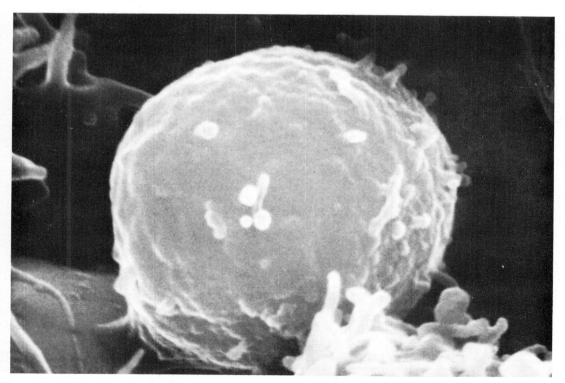

Figure 14–5 Scanning electron micrograph of a human T lymphocyte circulating in the blood. Except for a few short microvilli, the cell surface is smooth. ×21,000. (Courtesy of A. Polliak et al., J. Exp. Med., *138*:607, 1973.)

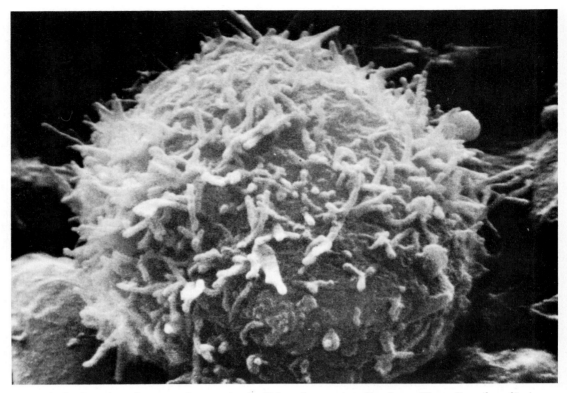

Figure 14-6 Scanning electron micrograph of a B lymphocyte in cell culture. The cell surface displays numerous and long microvilli. ×9500. (Courtesy of A. Polliak et al., J. Exp. Med., *138*:607, 1973.)

same species but with a slightly different genetic constitution, they elicit production of antibodies which combine with T but not with B lymphocytes. Thus, murine T cells possess a surface antigenic determinant called *theta,* which is lacking on B cells. Anti-theta antibodies, when injected into mice belonging to the strain whose T lymphocytes carry the theta antigen, lead to specific complement-mediated destruction of T cells. It is thus possible to study the distribution of T lymphocytes in the immune system and the functional impairment caused by their selective elimination. Furthermore, anti-theta antibody conjugated to a visible marker, such as fluorochrome or ferritin, or labeled with radioiodine, binds to the surface of T lymphocytes and permits their morphological identification. The functional significance of the chemical groupings at the surface of T cells which elicit the formation of anti-theta antibodies is unknown.

B cells have lower electrophoretic mo-

bility and lower density than T cells, and they adhere preferentially to nylon wool at 37° C. in the presence of serum. These properties have been exploited in attempts to separate the B from the T cell component of a mixed lymphocyte population. The different reactivity of T and B lymphocytes to various mitogens, to x-ray irradiation, and to cortisone, their distinctive distribution in the organs of the immune system, and their different pattern of recirculation are discussed on pages 444, 445, and 451.

Response of T Lymphocytes to Antigen

Both T and B lymphocytes manifest immunological specificity, that is, both are genetically programmed to respond to an antigen that is specific for each individual cell. This commitment is expressed by the presence of receptors on the lymphocyte plasma membrane, which combine with the antigenic determinants. This process of specific binding is called *antigen recognition.* Antigen binding by T lymphocytes can be studied in laboratory rodents by mixing lymphocyte suspensions with foreign erythrocytes, usually those of sheep. This technique cannot be applied to human T cells because most of them bind sheep erythrocytes nonspecifically. Antigen binding cells of laboratory rodents can also be studied by combined autoradiography and immunofluorescence, using radioiodine labeled antigen and fluorochrome-conjugated anti-theta antibody. It has been shown by these experimental strategies that antigen-binding T lymphocytes in animals not previously exposed to the antigen are very few in number and belong to the category of the small or medium-sized lymphocytes. They increase in number following immunization,

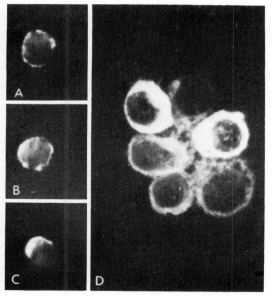

Figure 14-7 A, B, C, B lymphocytes from the mouse spleen stained with anti-immunoglubulin antibody conjugated to fluorescein isothyocyanate and photographed with the fluorescence microscope. In *A,* the lymphocyte was reacted with the labeled antibody at 4° C. The anti-immunoglobulin is dispersed over the entire cell surface, although some patching of the marker is already in progress. *B* and *C,* Upon warming at 37° C., the fluorescent antibody becomes concentrated over one pole of the cell (capping). For comparison, *D* illustrates the intense staining of the antibody in the cytoplasm of splenic plasma cells treated with fluorescent anti-immunoglobulin. ×1200. (Courtesy of E. R. Unanue.)

probably because the challenge with the antigen induces amplification of that small fraction of the lymphocyte population that carries surface receptors specific for the particular antigen. The number of receptor sites for antigen on the membrane of T lymphocytes is very small, probably a few hundred, in contrast to the several thousands on B lymphocytes. The immunoglobulin nature of these sites has been suggested but not proved beyond doubt.

The sequence of events following antigen binding of T lymphocytes is not fully understood. However, circumstantial evidence favors the view that antigen, upon combining with its receptor at the cell surface, somehow triggers the transformation of the small lymphocyte into a proliferating lymphoblast (Figs. 14–1*A* through *F*). The size of the cell increases, its nucleus becomes euchromatic, the nucleolus enlarges, a great number of polyribosomes appears in the cytoplasm, and the Golgi apparatus becomes more prominent. Probably related to antigen recognition are the behavioral phenomena called *peripolesis* and *emperipolesis* — that is, the tendency of lymphocytes in cell culture to move about, indenting and even penetrating other cells. Only antigen deployed on the surface of cells can stimulate T lymphocytes directly. Most soluble and particulate antigens, and even certain foreign cells, such as erythrocytes, require the participation of macrophages for effective immunization. The functions of macrophages in the immune response are discussed in a later section of this chapter.

After combining with antigens that elicit an antibody response, the stimulated T lymphocyte, at some unknown stage of its transformation into a lymphoblast, interacts with B lymphocytes and triggers their differentiation into antibody secreting cells. Furthermore, lymphoblast proliferation leads to amplification of the response and to the differentiation of memory T cells, which revert to the state of small lymphocytes.

With antigens such as tissue grafts, which elicit a cell-mediated response, lymphoblast proliferation and differentiation lead to the appearance of both cytotoxic lymphocytes and memory cells. Cytotoxic lymphocytes have the ability to impair the viability of the graft either through direct interaction with the foreign cells or through synthesis and release of soluble factors (*mediators* or *lymphokines*). The mechanism of

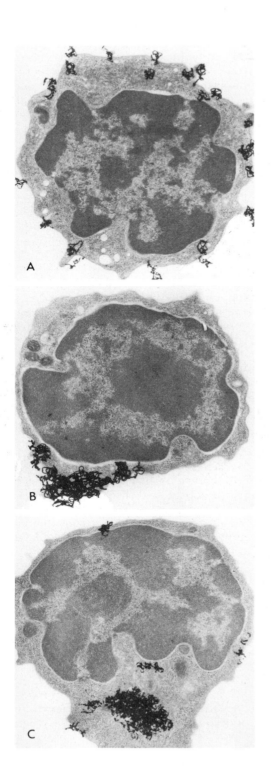

direct cytotoxicity is poorly understood. It is specific for the cells which caused immunization, for nearby cellular elements are not affected, and it requires close cell-to-cell contact. As a consequence of this puzzling interaction, the normal permeability properties of the plasma membrane of the target are altered, and cell lysis follows. Soluble mediators released by activated T lymphocytes are molecules of 8000 to 80,000 daltons in molecular weight, which display a great variety of pharmacological activities. They are not immunoglobulins, and most of them have been extracted from the supernatant of lymphocyte cultures stimulated by mitogens (see p. 444). They lack antigenic specificity, that is to say, they are also effective on cells other than those used for immunization. The best known of the several mediators identified to date is the *migration inhibiting factor (MIF)*, which immobilizes macrophages and may possibly lead to accumulation of these cells at the site of the antigen. Another mediator, *lymphotoxin (LT)* causes cell lysis. The *lymphocyte transforming factor (LTF)* or *blastogenic factor (BF)* causes transformation and clonal expansion of nonsensitized lymphocytes, apparently acting like a mitogen (see p. 444). The *cloning* and *proliferation inhibiting factors (CIF and PIF)* inhibit mitosis in tissue culture cells. It is not known at present whether all these mediator effects are attributable to different substances or represent different actions of one or a few molecules. A noteworthy exception is a *transfer factor (TF)*, which seems to be antigen specific; in fact, it seems capable of conferring antigen specificity to quiescent, circulating lymphocytes. Moreover, it is extracted from lymphocytes immediately after contact with the antigen, rather than following their differentiation into effector cells.

Thus, T lymphocytes, upon stimulation by antigen, do not secrete conventional anti-

Figure 14-8 Electron microscope autoradiography of mouse spleen B lymphocytes treated with ^{125}I-labeled rabbit anti-immunoglobulin antibody. *A,* At 4° C. the marker is randomly distributed over the entire cell membrane. *B,* When the lymphocytes are incubated at 37° C., the label becomes concentrated at one pole of the cell, forming a cap. *C,* Finally, the label is interiorized by endocytosis. ×15,000. (Courtesy of E. R. Unanue et al., J. Exp. Med., *136*:885, 1972.)

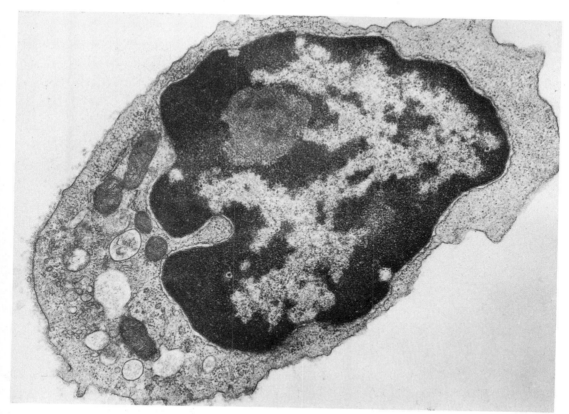

Figure 14-9 B lymphocyte of the mouse spleen treated with rabbit anti-immunoglobulin antibody conjugated with hemocyanin, a respiratory pigment present in the hemolymph of many invertebrates. The hemocyanin molecule has the shape of a short cylinder and is readily recognized with the electron microscope. This lymphocyte was reacted with the labeled anti-immunoglobulin at 4° C. and then warmed to 37° C. for 10 min. The label is concentrated in a cap over the cell pole in which the Golgi apparatus is contained. ×23,000. (Courtesy of M. J. Karnovsky et al., J. Exp. Med., *136*:907, 1972.)

body, but instead acquire the ability to release soluble mediators which have a short-range effect on B lymphocytes and macrophages, or which are toxic in a nonspecific manner to neighboring cells. Some of these lymphocytes became capable of directly and specifically damaging the membrane of the cells which triggered their differentiation.

Response of B Lymphocytes to Antigen

Antigen receptors on the surface of B lymphocytes are clearly immunoglobulins, for it can be shown that specific binding of radioactive antigen to the cell membrane is blocked by anti-immunoglobulin antibody. The number of immunoglobulin receptors varies between 50,000 and 150,000 per cell;

thus the number of sites is much higher than on T lymphocytes. Despite the abundance of binding sites at the cell surface, direct stimulation of B lymphocytes is only possible by polymeric antigens—that is, by molecules which display identical groupings in a linear, repetitive sequence such as the pneumococcal polysaccharide. Furthermore, the response only occurs within a narrow range of antigen dose and results predominantly, if not solely, in production of IgM antibodies. With most antigens that elicit a humoral response, B cell stimulation also requires the participation of stimulated T lymphocytes and the presence of a third partner cell, the macrophage. In this cooperative interaction, both T and B lymphocytes are committed to react specifically with a given antigen, but the influence of stimulated T cells is necessary for efficient production of IgG antibodies by B lympho-

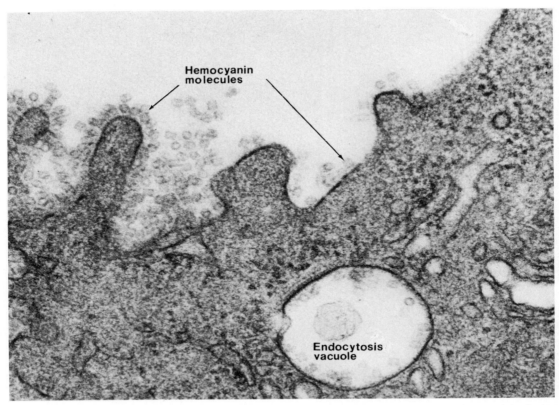

Figure 14–10 Same specimen as in Figure 14–9. Hemocyanin labeled anti-immunoglobulin antibody is attached to the membrane immunoglobulins of the B lymphocyte. The cell has begun to interiorize the label in endocytotic vacuoles. ×95,000. (Courtesy of M. J. Karnovsky et al., J. Exp. Med., *136*:907, 1972.)

cytes and for the differentiation of memory cells within the B cell population. The mechanism of the "helper activity" of T cells is very poorly understood; various theories have been proposed, and they may not be mutually exclusive. The T lymphocytes might conceivably concentrate antigen at their surface or cause antigen to concentrate at the surface of macrophages, thus generating the repetitive sequence of determinants that is effective in B cell stimulation. It has also been speculated that T lymphocytes may elaborate and release soluble mediators, either nonspecific or antigen-specific, which might regulate B cell function.

The morphological events underlying lymphocyte cooperation are still largely unknown. Experiments in which the primary response to foreign red blood cells has been reproduced in vitro show that the three cell types required for production of anti-erythrocyte antibody, T and B lymphocytes and macrophages, intimately adhere to each other in small clusters. It is not yet clear, however, whether cluster formation is essential for antibody production.

As a result of the cooperation between stimulated T and B lymphocytes, antibody is secreted and plasma cells appear. That plasma cells synthesize and release antibody, has been firmly established by comparative immunological and histological studies, by immunofluorescent (Figs. 6–25 and 14–7D) and autoradiographic technique, and by antibody assay in microdroplets containing individual plasma cells. In recent years, however, it has been clearly shown that certain lymphocytes are also capable of synthesizing and releasing antibody. Evidence for this was obtained from antibody assay in microdroplets containing single cells and from electron microscopic identification of single cells that had demonstrated their capacity to produce hemolytic antibody by forming a plaque of lysis in a layer of erythrocytes dispersed in agar (Figs. 14–11 and 14–12).

Antibody producing lymphocytes are typical lymphoblasts or large cells which in addition to polyribosomes contain a small amount of cisternae of the granular endoplasmic reticulum. These cells have been regarded as transitional forms between lymphocytes and immature plasma cells.

Two schools of thought have developed on the interrelationships between lymphocytes and plasma cells, one regarding the lymphocyte as the ancestor of the plasma cell, the other considering plasma cells as a separate cell line arising from independent, still unidentified, stem cell precursors. Although proof is lacking, a great deal of circumstantial evidence favors the view that lymphocytes represent the precursors of the plasma cells. Especially persuasive are the fact that lymphocytes can also secrete antibody and the observation that during the immune response, transitional forms having cytological characteristics intermediate between lymphoblasts and immature plasma cells are found

consistently. Furthermore, all experiments in which lymphocyte populations have been transferred from immunized animals into syngeneic* unprimed recipients, or from unprimed donors into allogeneic recipients, have led to the appearance of plasma cells in the recipient.

It is thus widely accepted that the small lymphocytes of the B type, stimulated by antigen under the influence of T lymphocytes, undergo transformation into lymphoblasts. During this process, antibody having identical specificity to that deployed on the cell surface is synthesized in increasing amounts and is released as a secretory product instead of simply being inserted into the plasma membrane. Antibody secreting

---

Syngeneic in the field of transplantation immunity refers to individuals of the same species which are genetically identical, such as monozygotic twins or inbred laboratory animals. *Allogeneic* refers to individuals of the same species which are not genetically identical.

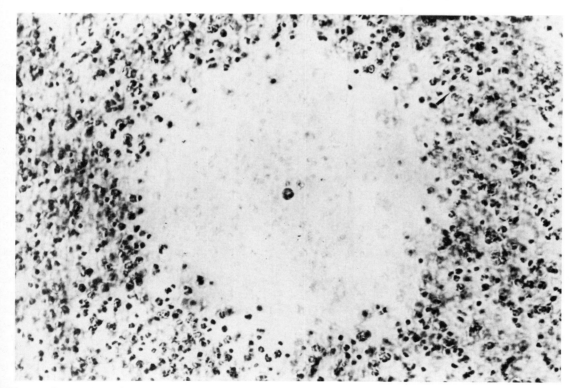

Figure 14–11 Hemolytic plaque-forming cell. A diluted suspension of lymphoid cells from an animal immunized with foreign erythrocytes was plated in agar along with the erythrocytes that served as antigen. The lymphoid cell at the center has synthetized and released hemolytic antibody into the surrounding agar, and the antibody has combined with the erythrocytes embedded in it. Complement has subsequently been added and the erythrocytes carrying the antibody have lysed, leaving a clear halo or plaque around the antibody-secreting cell. ×200. (Courtesy of A. A. Nordin and N. K. Jerne.)

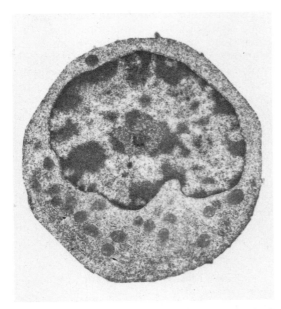

Figure 14–12 Electron micrograph of an antibody secreting cell from the rabbit popliteal lymph node identified by the hemolytic-antibody plaque technique illustrated in Figure 14–11. The cell has the morphology of a large lymphocyte with euchromatic nucleus, prominent nucleolus, and abundant cytoplasm lacking an organized granular endoplasmic reticulum. ×10,000. (Courtesy of T. N. Harris et al., J. Exp. Med., *123*:161, 1966.)

lymphoblasts are actively proliferating cells; their progeny include (1) memory B cells, which revert to the state of small lymphocytes, and (2) transitional elements, which display an enlarged Golgi apparatus and increasing amounts of granular endoplasmic reticulum. These transitional cells, in turn, undergo further differentiation into plasma cells, passing through the stages in which they are identified as plasmablasts and proplasmacytes. Differentiation into plasma cells is accompanied by decrease in amount of the surface membrane-bound immunoglobulins, loss of proliferative capacity, and loss of motility. Experiments involving labeling with ³H-thymidine indicate that the process of differentiation of lymphocytes into plasma cells takes about one day. The life span of plasma cells is of the order of a few weeks. Lymphoblasts and immature plasma cells also have the capacity to enter the efferent lymph of the lymph nodes draining the site of antigen injection and to colonize additional lymph nodes along the same path of lymphatic drainage. There are also indi-

cations that they may transform into smaller cells with condensed, central nucleus, scanty cytoplasm, but abundant granular endoplasmic reticulum, and that these small cells enter the blood and propagate the response throughout the body.

During the primary response to antigen, the first antibody to appear in the blood belongs to the IgM type; later, much larger amounts of the more efficient IgG are produced. The switch from IgM to IgG production is dependent upon the regulatory influence of T lymphocytes. Both types of immunoglobulins can be produced by either lymphocytes or plasma cells. Whether lymphocytes produce predominantly IgM and plasma cells produce IgG, or whether IgG producing plasma cells arise from IgM producing lymphocyte precursors, are still subjects of controversy. There is no doubt, however, that each individual element, either lymphocyte or plasma cell, produces immunoglobulins of a single class and with unique antigenic specificity.

The intracellular secretory pathway of immunoglobulins has not yet been fully elucidated. The heavy and light chains are transcribed from separate messengers on polyribosomes bound to the membranes of the granular endoplasmic reticulum. They are subsequently transferred into the lumen of the cisternae, either free or combined with each other. In lymphocytes, the first detectable antibody appears in the perinuclear cisterna and later, as differentiation to plasma cells proceeds, antibody is produced and stored throughout the granular endoplasmic reticulum. In mature plasma cells, antibody is no longer detected in the space within the nuclear envelope and it disappears from some of the cisternae of the granular endoplasmic reticulum. Some carbohydrate components of the antibody molecules (e.g., N-acetylglucosamine) are incorporated into the nascent H chain. The polypeptide backbone, carrying part of the carbohydrate moiety, is subsequently transported to the Golgi apparatus, where additional saccharides (e.g., galactose) are added. From the Golgi, antibody is carried to the cell surface by some unknown mechanism and is released from the cell. According to this view, antibody synthesis and release involve an intracellular pathway that has been found to be typical of all other protein secreting cells studied to date.

The amount of antibody produced by

lymphocytes may be smaller than that produced by plasma cells, but it is released at an early stage of the response and at the very site of antigen stimulation, where it can be much more effective than the circulating antibody, which is confined largely to the intravascular space. Plasma cells may synthesize much larger amounts of antibody, but they store a large proportion of this immunoglobulin in the distended cisternae of their granular reticulum and may release it only upon cell death and disintegration.

The Role of Macrophages in Immune Responses

Optimal response to most antigens requires the collaboration of macrophages, which participate in both the initial phase of lymphocyte stimulation by antigen and the terminal events of antigen disposal. However, the specificity of the immune response is determined by the lymphocytes, because macrophages are not able to distinguish foreign determinants from the normal body constituents. There is a special need of macrophage assistance in the immune responses which depend on collaborative interaction of B and T lymphocytes. On the other hand, the response to certain polymeric antigens that directly stimulates B cells does not require macrophage participation, nor is macrophage function necessary in T lymphocyte stimulation by antigenic determinants deployed on the surface of eukaryotic cells. A noteworthy exception to this rule is the response to foreign red blood cells, which involves cooperation between the two types of lymphocytes.

Although macrophages engulf a great variety of substances, regardless of whether or not they are immunogenic, they are not capable of taking up all antigenic materials. Phagocytosis follows only when the macrophage membrane is able to bind the antigen either in its native form or after opsonization. Thus, polymeric antigens interact with the macrophage membrane more easily than their monomeric forms do. Certain bacteria, such as pneumococci, are not engulfed because their carbohydrate capsule does not bind to the macrophage membrane, whereas most protein antigens are easily phagocytized. The need for macrophage participation in the inductive phase of the immune response has emerged clearly from a wide variety of experiments, all showing that antigens which

are avidly taken up by macrophages are good immunogens, whereas those which are not phagocytized are poor immunogens. Blockade of the macrophages of the body by administration of inert particulate suspensions significantly depresses the immune response. If a donor animal is injected with an antigen that is feebly immunogenic, and its macrophages are then transferred to a syngeneic recipient, this latter responds with a vigorous immune response possibly because the small amount of antigen bound to the surface of the macrophages is a much stronger immunogen then the antigen in its original dispersed form. The strongest evidence for macrophage participation in lymphocyte stimulation comes from experiments in which the response to foreign red blood cells has been reproduced in vitro; in this system, it has been clearly shown that in addition to T and B lymphocytes, a third partner cell is required. This cell has all the properties of macrophages; it is phagocytic, is radioresistant, adheres to glass surfaces, is inactivated by all treatments which affect macrophages in vivo, and does not synthesize antibodies.

The precise mechanism of macrophage function in the induction of an immune response by lymphocytes is obscure. Macrophages certainly act in general by removing and digesting excess of antigen. If antigen interacts indiscriminately with lymphocytes in a location unfavorable for cell cooperation, tolerance is induced instead of immunity. Thus, only a small fraction of the antigen escapes destruction by macrophages and triggers immunization. Macrophages, however, seem to play a more intimate and important role in lymphocyte stimulation by antigen. According to a widely accepted hypothesis, in addition to ingesting and destroying antigen, macrophages retain a small amount of antigen bound to their surface and present it in a concentrated form to lymphocytes (a phenomenon referred to as *antigen presentation*). This function implies close topographical relationships between macrophages and lymphoid cells, and this intimate association has been demonstrated with the electron microscope in the cell clusters that produce antibody against foreign red blood cells in vitro.

In most cases, the antigen must retain its native configuration to elicit an appropriate immune response, although with particulate substances, it has been postulated that macrophages partially degrade the antigen and couple it to RNA (*antigen processing*). This idea is in conflict with studies indicating that the membrane of the digestive vacuoles is impermeable to large molecules; furthermore, the alleged association of antigen with RNA may well be a technical artifact.

The role of macrophages in antigen disposal includes removal of foreign cells or bacteria whose viability has been impaired by cytotoxic lymphocytes or by lytic antibody in presence of complement. Furthermore, phagocytosis of foreign material, cells, and bacteria is powerfully enhanced when the antigenic determinants are opsonized, that is, complexed with antibody or with antibody and complement. Opsonization depends on the presence of receptors on the macrophage membrane which bind the Fc part of the antibody molecule or the $C'3$ component of the complement system. Only certain classes of immunoglobulins bind directly to the macrophage surface (IgG in humans, IgG and IgM in mice), and the interaction is especially strong when they are combined with antigen. IgM, which does not bind to the membrane of human macrophages directly, becomes cytophilic in the presence of complement.

The enhancement of phagocytosis by antibody and complement is not an exclusive property of macrophages; granulocytes also have an enhanced capacity for engulfing bacteria when the bacteria are complexed with antibody and complement.

Nonspecific Stimulation of Lymphocytes

A number of agents besides antigen, commonly referred to as *mitogens*, stimulate lymphocytes, inducing their transformation into actively proliferating lymphoblasts. The major difference between antigen and mitogens resides in the fact that the former reacts with individual lymphocytes that on a genetic basis have developed membrane receptors specific for its surface determinants, whereas mitogens are effective on much larger lymphocyte populations. Mitogens include a variety of substances extracted from plants or seeds, constituents of bacteria or products of their metabolism, and antilymphocyte sera, produced by immunizing animals with exogenous lymphocytes. All mitogens whose mechanism of action has been studied in detail have the capacity to bind chemical groupings on the plasma membrane of lymphocytes; many of them also combine with the surface of other cells, but only lymphocytes respond with transformation and mitosis. As agents also exist which bind to the surface of lymphocytes without stimulating them, mitogens can be regarded as belonging to a larger class of substances, whose common property is an affinity for chemical groupings on the surfaces of cells, and which are therefore generically named *ligands*. The effects of mitogenic ligands on lymphocytes has great theoretical importance, because their mechanism of action, although nonspecific, appears to be identical to that of antigens. Therefore, they have recently become a useful laboratory tool in studies aimed at an understanding of lymphocyte stimulation. Especially well studied are the chemical and biological properties of extracts of certain plants or seeds, which have long been known to cause agglutination of erythrocytes and leukocytes. These substances are called *lectins*. Agglutination depends on the fact that lectins are multivalent ligands and thus form bridges between neighboring cells, causing formation of clumps. Plant lectins are proteins or glycoproteins that have strong chemical affinity for the oligosaccharide residues on the plasma membrane of mammalian cells. They can be conjugated to an ultrastructural marker such as ferritin or hemocyanin, and in this way the distribution of the lectin-binding oligosaccharides at the cell surface can be visualized with the electron microscope.

Ligands do not stimulate all lymphocytes indiscriminately. Phytohemagglutinin (PHA), a lectin extracted from the red kidney bean (*Phaseolus vulgaris*) and concanavalin A (Con A), extracted from the jackbean (*Canavalia ensiformis*) stimulate T lymphocytes. Pokeweed mitogen (PWM), extracted from the root of *Phytolacca americana* activates both T and B cells, whereas a lipopolysaccharide extracted from the bacterium *Escherichia coli* (LPS) is specific for B cells.

T lymphocyte stimulation by PHA has been studied in great detail and provides a satisfactory means of imitating the morphological and biochemical phenomena that follow combination of antigen with T cells. The earliest event after addition of PHA to a culture of small lymphocytes (15 min.) is enhanced endocytotic activity, as evidenced by increased uptake of neutral red, and increased synthesis of RNA (15 to 30 min.).

Soon afterward, the nucleolus begins to enlarge (4 hours). At 24 to 36 hours, the nucleus becomes more euchromatic, the nucleolonema is clearly visible in the nucleolus, and the cell volume increases. The cell begins DNA synthesis, thus entering the S phase of the cell cycle, which lasts 6 to 10 hours. Then, it enters the G2 phase, characterized by active RNA and protein synthesis. There is a striking concomitant increase in cytoplasmic polyribosomes, whereas the granular endoplasmic reticulum remains relatively sparse. The Golgi apparatus enlarges and the lysosomes are moderately increased in number. At the end of G2, which lasts 2 to 4 hours, the lymphocyte has undergone a fourfold increase in volume and enters mitosis. DNA synthesis in cultures of PHA stimulated lymphocytes reaches a peak at 72 to 120 hours, then slowly declines over a period of 5 to 7 days. Beginning at about 24 hours after PHA exposure, the T lymphocyte develops cytotoxicity; that is, it acquires the capacity to impair nonspecifically the viability of other cells, such as fibroblasts. This property is mediated by production and release into the culture medium of various lymphokynes. The effects of lectins on B lymphocytes are poorly understood, but there is evidence that in 7 to 10 day old cultures of PWM stimulated lymphocytes, plasma cells develop. Furthermore, both PWM and LPS induce the synthesis of proteins having the same sedimentation coefficient as IgM antibody.

From all the above-mentioned studies, it is evident that binding of molecules to the plasma membrane is not effective per se in causing lymphocyte stimulation, but saturation of specific chemical groupings at the cell surface is probably required. Once a mitogenic ligand has bound to the plasma membrane, it somehow triggers lymphocyte transformation. Lymphocytes are unique among mammalian cells in that they respond with cell division and differentiation to a variety of exogenous substances, including the antigen for which they carry specific receptors. The events following stimulation are a stereotyped response, imprinted on the lymphocyte genome during the cell's developmental history. T lymphocytes become cytotoxic and B lymphocytes secrete antibody, regardless of whether the stimulus for transformation was antigen or a nonspecific ligand.

Recent studies using ligands conjugated to a visible marker have cast some light upon the cellular events that immediately follow the ligand's combination with the lymphocyte membrane (Figs. 14–7 through 14–10). When anti-immunoglobulin antibody conjugated to a fluorescent dye (or to ferritin or hemocyanin) is reacted at 4°C. with a B lymphocyte bearing the immunoglobulin, the label appears uniformly dispersed over the entire cell surface. This demonstrates that antibody molecules on B cells are uniformly distributed throughout the plasma membrane. With the passage of time, the marker becomes aggregated, resulting in formation of interconnected patches. This phenomenon, called *patching*, depends upon the fact that surface immunoglobulins move randomly in the fluid domain of the plasma membrane and that when they approach sufficiently close to one another, they are cross linked by the multivalent anti-immunoglobulin antibody. However, if the cell suspension is warmed to 37°C., the marker molecules become aggregated to form a continuous cap localized in the region of the cell surface overlying the Golgi apparatus, a behavior called *capping*. That portion of the plasma membrane bearing the marker subsequently becomes interiorized by endocytosis, or the label is shed from the cell surface. This process leaves the B lymphocyte denuded of its surface immunoglobulins and antigen receptors for several hours. Similar phenomena have also been described in T cells treated with ligands.

Capping is an energy-dependent process by which the cell eliminates the ligand bound to its surface; its relationship to lymphocyte stimulation is still poorly understood. However they seem to represent independent phenomena, for capping is not sufficient to trigger lymphocyte activation, nor does it inactivate the cell.

Other Functional Properties of Lymphocytes

Lymphocyte heterogeneity is not limited to the two classes of T and B cells. Within each class, lymphocytes may differ considerably in other functional properties, such as immunocompetence, life span, and sensitivity to ionizing radiation or to adrenal steroids. In T lymphocytes, which have been more thoroughly studied, these functional differences are related to the degree of cell differentiation. Most lymphocytes of the thymus, which represent the precursors of the T lymphocyte, are not immunocompetent—that is, they lack the capacity·to respond to antigen or to lectins such as PHA by transformation and proliferation. They are also readily destroyed by x-ray irradiation or administration of cortisone; furthermore, some of the thymic lymphocytes have a very short life span (see Chapter 15). Upon leaving the thymus, T lymphocytes become immunocompetent and more resistant to irradiation and cortisone. Their life span is unknown, but upon interaction with antigen, they can give rise to memory cells, which have the morphology of small lymphocytes and a life span in man of up to several years.

The changes in functional properties of B lymphocytes during their development are still poorly understood. There is evidence, however, that their bone marrow precursors are resistant to corticosteroids, whereas peripheral B lymphocytes are sensitive to both x-ray irradiation and adrenal steroids. Memory cells of the B type also have a long life span.

An important property of lymphocytes is their motility, which enables them to cross the walls of the postcapillary venules in order to enter or leave the bloodstream. They also move about in the parenchyma of lymph nodes and can leave the nodes by migrating into the lymph. They penetrate epithelia and freely wander through the connective tissues of the body. Differentiation into plasma cells is accompanied by a loss of motility.

LYMPHOID TISSUE

Lymphocytes occur as individual cells in blood, lymph, and throughout the connective and epithelial tissues of the body. However, in most organs, but especially in the lamina propria of the digestive and respiratory tracts, they occur together with plasma cells and macrophages as densely packed masses in loose connective tissue. Furthermore, the thymus, lymph nodes, white pulp of the spleen, and tonsils consist mainly of lymphocytes. The terms "lymphoid" and "lymphatic tissue" have been widely employed to define the common features of all aggregates of lymphocytes and lymphocyte-rich organs. Although in the past these terms were often used with quite different connotations, modern advances in immunology have rendered the traditional distinctions obsolete. On the other hand, our knowledge of the cell to cell interactions at a tissue or organ level is still largely incomplete, and a solid basis for a rational classification of the lymphocyte collections of the body is lacking. The term "lymphoid tissue" or "lymphoid organ" will be used here to define regions of the body in which lymphocytes, with or without associated plasma cells, represent the chief cellular constituent. It must be emphasized, however, that this definition is purely descriptive and includes cell aggregates that may have very different functions.

One morphologically and functionally distinct type of lymphoid tissue is that found in the thymus and in the medulla of the nodules of the avian bursa of Fabricius. It consists of lymphocytes and a few macrophages, contained in the meshes of a tridimensional network of stellate cells joined by desmosomes. These stellate stromal elements are called *reticular cells* simply because they form a network. Unlike the mesenchymal stroma of most other organs, these cells arise from an epithelial outgrowth of the endoderm, which becomes secondarily invaded by lymphopoietic stem cells. Reticular fibers are scarce in this variety of lymphoid tissue.

A much more common type of lymphoid tissue makes up the bulk of the lymph nodes, the white pulp of the spleen, and the tonsils and forms more or less discrete masses scattered in the connective tissues of the body. From a descriptive point of view, "diffuse" and "nodular" subvarieties of this second type of lymphoid tissue can be distinguished (Fig. 14–13).

Diffuse Lymphoid Tissue

Lymphoid tissue of this description is typically found in the internodular, deep cortical, and medullary regions of lymph nodes, in the periarterial lymphoid sheaths of the spleen, in the internodular regions of the tonsils, and Peyer's patches. It consists of a sponge-like stroma with lymphocytes in the meshes. The stroma, in turn, is made up of reticular fibers and reticular cells of mesenchymal origin (Fig. 14–14). Reticular fibers, best shown by the silver impregnation methods, are intimately associated with the reticular cells and often occupy deep recesses or grooves in their surface. In ordinary histological preparations the reticular cells appear as stellate or elongate elements with oval, euchromatic nucleus and scanty acidophilic

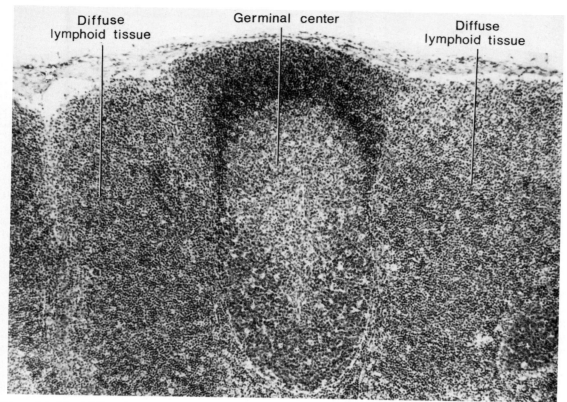

Figure 14-13. Diffuse lymphoid tissue and a germinal center in the outer cortex of a mesenteric lymph node of a dog. Hematoxylin-eosin.

cytoplasm. In vitally stained animals, some of the reticular cells take up colloidal dyes avidly while others do not. By this functional criterion, some of them can actually be regarded as macrophages. With the electron microscope, reticular cells display cisternae of granular endoplasmic reticulum in varying amounts and a moderately well developed Golgi apparatus, whereas the other cell organelles are inconspicuous. The cell periphery is often devoid of organelles and inclusions and contains many delicate filaments. Thus, some of the reticular cells of the diffuse lymphoid tissue are fixed macrophages, while others are not very different from the fibroblasts of the connective tissues elsewhere in the body. Experiments involving labeling with ^{3}H-thymidine have shown that in lymph nodes, reticular cells have a very slow turnover rate. Moreover, during the regeneration of the lymph node following irradiation, no transformation of labeled reticular cells to the free elements of the lymphoid parenchyma is seen. Thus, contrary to the traditional teach-ing, it seems unlikely that reticular cells can give rise to other cell types. There seems to be no evidence supporting the time-honored view that reticular cells are primitive or undifferentiated elements, capable of giving rise to lymphoblasts or other connective tissue elements. It now appears that reticular cells, as seen with the light microscope, represent either fibroblasts, concerned with the synthesis and maintenance of the reticular fibers, or occasional fixed phagocytes, belonging to the monocyte-macrophage system. The free cells of the diffuse lymphoid tissue are lymphocytes of various sizes, macrophages, and a variable number of plasma cells.

Lymphoid Nodules

Lymphoid nodules are compact, circumscribed collections of cells within the diffuse lymphoid tissue. They are typically found in the cortex of lymph nodes, at the periphery of the white pulp of the spleen, and in the lamina propria of the digestive and respiratory passages. They are very numerous in the

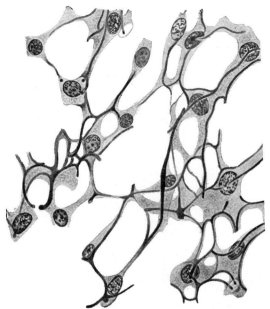

Figure 14-14 Section of a lymph node after the lymphocytes have been removed, showing the network of reticular cells and their intimate relations with the reticular fibers. Mallory-azan stain. (Redrawn after Heidenhain.)

tonsils, Peyer's patches, and appendix. There is much disagreement in the literature as to the nomenclature for lymphoid nodules, since the terms "primary" and "secondary nodule" and "germinal center" have been used to define different entities. *Primary nodule* is most commonly employed to designate a rounded collection of tightly packed small lymphocytes, whereas *secondary nodule* (also called *germinal center*) describes ovoid structures consisting of a spherical cluster of larger, pale staining cells invested by a cap of small lymphocytes.

The precise organization of primary nodules is unknown; moreover, it is not clear whether they represent functionally significant entities. What are interpreted as primary nodules in young adult subjects may merely represent tangential sections through the lymphocyte cap of germinal centers or secondary nodules. There is no evidence that secondary nodules, with their cap of small lymphocytes, arise by transformation of preexisting primary nodules, as the terms would imply. Thus the term "secondary nodule" does not seem to be justified experimentally and should be discarded in favor of "germinal center."

Germinal centers are a highly organized, widely distributed component of the lymphoid tissue absent only in the normal thymus (Figs. 14-13 and 14-15). In their fully developed form, the germinal centers appear as a spherical mass with a dark, or densely populated, pole and a pale, or less densely populated, pole. The germinal center is surrounded by a capsule of elongated cells, which is in turn partially invested by a crescentic cap of small lymphocytes. Germinal centers display a clear-cut morphological polarity, inasmuch as the lymphocyte cap is especially thick over the light region and becomes gradually thinner toward the darker pole. Furthermore, they show a consistent orientation with respect to the neighboring structures. In the lymph nodes, the light region and lymphocyte cap of the germinal centers are directed toward the marginal sinus; in the spleen they are directed toward the red pulp. In the digestive and respiratory passages they are oriented toward the nearest epithelial surface. When the plane of a histological section passes through a germinal center in a direction perpendicular to its axis of symmetry, the polarity just described is not seen, for the cap of small lymphocytes appears as a circular rim of uniform width surrounding the germinal center. For this reason, the cap has often been described as a mantle or corona.

In the dark region of the germinal center (Fig. 14-16), the intense staining results from the nuclei and basophilic cytoplasm of numerous closely packed elements of the lymphoid cell line—namely, lymphoblasts, large and medium-sized lymphocytes, and cells in transition to the plasma cell line. All these cells are actively proliferating and they contain antibody within the perinuclear space and occasional cisternae of the granular endoplasmic reticulum. In the dark zone, macrophages are also found consistently, loaded with debris of phagocytized lymphocytes. The free cells are contained in the meshes of a cellular framework composed of stellate elements joined by desmosomes. These cells display little cytoplasmic specialization; they are stained by silver methods and were called dendritic cells because of their numerous radiating processes. The transition between the light and the dark region at the equator of the germinal center is a gradual one; the large basophilic cells of the lymphoid line progressively give way to small lymphocytes, mitotic figures disappear, and macrophages decrease in number. The dendritic cells acquire abundant eosinophilic cytoplasm and myriad peripheral interdigitating processes.

The capsule of the germinal center consists of a few layers of flattened reticular cells joined by desmosomes. This investment is disorganized over the light pole because of the presence of many highly deformed small lymphocytes, allegedly fixed in the course of their migration toward or from the overlying small lymphocyte cap. Mature plasma cells are scarce in germinal centers except in those of the tonsils. Reticular fibers are sparse within the center, but they form a concentric envelope around its periphery.

Germinal centers are thought to pass through a sequence of developmental changes and ultimately to involute and disappear. They seem to arise from small nests of large lymphocytes or lymphoblasts, which progressively gain in size and complexity to form aggregations, up to 1 mm. in diameter. In very large germinal centers lymphocyte phagocytosis is intense; thus, they acquire a characteristic appearance with the light microscope, because the macrophages loaded with residual bodies are seen as light areas on a background of tightly packed nuclei (starry sky). The life span of germinal centers and the precise sequence of events leading to their disappearance are unknown.

Very little is understood about the function of germinal centers. They are the site of active production of lymphocytes, but a proportion of the newly formed cells die locally and are disposed of by macrophages; the fate of the survivors is unknown. On the one hand, autoradiographic studies on the tonsil after ³H-thymidine injection seem to indicate that lymphocytes arise in the germinal center,

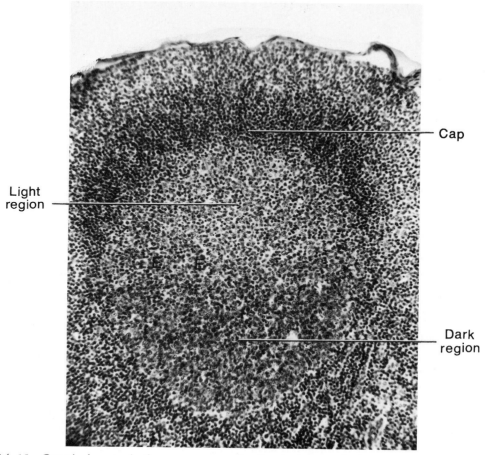

Cap

Light region

Dark region

Figure 14-15   Germinal center in the outer cortex of an inguinal node of a dog. Hematoxylin-eosin.

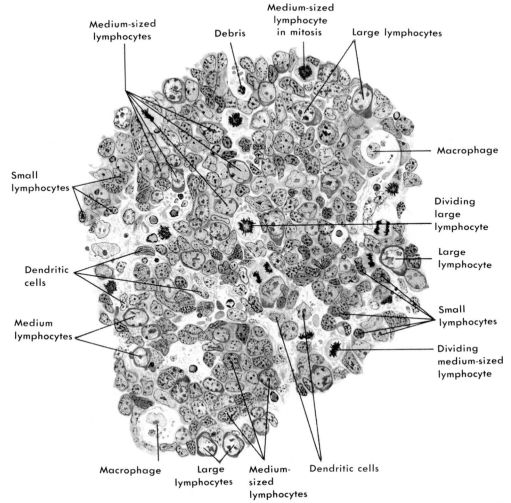

Figure 14-16 Portion of a germinal center of a human lymph node. Hematoxylin-eosin-azure II. ×750. (After A. A. Maximow.)

move outward entering the small lymphocyte cap, and finally migrate into the overlying epithelium. On the other hand, in the germinal centers of lymph nodes and spleen, no such centrifugal cell movement is observed and the small lymphocytes of the cap seem to belong to the long-lived variety.

The functional significance of the dendritic cells and their relationships with the reticular cells of the diffuse lymphoid tissue is not clear. They do not seem to be capable of phagocytosis, for which reason the term "dendritic macrophages" originally applied to these cells is no longer tenable. However, they have been shown to trap antigen in the presence of antibody and to retain the antigen-antibody complex for long periods of time. It has been suggested that the numerous peripheral processes of these cells bind the complex to their surface membrane, but inert particles, such as carbon, titanium oxide, and saccharated iron oxide are also retained.

Germinal centers also develop in rodents thymectomized at birth and in patients with congenital thymic aplasia. In birds, their appearance is prevented by bursectomy, and they are absent in humans with congenital agammaglobulinemia. Intravenously injected B lymphocytes, but not T lymphocytes, localize both in germinal centers and in their small lymphocyte cap. Thus, they are probably involved in some stage of the development or functional differentiation of B lymphocytes.

The appearance of germinal centers is closely correlated with the evolution of humoral immunological responses. They are formed *de novo* during the primary response to antigen and increase explosively in number during the secondary response, whereas they are very few in animals reared in a germ-free environment. Furthermore, their lymphoid cells synthesize antibody of the IgG variety, although they do not differentiate into plasma cells or do so only to a very limited extent. Each germinal center seems to produce monospecific antibody; thus, the suggestion has been advanced that the whole lymphoid population of an individual germinal center may represent a clone of cells, all committed in the response to a single antigen. Despite the good correlation between the appearance of germinal centers and the humoral response to antigen, germinal centers are not essential for antibody production nor for plasma cell formation. In the human fetus, there is antibody secretion before germinal centers develop; in the course of the primary response to antigen, antibody appears in the blood and plasma cells develop before antibody producing germinal centers can be demonstrated. It has been claimed, however, that during the secondary response, germinal center formation precedes the rise of circulating antibody. On the basis of this observation and experiments on antibody secretion in vitro, transfer of immune responses, and effects of drugs or x-ray irradiation, it has been speculated that germinal centers develop following repeated contact with antigens eliciting antibody secretion and that they may therefore be involved in the long-term memory of the IgG response. At the present state of our knowledge, however, it must be admitted that the precise function of the germinal center, a conspicuous and ubiquitous component of the lymphoid tissue, is still unknown.

HISTOPHYSIOLOGICAL OVERVIEW OF THE IMMUNE SYSTEM

LYMPHOCYTE CIRCULATION

The immune system consists of: (1) specific lymphoid organs, (2) masses of lymphoid tissue embedded in other organs, (3) isolated lymphoid cells infiltrating the epithelial and connective tissues of the body, and (4) lymphocytes circulating with blood and lymph. Among the organs of the immune system, the thymus and lymph nodes are composed exclusively of lymphoid tissue, whereas the spleen possesses an additional component, the red pulp, which is primarily concerned with nonimmune functions. Aggregates of lymphoid tissue and lymphoid cells can be found anywhere in the body, with the single exception of the central nervous system. A special situation is found in the bone marrow, which *in sensu stricto* does not belong to the immune system, but which represents the only source for the stem cell precursors of lymphocytes in late fetal and postnatal life. The various regions of the immune system have precise functional interrelationships and are interconnected by an orderly traffic of lymphocytes, which exploit blood and lymph as circulatory pathways. To understand these relationships, one must first recapitulate the developmental history of the lymphocyte; stem cell precursors arising from the yolk sac in the embryo and from the bone marrow in the adult migrate through the bloodstream into the thymus and the unknown mammalian analogue of the avian bursa of Fabricius Under the influence of thymus and bursa equivalent, these stem cell precursors undergo antigen-independent proliferation and differentiate into immunocompetent T and B lymphocytes, respectively. These reenter the bloodstream and populate the lymph nodes, the spleen, and the connective tissues of the body. Upon meeting their appropriate antigen, T and B lymphocytes are stimulated to transform, proliferate, and differentiate, thus giving rise to cytotoxic T lymphocytes and antibody secreting B lymphocytes and plasma cells. As a result of antigen stimulation, lymphocytes also arise which propagate the response throughout the immune system or carry memory of the primary response, and these are capable of mounting an enhanced reaction upon successive exposures to the same antigen.

An efficient immunological surveillance of the body is only possible if lymphocytes, each endowed with the property to respond to a single antigen, are able to move freely throughout the body, thus increasing the chance for them to encounter their appropriate antigen. That this is the case has been proved by a series of elegant studies which have disclosed the existence of a continuous traffic of lymphocytes between the various lymphoid organs via the blood and lymph. There are two main patterns of migration of lymphocytes through the body — slow and fast. The movement of stem cells from bone marrow to thymus and bursa and the subsequent seeding of lymphocytes to the peripheral lymphoid organs are measured in weeks, during which cells undergo sequential steps of differentiation. Superimposed upon this slow traffic is a second type of migratory phenomenon, by which long-lived small lymphocytes rapidly move from blood to peripheral lymphoid organs and tissues and back into the blood. This latter process, called *recirculation*, does not involve lymphocyte proliferation and is measured in hours. Finally, there are hints of a third pattern of cell migration, which may be especially prominent in the course of an acute immune response; effector lymphocytes and plasma cell precursors are seeded by lymph and blood throughout the immune system and connective tissues of the body, thus bringing about a propagation of the immune response. The plasma cell precursors localize in great numbers in the lamina propria of the mucosa of the gut, where they undergo differentiation into mature plasma cells; a proportion of them may be involved in synthesis and release of immunoglobulins A.

Recirculation was demonstrated by experimental drainage of lymphocytes from a chronic fistula of the thoracic duct. This lymphatic channel collects most of the lymph of the body and returns it to the bloodstream; the thoracic duct lymph contains variable numbers of cells in different mammals (2 to $30 \times 10^3/\text{mm}^3$ in man) predominantly represented by small lymphocytes (90 to 95 per cent) (Fig. 14–1*A*). The remaining cells are large lymphocytes that do not recirculate and possibly represent plasma cell precursors which are released into the blood and later selectively localize in the mucosa of the gut. The output of small lymphocytes from the thoracic duct is sufficient to replace all blood lymphocytes several times daily; thus, since the number of blood lymphocytes remains constant, they must continuously leave the blood at the same rate as they enter it through the thoracic duct.

Prolonged drainage of the thoracic duct lymph causes pronounced lymphopenia and extreme depletion of the lymphocyte population of the spleen, lymph nodes, and gut-associated lymphoid tissue. The bone marrow

is not affected; the thymus responds with a decrease in weight, but this effect seems to be nonspecific.

If thoracic duct lymphocytes are recovered, labeled radioactively in vitro, and injected intravenously into a syngeneic recipient, it can be shown that they rapidly leave the bloodstream and localize in the peripheral lymphoid organs. They do not enter either the thymus or the bone marrow. The idea therefore emerged that a pool of small lymphocytes continuously migrate from the blood into the peripheral lymphoid organs and tissues, but leave them again to reenter the blood, either directly or through the lymphatic system. This being true, it should be possible to deplete the recirculating pool by destroying lymphocytes at any point along their migratory pathway. This has been shown to be the case through local irradiation of the hilus of the spleen.

Recirculation is very rapid, as the average transit time of the small lymphocytes through the blood is 0.6 hours; transit time through the spleen is 5 to 6 hours, and through the lymph nodes 15 to 20 hours. Recirculating lymphocytes represent a substantial fraction of the body's small lymphocyte population (about half of it in rats); most, if not all, of these cells are long-lived (Fig. 14–1*B*). Since the blood contains a much higher proportion of short-lived small lymphocytes (30 to 50 per cent in rats) than the thoracic duct lymph, only part of the blood lymphocytes must belong to the recirculating pool. The origin and fate of these short-lived blood lymphocytes are poorly understood. The vast majority of the recirculating lymphocytes belongs to T variety (85 per cent in mice), the remaining being B lymphocytes. These latter seem to recirculate at a slower rate than T cells and are mobilized with difficulty by prolonged drainage of the thoracic duct lymph, possibly because they are inherently sluggish or because they are somewhat segregated from the main recirculatory pathway.

Drainage of the thoracic duct lymph causes a selective lymphocyte depletion in specific territories of the lymphoid organs and tissues: at the beginning of the experiment, lymphocytes disappear from the deep cortex of the lymph nodes, the central region of the periarterial lymphoid sheaths of the spleen, and the internodular regions of Peyer's patches. These territories are the same which appear devoid of lymphocytes in

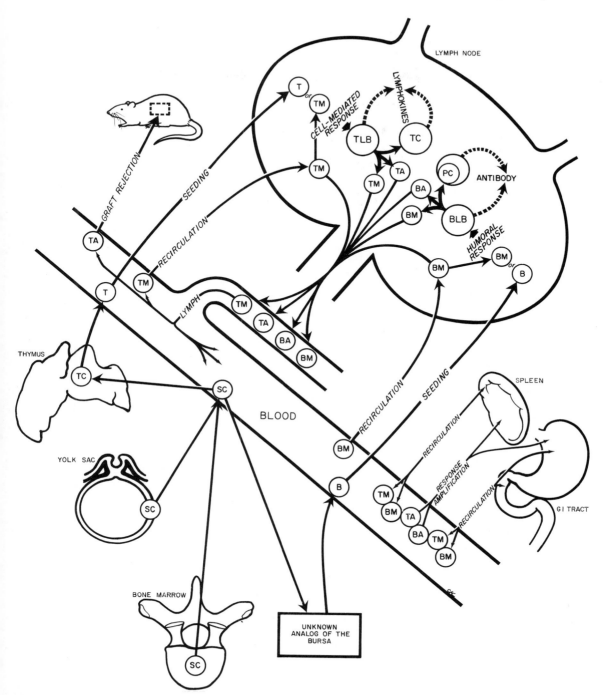

Figure 14-17   Diagram of lymphocyte circulation and differentiation. Stem cell precursors arising from the yolk sac in the embryo or the bone marrow in the adult enter the blood and migrate into the thymus and the unknown mammalian analogue of the avian bursa. Here they proliferate and differentiate into T and B lymphocytes. These enter the blood and seed the peripheral lymphoid organs (lymph nodes, spleen, gut-associated lymphoid tissue), where they undergo antigen-dependent proliferation and differentiation. SC, stem cell; TC, thymic lymphocyte; T, Thymus-dependent lymphocyte; B, bursa-dependent lymphocyte; TLB and BLB, thymus- and bursa-dependent lymphoblasts; TM and BM, thymus- and bursa-dependent memory lymphocytes; TC, cytotoxic T lymphocyte; PC, plasma cell; TA and BA, T and B effector lymphocytes, which propagate the immune response throughout the body.

neonatally thymectomized rodents and which were therefore designated *thymus-dependent*. This observation can be explained by the fact that T lymphocytes represent the main component of the recirculating pool and that they are rapidly mobilized from the peripheral lymphoid organs. More prolonged drainage of the thoracic duct lymph leads to lymphocyte depletion of the *thymus-independent* territories of the peripheral lymphoid organs: namely, the superficial cortex and medullary cords of lymph nodes and the peripheral regions of the white pulp of the spleen. This finding may reflect the late mobilization of the recirculating B lymphocytes. The recirculating T and B lymphocytes, labelled in vitro and injected into a syngeneic recipient, localize respectively in the thymus-dependent and thymus-independent (or bursa-dependent) territories of the peripheral lymphoid organs. The mechanism by which recirculating small lymphocytes leave and subsequently reenter the bloodstream in the spleen or leave the blood and enter the lymph in lymph nodes will be discussed in the chapters devoted to these organs (Chapters 16 and 17).

In normal subjects, despite the continuous exchange of lymphocytes between the various districts of the immune system, a steady state is reached which ensures a consistent proportion of T and B lymphocytes in blood, lymph, and major lymphoid organs. Thus, in the mouse, 65 to 85 per cent of the small lymphocytes of the lymph nodes and thoracic duct lymph and 30 to 50 per cent of those in the spleen belong to the T variety. In the human blood, 69 to 82 per cent of the lymphocyte population are T and the remaining 20 to 30 per cent are B lymphocytes. The significance of the recirculation of the small lymphocytes is still open to investigation, but it has been speculated that they represent, at least in part, memory cells "patrolling" the immune system, ready quickly and efficiently to set up a secondary response upon meeting their appropriate antigen.

REFERENCES

Symposia, Journals and Books

In seeking detailed information on lymphocyte physiology, the student should consult a modern textbook of immunology. Topics of current interest on the cells of the immune system are reviewed in specific journals such as *Advances in Immunology* and *Transplantation Reviews*. Additional books and symposia are listed below:

Burnet, Sir F. McF.: Cellular Immunology. Melbourne, Australia, Melbourne University Press, 1969.

Cottier, H., N. Odartchenko, R. Schindler, and C. C. Congdon (eds.): Germinal Centers in Immune Responses. New York, Springer, 1967.

Good, R. A., and D. W. Fisher (eds.): Immunobiology. Stamford, Conn., Sinauer Associates, Inc., 1971.

Lawrence, H. S., and M. Landy: Mediators of Cellular Immunity. New York, Academic Press, 1969.

Weiss, L.: The Cells and Tissues of the Immune System: Structure, Functions, Interactions. Englewood Cliffs, N.J., Prentice-Hall, 1972.

Reviews and Original Articles

Ada, G. L.: Antigen binding cells in tolerance and immunity. Transplant. Rev., 5:105, 1970.

Andersson, J., O. Sjöberg, and G. Möller: Mitogens as probes for immunocyte activation and cellular cooperation. Transplant. Rev., *11*:131, 1972.

Aoki, T., U. Hämmerling, E. de Harven, E. A. Boyse, and L. J. Old: Antigenic structure of cell surfaces: an immunoferritin study of the occurrence and topology of H-2, θ, and TL alloantigens on mouse cells. J. Exp. Med., *130*:979, 1969.

Attardi, G., M. Cohn, K. Horibata, and E. S. Lennox: Antibody formation by rabbit lymph node cells. II. Further observations on the behavior of single antibody-producing cells with respect to their synthetic capacity and morphology. J. Immunol., 92:346, 1964.

Avrameas, S., and E. H. Leduc: Detection of simultaneous antibody synthesis in plasma cells and specialized lymphocytes in rabbit lymph nodes. J. Exp. Med., *131*:1137, 1970.

Balfour, B. M., E. H. Cooper, and E. L. Alpen: Morphological and kinetic studies on antibody-producing cells in rat lymph nodes. Immunology, 8:230, 1965.

Baney, R. N., J. J. Vazquez, and F. J. Dixon: Cellular proliferation in relation to antibody synthesis. Proc. Soc. Exp. Biol. Med., 109:1, 1962.

Berenbaum, M. C.: The autoradiographic localization of intracellular antibody. Immunology, 2:71, 1959.

Björneboe, M., and H. Gormsen: Experimental studies on the role of plasma cells as antibody producers. Acta Path. Microbiol. Scand., 20:649, 1943.

Bussard, A. E., and J. L. Binet: Electron micrography of antibody-producing cells. Nature, 205:675, 1965.

Carr, I.: The fine structure of the mammalian lymphoreticular system. Int. Rev. Cytol., 27:283, 1970.

Cerottini, J. C., and K. T. Brunner: Cell-mediated cytotoxicity, allograft rejection, and tumor immunity. Adv. Immunol., 18:67, 1974.

Chang, T. S., B. Glick, and A. R. Winter: The significance of the bursa of Fabricius of chickens in antibody production. Poultry Sci., 34:1187, 1955.

Chen, L.-T., A. Eden, V. Nussenzweig, and L. Weiss: Electron microscopic study of the lymphocytes capable of binding antigen-antibody-complement complexes. Cell. Immunol., 4:279, 1972.

Clark, S. L., Jr.: The synthesis and storage of protein by isolated lymphoid cells, examined by autoradiography with the electron microscope. Am. J. Anat., 119:375, 1966.

Cohn, Z. A.: The structure and function of monocytes and macrophages. Adv. Immunol., 9:163, 1968.

Coons, A. H.: Some reactions of lymphoid tissues to stimulation by antigens. Harvey Lectures, Ser. *53*:113, 1957–58.

Coons, A. H., E. H. Leduc, and J. M. Connolly: Studies on antibody production. I. A method for the histochemical demonstration of specific antibody and its application to a study of the hyperimmune rabbit. J. Exp. Med., *102*:49, 1955.

Cooper, M. D., R. D. A. Peterson, M. A. South, and R. A. Good: The function of the thymus system and bursa system in the chicken. J. Exp. Med., *123*:75, 1966.

Craddock, C. G., R. Longmire, and R. McMillan: Lymphocytes and the immune response. New Eng. J. Med., *285*:324, 378, 1971.

de Petris, S., G. Karlsbad, and B. Pernis: Localization of antibodies in plasma cells by electron microscopy. J. Exp. Med., *117*:849, 1963.

Dougherty, T. F., J. H. Chase, and A. White: The demonstration of antibodies in lymphocytes. Proc. Soc. Exp. Biol. Med., *57*:295, 1944.

Douglas, S. D.: Human lymphocyte growth *in vitro:* morphologic, biochemical, and immunologic significance. Int. Rev. Exp. Pathol., *10*:41, 1971.

Dutton, R. W.: *In vitro* studies of immunological responses of lymphoid cells. Adv. Immunol., *6*:253, 1967.

Everett, N. B., and R. W. Tyler: Lymphopoiesis in the thymus and other tissues: functional implications. Int. Rev. Cytol., *22*:205, 1967.

Fagraeus, A.: Antibody production in relation to the development of plasma cells; *in vivo* and *in vitro* experiments. Acta Med. Scand., *130*(Suppl. 204):3, 1948.

Feldman, J. D.: Ultrastructure of immunologic processes. Adv. Immunol., *4*:175, 1964.

Fitch, F. W., D. A. Rowley, and S. Coulthard: Ultrastructure of antibody-forming cells. Nature, *207*:994, 1965.

Ford, W. L., and J. L. Gowans: The traffic of lymphocytes. Sem. Hematol., *6*:67, 1969.

Gengozian, N.: Heterotransplantation of human antibody-forming cells in diffusion chambers. Ann. N.Y. Acad. Sci., *120*:91, 1964.

Gowans, J. L.: The effect of the continuous reinfusion of lymph and lymphocytes on the output of lymphocytes from the thoracic duct of unanesthetized rats. Brit. J. Exp. Path., *38*:67, 1957.

Gowans, J. L.: The recirculation of lymphocytes from blood to lymph in the rat. J. Physiol., *146*:54, 1959.

Gowans, J. L., and E. J. Knight: The route of recirculation of lymphocytes in the rat. Proc. Roy. Soc. B, *159*:257, 1964.

Green, N. M.: Electron microscopy of the immunoglobulins. Adv. Immunol., *11*:1, 1969.

Gudat, F. G., T. N. Harris, S. Harris, and K. Hummeler: Studies on antibody-producing cells. I. Ultrastructure of 19S and 7S antibody-producing cells. J. Exp. Med., *132*:448, 1970.

Gudat, F. G., T. N. Harris, S. Harris, and K. Hummeler: Studies on antibody-producing cells. II. Appearance of ^{3}H-thymidine-labeled rosette-forming cells. J. Exp. Med., *133*:305, 1971.

Gudat, F. G., T. N. Harris, S. Harris, and K. Hummeler: Studies on antibody-producing cells. III. Identification of young plaque-forming cells by thymidine-^{3}H labeling. J. Exp. Med., *134*:1155, 1971.

Hall, J. G., B. Morris, G. D. Moreno, and M. C. Bessis: The ultrastructure and function of the cells in lymph following antigenic stimulation. J. Exp. Med., *125*:91, 1967.

Harris, S., and T. N. Harris: Influenzal antibodies in lymphocytes of rabbits following the local injection of virus. J. Immunol., *61*:193, 1949.

Harris, T. N., E. Grimm, E. Mertens, and W. E. Ehrich: The role of the lymphocyte in antibody formation. J. Exp. Med., *81*:73, 1945.

Harris, T. N., and S. Harris: The genesis of antibodies. Am. J. Med., *20*:114, 1956.

Harris, T. N., K. Hummeler, and S. Harris: Electron microscopic observations on antibody-producing lymph node cells. J. Exp. Med., *123*:161, 1966.

Holub, M.: Potentialities of the small lymphocyte as revealed by homotransplantation and autotransplantation experiments in diffusion chambers. Ann. N.Y. Acad. Sci., *99*:477, 1962.

Hummeler, K., T. N. Harris, N. Tomassini, M. Hechtel, and M. B. Farber: Electron microscopic observations on antibody-producing cells in lymph and blood. J. Exp. Med., *124*:255, 1966.

Ingraham, J., and A. Bussard: Application of localized hemolysin reaction for specific detection of individual antibody-forming cells. J. Exp. Med., *119*:667, 1964.

Jerne, N. K., and A. A. Nordin: Plaque formation in agar by single antibody-producing cells. Science, *140*:405, 1963.

Karnovsky, M. J., E. R. Unanue, and M. Leventhal: Ligand-induced movement of lymphocyte membrane macromolecules. II. Mapping of surface moieties. J. Exp. Med., *136*:907, 1972.

Katz, D. H., and B. Benacerraf: The regulatory influence of activated T cells on B cell responses to antigen. Adv. Immunol., *15*:1, 1972.

Leduc, E. H., S. Avrameas, and M. Bouteille: Ultrastructural localization of antibody in differentiating plasma cells. J. Exp. Med., *127*:109, 1968.

Leduc, E. H., A. H. Coons, and J. M. Connolly: Studies on antibody production. II. The primary and secondary responses in the popliteal lymph node of the rabbit. J. Exp. Med., *102*:61, 1955.

Lin, P. S., A. G. Cooper, and H. H. Wortis: Scanning electron microscopy of human T-cell and B-cell rosettes. New Eng. J. Med., *289*:548, 1973.

Mäkelä, O., and G. J. V. Nossal: Bacterial adherence: a method for detecting antibody production by single cells. J. Immunol., *87*:447, 1961.

McGregor, D. D., and J. L. Gowans: The antibody response of rats depleted of lymphocytes by chronic drainage from the thoracic duct. J. Exp. Med., *117*:303, 1963.

McIntyre, J. A., and C. W. Pierce: Immune responses *in vitro.* IX. Role of cell clusters. J. Immunol., *111*: 1526, 1973.

McMaster, P. D., and S. S. Hudack: The formation of agglutinins within lymph nodes. J. Exp. Med., *61*:783, 1935.

Miller, J. F. A. P., and G. F. Mitchell: Thymus and antigen-reactive cells. Transplant. Rev., *1*:3, 1969.

Millikin, P.: Anatomy of germinal centers in human lymphoid tissue. Arch. Pathol., *82*:499, 1966.

Mills, J. A., and S. R. Cooperband: Lymphocyte physiology. Ann. Rev. Med., *22*:185, 1971.

Mishell, R. I., and R. W. Dutton: Immunization of dissociated spleen cell cultures from normal mice. J. Exp. Med., *126*:423, 1967.

Moore, M. A. S., and J. J. T. Owen: Experimental studies on the development of the bursa of Fabricius. Develop. Biol., *14*:40, 1966.

Moore, M. A. S., and J. J. T. Owen: Experimental studies on the development of the thymus. J. Exp. Med., *126*:715, 1967.

Mosier, D. E., and L. W. Coppleson: A three-cell interaction required for the induction of the primary immune response *in vitro*. Proc. Nat. Acad. Sci. (U.S.A.), *61*:542, 1968.

Movat, H. Z., and N. V. P. Fernando: The fine structure of lymphoid tissue. Exp. Mol. Pathol., *3*:546, 1964.

Movat, H. Z., and N. V. P. Fernando: The fine structure of the lymphoid tissue during antibody formation. Exp. Mol. Pathol., *4*:155, 1965.

Murphy, M. J., J. B. Hay, B. Morris, and M. C. Bessis: Ultrastructural analysis of antibody synthesis in cells from lymph and lymph nodes. Am. J. Pathol., *66*:25, 1972.

Neil, A. L., and F. J. Dixon: Immunohistochemical detection of antibody in cell-transfer studies. Arch. Path., *67*:643, 1959.

Nossal, G. J. V.: Antibody production by single cells. III. The histology of antibody production. Brit. J. Exp. Path., *40*:25, 1959.

Nossal, G. J. V.: Cellular genetics of immune responses. Adv. Immunol., *2*:163, 1962.

Ortega, L. G., and R. C. Mellors: Cellular sites of formation of gamma globulin. J. Exp. Med., *106*:627, 1957.

Perkins, W. D., M. J. Karnovsky, and E. R. Unanue: An ultrastructural study of lymphocytes with surface-bound immunoglobulin. J. Exp. Med., *135*:267, 1972.

Pernis, B., L. Forni, and L. Amante: Immunoglobulin spots on the surface of rabbit lymphocytes. J. Exp. Med., *132*:1001, 1970.

Polliack, A., N. Lampen, B. D. Clarkson, and E. de Harven: Identification of human B and T lymphocytes by scanning electron microscopy. J. Exp. Med., *138*:607, 1973.

Rabellino, E., S. Colon, H. M. Grey, and E. R. Unanue: Immunoglobulins on the surface of lymphocytes. I. Distribution and quantitation. J. Exp. Med., *133*:156, 1971.

Raff, M. C.: Theta isoantigen as a marker of thymus-derived lymphocytes in mice. Nature, *224*:378, 1969.

Raff, M. C.: Two distinct populations of peripheral lymphocytes in mice distinguishable by immunofluorescence. Immunology, *19*:637, 1970.

Raff, M. C., M. Sternberg, and R. B. Taylor: Immunoglobulin determinants on the surface of mouse lymphoid cells. Nature, *255*:553, 1970.

Reiss, E., E. Mertens, and W. E. Ehrich: Agglutination of bacteria by lymphoid cells *in vitro*. Proc. Soc. Exp. Biol. Med., *74*:732, 1950.

Roelants, G.: Antigen recognition by B and T lymphocytes. Curr. Top. Microbiol. Immunol., *59*:135, 1972.

Saunders, G. C., and W. S. Hammond: Ultrastructural analysis of hemolysin-forming cell clusters. I. Preliminary observations. J. Immunol., *105*:1299, 1970.

Sordat, B., M. Sordat, M. W. Hess, R. D. Stoner, and H. Cottier: Specific antibody within lymphoid germinal center cells of mice after primary immunization with horseradish peroxidase: a light and electron microscopic study. J. Exp. Med., *131*:77, 1970.

Sprent, J.: Circulating T and B lymphocytes of the mouse. I. Migratory properties. Cell. Immunol., 7:10, 1973.

Sprent, J., and A. Basten: Circulating T and B lymphocytes of the mouse. II. Lifespan. Cell. Immunol., 7:40, 1973.

Stackpole, C. W., T. Aoki, E. A. Boyse, L. J. Old, J. Lumley-Frank, and E. de Harven: Cell surface antigens: serial sectioning of single cells as an approach to topographical analysis. Science, *172*:472, 1971.

Taylor, R. B., P. H. Duffus, M. C. Raff, and S. de Petris: Redistribution and pinocytosis of lymphocyte surface immunoglobulin molecules induced by anti-immunoglobulin antibody. Nat. New Biol., *233*:225, 1971.

Uhr, J. W.: Intracellular events underlying synthesis and secretion of immunoglobulin. Cell. Immunol., *1*:228, 1970.

Unanue, E. R.: The regulatory role of macrophages in antigenic stimulation. Adv. Immunol., *15*:95, 1972.

Unanue, E. R., W. D. Perkins, and M. J. Karnovsky: Ligand-induced movement of lymphocyte membrane macromolecules. J. Exp. Med., *136*:885, 1972.

Unanue, E. R., W. D. Perkins, and M. J. Karnovsky: Endocytosis by lymphocytes of complexes of anti-Ig with membrane-bound Ig. J. Immunol., *108*:569, 1972.

Urso, P., and T. Makinodan: The roles of cellular division and maturation in the formation of precipitating antibody. J. Immunol., *90*:897, 1963.

van Furth, R., Z. A. Cohn, J. G. Hirsch, J. H. Humphrey, W. G. Spector, and H. L. Langevoort: The mononuclear phagocyte system: a new classification of macrophages, monocytes, and their precursor cells. Bull. WHO, *46*:845, 1972.

White, R. G., A. H. Coons, and J. M. Connolly: Studies on antibody production. III. The alum granuloma. J. Exp. Med., *102*:73, 1955.

Wybran, J., and H. H. Fudenberg: Thymus-derived rosette-forming cells. New Eng. J. Med., *288*:1072, 1973.

Zagury, D., J. W. Uhr, J. D. Jamieson, and G. E. Palade: Immunoglobulin synthesis and secretion. II. Radioautographic studies of sites of addition of carbohydrate moieties and intracellular transport. J. Cell Biol., *46*:52, 1970.

Zlotnik, A., J. J. Vazquez, and F. J. Dixon: Mitotic activity of immunologically competent lymphoid cells transferred into X-irradiated recipients. Lab. Invest., *11*:493, 1962.

15
Thymus

by Elio Raviola

The thymus is a median organ situated in the superior mediastinum anterior to the great vessels as they emerge from the heart. It extends from the pericardial sac, caudally, to the root of the neck, cranially. It consists of two lobes, arising in the embryo as separate primordia on each side of the midline, but later becoming closely joined by connective tissue. The thymus attains its greatest relative weight at the end of fetal life, but its absolute weight continues to increase, reaching 30 to 40 g. at about the time of puberty. It then begins to undergo an involution which progresses rapidly until in the adult the organ becomes largely replaced by adipose cells.

The thymus is the only primary lymphoid organ thus far identified in mammals. It is the first organ to become lymphoid during embryonic life, being seeded by blood-borne stem cells from the yolk sac, which then differentiate into lymphocytes within the special environment of the thymus. Thymic lymphocytes undergo intensive, antigen-independent proliferation. For reasons that are not understood, a portion of them degenerate within the organ, while the remainder enter the bloodstream, populate the peripheral lymphoid organs and ultimately differentiate into thymus-dependent or T lymphocytes. These are capable of performing a variety of immunological functions that collectively constitute the cell-mediated immune response and also of cooperating with B lymphocytes in humoral responses. Germinal centers are lacking in the thymus and there is no antibody production. Although the majority of the thymic lymphocytes have not yet acquired immunological competence, the removal of the organ before the immune system has completed development causes a specific irretrievable impairment of the body's immunological defenses.

HISTOLOGICAL ORGANIZATION

Each thymic lobe is invested by a thin capsule of loose connective tissue and is subdivided by primary connective tissue septa that carry blood vessels into a number of parenchymal lobules which appear polyhedral in shape and are 0.5 to 2 mm. in diameter (Figs. 15–1*A* and 15–2). The thymic lobules are not, however, completely independent of one another. By serial sectioning, one can demonstrate continuity from lobule to lobule via narrow parenchymal bridges. Thus, each lobe of the thymus actually consists of a convoluted parenchymal strand with irregular expansions corresponding to the lobules.

The principal cellular constituents of the thymus are lymphocytes (thymocytes), reticular cells, and a smaller number of macrophages. At the periphery of the lobule, small lymphocytes are numerous and densely packed, whereas at the center of the lobule, lymphocytes are fewer in number and reticular cells have more abundant acidophilic cytoplasm. Thus, each lobule comprises a darkly stained, peripheral region, the *cortex*, and a lighter staining central portion, the *medulla* (Figs. 15–2 and 15–3). Secondary connective tissue septa, carrying blood vessels, extend inward from the surface of the cortex and reach as far as the corticomedullary boundary.

The thymic parenchyma consists of a tridimensional network of stellate reticular cells bounding irregular compartments filled with

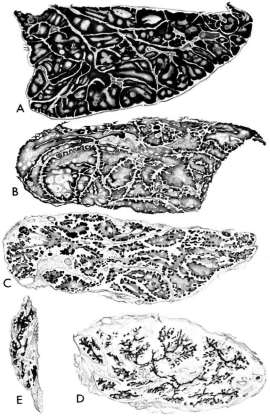

Figure 15-1 Sections of human thymuses, showing age and accidental involution. *A,* From a newborn (15 gm. gland); *B,* from a 7 year old boy (35 gm. gland); *C,* from a 17 year old boy (35.2 gm. gland), showing the beginning of age involution; *D,* from a 17 year old boy (8.8 gm. gland), high grade accidental involution, the dark parenchyma being surrounded by fat and connective tissue; *E,* from a 17 year old boy (1.65 gm. gland), extensive accidental involution. (Redrawn and slightly modified from Hammar, 1906.)

lymphocytes that are closely aggregated and in direct contact with each other, without intervening connective tissue. This compact cellular mass is comparable to an epithelium or to the brain in its paucity of intercellular substance, but small blood vessels do thread their way through it bringing a minimal amount of connective tissue in their adventitia.

The reticular cells of the thymus, like those of the lymph nodes and spleen, are stellate in shape, but their embryonal origin is endodermal instead of mesenchymal. They are rarely associated with connective tissue fibers of the reticular type. They occasionally display more obvious epithelial features in the medulla of the lobule, where they may

bound cysts or be organized into concentric arrays of squamous epithelial cells, comprising the *Hassall's bodies* or *thymic corpuscles.* The thymic reticulum is often referred to as cytoreticulum, to emphasize the cellular nature of the parenchymal framework of the thymic lobules. Thymic lymphocytes are morphologically indistinguishable from the lymphocytes of the blood, lymph, and peripheral lymphoid organs.

The thymic lobule is a highly dynamic structure. Lymphocytes are continuously produced in the cortex; some of them die and are destroyed by macrophages, others migrate toward the medulla and enter the bloodstream through the walls of the postcapillary venules.

The Cortex

The stellate reticular cells in the cortex have a scanty acidophilic cytoplasm and a large, oval nucleus, 7 to 11 μm. in diameter, which is smooth-contoured, lightly staining, and contains one or two small nucleoli. In electron micrographs (Figs. 15–4 and 15–5), the processes of the reticular cells are seen to be joined by small desmosomes. Their cytoplasm contains bundles of filaments, some of which seem to insert on the desmosomes. Their cytoplasmic organelles are unremarkable: sparse mitochondria, a few ribosomes, either free or attached to rare cisternae of the granular endoplasmic reticulum, and a small Golgi apparatus. Membrane bounded vacuoles which contain a transparent matrix and a variable amount of debris are also found. Although these are scarce in the fetal thymus and in the superficial cortex, they increase in number with age, especially in the deep cortical regions of the lobule. They are probably lysosomes, but their significance is obscure, inasmuch as reticular cells are believed to be incapable of phagocytosis and possess remarkably few plasmalemmal vesicles.

At the periphery of the cortex (Fig. 15–4) and around the blood vessels, attenuated reticular cell processes form a continuous limiting sheath that separates the thymic parenchyma from the interlobular and adventitial connective tissue. A boundary layer of amorphous material analogous to the basal lamina of epithelia intervenes between this limiting cellular sheath and the connective tissue.

The vast majority of the cell population of the cortex is made up of lymphocytes. These include large, medium-sized, and small forms. The largest lymphocytes have a round or oval nucleus, 9 μm. in diameter, rich in euchromatin, and containing one or two prominent nucleoli. The cytoplasm is relatively abundant and strongly basophilic. In electron micrographs (Fig. 15–4), the most prominent feature of the cytoplasm of large lymphocytes is the abundance of free poly-ribosomes, whereas cisternae of the granular endoplasmic reticulum are exceedingly rare. A diplosome surrounded by a small Golgi apparatus is located near a slight indentation of the nuclear envelope. Mitochondria are few and tend to be grouped near the Golgi apparatus. Multivesicular bodies, small dense granules and lipid droplets are seen only exceptionally. The small lymphocytes (Fig. 15–5) have a round, darkly staining nucleus, 4 to 5 μm. in diameter, with a small nucleolus. The rim of cytoplasm is very thin and contains a few free ribosomes, mostly dispersed as single units. The cytocentrum and associated minute Golgi apparatus slightly indent the nucleus. Mitochondria and granular endoplasmic reticulum are encountered even less often than in large lymphocytes.

Occasional multivesicular bodies, a rare lipid droplet, and small dense granules complete the list of cytoplasmic organelles. Large and small lymphocytes are at the extremes of a continuous spectrum of cells displaying intermediate gradations of nuclear and cytoplasmic organization. A consistent feature of cortical lymphocytes is their smooth surface contour, the paucity of plasmalemmal vesicles, and their polyhedral shape, due to mutual deformation.

Large lymphocytes make up only a small proportion of the lymphoid population of the lobule and tend to be concentrated at the periphery of the cortex; progressively smaller forms are found in increasing number toward the center of the lobule and the deep cortex consists chiefly of tightly packed small lymphocytes. Both dividing and degenerating lymphocytes are commonly found in the cortex. Mitoses are more frequent at the periphery of the lobule, whereas degenerating cells with pyknotic nuclei are most abundant in the deep cortical areas.

The macrophages represent a minor, but consistent component of the cell population

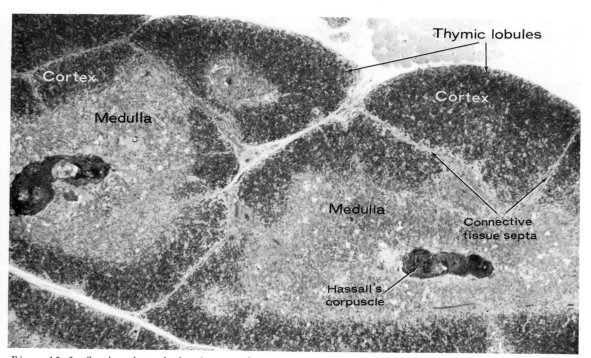

Figure 15–2 Section through the thymus of a guinea pig. The thymic lobes consist of polyhedral lobules separated from each other by connective tissue septa. Each lobule comprises a densely staining peripheral region or cortex and a lighter staining central portion, the medulla. The dark areas in the medulla are Hassall's bodies or corpuscles. Toluidine blue. ×75. (Courtesy of G. B. Schneider and S. Clark, Jr.)

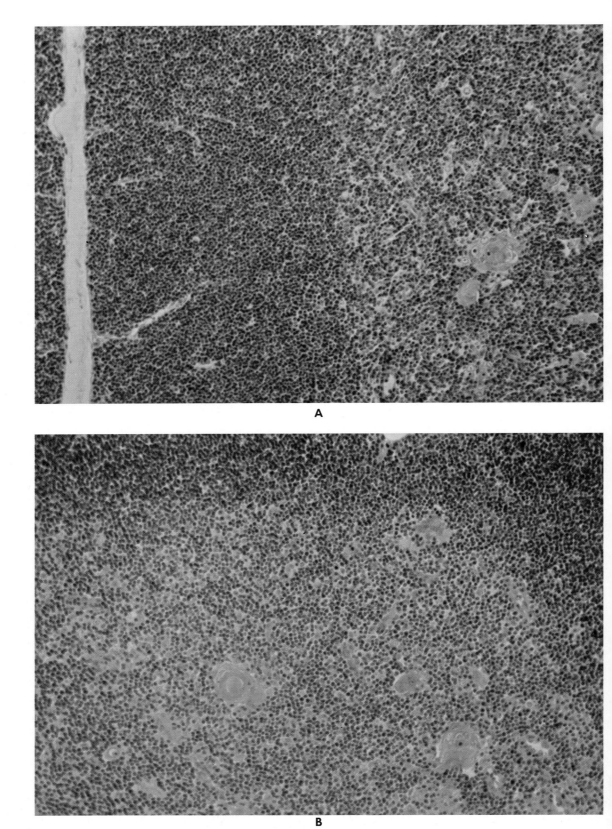

Figure 15–3 Sections through the thymus of monkey. *A,* On the left is the cortex of a lobule with densely packed lymphocytes. On the right, and in *B,* is the medulla: the lymphocytes are fewer in number and the reticular cells have more abundant acidophilic cytoplasm. The pink, homogenous areas are Hassall's bodies. Hematoxylin-eosin.

of the cortex. They are scattered throughout the cortex, and in most mammals except the mouse, they increase in number at the boundary region between the cortex and the medulla. With the light microscope, they are distinguished from reticular cells with some difficulty, but with the electron microscope, they can be easily recognized by their lack of desmosomes and the presence within the cytoplasm of phagocytized lymphocytes or the remnants of their digestion. The cells that have been described by light microscopists as containing PAS-positive inclusions are actually macrophages loaded with residual bodies.

A few plasma cells are present within the parenchyma and the interstitial connective tissue of the involuting thymus. They occur at the extreme periphery of the cortex and along the blood vessels; their significance is not known. Mast cells may also be found, but they are mainly extralobular.

The Medulla

In the medulla, the reticular cells are extremely pleiomorphic. In some areas they maintain a stellate shape and contain numerous bundles of cytoplasmic filaments (Fig. 15–6); in other areas, they are much larger, have a pale cytoplasm and myriad cytoplasmic processes. Some of them contain granules of unknown nature; others are filled with vacuoles. Some are rounded; others are flattened and wrapped around one another, giving rise to the structures known as thymic corpuscles or Hassall's bodies (Fig. 15–7). These may reach 100 μm. or more in diameter and consist of a concentric array of squamous cells joined by many desmosomes and containing keratohyalin granules and conspicuous bundles of cytoplasmic filaments. The cells in the central part of a Hassall's corpuscle may degenerate or become calcified.

Lymphocytes are much less abundant

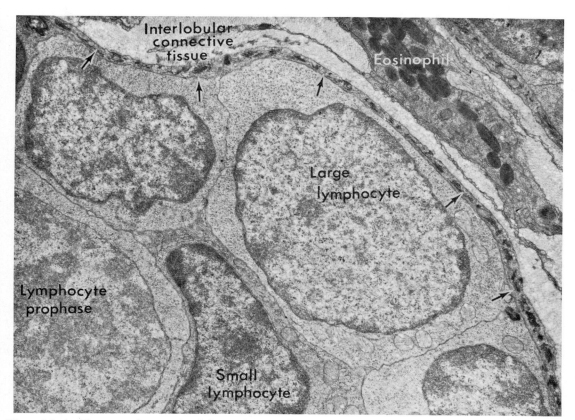

Figure 15–4 Electron micrograph of the periphery of a rat thymic lobule. Large and small lymphocytes are seen in the superficial portion of the cortex. These are separated from the connective tissue of the interlobular septum by a continuous layer of attenuated processes of the reticular cells, indicated here by the arrows. ×9600. (Courtesy of E. Raviola.)

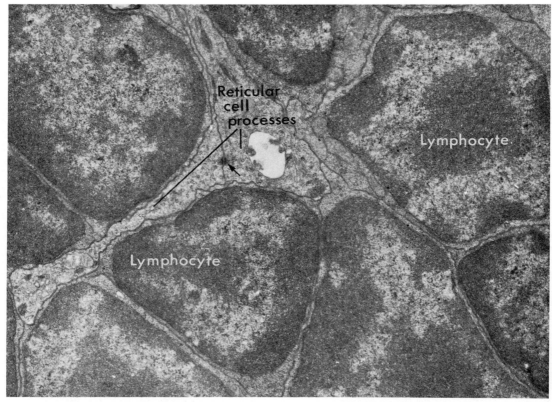

Figure 15-5 Electron micrograph from the deep cortex of a rat thymic lobule, showing among the crowded small lymphocytes two reticular cell processes joined by a desmosome (at arrow). × 14,000. (Courtesy of E. Raviola.)

than in the cortex and are predominantly of the small variety. They also differ from cortical small lymphocytes in their irregular shape and have a somewhat greater amount of cytoplasm containing relatively few ribosomes.

Macrophages are only rarely found in the medulla of the thymus. Granulocytes, especially eosinophils, may be found in small numbers. Plasma cells are absent from the medulla.

The significance of the pleiomorphism of reticular cells in the medulla is not understood. It may well represent an abnormal, local response of the thymic reticulum to the loss of surface relationships with the lymphocytes.

In the thymus of nonmammalian vertebrates, especially reptiles and birds (and also rarely in mammals), the medulla of the thymic lobules displays an extraordinary congeries of seemingly extraneous components, such as striated muscle cells (Hammar's myoid cells); cysts lined by epithelial cells provided with a brush border or with cilia; mucus secreting

cells; and reticular cells with large vacuoles lined by microvilli. It is not clear whether these unusual constituents have functional significance or are simply embryonic rests or errors of differentiation.

Germinal centers may appear in the medullary region of the lobules as a consequence of certain diseases for which an autoimmune pathogenesis has been postulated.

Vessels and Nerves

The arteries supplying the thymus arise from the internal thoracic arteries and their mediastinal and pericardiophrenic branches. They ramify in the interlobular connective tissue, and their ultimate subdivisions follow the secondary connective tissue septa, which extend inward from the surface of the lobules; thus, they penetrate the lobule at the corticomedullary boundary, without coursing through the cortex. The arterioles, following the boundary between the cortex and medulla, give off capillaries that ascend into the cortex, joined to each other by collateral anastomoses. At the periphery of the cortex, but still within the cortical parenchyma, the capillaries form a network of branching and anastomosing arcades and turn back toward the interior of the lobe. In their recurrent course through the cortex, the capillaries join to form larger vessels, which can still be classified as capillaries on the basis of their fine structure. These vessels are confluent with postcapillary venules at the corticomedullary boundary and in the medulla. As an exception to this basic pattern, capillaries may leave the periphery of the cortex and join superficial veins coursing within the interlobular connective tissue. The postcapillary venules of the corticomedullary boundary and medulla leave the thymic parenchyma via the secondary connective tissue septa and join to form interlobular veins. The majority of these are ultimately drained by a single thymic vein, a tributary of the left brachiocephalic vein.

Because of the peculiar arrangement of the parenchymal blood vessels, the various segments of the vascular tree appear to be spatially segregated within the lobules, the cortex being exclusively supplied by capillaries, and the corticomedullary boundary and the medulla also containing arterioles and venules. There is very little movement of macromolecules from blood to thymic parenchyma across the capillary walls in the cortex (Fig. 15–8), whereas the large medullary vessels are highly permeable to substances in the plasma. Thus, only the lymphoid population of the cortex is protected from the influence of circulating macromolecules. This is the structural basis for the so-called *blood-thymus barrier* to antigens.

Great numbers of lymphocytes enter the bloodstream by traversing the walls of the postcapillary venules of the corticomedullary junction and those of the medulla. Thus these vessels functionally resemble the postcapillary venules in lymph nodes, but they lack the characteristic cuboidal endothelium.

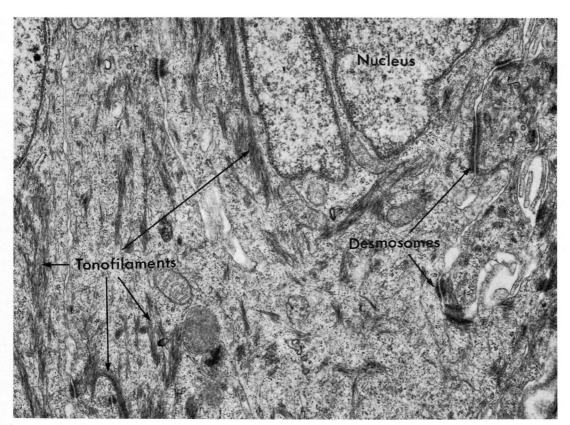

Figure 15–6 Electron micrograph from the medulla of rat thymus, showing portions of several reticular cells joined by desmosomes and containing conspicuous bundles of tonofilaments. ×11,000. (Courtesy of E. Raviola.)

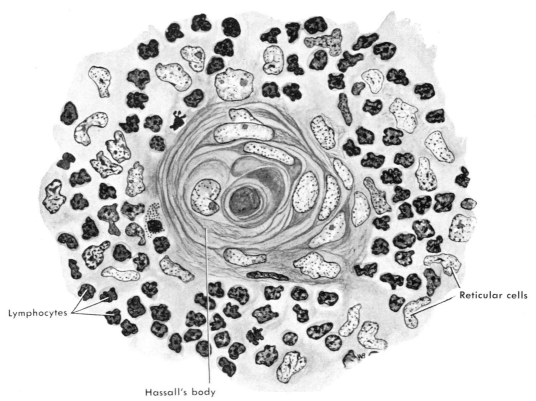

Lymphocytes

Reticular cells

Hassall's body

Figure 15–7 Hassall's body in the medulla of the thymus of an 8 year old boy. It consists of a concentric array of squamous reticular cells. Eosin-azure. ×970.

Lymphatics are found in the connective tissue septa, but they seem to be lacking within the lobular parenchyma; their lymph is drained by the sternal, tracheobronchial, and anterior mediastinal nodes.

The thymus receives branches from the vagus and sympathetic nerves. Sympathetic fibers are distributed to the blood vessels, but the manner of termination of the vagal fibers is unknown.

Histogenesis

In man, the thymus arises from an outgrowth of the endodermal lining of the third branchial pouch on each side of the midline; the fourth branchial pouch often gives rise to some thymic tissue. The primordium has a cleft-like lumen continuous with that of the embryonic pharynx and a wall composed of several layers of columnar epithelium. The lumen disappears as the endodermal bud proliferates, giving rise to solid epithelial outgrowths that invade the surrounding mesenchyme. Round, basophilic cells have been described in the mesenchyme surrounding the thymic rudiment at very early stages of development.

The two separate primordia, after considerable elongation caudally and medially, meet in the midline in embryos of about 8 weeks and acquire a common mesenchymal investment. At about the same time, lymphocytes appear within the epithelium. Lymphocytes subsequently increase in number, blood vessels penetrate the rudiment, and the parenchyma is gradually converted into a meshwork of stellate cells of endodermal origin attached by desmosomes and bounding a labyrinthine system of spaces occupied by proliferating lymphocytes. The medulla arises relatively late in the deep region of the lobules, by disappearance of many lymphocytes and an enlargement of the reticular cells.

Although some students of the histogenesis of the thymus believed that its lymphocytes arose from the epithelium of the primitive endodermal rudiment, it was widely accepted for five decades that the lymphocytes were cells of mesenchymal origin that wandered into the epithelium and proliferated there. A few years ago this view was vigorously challenged when experiments with tissue cultures and transplantation of thymic rudiments appeared to show that the thymic lymphocytes could arise from the endodermal epithelium. More recently, however, studies using both the chromosomal marker technique and antisera to surface antigens on thymic lymphocytes have clearly shown that blood-borne stem cells, originating from the yolk sac in the embryo or from the bone marrow during postnatal life, migrate into the thymic primordium and there differentiate into lymphocytes.

In man, the thymus is the first organ of the immune system in which lymphocytes appear, and it continues to be the most active lymphopoietic tissue of the body throughout embryonal life. The rate of growth of the thymus, when expressed in relation to the body weight, levels off at the beginning of the third fetal trimester; a gradual decline follows, which is already perceptible at birth, and continues thereafter. In laboratory rodents, on the other hand, the thymus continues to grow until the second week of postnatal life.

NORMAL, ACCIDENTAL, AND EXPERIMENTAL INVOLUTION

The thymus undergoes a slow physiological process of involution with age; lymphocyte production declines, the cortex becomes thinner, and the parenchyma shrinks and becomes replaced by adipose tissue, which is thought to arise from precursors in the interlobular connective tissue (Fig. 15–1*A*, *B*, and *C*). It is generally assumed that the onset of this normal process of *age involution* is coincidental with puberty, but if relative reduction of the cortical parenchyma is taken as an index of declining functional activity, age involution in humans actually begins in early childhood. In adults, the thymus is transformed into a mass of adipose tissue, containing scattered islands of parenchyma consisting mainly of enlarged reticular cells. The parenchyma, however, does not disappear completely, even in old age. Moreover, experiments involving thymectomy in adult rodents that have been deprived of their lymphoid population show that the thymus maintains its functional competence throughout life and can reacquire full lymphocytopoietic capacity. The same may be true of man, although it has not been demonstrated.

The process of gradual age involution can be complicated or accelerated by acute involutional changes constituting the so-called *accidental involution* (Fig. 15–1*D* and *E*), which occurs in response to a wide variety of stimuli, such as disease, severe stress, dietary deficiencies, ionizing radiation, injection of colloidal substances, bacterial endotoxin, adrenocorticotrophic hormone, and adrenal and gonadal steroids. Under these conditions, the thymus rapidly diminishes in size, primarily because of massive death of cortical small lymphocytes and their destruction by macrophages. Medullary lymphocytes are less sensitive, so that the usual pattern of the lobule, with a densely staining cortex and a lighter medulla, may be reversed. Acute involution in experimental animals is followed by intensive regeneration, so that the thymus rapidly returns to its former size.

HISTOPHYSIOLOGY

The thymus is essential to the development of the class of lymphocytes that is responsible for homograft rejection, for delayed cutaneous reactions to protein antigens (delayed hypersensitivity), for immune attack of a nonresponsive host (graft-versus-host reaction), and for immune response to fungi, certain microorganisms, and certain viruses. Thymus-dependent lymphocytes do not release conventional antibody, but act as helper cells in humoral responses. All of these functions depend upon a property of the lymphocytes that are circulating in the blood and lymph or residing in the spleen, lymph nodes, and connective tissues of the body. The vast majority of the lymphocytes located in the thymus are functionally inert. There is evidence that thymic lymphocytes become immunocompetent when they move into the blood or peripheral lymphoid organs, but the mechanism triggering this further differentiation is unknown. Thus, the thymic lymphocyte or thymocyte must be regarded as a type of cell functionally distinct from the

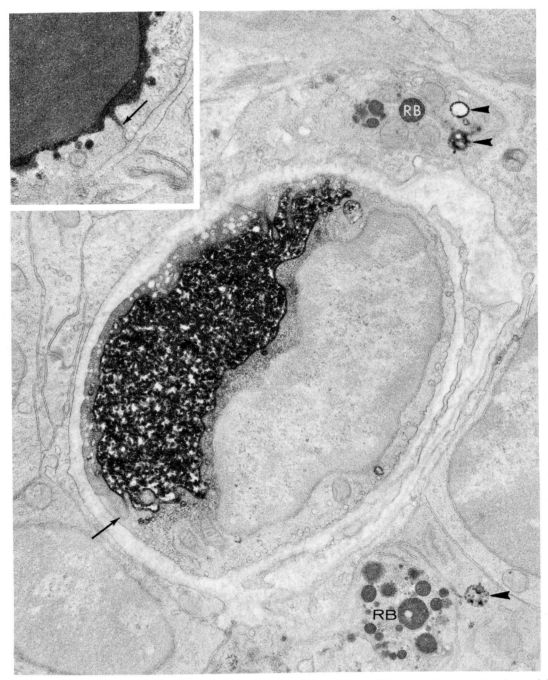

Figure 15-8 Cortical capillary in the mouse thymus. When horseradish peroxidase (molecular weight, 40,000 daltons) is injected as a tracer into the bloodstream, its progression along the intercellular clefts of the capillary endothelium is blocked by an impermeable tight junction (*arrow*). Very little tracer is transported across the endothelium by micropinocytotic vesicles, and this is readily sequestrated by perivascular macrophages (*arrowheads*). *RB,* residual bodies. ×18,500. *Inset.* In addition, a much smaller molecule, such as cytochrome *c* (molecular weight, 12,000 daltons), is arrested by the interendothelial junctions (*arrow*). ×26,500. (Courtesy of E. Raviola and M. J. Karnovsky, J. Exp. Med., *136*:466, 1972.)

peripheral thymus-dependent (T) lympho-cyte, but it may possibly be the immature precursor of the latter.

Much of the current knowledge on the functions of the thymus began with experi-ments in rodents involving thymectomy at a critical stage of the development of the im-mune system. The removal of the thymus in adult animals has but little effect on periph-eral lymphocyte populations or immune re-sponsiveness, but in newborn rodents, thy-mectomy causes lymphocytopenia, marked decrease in the population of long-lived re-circulating lymphocytes, impairment of cell-mediated immune reactions, and severe de-pression of those antibody responses requiring the cooperative participation of the thymus-dependent lymphocyte. The inner cortex of the lymph nodes and the periarterial lym-phoid sheaths in the spleen fail to develop, but plasmacytopoiesis and germinal center formation are not affected.

In neonatal rodents, the thymus has completed development, but the peripheral population of thymus-dependent lympho-cytes has not yet been established. The ap-pearance of this population is therefore pre-vented by removal of the thymus. Once the periphery has become populated with T lym-phocytes, thymectomy is no longer followed by a dramatic deficiency of cell-mediated im-mune responses, unless the peripheral stock of thymus-dependent lymphocytes is de-stroyed by sublethal, total body irradiation. In other mammals, including man, the immune system is fully mature at birth and therefore less dependent upon the integrity of the thy-mus.

In neonatally thymectomized rodents, the immunological defect can be corrected by grafting a thymus or injecting lymph node or spleen cells. Injection of thymic cell suspen-sions, on the other hand, is relatively ineffec-tive, probably because very few mature lym-phocytes are present in the thymus. Experiments in animals which were thymec-tomized, irradiated, "reconstituted" with bone marrow cells bearing a chromosomal marker, and grafted with an unmarked thymus have shown that the original lymphocyte popula-tion of the grafted thymus is replaced by a new population of cells bearing the bone mar-row karyotype; this provides further evidence that the lymphocyte population of the thymus arises from immigration and differentiation of blood-borne stem cell precursors, arising in this instance from the bone marrow.

Two possible explanations exist for the results of the reconstitution experiments: (1) The thymus may provide stem cell precursors immigrating from the embryonic yolk sac or postnatal marrow with a uniquely favorable environment for differentiation into periph-eral, thymus-dependent lymphocytes. The thymus would therefore seed the immune system with lymphocytes capable of express-ing the thymus-dependent immune func-tions. (2) Alternatively, the thymus may pro-duce one or more factors which act at the periphery on stem cell precursors, triggering their differentiation into thymus-dependent lymphocytes. Whereas little doubt exists that the thymus seeds the peripheral lymphoid organs with lymphocytes, no definitive evi-dence is available so far that thymic factors are released into the circulation and act on a peripheral target.

Once stem cells have migrated into the thymus, they differentiate into thymic lym-phocytes, possibly under local inductive influ-ences, and begin a sustained proliferation. At the peak of its activity, which corresponds to the perinatal period in laboratory rodents, the thymus has the highest rate of lymphocyte production in the whole immune system. Larger lymphocytes proliferate in the super-ficial cortex and give rise to generations of smaller cells that accumulate in the deep cor-tical areas of the lobule. This lymphocyte pro-liferation does not depend on antigen stimu-lation, in contrast with the situation in periph-eral lymphoid organs. However, the mechan-ism controlling the rate of lymphocyte pro-duction is unknown.

The intrathymic life span of the newly formed small lymphocytes has been shown to be very short (2 to 3 days). It follows that ei-ther lymphocytes die within the organ or mi-grate out of the thymus. Lymphocyte death does occur in the cortex, and these cells are disposed of by macrophages. The extent of this cell death and its physiological signifi-cance are not understood. However, evidence coming from autoradiographic and chromo-some marker labeling, from experiments in-volving thymectomy, and from lymphocyte counts in arterial and thymic venous blood shows that a proportion of the thymic lym-phocytes do migrate from the cortex to the medulla of the lobule and there enter the bloodstream through the walls of the post-capillary venules.

The lymphocytes that leave the thymus "home in" to the so-called thymus-dependent regions of the peripheral lymphoid organs, namely, the inner cortex of lymph nodes, the periarterial lymphoid sheaths of the spleen, the internodular areas of the tonsils, appendix, and Peyer's patches. All these regions represent the portal of entry of blood-borne lymphocytes into the peripheral stations of the immune system and the sites in which the thymus-dependent lymphocytes are preferentially concentrated.

Despite the essential role of the thymus in the development of cell mediated immune responses, the vast majority of the lymphocytes that populate the thymus are incapable of restoring competence to animals experimentally deprived of the thymus-dependent immune mechanisms. In suspensions of thymic cells, only a small proportion of thymic small lymphocytes seem to be capable of transformation upon interaction with phytohemagglutinin or allogeneic cells.* These lymphocytes are less sensitive to x-ray irradiation and to the cytolytic effect of adrenal steroids, and they have therefore been identified with the lymphocytes located in the medulla of the lobule. These observations seem to suggest that the small lymphocytes of the cortex of the lobule are functionally inert and acquire immunological competence as they migrate to the medulla.

Indirect evidence supporting this hypothesis comes from a growing body of animal experiments with antisera to surface antigens on the thymic or thymus-derived lymphocytes. Thymic lymphocytes possess membrane constituents, such as the *theta* and *TL antigens* in mice, which can be detected by immunological methods; their nature and significance are unknown, but they can be usefully employed as cell markers for investigating cell interactions, differentiation, and migration. These specific surface antigens appear on thymic lymphocytes as the latter differentiate from stem cell precursors, and they disappear again or become reorganized upon migration of the lymphocytes out of the thymus and their differentiation into peripheral immunocompetent T cells. From these studies, the hypothesis has emerged that the differentiation of thymic lymphocytes into peripheral, thymus-dependent lymphocytes consists of an orderly succession of maturational steps: first undifferentiated stem cell

precursors of yolk sac or bone marrow origin enter the thymus and differentiate into thymic lymphocytes. These proliferate in the cortex, then move to the medulla and acquire immunocompetence either at the very moment of leaving the organ or after they have entered the bloodstream through the wall of the postcapillary venules.

It has been claimed that immunological responsiveness can be partially restored in thymectomized animals by grafts of thymus enclosed in chambers which are permeable to molecules but not to cells. On this basis, it was postulated that the thymus induces the differentiation of stem cell precursors to immunocompetent T lymphocytes by releasing one or more factors into the bloodstream. Cell-free extracts of the organ were prepared and purified. These seemed to simulate the function of the thymus both in vivo and in vitro, and the existence of a thymic hormone or *thymosin* was postulated. However, the evidence supporting the putative endocrine function of the thymus is still controversial. The reconstitution experiments have proved difficult to repeat regularly, and criticisms were raised on the specificity of the thymic extracts. Furthermore, the various thymic factors might act within the organ as mediators of short-range cellular interactions rather than as circulating hormones.

REFERENCES

Abe, K., and T. Ito: Fine structure of small lymphocytes in the thymus of the mouse: qualitative and quantitative analysis by electron microscopy. Z. Zellforsch., *110*:321, 1970.

Bach, J. F., and M. Dardenne: Studies on thymus products. II. Demonstration and characterization of a circulating thymic hormone. Immunology, *25*:353, 1973.

Bargmann, W.: Der Thymus. *In* von Mollendorff, W., and Bargmann, W. (eds.): Handbuch der mikroskopischen Anatomie des Menschen. Berlin, Julius Springer, 1943, Vol. 6, Part 4, p. 1.

Blomgren, H., and B. Andersson: Evidence for a small pool of immunocompetent cells in the mouse thymus. Exp. Cell Res., *57*:185, 1969.

Cantor, H., M. A. Mandel, and R. Asofsky: Studies of thoracic duct lymphocytes of mice. II. A quantitative comparison of the capacity of thoracic duct lymphocytes and other lymphoid cells to induce graft-versus-host reactions. J. Immunol., *104*:409, 1970.

Claman, H. N., and F. H. Brunstetter: The response of cultured human thymus cells to phytohemagglutinin. J. Immunol., *100*:1127, 1968.

Claman, H. N., and F. H. Brunstetter: Effects of anti-lymphocyte serum and phytohemagglutinin upon cultures of human thymus and peripheral blood lymphoid cells. I. Morphologic and biochemical studies

---

*See footnote on page 441.

of thymus and blood lymphoid cells. Lab. Invest., *18*:757, 1968.

Clark, S. L., Jr.: The thymus in mice of strain 129/J studied with the electron microscope. Am. J. Anat., *112*:1, 1963.

Clark, S. L., Jr.: Incorporation of sulfate by the mouse thymus: its relation to secretion by medullary epithelial cells and to thymic lymphopoiesis. J. Exp. Med., *128*:927, 1968.

Cohen, M. W., G. J. Thorbecke, G. M. Hochwald, and E. B. Jacobson: Induction of graft-versus-host reaction in newborn mice by injection of newborn or adult homologous thymus cells. Proc. Soc. Exp. Biol. Med., *114*:242, 1963.

Colley, D. G., A. Malakian, and B. H. Waksman: Cellular differentiation in the thymus. II. Thymus-specific antigens in rat thymus and peripheral lymphoid cells. J. Immunol., *104*:585, 1970.

Colley, D. G., A. Y. Shih Wu, and B. H. Waksman: Cellular differentiation in the thymus. III. Surface properties of rat thymus and lymph node cells separated on density gradients. J. Exp. Med., *132*:1107, 1970.

Dardenne, M., and J. F. Bach: Studies on thymus products. I. Modification of rosette-forming cells by thymic extracts. Determination of the target RFC subpopulation. Immunology, *25*:343, 1973.

Davies, A. J. S., E. Leuchars, V. Wallis, R. Marchant, and E. V. Elliott: The failure of thymus-derived cells to produce antibody. Transplantation, *5*:222, 1967.

Defendi, V., and D. Metcalf (eds.): The Thymus. The Wistar Institute Symposium, Monograph No. 2, Philadelphia, The Wistar Institute Press, 1964.

Doenhoff, M. J., A. J. S. Davies, E. Leuchars, and V. Wallis: The thymus and circulating lymphocytes of mice. Proc. Roy. Soc. B, *176*:69, 1970.

Ernström, U., and B. Larsson: Thymic export of lymphocytes 3 days after labelling with tritiated thymidine. Nature, *222*:279, 1969.

Ford, W. L., and J. L. Gowans: The traffic of lymphocytes. Sem. Hematol., *6*:67, 1969.

Goldschneider, I., and D. D. McGregor: Migration of lymphocytes and thymocytes in the rat. I. The route of migration from blood to spleen and lymph nodes. J. Exp. Med., *127*:155, 1968.

Goldstein, A. L., F. D. Slater, and A. White: Preparation, assay, and partial purification of a thymic lymphocytopoietic factor (thymosin). Proc. Nat. Acad. Sci. (U.S.A.), *56*:1010, 1966.

Good, R. A., and A. E. Gabrielsen (eds.): The Thymus in Immunobiology. New York, Hoeber Medical Division, Harper and Row, 1964.

Haelst, U. van: Light and electron microscopic study of the normal and pathological thymus of the rat. I. The normal thymus. Z. Zellforsch., *77*:534, 1967.

Hoshino, T., M. Takeda, K. Abe, and T. Ito: Early development of thymic lymphocytes in mice, studied by light and electron microscopy. Anat. Rec., *164*:47, 1969.

Ishidate, M., and D. Metcalf: The pattern of lymphopoiesis in the mouse thymus after cortisone administration or adrenalectomy. Aust. J. Exp. Biol. Med. Sci., *41*:637, 1963.

Izard, J.: Ultrastructure of the thymic reticulum in guinea pig. Cytological aspects of the problem of the thymic secretion. Anat. Rec., *155*:117, 1966.

Kennedy, J. C., L. Siminovitch, J. E. Till, and E. A. McCulloch: A transplantation assay for mouse cells responsive to antigenic stimulation by sheep erythrocytes. Proc. Soc. Exp. Biol. Med., *120*:868, 1965.

Leckband, E., and E. A. Boyse: Immunocompetent cells among mouse thymocytes: a minor population. Science, *172*:1258, 1971.

Lundin, P. M., and U. Schelin: Ultrastructure of the rat thymus. Acta Path. Microbiol. Scandinav., *65*:379, 1965.

Mandel, T.: The development and structure of Hassall's corpuscles in the guinea pig. Z. Zellforsch., *89*:180, 1968.

Mandel, T.: Ultrastructure of epithelial cells in the cortex of guinea pig thymus. Z. Zellforsch., *92*:159, 1968.

Miller, H. C., S. K. Schmiege, and A. Rule: Production of functional T cells after treatment of bone marrow with thymic factor. J. Immunol., *111*:1005, 1973.

Miller, J. F. A. P., and P. Dukor: Die Biologie des Thymus nach dem heutigen Stande der Forschung. Basel, Karger, 1964.

Miller, J. F. A. P., and D. Osoba: Current concepts of the immunological function of the thymus. Physiol. Rev., *47*:437, 1967.

Mitchell, G. F., and J. F. A. P. Miller: Immunological activity of thymus and thoracic-duct lymphocytes. Proc. Nat. Acad. Sci. (U.S.A.), *59*:296, 1968.

Moore, M. A. S., and J. J. T. Owen: Experimental studies on the development of the thymus. J. Exp. Med., *126*:715, 1967.

Murray, R. G., A. Murray, and A. Pizzo: The fine structure of the thymocytes of young rats. Anat. Rec., *151*:17, 1965.

Order, S. E., and B. H. Waksman: Cellular differentiation in the thymus. Changes in size, antigenic character, and stem cell function of thymocytes during thymus repopulation following irradiation. Transplantation, *8*:783, 1969.

Owen, J. J. T., and M. C. Raff: Studies on the differentiation of thymus-derived lymphocytes. J. Exp. Med., *132*:1216, 1970.

Owen, J. J. T., and M. A. Ritter: Tissue interaction in the development of thymus lymphocytes. J. Exp. Med., *129*:431, 1969.

Parrott, D. M. V., M. A. B. de Sousa, and J. East: Thymus-dependent areas in the lymphoid organs of neonatally thymectomized mice. J. Exp. Med., *123*:191, 1966.

Raff, M. C.: Evidence for subpopulation of mature lymphocytes within mouse thymus. Nat. New Biol., *229*:182, 1971.

Raviola, E., and M. J. Karnovsky: Evidence for a blood-thymus barrier using electron-opaque tracers. J. Exp. Med., *136*:466, 1972.

Raviola, E., and G. Raviola: Striated muscle cells in the thymus of reptiles and birds: An electron microscopic study. Am. J. Anat., *121*:623, 1967.

Sainte-Marie, G., and F. S. Peng: Emigration of thymocytes from the thymus: A review and study of the problem. Rev. Canad. Biol., *30*:51, 1971.

Sanel, F. T.: Ultrastructure of differentiating cells during thymus histogenesis. Z. Zellforsch., *83*:8, 1967.

Schwarz, M. R.: Transformation of rat small lymphocytes with allogeneic lymphoid cells. Am. J. Anat., *121*:559, 1967.

Small, M., and N. Trainin: Contribution of a thymic humoral factor to the development of an immunologically competent population from cells of mouse bone marrow. J. Exp. Med., *134*:786, 1971.

Warner, N. L.: The immunological role of different lymphoid organs in the chicken. II. The immunological competence of thymic cell suspensions. Aust. J. Exp. Biol. Med. Sci., *42*:401, 1964.

Weber, W. T.: Difference between medullary and cortical

thymic lymphocytes of the pig in their response to phytohemagglutinin. J. Cell Physiol., 68:117, 1966.

Weiss, L.: The Cells and Tissues of the Immune System. Structure, Functions, Interactions. Englewood Cliffs, N.J., Prentice-Hall, Inc., 1972.

Weissman, I. L.: Thymus cell migration. J. Exp. Med., 126:291, 1967.

Williams, R. M., A. D. Chanana, E. P. Cronkite, and B. H. Waksmann: Antigenic markers on cells leaving calf thymus by way of the efferent lymph and venous blood. J. Immunol., 106:1143, 1971.

Winkelstein, A., and C. G. Craddock: Comparative response of normal human thymus and lymph node cells to phytohemagglutinin in culture. Blood, 29:594, 1967.

Wolstenholme, G. E. W., and R. Porter (eds.): The Thymus: Experimental and Clinical Studies. A Ciba Foundation Symposium. Boston, Little, Brown and Co., 1966.

16

Lymph Nodes

By Elio Raviola

Lymph nodes are small organs occurring in series along the course of lymphatic vessels. Their parenchyma consists of a highly organized accumulation of lymphoid tissue, which recognizes antigenic materials in the lymph that percolates through the node, and builds up against them a specific immune reaction. Lymph nodes are also very rich in macrophages, which clear the lymph of undesirable cells, invading microorganisms, and other particulate matter.

Large numbers of lymph nodes occur, usually in groups, scattered throughout the prevertebral region, along the large blood vessels of the thoracic and abdominal cavities, between the leaves of the mesentery, and in the loose connective tissue of the neck, axilla, and groin. They are commonly flattened and ovoid or reniform in shape, varying from 1 to 25 mm. in diameter, with a slight indentation, the *hilus,* where blood vessels enter or leave the organ. In most mammals, as *afferent lymphatic vessels* approach the node they give rise to a number of branches which enter the node at multiple sites over its convex surface (Fig. 16–2). A smaller number of *efferent lymphatic vessels* leave the node at the hilus. The afferent vessels are provided with valves that open toward the node, whereas the valves of the efferent lymphatics point away from the hilus. This arrangement of valves ensures unidirectional lymph flow through the node.

Lymph nodes vary somewhat in their structure from species to species, but their variation in appearance within species depends primarily upon their state of activity. In a healthy subject, each lymph node reflects in its organization both the background activity of the immune system as a whole and the local response of the node to small amounts of antigens reaching it from the body territory drained by its afferent lymphatics. Resting lymph nodes therefore show pronounced structural differences according to their location in the body. Extreme examples are, on the one hand, the small, poorly developed popliteal node of unstimulated laboratory rodents and, on the other hand, the highly organized human mesenteric nodes, which are continuously bombarded by a variety of antigens of intestinal origin. If, however, microorganisms or a high dose of any foreign macromolecule is injected subcutaneously, or if a foreign tissue is transplanted into the body, the lymph nodes draining the site of injection or grafting undergo profound structural changes typical of an acute primary or secondary immune response.

HISTOLOGICAL ORGANIZATION

The lymph node consists basically of a parenchymal mass of lymphoid tissue, traversed by specialized lymph vessels or *sinuses* (Figs. 16–1 and 16–2). Its collagenous framework consists of a *capsule,* which invests the whole organ, but which is greatly thickened at the hilus. From the capsule a variable number of branching connective tissue *trabeculae* extend into the substance of the node. The lymphoid parenchyma between the trabeculae is supported by a tridimensional network of reticular fibers with associated reticular cells. The meshes of this network are filled with lymphocytes, plasma

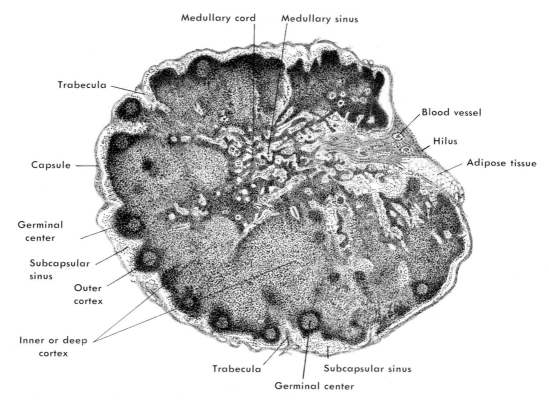

Medullary cord   Medullary sinus

Trabecula

Blood vessel

Hilus

Capsule

Adipose tissue

Germinal center

Subcapsular sinus

Outer cortex

Inner or deep cortex

Trabecula   Subcapsular sinus

Germinal center

Figure 16–1   Section through small jugular lymph node of man. × 18. (Redrawn and slightly modified from Sobotta.)

cells, and macrophages. The lymph sinuses are irregular channels transformed into a labyrinth of intercommunicating chambers by a loose network of tissue strands that traverse their lumen.

Under low magnification, the sectioned lymph node is seen to have an outer, densely staining *cortex* and an inner, paler *medulla.* The difference in appearance of these two regions is due mainly to differences in number, diameter, and arrangement of the lymph sinuses. The relative amounts of cortical and medullary substance and their distribution vary within wide limits. The nodes of the abdominal cavity are especially rich in medullary substance. The cortical substance in some nodes may surround the medulla completely but in others, the medullary substance may border directly on the capsule for long distances. In some cases the medulla and cortex may accumulate at opposite poles of the node. In the pig, the "cortical" substance is collected in the central portion of the node, while "medullary" tissue may occupy only small portions of the periphery. In the

ox, the cortex is extensively compartmentalized by numerous trabeculae, whereas in man trabeculae are poorly developed and the cortex appears as a diffuse, continuous mass. The trabeculae are prominent in large lymph nodes, but in small nodes they are thin and frequently interrupted. Nodes deep in the body, as in the abdominal cavity, are distinguished by the relatively poor development of their trabeculae compared with that of the more peripheral nodes. In some cases, a hilus may be absent; in others, it is highly developed, with its connective tissue penetrating far into the node and partitioning it extensively.

Lymph Sinuses

The afferent lymphatic vessels approach the convex surface of the node, pierce its capsule obliquely and open into the *marginal* or *subcapsular sinus* (Figs. 16–3 and 16–4). This is not a cylindrical channel, but a bowl-shaped cavity, which separates the capsule from the cortical parenchyma. It is traversed

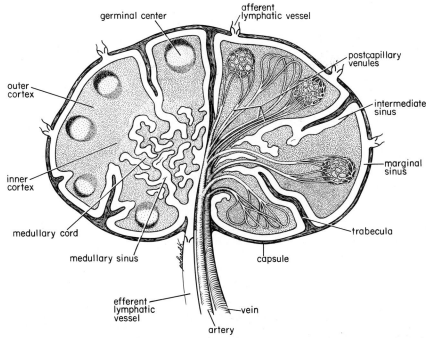

germinal center

afferent lymphatic vessel

postcapillary venules

outer cortex

intermediate sinus

inner cortex

marginal sinus

medullary cord

trabecula

medullary sinus

capsule

efferent lymphatic vessel

vein

artery

Figure 16-2 Diagram of lymph node. Blood supply is depicted on the right side.

by the collagenous trabeculae and communicates at the hilus with the lumen of the efferent lymph vessels. Arising from the marginal sinus are radially directed lymph channels called the *intermediate* or *cortical sinuses*, which penetrate the cortical parenchyma, usually following along the collagenous trabeculae. The compact appearance of the cortex is primarily due to the relatively small number and narrow lumen of the intermediate sinuses. These continue into the medulla as *medullary sinuses* — large, tortuous, irregular channels, that branch and anastomose repeatedly, thus fragmenting the lymphoid parenchyma into a number of *medullary cords* (Figs. 16–3 and 16–5). The sinuses of the medullary substance are confluent with the marginal sinus at the hilus and form there a plexus of tortuous vessels, which penetrate the thickened capsule of this region and continue into the efferent lymphatics.

Seen with the scanning electron microscope (Fig. 16–6), the sinuses appear as tunnels lined by a layer of attenuated cells, but their lumens are bridged by a meshwork of stellate cells, which are connected to each other and to the opposite walls of the sinus

via slender cell processes. Projecting from the sinus walls and luminal network of stellate elements are rounded macrophages, hirsute with myriad surface protrusions. Also present are smaller cells, probably lymphocytes. The framework of the sinus walls is a layer of reticular fibers, continuous with the parenchymal reticulum. These fibers directly underlie the sinus lining cells without any intervening basal lamina. The intraluminal network of cell processes is also supported by a skeleton of reticular fibers anchored to the reticulum of the sinus walls and suspended from the collagenous framework of the capsule and the trabeculae. The fibers traversing the sinuses are not directly exposed to the lymph, but are completely invested by the luminal stellate cells, often lying embedded in deep invaginations of the cell surface.

There is no doubt that the wall of the sinuses is freely permeable to the constituents of the lymph and is continually crossed by wandering cells, which move freely between lymph and lymphoid parenchyma. However, the nature and physiological properties of the cells lining the walls of the sinuses and those traversing their lumens have long been subjects of controversy and are far from being settled satisfactorily. Traditionally, these cells were identified with the "reticular cells" of the lymphoid parenchyma and were thought to be capable of phagocytosis. At present, however, there are indications that there are two distinct categories of lining cells: macrophages and flattened or stellate endothelial cells. These latter have an inconspicuous complement of cell organelles. They are connected to each other by specialized junctions and they take up only small amounts of particulate matter by endocytosis, like the endothelium of blood vessels generally. The precise structural relationships between these two categories of cells are not known, but may be similar to those recently reported for the lining of the sinusoids of the liver. The source of the macrophages is still unknown. Nor is it clear whether they are permanently associated with the endothelium (fixed macrophages), having migrated from the parenchyma into the sinuses, or are lymph-borne elements that secondarily took up residence in the sinus walls and acquired phagocytic properties. Evidence is also lacking as to whether the endothelial cells synthesize the collagen of the reticular framework of the lymph sinuses.

The relative proportions of macrophages and endothelial cells seem to vary in different regions of the node. The capsular wall of the marginal sinus and the wall of the intermediate sinuses adjacent to the collagenous trabeculae are composed exclusively of flattened endothelial cells, whose outlines are easily stained by treatment with silver nitrate. On the other hand, macrophages are especially numerous in medullary sinuses, and there the outlines of endothelial

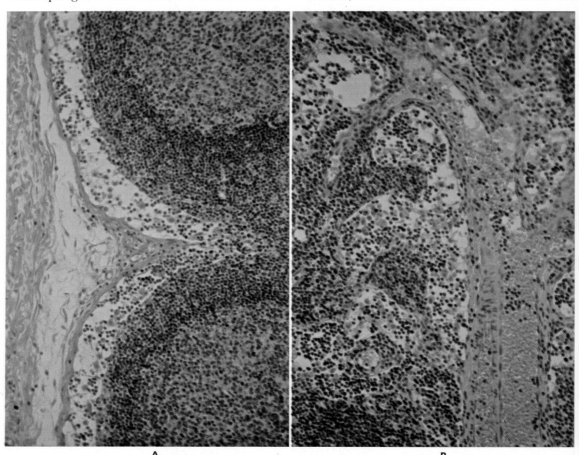

Figure 16–3   A, Capsule, marginal sinus and part of two germinal centers in a mesenteric lymph node of a dog. *B,* Medullary sinuses and cords from a mesenteric lymph node of a dog. A trabecula is seen on the right carrying an artery and a vein; the vein receives tributaries from neighboring medullary cords. Hematoxylin-eosin.

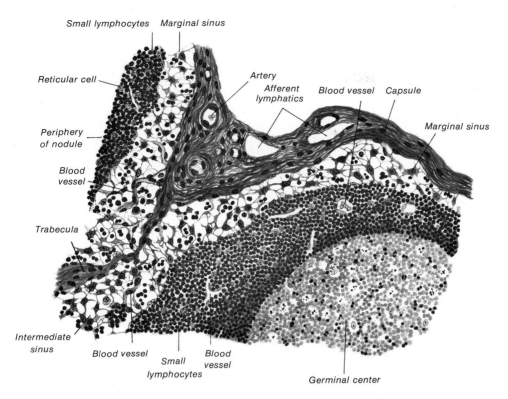

Small lymphocytes   Marginal sinus

Reticular cell

Artery
Afferent
lymphatics   Blood vessel   Capsule

Periphery
of nodule

Marginal sinus

Blood
vessel

Trabecula

Intermediate
sinus   Blood vessel   Small
lymphocytes   Blood
vessel

Germinal center

Figure 16–4   Diagram of the marginal sinus in a lymph node of a dog. Hematoxylin-eosin-azure II. × 187. (After A. A. Maximow.)

cells usually cannot be demonstrated by silver nitrate.

The organization of the lymph sinuses is well suited to the filtering function of the lymph node. The lymph entering the organ through the afferent vessels floods the marginal sinus and slowly percolates through the intermediate and medullary sinuses, freely exchanging with the lymphoid parenchyma substances in solution, particulate matter, and cells. The system of sinuses functions as a "trap" or "settling chamber," with the intraluminal tissue strands acting as a multitude of microscopic baffles which increase the surface exposed to the lymph, generate turbulence, and facilitate the monitoring function of the macrophages deployed along the sinus walls.

Cortex

The cortical parenchyma appears with the light microscope as a dense mass of lym-

phoid cells, traversed in places by the collagenous trabeculae and intermediate sinuses. It has been customary to classify certain regional differentiations in the cortical parenchyma as *primary lymphoid nodules, secondary nodules,* and *diffuse lymphoid tissue.* Secondary nodule is a term which has been used to describe either the *germinal centers* proper or the germinal centers together with their cap of small lymphocytes. Primary nodules and germinal centers are usually located at the periphery of the node and together comprise the *outer cortex,* whereas the *inner* or *deep cortex* (also called the paracortical area) consists of diffuse lymphoid tissue (Fig. 16–7).* No clear-cut boundary exists between outer and deep

---

*Tertiary nodule is a term which has been variously employed to indicate the germinal centers located deep in the cortex, the deep cortex itself, or the pseudo-follicles of Ehrich (large aggregates of small lymphocytes of unknown significance located in the deep cortex).

cortex, and the latter continues without demarcation into the medullary cords. Furthermore, the relative proportions of the two zones are quite variable in different lymph nodes and in various functional states. This rather arbitrary and artificial subdivision does, however, have considerable physiological importance, because only the deep cortex is populated by lymphocytes of the recirculating pool and it contains postcapillary venules with cuboidal endothelium, which represent the portal of entry of blood-borne lymphocytes into the node.

Primary nodules are not clearly defined morphological entities. In man and laboratory rodents, they consist merely of the lymphoid tissue intervening between the germinal centers of the outer cortex. Only in species such as the ox, whose lymph nodes possess a well developed system of trabeculae and intermediate sinuses, does the parenchyma of the outer cortex appear subdivided into discrete, rounded aggregates, projecting slightly at the surface of the organ. The stroma of the primary nodules consists of a rather loose network of reticular fibers and associated reticular cells. The labyrinthine interstices of this reticulum are occupied by small lymphocytes. Both large lymphocytes and macrophages are rare; mature plasma cells are usually lacking. On the basis of electron micrographs, the reticular cells have been described as having a pale nucleus and numerous cytoplasmic

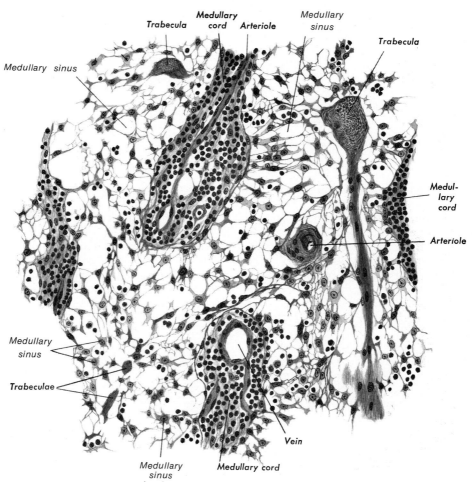

Figure 16–5 Diagram of a medulla in a lymph node of a dog. Hematoxylin-eosin-azure II. × 187. (After A. A. Maximow.)

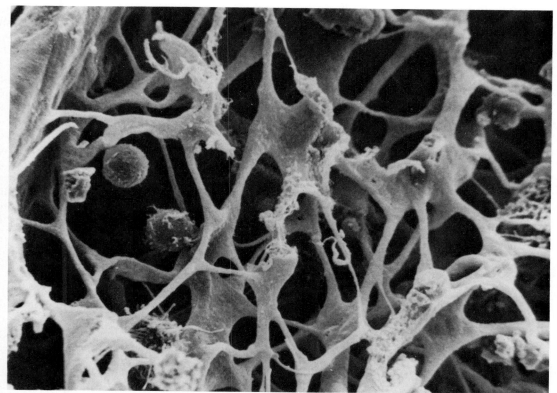

Figure 16-6 Scanning electron micrograph of the lumen of a sinus in a mesenteric lymph node of a dog. The spider web of luminal stellate cells acts as a multitude of microscopic baffles which generate turbulence in the lymph and facilitate the monitoring function of the macrophages deployed along the sinus walls. On the left, two rounded cells, probably lymphocytes, were trapped in the lumen of the sinus. × 2000. (Courtesy of T. Fujita et al., Z. Zellforsch., *133*:147, 1972.)

processes. In some places, they are wrapped around the reticular fibers and, like fibroblasts, they may display a prominent granular endoplasmic reticulum. In other locations, they have a rather sparse complement of cytoplasmic organelles, but they are joined to each other by desmosomes and show myriad peripheral processes that interdigitate with processes of neighboring lymphocytes and reticular cells. Thus, they resemble the dendritic cells of the germinal centers (see page 448). It is not known whether dendritic cells and the fibroblast-like elements represent two different classes of cells or are merely different functional states of a single cell type.

Germinal centers occur in variable numbers in the outer cortex, are less commonly found deeper in the cortex, and are only exceptionally present in the medullary cords. Those located at the lymph node periphery are polarized in such a way that their light regions, invested by the small lymphocyte cap, point toward the marginal sinus which receives the incoming lymph (Fig. 16-8). In the lymph nodes of the pig, these relationships are reversed, with the germinal centers pointing toward the central sinus, which in this species receives the incoming lymph. In germinal centers situated deep in the cortex, the orientation of the light pole and lymphocytic cap is either random or toward a neighboring intermediate sinus. The structure of germinal centers conforms to the general description provided on page 448.

In the deep cortex, cells are more loosely packed than in the outer cortex. Small lymphocytes predominate, while large lymphocytes, macrophages, and plasma cells are found only occasionally. Dendritic cells are lacking. Reticular fibers are more abundant than in the outer cortex and increase additionally in number at the junction of the cortex with the medulla.

Medulla

The medullary cords consist of aggregations of lymphoid tissue organized around small blood vessels. The cords branch and anastomose freely with one another, and near the hilus they terminate blindly or, more frequently, they form loops that continue into other cords. The medullary cords are not very prominent in resting lymph nodes. They consist of a rich network of reticular fibers and reticular cells, enclosing small lymphocytes, mature plasma cells, and macrophages. Dendritic cells are lacking.

The lymph node parenchyma contains variable, but usually small numbers of granulocytes and erythrocytes. The number of these cellular elements may, however, be greatly increased upon stimulation or in pathological states.

Capsule and Trabeculae

The capsule of the lymph node consists of dense collagenous fibers with a few fibro-blasts and, especially on its inner surface, networks of thin elastic fibers. A few smooth muscle cells are also found in the capsule around the points of entry and exit of the afferent and efferent lymph vessels. The outer aspect of the capsule blends into the fat or loose connective tissue surrounding the lymph node, whereas its inner aspect is more sharply defined and is lined by the endothelium of the marginal sinus, except where it gives rise to the cortical trabeculae. The trabeculae do not represent complete septa, but cylindrical or flattened beams of dense connective tissue; they traverse the node completely ensheathed by the intermediate and medullary lymph sinuses, and, near the hilus, they carry the major blood vessels.

Blood Vessels and Nerves

Almost all the blood vessels destined for the lymph node enter the organ through the hilus, with only occasional small ones entering through the rest of the capsule (Fig. 16–2). The larger arterial branches initially run

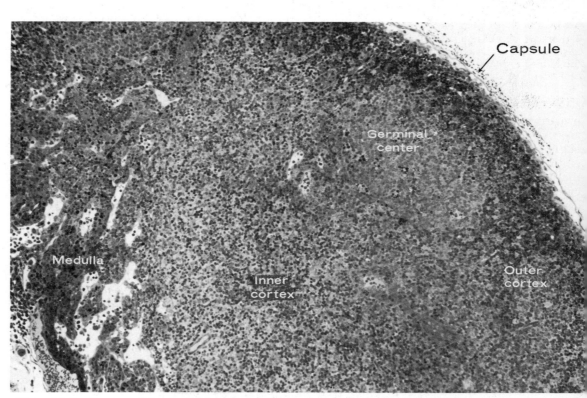

Figure 16–7 Portion of the auricular lymph node of a mouse. Notice the considerable thickness of the inner cortex. Toluidine blue. × 140. (Courtesy of G. B. Schneider.)

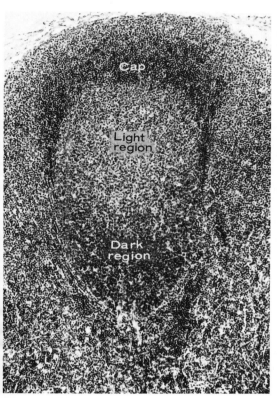

Figure 16–8 Germinal center in the outer cortex of a mesenteric lymph node of a dog. Hematoxylin-eosin.

lymph node parenchyma either by perforating the endothelial cells or by insinuating themselves into the interendothelial clefts. Similar vessels occur in certain segments of the vascular tree of the tonsils, Peyer's patches, and appendix. The exact significance of the cuboidal endothelium is obscure, but it has been suggested that the compliant endothelial cells adapt their surface contours to the shape of the wandering lymphocytes, thus limiting the plasma loss which might otherwise be associated with cell migration. Circulating lymphocytes seem to be capable of specifically recognizing this segment of the vascular tree as the portal of entry into the lymph node parenchyma. The mechanism of this remarkable phenomenon is unknown, but it may imply some sort of specific surface interaction between lymphocytes and cuboidal endothelial cells. Experiments involving enzymatic digestion suggest that carbo-

within the trabeculae, but they soon enter the medullary cords and supply their capillary networks. Passing along the cords, the arteries reach the cortex, where they distribute to capillary plexuses of the diffuse cortical parenchyma and around the germinal centers. Special *postcapillary venules* with cuboidal endothelium arise from these peripheral capillary plexuses and course radially through the deep cortex to enter the medullary cords. Here they give rise to small veins lined with normal endothelium. These in turn are tributaries of the larger venous channels that accompany the major arterial trunks in the interior of the collagenous trabeculae.

The postcapillary venules of the deep cortex are of special interest (Figs. 16–9 and 16–10). They have tall endothelial cells and no muscular coat, and their wall is traversed by great numbers of blood-borne small lymphocytes, which migrate into the

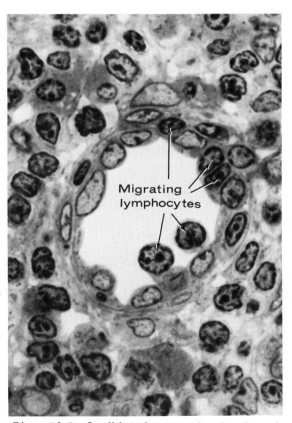

Figure 16–9 Small lymphocytes migrating through the endothelium of a postcapillary venule in the popliteal lymph node of a rabbit. Toluidine blue. (Courtesy of C. Compton.)

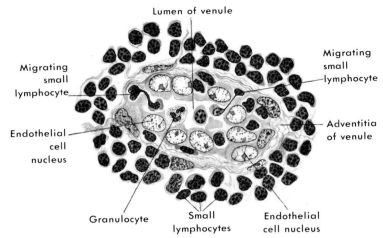

Figure 16–10 Diagram of lymphocyte migration through the walls of the postcapillary venules. (After A. A. Maximow.)

hydrate moieties of membrane glycoproteins are the essential component of the recognition sites on the surface of the lymphocytes. On the other hand, immunoglobulins have been demonstrated at the surface of the endothelial cells, and these might also be the basis for selective capture of circulating lymphocytes.

Nerves enter the hilus of the node with the blood vessels, forming perivascular plexuses. In the trabeculae and medullary cords, nerve fibers are observed which are independent of the vessels, but in the cortex all nerves are probably of vasomotor type.

Histogenesis

There is no unanimity on the mode of development of lymph nodes or the source of their lymphocytes. The earliest or primary nodes seem to develop by transformation of embryonic lymphatic sacs, which are subdivided into networks of lymphatic vessels by invasion of the surrounding mesenchyme. Bars or partitions are thus generated, which originally consist of mesenchymal cells. Inasmuch as the lymphatic sacs are at first the centers of outgrowth of the lymphatic vessels in a particular region of the body, all the lymph collected from that region is ultimately carried back into the corresponding group of deep primary nodes. The deep jugular nodes and the retroperitoneal nodes are examples of primary nodes. The second-

ary nodes, such as the popliteal, the inguinal and the like, appear late in embryonic development along the course of lymphatic vessels, presumably developing by a similar mechanism. Many smaller nodes are apparently formed after birth.

According to a different interpretation, nodes arise as a result of joining of lymphatic vessels into a network or plexus; mesenchyme is thus trapped within the primordium. Another contention has been that the lymphatic sinuses arise as irregular, anastomosing spaces, lined from the beginning by flattened mesenchymal cells, and that only secondarily do they become confluent with the endothelium-lined afferent and efferent vessels.

The newly formed lymph node is the primordium common to the lymphoid tissue of the cortex and medulla. The medullary substance arises first and the true cortical substance appears much later, when the medullary cords at the periphery of the node gradually develop club-shaped thickenings that bulge into the marginal sinus.

The source of the lymphocytes that populate the lymph node anlage is unknown. Local origin from mesenchymal cells and emigration from the bloodstream have both been suggested. There is no doubt, however, that later on in fetal development a large proportion of lymph node lymphocytes are thymic in origin. The germinal centers of the cortex usually appear after birth, concurrently with antigenic stimulation.

HISTOPHYSIOLOGY OF LYMPH NODES

The delicate walls of the lymphatic capillaries are easily penetrated by macromolecules, particulate matter, and wandering cells of the connective tissue. Thus, there is essentially no barrier to prevent entry into the lymph of endogenous or exogenous immunogenic substances. Furthermore, bacterial cells may cross the epidermis or the epithelium of the mucous membranes lining the body cavities. Escaping destruction by local or blood-borne phagocytes, they may proliferate and release toxins. Both microorganisms and their toxins easily gain access to the lymph. Lymph nodes intercalated along the path of lymph drainage prevent entry into the bloodstream of potentially harmful macromolecules, particulate matter, and bacteria carried by the lymph and exert immunological surveillance on their antigenic determinants.

The filtering capacity of the lymph nodes, recognized long ago by Virchow and substantiated by experiments involving perfusion with particulate matter and bacterial cells, is based on both mechanical and biological mechanisms. The labyrinthine configuration of the sinuses favors arrest of the particles suspended in the lymph and the macrophages of the sinus walls remove them by phagocytosis (Fig. 16–11). Lymph nodes, however, represent a much less efficient barrier for lymph-borne cells and may even facilitate dissemination of certain viruses. Erythrocytes injected into the afferent lymphatic vessels are effectively retained by the node, although the filtering efficiency decreases when very large numbers of red blood cells are infused. On the other hand, lymph nodes retain only a small proportion of lymph-borne cancer cells. Viruses which are capable of proliferating in the lymph node cells are quickly disseminated throughout the body, possibly carried by the recirculating lymphocytes.

The function of the lymph nodes in the immunological defenses of the body is a property of their lymphocyte and plasma cell

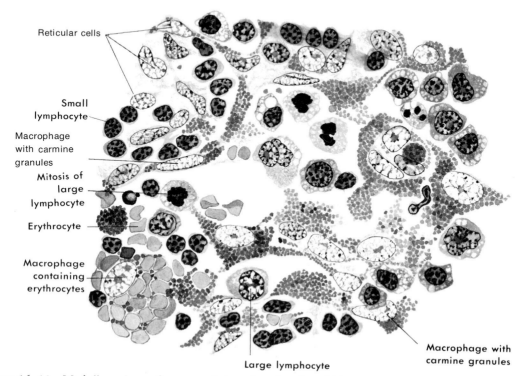

Reticular cells

Small lymphocyte

Macrophage with carmine granules

Mitosis of large lymphocyte

Erythrocyte

Macrophage containing erythrocytes

Large lymphocyte

Macrophage with carmine granules

Figure 16–11 Medullary sinus of mesenteric lymph node of a rabbit which had repeated intravenous injections of lithium carmine. Hematoxylin-eosin-azure II stain. × 950. (After A. A. Maximow.)

populations, assisted by the macrophages in both the preliminary phase of antigen recognition and the terminal phase of antigen disposal. To initiate a primary immune response, uncommitted T and B lymphocytes must be present in the resting lymph node, whereas memory cells are required for a secondary response. Upon interaction with antigens which elicit a humoral response, lymphocytes are activated and undergo antigen-dependent proliferation and differentiation. As a consequence, plasma cells appear in the node and antibody is synthesized and released into the efferent lymph, together with lymphoid cells that propagate the response throughout the body. In cell-mediated immune responses, lymphocyte activation and differentiation lead to the development and systemic dissemination of cytotoxic lymphocytes. Although these events are known to occur in the lymph node, the precise location of the relevant cell populations within the organ and the ultrastructural details of their antigen-dependent differentiation are poorly understood.

In resting peripheral lymph nodes, such as the popliteal node of the sheep which has been studied in some detail, the afferent lymph contains very few cells. Among these are lymphocytes, macrophages and occasional granulocytes. The efferent lymph contains 20 to 75 times more cells than the afferent lymph, and these are predominantly small lymphocytes (98 per cent). Only a very small fraction of the small lymphocytes emerging with the efferent lymph actually arise from division of precursors in the node, the vast majority (95 per cent) being derived from the bloodstream. These lymphocytes belong to the recirculating pool and enter the node through the cuboidal endothelium of the postcapillary venules in the deep cortex. Blood-borne small lymphocytes are selectively trapped by these vessels, whereas granulocytes and monocytes are specifically excluded. Most of the recirculating lymphocytes are thymus-dependent and, upon entering the node, they localize in the deep cortex. Shortly thereafter, they migrate into the sinus lymph and leave the organ through the efferent lymphatic vessels. The fate of the small component of the recirculating pool that consists of B lymphocytes is poorly understood. B cells recirculate at a slower rate than T cells, either because they are inherently sluggish or because they are somehow separated from the main recirculatory pathway. Thoracic duct cells of animals congenitally or experimentally deprived of T lymphocytes "home in" to the outer cortex and medullary cords, but the majority of the lymphocyte population of these two regions seem to lack the mobility typical of the elements located in the deep cortex.

Lymph nodes are also likely to be seeded with cells that have just emerged from the thymus or the bone marrow. Neonatal thymectomy is followed by a deficit of small lymphocytes in the deep cortex of lymph nodes, whereas outer cortex and medullary cords are unaffected; furthermore, experiments involving careful infusion of radioactive label into the thymus show that thymic lymphocytes specifically "home in" to the deep cortex. Lymphocytes of bone marrow origin also appear to migrate continuously into the resting lymph node; they do not seem to localize in specific regions of the organ, but instead become distributed throughout cortex and medulla. It is still a matter of conjecture whether or not this direct inflow of lymphocytes from thymus and bone marrow endows the lymph node with a complement of newly formed, uncommitted elements, capable of reacting to antigens never experienced previously by the immune system. Also unknown is the life span of these cells and their contribution to the recirculating pool.

Observations on the effects of thymectomy and the selective "homing" of both thymic and thoracic duct lymphocytes have given rise to the concept that the parenchyma of the lymph nodes consists of a thymus-dependent area, the deep cortex, and a bursa-dependent area, which includes the medullary cords and the outer cortex with its germinal centers. This postulated compartmentalization of the lymph node is easily understood in view of the facts that the deep cortex is the major traffic area of the lymph node and that the vast majority of the recirculating lymphocytes are thymus-dependent. Less compelling evidence exists for the bone marrow ancestry of the lymphocytes of the outer cortex and medullary cords, regions which seem to be inhabited by a population of lymphocytes which are either sessile or sluggishly migratory, and whose functional properties are still poorly understood.

The lymphopoietic activity of a quiescent lymph node seems to be slight; in fact, 75 per cent of the lymphocytes of the mesenteric nodes of the rat belong to the long-lived variety. The only sites of sustained lymphocyte proliferation in the lymph nodes are the germinal centers, but the fate of the lymphocytes produced by these enigmatic structures is still not known. Of the remaining cellular elements of the resting node, the plasma cells located in the medulla are sessile, effete elements, which either arose locally as a consequence of a previous antigenic stimulation or differentiated from ancestors seeded throughout the body from a distant focus of immune activity. The macrophages of the lymph node parenchyma are probably of monocytic origin, although definitive evidence on this point has not yet been obtained. In contrast to the ideas prevailing in the past, autoradiographic studies show that the turnover of the reticular cells is extremely slow and not influenced by experimental procedures which deplete the lymphocyte population of the node. Thus, the claim that they represent primitive precursors of lymphocytes, plasma cells, or macrophages is devoid of experimental foundation. Detailed and systematic studies on the ultrastructure and functional properties of the reticular cells are still lacking. They probably are not a homogeneous class of cells but may include the fibroblasts responsible for the synthesis of the reticular fibers, the dendritic cells of the lymphoid nodules, and the fixed macrophages of the node. The dendritic cells seem to have the property of retaining for long periods of time soluble antigen and antibody in the labyrinth of clefts bounded by their interdigitating processes, but they retain inert particulate matter as well.

After administration of an antigen that elicits antibody production, the primary response of the lymph node draining the site of injection is characterized, during the first day, by an increase in number of granulocytes in both the parenchyma and lymph sinuses. Simultaneously, large and medium-sized basophilic mononuclear cells appear in the deep cortex. The antigen can be demonstrated in phagocytic vacuoles of the macrophages lining the sinuses of the medulla and is retained in the intercellular clefts of the outer cortex. On days 2 and 3, granulocytes usually disappear and the large basophilic or pyroninophilic cells proliferate and greatly increase in number. The lymph node enlarges, and the deep cortex seems to spread, invading the whole organ. Preexisting germinal centers usually disappear and the medul-

lary cords are greatly reduced in length or are no longer evident. With the electron microscope, the newly formed population of basophilic cells appears to include lymphoblasts and transitional forms between the lymphocytic and plasmocytic lines. The lymphoblasts have a pale nucleus, a prominent nucleolus, and a profusion of cytoplasmic polyribosomes. Cisternae of the granular endoplasmic reticulum are only exceptionally found in these cells, and mitochondria are few, whereas the Golgi apparatus is well developed but lacking the dense granules typical of this organelle in cells of the plasmocytic series. The transitional cells display increasing amounts of granular endoplasmic reticulum, suggestive of a differentiation into immature plasma cells. Both the lymphoblasts and the transitional elements have been shown to produce antibody.

Later on, immature members of the plasma cell family become more and more numerous, with their eccentric nucleus, condensed chromatin and large amounts of granular endoplasmic reticulum. Antibody is actively synthesized at this stage and appears in both efferent lymph and blood. Furthermore, well circumscribed nests of small to large lymphocytes appear near the surface of the node. These probably represent early developmental stages of new germinal centers.

Toward the end of the first week after the injection, the lymph node begins to reacquire its normal architecture. Numerous, newly formed germinal centers have appeared in the cortex; medullary cords are prominent again near the hilus and contain abundant immature and mature plasma cells.

During the second week after antigenic challenge, plasma cells begin to decrease in number and become exclusively confined to the medullary cords. Antigen is still present in the node, confined both to the residual bodies of medullary macrophages and to the intercellular clefts between the dendritic cells of the germinal centers.

These events in the lymph node are accompanied by characteristic changes in the efferent lymph. After antigen administration, lymphocyte recirculation is temporarily arrested and the output of cells from the node decreases. Later on, cell release by the node doubles and the newly emerging population contains a large proportion (20 to 40 per cent) of large lymphocytes, with euchromatic nucleus, prominent nucleoli, and abundant cytoplasm very rich in polyribosomes. These cells have only a few elements of the granular endoplasmic reticulum even though they are actively producing antibody; they are motile and capable of incorporating DNA precursors into their chromatin. The remaining cells leaving the stimulated node include antibody producing small lymphocytes and immature elements of the plasma cell line. The antibody producing cells of the efferent lymph are thought to colonize successive lymph nodes along the chain and, by entering the bloodstream through the thoracic duct, may propagate the immune response throughout the body. In fact, if the efferent lymphatic vessel of a locally stimulated node is cannulated and its lymph drained off, antibody fails to appear in the blood and the dissemination of the immune response is prevented. If the cells leaving a stimulated node are recovered from the efferent lymph, labeled radioactively in vitro and reinfused into an afferent lymphatic of a quiescent node, they localize in the medullary cords, proliferate and finally differentiate into mature plasma cells. Antibody producing cells have also been demonstrated in the thoracic duct lymph. The fate of these cells has been studied after in vitro labeling and intravenous injection into a syngeneic animal (see footnote on page 441). They are retained transiently in the lung, liver, and spleen, but later they localize in the spleen, lymph nodes, gut-associated lymphoid structures and especially in the lamina propria of the small intestine.

The antibody producing cells appearing in the thoracic duct lymph after local stimulation of a lymph node seem to undergo further modulation as they enter the bloodstream. Here, they appear as small elements with a central nucleus, an inconspicuous nucleolus, and a narrow rim of cytoplasm, filled by parallel arrays of cisternae of the granular endoplasmic reticulum. With the light microscope, these cells would be hard to distinguish from small lymphocytes.

During the secondary response, the lymph node undergoes changes that resemble those following the first exposure to antigen, but they occur earlier and are much more pronounced.

When a lymph node is involved in a cell-mediated immune response, it undergoes morphological changes that are not strikingly different from those typical of a humoral response. A reason for this similarity is that antibody production is consistently superimposed on the cell-mediated events. If skin is grafted from a donor onto an allogeneic recipient (allograft or homograft) or if delayed hypersensitivity is induced by application of a chemical sensitizing agent to the skin, the draining node enlarges markedly and the deep cortex becomes very thick. Lymphoblasts with pale nucleus, prominent nucleoli, and abundant basophilic cytoplasm (large pyroninophilic cells) appear in the deep cortex. With the electron microscope, they display abundant cytoplasmic polyribosomes, minimal amounts of granular endoplasmic reticulum, a small Golgi apparatus, and a few mitochondria. These are actively dividing cells, and their number in the deep cortex increases rapidly, reaching a maximum toward the end of the first week. At the beginning of the second week, the number of lymphoblasts declines rapidly and a second phase in the response becomes apparent: newly formed germinal centers appear in the outer cortex and immature and mature plasma cells become localized in the medullary cords. At the same time, humoral antibody is detected in the blood.

With a slight time lag with respect to the appearance of the lymphoblasts in the deep cortex of the draining node, lymphocytes and macrophages begin to infiltrate the graft or the sensitized skin region. The peripheral response reaches its peak and the graft is rejected when the number of lymphoblasts has already begun to decline in the draining node, but before antibody is produced in significant amounts.

The mechanism of the cell-mediated response is poorly understood. Antigens from the homograft or the site of application of the sensitizing agent may reach the regional lymph node through the afferent lymph. Small lymphocytes in the deep cortex may react with the antigens and differentiate into proliferating lymphoblasts; these in turn again produce lymphocytes of decreasing size, which emigrate from the regional node, circulate in the blood, and are disseminated throughout the immune system. They invade the graft and destroy it or cause the skin lesion typical of a delayed hypersensitivity reaction (contact dermatitis or erythematous papule). The antibody response which accompanies the cell-mediated immune reaction seems to contribute but little to the rejection process, at least in laboratory rodents.

Neonatal thymectomy prevents the appearance of the lymphoblasts in the deep cortex in response to homologous transplantation and prolongs the survival of the graft, but it does not suppress germinal center and plasma cell formation. Normal reactivity is restored if thymectomized animals are restored to normal with a thymus graft. Thus, the lymphoblasts appearing in the deep cortex are likely to be thymus-dependent.

Hemal Nodes

Even in normal lymph nodes, varying numbers of erythrocytes are found. These have either entered the lymph from the afferent vessels or come from the blood vessels of the node. Some of them pass with the lymph into the efferent vessels, but most of them are engulfed by macrophages. Some nodes, however, called *hemal nodes*, are characterized by the exceptionally high content of erythrocytes. They are most numerous and best defined in the ruminants (sheep); they probably do not occur in man. They vary from minute bodies scarcely noticeable to the size of a pea or larger, and are scattered along large blood vessels from the neck to the pelvic inlet. They are also found near the kidneys and spleen, where they are believed by some to be accessory spleens. Each hemal node is covered by a dense capsule loosely connected to the surrounding tissue. At the hilus a small artery and a large vein enter and leave. The nodes are devoid of afferent lymphatics and have postcapillary venules with walls infiltrated by migrating lymphocytes. In the pig, a special type of hemal node has characteristics intermediate between the ordinary lymph node and the typical hemal node. It has blood vessels as well as lymphatic vessels, and the contents of both types of vessels mix in the sinuses. The functions of the hemal nodes are probably comparable to those of the spleen.

REFERENCES

Ada, G. L., G. J. V. Nossal, and J. Pye: Antigens in immunity. III. Distribution of iodinated antigens following injection into rats via the hind footpads. Aust. J. Exp. Biol. Med. Sci., 42:295, 1964.

Borum, K., and M. H. Claesson: Histology of the induction phase of the primary immune response in lymph nodes of germfree mice. Acta Path. Microbiol. Scand. [A], 79:561, 1971.

Brahim, F., and D. G. Osmond: The migration of lymphocytes from bone marrow to popliteal lymph nodes demonstrated by selective bone marrow labeling with ³H-thymidine *in vivo*. Anat. Rec., 175:737, 1973.

Caffery, R. W., N. B. Everett, and W. O. Rieke: Radioautographic studies of reticular and blast cells in the hemopoietic tissues of the rat. Anat. Rec., 155:41, 1966.

Carr, I.: The fine structure of the mammalian lymphoreticular system. Int. Rev. Cytol., 27:283, 1970.

Claësson, M. H., O. Jørgensen, and C. Röpke: Light and electron microscopic studies of the paracortical postcapillary high-endothelial venules. Z. Zellforsch., 119:195, 1971.

Clark, S. L., Jr.: The reticulum of lymph nodes in mice studied with the electron microscope. Am. J. Anat., 110:217, 1962.

Cohen, S., P. Vassalli, B. Benacerraf, and R. T. McCluskey: The distribution of antigenic and nonantigenic compounds within draining lymph nodes. Lab. Invest., 15:1143, 1966.

Conway, E. A.: Cyclic changes in lymphatic nodules. Anat. Rec., 69:487, 1937.

Dougherty, T. F., M. L. Berliner, G. L. Schneebell, and D. L. Berliner: Hormonal control of lymphatic structure and function. *In* Bierman, H. R., (ed.): Leukopoiesis in Health and Disease. Ann. N. Y. Acad. Sci., 113:511, 1964.

Downey, H.: The structure and origin of the lymph sinuses of mammalian lymph nodes and their relations to endothelium and reticulum. Haematologica, 3:431, 1922.

Downey, H. (ed.): Handbook of Hematology. New York, Paul B. Hoeber, Inc., 1938.

Drinker, C. K., M. E. Field, and H. K. Ward: The filtering capacity of lymph nodes. J. Exp. Med., 59:393, 1934.

Fisher, B., and E. R. Fisher: Barrier function of lymph node to tumor cells and erythrocytes. I. Normal nodes. Cancer, 20:1907, 1967.

Ford, W. L., and J. L. Gowans: The traffic of lymphocytes. Sem. Hematol., 6:67, 1969.

Fujita, T., M. Miyoshi, and T. Murakami: Scanning electron microscope observation of the dog mesenteric lymph node. Z. Zellforsch., 133:147, 1972.

Goldschneider, I., and D. D. McGregor: Migration of lymphocytes and thymocytes in the rat. I. The route of migration from blood to spleen and lymph nodes. J. Exp. Med., 127:155, 1968.

Gowans, J. L., and E. J. Knight: The route of recirculation of lymphocytes in the rat. Proc. Roy. Soc. B, 159:257, 1964.

Hall, J. G., and B. Morris: The output of cells in lymph from the popliteal node of sheep. Quart. J. Exp. Physiol., 47:360, 1962.

Hall, J. G., and B. Morris: The lymph-borne cells of the immune response. Quart. J. Exp. Physiol., 48:235, 1963.

Hall, J. G., B. Morris, G. D. Moreno, and M. C. Bessis: The ultrastructure and function of the cells in lymph following antigenic stimulation. J. Exp. Med., 125:91, 1967.

Han, S. S.: The ultrastructure of the mesenteric lymph node of the rat. Am. J. Anat., 109:183, 1961.

Harris, T. N., K. Hummeler, and S. Harris: Electron microscopic observations on antibody-producing lymph node cells. J. Exp. Med., 123:161, 1966.

Hay, J. B., M. J. Murphy, B. Morris, and M. C. Bessis: Quantitative studies on the proliferation and differentiation of antibody-forming cells in lymph. Am. J. Pathol., 66:1, 1972.

Hostetler, J. R., and G. A. Ackerman: Lymphopoiesis and lymph node histogenesis in the embryonic and neonatal rabbit. Am. J. Anat., 124:57, 1969.

Hummeler, K., T. N. Harris, N. Tomassini, M. Hechtel, and M. B. Farber: Electron microscopic observations on antibody-producing cells in lymph and blood. J. Exp. Med., 124:255, 1966.

Leduc, E. H., A. H. Coons, and J. M. Connolly: Studies on antibody production. II. The primary and secondary responses in the popliteal lymph node of the rabbit. J. Exp. Med., 102:61, 1955.

Marchesi, V. T., and J. L. Gowans: The migration of lymphocytes through the endothelium of venules in lymph nodes: an electron microscope study. Proc. Roy. Soc. B, 159:283, 1964.

Mikata, A., and R. Niki: Permeability of postcapillary venules of the lymph node. An electron microscopic study. Exp. Mol. Pathol., 14:289, 1971.

Miller, J. J., and G. J. V. Nossal: Antigens in immunity. VI. The phagocytic reticulum of lymph node follicles. J. Exp. Med., 120:1075, 1964.

Millikin, P. D.: Anatomy of germinal centers in human lymphoid tissue. Arch. Pathol., 82:499, 1966.

Moe, R. E.: Fine structure of the reticulum and sinuses of lymph nodes. Am. J. Anat., 112:311, 1963.

Moe, R. E.: Electron microscopic appearance of the parenchyma of lymph nodes. Am. J. Anat., 114:341, 1964.

Mori, Y., and K. Lennert: Electron Microscopic Atlas of Lymph Node Cytology and Pathology. Berlin, Springer Verlag, 1969.

Movat, H. Z., and N. V. P. Fernando: The fine structure of lymphoid tissue. Exp. Mol. Pathol., 3:546, 1964.

Movat, H. Z. and N. V. P. Fernando: The fine structure of the lymphoid tissue during antibody formation. Exp. Mol. Pathol., 4:155, 1965.

Murphy, M. J., J. B. Hay, B. Morris, and M. C. Bessis: Ultrastructural analysis of antibody synthesis in cells from lymph and lymph nodes. Am. J. Anat., 66:25, 1972.

Nopajaroonsri, C., S. C. Luk, and G. T. Simon: Ultrastructure of the normal lymph node. Am. J. Pathol., 65:1, 1971.

Nopajaroonsri, C., and G. T. Simon: Phagocytosis of colloidal carbon in a lymph node. Am. J. Pathol., 65:25, 1971.

Nossal, G. J. V., A. Abbot, and J. Mitchell: Antigens in immunity. XIV. Electron microscopic radioautographic studies of antigen capture in the lymph node medulla. J. Exp. Med., 127:263, 1968.

Nossal, G. J. V., A. Abbot, J. Mitchell, and Z. Lummus: Antigens in immunity. XV. Ultrastructural features of antigen capture in primary and secondary lymphoid follicles. J. Exp. Med., 127:277, 1968.

Nossal, G. J. V., G. L. Ada, and C. M. Austin: Antigens in immunity. IV. Cellular localization of ^{125}I- and ^{131}I-labelled flagella in lymph nodes. Aust. J. Exp. Biol. Med. Sci., 42:311, 1964.

Nossal, G. J. V., G. L. Ada, C. M. Austin, and J. Pye: Antigens in immunity. VIII. Localization of ^{125}I-labelled antigens in the secondary response. Immunology, 9:349, 1965.

Parrott, D. M. V., M. A. B. de Sousa, and J. East: Thymus-dependent areas in the lymphoid organs of neonatally thymectomized mice. J. Exp. Med., 123:191, 1966.

Röpke, C., O. Jørgensen, and M. H. Claësson: Histochemical studies of high-endothelial venules of lymph nodes and Peyer's patches in the mouse. Z. Zellforsch., 131:287, 1972.

Sainte-Marie, G., and Y. M. Sin: Structures of the lymph node and their possible function during the immune response. Rev. Can. Biol., 27:191, 1968.

Schoefl, G. I.: The migration of lymphocytes across the vascular endothelium in lymphoid tissues. A reexamination. J. Exp. Med., 136:568, 1972.

Sordat, B., M. W. Hess, and H. Cottier: IgG immunoglobulin in the wall of post-capillary venules: possible relationship to lymphocyte recirculation. Immunology, 20:115, 1971.

Sorenson, G. D.: An electron microscopic study of popliteal lymph nodes from rabbits. Am. J. Anat., 107:73, 1960.

Straus, W.: Localization of the antigen in popliteal lymph nodes of rabbits during the formation of antibodies to horseradish peroxidase. J. Histochem. Cytochem., 18:131, 1970.

Sprent, J.: Circulating T and B lymphocytes of the mouse. I. Migratory properties. Cell. Immunol., 7:10, 1973.

Weiss, L.: The Cells and Tissues of the Immune System. Structure, Functions, Interactions. Englewood Cliffs, N.J., Prentice-Hall, Inc., 1972.

Yoffey, J. M., and F. C. Courtice: Lymphatics, Lymph and Lymphoid Tissue. Cambridge, Harvard University Press, 1956.

Zimmermann, A. A.: Origin and development of the lymphatic system in the opossum. Illinois Medical and Dental Monographs, Vol. 3, Nos. 1 and 2, 1940.

17

Spleen

By Elio Raviola

The spleen is an abdominal organ situated in the left hypochondrium beneath the diaphragm; largely invested by visceral peritoneum, it is connected to the stomach, diaphragm, and left kidney by peritoneal folds, called gastrolienal, phrenicolienal, and lienorenal ligaments. The lienorenal ligament carries the splenic blood vessels, lymphatics, and nerves. The spleen is a complex filter interposed in the bloodstream. It is concerned with clearing the blood of particulate matter and effete cells, and with immune defense against blood-borne antigens. In many vertebrates, but not in man, the spleen is also involved in formation of erythrocytes, granulocytes, and platelets, and in certain mammals it acts as a reservoir for mature erythrocytes that can be added to the circulation in response to unusual demands. The spleen contains a large amount of lymphoid tissue and possesses a peculiar type of blood vessel that allows the circulating blood to come into contact with great numbers of macrophages.

HISTOLOGICAL ORGANIZATION

On the freshly sectioned surface of the spleen, elongate or rounded gray areas, 0.2 to 0.7 mm. in diameter are visible with the naked eye (Fig. 17–1). Together these compose the *white pulp*; they are scattered throughout a soft, dark red mass, the *red pulp*, which can easily be scraped from the cut surface of the organ. The white areas, often called *Malpighian bodies*, consist of diffuse and nodular lymphoid tissue. The red pulp consists of irregularly shaped blood vessels of large caliber (the *venous sinuses*) and the tissue

occupying the spaces between them (the *splenic cords of Billroth*). The color of the red pulp is due to the abundance of the erythrocytes which fill the lumen of the sinuses and infiltrate the splenic cords.

The spleen, much like the lymph nodes, has a collagenous *capsule* with inward extensions called *trabeculae* (Fig. 17–1). This capsule is continuous with a delicate reticular framework that occupies the rest of the interior of the organ and holds in its meshes the lymphocytes and other free cells of the splenic tissue. The *capsule* is thickened at the hilus of the organ, where it is attached to the peritoneal ligaments and where arteries and nerves enter and veins and lymphatic vessels leave the viscus.

The structure of the spleen and the relationships between the red and white pulp depend on the distribution of the blood vessels. They differ markedly in different animal species and change in the course of immune responses or disturbances of blood cell formation and destruction. Animal species with a large blood volume (horse, ruminants, carnivores) have scanty white pulp and a robust connective tissue and muscular framework. Species with a relatively small blood volume (man, rabbit, laboratory rodents) have abundant white pulp, a less prominent connective tissue framework, and poorly developed smooth musculature. In the splenic parenchyma, the white pulp is organized around the arteries and the red pulp fills the interstices among the venous sinuses.

White Pulp

The white pulp forms periarterial lymphoid *sheaths* (PALS) about the arteries

487

where these leave the trabeculae to penetrate the parenchyma (Figs. 17–1 and 17–6). The periarterial lymphoid sheaths follow peripherally along the vessels almost to the point where they break up into capillaries. In many places along their course the sheaths contain germinal centers. Although both the periarterial lymphoid sheaths and the germinal centers consist of lymphoid tissue, they differ in their physiological significance; the former, in fact, consist predominantly of lymphocytes belonging to the recirculating pool, whereas the germinal centers are bursa-dependent structures, whose function is still poorly understood.

The periarterial lymphoid sheaths display an organization similar to the deep cortex of the lymph nodes. They have a loose, irregular framework of reticular fibers with associated reticular cells. At the periphery of the sheath, the reticular fibers become circumferentially arranged, and flattened reticular cells form concentric layers that delimit the lymphoid tissue from the surrounding red pulp. Near the central artery, a few elastic fibers are interspersed among the reticular fibers. The meshes of the reticular framework are occupied by lymphocytes, predominantly belonging to the small and medium-sized variety. Plasma cells and macrophages

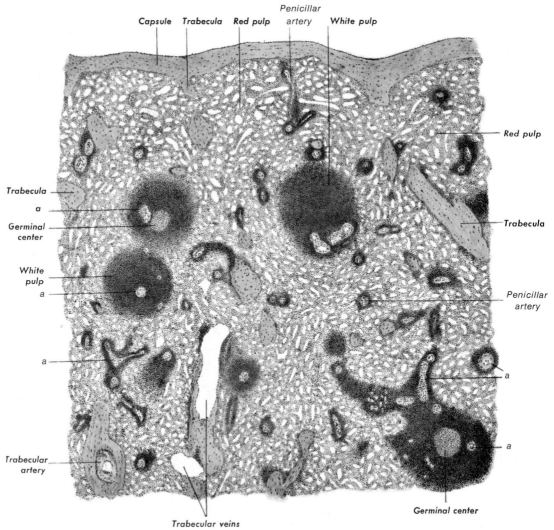

Figure 17–1   Section of human spleen. *a*, central arteries of the white pulp. × 32. (After A. A. Maximow.)

A

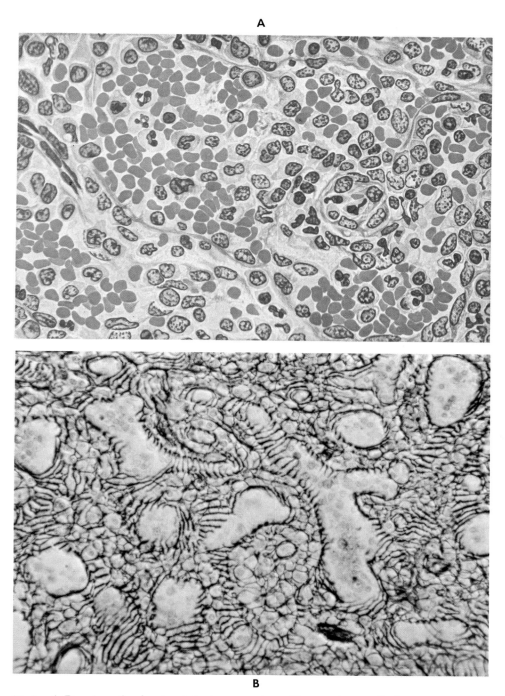

B

Figure 17-2   *A*, Drawing of red pulp of the human spleen. Venous sinuses filled with erythrocytes are separated from each other by the pulp cords. Hematoxylin-eosin. × 600. (After W. Bloom.) *B*, Photomicrograph of a silver impregnation of the reticular fibers of the spleen. The regularly spaced, circumferential ribs encircling the sinus endothelium are readily distinguished from the randomly distributed reticular fibers of the surrounding splenic cords. (Preparation by K. Richardson.)

are only occasionally found but increase in number toward the periphery of the sheath. Erythrocytes are rare, but they may occur at the boundary between white and red pulp. In the course of immune responses to blood-borne antigens, great numbers of large lymphocytes, lymphoblasts, and immature plasma cells appear in the periarterial lymphoid sheaths and soon become concentrated at their periphery.

The germinal centers display the usual architecture (see page 448); they are eccentrically situated within the sheath and, when fully developed, their light region and cap of small lymphocytes are directed toward the red pulp. Their number varies in different animal species and tends to decrease progressively with age.

Red Pulp

The red pulp consists of a network of branching and anastomosing, tortuous sinuses, separated from each other by highly cellular partitions, the splenic or pulp cords (Figs. 17–2 and 17–3). The venous sinuses are discussed with the blood vessels of the spleen. The splenic cords vary in thickness but typically form a spongy cellular mass supported by a framework of reticular fibers (Fig. 17–2). The collagenous fibers of the trabeculae continue directly into the reticular fibers of the red pulp. As elsewhere in the body, the reticular fibers as seen with the electron microscope consist of collagen fibrils embedded in a finely filamentous matrix. They are completely invested by stellate reticular cells (Fig. 17–4), which resemble fibroblasts in their complement of cytoplasmic organelles except for an uncommon abundance of filaments in their peripheral cytoplasm. Some of the reticular cells, as seen with the light microscope, may actually represent fixed macrophages of monocytic origin. The reticular fibers of the red pulp merge with ribs of basal lamina-like material that support the sinus endothelium. Their investing reticular cells are in turn anchored to the sinus walls through footlike processes, which are directed perpendicularly to the long axis of the sinuses.

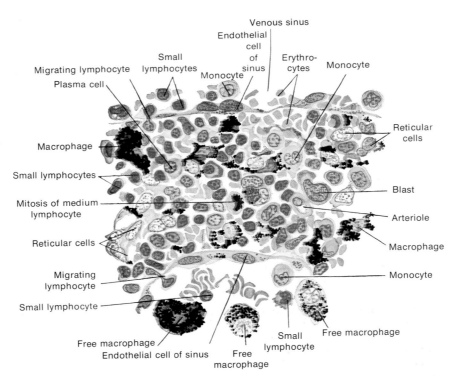

Figure 17–3 Cross section of splenic cord lying between two venous sinuses, from spleen of a rabbit injected with lithium carmine and India ink. Hematoxylin-eosin-azure II. × 560. (After A. A. Maximow.)

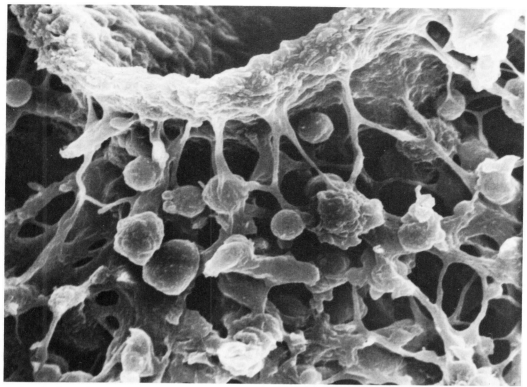

Figure 17–4 Scanning electron micrograph of a splenic cord adjacent to a pulp vein in the dog. Spleen perfusion with physiological salt solution has removed the majority of the free cells, thus exposing the three dimensional network formed by the reticular cells. × 2600. (Courtesy of M. Miyoshi and T. Fujita, Arch. Histol. Jap., *33*:225, 1971.)

The meshes of reticulum in the pulp cords are filled with great numbers of free cells, which include: macrophages, all the cellular elements circulating in the blood, including great numbers of erythrocytes and platelets, and a few plasma cells (Figs. 17–3 and 17–8). With the light microscope the macrophages are readily recognized as large, rounded, or irregularly shaped cells, with a vesicular nucleus and abundant cytoplasm. They often contain engulfed erythrocytes, neutrophils, and platelets or are loaded with masses of a yellowish-brown pigment that stains for iron with the Prussian blue reaction and gives a positive reaction for the lysosomal enzyme acid phosphatase. This pigment represents the undigestible residues of phagocytized materials, especially red blood cells. Its iron, in the form of ferritin or hemosiderin, comes from the degradation of hemoglobin. In many mammalian species (laboratory rodents, hedgehog) and in the embryonic spleen, the red pulp contains groups of erythroblasts of various sizes, myeloblasts, myelocytes, and megakaryocytes. In adult man, these islands of hemopoietic tissue are lacking, but in certain infections, in some of the anemias, in leukemias, and in poisoning with certain blood-destroying agents, they may reappear, a condition described as *myeloid metaplasia.*

Immediately peripheral to the white pulp is an 80 to 100 μm. transitional region between lymphoid tissue and red pulp, called the *marginal zone*; it contains smaller venous sinuses, circumferentially oriented around the white pulp. In the marginal zone, the reticular fibers of the cords form a closely knit concentric network, and the meshes of the cords have a greater content of small lymphocytes and plasma cells than the rest of the red pulp. The marginal zone is the region of the red pulp that receives the incoming arterial blood; thus, it is the site where blood-borne cells and particulate matter first contact the splenic parenchyma. Here, the lymphocytes of the recirculating pool leave the blood of the sinuses to enter the periarterial lymphoid sheaths.

Capsule and Trabeculae

The capsule and the trabeculae of the spleen consist of dense connective tissue, smooth muscle cells, and elastic networks. The external surface of the capsule is covered by a layer of flattened mesothelium, which is part of the general peritoneum. In man, rabbits and laboratory rodents, the capsule is rich in elastic fibers, especially in its deep layers, and in addition to typical fibroblasts, it contains a small number of stellate elements that display cytological characteristics intermediate between smooth muscle cells and fibroblasts, having filamentous cytoplasm and abundant glycogen. Smooth muscle cells are especially abundant in the splenic capsule of the horse, ruminants, and carnivores.

The trabeculae are flattened or cylindrical strands that carry arteries, veins, and lymphatics. They contain a larger number of elastic fibers than the capsule and varying amounts of smooth muscle cells (Fig. 17–5). Smooth muscle cells are sparse in the human spleen. In those species in which muscle is prominent, changes in the volume of the organ, either spontaneous or induced by injection of epinephrine, are due to contraction of the smooth muscle in the capsule and trabeculae, as well as to the vasomotor changes in the amount of blood in the organ.

Arteries

The branches of the splenic artery enter the hilus and pass along the trabeculae, within which they branch repeatedly, becoming smaller in diameter (Fig. 17–6). They are muscular arteries of medium caliber and have a loose tunica adventitia surrounded by the dense connective tissue of the trabeculae. When the arterial branches have been reduced by progressive dichotomous branching to a diameter of approximately 0.2 mm., they leave the trabeculae. At this point, the tunica adventitia is replaced by a cylindrical sheath of lymphoid tissue, and the artery is designated the *central artery*. Where germinal centers are embedded in the periarterial lymphoid sheath, the artery is displaced to one side, thus losing its central position. It almost never passes through the center of the nodules. The central artery is a muscular artery with tall endothelial cells and one or two layers of smooth muscle cells. Throughout its course within the white pulp, the artery gives off numerous collateral capil-

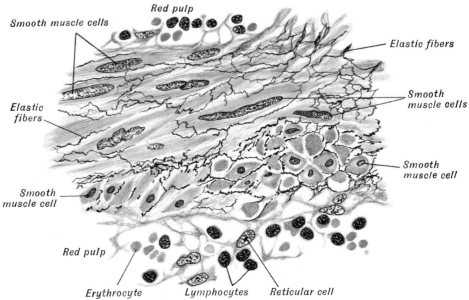

Figure 17-5 Portion of a trabecula from spleen of a cat. Elastic fiber stain. × 750. (After A. A. Maximow.)

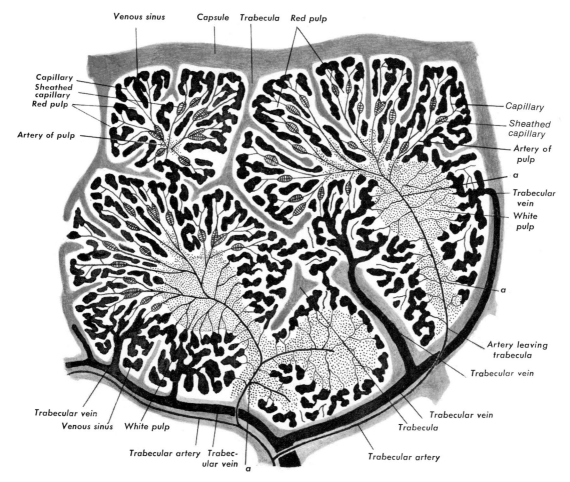

Figure 17–6 Diagram of the vascular tree of the spleen. Capillaries are depicted as communicating with the venous sinuses, according to the "closed circulation" theory. *a,* Central arteries. (After A. A. Maximow.)

laries, which supply the lymphoid tissue of the sheath. Initially, the capillary wall consists of tall endothelial cells, basal lamina, and an investment of pericytes; farther on, the endothelium becomes low and the pericytes disappear. Around the capillaries, the reticular meshwork of the white pulp is condensed and contains a few elastic fibers. These collateral capillaries, after coursing through the white pulp, pass into the surrounding marginal zone; how they end is uncertain.

The central artery continues to branch and becomes thinner. On reaching a diameter of 40 to 50 μm., its lymphoid sheath appears greatly reduced in thickness and the artery suddenly branches into two to six vessels, called *penicillar arteries* (Latin, penicillus = a painter's brush) or *arteries of the red pulp.*

These pursue a radiating course still invested by one or two layers of lymphocytes that represent a greatly attenuated terminal extension of the periarterial lymphoid sheaths. The penicillar arteries are 0.6 to 0.7 mm. in length, and have a tall endothelium resting on a continuous basal lamina, but they lack an elastica interna. Their media consists of one layer of smooth muscle cells; they lack an elastica externa and have a thin adventitia of collagenous and elastic fibers.

Upon entering the red pulp, each penicillar artery as a rule branches into two to three capillaries, which may exhibit a characteristic thickening of their walls, called the Schweigger-Seidel sheath (Fig. 17–7). The capillaries are therefore named *sheathed capillaries.* The endothelium of these vessels consists of tall, fusiform cells arranged parallel to the long axis of the vessel. They are connected by intercellular junctions, contain abundant cytoplasmic filaments, and rest on a thin, continuous basal lamina. In man, the sheath is tubular and fairly thin (50 to 100 μm. in length and 20 to 30 μm. in diameter), but in certain species it is very prominent and ellipsoidal or spherical in shape (pig and cat). Sheathed capillaries are lacking in the spleen of laboratory rodents. Not all capillaries arising from a penicillar artery are sheathed, and most commonly only one sheath is associated with the terminal branches of a penicillar artery. Occasionally, multiple vessels (two to five) are invested by a single sheath, and sometimes two to three sheaths are arranged in series along a single branch of a penicillar artery. The sheath consists of a closely knit network of fibers and cells. The cells are rounded near the capillary and stellate toward the periphery; they have finely dispersed chromatin and an acidophilic cytoplasm, rich in acid phosphatase (presumably residing in lysosomes). With the electron microscope, their cytoplasm displays numerous residual bodies and occasional phagocytized red blood cells. Upon intravenous injection of particulate matter, these cells become avidly phagocytic; thus they appear to belong to the macrophage-monocyte system. It is unknown, however, why phagocytes specifically congregate around the initial segment of certain splenic capillaries. Red blood cells are always present, in large or small numbers, among the cells of the sheath.

The sheathed capillaries continue as simple capillaries that either do not divide or bifurcate only once. Their mode of termination is unknown and will be discussed below after the venous sinuses have been described.

Venous Sinuses and Veins

The venous sinuses permeate the entire red pulp and are especially numerous around the white pulp (Fig. 17-8). These vessels are called sinuses because they have a wide (12 to 40 μm.), irregular lumen, which varies in size depending upon the amount of blood in the

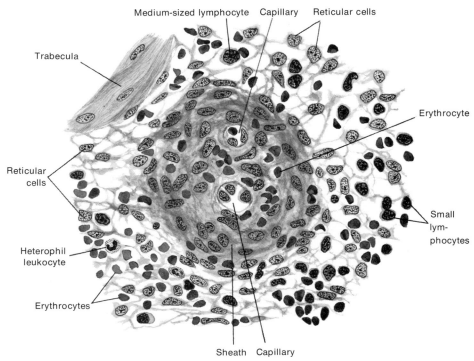

Medium-sized lymphocyte Capillary Reticular cells

Trabecula

Erythrocyte

Reticular cells

Small lymphocytes

Heterophil leukocyte

Erythrocytes

Sheath Capillary

Figure 17-7 Cross section of a Schweigger-Seidel sheath surrounding two capillaries in the spleen of a dog. Eosin-azure stain. × 500. (After A. A. Maximow.)

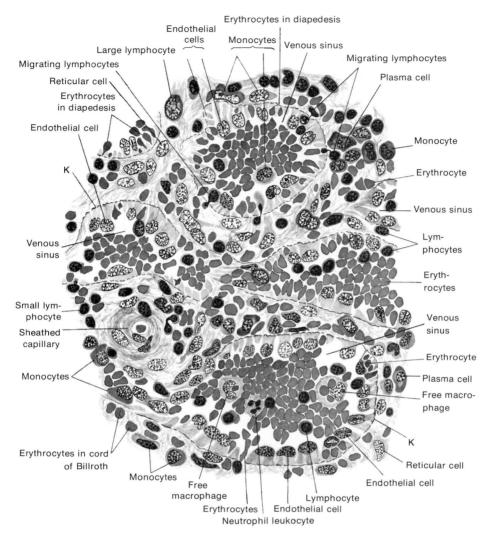

Figure 17–8 Venous sinuses in the red pulp of the human spleen. Notice the cuboidal shape of the cross sectioned endothelial cells. The cytoplasmic densities at the base of the cells *(K)* probably correspond to the condensations of finely filamentous material revealed by the electron microscope. Eosin-azure stain. × 750. (After A. A. Maximow.)

organ. The sinuses, even when only moderately distended, occupy more space than the splenic cords between them. Venous sinuses are said to be missing in the mouse spleen.

Unlike true veins, the walls of the sinuses lack a muscular coat and display a unique arrangement of endothelium and basal lamina. The endothelial cells are fusiform elements, about 100 μm. long, oriented parallel to the longitudinal axis of the sinus (Fig. 17–9). The central nuclear region of the cell body is thick and tapers toward the ends; they

are in contact with each other laterally but lack typical intercellular junctions. Micropinocytotic vesicles are plentiful on both the luminal and lateral surfaces, and the cytoplasm contains, in addition to the usual complement of organelles, two types of filaments, both oriented parallel to the long axis of the cells. There are loosely packed filaments, free in the cytoplasmic matrix, and denser bands of finely filamentous material in the basal region of the cell. These latter seem to run from one rib of the basal lamina to the next, where they insert on the inner aspect of the plasma membrane; they are probably responsible for the longitudinal basal striations of the endothelium which are seen in specimens stained with iron hematoxylin. Except for their unusual shape, lack of intercellular junctions and abundance of filaments, the sinus-lining cells resemble endothelial cells elsewhere in the body. Like other endothelial cells, they display only a limited capacity to take up particulate matter injected into the bloodstream. Thus, the traditional interpretation of the sinus-lining cells of the spleen as fixed macrophages is no longer tenable.

Outside the endothelium, the wall of the sinuses is supported by a system of circumferential ribs, about 1 μm. in thickness, encircling the endothelial cells as the hoops embrace the staves of a barrel (Fig. 17–2). The ribs are spaced 2 to 5 μm. apart and are interconnected by relatively few, thin longitudinal strands. At the light microscope level, they are observed to stain with silver impregnation methods and with histochemical methods for carbohydrates. In electron micrographs, they appear to consist of finely filamentous material with a few embedded collagen fibrils. Thus, in their fine structure, they correspond to an unusually thick, fenestrated basal lamina. The ribs are continuous with the reticular fibers of the splenic cords and are interposed between the endothelium on one side and the foot processes of the reticular cells of the cords on the other. Cellular elements of the circulating blood can easily migrate through the sinus wall, traversing the interendothelial clefts and the fenestrations of the basal lamina. Furthermore, cordal macrophages are frequently seen extending processes through the sinus walls into the lumen and they may also migrate into the blood within the sinus.

The venous sinuses empty into the *veins of the pulp*, whose walls consist of elongated, slender endothelial cells, a continuous basal lamina, and a thin layer of smooth muscle. They are supported externally by a condensa-

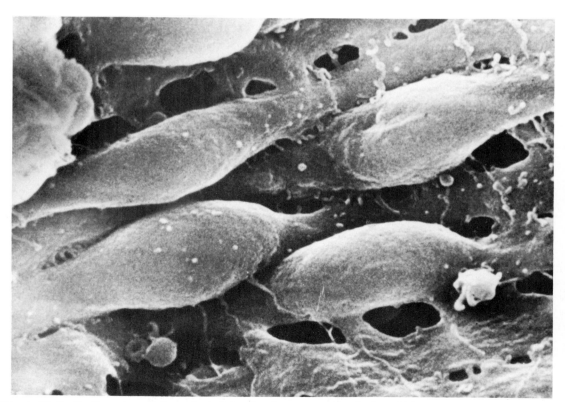

Figure 17–9 Surface view of the endothelial cells of a venous sinus in the rabbit spleen as seen with the scanning electron microscope. As the specimen was air dried, cells have pulled apart, thus exposing the fenestrations of the basal lamina. × 4800. (Courtesy of M. Miyoshi et al., Arch. Histol. Jap., *32*:289, 1970.)

tion of the stroma of the red pulp and by a few elastic fibers. The pulp veins coalesce to form the veins of the trabeculae; in turn, these are drained by the veins at the hilus of the spleen, which are tributaries of the splenic vein.

Union of the Arteries with the Veins

In almost all other organs of the body, the arterial is joined to the venous system by a continuous capillary network, in which the vascular lumen is completely enclosed. In the spleen, however, the connection of arterial and venous systems may be different, and its details are still subject to dispute. There are three main theories as to how blood gets from the arteries to the venous sinuses (Fig. 17–10). (1) The "open circulation" theory holds that the capillaries open directly into the spaces among the reticular cells of the splenic cords, and that the blood gradually filters into the venous sinuses. (2) The "closed circulation" theory holds that the capillaries communicate directly with the lumen of the venous sinuses. (3) A compromise interpretation holds that both types of circulation are present at the same time. One of the variants of this theory contends that a "closed" circulation in a contracted spleen may become an "open" circulation when the organ is distended.

The opposing theories are based on the following observations: (1) There are always many erythrocytes scattered throughout the tissue spaces of the splenic cords. Since in most species there is little or no erythropoiesis in the cords, it is concluded that the red blood cells have come from the circulating blood through gaps in the vascular segment between the arterioles and the venous sinuses. Those who maintain that the circulation is "closed" hold that the number of erythrocytes in the splenic cords is much smaller than it would be if the capillaries opened directly into the pulp. They argue that if the capillaries were open, the red pulp would be completely filled with blood, as in hemorrhages of the spleen. (2) When the splenic arteries are injected even at low pressures with dye solutions, India ink, or avian erythrocytes, the foreign materials readily gain access to the tissue spaces of the splenic cords, particularly in the marginal zone. Only later do they reach the venous sinuses. When the splenic vein is injected, the venous sinuses and the meshes of the stroma can be filled easily, but the arteries cannot.

Those who favor a closed circulation believe that this injection of the red pulp by foreign materials is an artificial situation resulting from the rupture of the delicate vascular walls. (3) In every freshly fixed spleen, granulocytes, lymphocytes and erythrocytes can be found passing through the walls of the

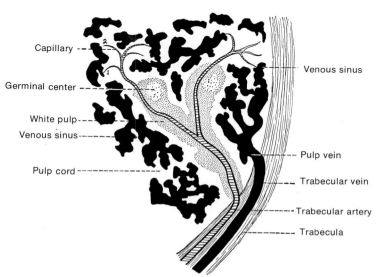

Figure 17–10 Diagram to show closed (1) and open (2) circulation through the spleen.

venous sinuses. According to the "open" circulation theory, these cells are returning to the bloodstream from the extravascular spaces of the splenic cords. According to the "closed" circulation theory, both plasma and cells of the blood are believed to pass into the cordal spaces at the arterial end of the sinuses and to return to the circulation at their venous end, driven by a pressure gradient which may exist between the two ends of these blood vessels.

The problem of the circulation in the spleen would seem to be an ideal one for solution by direct observation of the living organ. Unfortunately, the techniques available for this are difficult, and the reports made on such studies are contradictory. According to one group, the circulation in the spleen appears to be closed, there is a marked intermittency of circulation, there is extensive filtering of the liquid portion of the blood from the sinuses into the splenic cords, and erythrocytes normally leave the sinuses by diapedesis.

These conclusions are contradicted by another group of observers that report the circulation to be open—that is, without preformed connections between the arterial and venous systems, so that the blood from the terminations of the arterial tree percolates between the reticular cells and macrophages of the splenic cords and finds its way through openings in the wall of the sinuses. According to these observations, erythrocytes may be stored in the interstices among the reticular cells. The channels in the splenic cords vary from time to time with the degree of engorgement of that part of the organ, so that a channel which previously had been a tortuous passage between reticular cells may appear as a direct communication to the lumen of a venous sinus when the spleen is contracted. From the foregoing, it is obvious that the connection of arterioles and venules in the spleen requires further investigations.

Lymphatic Vessels and Nerves

In man, lymphatic vessels are poorly developed and are found only in the capsule of the spleen and in the thickest trabeculae, particularly those in the vicinity of the hilus. In some mammals, true lymphatic vessels follow the arteries of the white pulp. Networks of nerves that originate from the celiac plexus and which consist almost entirely of unmyelinated fibers accompany the splenic artery and penetrate into the hilus of the spleen. In the sheep and ox, these nerves form trunks of considerable thickness. The nerve bundles mainly follow the ramifications of the arteries and form networks that can be followed as far as the central arteries of the white pulp and even along the branches of the penicillar arteries. The terminal branches usually end with button-like thickenings on the smooth muscles of the arteries and of the trabeculae. Apparently many branches penetrate into the red as well as the white pulp, but their endings here are not definitely established.

HISTOGENESIS AND REGENERATION OF THE SPLEEN

The primordium of the spleen appears, in human embryos of 8 to 9 mm., as a small thickening of the dorsal mesogastrium, consisting of a closely aggregated mass of mesenchymal elements.

The mesenchymal cells which compose this first primordium of the spleen multiply by mitosis, and the primordium grows. It has been supposed that it also increases in size by apposition of new cells from the mesothelium of the body cavity covering the primordium. After the embryo (pig) has reached a length of 15 mm., it receives no more cells from the mesothelium.

The elements of the primary mesenchymal primordium remain connected with one another by means of processes and form the reticular framework of the white as well as of the red pulp. According to the traditional view, some of the mesenchymal elements soon become isolated from the rest and differentiate into free cells, located in the meshes of the framework. At first they all have the character of basophilic wandering elements; later on, they give rise to red corpuscles, granular myelocytes and leukocytes, and megakaryocytes. More recent evidence, however, has indicated that the primitive basophilic elements arise from stem cell precursors of yolk sac, liver, or bone marrow origin. Splenic lymphocytes are in part of thymic origin (T lymphocytes) and in part arise from the bone marrow; these latter are possibly preconditioned in the unknown mammalian analogue of the avian bursa (B lymphocytes). Splenic macrophages also seem to derive from bone marrow precursors. In the lower vertebrates, up to the urodele amphibians, the erythropoietic function is retained in the spleen throughout life; in the higher vertebrates the myeloid function stops sooner or later and is replaced by an erythrolytic function, although the formation of lymphocytes persists throughout life. In man there seems to be very little hemopoiesis even in the embryonal spleen.

In mammals (pig), the mesenchymal primordium contains a capillary network connected with the afferent arteries and efferent veins. Irregular spaces, the precursors of the venous sinuses, subsequently appear (pig embryos of 4 to 6 cm.) and become connected, in 6 to 7 cm. embryos, with the preexisting vessels. The embryonic mammalian spleen has, at first, a myeloid character and cannot be compared with either the red or the white pulp. At the end of fetal life (in the rat) the adventitia of the arteries begins to be infiltrated with large numbers of lymphocytes, and in this manner the white pulp originates; typical lymphoid nodules appear after birth following antigen stimulation. The myeloid elements, which in the rat had reached their maximum development three weeks after birth, gradually disappear and the tissue of the spleen located between the accumulations of white pulp can then be called the red pulp.

When the spleen is removed, its functions are taken over by other organs, and the formation of a new spleen has never been observed, although a compensatory hypertrophy of the so-called "accessory spleens" has been described. Local injuries and wounds of the spleen are followed by a temporary myeloid metaplasia of the red pulp. They subsequently heal with a simple scar. In the amphibians, particularly in larval stages, a certain degree of regeneration is possible. In birds, the spleen shows marked regenerative powers.

HISTOPHYSIOLOGY

The filtering function of the spleen depends upon the abundant population of macrophages of the splenic cords, which probably arise from blood monocytes. Upon intravenous injection, particulate matter or macromolecular antigen first localize in the macrophages of the marginal zone and subsequently spread to the phagocytes of the rest of the red pulp. Neither the endothelial cells of the sinuses nor the fibroblast-like reticular cells of the splenic cords contribute significantly to clearing the blood of foreign material. Very little particulate matter enters the white pulp, but in the presence of antibody, antigen may be trapped for long periods of time in the germinal centers. When lipid in the blood is increased in amount, the macrophages of the spleen, like the other phagocytes of the body, have the capacity to remove it from the circulation. In this process, the macrophages enlarge and become filled with lipid droplets, thus acquiring a foamy appearance. This phenomenon is observed in diabetic hyperlipemia in man and in experimental hypercholesterolemia of rabbits.

The destruction of aged, abnormal, or damaged blood cells and platelets takes place in the meshes of the cords of the red pulp. How blood-borne elements and especially erythrocytes, which lack motility, reach the tissue spaces of the cords still is a matter of controversy. According to the "open" circulation theory, the capillaries deliver the blood directly to the pulp cords; this being true, the constituents of the plasma and the cells of the blood can freely percolate through the interstitial spaces between cord macrophages and reticular cells and finally reenter the blood through the walls of the venous sinuses. In a "closed" vascular system, one must postulate either that the pressure gradient between the arterial and venous ends of the sinuses drives plasma and erythrocytes into the cord spaces and then back into the blood, or that rhythmic contractions of the sinus endothelium squeeze the blood out of the vascular bed; this latter hypothesis implies the existence of a sphincteric mechanism at the venous end of the sinuses. With either theory, both plasma and blood cells establish extensive contact with the macrophages of the cords, which can then remove any undesirable component. Unphagocytosed cells can freely return to the intravascular compartment through the fenestrations of the basal lamina and the interendothelial clefts of the sinuses. The precise role of the spleen in removing aged erythrocytes, as well as the extent to which this function is shared with bone marrow and liver, is poorly understood. Splenectomy does not seem to affect the average life span of red blood cells significantly. There is no doubt, however, that the spleen plays a major role in destroying pathologic or defective blood elements. When abnormal or experimentally damaged erythrocytes are perfused through the spleen, they are retained by this organ, whereas normal erythrocytes are not. Granulocytes damaged by endotoxin have also been shown to be destroyed in the spleen. Moreover, splenectomy is followed by the appearance in the bloodstream of defective erythrocytes containing remnants of the nucleus or cytoplasmic organelles. The mechanism by which macrophages recognize old or abnormal blood cells is unknown. It has been postulated that the immune system may react to changes in the erythrocyte surface and tag pathologic cells with opsonizing antibody. In normal subjects, no lysis or fragmentation of red blood cells is observed either in the lumen of the sinuses or in the cord spaces, and erythrocytes seem to be phagocytized intact by macrophages. In pathologic conditions, however, extracellular disintegration of red blood cells has been described.

Closely connected with erythrocyte destruction by the macrophages is the function of the spleen in hemoglobin degradation and iron metabolism. In the lysosomes of the macrophages, the iron of hemoglobin is freed and stored by the cell as ferritin or hemosiderin, readily available to the body for synthesis of new hemoglobin by bone marrow erythroblasts. The heme moiety of hemoglobin is degraded by macrophages to bilirubin, which enters the plasma, where it binds to albumin. It is then captured by the liver, conjugated to glucuronic acid, and secreted in the bile.

In animal species in which the capsule and trabeculae are rich in smooth muscle cells, the spleen can act as a store for red blood cells; large numbers of them can in fact be retained in the red pulp and then given up to the bloodstream when they are needed in the circulation. This may also occur experimentally following injection of drugs, such as epinephrine, that induce contraction of the splenic smooth muscle. The human spleen has little storage capacity (about 30 to 40 ml. of erythrocytes), but it traps a large fraction of blood platelets in a reserve pool available to meet physiologic demands or emergency conditions.

Although in the embryo the spleen contains immature precursors of the circulating blood elements, the erythrocytes found in the red pulp in the normal, adult human are never formed there. In some pathologic conditions, especially myeloid leukemia, the red pulp of the spleen undergoes myeloid metaplasia, after which a large number of erythroblasts, megakaryocytes, and myelocytes appear in the tissue, so that the red pulp acquires a structure resembling that of the red bone marrow. In many other adult mammals, some myelocytes and erythroblasts may be found normally in the red pulp, and megakaryocytes are consistently present in the spleen of rats and mice.

The spleen has great physiological importance in the immune response to bacteria, viruses, and foreign macromolecules which have invaded the circulation. In an animal not involved in an acute response to antigen, it is evident from the small arteriovenous difference in lymphocyte counts on splenic blood that only a small fraction of the lymphocytes that leave the spleen via the veins arise from division of precursors in that organ. A large fraction of splenic lymphocytes belong to the recirculating pool and they are specifically localized in the periarterial lymphoid sheaths. This has been shown by experiments involving drainage of the thoracic duct lymph and reinjection of thoracic duct lymphocytes after labeling in vitro. Drainage of the thoracic duct lymph initially affects the central region of the periarterial lymphoid sheaths; only after prolonged drainage do the peripheral regions of the white pulp also become depleted of lymphocytes. This finding has been interpreted as an evidence favoring the idea that the rapidly recirculating T lymphocytes localize close to the central artery, whereas the sluggishly migrating B cells assume a more peripheral position in the periarterial lymphoid sheaths. After intravenous injection, labeled thoracic duct cells first localize throughout the marginal zone of the red pulp, but a few hours later they have migrated into the periarterial lymphoid sheaths. Labeled thoracic duct lymphocytes from mice congenitally lacking T cells "home in" preferentially in the peripheral regions of the sheaths; thus, the suggestion has been advanced that the periarterial lymphoid sheaths consist of a central, thymus-dependent region and a peripheral, bursa-dependent region. In neonatally thymectomized rodents, the periarterial lymphoid sheaths are poorly populated with lymphocytes; thus, the vast majority of their lymphocytes are represented by T cells.

The transit time of the recirculating lymphocytes through the spleen is very short and may be as brief as two hours. The pathway followed by the lymphocytes in entering and leaving the periarterial lymphoid sheaths is poorly understood. They probably enter the cords of the marginal zone by crossing the walls of the venous sinuses and subsequently migrate into the white pulp. The route by which the lymphocytes reenter the blood is unknown; it has been suggested that they follow the lymphatic vessels which accompany the central artery, but these vessels do not seem to be found consistently in the splenic white pulp of all mammals.

For the significance of the germinal centers which are scattered along the periarterial lymphoid sheaths, see the general discussion of these structures on page 449.

Upon introduction into the bloodstream of an antigen that elicits a humoral response, morphological changes are first seen in the periarterial lymphoid sheaths. One day after the injection, proliferating lymphoblasts appear, scattered throughout the sheaths. They increase in number during the following one or two days and become more concentrated toward the periphery of the sheaths. At the same time, antibody first appears in the bloodstream. Lymphoblasts also occur around the small arteries of the red pulp. These may have developed from the terminal extensions of the periarterial lymphoid sheaths which surround the penicillar arteries. On days four to six, an increasing number of immature plasma cells appears at the periphery of the periarterial lymphoid sheaths and along the penicillar arteries; mature plasma cells are also found, but in very small numbers. At this stage, morphological changes in germinal centers are first seen; they contain many proliferating lymphoblasts and macrophages loaded with debris of phagocytized lymphocytes. At the end of the first week, lymphoblasts and immature plasma cells begin to decrease in number in the periarterial lymphoid sheaths, mature plasma cells are more numerous at the boundary between white and red pulp and along the penicillar arteries. They also occur in the cords of the red pulp and not infrequently free in the sinus lumen. During the second week after the introduction of the antigen, the structure of the spleen reverts to normal, except for the germinal centers, which continue to remain prominent for about one month.

During the secondary response, the spleen undergoes changes that resemble those following the first exposure to antigen, but they occur earlier and are much more dramatic. At the beginning of the response the spleen is, per unit weight, the most active organ of the body in antibody secretion, but it rapidly falls off in production as the response becomes propagated throughout the other peripheral lymphoid tissues and organs of the body.

Inasmuch as macrophages and lymphocytes are not restricted to the spleen, it is not surprising that the effects of splenectomy are transient and largely disappear as splenic functions are assumed by other organs.

REFERENCES

Burke, J. S., and G. T. Simon: Electron microscopy of the spleen. I. Anatomy and microcirculation. Am. J. Pathol., 58:127, 1970.

Burke, J. S., and G. T. Simon: Electron microscopy of the spleen. II. Phagocytosis of colloidal carbon. Am. J. Pathol., 58:157, 1970.

Carr, I.: The fine structure of the mammalian lymphoreticular system. Int. Rev. Cytol., 27:283, 1970.

Chen, L-T., and L. Weiss: Electron microscopy of the red pulp of human spleen. Am. J. Anat., 134:425, 1972.

Coons, A. H.: Some reactions of lymphoid tissues to stimulation by antigen. Harvey Lectures, 53:113, 1959.

Edwards, V. D., and G. T. Simon: Ultrastructural aspects of red cell destruction in the normal rat spleen. J. Ultrast. Res., 33:187, 1970.

Ernstrom, U., and G. Sandberg: Migration of splenic lymphocytes. Acta Path. Microbiol. Scandinav., 72:379, 1968.

Ford, W. L., and J. L. Gowans: The traffic of lymphocytes. Sem. Hematol., 6:67, 1969.

Galindo, B., and T. Imaeda: Electron microscope study of the white pulp of the mouse spleen. Anat. Rec., 143:399, 1962.

Goldschneider, I., and D. D. McGregor: Migration of lymphocytes and thymocytes in the rat. I. The route of migration from blood to spleen and lymph nodes. J. Exp. Med., 127:155, 1968.

Hanna, M. G., Jr., and A. K. Szakal: Localization of ^{125}I-labeled antigen in germinal centers of mouse spleen: histologic and ultrastructural autoradiographic studies of the secondary immune reaction. J. Immunol., 101:949, 1968.

Jacobsen, G.: Morphological-histochemical comparison of dog and cat splenic ellipsoid sheaths. Anat. Rec., 169:105, 1971.

Jacobson, L. O., E. K. Marks, M. J. Robson, E. Gaston, R. E. Zirkle: The effect of spleen protection on mortality following x-irradiation. J. Lab. Clin. Med., 34:1538, 1949.

Klemperer, P.: The Spleen. *In* Downey, H. (ed.): Handbook of Hematology. New York, Paul B. Hoeber, Inc., 1938.

Knisely, M. H.: Spleen studies. I. Microscopic observations of the circulatory system of living unstimulated mammalian spleens. Anat. Rec., 65:23, 1936.

Langevoort, H. L.: The histophysiology of the antibody response. I. Histogenesis of the plasma cell reaction in rabbit spleen. Lab. Invest., 12:106, 1963.

Lewis, O. J.: The blood vessels of the adult mammalian spleen. J. Anat., 91:245, 1957.

MacKenzie, D. W., Jr., A. O. Whipple, and M. P. Wintersteiner: Studies on the microscopic anatomy and physiology of living transilluminated mammalian spleens. Am. J. Anat., 68:397, 1941.

Miyoshi, M., and T. Fujita: Stereo-fine structure of the splenic red pulp. A combined scanning and transmission electron microscope study on dog and rat spleen. Arch. Histol. Jap., 33:225, 1971.

Miyoshi, M., T. Fujita, and J. Tokunaga: The red pulp of the rabbit spleen studied under the scanning electron microscope. Arch. Histol. Jap., 32:289, 1970.

Mollier, S.: Uber den Bau der Capillaren Milzvenen (Milzsinus). Arch. f. mikr. Anat., 76:608, 1911.

Movat, H. Z., and N. V. P. Fernando: The fine structure of lymphoid tissue. Exp. Mol. Pathol., 3:546, 1964.

Movat, H. Z., and N. V. P. Fernando: The fine structure of the lymphoid tissue during antibody formation. Exp. Mol. Pathol., 4:155, 1965.

Peck, H. M., and N. L. Hoerr: The intermediary circulation in the red pulp of the mouse spleen. Anat. Rec., 109:447, 1951.

Pictet, R., L. Orci, W. G. Forssmann, and L. Girardier: An electron microscope study of the perfusion-fixed spleen. I. The splenic circulation and the RES concept. Z. Zellforsch., 96:372, 1969.

Robinson, W.: The vascular mechanism of the spleen. Am. J. Path., 2:341, 1926.

Simon, G. T., and J. S. Burke: Electron microscopy of the spleen. III. Erythroleukophagocytosis. Am. J. Pathol., 58:451, 1970.

Snodgrass, M. J.: A study of some histochemical and phagocytic reactions of the sinus lining cells of the rabbit's spleen. Anat. Rec., 161:353, 1968.

Snook, T.: A comparative study of the vascular arrangements in mammalian spleens. Am. J. Anat., 87:31, 1950.

Solnitzky, O.: The Schweigger-Seidel sheath (ellipsoid) of the spleen. Anat. Rec., 69:55, 1937.

Sprent, J.: Circulating T and B lymphocytes of the mouse. I. Migratory properties. Cell. Immunol., 7:10, 1973.

Stutte, H. J.: Nature of human spleen red pulp cells with special reference to sinus lining cells. Z. Zellforsch., 91:300, 1968.

Sussdorf, D. H., and L. R. Draper: The primary hemolysin response in rabbits following shielding from x-rays or x-irradiation of the spleen, appendix, liver or hind legs. J. Infect. Dis., 99:129, 1956.

Szakal, A. K., and M. G. Hanna, Jr.: The ultrastructure of antigen localization and virus-like particles in mouse spleen germinal centers. Exp. Mol. Pathol., 8:75, 1968.

Thiel, G. A., and H. Downey: The development of the mammalian spleen, with special reference to its hematopoietic activity. Am. J. Anat., 28:279, 1921.

Weidenreich, F.: Das Gefässsystem der menschlichen Milz. Arch. mikr. Anat., 58:247, 1901.

Weiss, L.: An experimental study of the organization of the reticuloendothelial system in the red pulp of the spleen. J. Anat., 93:465, 1959.

Weiss, L.: The structure of fine splenic arterial vessels in relation to hemoconcentration and red cell destruction. Am. J. Anat., 111:131, 1962.

Weiss, L.: The structure of intermediate vascular pathways in the spleen of rabbits. Am. J. Anat., 113:51, 1963.

Weiss, L.: The Cells and Tissues of the Immune System: Structure, Functions, Interactions. Englewood Cliffs, N.J., Prentice-Hall, Inc., 1972.

Weiss, L.: The development of the primary vascular reticulum in the spleen of human fetuses (38 to 57 mm. crown-rump length). Am. J. Anat., 136:315, 1973.

Weiss, L., and M. Tavassoli: Anatomical hazards to the passage of erythrocytes through the spleen. Sem. Hematol., 7:372, 1970.

Wennberg, E., and L. Weiss: The structure of the spleen and hemolysis. Ann. Rev. Med., 20:29, 1969.

18

Hypophysis (Pituitary Gland)

The hypophysis or pituitary is an endocrine gland located at the base of the brain. It is about 1 cm. in length, 1 to 1.5 cm. in width, and about 0.5 cm. deep. It weighs about 0.5 gm. in men and slightly more in women. Despite its small size it is one of the most important organs in the body, producing at least nine hormones and having many reciprocal relations with other endocrine glands. It also has neural and vascular connections with the brain, to which it is attached by a slender stalk. By virtue of these connections, the hypophysis occupies a key position in the interplay of the nervous system and the endocrine system—the two great integrating systems of the body.

The hypophysis has two major subdivisions, the *neurohypophysis*, which develops as a process growing downward from the floor of the diencephalon, and the *adenohypophysis*, which originates in the embryo as a dorsal outpocketing of the roof of the embryonic pharynx. There are three subdivisions of the adenohypophysis: the *pars distalis* or anterior lobe, the *pars infundibularis (pars tuberalis)*, and the *pars intermedia*. The neurohypophysis generally is divided into three regions: the *median eminence*, a funnel-shaped extension of the tuber cinereum; the *infundibular stalk;* and the *infundibular process*. The relations of these components are depicted in Figure 18–3. In many species, the pars intermedia is closely adherent to the infundibular process to form the so-called *posterior lobe,* separated by a cleft from the pars distalis or anterior lobe. In man the cleft is largely obliterated in late fetal and postnatal life, so that the anterior and posterior lobes

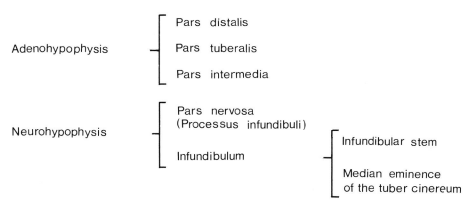

Figure 18–1 Terminology of the divisions and subdivisions of the hypophysis. In addition, the pars intermedia and pars nervosa together are sometimes called the posterior lobe, and the pars distalis and pars tuberalis are collectively called the anterior lobe.

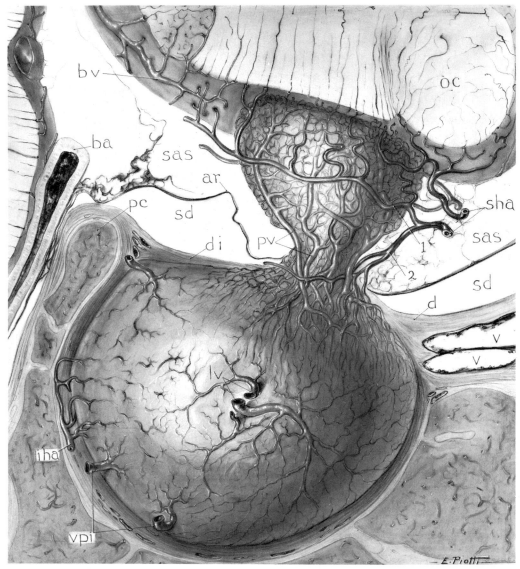

Figure 18-2 Schematic drawing of the hypophysis of an adult rhesus monkey, showing its relation to the sella turcica of the sphenoid bone. Also depicted are the superior and inferior hypophyseal arteries (*sha* and *iha*) and the important portal venules (*pv*) coursing down the infundibular stalk. The superior hypophyseal artery usually sends an ascending branch (*1*) to the proximal part of the infundibular stalk and median eminence and a descending branch (*2*) coursing distally. *ar,* Arachnoid membrane; *ba,* basilar artery; *bv,* basilar veins; *d,* dura; *di,* sellar diaphragm; *lv,* lateral hypophyseal veins; *oc,* optic chiasm; *pc,* posterior clinoid process; *sas,* subarachnoid space; *sd,* subdural space; *v,* dural vein; *vpi,* veins of the infundibular process. (After G. B. Wislocki, Proc. Assoc. Res. Nervous and Mental Diseases, *17*:48, 1936.)

are in continuity. The subdivisions of the hypophysis and the accepted descriptive terminology are presented in tabular form in Figure 18–1.

The hypophysis is lodged in a deep depression in the sphenoid bone, the *sella turcica,*

and is covered by a tough diaphragm, the *diaphragma sellae.* This barrier between the sella turcica and the intracranial cavity is often incomplete, being penetrated by an opening 5 mm. or more in diameter around the hypophyseal stalk. Some of the pia-arachnoid may extend through this opening and occupy the narrow space between the diaphragm and the connective tissue capsule of the gland. Elsewhere the dense collagenous capsule is separated from the periosteum of the sphenoid bone by a looser layer of connective tissue containing numerous veins. This layer appears to be separate from the pia-arachnoid. In mammals other than man, the diaphragma sellae is commonly incomplete.

PARS DISTALIS

The pars distalis or anterior lobe is the largest subdivision of the hypophysis. It is composed of glandular cells arranged in irregular cords and clumps. These are intimately related to an extensive system of thin-walled sinusoids of the blood vascular system. The anterior lobe is largely enclosed by a dense collagenous capsule. The stroma of the gland is not abundant, but some collagenous fibers, which accompany the superior hypophyseal arteries and the portal venules, penetrate the anterior lobe at the pole adjacent to the pars tuberalis and fan out bilaterally, extending about a third of the way into the gland. There they become continuous with reticular fibers that surround the cords of parenchymal cells and support the small branches of the hypophyseal artery and the sinusoids. Although the endothelium lining the sinusoids has traditionally been regarded as phagocytic, like that of the liver, this has not been borne out by electron microscopy. Therefore, the sinusoids of the pituitary are no longer considered to be part of the reticuloendothelial system. The sinusoids at the periphery of the gland continue into collecting venules that join an extensive venous plexus in the capsule.

The glandular cells are classified as *chromophilic* or *chromophobic* on the basis of their avidity or lack of affinity for the dyes used in routine staining of histological sections. The chromophilic cells were originally subdivided into *acidophilic cells* or *basophilic cells*, according to the tinctorial reactions of their specific granules in sections stained with eosin and alum-hematoxylin or with other combinations of an acidic and a basic dye.

It is important to realize that the terms acidophilic and basophilic as used by the pituitary cytologist do not have the same con-

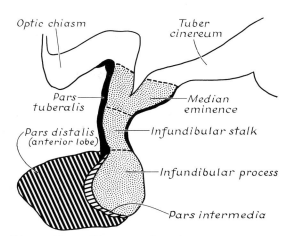

Figure 18-3 Diagram of midsagittal section of hypothalamus and hypophysis of man to show relations of major divisions and subdivisions of the gland to the hypothalamus. (Modified from Tilney.)

notation with respect to the chemistry of the cytoplasm that they generally have in other fields of cytology. The basophilia of the granules in the pituitary basophilic cell is not to be confused with that resulting from ribonucleoprotein in other glandular cells. In the naming of the pituitary cells, *acidophilic* and *basophilic* refer only to the staining affinities of the specific granules. Historically these terms were reasonable and adequate in that they served to distinguish two major classes of chromophilic cells at a time when there were only a few empirically developed staining combinations in routine use, and when the great diversity of pituitary functions was not yet appreciated. As time has passed, the number of hormones known to be secreted by the adenohypophysis has increased to seven. The effort to identify cell types to which synthesis of each of these hormones could be attributed led to the development of numerous staining methods. The terminological problem has been greatly aggravated by the fact that most of the staining procedures now considered useful for the study of the adenohypophysis do not make use of an acid and a basic dye but involve mixtures of acid dyes. With many of these methods, staining does not depend on the binding of a dye by a tissue component of opposite charge, and no conclusion as to the chemical nature of the granules can be drawn from their color in sections stained in this way. The color of specific granules of the same cell type may be red, orange, purple, or blue, depending on the combination of acid dyes used. With the trichrome staining methods, it has been necessary to establish the relation of the cell types to the traditional acidophilic, basophilic, and chromophobic categories by comparison of the same cells in consecutive sections stained with trichrome mixtures and with hematoxylin and eosin.

The most meaningful histochemical method for identification of cell categories is the periodic acid–Schiff (PAS) reaction, which selectively stains the granules of basophils because of their content of glycoprotein. Another approach of proved value for identification of the cell of origin of various hormones involves the use of immunohistochemical procedures. In these methods, antibodies to a specific hormone are induced in another species and are conjugated with fluorescent dyes or with horseradish peroxidase. These labeled antibodies are then reacted with sections of hypophysis and the sites of the antigen in the tissue are localized by fluorescence microscopy or by the histochemical method for peroxidase.

Electron microscopic studies have shown that the specific granules of the cells in the adenohypophysis differ significantly in their size. Granule size and shape are therefore valuable criteria for distinguishing cell types in electron micrographs.

Various systems of nomenclature based on Greek letter designations have been proposed to avoid the inconsistency involved in continued use of "acidophilic" and "basophilic," but none of these has gained widespread acceptance. The terminology now in

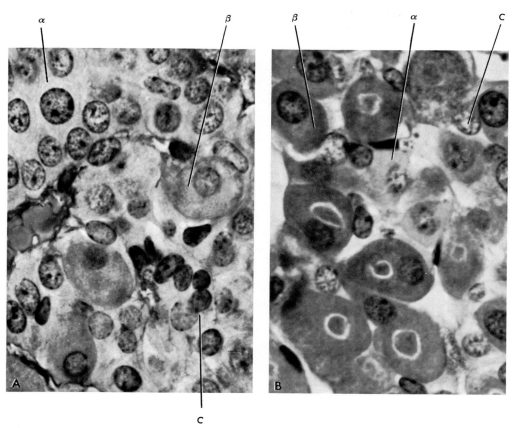

Figure 18–4 Photomicrographs of anterior lobe of hypophysis of adult rats. *A*, Normal female rat. *B*, Castrated female rat of same age. Hypertrophy of basophil cells (β), with enlargement of the Golgi complexes (here shown next to each nucleus as a negative image and appearing as a clear halo), and reduction in acidophil (α) and chromophobe (C) cells follow castration. Zenker-formol, Mallory-azan. × 1300. (Courtesy of I. Gersh.)

general use is therefore a confusing mixture of terms in which acidophilic, basophilic, and chromophobic are used to designate three major classes of cells in the adenohypophysis, while various Greek letters or adjectives referring to distinctive tinctorial reactions are used to identify specific cell types within these classes. There has been a trend in recent years to substitute terms that identify the hormone secreted or the end-organ stimulated (e.g., gonadotrope, thyrotrope, corticotrope).

The description of the fine structure of the cell types which follows is based mainly upon the laboratory rat, because comparable studies of human hypophysis are not yet available. The general principles will be the same, although some interspecific differences will no doubt be found.

ACIDOPHILS (ALPHA CELLS)

These cells, 14 to 19 μm. in diameter in the human, are rounded or ovoid, with a well-developed juxtanuclear Golgi apparatus and small rod-shaped mitochondria. Their refractile granules are large enough to be resolved with the light microscope if adequately separated. In routine preparations, they stain with eosin, so that this category of cells is easily identified in routine preparations.

Two types of acidophils can be distinguished in a number of mammalian species, on the basis of special staining methods, granule size, and other criteria.

Somatotrope

The acidophils that are usually arranged in groups along the sinusoids, and which stain preferentially with orange G, are believed to produce growth hormone *(somatotropin)*, and are therefore called *somatotropes*. They have numerous dense, spherical granules 350 to 400 nm. in diameter (Figs. 18–5 and 18–6). Cisternae of the granular endoplasmic reticulum are often parallel to the cell surface, but occasionally they form concentric systems.

The conclusion that these are the cells that are responsible for growth hormone production is based upon several independent kinds of evidence. Human pituitary gigantism resulting from an excess of growth hormone is associated with tumors of the pars distalis that are composed of acidophils. Immunohistochemical studies involving use of fluorescein-labeled antibody to purified growth hormone have localized the hormone in acidophils of the human hypophysis (Leznoff et al.). It has been possible to dissociate the cells of the rat anterior pituitary with mild trypsin treatment and to separate the cell types. Growth hormone was found to be associated with cells that exhibited the granule size and other cytological characteristics described above (Malamed et al.). Differential centrifugation of homogenates of the anterior lobe has yielded a number of granule fractions. One type of rapidly sedimenting granules, which are acidophilic and in the size range of 325 to 600 nm., have been shown to contain somatotropin and prolactin (Hymer and McShan). Other evidence indicates that the prolactin resides in the larger granules that come from the other type of acidophil, the mammatrope.

Mammatrope (Luteotrope, Prolactin Cell)

Acidophils of the second category tend to be distributed individually in the interior of the cell cords. They have an affinity for azocarmine, in a modified Heidenhain's azan trichrome stain (Dawson) or for erythrosin in a tetrachrome stain (Herlant and Pasteels). Their granules are 550 to 615 nm. in diameter and often irregular in outline (Fig. 18–7). These cells are believed to secrete *prolactin* or *luteotropin* (LTH). In the nonlactating sexually mature female, the endoplasmic reticulum occurs in the form of short cisternae near the cell periphery. During lactation, these cells hypertrophy. Their Golgi apparatus enlarges and their reticulum becomes more extensive, forming multiple layers parallel to the plasmalemma. The mammatropes also have a moderate number of lysosomes.

The period of greatest activity of the mammatropes is during the postpartum prolactin secretion necessary to initiate and maintain lactation. When suckling is terminated, the lysosomes appear to have an important role in the elimination of excess secretory granules and in the involution of the hypertrophied cellular organelles involved in the earlier period of active protein synthesis. The secretory granules fuse with lysosomes to form autophagic vacuoles in which they are degraded by hydrolytic enzymes (Fig. 18–8). This method of disposal of secretory granules that are no longer needed has been called *crinophagy*. Excess membranes and ribosomes of the reticulum are also enclosed in membranes and degraded by autophagy until the hypertrophied mammatropes have reverted to the relatively inactive state characteristic of the normal cycling female (Smith and Farquhar).

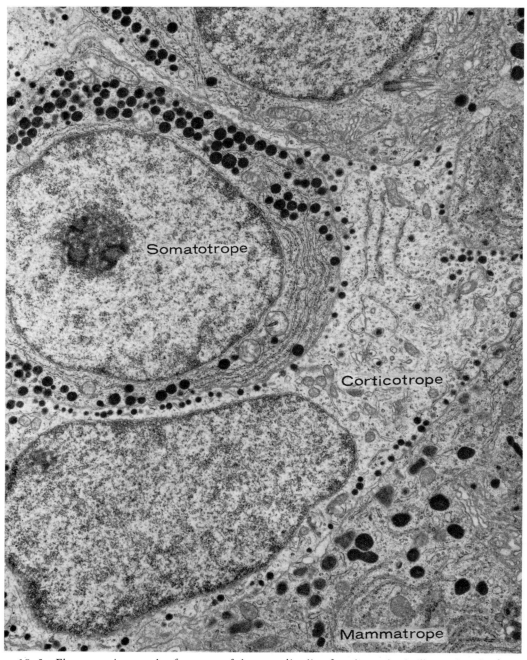

Figure 18–5 Electron micrograph of an area of the pars distalis of rat hypophysis illustrating the fine structure and relative size of the specific granules of a somatotrope, mammatrope, and corticotrope. (Micrograph courtesy of I. Nakayama, F. A. Nickerson, and F. R. Shelton, Lab. Invest. *21*:169, 1969.)

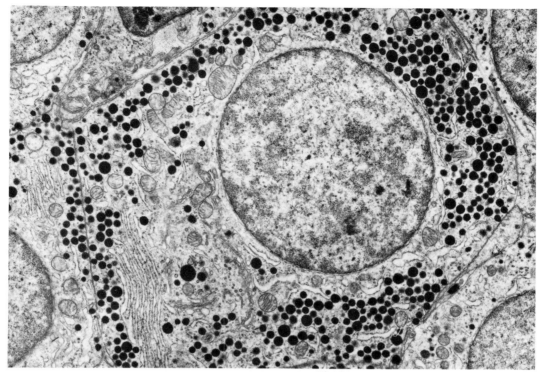

Figure 18-6   A typical somatotrope, showing numerous cisternae of endoplasmic reticulum, a well developed Golgi complex, and many specific granules about 350 nm. in diameter. (Micrograph courtesy of M. Farquhar.)

BASOPHILS (BETA CELLS)

This group of cellular elements of the anterior pituitary stains poorly with hematoxylin and is less easily identified in routine preparations than are the acidophils. Basophils stain very well with the aniline blue of Mallory's trichrome and with resorcin-fuchsin. The basophils are most easily distinguished from acidophils by their pink staining with the PAS reaction for carbohydrates. The basophils seem to comprise at least two distinct cell types: the *thyrotropes* and *gonadotropes*. Centrifugally isolated basophilic granules have been shown to contain thyrotropin and gonadotropin.

Thyrotropes (Beta Basophils)

These are elongated or polygonal cells arranged in clusters in the center of the anterior hypophysis. They are usually not in contact with the sinusoids but are more deeply situated in the cords. The thyrotropes

can be distinguished from other basophils by the selective staining of their granules with aldehyde fuchsin. In electron micrographs, their granules are among the smallest in the pituitary, being 140 to 160 nm. in diameter, somewhat irregular in outline, and less dense than the granules of other types of basophils. The granules tend to congregate at the periphery of the cell.

Evidence for assignment of thyrotropin secretion to this cell type depends upon the experimental observation that they hypertrophy following thyroidectomy and atrophy after thyroxin administration. Immunohistochemical studies using peroxidase-labeled antibody against thyrotropic hormone localize the hormone in cells with the characteristics just described.

Gonadotropes (Delta Basophils)

Basophils of this type are larger than the others and rounded in outline. They are usually situated adjacent to sinusoids. They are PAS-positive but do not stain with aldehyde-fuchsin. There is a prominent juxtanuclear Golgi apparatus and a well-developed endoplasmic reticulum with meandering cisternae that are often distended with a homogeneous content of low density (Fig. 18–9). The granules are spherical and 150 to 250 nm. in diameter. Cells of this type secrete follicle stimulating hormone (FSH) and luteinizing hormone (LH). Some workers believe that the two hormones are synthesized by two distinct cell types, *FSH gonadotropes* and *LH gonadotropes*. There are some indications that two populations of gonadotropes respond differently to castration and to administration of LH and FSH, but the evidence for two distinct types of gonadotropes is not yet compelling. When sections of pituitary are exposed to separately labelled antibodies against LH and against FSH, the gonadotropes centrally located in the gland react mainly with antibody against LH, but some at the periphery of the gland appear to contain both FSH and LH (Nakane).

CHROMOPHOBES (RESERVE CELLS)

Chromophobes are usually small cells located in groups in the interior of the cell cords. They generally have less cytoplasm than the chromophilic cells but may rarely reach the dimensions of acidophils or basophils. Traditionally, chromophobes have been considered to be devoid of specific granules, but electron micrographs reveal relatively few cells with no specific granules. It seems likely that many of the cells identified as chromophobes with the light microscope are, in fact, partially degranulated chromophil cells.

Mitoses are relatively few in the anterior lobe. For this reason, it was formerly thought that the shifts in proportions of the three major cell categories were the result of transformations of one cell type to another. Investigations of these population shifts led to proposals of several cell lineages based upon observation of what were presumed to be morphological transition stages. The most

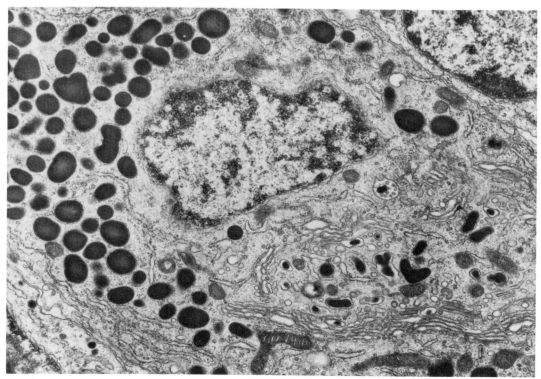

Figure 18–7 Electron micrograph of a rat mammatrope. Notice the relatively large size and irregular shape of the granules. A number of developing granules are associated with a large Golgi complex at the lower right of the figure. (Micrograph courtesy of M. Farquhar and T. Kanaseki.)

widely accepted of these schemes considered the chromophobes to be a reserve population of relatively undifferentiated cells capable of differentiating into either acidophils or basophils. It has become increasingly apparent that the cells classified as chromophobes by light microscopy are not a homogeneous population. Some are evidently chromophils degranulated to the point that their specific nature is not detectable. There seems to be a considerable degree of cytological specialization among the cells normally classified as chromophobes. Some are said to have a Golgi apparatus characteristic of acidophils, while in others the Golgi apparatus resembles that of basophils. It is probable that many of the apparent chromophobes are already determined and capable of differentiating into only one of the chromophil types. If chromophobes that are nonspecific stem cells exist at all, they are evidently much less numerous than they were formerly thought to be.

It is probable that some of the cells classified as chromophobes are actually cell types with a few granules that are of such small size that they are not resolved with the light microscope. Such a cell type is the *corticotrope*.

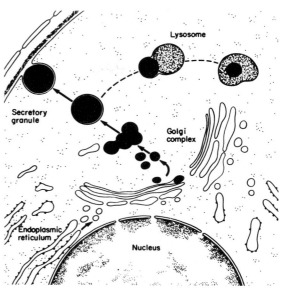

Figure 18–8 Diagram illustrating the secretory pathway of a mammatrope. Small granules are formed in the Golgi complex and subsequently fuse to form larger granules, often of irregular outline. During lactation, they are discharged by exocytosis, but after the young are weaned, excess granules fuse with lysosomes and are destroyed by autophagy. (After R. E. Smith and M. G. Farquhar, J. Cell Biol., 31:319, 1966.)

Corticotrope

This cell type is present in small numbers distributed throughout the gland. They are irregularly stellate in shape, with cell processes that extend between and partially surround neighboring cells to end on the walls of sinusoids. They stain very faintly with the PAS reaction. The cytoplasm in electron micrographs is of low density and has a rather sparse endoplasmic reticulum. Relatively few granules accumulate in these cells. Those that are present are 200 to 250 nm. in diameter and are located for the most part immediately beneath the cell membrane (Fig. 18–5). This peripheral location of the granules and the irregular shape of the cells are valuable identifying criteria (Siperstein; Nakayama and Shelton). These characteristics also account for the fact that efforts to achieve a distinctive staining of these cells have failed, and they have usually been identified as chromophobes.

Following adrenalectomy, cells of this nature become more numerous, are larger, and have more granules than the corresponding cells of control animals (Siperstein and Miller). Cells with the characteristics attributed to corticotropes are stained with peroxidase-labeled antibody against corticotropin. There is a profound reduction in their size and degree of staining after prolonged administration of cortisol, their size correlating directly with the assayed content of corticotropin in the pituitary gland (Baker et al.).

BLOOD SUPPLY

The blood supply of the hypophysis is unusual and is intimately involved in the control of the secretory activity of the gland. Two *inferior hypophyseal* arteries from the internal carotid arborize within the capsule of the gland, sending branches to the posterior lobe and to a lesser extent to the sinusoids of the anterior lobe. Several *superior hypophyseal* arteries arise from the internal carotid artery and posterior communicating artery of the circle of Willis and anastomose freely in the region of the median eminence of the hypothalamus and base of the pituitary stalk (Figs. 18–2 and 18–11). From these vessels, capillaries comprising the so-called *primary plexus* extend into the median eminence and are then returned to the surface, where they are collected into veins that run downward around the hypophyseal stalk to supply the sinusoids of the adenohypophysis below. The venules connecting capillaries in the median eminence with the sinusoidal capillaries of the anterior lobe constitute the *hypophyseoportal* system. The venous drainage of the hypophysis is chiefly through vessels that run in the vascular layer of the capsule to the diaphragm of the sella turcica and thence into adjacent dural sinuses. Some venous blood may also enter sinuses in the sphenoid bone. There is strong evidence that neurohumoral substances (*releasing factors* or *hypophyseotropic hormones*) released by nerves in the median eminence of the hypothalamus are carried in the blood via the hypophyseoportal system to the adenohypophysis, where they stimulate the cells to release their specific hormones.

HISTOPHYSIOLOGY OF THE PARS DISTALIS

Surgical removal of the anterior lobe results in cessation of growth in young animals; atrophy of the adrenal cortex, thyroid, testis, and ovaries; and disturbances of carbohydrate, protein, and lipid metabolism. These profound and potentially fatal effects of hypophysectomy are the collective consequences of eliminating the source of the following hormones, which have been isolated in nearly pure form from the anterior lobe.

Growth Hormone (Somatotropin, STH)

This is a protein hormone composed of about 188 amino acid residues, having a

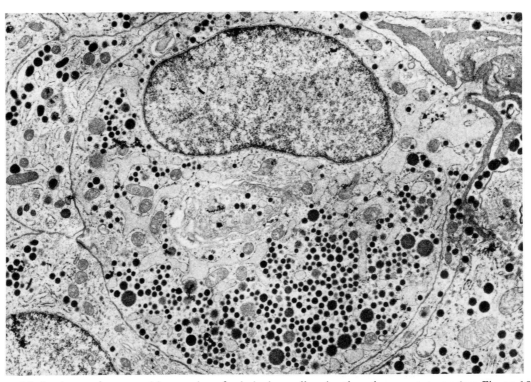

Figure 18-9 A gonadotrope with granules of relatively smaller size than the somatotrope (see Figure 18-6) but displaying considerable variability. The endoplasmic reticulum is typically distended with an amorphous material of low density. (Micrograph courtesy of M. Farquhar.)

Hormones	Cell Type		Staining reactions*		Electron microscopic description
	General	Specific	AF	PAS	
Growth or somato-tropic hormone (STH)	Acidophil	Somatotrope	–	–	350 nm. granules, cells columnar and arranged in groups on sinusoids
Lactogenic or luteo-tropic hormone (LTH)	Acidophil	Mammotrope or luteotrope	–	–	600 nm. elliptical gran-ules, cells located indi-vidually in interior of cell cords
Thyrotropic hormone (TSH)	Basophil	Thyrotrope	+	+	140 nm. granules, cells angular and not usually located on sinusoids
Follicle stimulating hormone (FSH)	Basophil	FSH Gonadotrope	–	+	200 nm. granules, cells located on sinusoids and are usually rounded
Luteinizing hormone (LH)	Basophil	LH Gonadotrope	–	+	200 nm. granules, cells usually located on sinusoids, rounded and contain bizarre cyto-plasmic formations
Adrenocorticotropic hormone (ACTH)	Chromophobe	Corticotrope	–	–	200–250 nm. granules, cells pale, stellate. Few granules at cell periphery
No specific hormone	Chromophobe	Acidophilic chromophobe Basophilic chromophobe	–	–	Few characteristic granules

*AF, Aldehyde fuchsin; PAS, periodic acid–Schiff.

Figure 18–10   A summary of current views of rat anterior pituitary cell types and their secretions. (Modified from McShan and Hartley, Ergebn. Physiol., 56:264, 1965.)

molecular weight of about 21,000, and which does not have any carbohydrate constituents. It plays an important part in the normal growth of the body. The cessation of growth that follows hypophysectomy is reversed by administration of this hormone, and gigan-tism may be produced experimentally by giving excessive doses. Dwarfism in certain strains of mice has been traced to a con-genital defect in the development of the hypophysis. The hormone has a nearly specific growth effect on epiphyseal cartilage. Simultaneous administration of thyroid extracts augments the action of the growth hormone, while simultaneous administration of adrenocorticotropic hormone inhibits its action. Certain tumors of the anterior lobe in children cause *gigantism* by inducing contin-ued growth in length of the bones. If such tumors arise after closure of the epiphyseal plates, they cause *acromegaly*, in which the bones become thicker, the hands and feet broader, the mandible heavier, and the cal-varia thicker.

Somatotropin also plays a significant role in the metabolism of proteins, fats, and car-bohydrates, and it appears to enhance the effectiveness of certain other hormones.

Follicle Stimulating Hormone (FSH)

FSH is a water soluble glycoprotein with molecular weight of about 30,000. It has not yet been isolated in pure form. It promotes the growth of ovarian follicles in the female and stimulates the seminiferous tubules of the testis in the male. The atrophy of the female sex organs that follows hypophysectomy is largely reversed by administration of this hormone. Luteinizing hormone is also required for secretion of adequate amounts of estrogen by the follicles and for maintenance of spermatogenesis in the male.

Luteinizing Hormone (LH or ICSH)

This glycoprotein hormone has a molecular weight of about 26,000. It reverses the involution of the interstitial cells of the ovary in hypophysectomized animals, but causes luteinization of follicles only after they have been ripened by prior treatment with follicle stimulating hormone. Luteinizing hormone activates the interstitial cells of the testis and stimulates their production of androgenic steroid hormones.

Prolactin (Lactogenic Hormone)

Prolactin is a protein hormone consisting of a single chain of 205 amino acids having a molecular weight of about 25,000. It has diverse functions in different species. In rodents and possibly other mammals it has a "luteotropic" effect—that is, it promotes the secretion of progesterone by the corpus luteum of the ovary. It is also involved in causing secretion of milk after the ducts and secretory portions of the mammary gland have been developed in response to ovarian hormones.

Procedures that can be used for isolation of prolactin from domestic animal pituitaries

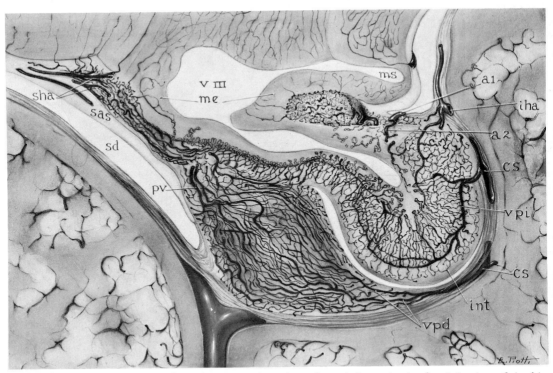

Figure 18–11 Drawing of a thick median sagittal section of a cat's hypophysis after injection of the blood vascular system with India ink. The main blood supply is via the superior hypophyseal artery (*sha*) and inferior hypophyseal arteries (*iha*). The venous drainage is via systemic veins from the pars distalis (*vpd*) and the pars nervosa (*vpi*). Portal veins arising in capillaries in the median eminence and pars tuberalis (*pv*) carry the neurohumoral releasing hormones from the median eminence of the hypothalamus (*me*) to the pars distalis. *sas*, Subarachnoid space; *sd*, subdural space; *viii*, third ventricle; *a1* and *a2*, branches of inferior hypophyseal artery; *cs*, capsular venous sinuses; *int*, pars intermedia. (G. B. Wislocki, Anat. Rec., 69:361, 1937.)

are less satisfactory for the human gland. Fractions possessing prolactin activity have all been rich in growth hormone as well. Thus it has yet to be clearly established that the prolactin activity of human pituitary resides in a unique protein distinct from growth hormone.

Adrenocorticotropic Hormone (ACTH, Corticotropin)

This is a straight chained polypeptide with 39 amino acid residues and a molecular weight of about 4500. Its complete synthesis has been accomplished. The minimum requirement for its biological activity resides in the first 13 amino acids from the N-terminal end. When given to hypophysectomized animals, ACTH repairs the atrophy of the adrenal cortex, particularly the zona fasciculata and reticularis, and stimulates the production of adrenal glucocorticoids.

Thyrotropic Hormone (TSH, Thyrotropin)

Thyrotropic hormone appears to be a basic glycoprotein of molecular weight of about 25,000. The atrophic thyroid of hypophysectomized animals is restored to normal by administration of TSH. It stimulates hypertrophy of thyroid cells and promotes their secretion.

Other Possible Hormones

A number of other functions have been attributed to the anterior lobe of the pituitary, but these are less well established than those enumerated above. Some of them may prove to be the result of combined action of two or more of the hormones already mentioned or may be mediated by effects on other endocrine glands.

Histophysiological Correlations

The cell types believed to be responsible for secretion of these hormones have already been identified. Elaboration of somatotropin and prolactin are attributed to two morphologically distinct types of acidophil. The glycoprotein gonadotropic hormones FSH and LH are assigned to the PAS positive basophils. There is reason to believe that basophils that also stain with aldehyde-fuchsin are respon-

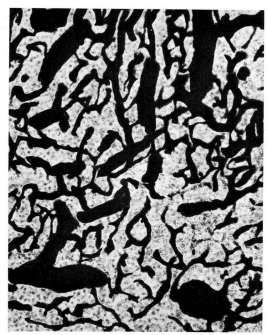

Figure 18–12 Photomicrograph of anterior lobe of hypophysis of monkey injected intravenously with India ink to show the irregular, richly anastomotic sinusoids. × 165. (Courtesy of I. Gersh.)

sible for secretion of thyrotropin. In addition to the histochemical and biochemical evidence relating these hormones to the basophils, there is experimental evidence based upon the negative feedback mechanisms that operate in the regulation of hormone release.

Endocrine glands that are under the direct control of the anterior lobe hormones usually exert a reciprocal inhibiting effect upon hypophyseal function via the hypothalamus. Removal of the target organ therefore results in hypertrophy of those cells in the adenohypophysis responsible for elaboration of the corresponding tropic hormone. After castration, the rat hypophysis contains increased amounts of gonadotropic hormones, and at the same time the basophils become markedly enlarged and vacuolated in a characteristic way (*castration cells*, Fig. 18–4). Thyroidectomy also results in an increase in the percentage of another type of basophil, *thyroidectomy cells*.

Releasing Hormones

The adenohypophysis has long been regarded as the "master gland" because of its role in regulation of other endocrine glands, but recently it has become apparent that the adenohypophysis in turn is regulated by centers in the hypothalamus. Neurosecretory cells in that region of the brain produce *releasing factors (releasing hormones)*. These are liberated in the perivascular spaces and carried via the hypophyseoportal vessels to the pars distalis, where they cause release of specific pituitary hormones. The releasing hormones are relatively small peptides and most of them have been sequenced and the structure confirmed by synthesis. There are believed to be six chemically distinct releasing factors, one for each of the six anterior pituitary hormones: corticotropin releasing hormone (CRH), thyrotropin releasing hormone (TRH), somatotropin releasing hormone (GHRH), and so forth. The mechanism of gonadotropin release is complex and it is not certain that there are separate hormones for

release of FSH and LH. A common designation used therefore is FSH/LH-RH or Gn-RH.

The releasing hormones increase the concentration of cyclic AMP in anterior pituitary tissue incubated in vitro. Moreover, upon addition of cyclic AMP to the incubation medium of intact pituitary tissue or isolated cells, there is a rapid release of growth hormone and prolactin. Electron micrographs of pituitaries or dissociated cells fixed at this time show active exocytosis of specific granules, and at later times hypertrophy of the Golgi apparatus.

PARS INTERMEDIA

In many mammals, the pars distalis is separated from the neurohypophysis by a cleft, lined on the juxtaneural side by a

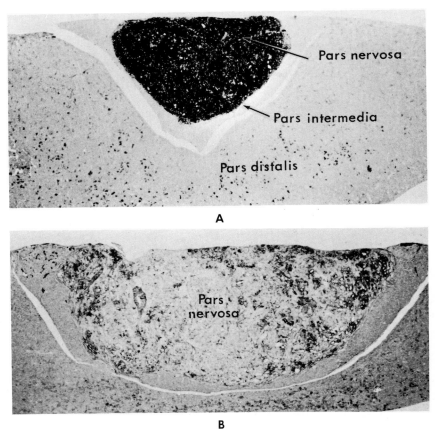

Figure 18–13 Photomicrograph of cross sections of rat hypophysis stained with paraldehyde-fuchsin. *A,* Hypophysis of a normal control rat showing abundant densely stained neurosecretory material in the neurohypophysis. *B,* Hypophysis of a rat of the Brattleboro strain with hypothalamic diabetes insipidus. The neurohypophysis is unusually large but contains very little neurosecretion (black). × 40. (After H. W. Soko and H. Valtin, Endocrinology, 77:692, 1965.)

multilayered epithelium of basophilic cells comprising the pars intermedia. In the human embryo there is a distinct cleft, and the pars intermedia is represented by a typical stratified epithelium adjacent to the infundibular process. The cleft may persist in young children and, rarely, in adults. In such cases the posterior wall consists of several layers of small basophilic cells forming a discrete pars intermedia. In the great majority of humans, however, the cleft becomes discontinuous in postnatal life and is represented in the adult by a zone of cysts (Rathke's cysts). These are often lined by ciliated epithelium and contain a colorless to yellow colloidal material that varies in consistency from a thin to a highly viscous fluid. With the disappearance of the cleft, the epithelium of the pars intermedia adjacent to the neural lobe becomes an inconspicuous, discontinuous layer, and its basophilic cells not infrequently extend some distance into the neural tissue of the infundibular process. Thus, the pars intermedia of man differs from that of most mammals in several respects: the cleft is rarely complete; cysts are of common occurrence; and the basophilic cells extend into the neural lobe, sometimes to a surprising degree. Whereas in rodents such as the mouse the pars intermedia constitutes some 19 per cent of the hypophysis, it forms only 2 per cent in man. In the whale, porpoise, manatee, and some birds, the intermediate lobe is entirely lacking.

The cells of the pars intermedia are polygonal or prismatic and are basophilic in their staining properties. At the light microscope level their nucleus and cytoplasmic organelles are in no way unusual and resemble those of the basophils of the pars distalis. In the cytoplasm there are small granules (200 to 300 nm.), barely visible with the light microscope but clearly seen in electron micrographs. The granules are often polarized toward the basal lamina, they consist of glycoprotein and stain with the PAS reaction and with aldehyde-fuchsin or resorcin-fuchsin. The carbohydrate staining reactions of the granules in this instance are not correlated with the chemical nature of the hormone. The only hormone known to be secreted by the pars intermedia is *melanocyte stimulating hormone* (MSH), a simple polypeptide having close structural affinities to adrenocorticotropin (ACTH). It is possible, however, that in the cell it is bound to glycoprotein in the granules.

In mammals generally the pars intermedia is rather poorly vascularized. In man, numerous anastomoses between the superior and inferior hypophyseal arteries traverse the pars intermedia, and it receives some supply from a rich capillary network in the connective tissue layer that incompletely separates it from the neural lobe. This plexus is continuous with the capillary bed of the neural lobe but also has some connections with the sinusoids of the pars distalis.

Nerve fibers enter the pars intermedia from the neural lobe and ramify among its cells. These nerves, originating in the hypothalamus, appear to have a mainly inhibitory effect. In some mammalian species, their interruption by stalk section results in hypertrophy of the intermedia. In amphibia, their interruption results in increased liberation of the hormone of the intermediate lobe. Neurosecretory material has been demonstrated in some of the nerves of the pars intermedia in amphibians and some mammals but has not been reported in man.

HISTOPHYSIOLOGY OF THE PARS INTERMEDIA

Melanocyte stimulating hormone (MSH) of the hypophysis appears to be produced mainly in the pars intermedia. The evidence for this is the demonstration that removal of the anterior and intermediate lobes of the hypophysis in frogs results in skin lightening, and when these lobes are then transplanted separately into tadpoles, only the intermediate lobe transplants produce skin darkening (Allen). The pars intermedia is anatomically associated with the neural lobe and comes away with it when the anterior and posterior lobes are separated. Assays of the separated portions show 10 times more MSH activity in the posterior and intermediate lobe portion.

A highly basic melanocyte stimulating polypeptide was first isolated in pure form by Lee and Lerner from pig pituitary glands. This is now designated α-MSH. A slightly acidic polypeptide isolated by Benfey and Purvis from the same source is called β-MSH. These two forms of MSH have since been isolated from pituitaries of other species, including man. α-MSH contains 13 amino acids in a sequence that is identical to one portion of the molecule of adrenocorticotropic hormone (ACTH). β-MSH contains 18 amino acids, of which seven are in a sequence similar to part of the ACTH molecule. The common structure of certain regions of MSH and ACTH is believed to account for the fact that ACTH shows some melanocyte stimulating activity.

The effect of MSH upon pigmentation in amphibian skin is to cause dispersion of the melanin granules in chromatophores and consequent darkening of the skin. There is evidence that it also affects the synthesis of melanin. In mammals whose melanocytes are not subject to expansion and contraction, as are the melanophores of lower animals, the effect of the hormone appears to be on melanin production. The pigmentation that occurs in humans suffering from deterioration of the adrenal cortex (Addison's disease) is apparently due to the release by the hypophysis of excess ACTH and MSH, both of which have melanocyte stimulating properties. The darkening of the skin during human pregnancy may also result from increased release of one or both of these hormones.

PARS INFUNDIBULARIS OR TUBERALIS

Like the pars intermedia, the pars tuberalis constitutes only a small part of the hypophysis. Both are adjacent to and continuous with the anterior lobe. The pars tuberalis is 25 to 60 μm. thick and forms a sleeve around the stalk, the thickest portion being on its anterior surface (Fig. 18–3). It is frequently incomplete on the posterior surface of the stalk. The distinctive morphological characteristic of the pars tuberalis is the longitudinal arrangement of its cords of epithelial cells, which occupy the interstices between the longitudinally oriented blood vessels.

The pars tuberalis is the most highly vascularized subdivision of the hypophysis, because it is traversed by the major arterial supply for the anterior lobe and the hypothalamohypophyseal venous portal system. The pars tuberalis is separated from the infundibular stalk by a thin layer of connective tissue continuous with the pia. On the outside, the connective tissue is typical arachnoidal membrane. Between these, the blood vessels and groups of epithelial cells are supported by reticular fibers.

The epithelial cells of the pars tuberalis include undifferentiated cells and some small acidophilic and basophilic cells. The main component is a cuboidal-columnar cell, which may reach 12 to 18 μm. in size and contains numerous small granules or sometimes fine colloid droplets. The mitochondria are short rods, and numerous small lipid droplets may be present. These are the only cells in the adult hypophysis containing large amounts of glycogen. The cells may be arranged to form follicle-like structures. Islands of squamous epithelial cells, 50 to 70 μm. in extent, may also be present. Despite the occurrence of a pars tuberalis in all vertebrates studied, the epithelial cells are not known to have any distinctive hormonal function.

NEUROHYPOPHYSIS

The median eminence of the tuber cinereum, the infundibular stalk, and infundibular process together comprise the neurohypophysis (Fig. 18–3). It consists of an intrinsic population of cells, the *pituicytes*, and the terminal portions of the axons belonging to extrinsic secretory neurons, whose cell bodies are located in the hypothalamus. The bulk of its substance is made up of a large bundle of approximately 100,000 unmyelinated nerve fibers comprising the *hypothalamohypophyseal tract*. This tract originates from the *supraoptic nucleus* of the hypothalamus close to the optic chiasm, and from the *paraventricular nucleus* in the wall of the third ventricle, with minor contributions from other hypothalamic areas. The fibers from these sources converge upon the median eminence and course down the infundibular stem into the infundibular process. There they do not terminate upon nerve cells or other effector cells but end blindly in intimate relation to the vessels of the rich capillary plexus of the pars nervosa.

Throughout the neurohypophysis—but particularly abundant in the infundibular process—are spherical masses of highly variable size that stain deeply with the chrome alum-hematoxylin stain. These are the so-called *Herring bodies* (Fig. 18–14). They were originally misinterpreted as a product of the pars intermedia and were thought to be situated in the extracellular spaces. They are now known to be local accumulations of neurosecretory material in the axoplasm of fibers of the hypothalamohypophyseal tract. Stainable neurosecretory material can be traced upward along the tract and can also be demonstrated in the cell bodies of the neurons in the hypothalamic nuclei. Electron microscope studies of these secretory neurons reveal cytological characteristics that are comparable to those of other protein secreting cells. Granular endoplasmic reticulum (Nissl substance) is abundant and is presumably the site of hormone synthesis. The hormone product, probably bound to some carrier protein, is segregated by the Golgi apparatus in membrane bounded electron-dense secretion granules 120 to 200 nm. in diameter. Granules of the same type are found in irregular accumulations along the length of axons destined for the neurohypophysis. In the pars nervosa, greatly dilated portions of axons are densely packed with granules. These undoubtedly correspond to the Herring bodies seen by light microscopy in sections stained with chrome alum-hematoxylin.

Surgical interruption of the hypophyseal stalk is followed by gradual disappearance of detectable hormone and of stainable neurosecretory substance in the infundibular process distal to the lesion, and by a concomitant accumulation of both in the stump proximal to the site of stalk section. From these observations, it is concluded that the Herring bodies of light microscopy and the 120 to 200 nm. dense granules seen in electron micrographs represent neurosecretory material that is formed in the cells of the supraoptic and paraventricular nuclei of the hypothalamus, transported along the nerve fibers, and stored in their terminals in the infundibular process.

Evidence for the association of the hormones with the stainable neurosecretory material and the electron-dense granules is of two kinds. Both stainable material and electron-dense granules disappear from the neurohypophysis under conditions of severe hormone depletion. Density gradient centrifugation of homogenates of neurohypophyseal tissue yields a fraction containing the neurosecretory granules, and this is very rich in hormone activity.

The terminal arborizations of the axons in the neural lobe abut on the basal lamina of capillaries (Fig. 18–15). The endothelial cells forming the walls of the capillaries of the pars nervosa, like those of the pars distalis and other endocrine glands, are extremely attenuated and penetrated by circular fenestrations closed only by thin diaphragms. In addition to the dense neurosecretory gran-

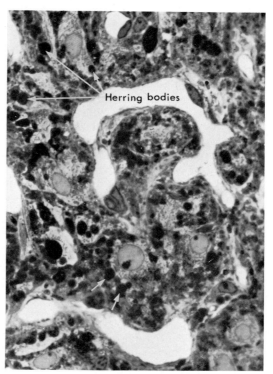

Figure 18–14 Photomicrograph of rat neurohypophysis fixed by perfusion. The large clear areas are capillaries. The dark rounded masses indicated by arrows are Herring bodies. In electron micrographs these are resolved as accumulations of neurosecretory material in dilatation of nerve axons. × 950. (Courtesy of P. Orkand and S. L. Palay.)

ules, the nerve endings contain aggregations of small vesicles similar to those found in synaptic terminals elsewhere in the nervous system. Secretion granules never appear free in the perivascular space and may not be released from the nerve endings as such. The hormones may possibly be released from the granules in the nerve terminals and traverse the perivascular space and the endothelium in molecular dispersion. The role of the small agranular vesicles in hormone release is unknown.

Distributed among the nerve fibers in the infundibular process are the *pituicytes*. In man they are highly variable in size and shape and commonly contain pigment granules that reduce silver directly or blacken with the methods of Bielschowsky and Hortega. These cells were extensively studied by Gersh and by Romeis, who distinguished several types and believed that one or more of them secreted the hormones of the neurohypophysis. The pituicytes are no longer believed to have a secretory function. Electron microscopic studies have greatly clarified their nature. Their structural relation to the nerve fibers is similar to that of the neuroglial cells of the central nervous system. The cytoplasmic processes meander among clusters of pre-terminal secretory axons and often intimately envelop their granule-filled expansions (Herring bodies). Many processes of pituicytes end upon the perivascular space, along with the nerve terminals. It is not known whether their only function is supportive or whether they have some metabolic role in the secretion process.

HISTOPHYSIOLOGY OF THE NEUROHYPOPHYSIS

The neural lobe of the hypophysis is the site of storage and release of two closely re-lated hormones, *oxytocin* and *vasopressin* (anti-diuretic hormone, ADH). Both have been isolated in pure form, their structure has been determined, and they have been synthe-sized (du Vigneaud). They are cyclic poly-peptides consisting of eight different amino acids.

In the pars nervosa they seem to be bound to a large protein carrier molecule, *neurophysin*, which may constitute the bulk of the Herring bodies. Oxytocin causes contrac-tion of uterine smooth muscle during coitus and at the time of delivery. It also causes con-traction of myoepithelial cells in the alveoli of the mammary gland, thus mediating the *milk ejection reflex* in response to suckling in lactating animals (Fig. 18–16).

Vasopressin raises the blood pressure by stimulating contraction of smooth muscle in the walls of small blood vessels, and conserves body water by promoting reabsorption of water in the distal convoluted tubules of the kidney (Fig. 18–17). The antidiuretic effect of the hormone is physiologically more im-

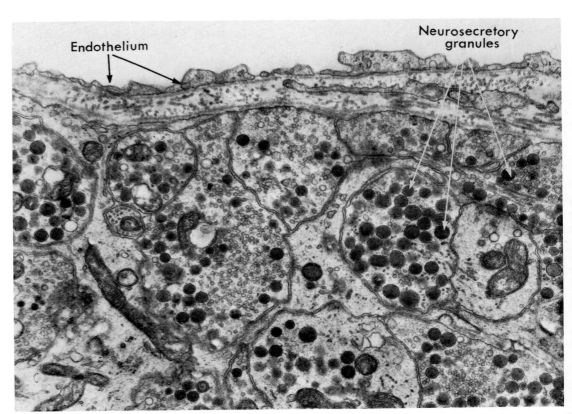

Figure 18–15 Electron micrograph of rat neurohypophysis, showing neurosecretory granules and small vesicles in the axoplasm of fibers of the hypothalamo-hypophyseal tract ending in close relation to a capillary × 22,000. (Courtesy of P. Orkand and S. L. Palay.)

portant than the pressor effect, and therefore vasopressin is often referred to as antidiuretic hormone.

Humans with tumor or injury to the hypothalamus may develop *diabetes insipidus,* a condition in which the capacity of the kidney to concentrate the glomerular filtrate is lost. A very large volume of urine is eliminated (polyuria) and the patient, driven by thirst, drinks a large quantity of water (polydipsia). A similar condition can be produced in experimental animals by hypothalamic lesions that destroy the supraoptico-hypophyseal tracts. A strain of rats with hereditary diabetes insipidus is now available for experimental study (Sokol). These animals are apparently unable to synthesize vasopressin and have a daily water consumption of 80 per cent of

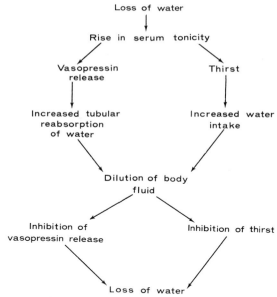

Figure 18–17 Diagram of the role of vasopressin or antidiuretic hormone of the neurohypophysis in regulation of the concentration of body fluids. Interaction of the neurohypophysis, the thirst center of the hypothalamus, and renal tubules results in maintenance of a constant osmolarity of the body fluids. (After A. Leaf and C. H. Coggins, in R. H. Williams, Textbook of Endocrinology. Philadelphia, W. B. Saunders Co., 1968.)

their weight and a urine output of 70 per cent of their weight. Sections of their hypophysis stained with aldehyde-fuchsin reveal little or no staining of neurosecretory material and a conspicuous compensatory hypertrophy of the neurohypophysis (Fig. 18–13). The neurons of the supraoptic nucleus also show hypertrophy and contain very few neurosecretory granules.

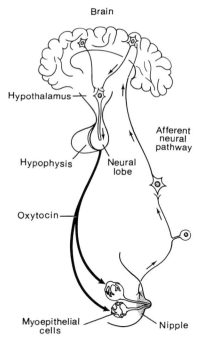

Figure 18–16 Diagram illustrating the role of oxytocin in the suckling reflex. Stimulation of the nipples generates sensory impulses that pass to the brain via dorsal root ganglia. In the brain, these impulses are relayed to the hypothalamus where they activate neurosecretory cells whose processes extend into the pars nervosa of the hypophysis. Stimulation of these cells results in release of the hormone oxytocin, which is carried in the blood to the mammary gland, where it causes contraction of myoepithelial cells, causing milk to be expressed.

REFERENCES

Allen, B. M.: Extirpation of the hypophysis and thyroid glands of *Rana pipiens.* Science, *44:*755, 1916.

Baker, B. L.: Studies on hormone localization with emphasis on the hypophysis. J. Histochem. Cytochem., *18:*1, 1970.

Baker, B. L., S. Pek, A. R. Midgley, Jr., and B. E. Gersten: Identification of the corticotropin cell in rat hypophysis with peroxidase-labelled antibody. Anat. Rec., *166:*557, 1969.

Barer, R., H. Heller, and K. Lederis: The isolation, identification and properties of the hormonal granules of the neurohypophysis. Proc. Roy. Soc. B., *158:*388, 1963.

Barer, R., and K. Lederis: Ultrastructure of the rabbit neurohypophysis with special reference to the release of hormones. Zeitschr. f. Zellforsch., 75:201, 1966.

Bargmann, W., A. Knoop, and A. Thiel: Elektronenmikroskopische Studie an der Neurohypophyse von *Tropidonotus natrix*. Zeitschr. f. Zellforsch., 47:114, 1957.

Bargmann, W., and E. Scharrer: The site of origin of the hormones of the posterior pituitary. Am. Scientist, 39:255, 1961.

Benfey, B. J., and J. L. Purvis: Purification and amino acid composition of melanophore-expanding hormone from hog pituitary gland. J. Amer. Chem. Soc., 77:5167, 1955.

Bergland, R.: The surgical significance of the anatomical variations surrounding the pituitary. Anat. Rec., 157:396, 1967.

Bodian, D.: Cytological aspects of neurosecretion in opossum neurohypophysis. Bull. Johns Hopkins Hosp., 113:57, 1963.

Bodian, D.: Herring bodies and neuroapocrine secretion in the monkey. An electron microscopic study of the fate of the neurosecretory product. Bull. Johns Hopkins Hosp., 118:282, 1966.

Bogdanove, E. M., and S. A. DiAngelo: The effects of hypothalamic lesions on goitrogenesis and pituitary TSH secretion in the propylthiouracil-treated guinea pig Endocrinology, 64:53, 1959.

Bogdanove, E. M., and N. S. Halmi: Effects of hypothalamic lesions and subsequent propylthiouracil treatment on pituitary structure and function in the rat. Endocrinology, 53:274, 1953.

Burgers, A. C. J.: Melanophore-stimulating hormones in vertebrates. Ann. N.Y. Acad. Sci., 100:669, 1963.

Dawson, A. B.: The demonstration by differential staining of two types of acidophile in the anterior pituitary gland of the rat. Anat. Rec., 120:810, 1954.

du Vigneaud, V.: Trail of sulfur research from insulin to oxytocin. Science, 123:967, 1956.

du Vigneaud, V., H. C. Lawler, and E. A. Popenoe: The synthesis of an oxtapeptide amine with the hormonal activity of ocytocin. J. Am. Chem. Soc., 75:4879, 1953.

Everett, J. W., and C. H. Sawyer: Estimated duration of the spontaneous activation which causes release of ovulating hormone from the rat hypophysis. Endocrinology, 52:83, 1953.

Farquhar, M. G.: Fine structure and function in capillaries of the anterior pituitary gland. Angiology, 12:270, 1961.

Farquhar, M. G., and J. F. Rinehart: Cytologic alterations in the anterior pituitary gland following thyroidectomy; an electron microscope study. Endocrinology, 55:857, 1954.

Furth, J.: Experimental pituitary tumors. *In* Pincus, G., ed.: Recent Progress in Hormone Research, Vol. XI, p. 221. New York, Academic Press, 1955.

Green, J. D.: The comparative anatomy of the portal vascular system and of the innervation of the hypophysis. *In* Harris, G. W., and B. T. Donovan, eds.: The Pituitary Gland. Vol. I, p. 127. Berkeley, University of California Press, 1966.

Green, J. D., and G. W. Harris: The neurovascular link between the neurohypophysis and adenohypophysis. J. Endocrinol., 5:136, 1947.

Greep, R. O.: Architecture of the final common path to the adenohypophysis. Fertil. Steril., 14:153, 1963.

Halmi, N. S.: Two types of basophils in the rat pituitary; "thyrotrophs" and "gonadotrophs" vs. beta and delta cells. Endocrinology, 50:140, 1952.

Harris, G. W.: Neural Control of the Pituitary Gland. London, Edward Arnold, Ltd., 1955.

Heller, H., ed.: The Neurohypophysis. New York, Academic Press, 1957.

Herbert, D. C., and T. Hayashida: Prolactin localization in the primate pituitary by immunofluorescence. Science, 169:378, 1970.

Herlant, M., and L. Pasteels: Histophysiology of the human anterior pituitary. Meth. Achievm. Exp. Path., 3:250, 1967.

Hopkins, C. R., and M. G. Farquhar: Hormone secretion by cells dissociated from rat anterior pituitaries. J. Cell Biol., 59:276, 1973.

Hume, D. M.: The neuroendocrine response to injury; present status of the problem. Ann. Surg., 138:548, 1953.

Hunt, T. E.: Mitotic activity in the anterior hypophysis of female rats. Anat. Rec., 82:263, 1942.

Hymer, W. C., and W. H. McShan: Isolation of rat pituitary granules and the study of their biochemical properties and hormonal activities. J. Cell Biol., 17:67, 1963.

Lederis, J.: An electron microscopical study of the human neurohypophysis. Zeitschr. f. Zellforsch., 65:847, 1965.

Lee, T. H., and A. B. Lerner: Isolation of melanocyte-stimulating hormone from hog pituitary gland. J. Biol. Chem., 221:943, 1956.

Lerner, A. B., and J. S. McGuire: Effects of alpha- and beta-melanocyte stimulating hormones on skin colour in man. Nature, 189:176, 1961.

Lerner, A. B., and Y. Takahashi: Hormonal control of melanin pigmentation. Rec. Prog. Hormone Res., 12:203, 1956.

Leznoff, A., J. Fishman, L. Goodfriend, E. McGarry, J. Beck, and B. Rose: Localization of fluorescent antibodies to human growth hormone in human anterior pituitary glands. Proc. Soc. Exper. Biol. Med., 104:232, 1960.

Malamed, S., R. Postanova, and G. Sayers: Fine structure of trypsin dissociated cells of the rat anterior pituitary gland. Proc. Soc. Exp. Biol. Med., 138:920, 1971.

McShan, W. H., and M. W. Hartley: Production, storage, and release of anterior pituitary hormones. Ergebn. Physiol. 56:264, 1965.

Midgley, A. R., Jr.: Immunofluorescent localization of human pituitary luteinizing hormone. Exper. Cell Res., 32:606, 1963.

Nakane, P.: Simultaneous localization of multiple tissue antigens using the peroxidase-labeled antibody method: A study on the pituitary gland of the rat. J. Histochem. Cytochem., 16:557, 1968.

Nakane, P. K.: Classification of anterior pituitary cell types with immunoenzyme histochemistry. J. Histochem. Cytochem., 18:9, 1970.

Nakayama, I., F. A. Nickerson, and F. R. Shelton: An ultrastructural study of the adrenocorticotrophic hormone secreting cell of the rat adenohypophysis during adrenal cortical regeneration. Lab. Invest., 21:169, 1969.

Palay, S. L.: The fine structure of the neurohypophysis. *In* Waelsch, H., ed.: Progress in Neurobiology. II. Ultrastructure and Cellular Chemistry of Neural Tissue. New York, Paul B. Hoeber, Inc., 1957.

Pelletier, G., A. LeMay, G. Béraud, and F. Labrie: Ultrastructural changes accompanying the stimulatory effect of monobutyryl adenosine 3'-5'-monophosphate on the release of growth hormone, prolactin, and adrenocorticotropic hormone in vitro. Endocrinology 91:1355, 1972.

Pickford, M.: Neurohypophysis and kidney function. *In* Harris, G. W., and B. T. Donovan, eds.: The Pituitary

Gland. Vol. 3, p. 374. Berkeley, University of California Press, 1966.

Pooley, A.: Ultrastructure and size of rat anterior pituitary secretory granules. Endocrinology, 88:400, 1971.

Purves, H. D.: Morphology of the hypophysis related to its function. *In* Young, W. C., ed.: Sex and Internal Secretions. 2nd ed. Vol. I, p. 161. Baltimore, Williams & Wilkins, 1961.

Purves, H. D.: Cytology of the adenohypophysis. *In* Harris, G. W., and B. T. Donovan, eds.: The Pituitary Gland. Vol. 1, p. 147. Berkeley, University of California Press, 1966.

Rennels, E. G.: Two tinctorial types of gonadotrophs in the rat hypophysis. Zeitschr. f. Zellforsch., 45:464, 1957.

Rinehart, J. F., and M. G. Farquhar: The fine vascular organization of the anterior pituitary gland; an electron microscopic study with histochemical correlations. Anat. Rec., 121:207, 1955.

Sawyer, W. H.: Comparative physiology and pharmacology of the neurohypophysis. Rec. Prog. Hormone Res., 17:437, 1961.

Sawyer, W. H.: Vertebrate neurohypophyseal principles. Endocrinology, 75:981, 1964.

Scharrer, E., and B. Scharrer: Hormones produced by neurosecretory cells. Rec. Prog. Hormone Res., 10:183, 1954.

Scharrer, E., and B. Scharrer: Neurosekretion. *In* von Möllendorff, W., and W. Bargmann, eds.: Handbuch der mikroskopischen Anatomie des Menschen. Vol. 6, Part 5, p. 953. Berlin, Springer Verlag, 1954.

Simpson, M. E., C. W. Asling, and H. M. Evans: Some endocrine influences on skeletal growth and differentiation. Yale J. Biol. Med., 23:1, 1950.

Simpson, M. E., H. M. Evans, and C. H. Li: The growth of hypophysectomized female rats following chronic treatment with pure pituitary growth hormone. Growth, 13:151, 1949.

Siperstein, E., and K. Miller: Further cytoplasmic evidence for the identity of the cells that produce ACTH. Endocrinology, 86:451, 1970.

Smith, P. E.: Hypophysectomy and replacement therapy in the rat. Am. J. Anat., 45:205, 1930.

Smith, R., and M. Farquhar: Lysosome function in the regulation of the secretory process in cells of the anterior pituitary gland. J. Cell Biol., 31:319, 1966.

Smith, R. W., Jr., Gaebler, O. H., and C. N. H. Long, eds.: The Hypophyseal Growth Hormone, Nature and Actions. (International symposium, sponsored by Henry Ford Hospital and Edsel B. Ford Institute for Medical Research, Detroit.) New York, Blakiston Division, McGraw-Hill Book Co., 1955.

Sokol, H. W., and H. Valtin: Morphology of the neurosecretory system in rats homozygous and heterozygous for hypothalamic diabetes insipidus (Brattleboro strain). Endocrinology, 77:692, 1965.

Turner, C. D., and J. T. Bagnara: General Endocrinology. 5th ed. Philadelphia, W. B. Saunders Co., 1971.

Wislocki, G. B.: The vascular supply of the hypophysis cerebri of the rhesus monkey and man. Proc. Assoc. Res. Nervous Mental Diseases, 17:48, 1938.

19

The Thyroid Gland

The thyroid gland situated in the anterior part of the neck weighs 25 to 40 gm. It consists of two *lateral lobes* connected by a narrow *isthmus*, which crosses the trachea just below the cricoid cartilage. In about one third of the persons examined, a *pyramidal lobe* extends upward from the isthmus near the left lobe.

The gland is enclosed in a connective tissue capsule that is continuous with the surrounding cervical fascia. This outer capsule is loosely connected on its deep surface to another layer of moderately dense connective tissue that is intimately adherent to the gland. This separation of the capsule into two layers creates a plane of cleavage between the two, which facilitates surgical removal of the gland.

The function of the thyroid is to elaborate, store, and release into the bloodstream *thyroid hormone*, which is concerned with the regulation of metabolic rate. The thyroid differs from other endocrine glands in that a mechanism for extracellular storage of its hormone is highly developed, whereas in other endocrine glands there are only rather limited provisions for intracellular storage.

Histological Organization

The gland is composed of spherical, cystlike follicles 0.02 to 0.9 mm. in diameter, lined with a simple epithelium and containing a gelatinous *colloid* (Figs. 19–1 and 19–2). This represents the stored product of secretory activity by the epithelium lining the follicle. In man there is great variability in the size of the follicles, but the small predominate over the large. In animals other than man, the follicles are of more uniform size. In the rat and guinea pig, those at the periphery of the gland are larger than those more centrally situated.

The follicles are surrounded by an extremely thin basal lamina, which usually is not resolved with the light microscope. With silver stains the follicles are seen to be enclosed by a delicate network of reticular fibers. A close-meshed plexus of capillaries surrounds each follicle (Fig. 19–3). Between the capillary nets of adjacent follicles are the blind terminations of lymphatic vessels, and in some rodent species lymphatics form extensive perifollicular sinusoids. Numerous nerve fibers accompany the blood vessels as they ramify among the follicles. These seem to terminate mainly along the vessels, but in some instances they appear to end in direct contact with the base of the thyroid epithelial cells. The nerves entering the thyroid are postganglionic sympathetic fibers originating in the middle and superior cervical ganglia. There are also preganglionic parasympathetic fibers, and ganglion cells may occasionally be encountered within the thyroid. The nerves to the thyroid are presumed to be mainly vasomotor, inasmuch as transplanted thyroid tissue functions adequately, suggesting that an intact nerve supply is not necessary for secretion.

Follicular Epithelial Cells. The epithelial cells vary in height but are commonly low cuboidal to squamous. In general, the epithelium tends to be squamous when the gland is underactive and columnar when it is overactive, but there are many exceptions, and an accurate assessment of the functional activity of the gland cannot be based upon histological examination alone.

The nucleus of the gland cell is spheroidal, centrally situated, poor in chromatin, and contains one or more nucleoli. The cytoplasm is basophilic; the mitochondria are thin rods and the Golgi apparatus is usually supranuclear. Lipid droplets are common, and

524

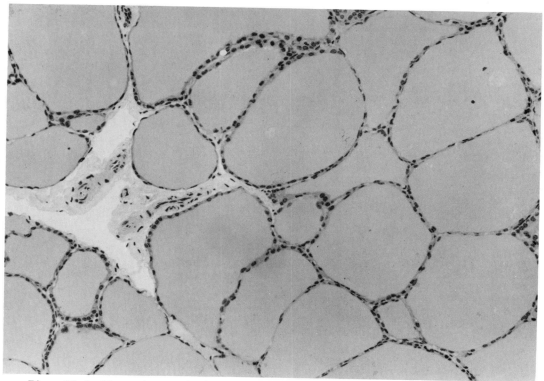

Figure 19–1   Photomicrograph of monkey thyroid showing variations in size of the follicles.

"clear droplets" have been described by various workers using the light microscope and interpreted as globules of colloid. They stain with aniline blue and with the periodic acid–Schiff reaction in much the same way as the colloid in the lumen of the follicle. Granules of varying size, located mainly in the apical cytoplasm, give positive staining reactions for acid phosphatase and esterase and are therefore considered to be lysosomes.

The fresh colloid is optically homogeneous, except for occasional desquamated cells and rare macrophages. After fixation the colloid stains with either acid or basic dyes, and with the trichrome stains it is not uncommon for different follicles or even different areas of the colloid in the same follicle to be colored differently. Although physiological significance has been erroneously ascribed to this multiple staining, the varied patterns observed appear to be due to local differences in concentration of protein that depend upon the direction and rate of penetration of fixative into the tissue block (Mayer). The colloid stains intensely with the

periodic acid–Schiff reaction, because the *thyroglobulin* secreted by the thyroid is a glyco-protein containing 2 to 4 per cent hexos-amine, as well as galactose, mannose, fucose, and other carbohydrates. The thyroglobulin of the colloid also contains various iodinated amino acids. Among these are *thyroxin* (tetra-iodothyronine) and *triiodothyronine*, which when released into the blood, constitute the *thyroid hormone*. The presence of these compounds in the colloid has been demonstrated by microchemical analysis, by ultraviolet absorption spectrophotometry, and by the use of radioactive ^{131}I (Fig. 19–5). The follicle cells were formerly believed to secrete into the colloid a protease that splits thyroglobulin into smaller molecules and liberates the biologically active iodinated derivatives of tyrosine, of which thyroxin is the principal circulating hormone. It is now widely accepted that the proteases act within the thyroid cells upon thyroglobulin taken up from the lumen of the follicle.

In electron micrographs the follicles of the human thyroid are found to be composed of a single layer of low cuboidal cells surrounding a homogeneous, moderately dense colloid. A thin, continuous basal lamina about 500 Å thick surrounds the entire follicle. In the interfollicular spaces are numerous capillaries of the fenestrated type, occasional fibroblasts, and small bundles of collagen fibrils. The follicle cells are joined laterally by typical junctional complexes, and the free surfaces bear a small number of short, irregularly oriented microvilli. In follicles with cuboidal epithelium, the microvilli are somewhat more numerous. The basal plasma membrane is smoothly contoured and not infolded. The relatively large nucleus is centrally placed and has an eccentric nucleolus. The mitochondria are relatively few and uniformly distributed. Their cristae are not especially numerous. The endoplasmic reticulum varies in its degree of development. In the flattened cells there are only a few elongated cisternal profiles, but in the cuboidal cells the reticulum is well developed (Fig. 19–6). The Golgi apparatus is in a supranuclear or paranuclear position and is composed of flattened or dilated saccules, vacuoles, and small vesicles. Small vesicles similar to those of the Golgi apparatus are present in abundance throughout the cytoplasm. Multivesicular bodies are also common. Membrane limited dense bodies 0.5 to 0.7 μm. in diameter are plentiful in the apical cytoplasm. These are lysosomes.

Parafollicular Cells. In addition to the principal cells of the thyroid follicles, there is another, smaller population of cells, present both in the follicular epithelium and in the interfollicular spaces. These cells were first described by Baker (1877) and Hürthle (1894) and studied in greater detail by Nonidez (1931) (Figs. 19–7 and 19–8), but evidence permitting assignment of a function to them was not forthcoming until 30 years later. They are variously designated as *parafollicular cells, light cells, mitochondria-rich cells, C-cells,* and *ultimobranchial cells.* The term

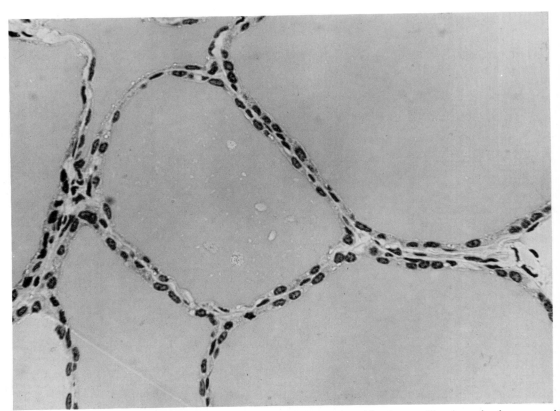

Figure 19–2 Photomicrograph of monkey thyroid at higher magnification to illustrate the homogenei of the colloid and the character of the epithelium.

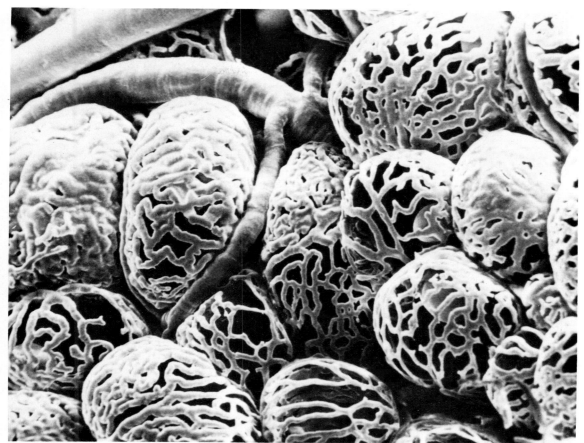

Figure 19-3 Scanning electron micrograph of a monkey thyroid in which the blood vessels have been injected with plastic and the tissue digested away. Each spherical follicle is surrounded by a dense network of capillaries. (Micrograph by courtesy of H. Fujita and T. Murakami, from Archivum Histologicum Japonicum 36:181, 1974.)

"parafollicular cell" was introduced to distinguish these cells from other interfollicular cells, some of which may be undifferentiated embryonal elements or connective tissue cells. They arise during embryonic life from the last pair of pharyngeal pouches. In fishes, amphibians, reptiles, and birds, they form discrete epithelial cell masses called *ultimobranchial bodies*, located in the neck or mediastinum. In mammals, they are incorporated into the thyroid. They are often larger than the principal cells and in routine histological preparations, they stain less deeply. They can be selectively stained by the silver nitrate method of Cajal, which reveals the presence of brown or black cytoplasmic granules (Figs. 19–7 and 19–8). The granules exhibit an affinity for aniline blue in trichrome stains. Cytochemically they are distinguished from follicular cells by their high level of activity of the mitochondrial enzyme α-glycerophosphate dehydrogenase (Pearse).

Where the parafollicular cells are intercalated among the principal cells· of the follicles, they are closer to the base of the epithelium; evidently, they never border directly on the lumen but are separated from it by overarching processes of neighboring principal cells (Fig. 19–9). The secretory granules are not easily preserved and had been extracted during preparation of the specimens that formed the basis of the early descriptions of parafollicular cell ultrastructure. They are adequately preserved by aldehyde fixatives and appear as membrane-limited, dense, spherical granules 0.1 to 0.4 μm. in diameter (Fig. 19–9). The parafollicular cells elaborate and secrete the blood calcium lowering hormone, *calcitonin.*

HISTOPHYSIOLOGY OF THE THYROID GLAND

The function of the thyroid gland is to synthesize, store, and release hormones concerned with the regulation of metabolic rate (thyroxin and triiodothyronine) and with maintenance of blood calcium levels within tolerable limits (calcitonin). The function related to metabolic rate resides in the follicular epithelial cells, whereas the calcium regulating action resides in the parafollicular cells.

THE PRINCIPAL CELLS

The thyroid is perhaps the only endocrine gland that stores its product extracellularly (in the lumen of the follicle). The secretory process is therefore somewhat more

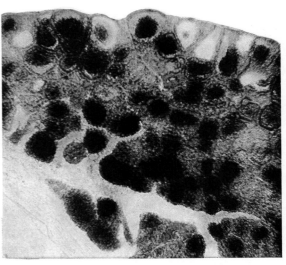

Figure 19–5 Low-power photomicrograph of autoradiograph of thyroid gland of rat previously injected with [131]I. The blackened areas represent sites of deposition of the radioactive material. There is great variability in the content of the isotope in the several follicles. In a few places the epithelium is blackened. (Courtesy of C. P. Leblond, D. Findlay, and S. Gross.)

complex than that in other glands. It involves (1) synthesis of the large protein thyroglobulin; (2) iodination of tyrosine molecules that are important constituents of thyroglobulin; (3) release of thyroglobulin into the lumen of the follicle for storage; (4) reabsorption of thyroglobulin into the follicular epithelial cells; (5) hydrolysis of thyroglobulin to liberate thyroxin and triiodothyronine; and (6) release of these hormones into the perifollicular capillaries and lymphatics.

Synthesis of thyroglobulin involves the same intracellular pathway described for other protein secreting cells. Amino acids are assembled into polypeptides on ribosomes of the endoplasmic reticulum, then transported to the Golgi complex. Since thyroglobulin is a glycoprotein, the Golgi apparatus no doubt plays a role in synthesis and conjugation of its carbohydrate components. From the Golgi complex, the product is transported in small vesicles to the apical surface of the cell, where it is discharged by exocytosis.

The thyroid has the capacity to concentrate iodine to several hundred thousand times the concentration of this element in the blood plasma. After an injection of inorganic iodide, 40 per cent of the circulating ion is

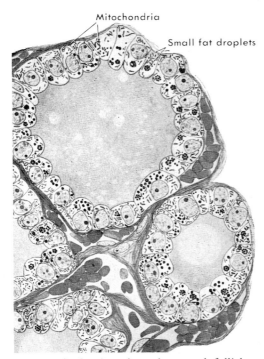

Mitochondria

Small fat droplets

Figure 19–4 Section through several follicles of human thyroid. Aniline–acid fuchsin. (Courtesy of R. R. Bensley.)

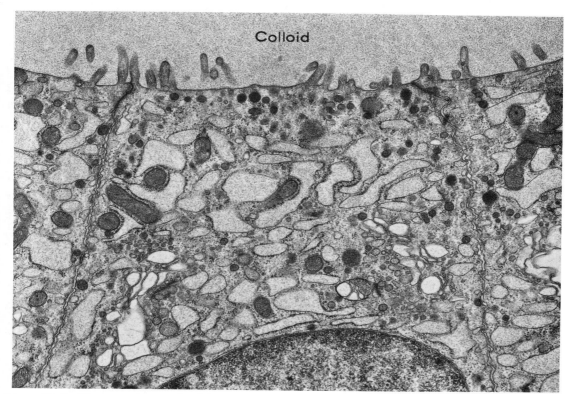

Figure 19-6   Electron micrograph of the apical half of an epithelial cell from rat thyroid gland. The free surface of the cell is provided with numerous short microvilli that project into the colloid of the follicle. The endoplasmic reticulum is well developed and its cisternae are distended with an amorphous content of low density. The small dense granules are lysosomes. (Micrograph courtesy of S. Wissig.)

concentrated in the thyroid gland within 10 minutes. The iodine is used to iodinate tyrosine molecules that are ultimately incorporated into the thyroglobulin. The synthesis of thyroglobulin and its iodination are apparently independent, and while the sites of synthesis of the glycoprotein are well known, the site of its iodination has been a subject of controversy—some believe that it takes place in the cells, whereas others contend that it occurs in the lumen of the follicle. After iodine is actively transported from the blood into the cells, it is oxidized in the presence of hydrogen peroxide to a different ionic species. The oxidized iodide ion subsequently iodinates the tyrosine residues of thyroglobulin to form mono- and diiodotyrosine. Triiodothyronine is formed when one molecule each of monoiodotyrosine and diiodotyrosine are coupled. Thyroxin is formed when two molecules of diiodotyrosine are joined. Since both the initial oxidation of iodide and the subsequent iodination of tyrosine may be catalyzed by the

enzyme peroxidase, histochemical localization of this enzyme seemed a reasonable approach for determining the site of iodination (Strum and Karnovsky, 1970). Peroxidase is found in the perinuclear cisternae, the endoplasmic reticulum, inner lamellae of the Golgi, apical vesicles, and the external surfaces of the microvilli projecting to the colloid. The reaction product observed in the membranous cell organelles is believed to represent continuous synthesis of peroxidase by the thyroid cells. Peroxidase transported along this pathway is no doubt incorporated into the cell surface membrane. It is believed that the principal site of iodination of thyroglobulin is probably the microvillous border of the thyroid cells, and possibly the apical vesicles. This interpretation is in agreement with autoradiographic studies localizing radioactive iodine at early time intervals over the interface between the epithelium and the colloid.

The uptake of colloid has been studied mainly in animals strongly stimulated to release hormone by administration of thyroid-stimulating hormone (TSH) of the hypophysis (Fig. 19–10). Under these conditions, large droplets containing colloid appear in the

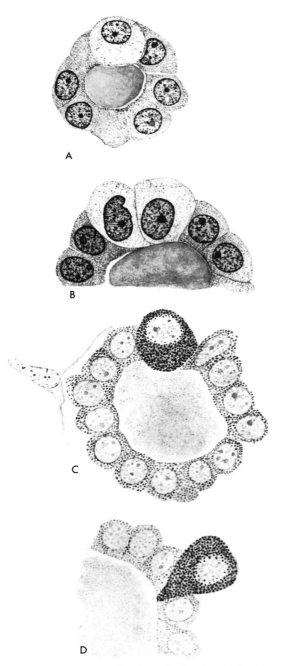

Figure 19–7 Parafollicular cells in thyroid follicles. A, B, Cat thyroid, Ehrlich's hematoxylin; C, D, dog thyroid (35 day old puppy), Cajal silver nitrate method. (After J. F. Nonidez, Amer. J. Anat., 49:479, 1932.)

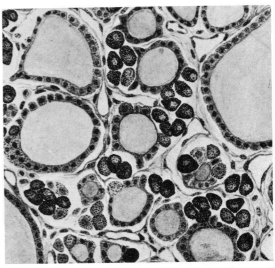

Figure 19–8 Drawing of an area occupied by small and medium-sized follicles in the thyroid of an adult dog. Numerous parafollicular cells are seen in clusters in the interfollicular spaces. Cajal stain. (After J. F. Nonidez, Anat. Rec., 53:339, 1932.)

apical cytoplasm. By microinjection of ferritin into follicles before administration of TSH, it was shown that the large colloid droplets which appeared in the cells after stimulation contained ferritin and hence represented colloid taken up from the lumen, not newly synthesized thyroglobulin (Seljelid).

The hydrolysis of thyroglobulin, formerly attributed to proteases in the lumen of the follicles, is now known to be a function of lysosomes in the epithelial cells. Lysosomes coalesce with the endocytosis vacuoles containing reabsorbed colloid, and add to their contents cathepsins that hydrolyze thyroglobulin (Wolman; Seljelid). The tetraiodothyronine (thyroxin) and triiodothyronine liberated apparently diffuse into the cytoplasmic matrix and through the cell base to enter the blood. This phase of the process cannot be visualized with the electron microscope. As in other endocrine glands, the capillaries of the thyroid are of the fenestrated type and offer little or no barrier to access of hormones to the blood. Whereas the blood vascular system is undoubtedly the most important avenue of egress of thyroid hormone because of the high rate of blood flow, it has been shown that concentration of hormone in the lymph draining the gland is as much as 100 times greater than the concentration in venous blood. Thus

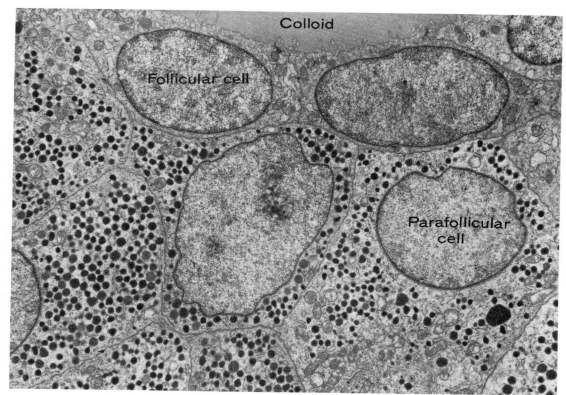

Figure 19-9 Electron micrograph of follicular and parafollicular cells of normal cat thyroid. The granular parafollicular cells do not border on the lumen but are usually separated from the colloid by follicular cells. When adequately fixed, the parafollicular cells contain many dense spherical secretory granules. (Micrograph courtesy of S. Wissig.)

the lymphatics must be considered a significant pathway for transport of hormone to the circulating blood (Daniel et al.).

The activity of the thyroid is regulated by the thyrotropic (or thyroid-stimulating) hormone (TSH) of the anterior lobe of the hypophysis, and this in turn is controlled by thyrotropin releasing factor (TRF) of the hypothalamus. Lowered levels of thyroid hormone in the blood stimulates the hypothalamus to secrete TRF, which results in increased thyrotropin secretion. Excess circulating thyroid hormone depresses thyrotropin secretion. Chronic hypersecretion of thyrotropin results in a highly vascular gland with columnar follicular epithelial cells and relatively little colloid. After hypophysectomy, the thyroid is no longer capable of accumulating significant amounts of ^{131}I and only traces of thyroid hormone appear in the blood.

The most striking effect of thyroid secretion is its control of the *metabolic rate* of the body. When a deficiency of thyroid hormone occurs, the metabolic rate falls below normal; when there is an excess, the metabolic rate rises above normal. When *hypothyroidism* begins in infancy and persists, it leads to *cretinism*, a condition attended by stunting of physical and mental development. When hypofunction begins in adulthood and persists, it leads to *myxedema*, a disorder characterized by a sallow, puffy appearance, dry sparse hair, lethargy and slow cerebration. In both conditions the basal metabolic rate is reduced, and in both, the symptoms may be suppressed through timely oral administration of dried thyroid gland.

Enlargement of the thyroid gland is called *goiter*, and any substance that causes enlargement of the thyroid is called a *goitrogen*. When iodine is deficient in the diet, as it tends to be in a number of geographical regions, there is an excess production and accumulation of colloid, but in the absence of sufficient iodine, relatively little active hormone is produced. This compensatory enlargement of the gland is called *colloid goiter*. Antithyroid substances occur naturally in some plants used for food. Excess consumption of these goitrogens may interfere with iodination in the thyroid and result in enlargement. A common form of *hyperthyroidism* in the human is *Graves' disease* or exophthalmic goiter. The follicles become enlarged, with tall cells and papillary projections into the lumen. The mitochondria increase in number, the Golgi apparatus hypertrophies, and colloid is diminished or absent. Such hyperplastic thyroids may secrete thyroxin at five to 10 times the normal rate. The patient suffers weight loss, nervousness, weakness, rapid heart rate, intolerance of heat, and tremor. The increased metabolic rate and associated symptoms return temporarily to normal after administration of iodine and of antithyroid agents, such as thiouracil. The exact cause of Graves' disease is poorly understood, but the blood of patients suffering from it often contains an immunoglobulin of the IgG type which is a long-acting thyroid stimulator (LATS). This substance may play a role in the pathogenesis of the disease.

THE PARAFOLLICULAR CELLS

Compelling evidence has now accumulated indicating that the parafollicular cells produce the hormone calcitonin, which lowers the level of blood calcium. In 1962, Copp and his collaborators, perfusing the thyroid and parathyroid glands of the dog with hypercalcemic blood, demonstrated release of a factor tending to lower blood calcium levels. They originally attributed this factor to the parathyroids and called it "calcitonin." In 1963, Hirsch and his collaborators confirmed the existence of the hypocalcemic factor, but demonstrated that it originated from the thyroid gland, and proposed the name "thyrocalcitonin." Calcium lowering activity has been demonstrated in thyroid tissue from many species, including the dog, rat, rabbit, ox, pig, goat, sheep, birds, and man.

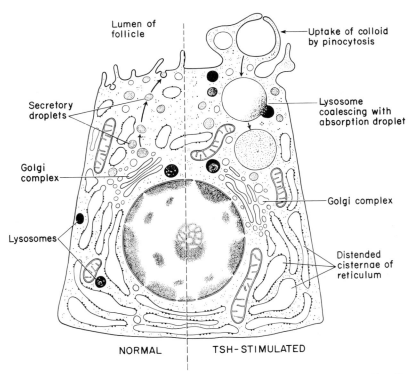

Figure 19-10 Left side: Diagram depicting the normal ultrastructure of the thyroid cell secreting thyroglobulin into the lumen of the follicle. Right side: The uptake of colloid by pinocytosis after stimulation with thyroid-stimulating hormone, and the lysosomal degradation of thyroglobulin to release thyroxin. (From D. W. Fawcett, J. A. Long, and A. L. Jones, Rec. Progr. Hormone Res. 25:315–380, 1969, Academic Press, New York.)

Several lines of evidence associated the calcium lowering factor with the parafollicular cells: (1) Sustained elevation of calcium results in degranulation of these cells; (2) extractable calcitonin correlates well with the presence and number of such cells; (3) human medullary carcinomas of the thyroid, which are thought to arise from the parafollicular or C-cells, contain 100 to 10,000 times as much calcitonin as normal thyroid tissue; (4) fluorescent antibodies to calcitonin are said to bind selectively to the C-cells.

The hormone was extracted in pure form from pig thyroid glands by 1968, and it was found to be a polypeptide consisting of a single chain of 32 amino acids. The sequence of the amino acids has been worked out, and the hormone has now been synthesized. Calcitonin of human thyroid origin differs slightly from the porcine hormone.

Calcitonin appears to exert its effect by suppressing release of calcium into the blood from resorption of bone. Bone is constantly undergoing internal remodeling (see Chapter 10). Parathyroid hormone tends to alter the balance between bone deposition and bone absorption so as to cause increased resorption. The calcium released from bone enters the blood, raising the blood calcium level. Parathyroid hormone acts upon osteocytes and osteoclasts, accelerating osteolysis. Calcitonin appears to have an opposite effect upon these cells, decreasing bone resorption and thus lowering the blood calcium level.

The role of calcitonin in normal human blood calcium regulation is less well established than in experimental animals. However, hypercalcitonism is thought to occur in medullary carcinoma and in certain adenomas of the human thyroid.

REFERENCES

Anast, C. S.: Thyrocalcitonin—A review. Clinical Orthopedics and Related Research, No. 47, p. 179, 1966.

Andros, G., and S. H. Wollman: Autoradiographic localization of iodine[125] in the thyroid epithelial cell. Proc. Soc. Exper. Biol. Med., 115:775, 1964.

Baghdiantz, A., G. V. Foster, A. Edwards, M. A. Kumar, E. Slack, H. A. Soliman, and I. MacIntyre: Extraction and purification of calcitonin. Nature, 203:1927, 1964.

Bargmann, W.: Schildrüse. In von Möllendorff, W., and W. Bargmann, eds.: Handbuch der mikroskopischen Anatomie des Menschen. Berlin, Julius Springer, 1939, Vol. 6, part 2, p. 2.

Bogdanove, E. M.: Regulation of TSH secretion. Federation Proc., 21:633, 1962.

Bussolati, G., and A. G. E. Pearse: Immunofluorescence localization of calcitonin in the C-cells of pig and dog's thyroid. J. Endocr., 37:205, 1967.

Copp, D. H., E. C. Cameron, B. A. Cheney, A. G. F. Davidson, and K. G. Henze: Evidence for calcitonin—a new hormone from the parathyroid that lowers blood calcium. Endocrinology, 70:637, 1962.

Daniel, P. M., Plaskett, L. G., and Pratt, O. E.: The lymphatic and venous pathways for the outflow of thyroxine, iodoprotein and inorganic iodide from the thyroid gland. J. Physiol. (London), 188:25, 1967.

Dempsey, E. W., and R. R. Peterson: Electron microscopic observations on the thyroid glands of normal, hypophysectomized, cold-exposed and thiouracil-treated rats. Endocrinology, 56:46, 1955.

Dempsey, E. W., and M. Singer: Observations on the chemical cytology of the thyroid gland at different functional stages. Endocrinology, 38:270, 1946.

Ekholm, R.: Thyroid gland. In Kurtz, S. M., ed.: Electron Microscopic Anatomy. New York, Academic Press, 1964.

Falck, B., B. Larsen, C. v. Mecklenburg, C. Rosengren, and K. Svenaeus: On the presence of a second specific cell system in mammalian thyroid gland. Acta Physiol. Scand., 62:491, 1964.

Foster, G. V., A. Baghdiantz, M. A. Kumar, E. Slack, H. A. Soliman, and I. MacIntyre: Thyroid origin of calcitonin. Nature, 202:1303, 1964.

Foster, G. V., I. MacIntyre, and A. G. E. Pearse: Calcitonin production and the mitochondrion-rich cells of the dog thyroid. Nature, 203:1029, 1964.

Fujita, H.: Outline of the fine structural aspects of synthesis and release of thyroid hormone. Gunma Symposium on Endocrinology, 7:49, 1970.

Fujita, H., and T. Murakami: Scanning electron microscopy on the distribution of the minute blood vessels of the dog, rat and Rhesus monkey. Arch. Histol. Jap., 36:181, 1974.

Gersh, I., and R. F. Baker: Total protein and organic iodine in the colloid of individual follicles of the thyroid gland of the rat. J. Comp. Physiol., 21:213, 1943.

Gittes, R. F., and G. L. Irvin: Thyroid and parathyroid roles in hypercalcemia: Evidence for a thyrocalcitonin releasing factor. Science, 148:1737, 1965.

Grollman, A.: Essentials of Endocrinology. Philadelphia, J. B. Lippincott Co., 1947.

Gross, J., and R. Pitt-Rivers: 3:5:3'-Triiodothyronine. 1. Isolation from thyroid gland and synthesis. 2. Physiological activity. Biochem. J., 53:645, 652, 1953.

Heimann, P.: Ultrastructure of the human thyroid. A study of normal thyroid, untreated and treated toxic goiter. Acta Endocr., 53(Suppl. 110):5, 1966.

Hilfer, R. S.: Follicle formation in embryonic chick thyroid. I. Early morphogenesis. J. Morphol., 115:135, 1964.

Hirsch, P. F., F. F. Gauthier, and P. L. Munson: Thyroid hypocalcemic principle and recurrent laryngeal nerve injury as factors affecting the response to parathyroidectomy in rats. Endocrinology, 73:244, 1963.

Hirsch, P. F., and Munson, P. L.: Thyrocalcitonin. Physiol. Rev., 49:548, 1969.

Kumar, M. A., E. Slack, A. Edwards, H. A. Soliman, A. Baghdiantz, G. V. Foster, and I. MacIntyre: A biological assay for calcitonin. J. Endocr., 33:469, 1965.

Leblond, C. P., and J. Gross: Thyroglobulin formation in the thyroid follicle visualized by the "coated autograph" technique. Endocrinology, 43:306, 1948.

MacIntyre, I., G. V. Foster, and M. A. Kumar: The thyroid origin of calcitonin. In Gaillard, P. J., R. V. Talmage, and A. M. Budy, eds.: The Parathyroid Glands: Ultra-structure, Secretion and Function. Chicago, University of Chicago Press, 1965.

Mayer, E.: Introduction to Dynamic Morphology. New York, Academic Press, 1963.

Nadler, N. J., S. K. Sarkar, and C. P. Leblond: Origin of intracellular colloid droplets in the rat thyroid. Endocrinology, 71:120, 1962.

Nadler, N. J., B. A. Young, C. P. Leblond, and B. Mitmaker: Elaboration of thyroglobulin in the thyroid follicle. Endocrinology, 74:333, 1964.

Nonidez, J. F.: The origin of the parafollicular cell, a second epithelial component of the thyroid gland of the dog. Am. J. Anat., 49:479, 1932.

Nonidez, J. F.: Further observations on the parafollicular cells of the mammalian thyroid. Anat. Rec., 53:339, 1932.

Pearse, A. G. E.: The cytochemistry of the thyroid C cells and their relationship to calcitonin. Proc. Roy. Soc. B., 164:478, 1966.

Pitt-Rivers, R.: Mode of action of antithyroid compounds. Physiol. Rev., 30:194, 1950.

Pitt-Rivers, R., and W. R. Trotter, eds.: The Thyroid. London, Butterworths, 1964.

Seljelid, R.: Electron microscopic localization of acid phosphatase in rat thyroid follicle cells after stimu-lation with thyrotropic hormone. J. Histochem. Cytochem., 13:687, 1965.

Seljelid, R.: Endocytosis in thyroid follicle cells. II. A micro-injection study of the origin of colloid droplets. J. Ultrastruct. Res., 17:401, 1967.

Strum, J. M., and M. J. Karnovsky: Cytochemical localization of endogenous peroxidase in thyroid follicular cells. J. Cell Biol., 44:655, 1970.

Turner, C. D., and J. T. Bagnara: General Endocrinology. 5th ed. Philadelphia, W. B. Saunders Co., 1971.

Welzel, B. K., S. S. Spicer, and S. H. Wollman: Changes in fine structure and acid phosphatase localization in rat thyroid cells following thyrotrophin administration. J. Cell Biol., 25:593, 1965.

Wissig, S. L.: The anatomy of secretion in the follicular cells of the thyroid gland; the fine structure of the gland in the normal rat. J. Biophys. Biochem. Cytol., 7:419, 1960.

Wissig, S. L.: The anatomy of secretion in the follicular cells of the thyroid gland. II. The effect of acute thyro-trophic hormone stimulation on the secretory apparatus. J. Cell Biol., 16:93, 1963.

Wolman, S. H., S. S. Spicer, and M. S. Burstone: Localization of esterase and acid phosphatase in granules and colloid droplets in rat thyroid epithelium. J. Cell Biol., 21:191, 1964.

20

Parathyroid Glands

The *parathyroid glands* are small, yellow-brown, oval bodies usually intimately related to the posterior surface of the thyroid gland. In man there are usually four glands, but accessory ones are common. Their total weight varies from 0.05 to 0.3 gm. They may range from 3 to 8 mm. in length, 2 to 5 mm. in width, and 0.5 to 2 mm. in thickness. Most of the glands are associated with the middle third of the thyroid, a smaller number with the inferior third. In 5 to 10 per cent of cases one or more parathyroids are associated with the thymus and may therefore be deep in the anterior mediastinum. This association of the parathyroid glands with the thymus stems from their common origin from the same pharyngeal pouch in the embryo.

Most parathyroid glands lie in the cap-sule of the thyroid, but they may be embedded within the gland. In either case, they are separated from the substance of thyroid by a thin connective tissue capsule. The capsular connective tissue extends into the parathyroid gland, and it is via these trabeculae that the larger branches of blood vessels, nerves, and lymphatics enter. Between the gland cells is a framework of reticular fibers. These support the rich capillary network and the nerve fibers. The connective tissue stroma may contain numerous fat cells.

The parenchyma of the parathyroid glands consists of densely packed groups of cells, which may form a compact mass or may be arranged as anastomosing cords, or less commonly as follicles with a small amount of colloidal material in the lumen. Two main

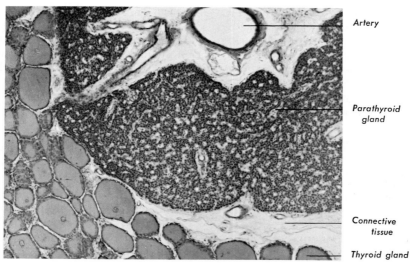

Figure 20–1   Photomicrograph of section of thyroid and parathyroid glands of *Macacus rhesus.* × 80.

535

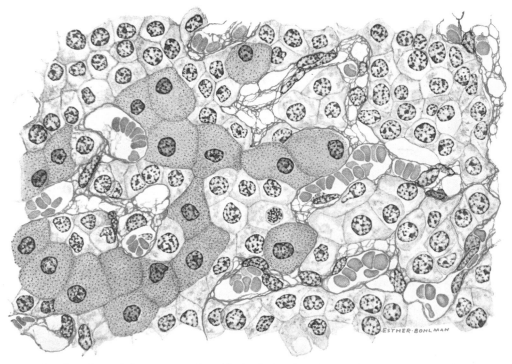

Figure 20–2   Section through human parathyroid gland showing the small principal cells, often vacuolated, and the large oxyphilic cells with fine purplish granules. Zenker-formol fixation. Mallory-azan stain. × 960.

types of epithelial cells have been described in man: *principal cells* and *oxyphilic cells* (Fig. 20–2).

The Principal Cells (Chief Cells)

The principal cells are polygonal and 7 to 10 μm. in diameter, with a centrally placed vesicular nucleus and a pale, slightly acidophilic cytoplasm that tends to shrink during fixation. There is a small juxtanuclear Golgi apparatus and a number of elongated mitochondria. Coarse granular deposits of fluorescent lipofuscin pigment are often present, and when the cells are appropriately stained, a considerable amount of glycogen is found. In addition to these components, small granules have been described that stain with iron-hematoxylin and exhibit argyrophilia with the Bodian stain. These have been interpreted by some investigators as secretory granules (Munger and Roth; Roth).

Electron microscopic studies reaffirm the presence of all of the components enumerated above and reveal, in addition, cisternal profiles of the granular endoplasmic reticulum, sometimes aggregated in conspicuous parallel ar-

rays. The argyrophilic granules at this level of resolution have irregular outlines, are limited by a membrane, and have a dense granular content. They appear to arise in the Golgi apparatus and tend to accumulate at the periphery of the cell. A single abortive cilium is often found projecting from the principal cell into the narrow intercellular space.

A second category of principal cells is distinguished at the electron microscope level. These have a smaller Golgi apparatus, few dense "secretory" granules, and large lakes of glycogen.

The Oxyphilic Cells

The oxyphilic cells are greatly in the minority and occur singly or in small groups. They are distinctly larger than the principal cells. They have a small, darkly staining nucleus and a strongly acidophilic cytoplasm. When stained by the aniline-acid fuchsin method, they are found to have many more mitochondria than the principal cells. This is borne out in electron micrographs, which show a remarkable concentration of elongated mitochondria with numerous closely spaced cristae. In the interstices among the mitochondria are numerous glycogen particles, but these do not form large masses as they do in the less active principal cell. The Golgi apparatus is inconspicuous and the endoplasmic reticulum sparse. The eosinophilic granulation formerly described by light microscopists must be attributed to the abundant mitochondria, for granules resembling secretory granules are rarely encountered in electron micrographs.

Another type of cell, intermediate between the oxyphilic and principal cells, has been described. It has a fine granular cytoplasm, which stains faintly with acid dyes, and a nucleus that is smaller and stains darker than that of the principal cells. Also, "water-clear" cells and "dark oxyphilic" cells have been described, but it is not clear to what extent these latter types are to be attributed to vagaries of fixation.

The parathyroid glands show certain changes with increasing age: (1) an increase in the amount of connective tissue, including increased numbers of fat cells; (2) the oxyphilic cells are said to appear at the age of 4½ to 7 years and to increase in number, especially after puberty; (3) in the closely packed masses of gland cells, some cords and follicles appear in the 1 year old infant, and they increase thereafter; colloid accumulation in the lumen of the follicles shows the same tendency.

When rats are given injections of a large dose of parathyroid extract, the cells of the parathyroid glands become smaller; the Golgi apparatus also becomes smaller and more compact. Both changes are suggestive of decreased functional activity. After two weeks the cells return to normal, both in size and in morphology of the Golgi apparatus, suggesting a resumption of normal secretory activity. During the hypertrophy of the parathyroid glands in rickets, the Golgi apparatus is described as undergoing changes that indicate great secretory activity in comparison with normal cells. It is not possible to extend these conclusions to the human gland, for it has yet to be clearly shown which cells in man are equivalent to those in laboratory animals.

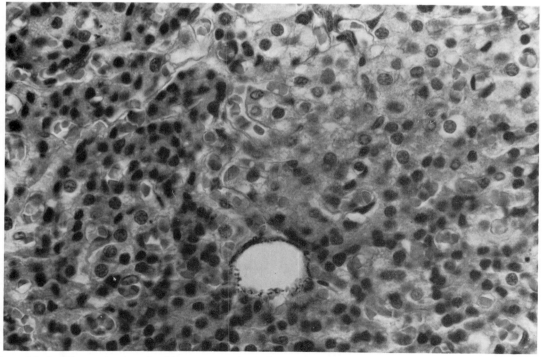

Figure 20–3 Photomicrograph of human parathyroid. Only one adipose cell is shown in this field, but such cells may be very numerous. (Courtesy of S. I. Roth.)

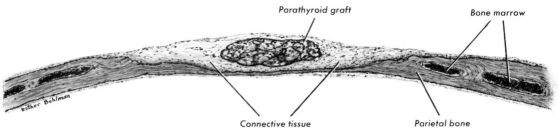

Figure 20-4 Section of parietal bone of rat 14 days after autogenous transplantation of parathyroid gland. The bone beneath the graft has been nearly completely resorbed. × 50. (From a preparation by H. Chang.)

HISTOPHYSIOLOGY

The parathyroid glands are essential for life. Their complete removal results in a precipitous fall in the level of blood calcium, leading to violent tonic spasm of skeletal muscle (tetany) and ultimately to death in most mammalian species. The glands elaborate *parathyroid hormone*, through which they exercise their control over calcium metabolism.

Although active extracts of bovine parathyroids have been available since 1925 there has been remarkable recent progress in our understanding of the chemistry

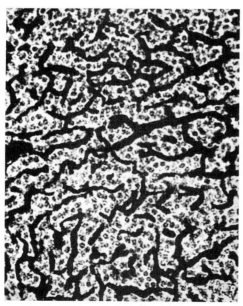

Figure 20-5 Photomicrograph of parathyroid gland of monkey injected intravenously with India ink to show the extensively anastomotic capillary network in intimate contact with the gland cells. × 165. (Courtesy of I. Gersh.)

and physiology of the hormone. A highly purified preparation with 200 times the activity of the earlier standard extract was prepared in 1961 (Rasmussen and Craig) and the amino acid sequence of the hormone was worked out in 1968 (Potts et al.). The hormone is a single chain polypeptide consisting of 84 amino acid residues, and it lacks cysteine. The amino terminal portion of the molecule consisting of 34 amino acids has been synthesized; it has been found to be qualitatively identical to the native hormone in its physiological effects and is nearly as active.

The secretion of parathyroid hormone is under feedback control by the blood calcium concentration. It is the ionized portion of the blood calcium that is the determinant of hormone release. The rate of hormone secretion may reach 50 to 100 times the normal level in response to a marked fall in blood calcium level.

The hormone acts directly upon bone cells, especially the osteocytes and osteoclasts. Its initial rapid effect is to increase the rate of release of calcium from bone mineral into the blood. This appears to be a result of hormonal stimulation of osteocytic osteolysis (see Chapter 10). If the increase in circulating parathyroid hormone continues for some time, there is an acceleration of the process of internal remodeling of bone, which is a function of the osteoclasts.

Parathyroid hormone also has a direct effect upon ion transport in the kidney. Within a very few minutes after administration of the hormone to parathyroidectomized animals, there is an increase in excretion of phosphate, sodium, and potassium in the urine, and a decrease in the clearance of calcium. There may also be an effect upon intestinal transport of calcium, but this is less well established.

The mechanism by which parathyroid hormone exerts its effect upon bone and kidney cells has yet to be completely worked out. There are strong indications, however, that activation of adenyl cyclase and elevated intracellular concentrations of cyclic AMP may be involved. The concentration of cyclic AMP in the urine rises within minutes after administration of the hormone to intact animals. In vitro, an increased activity of adenyl cyclase in kidney and bone can be demonstrated within 15 seconds after adding parathyroid hormone to the system.

The parathyroids may give rise to tumors in which the cells produce excessive amounts of hormone, resulting in *primary hyperparathyroidism*. Such patients have high blood calcium levels, rarefaction of their bones (osteitis fibrosa), low blood phosphate level, kidney stones, and deposits of calcium in other soft tissues. In *rickets*, calcium and phosphate are not adequately absorbed from the diet, owing to a deficiency of vitamin D. The resulting low blood calcium results in a compensatory activation of the parathyroids called *secondary hyperparathyroidism*. Similarly, in severe kidney disease, there may be phosphate retention, resulting in low blood calcium, and consequent hypertrophy of the parathyroids.

REFERENCES

Aurbach, G. D., R. Marcus, J. Heersche, S. Marx, H. Niall, G. W. Tregear, H. T. Keutmann, and J. T. Potts, Jr.: Hormones and other factors regulating calcium metabolism. *In* Robison, G. A., et al., eds.: Cyclic AMP and Cell Function. Ann. N.Y. Acad. Sci., *185*:386, 1971.

Bargmann, W.: Die Epithelkörperchen. *In* von Möllendorff, W., and W. Bargmann, eds.: Handbuch der mikroskopischen Anatomie des Menschen. Berlin, Julius Springer, 1939, Vol. 6, part 2, p. 137.

Barnicot, N. A.: The local action of the parathyroid and other tissues on bone in intracerebral grafts. J. Anat., *82*:233, 1948.

Bensley, S. H.: The normal mode of secretion in the parathyroid gland of the dog. Anat. Rec., *98*:361, 1947.

Chang, H. Y.: Grafts of parathyroid and other tissues to bone. Anat. Rec., *111*:23, 1951.

Copp, D. H., E. C. Cameron, B. A. Cheney, A. G. F. Davidson, and K. G. Henze: Evidence for calcitonin—a new hormone from the parathyroid that lowers blood calcium. Endocrinology, *10*:638, 1962.

Davis, R., and A. C. Enders: Light and electron microscope studies on the parathyroid gland. *In* Greep, R. O., and

R. V. Talmage, eds.: The Parathyroids. Springfield, Ill., Charles C Thomas, p. 76.

DeRobertis, E.: The cytology of the parathyroid gland of rats injected with parathyroid extract. Anat. Rec., *78*:473, 1940.

Gaillard, P. J.: Parathyroid gland tissue and bone *in vitro*. Exper. Cell Res., *3*(Suppl.):154, 1955.

Gaillard, P. J.: The influence of parathormone on the explanted radius of albino mouse embryos. J. Nederl. Akad. v. Wetensch., Amsterdam C, *63*:25, 1960.

Gaillard, P. J.: Parathyroid and bone in tissue culture. *In* Greep, R. O., and R. V. Talmage, eds.: The Parathyroids. Springfield, Ill., Charles C Thomas, 1961, p. 20.

Grafflin, A. L.: Cytological evidence of secretory activity in the mammalian parathyroid. Endocrinology, *26*: 857, 1940.

Greep, R. O.: Parathyroid glands. *In* The Parathyroids. Comparative Endocrinology. New York, Academic Press, 1963, Vol. I, p. 235.

Greep, R. O., and R. V. Talmage, eds.: The Parathyroids. Springfield, Ill., Charles C Thomas, 1961.

Habener, J. F., D. Powell, T. M. Murray, G. P. Mayer, and J. T. Potts, Jr.: Parathyroid hormone: Secretion and metabolism in vivo. Proc. Nat. Acad. Sci., *68*:2896, 1971.

Lange, R.: Zur Histologie und Zytologie der Glandula parathyroidea des Menschen: Licht und elektronenmikroskopische Untersuchungen an Epithelkörperadenomen. Zeitschr. f. Zellforsch., *53*:765, 1961.

Munger, B. L., and S. I. Roth: The cytology of the normal parathyroid glands of man and Virginia deer: A light and electron microscopic study with morphologic evidence of secretory activity. J. Cell Biol., *16*:379, 1963.

Potts, J. T., Jr., and L. J. Deftos: Parathyroid hormone, thyrocalcitonin, vitamin D and diseases of bone and bone mineral metabolism. *In* Bondy, P. K., ed.: Duncan's Diseases of Metabolism. 6th Ed. Philadelphia, W. B. Saunders Co., 1969.

Potts, J. T., Jr., T. Murray, M. Peacock, H. D. Niall, G. W. Tregear, H. T. Keutmann, D. Powell, and L. J. Deftos: Parathyroid hormone: sequence, synthesis, immunoassay studies. Am. J. Med., *50*:639, 1971.

Rasmussen, H.: Chemistry of parathyroid hormone. *In* Greep, R. O., and R. V. Talmage, eds.: The Parathyroids. Springfield, Ill., Charles C Thomas, 1961, p. 60.

Rasmussen, H., and L. C. Craig: Isolation and characterization of bovine parathyroid hormone. J. Biol. Chem., *236*:759, 1961.

Rosof, J. A.: An experimental study of the histology and cytology of the parathyroid glands in the albino rat. J. Exper. Zool., *68*:121, 1934.

Roth, S. I.: Pathology of the parathyroids in hyperparathyroidism with a discussion of recent advances in the anatomy and pathology of the parathyroid glands. Arch. Path., *73*:492, 1962.

Trier, J. S.: The fine structure of the parathyroid gland. J. Biophys. Biochem. Cytol., *4*:13, 1958.

Turner, C. D., and J. T. Bagnara: General Endocrinology. 5th ed. Philadelphia, W. B. Saunders Co., 1971.

Weymouth, R. J., and B. L. Baker: The presence of argyrophilic granules in the parenchymal cells of the parathyroid glands. Anat. Rec., *119*:519, 1954.

21

Adrenal Glands and Paraganglia

The paired *adrenal* or *suprarenal* glands of man are roughly triangular, flattened organs embedded in the retroperitoneal adipose tissue at the cranial pole of each kidney. They measure approximately 5 by 3 by less than 1 cm. and together weigh about 15 gm. Both weight and size may vary considerably, depending upon the age and physiological condition of the individual. The cut surface of the transected gland presents a bright yellow *cortex* in its outer part, with a reddish brown inner zone adjacent to the thin, gray *medulla*.

The adrenal glands comprise two distinct endocrine organs that differ in their embryological origin, type of secretion, and function—the *interrenal tissue* and the *chromaffin tissue*. In mammals these are arranged as cortex and medulla respectively, but in other vertebrate classes they may be intermingled in a variety of patterns or may be entirely dissociated.

THE ADRENAL CORTEX

The cortex, which forms the bulk of the gland, has three distinguishable concentric zones—a thin, outer *zona glomerulosa* adjacent to the capsule; a thick middle layer, the *zona fasciculata;* and a moderately thick, inner *zona reticularis* contiguous with the medulla (Figs. 21–1 and 21–2). In man these make up respectively 15 per cent, 78 per cent, and 7 per cent of the total cortical volume. The transition from one zone to another in histological sections is gradual but may appear sharper in preparations injected to show the vascular pattern.

The zona glomerulosa consists of closely packed clusters and arcades of columnar cells that are continuous with the cell columns of the zona fasciculata (Fig. 21–3). The spherical nuclei stain deeply and contain one or two nucleoli. The cytoplasm is less abundant than in the cells of the other zones and is generally acidophilic, but it contains some basophilic material, which is usually disposed in clumps. Lipid droplets are small and relatively scarce in this zone in most species but may be numerous in others. Mitochondria are filamentous. The compact Golgi apparatus is juxtanuclear and in some animals may be polarized toward the nearest vascular channel.

At the electron microscopic level, the most characteristic feature of the cytoplasm is its smooth surfaced endoplasmic reticulum, which forms an anastomosing network of tubules throughout the cell body. Profiles of granular endoplasmic reticulum are also present in limited numbers, and there are many polyribosomes free in the cytoplasmic matrix. There is nothing unusual in the organization of the Golgi complex or in the centrioles that are associated with it. The mitochondria as a rule have lamellar cristae like those of most other organs. The plasma membrane is smoothly contoured over most of the cell body but may have a few folds or microvilli on the surface bordering on a perivascular space and at the junctions where several cells meet.

The zona fasciculata consists of polyhedral cells considerably larger than those of the glomerulosa and arranged in long cords disposed radially with respect to the medulla (Fig. 21–4). The cords are usually one cell thick and separated by sinusoidal vessels. The nucleus is central, and binucleate cells are common. The cytoplasm is generally acidophilic but may contain basophilic masses, particularly in the peripheral portion of the zone. The cells are crowded with lipid droplets in the fresh condition, but after treatment with the organic solvents used in preparation of routine histological sections, the cytoplasm has a foamy appearance due to

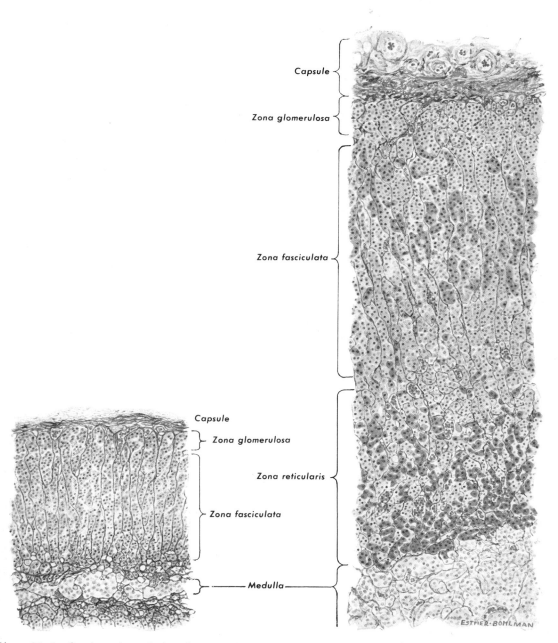

Capsule

Zona glomerulosa

Zona fasciculata

Capsule

Zona glomerulosa

Zona reticularis

Zona fasciculata

Medulla

ESTHER·BOHLMAN

Figure 21-1   Sections through the adrenal glands of a 6 month old infant (left) and of a man (right). Mallory-azan stain. × 110.

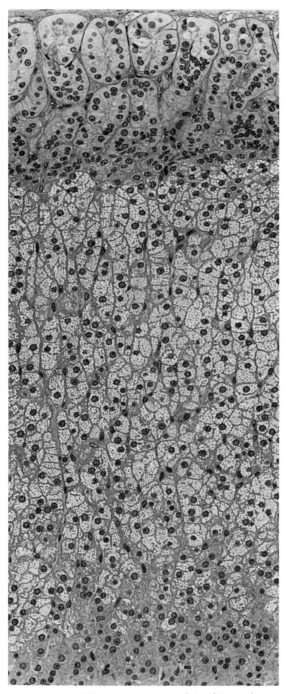

Figure 21-2 Photomicrograph of the full thickness of the adrenal cortex of a Rhesus monkey, showing from the top downward the zona glomerulosa, zona fasciculata, and zona reticularis.

the numerous clear vacuoles left by extraction of lipid (Fig. 21–4). In man, the zona glomerulosa may be absent in restricted areas of the cortex, and in such places the zona fasciculata is found immediately beneath the cortex, but this is not common. There may also be a thin transitional region between the zona glomerulosa and zona fasciculata which is relatively free of lipid droplets. Such a sudanophobic *zona intermedia* is particularly obvious in the rat adrenal.

When examined in electron micrographs, the nucleus of cells in the zona fasciculata is spherical and contains one or two nucleoli and small clumps of chromatin distributed around the periphery. The nuclear envelope has an obvious internal fibrous lamina. The smooth surfaced reticulum is much more elaborately developed than in the zona glomerulosa and occupies the bulk of the cytoplasm (Figs. 21–5 to 21–7). In man and other primates, parallel arrays of cisternae of the granular reticulum are also found, corresponding to the basophilic clumps seen with the light microscope (Figs. 21–5 and 21–6). These are less common in other species. The mitochondria appear to be less numerous and are more variable in size and shape than are those of the zona glomerulosa. Moreover, in rodents the mitochondria are spherical and the cristae are usually vesicular invaginations of the inner membrane or vesicles free in the mitochondrial matrix. In man and some other species they are long, tortuous tubules. The Golgi apparatus is considerably larger in this zone. Lysosomes are found in the Golgi region of the cell and deposits of lipochrome pigment are often present in abundance, particularly in older individuals.

In the zona reticularis, the regular parallel arrangement of cell cords gives way to an anastomosing network. The transition from the fasciculata is gradual, the cells differing but little. The cytoplasm contains fewer lipid droplets. Toward the medulla there is a variable number of "light" and "dark" cells. The nuclei of the light cells are pale-staining; those of the dark cells are hyperchromatic and shrunken. The physiological significance of these differences in staining affinity is not known. In other organs, this appearance is often a fixation artifact. It is so common in the zona reticu-

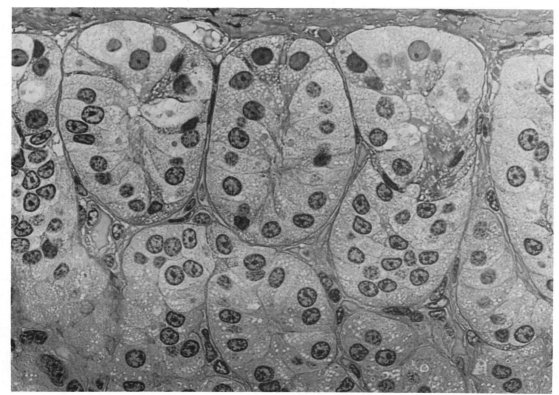

Figure 21–3 Photomicrograph of the monkey zona glomerulosa at higher magnification, showing the alveolar or glomerular arrangement of cells. These cells have relatively few vacuoles, representing extracted lipid.

laris, however, that some interpret these cells as degenerate. The cells of this zone, particularly the dark cells, contain large accumulations of lipofuscin pigment. Apart from the presence of light and dark cells and the greater amount of pigment, the cells of the zona reticularis resemble those of the fasciculata and, like them, have an abundance of agranular reticulum.

THE ADRENAL MEDULLA

The boundary between the zona reticularis and medulla is usually irregular in the human adult, with columns of cortical cells projecting some distance into the medulla. In other animals, the boundary may be quite sharp. The medulla is composed of large epithelioid cells arranged in rounded groups or short cords in intimate relation to blood capillaries and venules (Fig. 21–8). When the tissue is fixed in a solution containing potassium bichromate, these cells are seen to be filled with fine brown granules. This browning of the cytoplasmic granules with chromium salts is called the *chromaffin reaction* and is thought to result from the oxidation and polymerization of the catecholamines *epinephrine* and *norepinephrine* contained within the granules of the cells. The medulla is colored green after treatment with ferric chloride—apparently for the same reason. There are other cells in the body that give a similar reaction, notably some of the argentaffin cells of the gastrointestinal tract and the mast cells, which are reactive because of their content of 5-hydroxytryptamine. The chromaffin cells of the adrenal medulla, however, are derived from neuroectoderm, they secrete catecholamines, and they are innervated by preganglionic sympathetic fibers.

In most species the application of a group of histochemical methods to the chromaffin cells permits the identification of two types of cells, one containing norepinephrine and the other epinephrine. The norepinephrine storing cells are autofluorescent, give argentaffin and potassium iodate reactions, exhibit a low affinity for azocarmine, and give a negative acid phosphatase reaction. The epinephrine storing cells have a high staining affinity for azocarmine and a positive acid phosphatase reaction, and are not fluorescent or reactive with iodate or silver.

In electron micrographs, the most prominent feature of these cells is the presence of large numbers of membrane bounded dense granules 100 to 300 nm. in diameter (Fig. 21–9). The granules are bounded by a membrane separated from the dense content by an electron lucent gap. When tissue is fixed in glutaraldehyde, two populations of cells are distinguishable on the basis of the character of their granules. Cells that store norepinephrine have granules that contain a very electron dense core, often eccentric in its location within the membrane limited vesicle. Cells that store epinephrine have granules that are relatively homogeneous and less electron dense (Coupland). The mitochondria are not remarkable. The cisternae of the granular endoplasmic reticulum form small parallel arrays. The juxtanuclear Golgi apparatus frequently contains in its cisternae dense material interpreted as a precursor of the granules.

It has been established by cell fractionation and density gradient centrifugation that the hormones are contained within the secretory granules (Banks). The granules may contain as much as 20 per cent by weight of the hormone. Although they also contain a

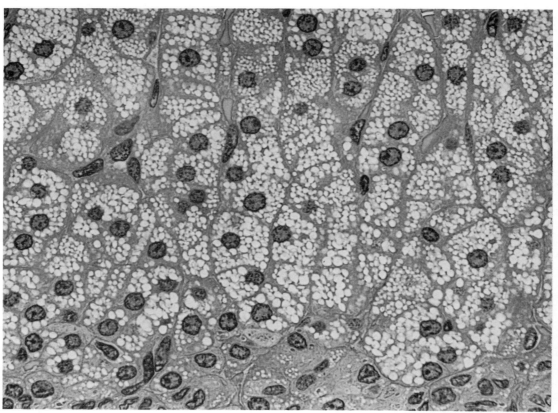

Figure 21–4 Photomicrograph of the zona fasciculata. This zone consists of cords of cells filled with spherical vacuoles resulting from extraction of the abundant lipid droplets characteristic of this zone.

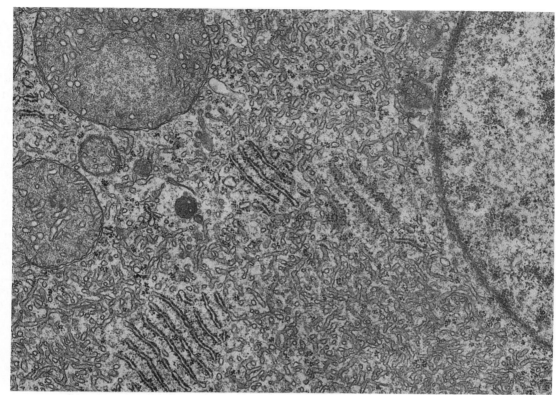

Figure 21–5   Electron micrograph of a portion of a cell from the human fetal adrenal cortex, showing large spherical mitochondria with tubular cristae, a few parallel arrays of cisternae of granular reticulum, and an extraordinary abundance of smooth endoplasmic reticulum. (Micrograph courtesy of A. L. Jones and S. McNutt.)

significant amount of protein, much of this is the soluble protein *chromogranin.* The catecholamines do not seem to be bound to a specific protein, as are the hormones of the neurohypophysis and other neurosecretory cells. Therefore, it is not entirely clear how such low molecular weight substances are retained in the granules. According to one hypothesis, the hormone forms high molecular weight aggregates with adenosine triphosphate (ATP) and divalent cations, both of which are present in the granules. The active uptake of catecholamine by the granules appears to be the result of an active transport mechanism dependent upon magnesium-activated ATPase in the limiting membrane. Thus, the ability of secretory granules in the adrenal medulla to retain hormones in vivo probably depends on (1) micelle formation between ATP and hormone, and (2) an active transport mechanism

in the membrane limiting the granules. The depletion of catecholamines by the pharmacologically active substance *reserpine* may be the result of inhibition of the active transport mechanism.

For some time there was a divergence of opinion as to whether the granules of the adrenal medulla are released by exocytosis, as are protein hormones, or whether the smaller molecules of catecholamines are released from the granules within the cytoplasm and diffuse out of the cell. It now seems to have been well established experimentally that all or nearly all of the hormones of the adrenal medulla are discharged by exocytosis. Evidence for this resides not only in morphological observations but in the physiological finding that a perfusate of a stimulated gland contains not only catecholamines but also soluble protein constituents of the granules (chromogranin) and ATP, in the same proportions that occur in a lysate of isolated granules, whereas the insoluble constituent associated with the membranes of the granules are retained within the gland (Smith and Winkler).

In addition to the chromaffin cells, sympathetic ganglion cells occur singly or in small groups in the adrenal medulla.

The adrenal is enclosed by a thick capsule of collagenous connective tissue that extends into the cortex to varying depths as trabeculae. Most of the rest of the supporting framework of the cortex consists of reticular fibers that lie between the sinusoids and the cell cords and penetrate to some extent between the gland cells. Reticular fibers also enclose the cell clusters in the medulla and support the capillaries, veins, and nerves. Collagenous fibers appear around the larger tributaries of the veins and merge with the capsular connective tissue.

BLOOD SUPPLY AND LYMPHATIC DRAINAGE OF THE ADRENAL

The gland is richly supplied by a number of arteries that enter at various points around the periphery. Three principal groups are recognized. The *superior suprarenal arteries* arising from the inferior phrenic artery appear to be the major source, but in addition there are the *middle suprarenals* arising from the aorta and the *inferior suprarenals*, which are branches of the renal artery. Arteries from these several sources form a plexus in the capsule. The *cortical arteries* arise from this capsular plexus and distribute to the anastomosing network of sinusoids surrounding the cords of parenchymal cells in the cortex (Fig. 21–10). The sinusoids of a given region converge in the zona reticularis

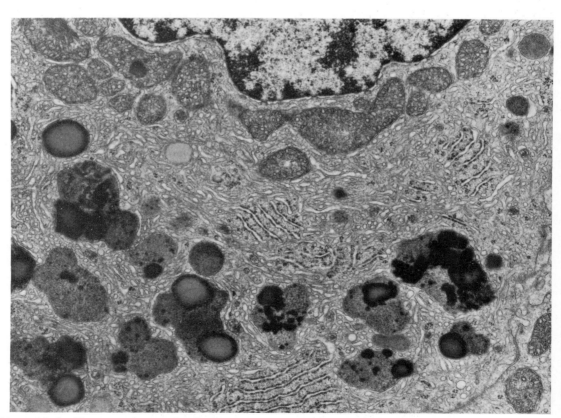

Figure 21–6 Electron micrograph of a juxtanuclear area of a cortical cell from an adult human adrenal. The smooth reticulum remains abundant, the mitochondria are variable in size and shape, and they generally have tubular cristae. There is a marked tendency for accumulation of irregular dense masses of lipochrome pigment. (Micrograph courtesy of J. Long.)

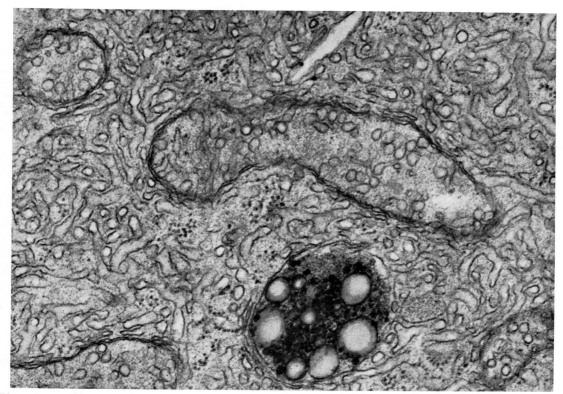

Figure 21–7   Electron micrograph of an area of cytoplasm of an adult adrenal cortical cell at higher magnification illustrating the tubular nature of the smooth reticulum and the fine structure of the mitochondria. (Micrograph courtesy of J. Long.)

upon a collecting vein at the corticomedullary junction. There is no venous system in the cortex.

Some major arterial branches from the capsule penetrate the connective tissue trabeculae and pass directly through the cortex, giving off few or no branches until they reach the medulla. In the medulla, they branch repeatedly to form the rich capillary net around the clumps and cords of chromaffin cells. The medulla thus has a dual blood supply—via the cortical sinusoids that anastomose with its capillary bed across the corticomedullary junction, and via the medullary arteries that course from the capsule directly to the medulla. The capillaries of the medulla empty into the same venous system that drains the cortex. The multiple venules ultimately join to form the large central veins of the medulla, which emerge from the gland as the *suprarenal vein.*

This pattern of vascularization has important physiological consequences. The blood reaching the medulla via the sinusoids has traversed the cortex, and is rich in cortical steroid hormones. There is evidence that high concentration of glucocorticoids may be required for induction and maintenance of the enzyme phenylethanolamine-N-methyl transferase, which is necessary for the synthesis of epinephrine. Thus, the adrenal cortical steroids have a local downstream effect on the medulla, as well as a general systemic effect. Indeed, whether a medullary cell secretes norepinephrine or epinephrine may be determined by where it is situated with respect to steroid rich blood from the cortex that regulates the synthesis of the enzyme necessary for conversion of norepinephrine to epinephrine (Wurtman and Pohorecky).

The cells lining the capillaries of the medulla are typical endothelium. The nature of the lining of the sinusoids in the cortex is still a subject of debate. These cells have been reported to take up colloidal vital dyes, such as lithium carmine and trypan blue, and on this basis they have been regarded as belonging to the reticuloendothelial system. More recent studies suggest that these substances simply adhere to the cell surface or that they are taken up by macrophages lying between the endothelium and the parenchymal cells. Electron microscopic observations have failed to reveal any evidence of phagocytosis by the endothelial cells of the sinusoids. Except in the regions occupied by the nucleus and cell center, the endothelium is extremely attenuated and interrupted at intervals by small circular pores or fenestrae closed only by a very thin diaphragm. There is a continuous basal lamina supported at intervals by small bundles of collagen fibrils corresponding to the reticulum of light microscopy.

Lymphatics are limited to the capsule and its cortical trabeculae, and to the connective tissue around the large veins.

NERVES OF THE ADRENAL

The cells of the adrenal cortex apparently are not innervated. Those of the zona fasciculata are stimulated by circulating adrenocorticotropic hormone (ACTH) of the pituitary; those of the glomerulosa are responsive to changes in extracellular fluid volume or changes in concentration of sodium and potassium in the blood, possibly acting indirectly via a hypothetical hormone of the diencephalon, *aldosterone-stimulating factor*.

Preganglionic sympathetic nerve fibers arising from cell bodies in the intermediolateral column of the spinal cord in the lower thoracic and lumbar regions of the spinal cord pass through the sympathetic chain and via splanchnic nerves to the capsule of the adrenal, where they form a rich nerve plexus, including a few sympathetic ganglion cells. From this plexus preganglionic nerves turn

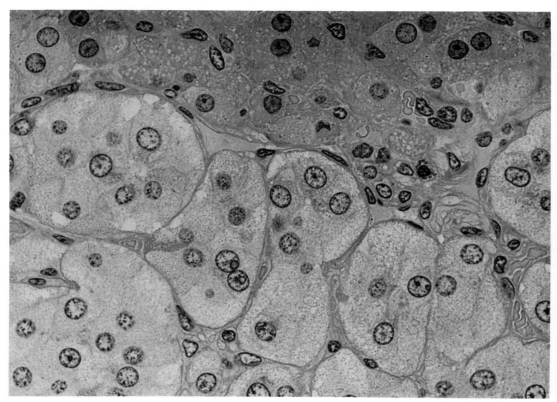

Figure 21–8 Photomicrograph of the junction of the zona reticularis (above) with the clusters of large pale cells of the adrenal medulla (below). Catecholamine granules ordinarily are not visible in the cells of the medulla with the light microscope.

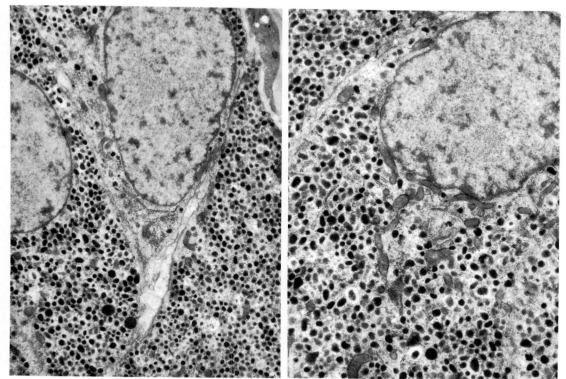

Figure 21–9   Electron micrographs of cells from the adrenal medulla of the cat, showing the abundant, membrane-limited, dense granules which are the sites of storage of catecholamines. ×9600 and ×13,600. (Courtesy of R. Yates.)

inward, traverse the cortex, and end in the medulla around the cells that secrete epinephrine and norepinephrine. These cells are derived embryologically from the nervous system in early development and are analogous to postganglionic neurons. The nerve terminals form typical synapses with the cells, in which the pre- and post-synaptic membranes are separated by a cleft of 150 to 200 Å. The nerve terminals are cholinergic and contain multiple clear synaptic vesicles.

HISTOPHYSIOLOGY OF THE ADRENAL CORTEX

The adrenal cortex is concerned with a wide variety of body functions, including maintenance of fluid and electrolyte balance, maintenance of carbohydrate balance, and maintenance of the normal function of certain cellular elements of the connective tissues. It is essential for life. Its removal or destruction

in man leads ultimately to death unless the patient is given exogenous adrenal cortical hormones.

The widely accepted zonal hypothesis of adrenal function affirms that different functions can be ascribed to the morphologically recognizable zones of the adrenal cortex. The zona glomerulosa secretes hormones collectively called *mineralocorticoids* (aldosterone and deoxycorticosterone), which are concerned with fluid and electrolyte balance, whereas the zona fasciculata and zona reticularis secrete hormones collectively referred to as *glucocorticoids* (cortisol, cortisone and corticosterone), which are concerned with metabolism of carbohydrates, proteins, and fat. The concept of a separate function of the zona glomerulosa and the inner zones of the cortex is supported by abundant experimental evidence. There is as yet no clear-cut evidence of qualitative functional differences between the zona fasciculata and zona reticularis.

The most important hormone of the

zona glomerulosa is *aldosterone*. When released in the body or administered exogenously, it has three basic effects: It increases reabsorption of sodium by the tubules of the kidney; it increases the excretion of potassium by the kidney; and it appears to increase both the movement of sodium into the cells of the body and the associated transfer of potassium out of the cells. If the secretion of this hormone is eliminated by disease or surgical removal of the adrenal, the sodium and chloride concentrations of the extracellular fluid decrease markedly, the volume of extracellular fluid is greatly diminished, and the patient goes into a shock-like state that is followed by death within a few days, unless he is treated by salt replacement or administration of exogenous mineralocorticoids.

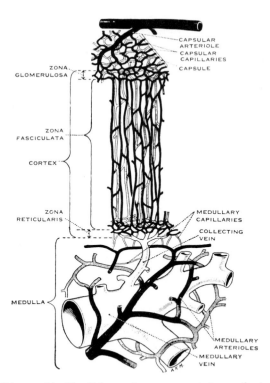

Figure 21-10 Schematic representation of the blood supply of the adrenal, showing how blood from capsular arterioles traverses the cortex and continues into capillaries and venules in the medulla. This arrangement carries blood rich in cortical steroids to the catecholamine synthesizing cells in the medulla. (From W. J. Hamilton, ed., *Textbook of Human Anatomy*. London, St. Martin's Press, Inc., Macmillan and Co., Ltd., 1957.)

As in other parts of the endocrine system, the secretion of aldosterone is carefully regulated to maintain constancy of the internal environment of the cells of the body. If for some reason the extracellular sodium concentration falls, or if potassium rises, or extracellular fluid volume is dangerously diminished, this is reflected in the concentration in the blood and detected by centers in the midbrain. These, in turn, release a hormone that stimulates the zona glomerulosa to release aldosterone, which acts upon the kidney tubules to increase sodium absorption and decrease potassium resorption, thus correcting the imbalance. If increased demands are placed upon the homeostatic mechanisms for maintaining electrolyte balance by giving an animal either an excess of potassium or a sodium deficient diet, there is a selective hypertrophy of the zona glomerulosa and an increase in the abundance of smooth endoplasmic reticulum in its cells (Long and Jones). Conversely, injection of large doses of aldosterone or deoxycorticosterone results in atrophy of this zone.

The glucocorticoids secreted by the two inner zones of the cortex are almost as important in sustaining life as are the mineralocorticoids. Secretion or administration of cortisol results in a great increase in the formation of glucose in the liver and its intracellular storage as glycogen. Excess glucose is also released into the blood, producing a condition comparable to diabetes. The hormone also causes a decrease in the rate of protein synthesis and an increase in the rate of protein breakdown in the cells of the body. Therefore the level of amino acids in the blood increases. Finally, cortisol acts upon adipose tissue, increasing both the rate at which lipid is accumulated in the fat cells, and the rate at which the lipids are mobilized from those cells.

The control of the secretion of glucocorticoids is quite independent of that of the mineralocorticoids. The maintenance of the inner zones of the cortex depends upon secretion of adrenocorticotropic hormone by the anterior lobe of the hypophysis. Hypophysectomy results in a marked atrophy of the zona fasciculata and zona reticularis but has little effect upon the zona glomerulosa. This atrophy of the inner zones can be prevented or reversed by injection of adrenocorticotropic hormone (ACTH). Conversely, administration of large doses of cortisol to an intact animal suppresses hypophyseal secretion of ACTH and results in atrophy of the inner zones of the adrenal cortex.

The mechanisms of control of glucocorticoid secretion have already been presented in Chapter 4 (see Fig. 4–29), but briefly restated, many different kinds of alarming or stressful situations, such as pain, fear, rage, etc., result in passage of nerve impulses to the hypothalamus that initiate secretion of corticotropin releasing factor (CRF) into the hypophyseoportal vessels. Carried to the anterior lobe of the hypophysis, this promotes adrenocorticotropin release which in turn causes discharge of glucocorticoids from the adrenal. The resulting increase in blood amino acid and glucose levels makes available to the cells the energy-rich substrates that may be needed for combat, flight, or other responses to stress.

The glucocorticoids also have effects upon inflammatory responses of the connective tissues and upon the immune system. The mechanisms of these actions are poorly understood but they are widely utilized in the treatment of allergies, arthritis, rheumatic fever, and many other inflammatory diseases. Cortisol somehow reduces the severity of allergic reactions and suppresses the inflammation. Among other effects it causes a destruction of lymphocytes, atrophy of lymphoid tissue, and a decrease in level of circulating eosinophils. Therefore, in surgical grafting of organs, cortisol is often given to suppress the rejection reaction.

There is also a relationship between the adrenal cortex and the reproductive system. Adrenalectomy is followed by loss of libido in the male and abnormal cycles in the female. Removal of the adrenal interrupts lactation. Whether or not these effects are mediated via the adenohypophysis is not clear. It is known that under normal conditions, small amounts of estrogens and androgens are produced in the two inner zones of the cortex. In the pathological condition known as *adrenogenital syndrome*, the inner zones of the cortex are hypertrophic and high levels of circulating androgens may result in precocious puberty, increased hirsutism, and other manifestations of virilism.

Hyperadrenocorticism or Cushing's disease is a condition in which the adrenal cortex is hyperplastic, as a result of stimulation by pituitary or other tumors producing excessive amounts of ACTH. It is characterized by obesity, particularly over the nape of the neck, hirsutism, impotence or amenorrhea, abdominal striae, and a characteristic round "moon face." *Hypoadrenocorticism* or *Addison's disease* is due to destruction of the adrenal cortex by tuberculosis or other infection of the gland, resulting in chronic insufficiency of hormone production. It is characterized by generalized weakness, weight loss, low blood pressure, and abnormal pigmentation, and leads ultimately to death if hormone replacement therapy is not undertaken.

HISTOPHYSIOLOGY OF THE ADRENAL MEDULLA

The adrenal medulla is not essential for life. Animals that have had their adrenal medullas removed can survive under ordinary circumstances but are unable to respond normally to emergency situations. The hormones of the medulla, *epinephrine* and *norepinephrine*, are catecholamines, and unlike the steroid hormones of the cortex, they accumulate in high concentration in the cells. The granules of the cells are the site of storage of catecholamines. The two hormones are produced in different proportions depending upon the species. Aggressive and predatory animals tend to secrete large amounts of norepinephrine, whereas the more timid and placid species produce relatively less.

Although the two hormones are very closely related chemically, there are important qualitative and quantitative differences in their physiological effects.

Epinephrine increases the heart rate and cardiac output without significantly increasing the blood pressure, and may increase the blood flow through some organs by as much as 100 per cent. It has effect on the cardiovascular system in very low concentrations. The denervated mammalian heart, for example, is accelerated by as little as one part epinephrine in 1.4 billion parts of fluid medium. Epinephrine also has a marked effect upon metabolism. It increases oxygen consumption and basal metabolic rate. It elevates the blood sugar level by mobilizing the carbohydrate stores of the liver; by promoting the conversion of muscle glycogen into lactic acid, from which new carbohydrate can be made in the liver; and by causing the release of ACTH from the hypophysis, which, in turn, affects gluconeogenesis by stimulating secretion of glucocorticoids from the adrenal cortex. The mobilization of glucose from the liver by epinephrine appears to result from its activation of the enzyme phosphorylase, which accelerates the first step in the breakdown of glycogen to glucose.

Norepinephrine has relatively little effect upon metabolism but causes a marked elevation of the blood pressure with very little effect upon heart rate or cardiac output. The effect of norepinephrine on the blood pressure is not due to an action upon the heart beat but is primarily a consequence of the vasoconstriction it brings about in the peripheral portion of the arterial system. Both epinephrine and norepinephrine cause lipolysis and release of unesterified fatty acid from adipose tissue isolated in vitro.

Norepinephrine is not confined to the adrenal medulla but is present in the brain and in most of the innervated peripheral tissues, where it is localized mainly in the sympathetic nerve endings. It has been established as the principal transmitter substance of adrenergic neurons. Thus it is a *neurohumor*. Neurohumors such as norepinephrine, acetylcholine, and serotinin are released by nerve cells, usually at their endings, and affect other neurons or muscles or glands. In general they act transiently and at very short range, being destroyed enzymatically before they reach effective concentrations in the circulation. The norepinephrine released into the bloodstream by the adrenal medulla is somewhat exceptional among neurohumors in that it does reach effective levels in the blood and acts at a distance. On the other hand, the *neurosecretory substances*, such as the oxytocin and vasopressin of the posterior lobe of the hypophysis, are long acting products of nerve cells that act at long range.

Although the adrenal medullary hormones are not essential for life, it appears that in times of stress they do help to maintain homeostasis and to prepare the organism to meet emergency situations. Epinephrine accomplishes this by elevating blood glucose levels, increasing cardiac output, and redistributing blood within the circulation to ensure continuing rapid flow to those organs vital for survival. Norepinephrine is less important in these emergency adjustments, but, as the mediator of adrenergic nerve impulses throughout the body, it acts continuously on the blood vessels of the normal animal to maintain blood pressure.

Hyperfunction of the adrenal medulla in man occurs with certain rare tumors of the medulla or of extramedullary chromaffin tissues. In such cases there may be attacks of sweating, mydriasis, hypertension, and hyperglycemia, terminating suddenly in death. The paroxysmal hypertension (acute high blood pressure) of adrenal medullary tumors is decreased or abolished by intravenous administration of a series of compounds that have an epinephrine inhibiting action.

The cells of the adrenal medulla are regarded as modified postganglionic neurons, and their secretory activity seems to be largely, if not entirely, under nervous control. Hormones of the medulla are increased in the blood of the adrenal veins after stimulation of the splanchnic nerves, and secretion is prevented by sectioning these nerves. After splanchnic nerve stimulation, about 75 per cent of the secretion is norepinephrine and 25 per cent epinephrine. Certain centers in the posterior hypothalamus are known to relay impulses to the adrenal medulla by way of the splanchnic nerves. In the intact animal, certain kinds of emotional stimuli are especially effective in releasing norepinephrine, and other kinds of stimuli, such as pain or hypoglycemia, promote the release of epinephrine. For this reason, it is believed that the cells producing epinephrine and those producing norepinephrine receive different innervation and secrete their hormones independently.

HISTOGENESIS OF THE ADRENAL GLANDS

The cortex develops from the coelomic mesoderm on the medial side of the urogenital ridge of the embryo. Mesothelial cells near the cranial pole of the mesonephros in 8 to 10 mm. human fetuses proliferate and penetrate the subjacent, highly vascular mesenchyme. These cells ultimately form the *fetal cortex*. A second proliferation of the coelomic mesothelium taking place in 14 mm. embryos later forms the definitive or *permanent cortex*. The adrenal gland in the fetus is relatively large, with the fetal zone composing about 80 per cent of the cortex. The cells of this zone are large and stain intensely with eosin. After birth the fetal cortex undergoes a rapid degeneration and the permanent cortex enlarges. Associated with these changes is a 50 per cent decline in the absolute weight of the adrenal during the first few postnatal weeks.

The adrenal in the fetus is functional and under the control of ACTH secreted by the hypophysis. Monstrous anencephalic fetuses, which lack a normal hypophysis, have very small adrenal glands with no *fetal zone*. The physiological role of this zone during intra-uterine life is not well understood. Progress in this area is hampered by the fact that none of the common laboratory animals has a comparable fetal zone. In the mouse, the so-called *X zone* differentiates postnatally and regresses at puberty in the male or at the time of the first pregnancy in the female. The hormonal factors controlling it appear to be different than those affecting the human fetal zone.

The medulla arises from the ectodermal neural crest tissue, which also gives rise to sympathetic ganglion cells. Strands of these sympathochromaffin cells migrate ventrally and penetrate the anlagen of the adrenal cortex on its medial side to take up a central position in the organ rudiment.

Cell Renewal and Regeneration in the Adrenal Cortex

There have long been divergent views as to the mode of growth and repair of the adrenal cortex. It was formerly believed that the cells arose either from fibroblast-like cells in the capsule or by division of the cells in the zona glomerulosa and that they gradually moved through the zona fasciculata and degenerated in the zona reticularis. The dark cells of this zone were interpreted as cells undergoing regressive changes. During their migration, the cells were believed to go through one cycle of secretion.

The bulk of the evidence now seems to favor the view that, once formed, the cells of the glomerulosa and fasciculata do not move appreciably and that replacement and repair take place as a result of local mitotic activity. After injection of colchicine to arrest cell division at metaphase, mitotic figures are not confined to any one region but are found throughout the cortex, the majority being in the zona fasciculata. Autoradiographic studies after administration of tritiated thymidine have produced equivocal results but, on the whole, they provide little evidence of extensive cell migration.

In experimental animals the adrenal cortex has a considerable capacity for regenera-tion. If the gland is incised and all of the tissue in its interior removed, leaving behind only the capsule and a few adherent granulosal cells, the whole cortex will be regenerated. The medulla is not restored. Studies of the steroids elaborated during regeneration of the cortex show that an adequate level of secretion of mineralocorticoids is established early, although the secretion of glucocorticoids does not occur until one to two weeks later. Thus, in the regenerating gland, cells functionally similar to those of the normal zona fasciculata and reticularis differentiate from cells of the zona glomerulosa.

Phylogeny of the Adrenal Gland

Chromaffin tissue which yields epineph-rine-like activity is present in the central nervous system of leeches; it is present also in the mantles of certain molluscs. In cyclostomes and teleosts, the *interrenal bodies* (which are homologous with the cortex) are separate from the discrete chromaffin bodies. In amphibians the two components are in juxtaposition, or they may be intermingled; in reptiles and birds they are commonly intermingled. The well known cortex and medulla relationship first appears in mammals, where this is the predominant form of organization.

THE PARAGANGLIA

The term *paraganglia* is used to describe small clusters of epithelioid cells that give a chromaffin reaction. They are found rather widely scattered in the retroperitoneal tissue. Some of them are associated with sympathetic ganglia, others with branches of the parasympathetic nerves. The cells of the paraganglia and those of the adrenal medulla are morphologically similar and of similar embryonic origin. Together they are said to make up the *chromaffin system*. In ordinary histological preparations the cells of paraganglia appear pale or clear, but they are stained by the chromaffin reaction.

These cells found in the ganglia and along the nerves of the sympathetic nervous system have now been studied electron microscopically (Elfvin; Yates) and by histochemical procedures for the identification of catecholamines (Nakata; Brudin). The paraganglia are surrounded by a rather thick investment of collagenous connective tissue that extends inward between clumps of parenchymal cells. Two types of parenchymal cells are distinguishable, the chief cells and supporting cells. The chief cells are irregular in shape, with a single nucleus and well developed juxtanuclear Golgi complex. The endoplasmic reticulum is sparse, but occasional parallel associations of cisternae are observed. Glycogen particles are present in small numbers scattered through the cytoplasmic matrix. In addition, there are numerous membrane limited electron opaque granules 50 to 200 nm. closely resembling those of the adrenal medulla (Fig. 21–11). Histochemical methods indicate that these granules contain catecholamines, principally if not exclusively norepinephrine. The supporting cells partially or completely surround each of the chief cells. The nucleus of these cells is elongated in section and frequently deeply infolded. The cytoplasm is devoid of secretory granules and is otherwise unremarkable.

The paraganglia are richly vascularized by capillaries lined by very attenuated endothelial cells, occasionally exhibiting fenestrated regions. The chief cells are usually separated from the blood by a barrier consisting of a thin, intervening supporting cell, two basal laminae, and the endothelium, but there are areas in which the supporting cell is absent and the chief cells are in close relation to the capillary wall (Mascorro and Yates). These vascular relationships are of some significance, for it is not yet clear whether the paraganglion cells have an endocrine function, releasing catecholamine into the blood, or whether the chief cells are essentially interneurons synapsing on sympathetic neurons and exerting an inhibitory effect on transmission in sympathetic ganglia.

The parasympathetic paraganglia often do not give a conspicuous chromafin reaction and they were formerly classified by light microscopists as "achromaffin paraganglia" to distinguish them from those associated with the sympathetic ganglia. It was even suggested by some that they probably elaborated acetylcholine. This distinction between chromaffin and achromaffin paraganglia receives no support from electron microscopic studies, and should probably be abandoned

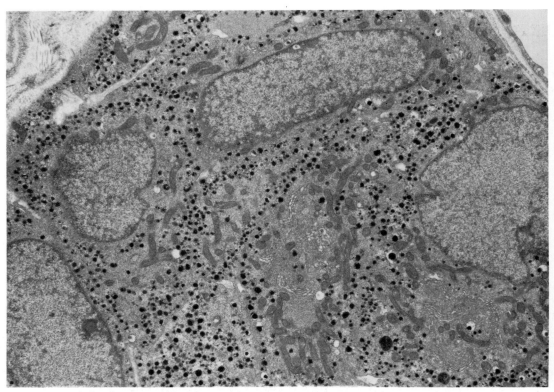

Figure 21–11 Cells of a paraganglion from rabbit, showing chief cells, which contain numerous catecholamine storing granules resembling those of the adrenal medulla. (Micrograph courtesy of R. Yates.)

(Chen and Yates). The chief cells of vagal paraganglia contain 50 to 200 nm. electron opaque granules that tend to be at the cell periphery or in its processes. The supporting cells are somewhat less numerous than in sympathetic paraganglia and chief cells may adjoin one another and be attached by desmosomes. Nerve terminals apposed to the surface of the chief cells contain numerous clear synaptic vesicles.

REFERENCES

Banks, P.: Adenosine-triphosphatase activity of adrenal chromaffin granules. Biochem. J., 95:490, 1965.

Baulieu, E. E., and P. Robel, eds.: Aldosterone. Philadelphia, F. A. Davis Co., 1964.

Benedeczky, I., and A. D. Smith: Ultrastructural studies on the adrenal medulla of the hamster: Origin and fate of secretory granules. Zeitsch. f. Zellforsch., 124:367, 1972.

Bennett, H. S.: Cytological manifestations of secretion in the adrenal medulla of the cat. Am. J. Anat., 69:333, 1941.

Brudin, T.: Catecholamines in the preaortal paraganglia of fetal rabbits. Acta Physiol. Scand., 64:287, 1965.

Bush, I. E.: Chemical and biological factors in the activity of adreno-cortical steroids. Pharmacol. Revs., 14:317, 1962.

Chen, I., and R. D. Yates: Ultrastructural studies of vagal paraganglia in Syrian hamsters. Zeitsch. f. Zellforsch. 108:309, 1970.

Coupland, R. E.: The Natural History of the Chromaffin Cell. London, Longmans, Green & Co., 1965.

Currie, A. R., T. Symington, and J. K. Grant, eds.: The Human Adrenal Cortex. Baltimore, Williams & Wilkins Co., 1962.

Deane, H. W., ed.: The adrenocortical hormones: Their origin, chemistry, physiology and pharmacology. *In* Eichler, O., and A. Farah, eds.: Handbuch der Experimentellen Pharmakologie. Berlin, Springer Verlag, 1962, Vol. 14, part 1.

Douglas, W. W.: Stimulus-secretion coupling: the concept and clues from chromaffin and other cells. Brit. J. Pharmacol., 34:451, 1969.

Elfvin, L. G.: A new granule-containing cell in the inferior mesenteric ganglion of the rabbit. J. Ultrastr. Res., 22: 37, 1968.

Ganong, W. F.: The central nervous system and the synthesis and release of adrenocorticotrophic hormone. *In* Nalbandov, A. V., ed.: Advances in Neuroendocrinology. Urbana, University of Illinois Press, 1963, p. 92.

Gorbman, A., and H. A. Bern: A Textbook of Comparative Endocrinology. New York, John Wiley & Sons, 1962.

Greep, R. O., and H. W. Deane: The cytology and cytochemistry of the adrenal cortex. Ann. N. Y. Acad. Sci., 50:569, 1948.

Hartman, F. A., and K. A. Brownell: The Adrenal Gland. Philadelphia, Lea & Febiger, 1949.

Hartroft, P. M., and W. S. Hartroft: Studies on renal juxtaglomerular cells; correlation of the degree of granulation of juxtaglomerular cells with width of the zona glomerulosa of the adrenal cortex. J. Exper. Med., 102:205, 1955.

Hechter, O., and I. D. K. Halkerston: On the action of

mammalian hormones. *In* Pincus, G., K. V. Thimann, and E. B. Astwood, eds.: The Hormones: Physiology, Chemistry and Applications. New York, Academic Press, 1964, Vol. 5, p. 697.

Hechter, O., and G. Pincus: Genesis of the adrenocortical secretion. Physiol. Rev., 34:459, 1954.

Hillarp, N. A., and B. Hökfelt: Cytological demonstration of noradrenaline in the suprarenal medulla under conditions of varied secretory activity. Endocrinology, 55:255, 1954.

Hillarp, N. A., S. Lagerstedt, and B. Nilson: The isolation of a granular fraction from the suprarenal medulla, containing the sympathomimetic catechol amines. Acta Physiol. Scand., 29:251, 1953.

Hoerr, N.: The cells of the suprarenal cortex in the guinea pig; their reaction to injury and their replacement. Am. J. Anat., 48:139, 1931.

Ingle, D.: Current status of adrenocortical research. Am. Scientist, 47:413, 1959.

Jones, I. C.: The Adrenal Cortex. London, Cambridge University Press, 1957.

Knigge, K. M.: The effect of acute starvation on the adrenal cortex of the hamster. Anat. Rec., 120:555, 1954.

Lanman, J. T.: The fetal zone of the adrenal gland. Medicine, 32:389, 1963.

Long, J. A., and A. L. Jones: Observations on the fine structure of the adrenal cortex of man. Lab. Invest., 17:355, 1967.

Mascorro, J. A., and R. D. Yates: Microscopic observations on abdominal sympathetic paraganglia. Texas Rep. Biol. Med. 28:59, 1970.

Mascorro, J. A., and R. D. Yates: Ultrastructural studies of the effects of reserpine on mouse abdominal sympathetic paraganglia. Anat. Rec. 170:269, 1971.

Moon, H. D., ed.: The Adrenal Cortex, New York, Paul B. Hoeber, Inc., 1961.

Nakata, Y.: Histochemical studies on catecholamines with reference to the paraganglia. Acta Neuroveg. 26:75, 1964.

Prunty, F. T. G., ed.: The Adrenal Cortex. Brit. Med. Bull., 18:89, 1962.

Prunty, F. T. G.: Chemistry and Treatment of Adrenocortical Diseases. Springfield, Illinois, Charles C Thomas, 1964.

Selye, H.: Textbook of Endocrinology. 2nd ed. Montreal, Acta Endocrinologica, Inc., 1949.

Smith, A. D.: Storage and secretion of hormones. The Scientific Basis of Medicine Annual Reviews, 1972.

Smith, A. D., and H. Winkler: *In* Blaschko, H., and E. Muschell, eds.: Catecholamines. Handbook of Experimental Pharmacology. Berlin, Springer Verlag, Vol. 33, p. 538, 1972.

Turner, C. D., and J. T. Bagnara: General Endocrinology. 5th ed. Philadelphia, W. B. Saunders Co., 1971.

Wolman, M.: Histochemistry of Lipids in Pathology. *In* Graumann, W., and K. Neumann, eds.: Handbuch der Histochemie. Stuttgart, Gustav Fischer Verlag, 1964, Vol. 5, part 2.

Wurtman, R. J., and L. A. Pohorecky: Adrenocortical control of epinephrine synthesis in health and disease. Adv. Metab. Disord. 5:53, 1971.

Yates, R. D.: A light and electron microscopic study correlating the chromaffin reaction and granule ultrastructure in the adrenal medulla of the Syrian hamster. Anat. Rec., 149:237, 1964.

Yates, R. D., J. G. Wood, and D. Duncan: Phase and electron microscopic observations on two cell types in the adrenal medulla of the Syrian hamster. Texas Rep. Biol. Med., 20:494, 1962.

22
Pineal
Gland

The *pineal body (epiphysis cerebri)* of the human brain is a somewhat flattened, conical gray body measuring 5 to 8 mm. in length, and 3 to 5 mm. in its greatest width. It lies above the roof of the diencephalon at the posterior extremity of the third ventricle. A small ependyma-lined recess of the third ventricle extends into a short stalk, which joins the pineal body to the diencephalic roof. The organ is invested by pia mater, from which connective tissue septa containing many blood vessels penetrate into the pineal tissue and surround its cords and follicles of epithelioid cells.

In sections stained with hematoxylin and eosin, the pineal body is seen to consist of cords of pale staining epithelioid cells. Their large nuclei are often irregularly infolded or lobulated and have prominent nucleoli. These cells, making up the bulk of the organ, are called *pinealocytes* or *chief cells.* When appropriately stained, the cytoplasm is moderately basophilic and often contains lipid droplets. As described by del Rio-Hortega, who used silver impregnation methods for their demonstration, human pinealocytes are cells with long tortuous processes, which radiate from the cords toward the connective tissue septa where they end in bulbous swellings on or near blood vessels (see Fig. 22–6). Such processes are seldom seen in routine preparations and are difficult to demonstrate by electron microscopy.

In electron micrographs the cytoplasm contains numerous free ribosomes and occasional short profiles of granular endoplasmic reticulum. Far more abundant are tubular and vesicular elements of an atypical agranular endoplasmic reticulum (see Fig. 22–7). The Golgi apparatus is not especially well developed or consistent in its location. Coated or alveolate vesicles are commonly associated with the Golgi, and some of these may have a dense content. Mitochondria are moderately abundant and not unusual in their structure. Centrioles are present, and the cells occasionally have a single flagellum. A distinctive feature of the cytoplasm is the presence of large numbers of microtubules. In the processes these may be aggregated in parallel bundles, but in the cell body they exhibit no consistent orientation. Lipid droplets, lipochrome pigment deposits, and structures resembling lysosomes are also present.

The second cell type of the pineal is the *interstitial cell.* These cells occur in the perivascular areas and between the clusters of pinealocytes. Their nuclei are elongated and stain more deeply than those of the parenchymal cells. The cytoplasm is somewhat more basophilic and drawn out into long processes. In electron micrographs the granular endoplasmic reticulum is well represented, and free ribosomes are numerous. In addition, occasional deposits of glycogen are found. Rare microtubules are present, but these are overshadowed by a profusion of cytoplasmic filaments 50 to 60 Å in diameter and of indeterminate length. They may occur in large bundles or as single randomly oriented filaments.

Some workers consider the interstitial cells, which represent about 5 per cent of the cells in the pineal, to be glial elements. The abundance of filaments in their cytoplasm is indeed reminiscent of the fine structure of

556

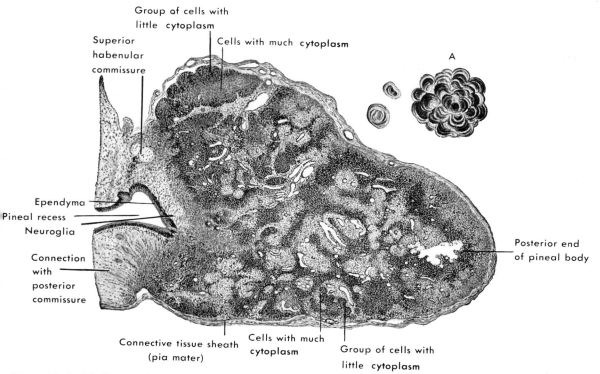

Figure 22–1 Median section through pineal body of a newborn child. Blood vessels empty. × 32. *A,* Corpora arenacea (sand granules) from the pineal body of a 69 year old woman. × 160. (After Schaffer.)

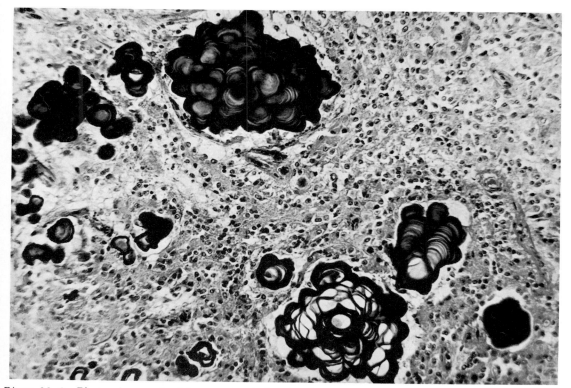

Figure 22–2 Photomicrograph of human pineal, showing the characteristic concretions (pineal sand). × 200.

astrocytes. The presence in rat pineal of stellate cells that stain strongly with the acid hematin method has been reported by Quay, but whether these represent a cell type distinct from interstitial cells is not yet clear.

The human pineal body often contains concretions called *corpora arenacea (psammoma bodies)* or brain sand (Fig. 22–2). They are extracellular and are composed of a mineralized organic matrix that often has a concentric organization. The concretions consist mainly of calcium phosphates and carbonates. They increase in number with age, but their exact manner of formation and their significance are not known.

Histogenesis

The pineal body first appears at about 36 days of gestation as a prominent thickening of the ependyma in the posterior part of the roof of the diencephalon. Cells migrate from this ependymal thickening to form a segregated mantle layer, whose cells tend to assume a follicular arrangement that is gradually transformed into the cordlike arrangement seen in later stages of development. By the end of the sixth month, interstitial (neuroglial) and pineal parenchymal cells have differentiated.

It is generally believed that the pineal body increases in size until about 7 years of age. Involution is said to begin at this time and to continue to 14 years of age. It is manifested by the development of hyaline changes in both the septa and the lobules, and by increasing numbers of corpora arenacea.

Innervation

Nerves are found throughout the organ in silver impregnated specimens. As the nerve fibers penetrate into the organ, their myelin sheaths terminate and the bare axons continue among the pinealocytes. Some of these contain many small vesicles in the size range of synaptic vesicles, suggesting that the nerves have functional endings in close relation to the parenchymal cells. The innervation appears to be exclusively via autonomic fibers originating in the superior cervical sympathetic ganglion.

Pineal System of Lower Vertebrates

In contrast to the single, relatively solid mass of tissue making up the pineal body in adult mammals, the organs in most lower vertebrates remain saccular throughout life and are somewhat more complex. The pineal system may consist of a single pineal sac (the intracranial epiphysis), as in most fishes and tailed amphibians, or it may be double. In the latter case (primitive fishes, tailless amphibians, and lizards) a second, *parapineal* organ results either from elaboration of an anterior end vesicle of the epiphysis, or from a separate evagination from the diencephalic roof situated more anteriorly. In frogs, the parapineal component (the frontal organ) comes to lie subepidermally and is discernible externally on the median dorsal aspect of the head. It is connected with the intracranial

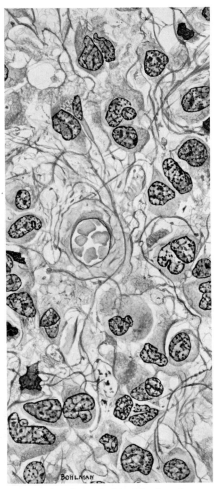

Figure 22-3 Section of pineal body of man stained with hematoxylin and eosin, showing irregularly shaped cells and their processes. Note the blood vessel in the center. Compare with Figure 22–6.

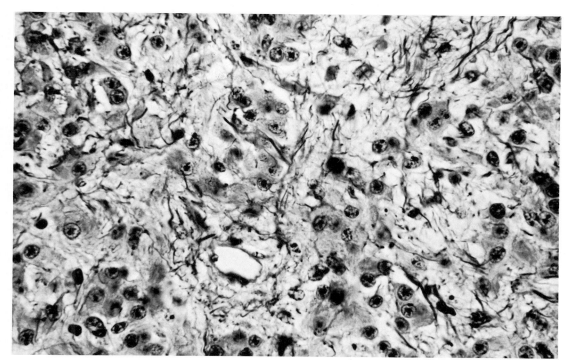

Figure 22-4 Photomicrograph of bovine pineal. The pinealocytes have large nuclei with prominent nucleoli. The outlines of the stellate cells are not easily distinguished. Many densely stained processes are visible in this preparation, but it is not possible to determine which belong to pinealocytes and which to interstitial cells. Iron hematoxylin stain. × 500. (Courtesy of E. Anderson.)

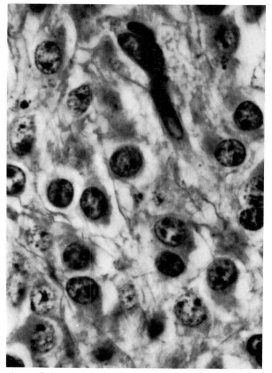

Figure 22-5 Histological section of sheep pineal. The pinealocyte nuclei are round or oval. The elongated nuclei in the upper part of the figure belong to interstitial glial cells. Heidenhain's iron-hematoxylin. × 700. (Courtesy of E. Anderson.)

epiphysis by a long pineal nerve. While many nerve fibers and their endings are readily demonstrable in pineal systems of lower vertebrates, no evidence exists suggesting that any are sympathetic.

Electron microscopic examination of adult saccular pineal systems reveals that, in most lower vertebrates, the principal cell type is an apparent photoreceptor. This cell closely resembles a retinal rod or cone, both in the form of the membranous lamellated modified flagellum that protrudes from the cell apex into the pineal lumen and in the presence of characteristic receptor synapses at the cell base. Physiological data indicate that, in these species, impulses course along pineal tracts to surrounding brain regions in response to darkness or to light of various wavelengths. The most elaborate pineal photoreceptor systems are found in certain lizards, such as the Tuatara (*Sphenodon*), in which, in addition to a photoreceptor-type intracranial epiphysis, the parapineal component (or parietal "eye") is specialized to the extent of possessing a distinct lens and a retina composed of photoreceptor cells backed by supportive cells containing pigment. Photoreceptor cells have not been distinguished in mammalian pineal systems.

Histophysiology

Opinions regarding the function of the mammalian pineal body have been widely divergent, some considering it a functionless vestigial organ and others regarding it as an important endocrine gland. Advances in recent years have brought a greater measure of agreement. Few would now insist that the pineal system of mammals and lower vertebrates is merely vestigial, but the physiological significance of its secretion and photoreception remains obscure.

The pineal has long been suspected of exerting an antigonadotropic effect. The principal basis for this was the clinical observation that boys with tumors that destroyed pineal parenchyma exhibited precocious puberty. Animal experimentation has, on the whole, substantiated this belief. Pinealectomy in young rats leads to enlargement of the reproductive organs and early onset of puberty. Injection of pineal extracts delays puberty and reduces ovarian weight. Other lines of evidence, none conclusive, have suggested relations to pituitary, adrenal, and thyroid function and a relation (possibly shared by the

nearby subcommissural organ) to water and salt balance. Work on experimental animals has shown that pineal physiology is influenced by diurnal variation in light and possibly by seasonal changes in day length.

Application of isotopic techniques has provided clear evidence of a surprising degree of metabolic activity. The pineal body of rodents displays a rapid uptake and turnover of radioactive phosphorus and a high rate of amino acid incorporation. The organ contains detectable amounts of a 5-hydroxyindole compound, *melatonin*, that is synthesized from serotonin, which is present in abundance (Ler-

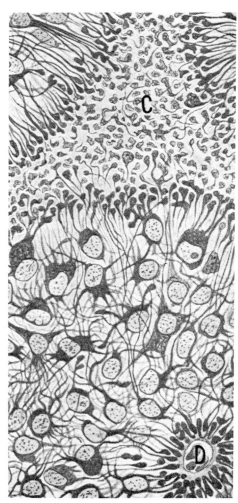

Figure 22-6 Specifically impregnated section of the pineal body of a young boy, showing interlobular tissue (*C*) and vessel (*D*) with club-shaped processes of specific cells in its adventitia. Note parenchymatous cells and their claviform processes bordering on *C*. (After del Rio-Hortega.)

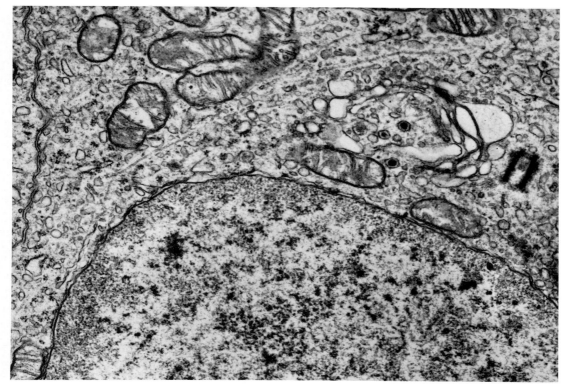

Figure 22-7   Electron micrograph of a juxtanuclear area of pinealocyte cytoplasm, showing a centriole and part of the Golgi complex, with associated vesicles with dense osmiophilic content. The cytoplasm generally contains abundant small vesicles and numerous microtubules. × 30,000. (Courtesy of E. Anderson.)

ner and Case). Both melatonin and the enzyme which is responsible for its formation (Axelrod and Weissbach), hydroxyindole-O-methyl transferase (HIOMT), are found exclusively in the pineal organ in white rats, but they are somewhat more widely distributed in the brain and retina of lower vertebrates possessing photoreceptor-type pineal systems.

Melatonin has been extracted primarily from mammalian pineal organs, but when applied in low concentrations to amphibian skin it causes marked aggregation of pigment granules in melanophores and hence results in blanching. It has therefore been suggested that melatonin is an antagonist of the melanophore stimulating hormone in the pigment regulation of lower vertebrates. No influence has been demonstrated on mammalian melanocytes. Some authors report, however, that melatonin seems to play an active role in the light-influenced reproductive cycles of rodents and birds. It is suggested that, in these forms, photic stimuli relayed from optic pathways to the pineal body via sympathetic nerves are translated by pineal activity into humoral gonadal control. Pineals from rats subjected to constant light weigh less and have smaller cells, exhibiting less basophilia and less lipid, than those from rats kept constantly in the dark (Roth). The activity of the specific enzyme for melatonin production (HIOMT) is also reduced in constant light. A diurnal rhythm of phosphorus uptake and serotonin content correlated with periods of daylight and darkness has also been reported. Extirpation of the superior cervical ganglion establishes that the responses to light are mediated by the autonomic nerves.

The physiology of the pineal is now a subject of intensive investigation. It appears that the pineal has a neuroendocrine function and that it participates in the regulation of the rhythmic activity of the endocrine system by elaborating specific methoxyindoles that serve as hormone-like mediators, but many of the details of its complex interrelationships have yet to be worked out.

REFERENCES

Anderson, E.: The anatomy of bovine and ovine pineals: Light and electron microscopic studies. J. Ultrastruct. Res., Suppl. 8, 1965.

Ariëns-Kappers, J., and J. P. Schadé, eds.: Structure and function of the epiphysis cerebri. *In* Progress in Brain Research. Amsterdam, Elsevier Publishing Co., 1965, Vol. 10.

Axelrod, J., and H. Weissbach: Purification and properties of hydroxyindole-O-methyl transferase. J. Biol. Chem., 236:216, 1961.

Bargmann, W.: Die Epiphysis Cerebri. *In* von Möllendorff, W., and W. Bargmann, eds.: Handbuch der mikroskopischen Anatomie des Menschen. Berlin, Springer, Verlag, 1943, Vol. 6, part 4, p. 309.

Fiske, V. M., J. Pound, and J. Putnam: Effect of light on the weight of the pineal organ in hypophysectomized, gonadectomized, adrenalectomized and thiouracil-fed rats. Endocrinology, 71:130, 1962.

Kelly, D. E.: Pineal organs: Photoreception, secretion and development. Am. Scientist, 50:597, 1962.

Kelly, D. E.: An ultrastructural analysis of the paraphysis cerebri in newts. Zeitschr. f. Zellforsch., 64:778, 1964.

Kelly, D. E.: Circumventricular organs. *In* Haymaker, W., and R. D. Adams, eds.: Histology and Neuropathology of the Human Nervous System. Springfield, Ill., Charles C Thomas, 1966.

Kitay, J. I., and M. D. Altschule: The Pineal Gland; a Review of the Physiologic Literature. Cambridge, Harvard University Press, 1954.

Lerner, A. B., and J. D. Case: Pigment cell regulatory factors. J. Invest. Derm., 32:221, 1959.

Quay, W. B.: Reduction of mammalian pineal weight and lipid during continuous light. Gen. Comp. Endocr., 1: 211, 1961.

Quay, W. B.: Experimental and cytological studies of pineal cells staining with acid hematin in the rat. Acta Morphol. Neerl. Scand., 5:87, 1962.

Quay, W. B.: Circadian rhythm in rat serotonin and its modifications by estrous cycles and photoperiod. Gen. Comp. Endocr., 3:473, 1963.

Quay, W. B.: Retinal and pineal hydroxyindole-O-methyl transferase activity in vertebrates. Life Sciences, 4: 983, 1965.

Reiter, R. J., et al.: Symposium on comparative endocrinology of the pineal. Amer. Zool., 10:187, 1970.

Roth, W. D.: Metabolic and morphologic studies on the rat pineal organ during puberty. *In* Ariëns-Kappens, J., and J. P. Schadé, eds.: Progress in Brain Research. Amsterdam, Elsevier Publishing Co., 1965, Vol. 10.

Roth, W. D., R. J. Wurtman, and M. D. Altschule: Morphologic changes in the pineal parenchymal cells of rats exposed to continuous light or darkness. Endocrinology, 71:888, 1962.

Wartenberg, H.: The mammalian pineal organ: Electron microscopic studies on the fine structure of pinealocytes, glial cells, and on the perivascular component. Z. Zellforsch., 86:74, 1968.

Wolfe, D. E.: The epiphyseal cell: An electron microscopic study of intercellular relationships and intracellular morphology in the pineal body of the albino rat. *In* Ariëns-Kappers, J., and J. P. Schadé, eds.: Progress in Brain Research. Amsterdam, Elsevier Publishing Co., 1965, Vol. 10.

Wolstenholme, G. E., and J. Knight (eds.): The pineal gland. Ciba Foundation Symposium, London, Churchill Ltd., 1971.

Wurtman, R. J.: Effects of light and visual stimuli on endocrine function. *In* Ganong, W. F., and L. Martini, eds.: Neuroendocrinology. New York, Academic Press, 1966.

Wurtman, R. J., W. D. Roth, M. D. Altschule, and J. J. Wurtman: Interactions of the pineal and exposure to continuous light on organ weights of female rats. Acta Endocr., 36:617, 1961.

23
Skin

The skin covers the surface of the body and consists of two main layers, the surface epithelium, or *epidermis,* and the subjacent connective tissue layer, the *corium* or *dermis* (Figs. 23–1 and 23–2). Beneath the dermis is a looser connective tissue layer, the superficial fascia, or *hypodermis,* which in many places is largely transformed into subcutaneous adipose tissue. The hypodermis is loosely connected to underlying deep fascia, aponeurosis, or periosteum. The skin is continuous which several mucous membranes at *mucocutaneous junctions.* Such junctions are found at the lips, nares, eyelids, vulva, prepuce, and anus.

The skin is one of the largest of the organs, making up some 16 per cent of the body weight. Its functions are several. It protects the organism from injury and desiccation; it receives stimuli from the environment; it excretes various substances; and, in warm-blooded animals, it takes part in thermoregulation and maintenance of water balance. The subcutaneous adipose tissue has an important role in fat metabolism.

The specific functions of the skin depend largely upon the properties of the epidermis. This epithelium forms an uninterrupted cellular investment covering the entire outer surface of the body, but it is also locally specialized to form the various skin appendages: *hair, nails,* and *glands.* Its cells produce the fibrous protein *keratin,* which is essential to the protective function of the skin, and *melanin,* the pigment that protects against ultraviolet irradiation. The epidermis gives rise to two main types of glands, one of which produces the watery secretion *sweat* and the other the oily secretion *sebum.*

The free surface of the skin is not smooth but is marked by delicate grooves or flexure lines, which create patterns that vary from region to region. They are deeper on non-hairy areas, such as knees and elbows, palms and soles. The most familiar of the surface patterns are those responsible for the fingerprints. It is well known that the complicated patterns of ridges found on the fingers are subject to such marked variations that their impressions are a dependable means for identification of individuals. The same degree of variation holds for skin patterns in other regions, but these are less commonly used.

The interface of the epidermis and the dermis is also uneven. A pattern of ridges and grooves on the deep surface of the epidermis fits a complementary pattern of corrugations on the underlying dermis. The projections of the dermis have traditionally been described as *dermal papillae* and those of the epidermis as *epidermal ridges,* owing to their respective appearances in vertical sections of skin. As will be seen later, these terms are not always accurately descriptive of their three dimensional configuration as seen in whole mounts.

Although the boundary between the epithelial and the connective tissue portions of the skin is sharp, the fibrous elements of the dermis merge with those of the hypodermis, so that there is no clear-cut boundary between these layers.

THE EPIDERMIS

The epidermis is a stratified squamous epithelium composed of cells of two distinct lineages. Those comprising the bulk of the epithelium undergo keratinization and form the dead superficial layers of the skin. They are derivatives of the ectoderm covering the embryo, and they constitute the *malpighian* or *keratinizing system.* There are also cells

563

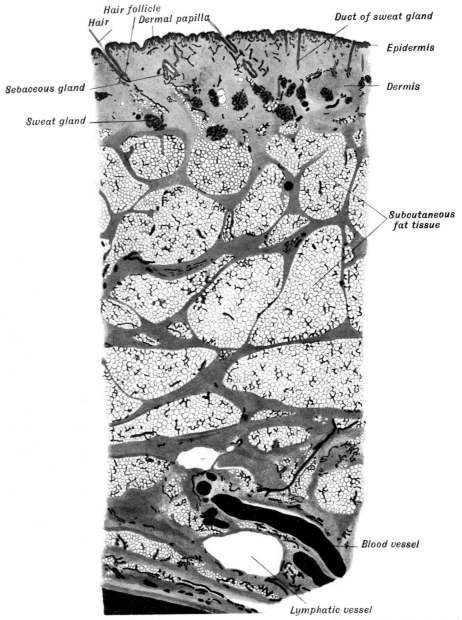

Figure 23-1 Section through human thigh perpendicular to the surface of the skin. Blood vessels are injected and appear black. Low magnification. (After A. A. Maximow.)

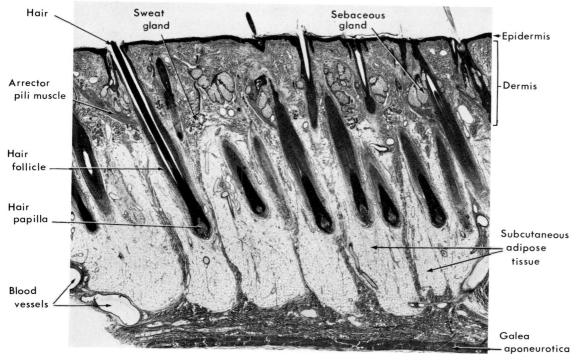

Figure 23-2 Section of the skin of the scalp. × 15. (Courtesy of H. Mizoguchi.)

in the deeper layers of the epidermis that do not keratinize but are capable of producing the pigment melanin. These are the *melanocytes*, which arise from the embryonic neural crest and invade the skin in the third to sixth months of intrauterine life. Collectively these cells comprise the *pigmentary system* of the skin. In addition, there are two other cell types, not part of the keratinizing system. These are the *Langerhans cells* and the *Merkel cells*. Their functions are obscure.

The epidermis varies from 0.07 to 0.12 mm. in thickness over most of the body, but it may reach a thickness of 0.8 mm. on the palms and 1.4 mm. on the soles. In the fetus, these sites are already appreciably thicker than other areas of skin, but continuous friction or pressure in postnatal life may cause considerable additional thickening of the outer layer of the epidermis on exposed areas of the body surface.

The superficial keratinized cells of the skin are continually exfoliated from the surface and are replaced by cells that arise from mitotic activity in the basal layer of the epidermis. The cells produced there are displaced to successively higher levels by the generation of new cells below them. As they move upward, they elaborate keratin, which accumulates in their interior until it largely replaces all metabolically active cytoplasm. The cell dies and its nucleus and other organelles disappear. It is finally shed as a flakelike, lifeless residue of a cell. This sequence of changes, referred to as the *cytomorphosis* of the malpighian cell, takes from 15 to 30 days, depending upon the region of the body and a number of other factors.

Epidermis of the Palms and Soles

The structural organization of the epidermis can be studied to advantage in those areas where it attains its greatest development—namely, the palm of the hand and the sole of the foot. In sections perpendicular to the surface, four layers can be distinguished (Figs. 23-3 and 23-4). The deepest of these is the *stratum malpighii*, which may be subdivided into the *stratum germinativum* (stratum basale), the layer of cells in contact with the dermis, and a layer of variable thickness above it called the *stratum spinosum* (prickle-cell layer). The next layer is the *stratum granulosum* or granular layer; then follow the *stratum lucidum* or clear layer and the *stratum corneum* or horny layer. The superficial keratinized portion of the epidermis consists of the stratum corneum and stratum lucidum.

The cells of the *stratum germinativum* adjacent to the dermis are cuboidal to columnar and have their cell axis perpendicular to the basal lamina. Mitotic figures are common in this layer but are by no means confined to it. As the cells move up into the stratum spinosum, they assume a flattened polyhedral form, with their long axis parallel to the surface and their nucleus somewhat elongated in this direction. All of the cells bear short processes or "spines" that are attached to similar projections from adjacent cells. Because the cell membranes at the sites of end to end junction of these processes cannot be resolved with light microscopy, these structures were formerly called "inter-

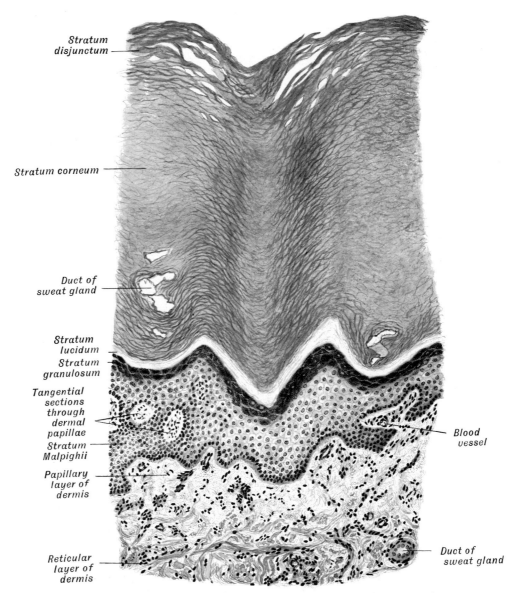

Figure 23-3   Section of human sole perpendicular to the free surface. × 100. (After A. A. Maximow.)

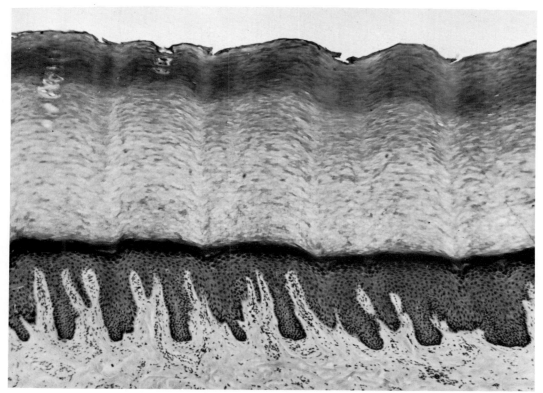

Figure 23–4 Skin of the human finger tip, illustrating a very thick stratum corneum. Hematoxylin and eosin. × 65.

cellular bridges" in the belief that they represented open communications between the epidermal cells (Fig. 23–5). The term is no longer appropriate and should be abandoned, since it has been shown by electron microscopy that there is no protoplasmic continuity between the cells. Instead, the processes or "prickles" simply meet end to end or side to side and are firmly attached by a well developed *desmosome*, which appeared in appropriately stained histological sections as a dense dot or granule in each "bridge" (Fig. 23–7). The cells of the malpighian layer are basophilic and show bundles of cytoplasmic fibrils called *tonofibrils*. These traverse the cytoplasm in various directions and extend into the cell processes to terminate in the desmosomes.

The *stratum granulosum* consists of three to five layers of flattened cells containing conspicuous granules of irregular shape that stain deeply with basic dyes and with hematoxylin. These are the *keratohyalin granules*.

They are not to be confused with granules of melanin pigment, which are most abundant in the basal layers of the epidermis. The origin and chemical nature of the keratohyalin granules have not been clearly established. They were formerly believed to be intimately associated with the process of keratinization, but they are not present in all keratinizing tissues. They are absent, for example, in nails but are abundant in epidermis of cattle hoofs.

The *stratum lucidum* is formed of several layers of flattened, closely compacted, eosinophilic cells. It appears in section as a wavy clear stripe interposed between the stratum granulosum and stratum corneum. The nucleus of the cells has disappeared.

The thick *stratum corneum* on the palms and soles consists of many layers of flat, cornified cells lacking a nucleus and with the cytoplasm replaced by keratin. The processes by which cells were joined in the spiny layer are no longer visible, and the lifeless cells are

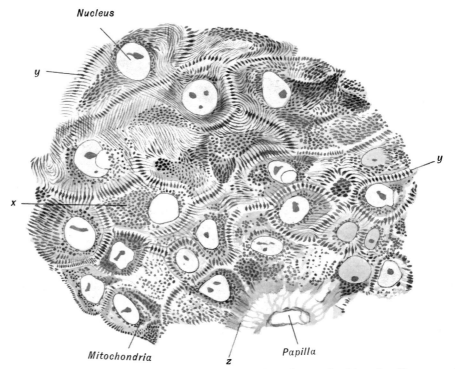

Nucleus

y

x

y

Mitochondria

z

Papilla

Figure 23–5   Section, tangential to the surface, of the malpighian layer of epidermis of human palm, showing fibrils and so-called "intercellular bridges" in cross section at *x* and in longitudinal section at *y*. The junction of the scalloped lower surface of the epithelial cells with the dermis is at *z*.

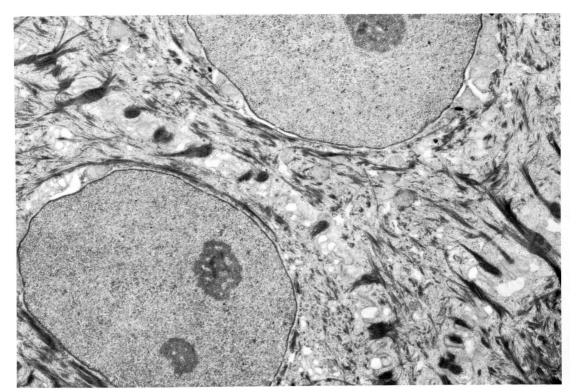

Figure 23–6   Electron micrograph of parts of three cells from the stratum germinativum of human epidermi × 12,000. (Courtesy of G. Odland.)

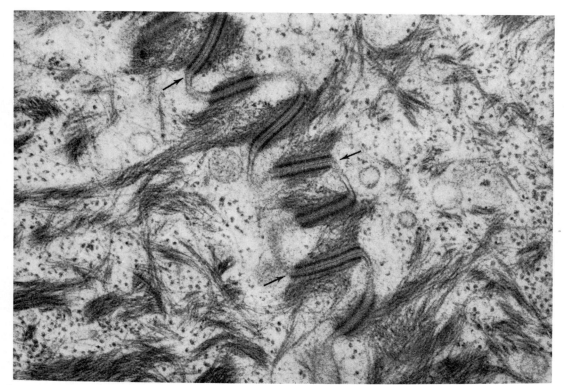

Figure 23–7 Electron micrograph of portions of two adjoining epidermal cells. The junction of the two cells runs diagonally across the figure. Desmosomes attaching the apposed cell surfaces are indicated by the arrows. Bundles of epidermal filaments run in various directions in the cytoplasm and terminate in desmosomes. × 50,000. (Courtesy of G. Odland.)

closely packed together without obvious interstices. In the most peripheral layers, where the dried horny cells are constantly being desquamated (*stratum disjunctum*), individual squamae or sheets of them may appear loosened and partially detached (Fig. 23–3).

The number of dividing cells in the malpighian layer corresponds to the intensity of desquamation of the stratum corneum in a given region.

Epidermis of the Body in General

On the rest of the body the epidermis is much thinner and simpler in its structure (Figs. 23–11 and 23–12). The stratum malpighii and stratum corneum are always present, although the latter may be relatively thin. A granular layer consisting of two or three layers of cells is usually identifiable, but a definite stratum lucidum is seldom seen in the thinner epidermis of the general body surface. The epidermis is entirely devoid of blood vessels; it is presumed to be nourished from capillaries in the underlying connective tissue by diffusion through tissue fluid, which occupies an extensive system of intercellular spaces of the malpighian layer. Human skin, unlike that of practically all other vertebrates, blisters after exposure to thermal and certain chemical stimuli, such as the vesicant gases. This reaction is apparently related to the many layers of cells in human epidermis.

Fine Structure of the Epidermis and the Process of Keratinization

In electron micrographs the cells of the malpighian layer are seen to be rich in free polyribosomes and to have occasional profiles of granular endoplasmic reticulum. The mitochondria are sparse and the Golgi apparatus poorly developed. The tonofibrils of light microscopy are resolved as bundles of 70 to 80 Å filaments called *tonofilaments*. In the basal layer of cells, these are loosely organized and randomly oriented, but in the spiny layer, they tend to be aggregated into conspicuous bundles (Fig. 23–7). In both layers the filaments converge upon the cell processes around the periphery and terminate in desmosomes where the processes of neighboring cells join.

In the uppermost cells of the stratum spinosum, there are numerous electron-dense spherical granules, 50 to 100 nm. in diameter (Odland). The exact nature of these granules is not known, but they gather at the uppermost cell surface. According to some authors they are secreted into the intercellular space, and their substance spreads upon the cell membrane, making it appreciably thicker than the lower surface. The term *membrane-coating granules* has therefore been applied to them (Matoltsy). Other workers prefer the term *keratinosomes*, and since they contain the enzyme acid phosphatase, it is suggested that they may be involved in the desquamation of the stratum corneum.

The cells of the granular layer differ from those of the spiny layer mainly in their more flattened shape and in the presence of irregular accumulations of dense material 1 to 5 µm. in diameter, among and around the bundles of tonofilaments. These correspond to the keratohyalin granules of light microscopy (Figs. 23–8 and 23–17). Although at low power they appear homogeneous, it is found at higher magnification that the epidermal filaments extend into and mingle with the dense matrix of the keratohyalin granules.

Above the granular layer, the cells undergo an abrupt change. In the stratum lucidum, they are very much elongated and flattened, and although the cell outlines are still discernible, all of the cell organelles including the nuclei have disappeared. The cells of this layer and of the overlying stratum corneum may appear homogeneous with the light microscope, but at higher magnification they are found to be completely

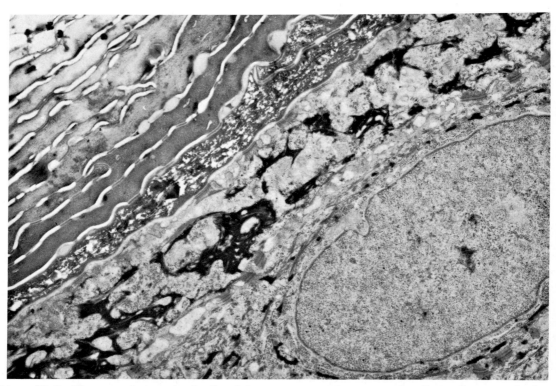

Figure 23-8 Electron micrograph of cells of the stratum granulosum, running diagonally across the figure and containing irregularly shaped keratohyalin granules. At the upper left are several cell layers of the stratum corneum. × 12,000. (Courtesy of G. Odland.)

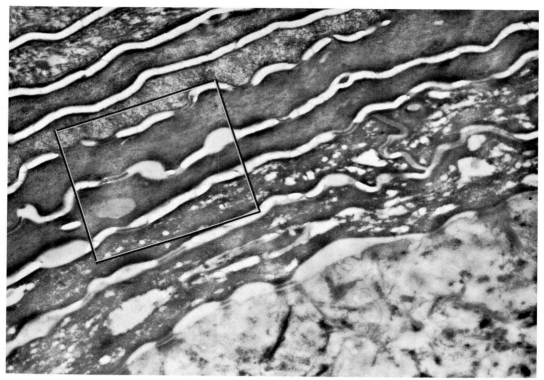

Figure 23-9 Electron micrograph showing a portion of a cell of the granular layer (*lower right*) and several layers of flattened cells of the stratum corneum (*upper left*). The area enclosed in the rectangle is shown at higher magnification in Figure 23-10. Osmium fixation. × 22,500. (Courtesy of G. Odland.)

filled with tightly packed 70 to 80 Å filaments embedded in an electron dense matrix (Figs. 23–9 and 23–10). Keratohyalin granules are no longer visible as such, but some authors believe that the interfibrillar matrix of the keratinized cell is of the same nature and may derive from the keratohyalin granules. As the cells move upward in the epidermis and become more flattened, their spines are effaced, but the desmosomes persist. Concurrent with the keratinization of the cells, there is a marked change in the character of the desmosomes. Instead of two thickened regions of the opposing membranes separated by a less dense intercellular cleft, the desmosome comes to be represented as a dense band of osmiophilic material that appears to be extracellular and to occupy the site of the intercellular cleft of the original desmosome (Fig. 23–10). The details of this transformation have not been worked out.

THE MELANOCYTE SYSTEM

The color of the skin is the resultant of three components. The tissue has an inherent yellowish color, attributable in part to *carotene*. The *oxyhemoglobin* in the underlying vascular bed imparts a reddish hue, and shades of brown to black are contributed by varying amounts of *melanin*. Of these three colored substances, only the melanin is produced in the skin. It is the product of specialized cells with elaborately branching processes called *melanocytes*, which are located in the malpighian layer of the epidermis or in the underlying connective tissue of the dermis. Although melanin granules are also found in the malpighian cells, they are formed only by the epidermal melanocytes, for these cells alone possess the enzyme tyrosinase that is necessary for synthesis of the pigment. The fully formed melanin granules are transferred from the melano-cytes to the malpighian cells by an unusual form of activity sometimes referred to as *cytocrine* secretion. The melanocytes are commonly located at the dermoepidermal junction with their pigment-containing proc-esses extending for long distances upward into the interstices among the malpighian cells. They are not attached to the other cells by desmosomes, and in specimen prepara-tion they may shrink away so that they are surrounded by a clear space. Because of their tendency to pass pigment to the malpighian cells, the melanocytes may actually contain less melanin than the neighboring epidermal cells, and their processes (or dendrites) are very difficult to identify in sections stained with hematoxylin and eosin. They are best studied in whole mounts of separated epi-dermis that have been treated with 1,3,4-dihydroxyphenylalanine (DOPA) (Fig. 23–13). In such preparations, the melanocytes

are blackened and appear as highly branched cells. The ratio of melanocytes to basal epidermal cells varies between 1 to 4 and 1 to 10, depending upon the region of the body. The melanocytes in the cheek and forehead and in the genital, nasal, and oral epithelium are about twice as numerous as in other parts of the body surface. It is also of interest that the number of melanocytes is approximately the same in all human races; differences in color are attributable to differences in the amount of pigment that these cells produce and transfer to the keratinocytes (Fig. 23–14).

Melanin is formed on a specific cell particle, the *melanosome*. In man it is an elongated body with rounded ends, measur-ing about 0.2 by 0.6 μm., with a fibrillar or lamellar internal structure exhibiting char-acteristic periodic density variations along its length in early stages of development. This internal structure tends to be obscured

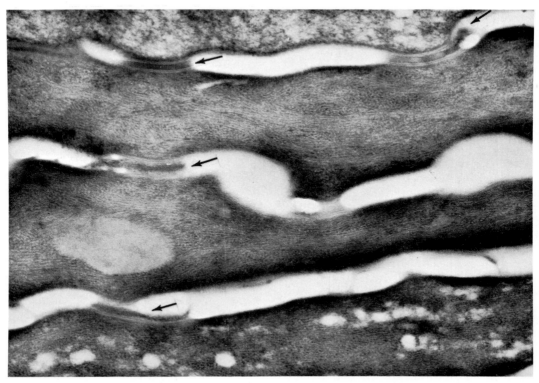

Figure 23–10 Electron micrograph of the area of stratum corneum of human epidermis enclosed in the rectangle in Figure 23–9. The cytoplasm of the flat keratinized cells appears devoid of organelles and seems to consist mainly of closely packed, fine filaments embedded in a rather dense matrix. The desmosomes, indicated by arrows, have an unusually thick, dense intermediate layer. The clear spaces between the cells are, in part, artifacts of specimen preparation. Osmium fixation. × 62,000. (Courtesy of G. Odland.)

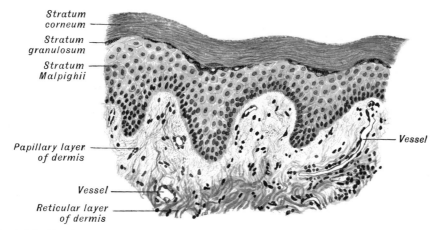

Figure 23–11 Section through skin of human shoulder. × 125. (After A. A. Maximow.)

by accumulation of dense melanin in the mature melanosome. The size, shape, and internal structure of the melanosomes vary with the animal species and are characteristic of particular genotypes within the same species. In man, however, melanosomes are uniformly elongated (Figs. 23–16 and 23–17) except in red-haired individuals, in whom they tend to be spherical. Melanosomes are somewhat larger in the skin of Australoids, Negroids, and Mongoloids than they are in

Caucasoids. Within the same individual they tend to be larger in the hair follicles than in the skin.

Lack of melanin in the epidermis of some areas of the skin of animals may be due either to absence of melanocytes or, as in *albinism*, to the inability of the melanocytes to form pigmented melanosomes. In man, the entire integument normally possesses functioning melanocytes. Their activity is influenced by hormones and by factors in the physical

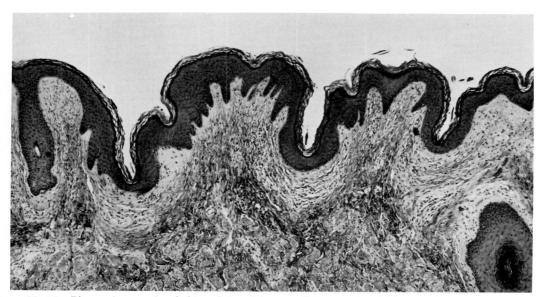

Figure 23–12 Photomicrograph of skin of the abdomen. Compare the thickness of the stratum corneum with that of the finger tip in Figure 23–4. × 60.

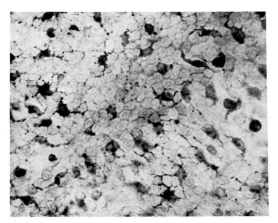

Figure 23-13 Photomicrograph of a whole mount of a sheet of epidermis from the thigh spread upon a slide and viewed from the underside to illustrate the melanocytes. The epidermis was separated from the dermis by treatment of the excised skin with trypsin. The epidermal sheet was then incubated in 1,3,4-dihydroxyphenylalanine (DOPA), which selectively stains the melanocytes. Notice their branching process. × 300. (Courtesy of G. Szabo.)

environment. During pregnancy, the pigmentation of the areola of the nipples increases. Freckles are intensified and some individuals develop *cloasma*, the so-called "mask of pregnancy," consisting of a pigmented area over the malar eminences and a brownish discoloration of the forehead. This gradually disappears after delivery. The phenomenon of *tanning* on exposure to sunlight results from an immediate darkening of the existing melanin and, after a few days, an enhanced tyrosinase activity in the melanocytes that leads to the formation of new melanin. The pigmentation of the skin is believed to protect the underlying tissues against the potentially harmful effects of solar radiation. In man small melanosomes often aggregate to form melanosome complexes within the keratinocytes (Fig. 23–16), whereas large melanosomes are usually individually distributed. A more effective protective layer against ultraviolet radiation results.

Melanin is also found in the retinal pigment epithelium of the eye (Fig. 23–15) and in dermal melanocytes and melanophores of cold-blooded vertebrates, where they constitute the pigmentary effector system responsible for rapid changes of color for purposes of camouflage and concealment. The "ink" of squid and other cephalopods consists of small spherical melanosomes, produced in a special ink gland, stored in the ink-sac, and squirted out to blacken the water and conceal the animal threatened by a predator (Szabo).

Throughout the epidermis, but particularly in the upper layers of the stratum malpighii, there are peculiar cells described by Langerhans in 1868. In routine hematoxylin and eosin preparations, they have dark staining nuclei surrounded by apparently clear cytoplasm. In sections stained by the gold chloride method, they are blackened and are revealed as stellate or dendritic cells (Fig. 23–18). Their slender processes penetrate the intercellular spaces among the prickle cells, but they themselves are devoid of desmosomes attaching them to neighboring cells. The Langerhans cells have been variously interpreted. One of the most persistent views has been that they are effete epidermal melanocytes that have given up their melanin and have lost the capacity to produce more (Masson). In favor of their relationship to melanocytes is their similar morphological appearance and some cytological and histochemical staining reactions that they have in common. Against their being degenerate or regressive forms is the fact that in the hyperplasia that follows ultraviolet irradiation of the epidermis, they exhibit a striking uptake of tritiated thymidine. Since the Langerhans cells are capable of active DNA synthesis they can no longer be regarded as worn-out melanocytes (Giacometti and Montagna). It has also been shown that Langerhans cells

SPECIES	AREA AND NUMBER OF INDIVIDUALS	NUMBER OF MELANOCYTES (PER mm.^{2} ± S.E.)
Man[1]		
Caucasoid	Thigh (35)	1000 ± 70
Mongoloid	Thigh (3)	1290 ± 45
Negroid	Thigh (7)	1415 ± 255
Guinea Pig[2]		
Black	Ear (8)	920 ± 145
Red	Ear (8)	865 ± 100
Mouse[3]		
C57 Black	Tail (4)	590 ± 65
DBL Dilute	Tail (4)	590 ± 165

[1] Szabo (1969) and Szabo; Gerald et al. (1971).
[2] Billingham and Medawar (1953).
[3] Gerson and Szabo (1969).

Figure 23-14 Comparison of melanocyte numbers among color variants of mammals.

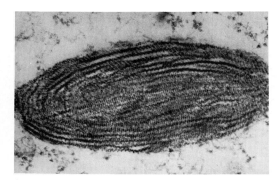

Figure 23–15 Electron micrograph of a developing human melanosome from the retina, showing the periodicity in its structural framework. When the melanosome is fully developed, its interior structure is obscured by the accumulated melanin. × 63,000. (Courtesy of A. Breathnach.)

are a highly constant population throughout the epidermis, whereas the numerical density of melanocytes exhibits marked regional variations (Wolff and Winkelmann). Their appearance in electron micrographs also is that of a healthy active cell. The nucleus is highly irregular in outline, and the cytoplasm is of relatively low density and lacks melanosomes and tonofilaments (Fig. 23–19). A Golgi complex, mitochondria, and endoplasmic reticulum are present but are unremarkable. The cytoplasm contains many small vesicles, rounded dense granules 0.3 μm. in diameter, and peculiar rod-shaped, membrane limited structures. These are 150 to 500 nm. long and 40 nm. wide with a central linear density (Fig. 23–20). Some of them seem to be continuous with the surface membrane. The so-called "vermiform bodies" of the Kupffer cells in the liver bear a superficial resemblance to these organelles. In neither case is their chemical nature or functional significance known. The Langerhans cells are capable of taking up ferritin by phagocytosis, but this activity bears no relation to the Langerhans granules described above. Moreover, the keratinocytes are much more active in uptake of ferritin. These results do not support the hypothesis that the Langerhans cell

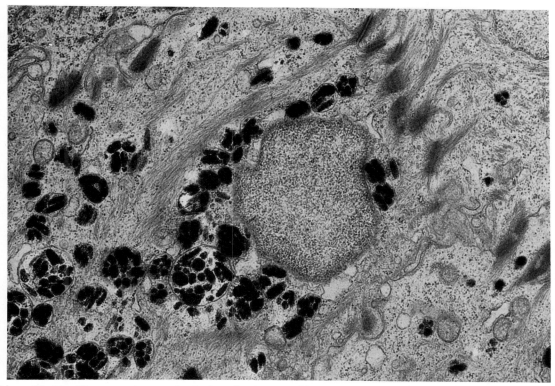

Figure 23–16 Electron micrograph of a heavily pigmented keratinocyte from the stratum malpighii of human skin. Whereas the melanosomes of melanocytes occur singly, those of keratinocytes are found in clusters of varying size enclosed by a membrane. ×20,000 (Courtesy of G. Szabo.)

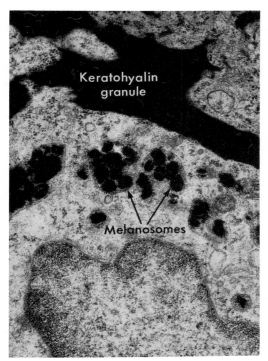

Figure 23-17 A micrograph of a portion of a cell from the stratum granulosum, showing dense keratohyalin granules and several clusters of melanosomes. × 8000. (Courtesy of G. Szabo.)

infrequently contains a peculiar inclusion consisting of a fascicle of straight parallel filaments (Winkelmann). The Merkel cells tend to be associated with areas where the dermis is especially well vascularized and richly innervated. Unmyelinated axons of what are presumed to be afferent sensory nerves are often found in close relationship to these cells. Although their appearance suggests that they are modified keratinocytes, their attachment to neighboring epithelial cells by desmosomes does not rule out the possibility that they may be of neurectodermal origin and may migrate into the epithelium with the nerves. No function has yet been established for the Merkel cells, but some suspect that they are involved in sensory reception.

MUCOCUTANEOUS JUNCTIONS

These are transitions between the mucous membranes and skin. Their epithelium is thicker than that of the adjacent skin and is more like that of the mucosa. They may have a thin, rudimentary, horny layer. Normally they do not contain sweat glands, hair follicles, hairs, or sebaceous glands, but are moistened by mucous glands situated within the body orifices. Since the horny layer

has a predominantly phagocytic function (Sagabiel).

The origin and function of the Langerhans cells remains obscure, but the bulk of the evidence seems to indicate that they are not related to the melanocytes. They have recently been shown to be present in skin grafts free of neural crest elements, hence lacking in melanocytes (Reams).

A third cell type in the epidermis is the *Merkel cell* (Fig. 23-21). It has a superficial resemblance to the keratinocytes to which it may be attached by desmosomes. The cytoplasm contains bundles of filaments in the perinuclear zone and in the peripheral cytoplasm, but these are less abundant than in keratinocytes. Their most distinctive feature in electron micrographs is the presence in their cytoplasm of small electron dense, membrane bounded particles resembling the catecholamine containing granules of the adrenal medulla or paraganglia (Fig. 23-22). They may occasionally contain transferred melanosomes (Hashimoto). The nucleus not

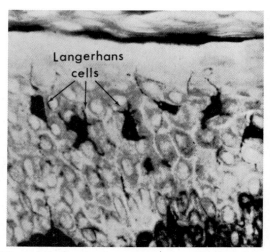

Figure 23-18 Section of human epidermis, showing gold impregnated Langerhans cells at a high level in the stratum malpighii. Gairn's gold chloride technique. × 610. (After A. S. Breathnach, Int. Rev. Cytol., *18*:1, 1965.)

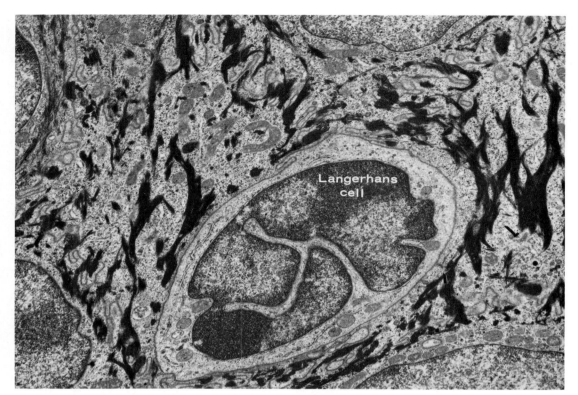

Figure 23–19   Electron micrograph of a Langerhans cell surrounded by keratinocytes containing dense bundles of filaments. The polymorphous appearance of the nucleus is typical. The stellate form of the cell is not evident here because none of the processes is included in the plane of section. (Micrograph by G. Szabo.)

is thin or may even be absent, the redness of the blood in the underlying capillaries shows through and gives the junction a red color.

THE DERMIS

The thickness of the dermis cannot be measured exactly, because it passes over into the subcutaneous layer without a sharp boundary. The average thickness is approximately 1 to 2 mm.; it is less on the eyelids and the prepuce (0.6 mm. or less) but reaches a thickness of 3 mm. or more on the soles and palms. On the ventral surface of the body and the appendages it is generally thinner than on the dorsal surface. It is thinner in women than in men.

The outer surface of the dermis in contact with the epidermis is usually uneven and is elevated into papillae that project into the concavities between the ridges on the deep surface of the epidermis. This sculptured surface of the dermis is called the *papillary layer,* and the deeper main portion of the dermis is called the *reticular layer.* The two cannot be clearly separated.

The reticular layer consists of rather dense connective tissue. Its collagenous fibers form a feltwork with bundles running in various directions but, for the most part, more or less parallel to the surface. Occasional bundles are oriented almost perpendicular to the majority. The papillary layer and its papillae consist of looser connective tissue with much thinner collagenous bundles.

The elastic fibers of the dermis form abundant, thick networks between the collagenous bundles and are condensed about the hair follicles and the sebaceous and sweat glands. In the papillary layer they are much thinner and form a continuous fine network in the papillae beneath the epithelium. The cells of the dermis are more abundant in the papillary than in the reticular layer and are similar to those of the subcutaneous layer except for the relative paucity of fat cells.

Within the deep parts of the reticular layer in the areolae, penis, perineum, and scrotum, numerous smooth muscle cells form a loose plexus. Such portions of the skin become wrinkled during contraction of these muscles. Smooth muscles, the so-called *arrector pili* muscles, are also connected with the hairs (Figs. 23–24 and 23–25). In many places in the skin of the face, cross striated muscle fibers terminate in the dermis. These are the *muscles of facial expression*. They are responsible for the voluntary movement of the ears and scalp. These represent vestiges, in man, of a more extensive subcutaneous layer of muscle that is present in many mammals, called the *panniculus carnosus*. This layer is responsible for the voluntary move-

ment of large segments of the integument, which can be observed when animals attempt to dislodge insects from their skin or to shake dry when they emerge from the water. The absence of this layer over most of the body in man is disadvantageous in that, after wounds, the skin is likely to become immobile and bound down to the underlying structures because of shrinkage of scar tissue. Greater disfigurement results than in other mammals with more mobile skin.

At various levels of the dermis are the hair follicles and the sweat and sebaceous glands, which are epidermal derivatives extending down into the dermis. Blood vessels, nerves, and nerve endings are also abundant.

Hypodermis

The subcutaneous layer consists of loose connective tissue and is a deeper continua-

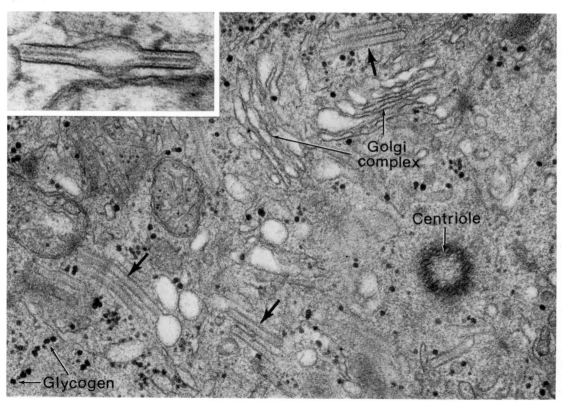

Figure 23-20 A small area of cytoplasm of a Langerhans cell, including one of the pair of centrioles, the Golgi complex, and several vermiform granules (at heavy arrows). One of these is shown at higher magnification in the inset. The dense granules in the cytoplasmic matrix are glycogen. (Micrograph by G. Szabo.)

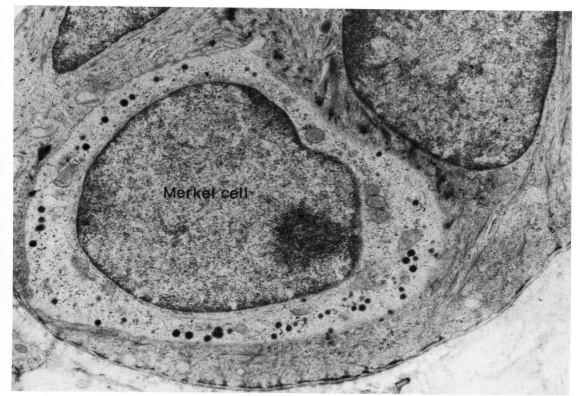

Figure 23-21   Electron micrograph of the base of the human epidermis, showing a Merkel cell surrounded by keratinocytes. Notice its pale cytoplasm and characteristic dense granules. (Micrograph by G. Szabo.)

tion of the dermis. Its collagenous and elastic fibers are directly continuous with those of the dermis and run in all directions but mainly parallel to the surface of the skin. Where the skin is flexible or freely movable, these fibers are few, but where it is closely attached to the underlying parts, as on the soles and palms, they are thick and numerous.

Depending on the portion of the body and the nutrition of the organism, varying numbers of fat cells develop in the subcutaneous layer. These are also found in clusters in the deep layers of the dermis. The fatty tissue of the subcutaneous layer on the abdomen may reach a thickness of 3 cm. or more, but in the eyelids and on the penis the subcutaneous layer does not contain fat cells.

The subcutaneous layer is penetrated everywhere by large blood vessels and nerve trunks and contains many nerve endings.

HAIRS

The hairs are slender keratinous filaments that develop from the matrix cells of follicular invaginations of the epidermal epithelium. They vary from several millimeters to over a meter in length and from 0.005 to 0.6 mm. in thickness. They are distributed in varying numbers (Fig. 23–40) and in variable thickness and length on the whole surface of the skin, except on the palms, the soles, the sides of fingers and toes, the side surface of the feet below the ankles, the lip, the glans penis, the prepuce, the clitoris, the labia minora, and the internal surface of the labia majora.

Each hair arises in a tubular invagination of the epidermis, the *hair follicle*, which extends down into the dermis, where it is surrounded by connective tissue (Figs. 23–2, 23–24, and 23–25). The active follicle has a

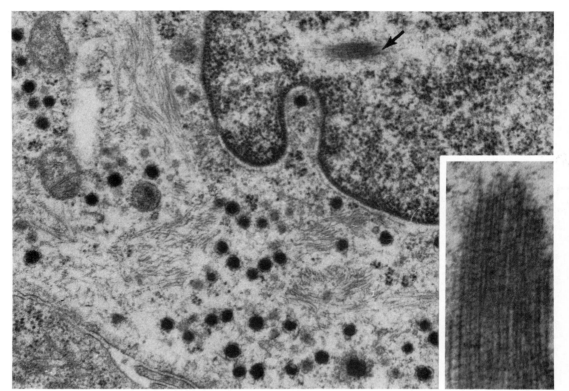

Figure 23-22 A portion of a Merkel cell from human gingival epithelium. The cytoplasm contains numerous dense granules and filaments. The nucleoplasm may contain an unusual inclusion consisting of paracrystalline aggregations of slender filamentous subunits (inset). (Micrograph courtesy of R. Winkelmann.)

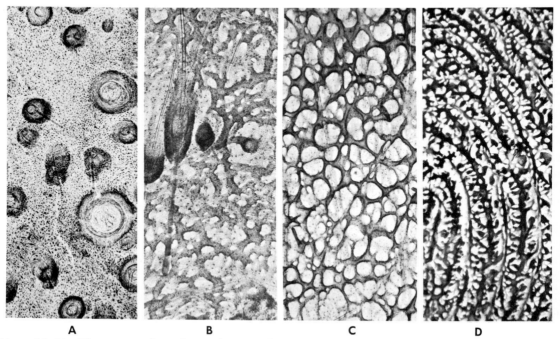

| A | B | C | D |

Figure 23-23 The pattern formed at a dermoepidermal junction shows marked regional variations. The figures shown here are views of the under surface of separated sheets of epidermis stained with carmine. The light areas are the depressions occupied in life by the dermal papillae. *A*, From the cheek; the under surface of the epidermis is smooth, except for the hair follicles. *B*, From the back. *C*, The breast. *D*, The elaborate pattern of concavities occupied by the dermal papillae of a finger pad. (Courtesy of G. Szabo.)

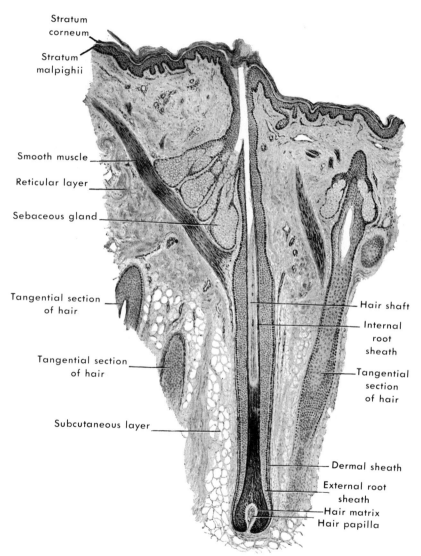

Stratum
corneum

Stratum
malpighii

Smooth muscle

Reticular layer

Sebaceous gland

Tangential section
of hair

Tangential section
of hair

Subcutaneous layer

Hair shaft

Internal
root
sheath

Tangential
section
of hair

Dermal sheath

External root
sheath

Hair matrix
Hair papilla

Figure 23-24 Section of the scalp of a man, showing the root of a hair in longitudinal section. × 32. (After Schaffer.)

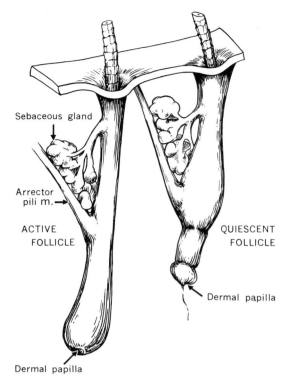

Sebaceous gland

Arrector
pili m.

ACTIVE
FOLLICLE

QUIESCENT
FOLLICLE

Dermal papilla

Dermal papilla

Figure 23–25 Diagrammatic representation of an actively growing and a quiescent hair follicle and the accessory structures. (Redrawn after W. Montagna, *in* Structure and Function of Skin. New York, Academic Press, 1956.)

bulbous terminal expansion with a concavity in its bottom occupied by a connective tissue *papilla* (Figs. 23–24 and 23–29). The papilla is covered by epithelial *matrix cells* of hair and root sheath. The cells on the dome of the convexity form the hair *root* which develops into the hair *shaft*. The free end of the shaft protrudes beyond the surface of the skin.

The hair is not a continuously growing organ but has phases of growth that alternate with periods of rest. The structure of the hair follicle varies markedly according to the stage of hair growth (Fig. 23–25). In the resting hair (club hair), the follicle is relatively short, its epithelium is more or less similar to the surface epidermis, and the hair shaft is firmly anchored into the follicle by fine filaments of keratin that penetrate between the follicular cells. A cluster of dermal cells attached to the end of the follicular epithelium is the remnant of the dermal papilla of the growing hair and will again develop into a typical dermal papilla at the next period of hair generation (Figs. 23–25 and 23–30).

In a phase of growth the follicle elongates and the epithelium again surrounds the dermal papilla. The epithelial cells around the papilla (the matrix) differentiate into several types. (1) In certain types of coarse hairs, the central matrix cells on top of the convexity of the papilla develop into the *medulla* of the hair shaft. The cells are large and vacuolated and eventually keratinize. This central part of the hair shaft is not demonstrable in thinner hairs. (2) The next concentric layer of matrix cells keratinize and develop into the *cortex* of the hair, the main constituent of the shaft. Its cells are heavily keratinized and tightly compacted, and they carry most of the pigment of the hair (Fig. 23–27). (3) Peripheral to the matrix cells of the cortex lie those of the *cuticle* of the hair (Figs. 23–27 and 23–28). These cells of the outermost layer are the most heavily keratinized and their imbrication (Fig. 23–26) prevents matting of the erupted hairs. These three layers of cellular components all undergo keratinization in the so-called *keratogenous zone* of the follicle, immediately above the dome of the dermal papilla, and form the solid hair shaft (Figs. 23–29 and 23–31).

The more peripheral concentric rows of matrix cells produce the *internal root sheath*, a transient structure surrounding the hair shaft below the level of the sebaceous glands, which is presumed to facilitate the movement of the growing hair shaft. It consists of three layers. The *cuticle of the internal root sheath*, like the cuticle of the hair, consists of overlapping thin scales with their free margins directed toward the bottom of the follicle. *Huxley's layer* consists of one to three layers of cornified cells and *Henle's layer* is a single layer of elongated cells closely adherent to the external sheath (Fig. 23–31). These three layers form "trichohyalin" granules and keratinize, but they do not form a compact enduring structure, and they finally desquamate at the level of the opening of the sebaceous glands.

The outermost layer of the follicle, the *outer root sheath*, is basically similar to the unspecialized epidermal epithelium and is continuous with it above. At the neck of the papilla it is one layer of flat cells. It becomes two-layered at the level of the middle third

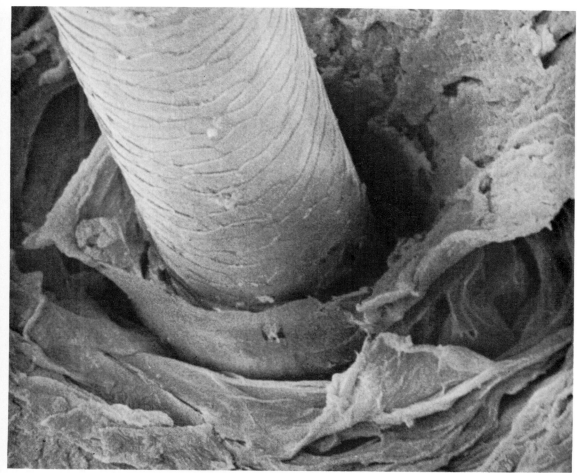

Figure 23–26 Scanning electron micrograph of hair shaft emerging from human scalp. (Micrograph by T. Fujita.)

of the papilla, and higher up it becomes stratified.

The glassy membrane, which is a part of the dermis, separates the epithelial from the connective tissue portion of the follicle. The latter portion is made up of two layers, a thin internal layer formed by circular fibers and an external, poorly outlined layer consisting of longitudinal collagenous and elastic fibers.

The hair matrix cells are analogous to the germinal cells of the epidermis insofar as the life cycle of each ends with formation of cornified cells. However, the epidermis produces a relatively soft keratinous material that is steadily shed, whereas the hair, the product of the matrix cells, is a hard, cohesive, nonshedding, keratinous structure consisting

of cells that accumulate in numerous concentric layers.

Since the hair is not perpendicular to the skin surface but inclined, it is very difficult to find a perfect longitudinal section of a follicle that displays these concentric layers well. The student will therefore have difficulty in identifying all of the structures described here. For this purpose the follicle needs to be reconstructed from serial sections.

It is well to bear in mind certain differences between the keratinizing epidermis and the keratinizing hair follicle. In the epidermis this process is general and continuous. In the case of the hair follicle it is intermittent and localized to a particular portion of the dermis —the dermal papilla, which has an inductive influence on the formation of the hair. If for any reason the dermal papilla is destroyed in postnatal life, no hair is formed. It is noteworthy, too, that there is a greater diversity of specialization and division of labor among the epidermal cells of the hair matrix with respect to their fate in the process of keratinization. In electron micrographs, the cells of the medulla, the cortex, and the internal and external root sheaths can all be distinguished by characteristic differences in their granules and their mode of keratinization.

The pigmentation of the hair is attributable to epidermal melanocytes located over the tip of the dermal papilla, a site corresponding to their location in the base of the epidermis generally (Fig. 23–30A). These melanocytes donate their pigment to the cells of the hair matrix and cortex. The melanosomes of the hair are usually larger than those found in the skin of the same individual. The melanocytes of the hair follicle function only at the beginning of the growing phase of the hair cycle, the onset of hair growth usually being heralded by increased melanogenic activity. In later stages of the growing phase or in the resting hair, melanocytes cannot be distinguished in the follicle.

In young rodents, hair growth is synchronized and spreads over the body in a *wave pattern*. Later in life, however, this process gives way to a *mosaic pattern*, hair growth beginning in isolated islands here and there. In man the mosaic growth pattern prevails, and the duration of the growing and resting phases varies from one region to another. In the case of scalp hair the growing phase is very long (several years), whereas the resting phase is of the order of three months.

Among mammals the human is excep-

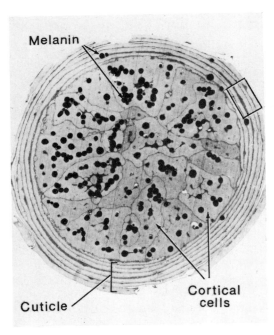

Figure 23–27

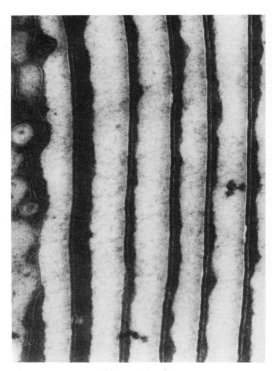

Figure 23–28

Figure 23–27 Electron micrograph of a mature black hair of a guinea pig in transverse section showing a few melanin granules in the concentrically arranged flattened cuticle cells, and a large number in the cortical cells in the interior of the hair. No medullary cells are present at this level in the hair. For higher magnification of the area in the rectangle, see Figure 23–28. (From R. Snell, J. Invest. Dermatol., 58:47, 1972.)

Figure 23–28 Higher magnification of the cuticle of a hair in area similar to that in the rectangle on Figure 23–27. The markedly flattened cuticle cells are separated with intercellular spaces filled with electron-dense amorphous material. (From R. Snell, J. Invest. Dermatol., 58:47, 1972.)

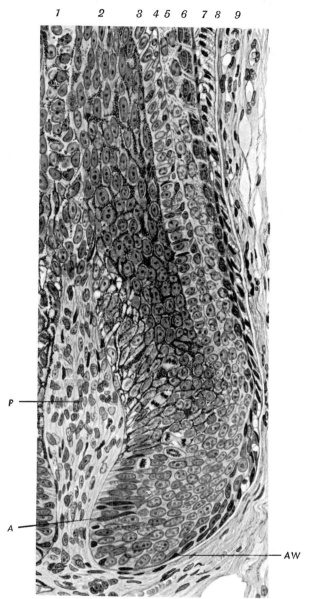

Figure 23-29 Longitudinal section through a hair from the head of a 22 year old man. *1*, Medulla; *2*, cortex; *3*, hair cuticle; *4*, inner sheath cuticle; *5*, Huxley's layer; *6*, Henle's layer; *7*, external root sheath; *8*, glassy membrane; *9*, connective tissue of the hair follicle; *A*, matrix; *AW*, external root sheath at the bulb; *P*, papilla. × 350. (After Hoepke.)

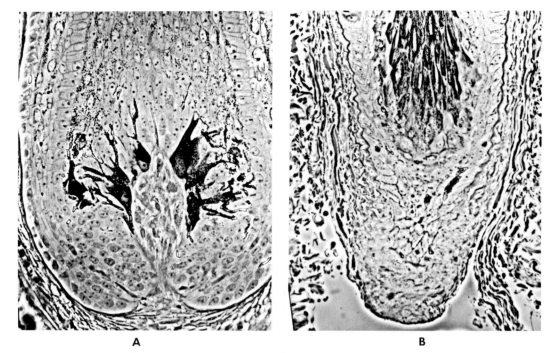

Figure 23–30 Unstained plastic sections of hair follicles. *A,* Active hair, showing large melanocytes and their processes contributing pigment to the hair. *B,* Inactive or club hair. × 200. (Courtesy of R. Mitchell and G. Szabo.)

tional in that its skin is not furry. It is by no means hairless, however (see Fig. 23–40 for numbers of hair follicles per square centimeter). In accordance with its relative paucity of hairs, the human epidermis is generally thicker than that of other mammals. The architectural pattern of the dermoepidermal junction varies greatly from region to region. It is almost flat on the cheek, whereas deep dermal ridges occur on the soles and palms (Fig. 23–23).

The human hairy coat also exhibits regional differences in the competence of the hair follicles to respond to male sex hormones. At the onset of puberty in males, the areas of the mustache and the beard produce strongly pigmented thick hairs. The same areas in the female, although they contain the same number of hair follicles, continue to produce fine hair. In other places, however, such as the axillae and the pubic regions, hair appears in both sexes at the onset of puberty. In males, there is often a characteristic regression of the scalp hair

with age, which varies in degree according to genotype. In its extreme form, this male pattern of changing hair distribution progresses so far that all the hair follicles are lost (baldness) or only a few are left and produce very fine hair.

One or more *sebaceous glands* are associated with each hair follicle. They discharge their holocrine secretory product through a short duct into the upper portion of the follicular canal.

A band of smooth muscle cells, the hair muscle or *arrector pili muscle,* is attached at one end to the papillary layer of the dermis and at the other to the connective tissue sheath of the hair follicle (Figs. 23–24 and 23–25). When this muscle contracts in response to cold, fear, or anger, it moves the hair into a more vertical position while depressing the skin in the region of its attachment and elevating the region immediately around the hair. This is responsible for the erection of hairs in animals and for the so-called "goose flesh" in man.

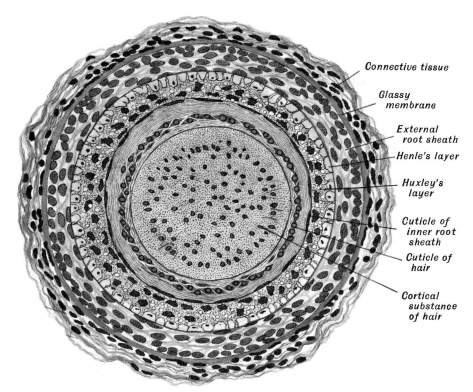

Connective tissue

Glassy membrane

External root sheath

Henle's layer

Huxley's layer

Cuticle of inner root sheath

Cuticle of hair

Cortical substance of hair

Figure 23–31   Cross section through a hair follicle in the skin of a pig embryo, at the level at which Henle's layer is completely cornified. × 375.

NAILS

The nails are horny plates on the dorsal surfaces of the terminal phalanges of the fingers and toes. The surface of the skin covered by them is the *nail bed.* It is surrounded laterally and proximally by a fold of skin, the *nail wall.* The slit between the wall and the bed is the *nail groove.* The proximal edge of the *nail plate* is the *root* of the nail. The visible part of the nail plate, called the *body of the nail,* is surrounded by the nail wall. The distal portion, becoming free of the nail bed, extends forward and is gradually worn off or is cut off. The nail is semitransparent and permits the color of the underlying tissue, rich in blood vessels, to show through. Near the root, the nail has a whitish color. This crescentic portion, the *lunula,* is usually covered by the proximal portion of the nail fold.

The nail plate consists of closely compacted horny scales, the dead residues of cornified epithelial cells so arranged that in section the nail appears longitudinally striated. The nail wall has the structure of skin, with all its layers. Turning inward into the nail groove, it loses its papillae, and the epidermis loses its horny, clear, and granular layers. Under the proximal fold, the horny layer spreads onto the free surface of the nail body as the *eponychium* (Fig. 23–32). The stratum lucidum and the stratum granulosum also reach far inside the groove but do not continue along the lower surface of the nail plate. On the surface of the nail bed only the malpighian layer of the epidermis is present.

In the nail bed the dermis is directly fused with the periosteum of the phalanx. The surface of the dermis under the proximal edge of the nail is provided with rather low papillae, but under the distal half of the lunula this surface is quite smooth. At the distal margin of the lunula, longitudinal, parallel ridges project instead of papillae. The boundary between the epithelium and the dermis of the nail bed is, therefore, scalloped in a perpendicular section (Fig. 23–33), whereas it is smooth in longitudinal sections. Beyond the free edge of the nail the dermal ridges are replaced by cylindrical papillae.

The epithelium of the nail bed distal to the lunula retains the typical structure of the malpighian layer. The epithelium is thicker between the ridges of the dermis than over them. The upper layer of cells, which touches the substance of the nail, is separated from it in places by an even line, while in others it is jagged. Under the free edge of the nail the usual horny layer again begins; it is thickened at this place and is called *hyponychium* (Fig. 23–32).

The epithelium that lines the proximal portion of the nail bed and corresponds roughly with the lunula is particularly thick; distally and upward it gradually passes over into the substance of the nail plate. Here the new formation of the nail substance proceeds; accordingly, this region of the epi-

thelium is called the *nail matrix* (Fig. 23–33). The cells of the deepest layer are cylindrical, and mitoses can be observed frequently in them. Above these are 6 to 10 layers of polyhedral cells joined by 3 to 12 layers of more flattened cells. This entire mass is penetrated by parallel fibrils of a special "onychogenic" substance. On passing into the proximal edge of the nail plate, these cells cornify and become homogeneous.

As new formation of the nail takes place in the matrix, the nail moves forward. Most authors deny the participation of the epithelium of the other portions of the nail bed in the formation of the nail substance, believing that the nail simply glides forward over this region.

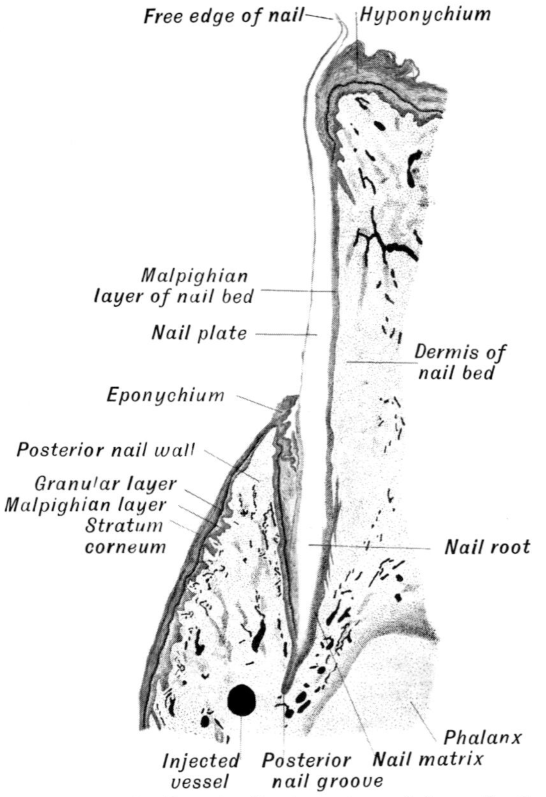

GLANDS

In man the glands of the skin include the sebaceous, sweat, and mammary glands. The last are described in Chapter 34.

Sebaceous Glands

The *sebaceous glands* are scattered over the surface of the skin (except in the palms, soles, and the sides of the feet, where there are no hairs). They vary from 0.2 to 2 mm. in diameter. They lie in the dermis, and their excretory ducts open into the necks of hair follicles. When several glands are connected with one hair, they lie at the same level. On the lips, about the corners of the mouth, on the glans penis and the internal fold of the prepuce, on the labia minora, and on the mammary papilla, the sebaceous glands are independent of hairs and open directly onto the surface of the skin. To this category also belong the *meibomian glands* of the eyelids. The sebaceous glands in mucocutaneous junctions are more superficial than those that are associated with hairs.

The secretory portions of the sebaceous glands are rounded sacs (alveoli). As a rule, several adjacent alveoli form a mass like a bunch of grapes, and all of them open into a short duct (Figs. 23–24 and 23–25). A simple branched gland results. Much less frequently, only one alveolus is present. In the meibomian glands of the eyelids there is one long, straight duct, from which a row of alveoli project.

The walls of the alveoli are formed by a

Free edge of nail — Hyponychium

Malpighian layer of nail bed

Nail plate

Dermis of nail bed

Eponychium

Posterior nail wall

Granular layer
Malpighian layer
Stratum corneum

Nail root

Phalanx

Injected vessel   Posterior nail groove   Nail matrix

Figure 23–32 Longitudinal section of the nail of a newborn infant. (After A. A. Maximow.)

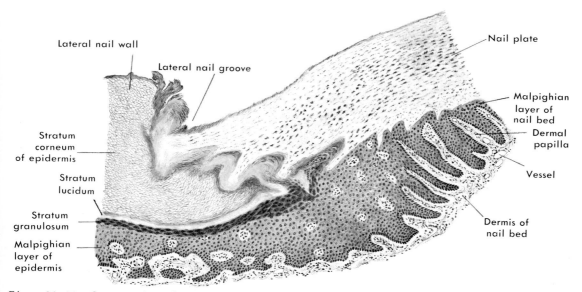

Lateral nail wall

Lateral nail groove

Nail plate

Stratum corneum of epidermis

Malpighian layer of nail bed

Dermal papilla

Stratum lucidum

Vessel

Stratum granulosum

Malpighian layer of epidermis

Dermis of nail bed

Figure 23–33 Cross section of the lateral edge of a nail and its surrounding parts. (After A. A. Maximow.)

basal lamina supported by a thin layer of fibrillar connective tissue. Along the internal surface is a single layer of thin cells with round nuclei. Toward the center of the alveoli a few cells keratinize, but most of them become larger and polyhedral, gradually fill with fat droplets, and resemble multilocular fat cells (Fig. 23–34). The nuclei gradually shrink and then disappear, and the cells break down into fatty detritus. This is the oily secretion of the gland, and it is secreted onto the hair and upon the surface of the epidermis. The ducts of sebaceous glands are lined by stratified squamous epithelium continuous with the external root sheath of the hair and with the malpighian layer of the epidermis.

In sebaceous glands, the secretion results from the destruction of the epithelial cells and is, therefore, of the holocrine type. It is accompanied by a regenerative multiplication of epithelial elements. In the body of the gland, mitoses are rare in the cells lying on the basal lamina. They are numerous, however, in the cells close to the walls of the ducts, whence the new cells move into the secretory regions.

The so-called *uropygial* or *preen glands* of birds, especially aquatic birds, are specialized sebaceous glands. They produce oily material that is spread with the beak over the

survace of the feathers to make them impervious to water.

Sweat Glands

The ordinary *eccrine* sweat glands are distributed along the surface of the skin, with the exception of the margins of the lips, the glans penis, and the nail bed. They are simple, coiled, tubular glands. The secretory portion is a simple tube convoluted in several unequal twists into a ball, and the duct is a narrow, unbranched tube (Figs. 23–35 and 23–36.

The bulk of the secretory portion is located in the dermis and measures 0.3 to 0.4 mm. in diameter. In the armpit and around the anus the secretory portions of some of the sweat glands may reach 3 to 5 mm. in diameter and are described as *apocrine sweat glands* because they are believed to shed the apical portion of their cells in the secretory process. They are connected with hair follicles and are located deep in the subcutaneous layer (Fig. 23–37).

The walls of the secretory portion rest on a thick basal lamina. Directly inside it are spindle-shaped and branching cells, 30 to 90 μm. long, with their long axis tangential to that of the glandular tube. They have an elongated nucleus and cytoplasmic myofilaments like those of smooth muscle (Fig. 23–38). It is supposed that, by contracting, these *myoepithelial cells* help to discharge the secretion. They are particularly numerous and highly developed in the large sweat glands of the axillary and perianal regions.

The truncated pyramidal cells that excrete sweat form a single internal layer resting upon the myoepithelial cells. At the base is a rather large, round nucleus; the cytoplasm contains mitochondria and, near the lumen, a number of secretory vacuoles, varying with the functional state of the cell. Sometimes there are also fat droplets, glycogen, and pigment granules. Glycogen diminishes in active cells. Pigment appears in the secretion of certain sweat glands, as in the axilla. The free surfaces of the cells in the apocrine glands often show protrusions of protoplasm that are believed to separate and become a part of the secretion. Between these glandular cells are typical secretory capillaries. The caliber and the shape of the free lumen of the secretory

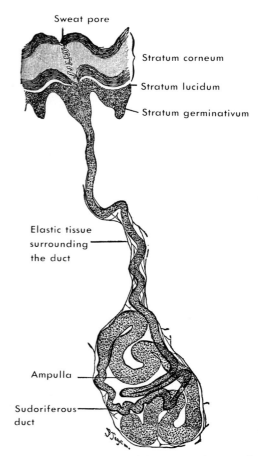

Figure 23-35 Sweat gland from the palmar surface of an index finger. The drawing was based on study of sections and a teased preparation. × 45. (Slightly modified from von Brunn.)

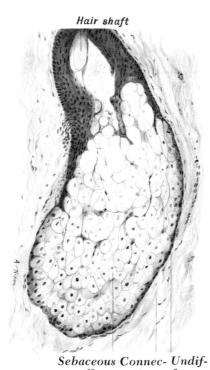

Figure 23-34 Section of human sebaceous gland. × 120.

portion fluctuate greatly with the functional state of the gland.

Two different cell types have been described in the secretory segment of human eccrine sweat glands, called respectively "dark" or mucoid cells and "clear" cells. It was not apparent with the light microscope whether they were merely stages of the physiological activity of the same cell type. At the electron microscope level, cells containing abundant ribosomes and numerous apical secretory vacuoles appear to correspond to the dark cells. Their shape is pyramidal, with the apical end being broader than the base. Glycoprotein has been identified both in the secretory vacuoles and in the lumen (Munger). The clear cells are associated with the inter-

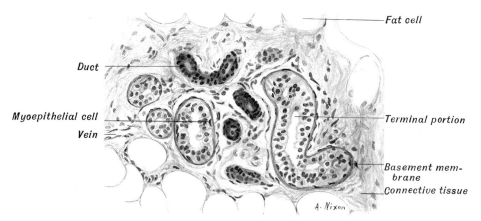

Figure 23–36 Section of human sweat gland. × 120.

cellular canaliculi. They have relatively few ribosomes but a considerable amount of glycogen. The endoplasmic reticulum is poorly developed. The basal plasma membranes, resting on the myoepithelial cells or basal lamina, are infolded in a complex manner. No secretory precursors are identified within their cytoplasm, but these cells are assumed to secrete into the intercellular canaliculi a product rich in water and various solutes.

The glandular tube, in passing over into the duct, suddenly becomes much narrower, and its lumen acquires a simple slitlike or starlike shape in cross section. The myoepithelial and glandular cells on the basal lamina are replaced by a double layer of cuboidal cells. The peripheral cells of the basal layer have comparatively large nuclei and rather abundant mitochondria (Fig. 23–39). The surface cells have large irregular nuclei and relatively little cytoplasm. The Golgi apparatus and other cytoplasmic membranes are poorly developed. Immediately beneath the free surface, the cytoplasm is specialized, with a rather remarkable condensation of filaments constituting a terminal web which, in the past, has been erroneously referred to as a "cuticular border." This structure is lacking in the basal cells, which otherwise resemble the cells of the surface layer.

As the duct passes through the dermis toward the epidermis, it is slightly twisted and curved. In the epidermis the lumen of the excretory duct is a twisted intercellular channel surrounded by concentrically arranged epidermal cells which, in the malpighian layer, have fine, keratohyalin granules in their cytoplasm. On the palms and soles and on the palmar surface of the fingers, the rows of ducts open on the ridges with funnel-shaped openings that can be seen easily with a magnifying glass.

In certain parts of the skin the sweat glands have a peculiar arrangement and function. Such are the glands that produce *cerumen* in the external auditory meatus. They reach a considerable size and extend to the perichondrium. The secretory portions of the *ceruminous glands* branch, and the ducts, which sometimes also branch, may open together with the ducts of the adjacent sebaceous glands into the hair sacs of the fine hairs. In the terminal portions are highly developed smooth muscle cells; the glandular cells located upon them are particularly rich in pigment granules containing lipid.

Moll's glands of the margin of the eyelid are also a special kind of sweat gland, with terminal portions that do not form a ball but are irregularly twisted and provided with a wide lumen. The excretory ducts open onto the free surface or into the hair sacs of the eyelashes. The secretion of the sweat glands is not the same everywhere. True sweat, a transparent, watery liquid, is excreted mainly by the small sweat glands, while a thicker secretion of complex composition is produced by those of the axilla and about the anus. In women, the apocrine sweat glands of the axilla show periodic changes with the menstrual cycle. These changes consist mainly in enlargement of the epithelial cells and of the lumens of the glands in the premenstrual period, followed by regressive changes during the period of menstruation (Fig. 23–37).

The differences between the eccrine and apocrine sweat glands are as follows. The eccrine glands have no connections with hair follicles; they function throughout life, producing a watery secretion; and they are innervated by cholinergic nerves. The apocrine glands are connected with hair follicles; they begin to function at puberty, producing a more viscous secretion; and they are supplied by adrenergic nerves.

The eccrine glands do not function simultaneously or under the same conditions on all parts of the body. When the human body is exposed to excessive heat, sweating begins on the forehead and spreads to the face, and then to the rest of the body. Finally, the palms and the soles will show increased sweat production. Under nervous strain, however, palms and soles may start to sweat first.

It has been shown that the glandular portion of the eccrine sweat gland excretes more electrolytes than are finally found at the surface of the skin. It is assumed that an absorption of electrolytes takes place in the duct portion of the gland.

BLOOD AND LYMPHATIC VESSELS

The arteries that supply the skin are located in the subcutaneous layer. Their branches, reaching upward, form a network (rete cutaneum) parallel to the surface on the boundary line between the dermis and the hypodermis. From one side of this network, branches are given off that nourish the subcutaneous stratum with its fat cells, sweat glands, and the deeper portions of the hair follicles. From the other side of this network,

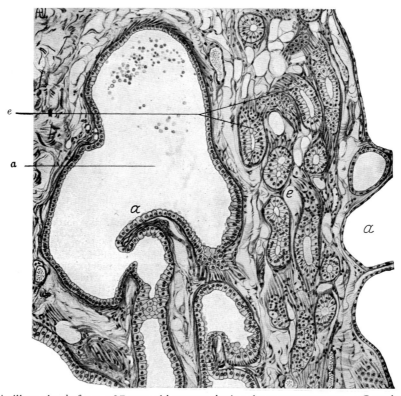

Figure 23–37 Axillary glands from a 37 year old woman during the premenstruum. *a,* Greatly enlarged glands that change with the menstrual cycle. *e,* Glands that do not change. Resorcin-fuchsin stain for elastic fibers. Preparation of Loescke. × 110. (After Hoepke.)

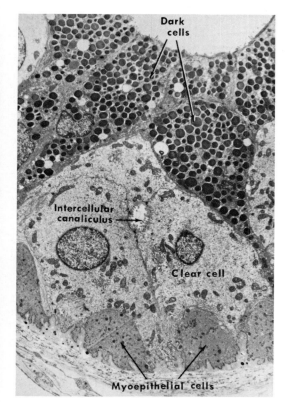

Figure 23–38 Electron micrograph of a sector of the secretory coil of a normal eccrine sweat gland. Muciginous, "dark" cells border the lumen, while "clear" serous cells are more deeply situated and surround intercellular canaliculi. The myoepithelial cells form an incomplete layer at the periphery of the tubule. × 3400. (Courtesy of R. E. Ellis.)

sebaceous and the sweat glands enter. From the deeper network the large, independent, subcutaneous veins pass, as well as the deep veins accompanying the arteries.

There are direct connections between the arterial and venous circulation in the skin without intervening capillary networks. These so-called "arteriovenous shunts" play a vital role in thermoregulation in the body.

Each hair follicle has its own blood vessels. It is supplied with blood from three sources: a special small artery that gives off a capillary network into the papilla; the rete subpapillare toward the sides of the hair sac; and several other small arteries that form a dense capillary network in the connective tissue layer of the follicle.

There is a dense network of capillaries outside the basal lamina of the sebaceous and, particularly, of the sweat glands.

The skin is rich in lymphatic vessels. In the papillary layer they form a dense, flat meshwork of lymphatic capillaries. They begin in the papillae as networks or blind outgrowths, which are always deeper than the blood vessels. From this peripheral network, branches pass to the deeper network, which lies on the boundary between the dermis and the hypodermis; under the rete cutaneum it has much wider meshes, and its vessels are provided with valves. From the deeper network, large, subcutaneous lymphatic vessels originate and follow the blood vessels. Lymphatic vessels are not connected with the hairs or glands of the skin.

vessels enter the dermis. At the boundary between the papillary and reticular layers they form the denser, subpapillary network or the rete subpapillare (Fig. 23–41). This gives off thin branches to the papillae. Each papilla has a single loop of capillary vessels with an ascending arterial and descending venous limb.

The veins that collect the blood from the capillaries in the papillae form the first network of thin veins immediately beneath the papillae. Then follow three flat networks of gradually enlarging veins on the boundary line between the papillary and reticular layers. In the middle section of the dermis and also at the boundary between the dermis and the subcutaneous tissue, the venous network is on the same level as the arterial rete cutaneum. Into this network the veins of the

NERVES

The skin, with its accessories, serves as an organ for receiving impulses from the external environment. It is, accordingly, abundantly supplied with sensory nerves. In addition, it contains nerves that supply the blood vessels, sweat glands, and arrector muscles.

In the subcutaneous stratum are rather thick nerve bundles that form networks composed mainly of myelinated and partly of nonmyelinated fibers. The branches given off by this reticulum form, in the dermis, several new thin plexuses. Among them, the network on the boundary between the reticular and papillary layers stands out clearly, as does the subepithelial one.

In all the layers of the hypodermis, dermis, and epidermis are many different kinds of nerve endings, which are discussed

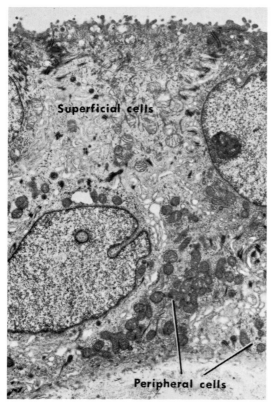

Superficial cells

Peripheral cells

Figure 23-39 Electron micrograph of a portion of the wall of the coiled duct of an eccrine sweat gland. The luminal margin of the superficial cells contains a concentration of filaments formerly described as a "cuticular border." The peripheral cells have elaborately convoluted surfaces and contain many mitochondria. × 4000. (Courtesy of R. A. Ellis.)

in Chapter 12. Among them, the sensory endings are probably all connected with the craniospinal myelinated fibers; the nonmyelinated fibers lead to the blood vessels, smooth muscles, and glands. There are also free endings of unmyelinated sensory fibers in or close to the epidermis. The abundant nerves at the base of hairs undoubtedly play an important part in the reception of tactile stimuli.

HISTOGENESIS OF THE SKIN AND ITS ACCESSORIES

The epidermis develops from the ectoderm, and the dermis arises from the mesen-

chyme. The *epidermis* in the human embryo, during the first two months, is a double layered epithelium. The basal layer, which lies on the mesenchyme, consists of cuboidal or cylindrical cells that multiply energetically. The peripheral layer consists of flat cells that are constantly formed anew from the elements of the deeper layer. Beginning with the third month, the epidermis becomes triple layered. The new intermediate layer above the basal cells consists of polygonal cells, which increase in number and develop the surface projections formerly interpreted as intercellular bridges. At the end of the third month, in the peripheral portions of the intermediate layer, cornification begins and leads to the formation of the layers found in the adult. The horny scales are desquamated and form part of the vernix caseosa.

The irregularities on the lower surface of the epidermis arise at the end of the third month on the inner surfaces of the fingers, palms, and soles as parallel ridges protruding into the dermis. From the beginning they show a characteristic pattern, and from them sweat glands develop. Protruding longitudinal cushions corresponding to the ridges are formed on the external free surface of the epidermis.

The regional specificity of the epidermis has been the subject of detailed embryological study. It has been shown by Billingham and Silvers that the maintenance of the adult specificity of the epidermis depends on the dermis. When the dermis and epidermis are separated and epidermis from the ear is grown together with dermis from the sole, thick epidermis will develop. If a composite graft from sole epidermis is maintained with ear dermis, the originally thick epidermis becomes thinner and hair follicles develop.

	AVERAGE NUMBERS, ± S.E. OF MEAN.		
	HAIR FOLLICLES PER SQUARE CENTIMETER	SWEAT GLANDS PER SQUARE CENTIMETER	MELANOCYTES PER SQUARE MILLIMETER
Face	700 ± 40	270 ± 25	2120 ± 90
Trunk	70 ± 10	175 ± 20	890 ± 70
Arm	65 ± 5	175 ± 15	1160 ± 40
Leg	55 ± 5	130 ± 10	1130 ± 60
Average	330 ± 20	212 ± 15	1560 ± 110

Figure 23-40 Regional anatomy of the human integument. (After G. Szabo.)

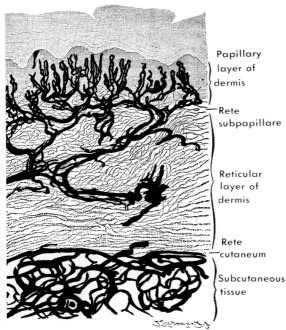

Papillary layer of dermis

Rete subpapillare

Reticular layer of dermis

Rete cutaneum

Subcutaneous tissue

Figure 23–41 Distribution of blood vessels in the skin. (Modified slightly from von Brunn.)

In the case of the tongue, however, the situation is different. There the epidermis remains tongue epidermis even when it is grown over dermis from the general body skin or the sole.

The *dermis* and *hypodermis* consist during the first six weeks of mesenchyme with wandering cells. From the second month on, the fibrillar interstitial substance appears, and elastic fibers follow. In still later stages, the mesenchyme divides into a peripheral dense layer with a compact arrangement of its elements—the dermis—and the deep loose layer, the future subcutaneous layer. In the dermis, in turn, the peripheral papillary layer differentiates.

In man, *hair* first appears in the eyebrows and on the chin and upper lip, at the end of the second month. At first, in the deep layer of the epidermis, a group of cylindrical dividing cells appear. These grow into the underlying connective tissue and produce a gradually elongating epithelial cylinder. This is the primordium of a hair follicle, the so-called "hair germ"; it is rounded and slightly flattened on its end. Under the latter an accumulation of condensed connective tissue appears early. From it the hair papilla

forms and protrudes into the epithelial mass of the bulb (or germ). The epithelial cells at the surface of the connective tissue papilla represent the matrix of the future hair. The connective tissue that surrounds the bulb later forms the connective tissue portions of the hair follicle. On the surface of the epithelial hair bulb, two projections arise. The upper represents the primordium of the sebaceous gland; its central cells early undergo a fatty transformation. The lower protuberance becomes the insertion of the arrector pili muscle on the hair sac. In the mass of the epithelium that forms the hair primordium, a layer of rapidly cornifying cells differentiates into the layers of matrix, cortex, and inner and outer root sheaths. The shaft of the new hair elongates, owing to the multiplication of the cells of the matrix on the summit of the papilla, and perforates the top of the hollow cone of Henle's sheath. The tip of the hair moves upward, pierces the epidermis, and protrudes above the surface of the skin.

The development of the *nails* begins in the third month by the formation, on the back of the terminal phalanx of each finger, of a flat area, the *primary nail field*, which is surrounded by a fold of the skin. In the region of the nail the epithelium has three or four layers. The true nail substance is laid down during the fifth month, and without the participation of keratohyalin, in the portion of the nail bed near the proximal nail groove. Here the deep layer of the epidermis is transformed into the nail matrix, and its cells are penetrated by the fibrils of onychogenic substance; they become flat, adjoin one another closely, and give rise to the true nail plate. In the beginning it is still thin and is entirely buried in the epidermis of the nail field or bed. It gradually moves in the distal direction. The layers of epidermis that cover the plate eventually desquamate.

The development of the eccrine *sweat glands* in man proceeds independently of that of the hairs. The first primordia appear during the fifth month on the palms and soles and the lower surface of the fingers. At first they are similar to the primordia of the hairs. An epithelial shaft with a terminal thickening grows into the underlying connective tissue. But, unlike that around the hairs, the connective tissue here does not condense about the epithelium. The shaft gradually elongates and becomes cylindrical, and its lower portion curls in the form of a ball. Beginning in the seventh month, an irregular lumen forms in this lower portion, which constitutes the secretory part; along the course of the future excretory duct another lumen develops and later unites with the first one. In the secretory portion, the epithelium around the lumen forms two layers, which differentiate into an external layer of myoepithelial elements and an internal layer of glandular cells.

Quantitative investigations have shown that in the embryo the density of the skin appendages, regardless of whether they are hair or eccrine glands, is originally the same. A large proportion of these appendages on the head, however, will become hairs and a large proportion of them on the rest of the body will become eccrine sweat glands. No hairs will be found on the palms and the soles. Due to the differential rate of growth of the body surface, the original uniform density changes because no new hair follicles or eccrine sweat glands form after the original population is established. These appendages subsequently become widely spaced in the trunk and in the extremities, which grow to a surface area about three times as great as that of the head. In wound healing, usually no new hair follicles are formed.

REFERENCES

Billingham, R. E.: Dendritic cells. J. Anat., 82:93, 1948.

Billingham, R. E., and P. B. Medawar: A study of the branched cells of the mammalian epidermis with special reference to the fate of their division products. Philos. Trans. Roy. Soc. B, 237:151, 1953.

Billingham, R. E., and W. K. Silvers: The melanocytes of mammals. Quart. Rev. Biol., 35:1, 1960.

Billingham, R. E., and W. K. Silvers: The origin and conservation of epidermal specificites. New Eng. J. Med., 268:477, 539, 1963.

Birbeck, M. S. C., and E. H. Mercer: Electron microscopy of the human hair follicle. J. Biophys. Biochem. Cytol., 3:203, 1957.

Breathnach, A. S.: The cell of Langerhans. Int. Rev. Cytol., 18:1, 1965.

Brody, I.: The keratinization of epidermal cells of normal guinea pig skin as revealed by electron microscopy. J. Ultrastruct. Res., 2:482, 1959.

Chase, H. B.: Growth of the hair. Physiol. Rev., 34:113, 1954.

Dole, V. P., and J. H. Thaysen: Variation in the functional power of human sweat glands. J. Exper. Med., 98:129, 1953.

Drochmans, P.: On melanin granules. Int. Rev. Exp. Pathol., 2:357, 1963.

Ellis, R. A.: Aging of the human male scalp. In Montagna, W., and R. A. Ellis, eds.: The Biology of Hair Growth. New York, Academic Press, 1958, p. 469.

Ellis, R. A.: Vascular patterns of the skin. In Montagna, W., and R. A. Ellis, eds.: Advances in Biology of the Skin. New York, Pergamon Press, 1961, Vol. 2, p. 20.

Felsher, Z.: Studies on the adherence of the epidermis to the corium. J. Invest. Derm., 8:35, 1947.

Fitzpatrick, T. B., P. Brunet, and A. Kukita: The nature of hair pigment. In Montagna, W., and R. A. Ellis, eds.: The Biology of Hair Growth. New York, Academic Press, 1958, p. 255.

Fitzpatrick, T. B., and G. Szabo: The melanocyte: Cytology and cytochemistry. J. Invest. Derm., 32:197, 1959.

Fitzpatrick, T. B., et al.: Dermatology in General Medicine. Part Two. Biology and Pathophysiology of Skin. New York, McGraw-Hill Book Co., 1971, p. 39.

Fortman, G. J., and R. K. Winkelman: A Merkel cell nuclear inclusion. J. Invest. Dermat., 61:334, 1973.

Giacometti, L.: The anatomy of the human scalp. In Montagna, W., and R. A. Ellis, eds.: Advances in Biology of the Skin. New York, Pergamon Press, 1965, Vol. 6, p. 97.

Giacometti, L., and W. Montagna: Langerhans cells: Uptake of tritiated thymidine. Science, 157:439, 1967.

Hashimoto, K.: Fine structure of the Merkel cell in human oral mucosa. J. Invest. Derm., 58:381, 1972.

Hibbs, R. G.: The fine structure of human eccrine sweat glands. Am. J. Anat., 103:201, 1958.

Hoepke, H.: Die Haut. In von Mollendorff, W., and W. Bargmann, eds.: Handbuch der mikroskopischen Anatomie des Menschen. Berlin. Julius Springer, 1927, Vol. 3, part 1, p. 1.

Jensen, H.: Two types of keratohyalin granules. J. Ultrastr. Res., 33:95, 1970.

Masson, P.: Les glomus cutanés de l'homme. Bull. Soc. franc. Dermat. Syph., 42:1174, 1935.

Matoltsy, A. G.: Chemistry of keratinization. In Montagna, W., and R. A. Ellis, eds.: The Biology of Hair Growth. New York, Academic Press, 1958, p. 135.

Matoltsy, A. G.: Membrane-coating granules of the epidermis. J. Ultrastruct. Res., 15:510, 1966.

Matoltsy, A. G., and P. F. Parakkal: Membrane-coating granules of keratinizing epithelia. J. Cell Biol., 24:297, 1965.

Matoltsy, A. G., and M. Matoltsy: The chemical nature of keratohyalin granules of the epidermis. J. Cell Biol., 47:593, 1970.

Medawar, P. B.: The micro-anatomy of the mammalian epidermis. Quart. J. Micr. Sci., 94:481, 1953.

Mercer, E. H.: Keratin and Keratinization. An Essay in Molecular Biology. New York, Pergamon Press, 1961.

Montagna, W., H. B. Chase, and W. C. Lobitz: Histology and cytochemistry of human skin. IV. The eccrine sweat glands. J. Invest. Derm., 20:415, 1953.

Montagna, W.: The Structure and Function of Skin. New York, Academic Press, 1956.

Munger, B. L.: The ultrastructure and histophysiology of human eccrine sweat glands. J. Biophys. Biochem. Cytol., 11:385, 1961.

Munger, B. L., and S. W. Brusilow: An electron microscopy study of eccrine sweat glands of the cat foot and toe pads. J. Biophys. Biochem. Cytol., 11:403, 1961.

Odland, G. F.: The fine structure of cutaneous capillaries. In Montagna, W., and R. A. Ellis, eds.: Advances in Biology of the Skin. New York, Pergamon Press, 1961, Vol. 2, p. 57.

Odland, G. F.: Tonofilaments and keratohyalin. In Montagna, W., and W. C. Lobitz, Jr., eds.: The Epidermis. New York, Academic Press, 1964, p. 237.

Quevedo, W. C., G. Szabo, J. Vicks, and S. J. Sinesi: Melanocyte populations in UV-irradiated human skin. J. Invest. Derm., 45:295, 1965.

Rawles, M. E.: Origin of pigment cells from the neural crest in the mouse embryo. Physiol. Zool., 20:248, 1947.

Rawles, M. E.: Skin and its derivatives. *In* Willier, B. J., P. A. Weiss, and V. Hamburger, eds.: Analysis of Development. Philadelphia, W. B. Saunders Co., 1955, p. 499.

Reams, W. M.: Ectodermal origin of epidermal Langerhans cells. Anat. Rec., 175:421, 1973.

Roth, S. I., and W. H. Clark, Jr.: Ultrastructural evidence related to the mechanism of keratin synthesis. *In* Montagna, W., and W. C. Lobitz, Jr., eds.: The Epidermis. New York, Academic Press, 1964, p. 303.

Rothman, S.: Physiology and Biochemistry of the Skin. Chicago, University of Chicago Press, 1954.

Sagabiel, R. W.: In vivo and in vitro uptake of ferritin by Langerhans cells of the epidermis. J. Invest. Derm., 58:47, 1972.

Seiji, M., T. B. Fitzpatrick, R. T. Simpson, and M. S. C. Birbeck: Chemical composition and terminology of specialized organelles (melanosomes and melanin granules) in mammalian melanocytes. Nature, 197:1082, 1963.

Southwood, W. F. W.: The thickness of the skin. Plast. Reconstr. Surg., 15:423, 1955.

Snell, R. S.: An electron microscopic study of melanin in the hair and hair follicles. J. Invest. Derm., 58:218, 1972.

Szabo, G.: Quantitative histological investigations on the melanocyte system of the human epidermis. *In* Gordon, M., ed.: Pigment Cell Biology. New York, Academic Press, 1959, p. 99.

Szabo, G.: Current state of pigment research with special reference to the macromolecular aspects. *In* Lyne, A. G., and B. F. Short, eds.: Biology of the Skin and Hair Growth. Sydney, Australia, Angus and Robertson, 1965, p. 705.

Szabo, G.: The regional anatomy of the human integument, with special reference to the distribution of hair follicles, sweat glands and melanocytes. Phil. Trans. Roy. Soc. Ser. B, 252:447, 1967.

Ugel, A. R.: Keratohyalin: Extraction and in vitro aggregation. Science, 166:250, 1969.

Wolff, K., and R. K. Winkelmann: Quantitative studies on the Langerhans cell population of guinea pig epidermis. J. Invest. Derm., 48:504, 1967.

Wolff, K., and E. Schreiner: Uptake, intracellular transport and degradation of exogenous protein by Langerhans cells. J. Invest. Derm., 54:37, 1970.

Zimmermann, A. A., and T. Cornbleet: The development of epidermal pigmentation in the Negro fetus. J. Invest. Derm., 11:383, 1948.

24
Oral Cavity and Associated Glands

The oral cavity is the entrance to the long tubular *digestive system*, which consists of the lips, mouth, pharynx, esophagus, stomach, small and large intestine, rectum, and anus. On its way through this tract, the food undergoes mechanical fragmentation and chemical digestion. Products of degradation of the food are absorbed through the wall of the intestine into the blood, which carries them to the tissues of the organism for utilization or storage. The undigested residue of the food is eliminated as feces.

The inner surface of the digestive tube is lined with a mucous membrane or *mucosa* consisting of a superficial layer of epithelium regionally specialized for different digestive functions and a supporting layer of loose connective tissue, the *lamina propria*. The peripheral layers of the wall of the digestive tube consist of smooth muscle making up the *muscularis externa* (Fig. 24–1). In most parts of the tract, the outer limit of the mucosa is demarcated by a thin layer of smooth muscle, the *muscularis mucosae*. Between it and the muscularis externa is a layer of loose connective tissue, the *submucosa*. Numerous blood vessels, nerves, lymphatics, and lymphoid nodules are to be found in this layer. Where a muscularis mucosae is absent, there is a gradual transition from the lamina propria to the submucosa.

The mucosa of the developing gastrointestinal tract evaginates to form *folds* and *villi* that project into the lumen and increase the surface area of the absorptive epithelium. It also invaginates to form tubular *crypts* or *glands* whose lining cells produce mucus, digestive enzymes, and hormones. The majority of these outgrowths remain confined to the thickness of the mucosa. Others proliferate to such an extent during embryonic development that they give rise to separate organs, the accessory glands of the gastrointestinal tract, such as the salivary glands, liver, and pancreas. However, these remain connected by long ducts to the epithelial surface from which they originated in embryonic life.

In the oral cavity, esophagus, and rectum, the wall of the digestive tube is surrounded by a layer of connective tissue that attaches it to the adjacent organs. The stomach and intestines, on the other hand, are suspended in the abdominal cavity by mesenteries, and their surface is covered by a moist serous membrane, the *serosa* or *peritoneum*, which permits these organs to slide freely over one another within the cavity during the peristaltic movements of the digestive tract.

The wall of the digestive tube is richly provided with blood vessels that bring to it oxygen and the metabolites necessary to sustain its secretory activities. The veins and lymphatics also carry away the absorbed products of digestion. In addition, the wall of the

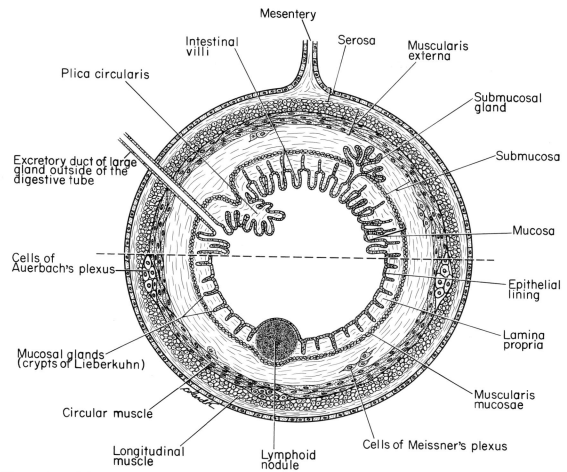

Figure 24-1 Schematic representation of the general features of organization in the gastrointestinal tract. The concentric layers of serosa, muscularis, and mucosa are common to virtually all regions of the tract. In the upper half of the drawing, the mucosa is depicted with glands and villi as in the small intestine; in the lower half it is shown with glands only, as in the colon.

digestive tract contains an intricate system of sympathetic ganglia and nerve plexuses which are concerned with coordination of the movements of the digestive tube.

THE ORAL CAVITY

The epithelium of the mucous membrane in the mouth is of stratified squamous type, like that of the skin. However, in man, it normally does not undergo complete keratinization. The nuclei of the cells of the superficial layers shrink and become metabolically inert, but do not disappear, and the cell bodies do not reach the same degree of flatness as in the epidermis. These superficial cells are continually exfoliating in great numbers and are found in the saliva. In some places they contain granules of keratohyalin, and glycogen is present in the superficial and middle layers of the epithelium. In many animal species, particularly ruminants, the epithelium of the oral cavity undergoes extensive keratinization.

The lamina propria, in most places, extends into concavities in the deep surface of the epithelium forming connective tissue papillae similar to those associated with the epidermis of the skin. Their structure is, however, more delicate, and the collagenous and elastic fibers are thinner than in the dermis. In the posterior region of the oral cavity the lamina propria contains many lymphocytes, which are often found migrating into and through the epithelium.

The arrangement of the blood vessels is similar to that in the skin. There is a deep submucous plexus of large vessels, from which arise branches that form a second plexus in the lamina propria. This in turn sends capillaries into the papillae. The lymphatics also show an arrangement similar to that in the skin, and begin with blind capillary outgrowths in the papillae.

The *oral mucous membrane* is very sensitive and is provided with many nerve endings belonging to the sensory branches of the trigeminal nerve. On that portion covering the tongue it also contains the specific end-organs of the sense of taste. In most places under the lamina propria, especially in the cheeks and on the soft palate, there is a loose submucosa, into which the denser connective tissue of the mucosa gradually merges. In regions with a well developed submucosa the mucous membrane can be easily lifted into folds, whereas in those places against which the food is crushed and rubbed, as on the hard palate, there is no submucosa, and the mucous membrane is firmly bound to the periosteum of the underlying bone.

The inner zone of the lip margin in the newborn is considerably thickened and provided with many high papillae and numerous sebaceous glands not associated with hairs (Fig. 24–2). These structural features seem to facilitate the process of sucking.

The soft palate consists of layers of striated muscle and fibrous connective tissue covered with mucous membrane. On the oral surface the latter has the structure typical of the oral cavity—a stratified squamous epithelium, with high papillae, and glands of the pure mucous type. The glands are surrounded by adipose tissue and are scattered

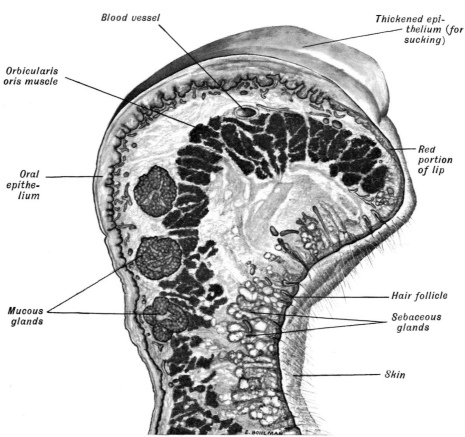

Figure 24–2 Camera lucida drawing of sagittal section through lip of a newborn infant. Stained with hematoxylin. × 10.

in a loose submucous layer separated from the lamina propria by dense elastic networks. This oral type of mucous membrane also covers the posterior margin of the soft palate and continues for some distance onto the nasal surface. On this surface, at varying distances from its posterior margin, the stratified epithelium is replaced by pseudostratified, ciliated, columnar epithelium, which rests on a thickened basal lamina. The lamina propria contains small glands of the mixed type, but no adipose tissue, and it is heavily infiltrated with lymphocytes. A dense layer of elastic fibers is found between the glands and the underlying muscle. A submucosa is not present.

Most of the structures in the oral cavity —the salivary glands, lining of the palate, the anterior two thirds of the tongue, and the vestibule—are derived from the embryonic ectoderm. The tooth enamel is said to be a neural crest derivative (Johnston), whereas the dentin and pulp originate from mesenchyme. Endodermal derivatives include the tonsils, the lining of the posterior third of the tongue, the pharyngeal tonsils, and the remainder of the gastrointestinal tract and its associated glands.

THE TONGUE

The tongue consists of interlacing bundles of striated muscle that run in three planes and cross one another at right angles. The muscular mass is covered by a tightly adherent mucous membrane. The dense lamina propria is continuous with the interstitial connective tissue of the muscle. A submucous layer is present only on the smooth ventral surface. The dorsal surface is covered in its anterior two thirds by a multitude of small excrescences—the *papillae*—whereas in its posterior one third it presents only irregular bulges of larger size. The boundary line between the two regions is V-shaped, with the opening of the angle directed forward (Fig. 24–3). At the apex of the angle is a small invagination, the *foramen caecum.* It is the rudiment of the thyroglossal duct, which in early embryonic stages connects the thyroid gland primordium with the epithelium of the oral cavity.

Papillae

Four types of papillae are present on the body of the tongue: filiform, fungiform, cir-

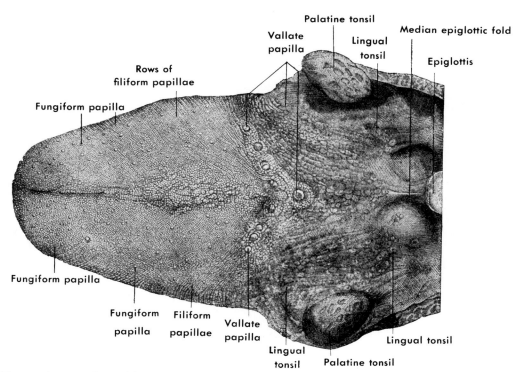

Figure 24–3 Surface of dorsum and root of human tongue. (After Sappey, from Schumacher.)

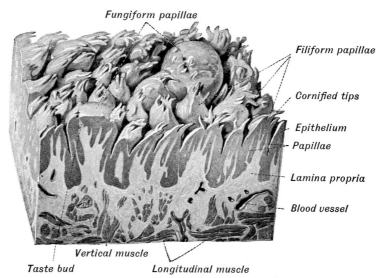

Fungiform papillae

Filiform papillae

Cornified tips

Epithelium

Papillae

Lamina propria

Blood vessel

Vertical muscle

Taste bud

Longitudinal muscle

Figure 24-4 Surface of dorsum of tongue, drawn from a combined study using the binocular microscope and from sections. The anterior cut surface corresponds with the long axis of the tongue—the tip of the tongue being to the reader's left. × 16. (After Braus.)

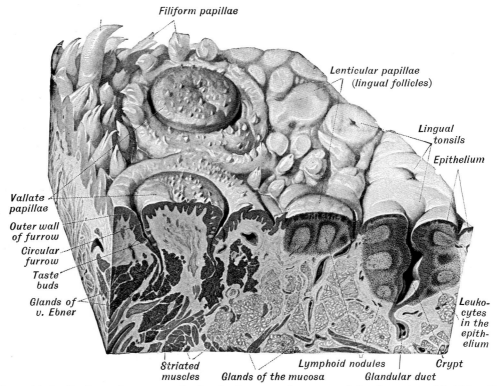

Filiform papillae

Lenticular papillae (lingual follicles)

Lingual tonsils

Epithelium

Vallate papillae

Outer wall of furrow

Circular furrow

Taste buds

Glands of v. Ebner

Leukocytes in the epithelium

Striated muscles

Glands of the mucosa

Lymphoid nodules

Glandular duct

Crypt

Figure 24-5 Surface of tongue at the border between the root and the dorsum. × 16. (After Braus.)

cumvallate, and foliate. The *filiform papillae* are arranged in more or less distinct rows diverging to the right and left from the middle line and parallel to the V-shaped region. The *fungiform papillae* are scattered singly among the filiform papillae and are especially numerous near the tip of the tongue. The *circumvallate papillae*, numbering only 10 to 12 in man, are distributed along the diverging arms of the V-shaped boundary between the anterior and posterior regions of the tongue (Fig. 24–3). The paired *foliate papillae* are found on the dorsolateral aspect of the posterior part of the tongue.

The filiform papillae are 2 to 3 mm. long. Their connective tissue core is beset with secondary papillae with pointed ends (Fig. 24–4). The epithelium covering these connective tissue outgrowths also forms short papillae, which taper into pointed processes (Fig. 24–6). In man the superficial squamous cells are transformed into hard scales containing shrunken nuclei. The axial parts of the scales at the point of the papilla are connected with its solid axial strand, and their lower edges project from the surface of the papilla like the branches of a fir tree. When digestion is disturbed in illness, the normal shedding of these scales is delayed. They then accumulate, in layers mixed with bacteria, on the surface of the tongue, which thus is covered with a gray film—the "coated" tongue.

The fungiform papillae have a short, slightly constricted stalk and a slightly flattened hemispherical upper part. The connective tissue core forms secondary papillae that project into recesses in the underside of the epithelium, which has a smooth free surface (Figs. 24–4 and 24–7). On many of the fungiform papillae the epithelium associated with the secondary papillae contains taste buds. Because the core is rich in blood vessels, the fungiform papillae have a distinct red color.

The circumvallate papillae are sunk into the surface of the mucous membrane, and each is surrounded by a deep, circular furrow. The connective tissue core forms secondary papillae only on the upper surface. The covering epithelium is smooth, whereas that of the lateral surfaces of the papillae contains many taste buds (Fig. 24–8). In vertical sections, 10 to 12 of them can often be seen aligned on the lateral surface of the papilla. A few may be present in the outer wall of the groove surrounding the papilla. The number of taste buds in a single papilla is subject to great variations, but it has been estimated to average 250. Connected with the circumvallate papillae are glands of the serous type (*glands of von Ebner*), whose bodies are embedded deep in the underlying muscular tissue and whose excretory ducts open into the bottom of the furrow.

In man foliate papillae are rudimentary, but in many animals they are the site of localization of the main aggregations of taste receptors (Fig. 24–9). The fully developed foliate papillae in the rabbit, for example, are oval bulgings on the mucous membrane, consisting of alternating parallel ridges and grooves. The epithelium of the sides of the ridges contains many taste buds. Small serous glands open into the bottom of the furrows.

Taste buds are also found on the glossopalatine arch, on the soft palate, on the posterior surface of the epiglottis, and on the posterior wall of the pharynx as far down as the inferior edge of the cricoid cartilage.

The nodular bulges on the root of the tongue are caused by lymphatic nodules, the *lingual tonsils* and *follicles* (Fig. 24–3). On the free surface of each lingual tonsil a small opening leads into a deep invagination, the *crypt*, lined with stratified squamous epithelium. The crypt is surrounded by lymphoid tissue. Innumerable lymphocytes infiltrate the epithelium and assemble in the lumen of the crypt, where they degenerate and form masses of detritus with the desquamated epithelial cells and bacteria. The lingual tonsils are often associated with mucous glands embedded in the underlying muscle tissue. The ducts of the latter open into the crypt or onto the free surface.

Taste Buds

The taste buds are seen in sections under low power as pale, oval bodies in the darker-stained epithelium (Fig. 24–9). Their long axis averages 72 μm. They extend from the basal lamina almost to the surface. The epithelium over each taste bud is pierced by a small opening—the *taste pore* (Figs. 24–10, 24–11 and 24–12).

Light microscopists distinguished two types of cells among the constituents of taste buds, the dark *supporting cells* (Type I) and the light *neuroepithelial cells* (Type II). Electron microscopists have confirmed the existence of two cell types but are not able to assign a functional role to them with any certainty and have therefore adopted the designation Type I and Type II to avoid functional implications. A Type III cell structurally comparable to the Type I cell has been identified in the taste buds of the rabbit. Typical synapses of nerves with the epithelial cells of taste buds have been observed only on Type III cells. *Basal cells* and *peripheral cells* have also been described, and these are believed to be progenitor cells of the taste buds.

Both Type I and Type II cells have large microvilli that projects into the taste pore or taste pit where they are embedded in a rather amorphous substance. Material of similar density and texture is found in membrane bounded vesicles in the apical region of Type I cells. It is presumed to be a secretory product of these cells. The *taste hairs* of traditional light microscopists were no doubt the clusters of coarse microvilli found in the pore region in electron micrographs. Zonulae occludentes are present on the boundaries between cells near the free surface. The lateral surfaces of the cells below the junctional complexes may be folded and interdigitated. The cytoplasm of the lighter Type II cells has

a rather extensive smooth endoplasmic reticulum, which is not observed in Type I cells.

There are only four fundamental taste sensations: sweet, bitter, acid, and salty. It has been shown by the application of substances to individual fungiform papillae that they differ widely in their receptive properties. Some do not give any taste sensations, whereas others give sensations of one or more of the four taste qualities. No structural differences in the various taste buds have been found, in spite of the differences in sensation mediated. There is, moreover, a general chemical sensitivity in regions of the mouth where there are no taste buds.

Nerves

The anterior two thirds of the tongue is innervated by the lingual nerve, which contains fibers of general sensibility from the fifth cranial nerve (trigeminal) and fibers of gustatory sensibility from the seventh cranial

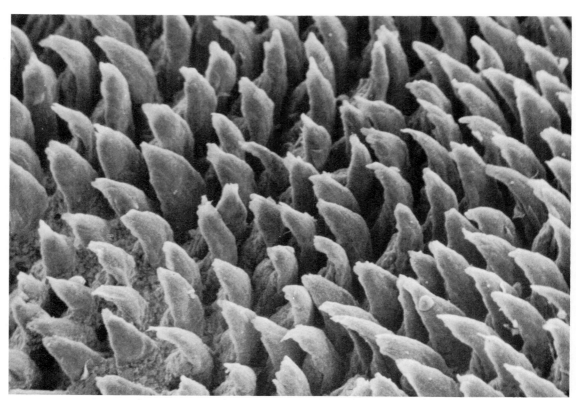

Figure 24-6 Scanning electron micrograph of the filiform papillae of rabbit tongue. (Micrograph courtesy of F. Fujita.)

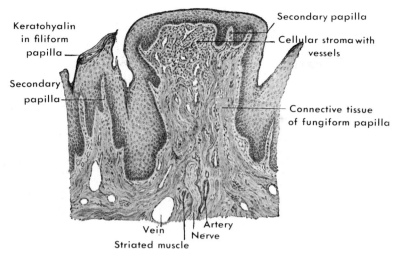

Figure 24-7 Perpendicular section through a fungiform papilla. × 46. (After Schaffer, from Schumacher.)

nerve (facialis). The latter enter the lingual nerve from the chorda tympani. The posterior third of the tongue is innervated by the glossopharyngeal nerve for both general and gustatory sensibility. Taste buds of the epiglottis and lower pharynx are innervated by the vagus. These nerve fibers are lightly myelinated. They branch profusely under the basal lamina, lose their myelin, and form a subepithelial plexus, from which fibers penetrate the epithelium. Some terminate as *intergemmal fibers* by free arborization between the taste buds. Others, the *perigemmal fibers,* closely envelop the taste buds; and still others, the *intragemmal fibers,* penetrate the

taste buds and end with small terminal enlargements in intimate contact with certain of the taste bud cells. The functional significance of these different nerve endings is unknown.

GLANDS OF THE ORAL CAVITY

General Description

Numerous *salivary glands* open into the oral cavity. Many of them are small glands in the mucosa or submucosa and are named according to their location. They seem to se-

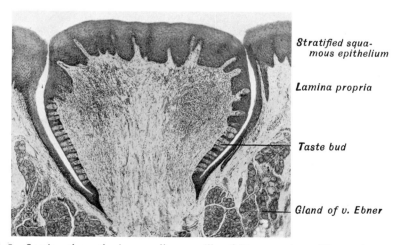

Figure 24-8 Section through circumvallate papilla of *Macacus rhesus.* Photomicrograph, × 42.

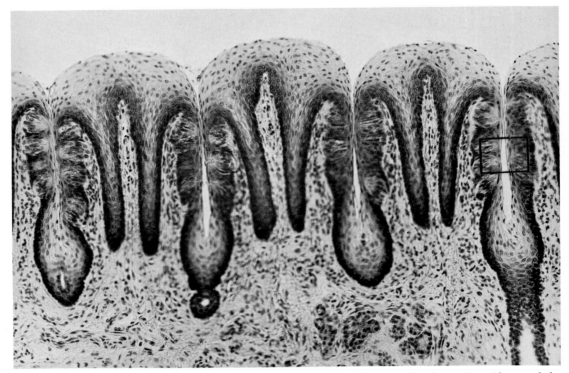

Figure 24–9 Photomicrograph of the foliate papillae of a rabbit, showing the alternating ridges and deep clefts with numerous taste buds on either side of the cleft. × 150. An area such as that enclosed in the rectangle is shown at higher magnification in Figure 24–10.

crete continuously and furnish a liquid, the *saliva*, which moistens the oral mucous membrane. In addition, there are three pairs of large glands, which constitute the salivary glands proper. They are the *parotid*, the *submandibular* (*submaxillary*), and the *sublingual* glands. They secrete only when mechanical, thermal, or chemical stimuli act upon the nerve endings in the oral mucous membrane, or as the result of certain psychic or olfactory stimuli.

The *saliva* collected from the oral cavity is a mixture of the secretions of the various salivary glands. It is a viscous, colorless, opalescent liquid which contains water, mucoprotein, immunoglobulins, carbohydrates, and a number of inorganic components, including calcium, phosphorus, sodium, potassium, magnesium, chloride, and traces of iron and iodine. Enzymes are also present, especially amylase (ptyalin), which splits starch into smaller, water-soluble carbohydrates. Saliva always contains desquamated squamous epithelial cells and the so-called *salivary cor-*

puscles. Most of the latter originate in the follicles of the tongue and in the tonsils, and are degenerating lymphocytes or granulocytes.

The quality of the saliva collected from the oral cavity varies, depending upon the degree of participation of the various salivary glands in its formation. But even the secretion of one gland may change considerably with variations in the stimuli acting upon the oral mucous membrane, as, for instance, with different kinds of food.

The salivary glands may be classified in three categories, according to the type of their secretory cells. The glands containing only *mucous* cells elaborate a viscid secretion that consists almost exclusively of mucin. In glands with only *serous* cells, the secretion is a watery liquid that lacks mucus but contains salts, proteins, and the enzyme ptyalin. In the *mixed glands*, containing serous and mucous cells, the secretion is a viscid liquid containing mucin, salts, and ptyalin.

All glands of the oral cavity have a system of branching ducts. The secretory portions or

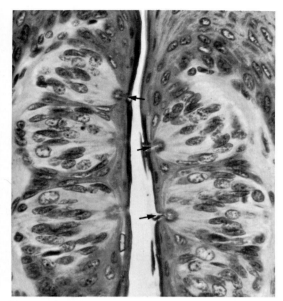

Figure 24-10 Photomicrograph of taste buds from the foliate papillae of a rabbit. × 450. See Figure 24–9 for location. The arrows indicate the taste pores.

compressed when there is a large accumulation of mucigen. The Golgi apparatus, mitochondria, and rough endoplasmic reticulum are usually located toward the cell base, below the mucigen granules. The amount of endoplasmic reticulum varies with the phase of the cell's secretory cycle. The free surface of the epithelium is usually provided with a network of occluding junctions. Secretory canaliculi are absent. Usually the lumen of the terminal portions of the glands is large and filled with masses of mucin.

When the secretion has been discharged, the cell collapses, and only a few granules of mucigen may remain near its free surface. In this depleted condition the mucous cells may be mistaken for serous cells, but the absence of secretory capillaries always distinguishes mucous from serous glands. The demonstration of these canaliculi, however, requires special staining methods or electron microscopy. With the initiation of the secretory cycle, the cell organelles undergo morphological changes correlated with the cell's activity. Rarely under physiological conditions do the mucous cells discharge all of their granules. The cells, as a rule, do not show any signs of degeneration and apparently recover completely from discharge of their secretion. Mitoses have occasionally been observed in them.

acini of the pure mucous glands are usually long, branching tubules. In the pure serous and mixed glands, the secretory portions vary from simple oval to tubuloacinar forms with irregular outpockeings.

The initial intralobular ducts are thin, branched tubules called the *necks*, or *intercalated ducts*. Branches of the next larger order, also located in the interior of the smallest lobules, have a vertically striated epithelium; these segments are called *striated ducts*. Then follow the larger branches. Among them lobular, interlobular, and primary ducts may be distinguished in the large glands.

Mucous Cells

In the pure mucous glands, the cells are arranged in a layer against the basal lamina and have an irregularly cuboidal form. In fresh condition their cytoplasm contains many pale droplets of *mucigen*, the antecedent of mucin. In fixed and stained sections, the droplets of mucigen are usually destroyed, so that the cell body appears clear and contains only a loose network of cytoplasm and traces of precipitated mucigen. This network stains red with mucicarmine, or metachromatically with thionine. The nucleus is at the base of the cell and usually appears angular and

Serous Cells

These cells are roughly cuboidal and surround a small tubular lumen. In an unfixed resting gland they contain numerous highly refractile secretion granules which accumulate between the nucleus and the free surface. After the gland has secreted for a certain period, the serous cells diminish in size and their few remaining granules are confined to the juxtaluminal cytoplasm. The Golgi complex is usually found in an apical or paranuclear position, and cisternae of endoplasmic reticulum are abundant toward the cell base. Mitochondria are scattered among the cisternae at the base and in the apical cytoplasm as well. The luminal surface of the serous cells has sparse microvilli, and intercellular canaliculi lined with microvilli are found between some of the cells. In human submandibular glands, the serous acinar cells have numerous basal processes that interdigitate to form a complex basal labyrinth.

The serous cells in the various oral glands have a similar microscopic structure even though they are not functionally identical. They are grouped together under a general heading because histological methods are not able to demonstrate differences corresponding to the variations in the nature of their secretions. In some instances, the secretory granules give a more or less distinct staining reaction with the old mucicarmine stain. Such cells are sometimes described as "mucoserous" or "mucoalbuminous."

Cells in the Mixed Glands

The relative numbers of the two kinds of glandular cells in the mixed glands vary within wide limits. In some cases the serous cells are far more numerous than the mucous cells, whereas in other cases the reverse is true. In still other instances both cell types are present in about equal numbers. The mucous and serous cells line different parts of the terminal secretory portion of the gland. In those mixed glands in which the serous cells predominate, some of the terminal portions may be exclusively serous (Fig. 24–15). In others a part of the secretory portion is lined with mucous cells and a part is lined with serous cells. In sections the mucous portions can usually be recognized by the clear, empty appearance of their cytoplasm, but they are identified more certainly by their color after specific staining of the mucus.

As a rule, the mucous cells are located nearer the ducts, whereas the serous cells are located at the blind end of the terminal secretory portion. It is quite probable that the mucous cells in mixed glands arise through the differentiation of the cells in the smallest ducts. Sometimes single mucous cells are scat-

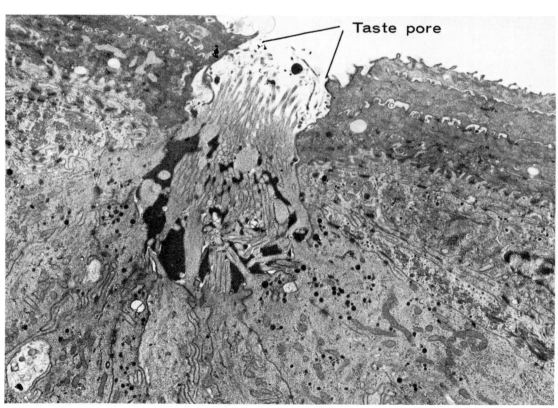

Figure 24-11 Electron micrograph of the pore region of a rabbit taste bud. Notice the large microvilli on the sensory cells, surrounded by a dense amorphous secretory product. For a surface view of the pore, see Figure 24-12. (Micrograph courtesy of M. Coppe.)

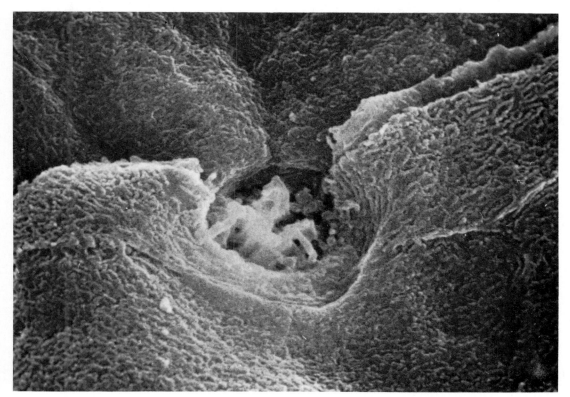

Figure 24-12 Scanning micrograph of the pore of a taste bud opening onto the surface of the epithelium. (Micrograph courtesy of M. Coppe.)

tered among the unspecialized cells of the neck of the gland. In other cases the part of the neck directly adjoining the terminal portion is lined exclusively with mucous cells. If the mucous transformation affects all the cells the neck of the duct ceases to exist as such. If the mucous cells are not numerous, the secretory portion of the gland will show an irregular mixture of the pale mucous and dark serous cells.

If the mucous cells predominate, the serous cells are displaced to the terminal portion or into saccular outpockets. Here they form small groups, which in sections appear as darkly staining crescents (*demilunes of Giannuzzi*) surrounding the ends of the tubules of mucous cells (Figs. 24–14 and 24–15). In them the serous cells are small and flattened and often seem to be entirely separated from the lumen by the large mucous cells. However, there are always secretory capillaries, which conduct the secretion through clefts between the mucous cells into the lumen (Fig. 24–14).

Basal Myoepithelial Cells (Basket Cells)

In all the glands of the oral cavity, the epithelium in the terminal portion, as well as in the ducts, is provided with basal cells. They lie between the glandular cells and the basal lamina and appear as slender, spindle-shaped elements. Usually only their nuclei can be discerned. When seen from the surface, they exhibit a stellate cell body with processes containing many cytoplasmic filaments. In their ultrastructure, they resemble smooth muscle cells.

The basal cells are presumed to be contractile and to facilitate the movement of the secretion into the ducts. They are considered to be myoepithelial cells and resemble those of the sweat glands and mammary gland.

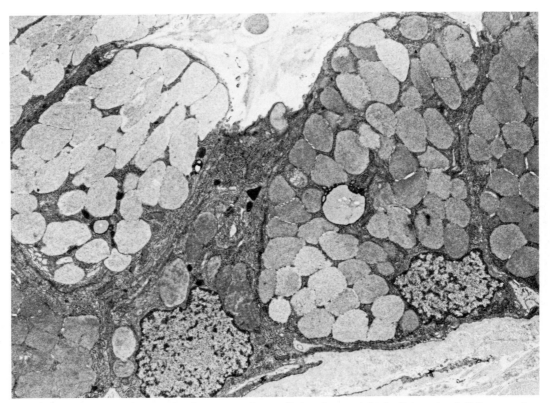

Figure 24-13 Electron micrograph of mucous acinar cells in a human labial salivary gland. (Micrograph courtesy B. Tandler.)

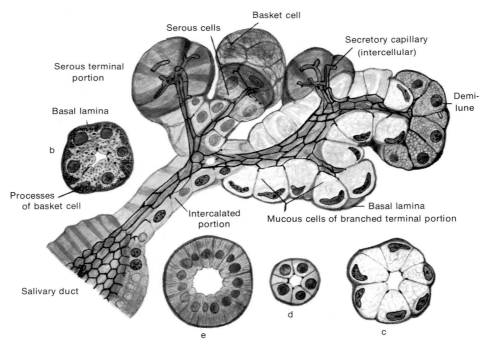

Figure 24-14 Reconstruction of a terminal portion of a submandibular gland with its duct. *b*, Cross section of a purely serous terminal portion, showing basal lamina; *c*, cross section through a purely mucous terminal portion; *d*, cross section through an intercalated portion; *e*, cross section through a salivary duct. (Redrawn and modified after a reconstruction by Vierling, from Braus.)

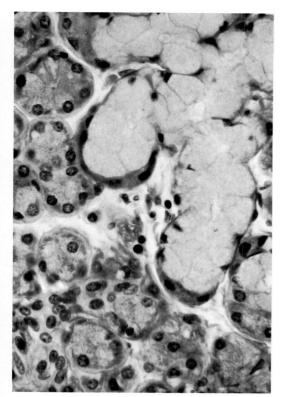

Figure 24-15 Photomicrograph of the human submandibular gland, a mixed gland, showing serous acini at the lower left and mucous acini with serous demilunes at the upper right. × 475.

Ducts of the Glands

The ducts of the glands of the oral cavity are of variable length and have a low cuboidal epithelium. Between the lining cells and the basal lamina are scattered myoepithelial cells. The epithelium of the necks often shows varying degrees of transformation to mucous cells.

In the columnar epithelium of the striated segments of the ducts, the lower parts of the cell bodies show a parallel striation, attributable to vertical orientation of mitochondria in slender compartments formed by infolding of the basal cell membrane. The numerous infoldings of the basal surface of the cells in the striated ducts are not resolved with the light microscope but are visible with the electron microscope, as they are in other epithelia in which there is rapid transport of water and ions (Figs. 24–18, 24–19, and 24–20).

In the larger ducts the epithelium is columnar and pseudostratified, and occasionally it contains goblet cells. Nearing the opening on the mucous membrane, it becomes stratified for a short distance and is then succeeded by stratified squamous epithelium.

Glands Opening into the Vestibule

Scattered in the mucous membrane of the upper and lower lips are small *labial glands* (Fig. 24–13). Similar glands associated with the mucous membrane of the cheeks are called *buccal glands.* Both of these are glands of mixed type. The secretory portion sometimes contains only seromucinous cells, but in most cases these are confined to the blind ends of the glands, with the remainder lined with mucous cells. Since the necks of the glands are short and branch very little, the mucous secretory portions often pass directly into striated ducts.

By far the largest salivary glands opening into the vestibule are the two *parotid glands.* Situated subcutaneously on either side of the face just in front of the ear, they extend from the zygomatic arch above to below the angle of the jaw. Each is connected to the vestibule by a long parotid duct (Stenson's duct) which emerges from the anterior border of the gland, courses forward and then through the cheek to open into the mouth opposite the second upper molar tooth. In adult man, the gland is a nearly pure serous gland. In the newborn, however, the glandular cells often give a positive staining reaction for mucus. Cells with such a staining reaction occur only in widely scattered small areas in adults.

The parotid is the gland specifically affected in mumps. It is also a frequent site of development of tumor.

Glands Opening on the Floor of the Mouth

In the space between the mandible and the muscles forming the floor of the mouth on either side is the large *submandibular gland.* Its duct (Wharton's duct) is about 5 cm. long; it leaves the deep surface of the gland and runs forward to open at the tip of the sublingual papilla on the floor of the mouth adjacent to the frenulum of the tongue. The secretory portion of the gland is mainly serous, but some parts are mucous, with serous cells at the blind ends. Typical serous demilunes (crescents of Gianuzzi) are less common in man than in other species. In some persons, many of the serous cells show a slight mucoid staining reaction. Striated ducts are numerous and long and have many branches.

Deep to the mucous membrane on the underside of the tongue, there is a large *sublingual gland*, 3 to 4 cm. long, on either side of the frenulum, and a number of smaller sublingual glands (Fig. 24–21). The ducts of the large glands open into the ducts of the submandibular gland. The small glands open separately along a fold of mucous membrane called the plica sublingualis. At the posterior end of these is another group of small glands called the *glossopalatine glands.*

In the sublingual glands, mucous cells are far more numerous than in the submandibular glands. Serous cells are in the minority and many of them are mucoserous in character. For the most part they are ar-

ranged in thick demilunes. The isthmuses are extremely variable in length. Some of these undergo a complete mucous transformation so that the terminal portions abut directly on the striated tubules. The latter are few and short and are sometimes represented only by small groups of basally striated cells in the epithelium of the interlobular ducts. The glossopalatine glands are pure mucous glands.

Glands of the Tongue

On either side of the midline near the tip of the tongue is an *anterior lingual gland* (gland of Blandin or Nuhn). The anterior portion of this gland contains secretory tubules with seromucinous cells only. Its posterior part consists of mixed branching tubules that contain mucous cells and, on their blind ends, thin demilunes of seromucinous cells.

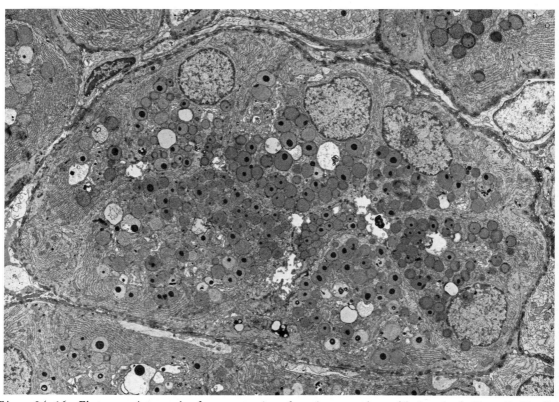

Figure 24–16 Electron micrograph of a serous acinus from human submandibular gland. (From B. Tandler and R. A. Erlandson, Am. J. Anat., *135:*419, 1972.)

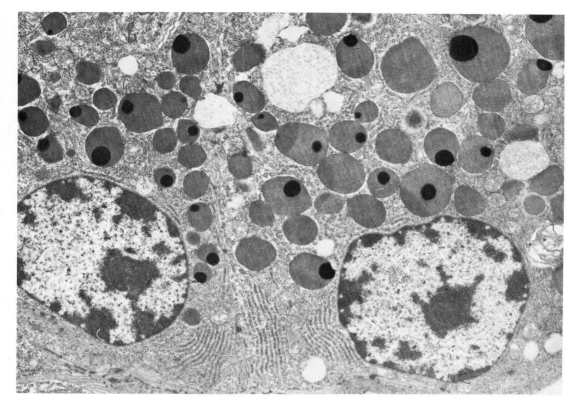

Figure 24-17 Electron micrograph of serous cells from submandibular gland of rhesus monkey. Notice the nonhomogeneity of the secretory granules, with dense and less dense regions. (Micrograph courtesy of A. Ichikawa.)

The posterior lingual glands comprise the *glands of von Ebner* that open into the groove around the circumvallate papillae and the *mucous glands of the root of the tongue.* The long secretory portions of von Ebner's glands are branching tubules that contain only serous cells. Rarely these show a slight reaction for mucus. The system of ducts is poorly developed; isthmuses are absent. These glands form a thin serous secretion that evidently serves to wash out the circumvallate groove and the associated taste buds.

The *glands of the root of the tongue* and the *palatine glands* are of the pure mucous variety. Short isthmuses have been found in the latter group.

Blood and Lymphatic Vessels

In the interstitial reticular connective tissue of the salivary glands are fibroblasts and macrophages, with fat cells scattered singly or in small groups. Plasma cells are of common occurrence and, occasionally, small lymphocytes are also found. The larger blood vessels follow the larger ducts. Loose capillary networks surround the ducts and the terminal portions. The lymph vessels are relatively scarce.

Nerves

Each salivary gland is provided with sensory nerve endings and two kinds of efferent secretory nerves, parasympathetic and sympathetic. The parasympathetic preganglionic fibers for the submandibular and sublingual glands run in the chorda tympani nerve to the submaxillary ganglion. The sympathetic preganglionic fibers go to the superior cervical ganglion. From here the postganglionic fibers follow along the carotid artery. The vasodilators are believed to be included in the chorda tympani, the vasoconstrictors in the sympathetic nerves.

The parotid gland receives its secretory

fibers from the glossopharyngeal nerve. In the interstitial tissue, along the course of its blood vessels, are found plexuses of myelinated (preganglionic and sensory) and nonmyelinated fibers, and groups of sympathetic multipolar nerve cells close to the larger ducts. On the outer surface of the terminal portions, nonmyelinated fibers form a network that sends small branches through the basal lamina. These branches form a second network, from which branches penetrate between the glandular cells, ramify, and end on the surfaces of the glandular cells with small, terminal thickenings.

Stimulation of the parasympathetic nerves of the submandibular gland causes the secretion of an abundant thin saliva, rich in water and salts but poor in organic substances. Stimulation of the sympathetic nerve, on the contrary, yields a small quantity of thick saliva, with a high content of organic substances. The mechanism of action of the nerves upon the glandular cells and the role of the vasodilators in secretion are not known. The presence of different kinds of nerve endings has not been proved. It is even doubtful whether the secretory fibers in the chorda tympani and in the sympathetic nerve are of different nature.

After sectioning of the chorda tympani nerve in the dog, the so-called "paralytic" secretion in the corresponding submandibular and retrolingual glands occurs. This secretion is accompanied by intense degeneration and atrophy of the gland cells, especially of the mucous elements in the retrolingual gland.

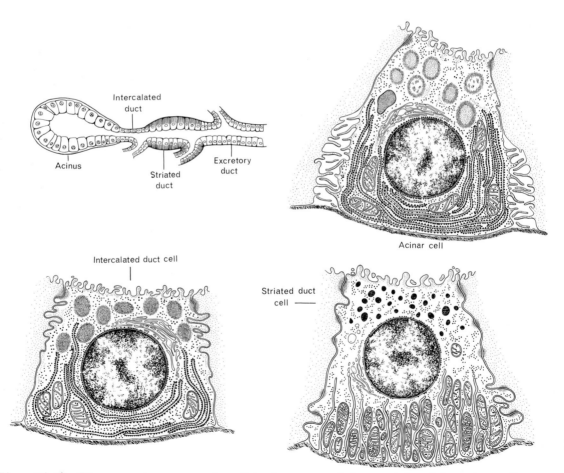

Figure 24–18 Diagrammatic representation of the fine structural characteristics of the various cell types in the mouse submandibular gland. (Redrawn after U. Rutberg.)

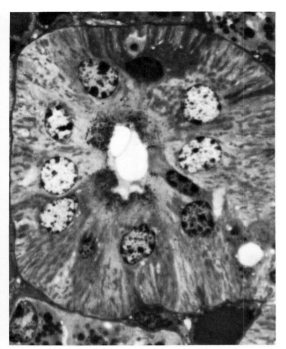

Figure 24-19 Photomicrograph of a striated duct from the parotid gland of a marmoset. Notice the orientation of mitochondria parallel to the cell axis, giving the basal cytoplasm a vertically striated appearance. (Micrograph courtesy of B. Tandler.)

TONSILS

The aperture through which the oral cavity communicates with the pharynx is called the *fauces*. In this region the mucous membrane of the digestive tract contains accumulations of lymphoid tissue. In addition to small infiltrations of lymphocytes, which may occur anywhere in this part of the mucous membrane, there are well outlined organs of lymphoid tissue. The surface epithelium invaginates into them, and they are called *tonsils*. The lingual tonsils have been described.

Between the glossopalatine and the pharyngopalatine arches are the *palatine tonsils*, two prominent, oval accumulations of lymphoid tissue in the connective tissue beneath the mucous membrane. The overlying epithelium invaginates to form 10 to 20 deep tonsillar *crypts*. The stratified squamous epithelium of the free surface overlies a thin layer of connective tissue. The crypts almost reach the connective tissue *capsule* and are of simple or branching form (Fig. 24–22).

The nodules with their prominent germinal centers are embedded in a diffuse mass of lymphoid tissue 1 to 2 mm. thick, and are usually arranged in a single layer under the epithelium. The epithelial crypts with their surrounding sheaths of lymphoid tissue are partially separated from one another by thin partitions of loose connective tissue which invaginate from the capsule. In this connective tissue there are always numerous lymphocytes of various sizes, mast cells, and plasma cells. The presence of large numbers of polymorphonuclear leukocytes is indicative of inflammation, which is very common in tonsils. Occasionally islands of cartilage or bone are found, which are probably late sequelae of earlier pathological processes in the tonsils. In the deeper portions of the crypts, the limit

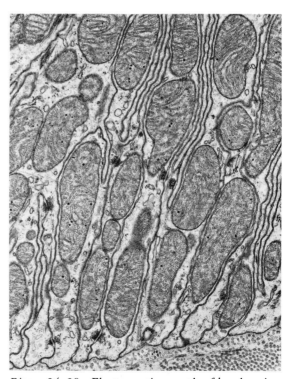

Figure 24-20 Electron micrograph of basal region of striated duct cells from cat submandibular gland. Notice the desmosomes joining interdigitating processes of neighboring cells. (Micrograph courtesy of B. Tandler.)

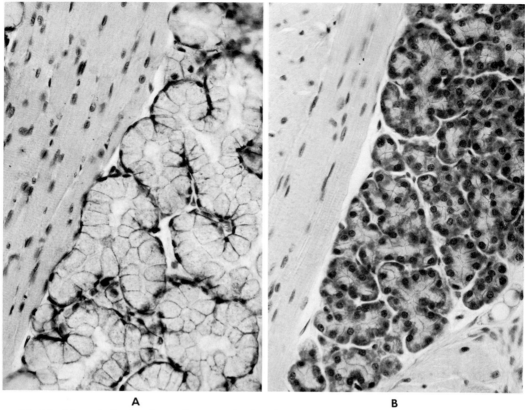

Figure 24–21 Lingual glands, situated among the bundles of striated muscle in rabbit tongue. *A*, Mucous glands. *B*, Serous glands. × 300.

between the epithelium and the lymphoid tissue is obscured by an intense infiltration of the epithelium with lymphocytes. The epithelial cells are pushed aside and distorted, so that only a few recognizable epithelial cells remain on the surface (Fig. 24–23). Plasma cells are common here.

The lymphocytes that pass through the epithelium are found in the saliva as the *salivary corpuscles.* They appear there as degenerating vesicular elements with a pyknotic nucleus surrounded by a clear vesicle containing granules that show Brownian movement. The salivary corpuscles that originate from polymorphonuclear leukocytes are recognized by the remnants of their specific granules and their polymorphous nucleus.

The lumen of the crypts may contain large accumulations of living and degen-erated lymphocytes mixed with desquamated squamous epithelial cells, granular detritus, and microorganisms. These masses may increase in size and form cheesy plugs, which are ultimately eliminated. If they remain for a long time, they may calcify. The microorganisms are sometimes the cause of inflammation and suppuration, and, carried to other parts of the body, they may be responsible for some general infections.

Many small glands are connected with the palatine tonsils. Their bodies are outside the capsule, and their ducts open for the most part on the free surface. Openings into the crypts seem rare.

In the roof and posterior wall of the nasopharynx is the unpaired *pharyngeal tonsil.* The epithelium on the surface of this tonsil is the same as in the rest of the respiratory passages—pseudostratified, cilated columnar

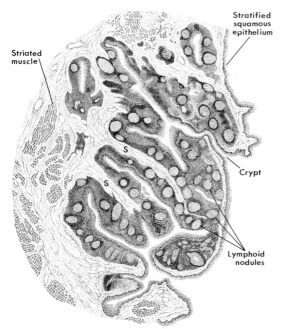

Striated muscle

Stratified squamous epithelium

Crypt

S

S

Lymphoid nodules

Figure 24-22 Section through palatine tonsil of man, showing crypts penetrating the tonsil from the free surface, and connective tissue septa (*S*) penetrating the lymphoid tissue from beneath. × 6. (Redrawn and modified from Sobotta.)

epithelium with many goblet cells. Small patches of stratified squamous epithelium are common, however. The epithelium is not invaginated to form crypts like those of the palatine tonsil but is plicated to form numerous surface folds. It is abundantly infiltrated with lymphocytes, especially on the crests of the folds. A 2 mm. thick layer of diffuse and nodular lymphoid tissue is found under the epithelium and participates in the formation of the folds. The lymphoid tissue of the tonsil is separated from the surrounding parts by a thin connective tissue capsule, which sends thin partitions into the core of each fold. Outside the capsule are small glands of mixed character. Their ducts—often markedly dilated—traverse the lymphoid tissue and empty into the furrows or on the folds.

Other small accumulations of lymphoid tissue occur in the mucous membrane of the pharynx, especially around the orifices of the eustachian tubes, behind the pharyngopalatine arches, and in the posterior wall.

Unlike the lymph nodes, the tonsils do not have lymphatic sinuses, and lymph is not filtered through them. However, plexuses of blindly ending lymph capillaries surround their outer surface.

The tonsils generally reach their maximal development in childhood. The involution of the palatine tonsils begins about the age of 15 or earlier, though the nodules on the root of the tongue persist longer. The pharyngeal tonsil is usually found in an atrophic condition in the adult, with its ciliated epithelium largely replaced by stratified squamous epithelium.

The participation of the tonsils in the new formation of lymphocytes is the only function that can definitely be ascribed to them. It is generally believed, but not proved, that infiltration of the tonsillar epithelium with lymphocytes has something to do with the protection of the organism against invasion by microorganisms. Pathogenic bacteria have been found in the lymphoid tissue of the tonsils and in the nodules of the intestine, and this is apparently a normal phenomenon. The bacteria penetrating the lymphoid tissue are made less virulent, and they act as antigens, stimulating the production of antibodies.

THE PHARYNX

The posterior continuation of the oral cavity is the pharynx. In this section of the digestive tract the respiratory passage and the pathway for the food merge and cross. The upper part of the pharynx is the *nasal*, the middle the *oral*, and the lower the *laryngeal* portion. In the upper part its structure resembles that of the respiratory system, whereas in the lower part it corresponds more closely to the general plan of the digestive tube.

Instead of a muscularis mucosae, the mucous membrane is provided with a thick, dense, elastic layer. A loose submucous layer is well developed only in the lateral wall of the nasal part of the pharynx and where the pharynx continues into the esophagus; here the elastic layer becomes thinner. In all other places, the mucous membrane is directly adjacent to the muscular wall, which consists of an inner longitudinal and an outer oblique or circular layer of striated muscle. The elastic layer fuses with the interstitial tissue of the muscle and sends strands of elastic fibers between the muscular bundles. In the fornix it is fused with the periosteum of the base of the skull.

The lamina propria mucosae consists of dense connective tissue containing fine elastic networks. Those areas covered with stratified squamous epithelium are provided with small papillae. In the area covered with pseudostratified ciliated columnar epithelium there are no papillae.

The two lower sections of the pharynx and a part of the nasal region have stratified squamous epithelium. Toward the roof of the pharynx its epithelium becomes stratified columnar ciliated, with many goblet cells. On the lateral sides of the nasopharynx this ciliated epithelium continues downward beyond the aperture of the eustachian tube. With age, the ciliated epithelium may be replaced by stratified squamous epithelium over large areas.

Glands of a pure mucous type are found in those places lined with stratified squamous epithelium (Fig. 24–24). They are always located under the elastic layer, sometimes penetrating deep into the muscle. Glands of mixed type, similar to those of the dorsal surface of the soft palate, are confined to the regions covered with ciliated epithelium.

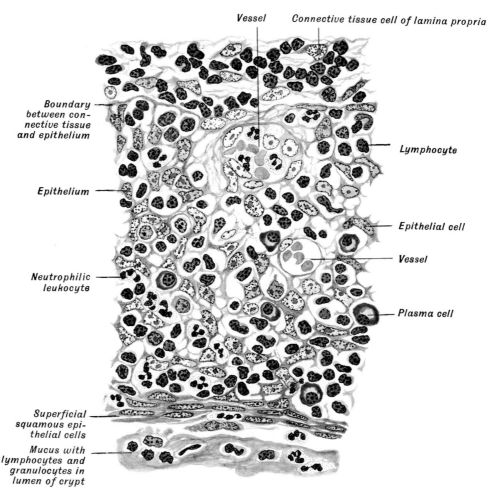

Figure 24-23 Human palatine tonsil, showing infiltration of the epithelium of the crypt with lymphocytes, neutrophilic (heterophilic) granular leukocytes, and plasma cells. Hematoxylin-eosin-azure stain. × 520. (After A. A. Maximow.)

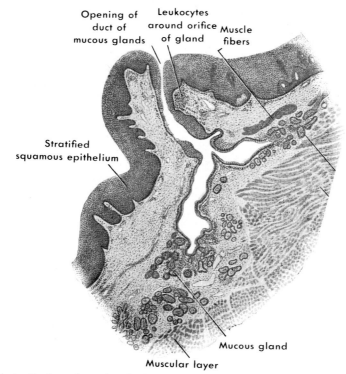

Opening of
duct of
mucous glands

Leukocytes
around orifice
of gland

Muscle
fibers

Stratified
squamous epithelium

Mucous gland

Muscular layer

Figure 24-24 Longitudinal section of wall of the pharynx of an 11 year old girl. × 27. (After Schaffer.)

REFERENCES

Amsterdam, H., I. Ohadu, and M. Schramm: Dynamic changes in the ultrastructure of the acinar cell of the rat parotid gland during the secretory cycle. J. Cell Biol., *41*:753, 1969.

Atkinson, W. B., F. Wilson, and S. Coates: The nature of the sexual dimorphism of the submandibular gland of the mouse. Endocrinology, *65*:114, 1959.

Beidler, L. M., and R. L. Smallman: Renewal of cells within taste buds. J. Cell Biol., *27*:263, 1965.

Farbman, A. I.: Fine structure of the taste bud. J. Ultrastruct. Res., *12*:328, 1965.

Farbman, A. I.: Electron microscope study of the developing taste bud in rat fungiform papilla. Develop. Biol., *11*:110, 1965.

Fujimoto, S., and R. G. Murray: Fine structure of degeneration and regeneration in denervated rabbit vallate buds. Anat. Rec., *168*:393, 1970.

Jacoby, F., and C. R. Leeson: The post-natal development of the rat submaxillary gland. J. Anat., *93*:201, 1959.

Jenkins, G. M.: Physiology of the Mouth. 3rd ed. Philadelphia, F. A. Davis Company, 1966.

Kolmer, W.: Geschmacksorgan. *In* von Möllendorff, W., and W. Bargmann, eds.: Handbuch der mikroskopischen Anatomie des Menschen. Berlin, Julius Springer, 1927, Vol. 3, Part 1, p. 154.

Lacassagne, A.: Dimorphisme sexuel de la glande sous-maxillaire chez la souris. Compt. rend. soc. biol., *133*: 180, 1940.

Langley, J. N.: On the changes in serous glands during secretion. J. Physiol., *2*:261, 1880.

Levi-Montalcini, R., and S. Cohen: Effects of the extract of the mouse submaxillary salivary glands on the sympathetic system of mammals. Ann. N.Y. Acad. Sci., *85*: 324, 1960.

Maximow, A. A.: Beiträge zur Histologie und Physiologie der Speicheldrüsen. Arch. f. mikr. Anat., *58*:1, 1901.

Murray, R. G., and A. Murray: Fine structure of taste buds of rabbit foliate papillae. J. Ultrastr. Res., *19*:327, 1967.

Murray, R. G., and S. Fujimoto: Fine structure of gustatory cells in the rabbit taste buds. J. Ultrastr. Res., *27*:444, 1969.

Oakley, B., and R. M. Benjamin: Neural mechanisms of taste. Physiol. Rev., *46*:173, 1966.

Parks, H. F.: Morphological study of the extrusion of secretory materials by the parotid glands of mouse and rat. J. Ultrastr. Res., *6*:449, 1962.

Pischinger, A.: Beiträge zur Kenntnis des Speicheldrüsen besonders der Glandula sublingualis und submaxillaris des Menschen. Zeitschr. f. mikr. Anat. u. Forsch., *1*:437, 1924.

Rauch, S.: Die Speicheldrüsen des Menschen. Stuttgart, Georg Thieme Verlag, 1959.

Rawinson, H. E.: The changes in the cells of the striated ducts of the cat's submaxillary gland after autonomic stimulation and nerve section. Anat. Rec., *63*:295, 1935.

Rutberg, V.: Ultrastructural and secretory mechanism of the parotid gland. Acta odontol. Scandinav., *19*:Suppl. 30, 1961.

Scheuer-Karpin, R., and A. Baudach: Cytology of the tonsils. Lymphology, *3*:109, 1970.

Schumacher, S.: Die Mundhöhle (p. 1), Die Zunge (p. 35),

Der Schlundkopf (p. 290). *In* von Möllendorff, W., and W. Bargmann, eds.: Handbuch der mikroskopischen Anatomie des Menschen. Berlin, Julius Springer, 1927, Vol. 5, Part 1.

Shackleford, J., and C. E. Klapper: Structure and carbohydrate histochemistry of mammalian salivary glands. Am. J. Anat., *111*:25, 1962.

Spicer, S. S., and L. Warren: The histochemistry of sialic acid containing mucoproteins. J. Histochem. Cytochem., *8*:135, 1960.

Tamarin, A., and L. Screenby: The rat submaxillary salivary gland. A correlative study by light and electron microscopy. J. Morph., *117*:295, 1965.

Tandler, B.: Ultrastructure of human submaxillary gland. I. Architecture and histological relationships of the secretory cells. Am. J. Anat., *111*:287, 1962.

Tandler, B.: Ultrastructure of human submaxillary gland. II. The base of the striated duct cells. J. Ultrastr. Res., *9*:65, 1963.

Tandler, B., C. R. Denning, I. D. Mandel, and A. H. Kutscher: Ultrastructure of human labial salivary glands. III. Myoepithelium and ducts. J. Morph., *130*: 227, 1970.

Tucker, D., and J. Smith: The chemical senses. In Mussen, P., and M. R. Rosenzweig (eds.): Annual review of Psychology, *50*:129, 1969.

Zimmermann, K. W.: Speicheldrüsen der Mundhöhle und die Bauchspeicheldrüse. *In* von Möllendorff, W., and W. Bargmann, eds.: Handbuch der mikroskopischen Anatomie des Menschen. Berlin, Julius Springer, 1927, Vol. 5, Part 1, p. 61.

25
The Teeth

The teeth are derivatives of the oral mucous membrane. They may be considered to be modified papillae whose surface is covered by a thick layer of calcified substance originating in part from epithelium and in part from connective tissue. The most primitive type of teeth, in which the character of cutaneous papillae is quite evident, is found in the placoid scales in the integument of elasmobranch fishes. Similar structures develop in many parallel rows in the mucous membrane of the oral cavity of the bony fishes, where they are subject to continuous renewal during life.

Two sets of teeth occur in man and most mammals. The first set forms the *primary* or *deciduous teeth* of childhood. Their eruption starts about the seventh month after birth, and they are shed between the sixth and the thirteenth year. They are gradually replaced by the *secondary* or *succedaneous teeth.* The microscopic structure of both kinds of teeth is basically similar, but the cusps of the permanent teeth have a more definitive form. Each of the various types of teeth in each set has a different form adapted to its specific functions; that is, the incisors are adapted for biting and the molars for crushing and grinding the food.

All teeth consist of two portions, the *crown* projecting above the gingiva (gum), and the tapering *root*, which fits into a socket, the *alveolus,* in the alveolar bone of the maxilla or the mandible. Where the crown and the root meet is sometimes called the *neck* or *cervix.* The lower molars have two, the upper molars three, roots. The tooth contains a small cavity which roughly corresponds in its shape with the outer form of the tooth. It is called the *pulp chamber* or *cavity* and continues downward into each root as a narrow canal that communicates with the *periodontal membrane* through one or more openings, the *apical foramina,* at the apex of the root.

The hard portions of a tooth consist of three different tissues: *dentin, enamel,* and *cementum* (Figs. 25–2 and 25–3). The bulk of the tooth is formed by the *dentin,* which surrounds the pulp chamber. It is thickest in the crown and gradually tapers as it reaches the apex of the root. Its outer surface is covered,

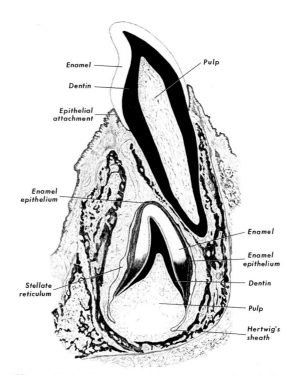

Figure 25–1 Diagram of deciduous tooth and the tooth germ (*below*) of its corresponding permanent tooth. Note the surrounding alveolar bone. × 5. (Redrawn from a photograph by B. Orban.)

621

in the region of the crown, by a layer of *enamel*, which is thinnest in the cervical region. On the root the tooth is covered by a thin layer of *cementum* which extends from the neck to the apical foramina.

The soft parts associated with the tooth are the *pulp*, which fills the pulp chamber; the *periodontal membrane*, which connects the cementum-covered surface of the root with the alveolar bone; and the *gingiva*, that portion of the oral mucous membrane surrounding the tooth. In young persons the gingiva is attached to the enamel; with increasing age it gradually recedes from the enamel, and in old people it is attached to the cementum.

Dentin

The dentin is yellowish and semitransparent in fresh condition. It is harder than compact bone, although it resembles bone in its structure, chemical nature, and development.

As in bone, the substance of dentin consists of an organic (20 per cent) and an inorganic (80 per cent) part. The organic part is 92 per cent collagen, and most of the inorganic components are incorporated into hydroxyapatite crystals. Upon decalcification in acids, the organic part remains and the substance of the tooth becomes soft. Upon incineration, only the inorganic material remains. The inorganic material is much the same as in bone, except that it is denser and less soluble. The organic part, like other collagen rich tissues, also contains glycosaminoglycan–protein complexes.

In a ground section passing through the axis of a macerated tooth, the dentin has a radially striated appearance (Fig. 25–2). This is attributable to the presence of innumerable minute canals, the *dentinal tubules*, which radiate from the pulp cavity toward the periphery and penetrate every part of the dentin. Apical cytoplasmic processes from the odontoblasts extend into these minute tubules. In the innermost part of the dentin, near the pulp, their diameter is 3 to 4 μm.; in the outer portions, they become narrower. In their outward course from the pulp cavity most of the tubules describe an S-shaped curve. The tubules branch, and, especially in the outer layers of dentin, frequently form loop-shaped anastomoses. The layer of dentin immediately surrounding each tubule, as a *sheath of Neumann*, differs from the rest of

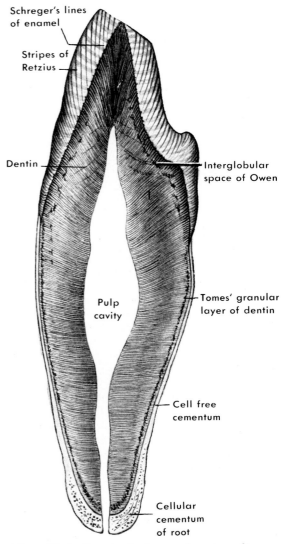

Figure 25–2 Longitudinal ground section of human cuspid. The top of the crown has been abraded. × 7. (After von Ebner, from Schaffer.)

the dentin in its high refringence and distinct staining in decalcified specimens.

Between the dentinal tubules are systems of collagenous fibrils arranged in bundles corresponding to the collagenous fibrils of bone. They are embedded in a ground substance consisting of glycosaminoglycans and protein. The course of the fibrillar bundles is, in general, parallel to the long axis of the tooth and perpendicular to the dentinal tubules. They also run obliquely and around the tubules. In the crown they

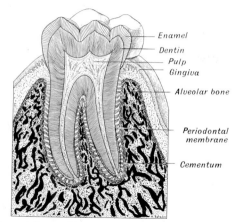

Figure 25–3 Diagram of sagittal section of adult human lower first permanent molar. (Courtesy of I. Schour.)

are tangential to the free surface. The fibrils in the adjacent layers form angles of varying degrees—more acute in the outermost portions of the dentin, and wider in the proximity of the pulp cavity. Some investigators distinguish a peripheral layer, the *cover* or *mantle dentin*, characterized by a branching pattern of dentinal tubules, and a thicker inner layer, the *circumpulpar dentin*, with thinner, straighter tubules.

The calcification of the developing dentin is not always complete and uniform. The deposits of calcium phosphate that appear during development in the organic ground substance have the form of spheres, which gradually gain in size and finally fuse. These nuclei of mineral are found initially in rows or chains on and within collagen fibrils. In incompletely calcified regions, between the calcified spheres, there remain angular "interglobular" spaces which contain only the organic matrix of the dentin (Fig. 25–11). The dentinal tubules continue without interruption through the spheres and interglobular spaces. In a macerated tooth from which all organic parts have disappeared, the tubules as well as the interglobular spaces are filled with air and appear dark in transmitted light. In many normal human teeth there are layers of large interglobular spaces in the deeper parts of the enamel covered dentin of the crown. Mineralization in dentin is not uniform, and as a result, curvilinear lines of appositional growth are apparent. These are called the *contour lines of Owen.* Immediately under the dentinocemental junction in the

root there is always a layer of small interglobular spaces, the *granular layer of Tomes* (Fig. 25–2).

In sections through a decalcified tooth, each dentinal tubule contains a slender cytoplasmic process, *Tomes' fiber*, which in life probably completely fills the lumen of the tubule, but which in fixed preparations appears shrunken. When the tubules are seen in cross section, each small oval contains a dark dot (Fig. 25–4). These Tomes' fibers are processes of the *odontoblasts*, the cells that elaborate the dentinal organic matrix. These cells persist in an epithelioid layer lining the wall of the pulp cavity, sending their protoplasmic processes into the dentinal tubules. Dentin continues to be formed very slowly throughout life, and the pulp cavity is therefore progressively narrowed with advancing age.

The dentin is sensitive to touch, to cold, to acid containing foods, and the like. Only occasional nerve fibers penetrate the dentin and extend for short distances. It has been suggested that the odontoblastic processes may transmit the sensory stimulation to the pulp, which contains many nerves.

With the aid of radioactive phosphorus it has been shown that there is an active interchange of calcium and phosphorus between dentin and enamel on the one hand and the blood on the other. The interchange persists on a diminished scale via the dentinocemental junction in teeth in which the pulp cavity has been filled.

The odontoblasts have been studied most thoroughly in the incisors of laboratory rodents, which differ from the incisors of man in that they continue to grow in length

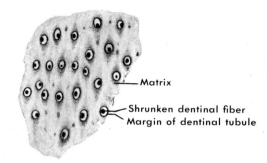

Figure 25–4 Tangential section though the root of a molar of an ape. The margin of the dentinal tubule is also called the sheath of Neumann. The dot in the center of each dentinal tubule is a somewhat shrunken Tomes' fiber. × 740. (After Schaffer.)

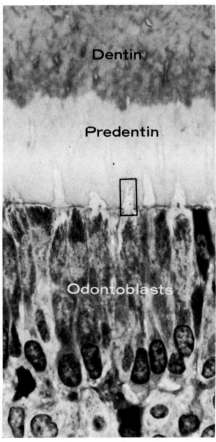

Figure 25–5 Photomicrograph from growing end of rat incisor, showing the relationship of the odontoblasts to the predentin and dentin. Notice the basal nuclei and the apical processes projecting into the predentin. An area such as that enclosed in the rectangle is shown at higher magnification in Figure 25–7. (From M. Weinstock and C. P. Leblond, J. Cell Biol., *60*:92, 1974.)

throughout adult life. The cytological characteristics and functions of human odontoblasts are generally similar to those of rodents during tooth development, but they become less active in the adult. The nucleus is near the base of these tall cells, and there is a large Golgi apparatus situated about midway between the nucleus and the cell apex (Fig. 25–5 and 25–6). The supranuclear region also contains many cisternal profiles of rough endoplasmic reticulum oriented more or less parallel to the long axis of the cell. Free ribosomes are also abundant. The cells are joined at their apices by junctional complexes, and there is a distinct terminal web. A light staining tapering odontoblastic process, extends beyond

the terminal web through the unmineralized predentin and into tubular channels in the mineralized dentin matrix (Fig. 25–7). A number of smaller lateral branches

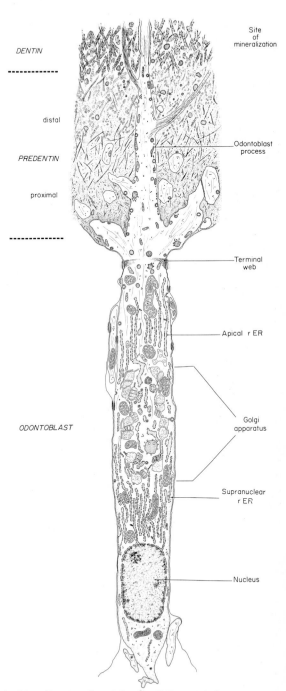

Figure 25–6. Drawing depicting the ultrastructure of a typical odontoblast from rat incisor. (From M. Weinstock and C. P. Leblond, J. Cell Biol., *60*:92, 1974.)

extend from the main process into the predentin. The cytoplasm of the odontoblastic processes is ordinarily devoid of membranous organelles. The cells actively synthesize and secrete precursors of the collagen and the amorphous glycosaminoglycans of the dentin matrix. Histochemical methods for detection of glycoproteins stain both large vesicles associated with the Golgi complex and membrane limited secretory granules scattered through the apical cytoplasm and in the odontoblast process. In electron micrographs, the contents of vesicles associated with the Golgi consist of randomly oriented thin filaments. When appropriately stained, bundles of parallel filaments in vesicles in the apical cytoplasm show periodic densities along their length. These bundles are believed to be parallel arrays of procollagen molecules.

When radioactively labeled precursors of collagen are given, the grains in autoradiographs of odontoblasts localize over the endoplasmic reticulum at very early time intervals (Fig. 25–8). They are later concentrated over the Golgi, then over the cell apex and in a few hours they are found over the predentin (Weinstock and Leblond). The intracellular pathway of protein synthesis in odontoblasts is thus similar to that of other secretory epithelial cells. Among collagen secreting cells, odontoblasts are exceptional in their polarization. In fibroblasts, the product seems to be released anywhere on the cell surface. Although the odontoblasts undoubtedly play a role in the nutrition of the dentin, the dentin does not become necrotic after odontoblasts are removed with the pulp.

In old age the dentinal tubules are often obliterated through calcification. The dentin then becomes more transparent. When the dentin is exposed by extensive abrasion of the enamel of the crown, or when the outside of the tooth is irritated, a production of new or "secondary" dentin of irregular structure may often be observed on the wall of the pulp chamber. This may be so extensive as to fill the chamber completely.

Enamel

This product of epithelial origin is the hardest substance found in the body; it gives sparks when struck with steel. It is bluish white and transparent in thin-ground sections. When fully developed, enamel consists almost entirely of calcium salts in the form of large apatite crystals; only 0.5 per cent comprises organic substance. The protein matrix of enamel, secreted by cells called *ameloblasts*, has been isolated, and oriented samples have

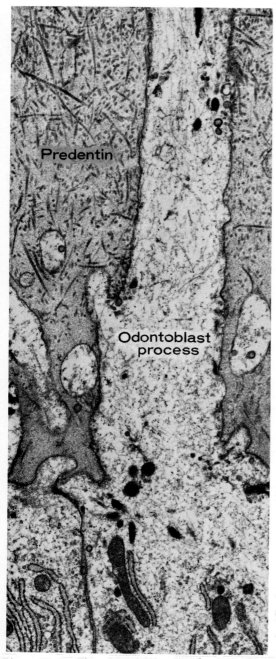

Figure 25–7 Electron micrograph of apical region of an odontoblast showing the appearance of the odontoblast process, and the fibrillar and amorphous components of the surrounding matrix of the predentin. (From M. Weinstock and C. P. Leblond, J. Cell Biol., *60*:92, 1974.)

been subjected to x-ray diffraction analysis. The protein was found to be in the cross-β configuration. Complete amino acid analysis revealed that between one fourth and one fifth of the amino acid residues are proline. The protein, accordingly, cannot be either keratin (as usually thought) or collagen. Relatively high concentrations of organic bound phosphorus have been found in bovine enamel organ matrix. This may play a role in the initiation of enamel calcification. After decalcification of a fully developed tooth, the enamel, as a rule, is completely dissolved.

As seen with the light microscope, the enamel consists of thin rods or prisms that stand upright on the surface of the dentin, usually with a pronounced inclination toward the incisal or occlusal edge. Between the rods is "interprismatic substance," which has a sub-

structure identical to that of the rods but is oriented in a different direction. Surrounding each rod is a clear area of organic matrix called the *enamel sheath* or *prismatic rod sheath*. Every rod runs through the whole thickness of the enamel layer. This, however, cannot be seen in sections of the enamel, because the rods are twisted and soon pass out of the plane of section. In a ground preparation, the substance of a rod in its longitudinal section seems homogeneous. However, after acid acts upon such a section, a distinct cross striation appears in the rods; this indicates that the calcification probably proceeds layer by layer.

Studies with the electron microscope show that the *enamel rods* or *prisms* and the interprismatic substance are both composed of apatite crystals and organic material. The

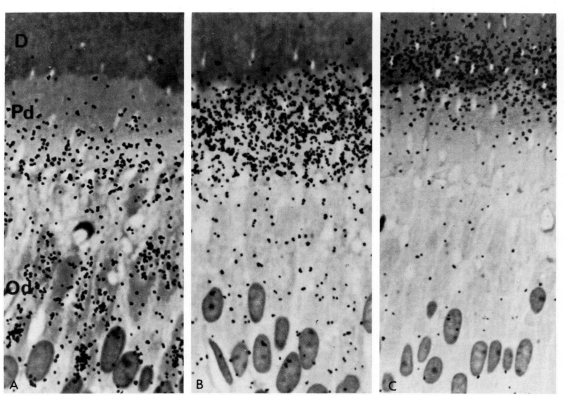

Figure 25-8 Autoradiographs of odontoblasts *(Od)*, predentin *(Pd)*, and dentin *(D)* from young rats killed at various times after administration of a single dose of ^{3}H proline. *A,* At 30 minutes, grains are located over the Golgi region, apical cytoplasm, and proximal predentin. *B,* At 4 hours, label is predominantly in the predentin and has largely left the cells. *C,* At 30 hours, the radioactive bond is over the dentin just beyond the predentin-dentin junction. Such autoradiographs clearly demonstrate the elaboration of dentin collagen precursors by the odontoblasts and the time course of their incorporation into the organic constituents of the teeth. (From M. Weinstock and C. P. Leblond, J. Cell Biol., 60:92, 1974.)

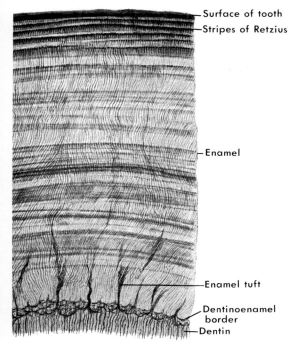

Surface of tooth
Stripes of Retzius

Enamel

Enamel tuft

Dentinoenamel border
Dentin

Figure 25–9 Portion of a ground cross section of crown of a human cuspid. × 80. (After Schaffer.)

relations of the crystals in the prisms and in the interprismatic substance are clearly shown in Figures 25–12 and 25–13.

In the human tooth, most of the rods in cross section have the form of fluted semicircles. The convex surfaces of all rods face the dentin, and their cross sections have a scale-like appearance (Fig. 25–10). The three dimensional configuration and arrangement of the enamel rods in human teeth is still controversial. Some investigators report that in electron micrographs the enamel rods in cross section have a keyhole shape, and that the asymmetrical projection is what others call interprismatic substance. This form and arrangement are explained by calcification beginning earlier on the side of the rods that lies nearest the dentin. This inner, harder side is supposed to press into the softer side of the adjacent rod, compressing it and leaving one or two groove-like impressions.

The exact course of the enamel rods is extremely complicated but seems to be perfectly adapted to the mechanical requirements of the grinding and crushing of food. Starting from the dentin, the rods run perpendicular to the surface; in the middle zone of the enamel they bend spirally, and in the

outer zone they again assume a direction perpendicular to the surface. In addition, the rods show numerous small, wavy curves. On the lateral surfaces of the crown the rods are arranged in zones that encircle the tooth in horizontal planes. The bends of the rods in two neighboring zones cross one another. In axial, longitudinal ground sections, the crossing of groups of rods appears in reflected light as light and dark lines, more or less perpendicular to the surface—the *lines of Schreger* (Fig. 25–2).

In a cross section of the crown, the enamel shows concentric lines, which are brown in transmitted light and colorless in reflected light. In longitudinal, undecalcified axial sections they are seen to run obliquely inward from the surface and toward the root. They are called the *lines of Retzius* or *incremental lines of Retzius* and are connected with the circular striation on the surface of the crown. They are believed to result from rhythmic deposition and mineralization of enamel matrix.

The free surface of the enamel is covered by two thin layers. The inner *enamel cuticle* (formerly called Nasmyth's membrane) is about a micron thick, and appears to be the final product of the activity of the enamel forming ameloblasts before they disappear. The outer is a keratinized acellular layer, probably derived from the keratinized remnants of the dental sac of the developing tooth. It is continuous with the cementum covering the root and is similar in composition and histological structure. This layer is tenaciously adherent to the tooth and is distinct from the connective tissue of the

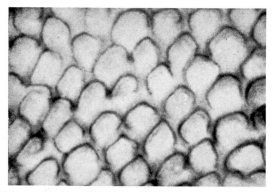

Figure 25–10 Enamel rods of human tooth in cross section. The dark lines are the cementing substance between the pale rods. Photomicrograph at high magnification. (Courtesy of B. Orban.)

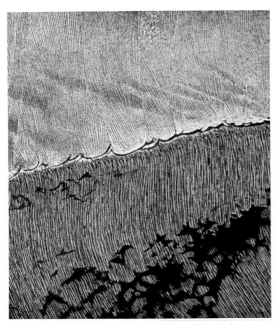

Figure 25–11 Dentinoenamel junction of a tooth of a man; ground section. The enamel prisms appear as a fine, wavy striation. The interglobular spaces in the dentin are black (air filled). Between these lacunae are the dentinal tubules. × 80. (After Braus.)

gingiva. It may persist for some time after eruption of the tooth (Levine et al.).

In an axial section of the tooth, the line of junction between the dentin and the enamel *(dentinoenamel junction)* is uneven and scalloped. Pointed or spindle-shaped processes of dentin penetrate the enamel and are separated from one another by excavations. Some dentinal tubules penetrate a short distance into the enamel and end blindly. The spindle-shaped processes of the dentinal matrix penetrating a short distance in the enamel are called *enamel spindles.*

Local disturbances of the enamel during development cause the so-called *enamel lamellae* and *tufts.* These lamellae, usually found in cervical enamel, are organic material extending from the surface of the enamel toward and sometimes into the dentin. The tufts extend from the dentinoenamel junction into the enamel for one third of its thickness. The tuftlike shape, however, is an optical illusion, due to the projection, into one plane, of fibers lying in different planes. They are groups of poorly calcified, twisted enamel rods with abundant cementing substance between them.

Cementum

The cementum covering most of the root is coarsely fibrillated bone substance. The periodontal ligament attaches to it and to the alveolar bone. Of all the dental hard tissues, cementum is the closest to bone in physical and chemical characteristics. In the adult the organic matrix is elaborated by the *cementocytes* embedded in the apical cementum. The cervical portion of the cementum is acellular, whereas at the apex there is only a thin layer of *acellular cementum* adjacent to the dentin. The remainder of the cementum in this region is *cellular cementum.* Canaliculi, haversian systems, and blood vessels are normally absent. The layer of cementum increases in thickness with age, especially near the end of the root, and then haversian systems with blood vessels may appear.

Coarse collagenous bundles from the periodontal membrane penetrate the cementum. These fibers, corresponding to Sharpey's fibers of bone, remain uncalcified and in ground sections of a macerated tooth appear as empty canals.

Not infrequently epithelial cells are found in cementum. These are thought to be remnants of *Hertwig's epithelial root sheath* (see page 637).

Unlike the dentin, which may remain unchanged even after the destruction of the pulp and the odontoblasts and after the "filling" of the pulp cavity, the cementum readily undergoes necrosis when the periodontal membrane is destroyed, and it may be resorbed by the surrounding connective tissue. On the other hand, new layers of cementum may be deposited on the surface of the root. This deposition is called *cementum hyperplasia* when it becomes excessive and is considered to be a reaction to irritation.

Pulp

The pulp occupies the pulp cavity of the tooth and is the connective tissue that formed the dental papilla during embryonic development. In the adult it has an abundant, gelatinous, metachromatic ground substance similar to that of mucoid connective tissue. It contains a multitude of thin collagenous fibrils running in all directions and not aggregated into bundles. Elastic fibers are found only in the walls of the afferent vasculature.

The odontoblasts previously described are the cells of the pulp adjacent to the den-

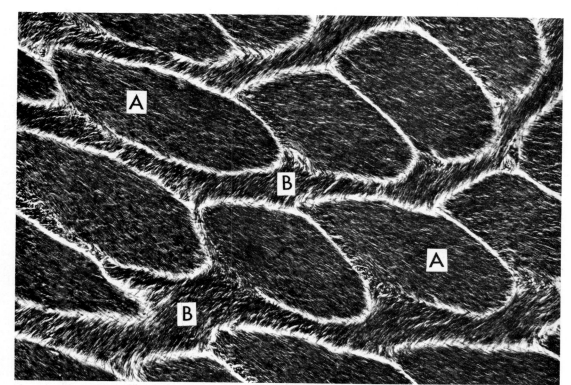

Figure 25-12 Slightly oblique section of undecalcified calf enamel, showing the roughly ovoid enamel prisms *(A)* and the interprismatic substance *(B)*. Note the remarkable orientation of the apatite crystals within the individual prisms, and the different orientation of the crystals in the interprismatic substance. Note, also, the clear areas that define the prisms. Embedded in methacrylate and sectioned with the diamond knife. Osmium fixation. × 18,000. (Courtesy of E. J. Daniel and M. J. Glimcher.)

tin. Beneath the layer of odontoblasts is a relatively cell-free area, *the zone of Weil.* With silver impregnation techniques, bundles of reticular fibers *(Korff's fibers)* are found in this zone (Fig. 25–21). These fibers, described by light microscopists, pass from the pulp into interstices between the odontoblasts and are incorporated in the dentinal matrix. Occasional cells are found in the zone of Weil, and capillaries and nerves are plentiful. Adjacent to this cell-poor zone, at the periphery of the pulp proper, is a cell-rich zone. Spindle-shaped or stellate fibroblasts are the predominant cell type of the pulp. Other cells present in limited numbers include mesenchymal cells, macrophages, lymphocytes, plasma cells, and eosinophils.

The pulp continues into the narrow canal of the root, where it surrounds the blood vessels and nerves, and continues through the openings in the root apex into the periodontal membrane. The pulp contains many blood vessels. Blood vessels and lymphatics enter and leave the pulp through the apical foramen. The circulation of the pulp consists of a system of arterioles and capillaries close to the bases of the odontoblasts. These drain into small veins, more centrally situated in the pulp. Arteriovenous anastomoses are readily demonstrable in the pulp. Numerous bundles of myelinated nerve fibers, which arise from small cells in the gasserian ganglion, enter the pulp cavity through the canals of the root. They form a plexus in the pulp, from which arises a finer plexus of nonmyelinated fibers in the peripheral layers. Nerve endings have been described between the odontoblasts.

Periodontal Membrane

The periodontal membrane, which also serves as periosteum to the alveolar bone, furnishes a firm connection between the root and the bone by way of intermediate fibrous networks. It differs from the usual periosteum by the absence of elastic fibers. It consists, in part, of thick collagenous bundles, that run from the alveolar wall into the cementum. The orientation of the fibers varies at different levels in the alveolus. From root tip to neck, there are the *cemento-alveolar fibers*, designated as *apical, oblique,* or *horizontal,* and *alveolar crest fibers*, the terms describing their direction or their attachments. The fiber bundles of the periodontal membrane have a slightly wavy course. When the tooth is not functioning, they are relaxed and permit it to move slightly on the application of stress. The ligament adjacent to the cementum contains only cementoblasts and the usual complement of connective tissue cells. On the alveolar bone side of the periodontal ligament, osteoblasts and osteoclasts may be found.

Scattered in many places in the periodontal membrane, especially near the surface of the cementum, are blood and lymph vessels and nerves embedded in a small amount of loose connective tissue, and small islands of epithelium. These islands are vestiges of the epithelial sheath of Hertwig. The epithelial rests frequently degenerate and undergo calcification, giving rise to the *cementicles.*

The Gingiva (Gum)

The gingiva is that part of the mucous membrane that is firmly connected with the periosteum at the crest of the alveolar bone. It is mainly a keratinized stratified squamous epithelium with numerous connective tissue papillae projecting into its base. It is also linked to the surface of the tooth by the *epithelial attachment of Gottlieb,* which gradually recedes with advancing age, moving toward the root.

Although the gingiva generally has high papillae, the epithelial attachment is devoid of papillae except when chronically inflamed. Between the epithelium and the enamel there is a small furrow surrounding the crown, the *gingival crevice,* which is lined by a non-keratinizing stratified squamous epithelium.

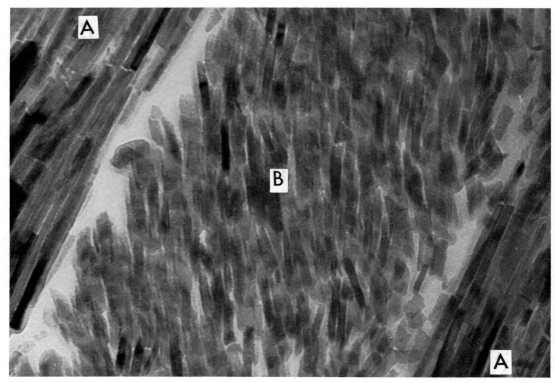

Figure 25-13 Higher magnification of an area of bovine dental enamel similar to that in Figure 25-12, showing longitudinally oriented prismatic crystals *(A)* with the interprismatic crystals *(B)* oriented approximately 30 degrees to the direction of the crystals within the prism. Osmium fixation. × 100,000. (Courtesy of E. J. Daniel and M. J. Glimcher.)

The crevicular margin of the epithelial attachment is the junction between the attached gingiva and the marginal gingiva, which surrounds the tooth like a collar about one millimeter wide.

The thinner portions of the gingival epithelium covering the papillae protrude slightly, giving a nubbled appearance to the otherwise smooth free surface. The free gingival margin does not have these surface irregularities, and the crevicular epithelium is also devoid of papillae except when chronically inflamed. Three groups of collagenous fibers are associated with the gingiva: the gingivodental group, the cuticular group, and the transseptal group, the latter usually being associated with the fibers of the periodontal ligament. Small aggregates of lymphocytes and plasma cells are usually found in the lamina propria at the base of the gingival crevice.

Alveolar Bone

As the teeth are formed, so is the bone that supports them, and it is to this bone that the principal fibers of the periodontal ligament attach. This *alveolar bone* consists of cancellous bone between two layers of cortical bone. The outer cortical plate is a continuation of the cortical layer of the maxilla or mandible. The inner cortical plate adjacent to the periodontal membrane is referred to by radiologists as the *lamina dura*. It surrounds the roots of the teeth to form the socket. The vessels and nerves to the teeth course through the alveolar bone to the apical foramina of the roots where they enter into the pulp chamber. Considerable resorption of alveolar bone can occur as a result of loss of permanent teeth or periodontitis—i.e., inflammation of the supporting tissues of the teeth. Alveolar bone is very labile and serves as a readily available source of calcium to maintain blood levels. The cancellous trabeculae buttressed by the labial and lingual cortical plates aid in support of the teeth during mastication.

Histogenesis of the Teeth

The enamel is a product of the neural crest epithelium, which is lined by a non-keratinizing stratified squamous epithelium. All the other parts are derivatives of the connective tissue.

In human embryos of the fifth week, the ectodermal epithelium lining the oral cavity presents a thickening along the edge of the future upper and lower jaws. The thickening consists of two solid epithelial ridges which extend into the subjacent mesenchyme. Of these, the labial ridge later splits and forms the space between lip and alveolar process of the jaw. The lingual ridge, nearer the tongue, produces teeth and is called the *dental lamina.* According to most investigators, both ridges are independent from the beginning.

The edge of the dental lamina extends into the connective tissue of the jaw and shows at several points budlike thickenings that are the primordia of the teeth, the *tooth germs.* There are ten tooth germs in each jaw, one for each deciduous tooth. In each germ a group of epithelial cells becomes conspicuous as the *enamel knot,* a temporary structure that later disappears. The cells of the mesenchyme under the enamel knot aggregate in a dense group to form the primordium of the papilla. The dental lamina then extends beyond the last deciduous tooth germ and slowly forms germs of the permanent molars, which are not preceded by corresponding deciduous teeth.

Beginning with the tenth to twelfth week, the remainder of the dental lamina again produces solid epithelial buds—the *germs for the permanent teeth*—one on the lingual side of each deciduous germ. After the formation of the permanent tooth germs, the dental lamina disappears. The germs of the permanent teeth undergo the same transformations as do those of the deciduous teeth.

The papilla enlarges and invaginates the base of the epithelial tooth germ (Figs. 25–14 and 25–15). The latter, while still connected by an epithelial strand with the dental lamina, becomes bell-shaped and caps the convex surface of the papilla. From now on it is called the *enamel organ,* because in its further development it produces the enamel. Both the papilla and the enamel organ gradually gain in height, and the latter soon acquires approximately the shape of the future tooth.

A concentric layer of connective tissue, the *dental sac,* develops around the tooth primordium and interrupts its epithelial connection with the oral cavity. Around the sac, and at a certain distance from it, the maxillary or mandibular bone develops (Fig. 25–16).

The peripheral cells of the enamel organ

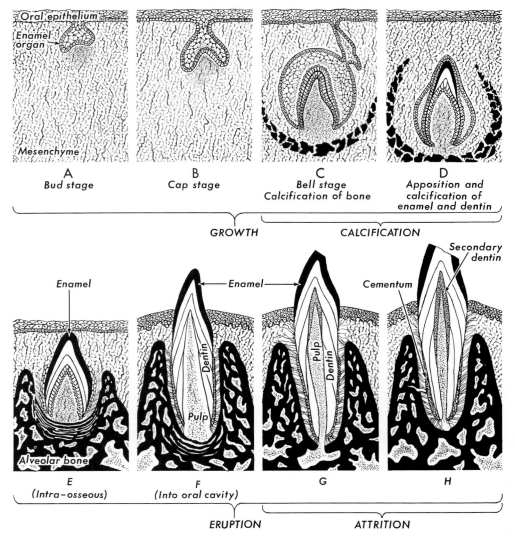

Figure 25-14 Diagram of life cycle of a human deciduous incisor. The normal resorption of the root is not indicated. Enamel and bone are drawn in black. (Redrawn and modified from Schour and Massler.)

are arranged in a regular, radial fashion. On the convex surface, the cells of the outer enamel epithelium remain small and cuboidal. On the invaginated base, the cells of the inner enamel epithelium become tall and regular. They play a major role in the elaboration of the enamel and are called *ameloblasts.* In the interior of the enamel organ a clear liquid accumulates between the cell bodies, which remain connected by long processes. The epithelium thus acquires a reticular appearance like that of connective tissue and forms the *stellate reticulum* of the enamel pulp (Figs. 25–16 and 25–17).

When the formation of the hard tooth substances begins (fetuses of about 20 weeks), the mesenchyme of the papilla contains numerous blood vessels and a few reticular fibrils between its cells. The cells adjacent to the layer of ameloblasts become transformed into odontoblasts (Figs. 25–16 and 25–17).

The dentin first appears as a thick limiting line between ameloblasts and odontoblasts, sometimes called the *membrana perforata.* The layer of dentin extends down the slopes of the dental papillae. It gradually grows thicker and is transformed into a solid cap of dentin by the apposition of new layers

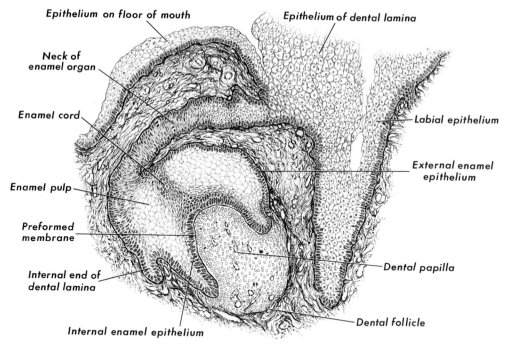

Epithelium on floor of mouth

Epithelium of dental lamina

Neck of enamel organ

Enamel cord

Enamel pulp

Preformed membrane

Internal end of dental lamina

Internal enamel epithelium

Labial epithelium

External enamel epithelium

Dental papilla

Dental follicle

Figure 25–15   Primordium of the right lower central incisor of a human fetus of 91 days, in sagittal section. Collagenous fibers are black. Mallory's connective tisue stain. × 80. (Redrawn and modified from Schaffer.)

on its concave surface. As the odontoblasts recede with the deposition of new dentin, thin processes of their cytoplasm remain in the mass of deposited dentin as the odontoblastic processes.

When the dentin first appears, it is a soft fibrillar substance—the *predentin*. The fibrils, as described by light microscopists, are continuations of the fibrils of the papilla. They are argyrophilic and are generally called *Korff's fibers* or *precollagenous fibers*. They enter the dentin, spread out fanlike, and are incorporated into the collagenous, fibrillated matrix of the dentin (Fig. 25–20). Mantle dentin is formed first, followed by formation of circumpulpar dentin.

In dentin formation, calcification follows closely the deposition of the fibrillar organic matrix. During the whole process, however, there is always a thin layer of uncalcified dentin adjacent to the odontoblasts.

The process of dentin formation is much the same as the formation of bone. Almost immediately after the appearance of the first calcified dentin on the convexity of the papilla, the ameloblasts begin the elaboration of enamel matrix. It is deposited layer by layer

on the surface of the calcifying dentin. On the slopes of the papilla the height of the ameloblasts decreases, and at the base of the papilla they continue into the outer enamel epithelium.

As the mass of enamel increases, the ameloblasts recede. Light microscopists believed that the enamel matrix was a specialization of the apical cytoplasm of the ameloblast and therefore intracellular, and that the calcified enamel prisms were essentially prolongations of the columnar cells. A distinct cell membrane has now been observed in electron micrographs between the cytoplasm and the calcified matrix. The ameloblasts are tall columnar cells with their elliptical nuclei located near the base (Fig. 25–18). They exhibit an unusual segregation of organelles in that most of the mitochondria are clustered between the nucleus and the cell base. A long cylindrical Golgi apparatus is situated in the supranuclear region and numerous cisternae of rough endoplasmic reticulum are found in the supranuclear and apical regions of the cytoplasm (Fig. 25–19). There is a diffuse terminal web and distal to this is a broad apical process (Tomes' process) embedded in the enamel matrix. Numerous spherical membrane limited secretory granules are found in the Golgi region, the apical cytoplasm, and the proximal portion of the apical cell process (Fig. 25–20). The secretory granules contain glycoprotein constituents of the enamel matrix. They are formed in the Golgi, transported to the cell process, and released there (Weinstock and Leblond).

Calcification of the enamel matrix starts at the periphery of each prism and proceeds toward its interior. When the organic matrix has fully calcified, so little organic material remains that the enamel is completely dissolved in decalcification. Complete calcification is not reached until late. That the cal-

cification is seldom absolutely uniform has been mentioned. One of the most striking causes of hypocalcification is parathyroid dysfunction. Schour (1936) studied the rate of deposition of enamel, with sodium fluoride, and of dentin, with vital injections of alizarin. He found that the daily thickening of dentin is about 4 μm. and that unusual increments (*neonatal lines*) appear in the enamel and dentin formed in the deciduous teeth at the time of birth.

When the definitive thickness and extent of the enamel are reached in the neck region of the tooth, the ameloblasts become small cuboidal cells and then atrophy. Before they disappear, they elaborate the enamel cuticle,

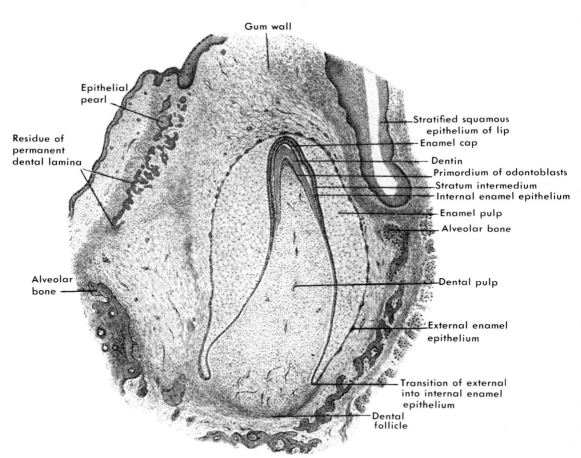

Gum wall

Epithelial pearl

Residue of permanent dental lamina

Alveolar bone

Stratified squamous epithelium of lip

Enamel cap

Dentin

Primordium of odontoblasts

Stratum intermedium

Internal enamel epithelium

Enamel pulp

Alveolar bone

Dental pulp

External enamel epithelium

Transition of external into internal enamel epithelium

Dental follicle

Figure 25–16 Primordium of lower central incisor of a 5 month fetus, in sagittal section. × 30. (After Schaffer.) Compare with photomicrographs in Figure 25–17.

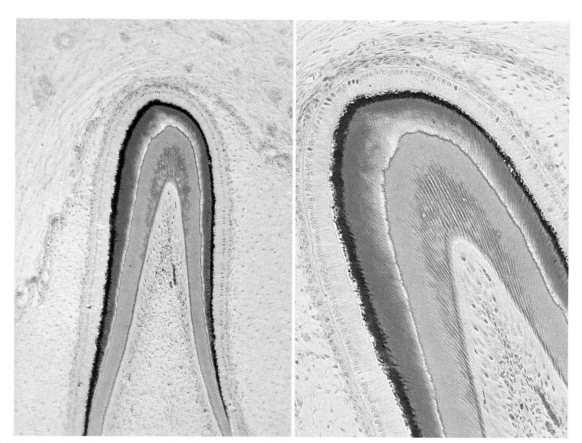

Figure 25–17 Photomicrographs of a portion of a developing tooth, showing the enamel stained red and dentin stained blue near the dental pulp and pink near the dentinoenamel junction. The columnar epithelium of ameloblasts is closely applied to the enamel. Peripheral to this epithelium are the stellate cells of the enamel pulp. The dental pulp is limited by an epithelial layer of odontoblasts depositing dentin. For further orientation see Figure 25–16.

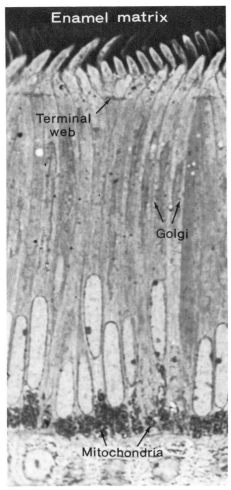

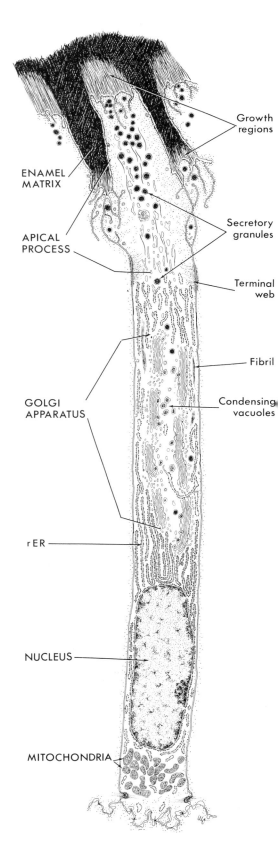

Figure 25-18 Photomicrograph of secretory ameloblasts in a region of enamel matrix secretion in rat maxillary incisor. Notice the clustering of mitochondria at the cell base, the basal location of the nuclei, and the apical processes extending into the enamel matrix. (From A. Weinstock and C. P. Leblond, J. Cell Biol., *51*:26, 1971.)

Figure 25-19 Diagrammatic representation of the ultrastructure of a secretory ameloblast from rat maxillary incisor. (From A. Weinstock and C. P. Leblond, J. Cell Biol., *51*:26, 1971.)

formerly known as Nasmyth's membrane, which covers the external surface of the enamel of recently erupted teeth.

At the end of the enamel organ, the outer and inner enamel epithelium form a fold, the *epithelial sheath of Hertwig.* The development of the root begins shortly before the eruption of the tooth, continues after the

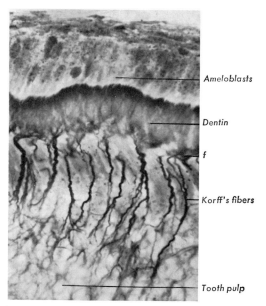

Figure 25–21 Continuation of Korff's fibers of the pulp into the matrix of the dentin at *f.* Photomicrograph. × 700. (Courtesy of B. Orban.)

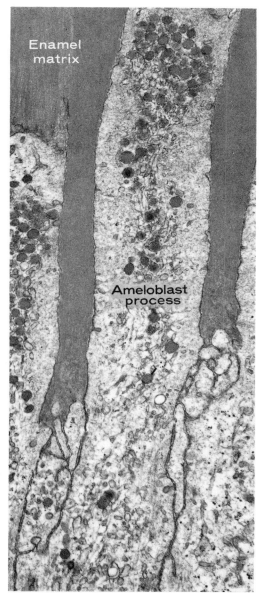

Figure 25–20 Electron micrograph of apical processes (Tomes' processes) of the ameloblasts and associated enamel matrix from rat incisor. (From A. Weinstock and C. P. Leblond, J. Cell Biol., *51*:26, 1971.)

crown has emerged from within the mucous membrane, and is not completed until much later. The epithelial sheath disappears when the root is completely developed. As mentioned previously, remnants of the epithelial sheath of Hertwig are found in cementum and in the periodontal ligament.

When the germ of the permanent tooth begins to develop, its growth pressure causes resorption, first of the bony partition between the two teeth, then of the root, and eventually even of a part of the enamel of the deciduous tooth. Osteoclasts are prominent in this process of destruction just as in the resorption of bone. The crown of the permanent tooth moving upward gradually takes the place of the crown of the former deciduous tooth.

REFERENCES

Becks, H., D. A. Collins, M. E. Simpson, and H. M. Evans: Changes in the central incisors of hypophysectomized female rats after different postoperative periods. Arch. Path., *41*:457, 1946.

Bélanger, L. F.: Autoradiographic visualization of the entry and transit of S[35] methionine nnd cystine in the soft and hard tissues of the growing rat. Anat. Rec., *124*:555, 1956.

Bevelander, G., and H. Nakahara: The formation and mineralization of dentin. Anat. Rec., *156*:303, 1966.

Bevelander, G., and H. Nakahara: The fine structure of the human peridental ligament. Anat. Rec., *162*:313, 1968.

Frank, R. M., and P. Cahan: Microscopie electronique de la pulpe dentaire humaine normale. Bull. Group Int. Rech. Sci. Stomatol., *13*:421, 1970.

Frank, R. M., and G. Cimasoni: Ultrastructure de l'epithélium cliniquement normal du sillon et de la jonction gingivo-dentaires. Zeitsch. f. Zellforsch., *109*:356, 1970.

Garant, P. R., G. Szabo, and J. Nalbandian: Fine structure of mouse odontoblast. Arch. Oral. Biol., *13*:857, 1968.

Greulich, R. C., and C. P. Leblond: Radioautographic visualization of the formation and fate of the organic matrix of dentin. J. Dent. Res., *33*:859, 1954.

Glimcher, M. J., L. C. Bonar, and E. J. Daniel: The molecular structure of the protein matrix of bovine dental enamel. J. Molec. Biol., *3*:541, 1961.

Glimcher, M. J., P. T. Levine, and L. C. Bonar: Morphological and biochemical considerations in structural studies of the organic matrix of enamel. J. Ultrastr. Res., *13*:281, 1965.

Glimcher, M. J., G. Mechanic, L. C. Bonar, and E. J. Daniel: The amino acid composition of the organic matrix of decalcified fetal bovine dental enamel. J. Biol. Chem., *236*:3210, 1961.

Hoffman, M. M., and I. Schour: Quantitative studies in the development of the rat molar; alveolar bone, cementum, and eruption (from birth to 500 days). Am. J. Orthodont., *26*:854, 1940.

Hoffman, R. L.: Formation of periodontal tissues around subcutaneously transplanted hamster molars. J. Dent. Res., *39*:781, 1960.

Höhling, H. J., R. Kreilos, G. Neubauer, and A. Boyde: Electron microscopy and electron microscopic measurement of collagen mineralization in hard tissues. Zeitsch. f. Zellforsch., *122*:36, 1971.

Jessen, H.: Ultrastructure of odontoblasts in perfusion fixed, demineralized incisors of adult rats. Acta Odont. Scand., *25*:491, 1967.

Katz, E. P., J. Seyer, P. T. Levine, and M. J. Glimcher: The comparative biochemistry of the organic matrix of developing enamel. II. Arch. Oral Biol., *14*:533, 1969.

Lehner, J., and H. Plenk: Die Zähne. *In* von Möllendorff, W., and W. Bargmann, eds.: Handbuch der mikroskopischen Anatomie des Menschen. Berlin, Julius Springer, 1936, Vol. 5, Part 3, p. 449.

Lester, K. S.: Incorporation of epithelial cells by cementum. J. Ultrastr. Res., *27*:63, 1969.

Levine, P. T., M. J. Glimcher, and L. C. Bonar: Collagenous layer covering the crown enamel of unerupted permanent human teeth. Science, *146*:1676, 1964.

Miles, A. E. W.: Structural and Chemical Organization of Teeth. Vols. I, II. New York, Academic Press, 1967.

Pannese, E.: Ultrastructure of the enamel organ. Int. Rev. Exp. Path., *3*:169, 1964.

Provenza, V. D.: Oral Histology, Inheritance and Development. Philadelphia, J. B. Lippincott Company, 1964.

Reith, E.: The stages of amelogenesis as observed in molar teeth of young rats. J. Ultrastr. Res., *30*:111, 1970.

Schour, I. (ed.): Noyes' Oral Histology and Embryology. 8th ed. Philadelphia, Lea & Febiger, 1960.

Schour, I., and Massler, M.: The effects of dietary deficiencies upon the oral structures. Physiol. Rev., *25*:442, 1945.

Seyer, J. M., and M. J. Glimcher: The isolation of phosphorylated polypeptide components of the organic matrix of embryonic bovine enamel. Bioch. Biophys. Acta, *236*:279, 1971.

Sicher, H. (ed.): Orban's Oral Histology and Embryology. 6th ed. St. Louis, C. V. Mosby, 1971.

Smukler, H., and C. J. Dreyer: Principal fibers of the periodontium. J. Periodont. Res., *4*:19, 1969.

Sognnaes, R. F.: Microstructure and histochemical characteristics of the mineralized tissues. Ann. N. Y. Acad. Sci., *60*:545, 1955.

Stahl, S. S., J. P. Weinmann, I. Schour, and A. M. Budy: The effect of estrogen on the alveolar bone and teeth of mice and rats. Anat. Rec., *107*:21, 1950.

Stern, I. B.: An electron microscopic study of the cementum: Sharpey's fibers and periodontal ligament in the rat incisor. Am. J. Anat., *115*:377, 1964.

Warshawsky, H.: A light and electron microscopic study of the nearly mature enamel of rat incisors. Anat. Rec., *169*:559, 1971.

Watson, M. L.: The extracellular nature of enamel in the rat. J. Biophys. Biochem. Cytol., 7:489, 1960.

Weidenreich, F.: Über den Bau und die Entwicklung des Zahnbeines in der Reihe der Wirbeltiere. Zeitschr. f. Anat. u. Entwicklungs., 76:218, 1925.

Weinstock, A., and C. P. Leblond: Elaboration of the matrix glycoprotein of enamel by the secretory ameloblasts of the rat incisor as revealed by radioautography after galactose-[3] H injection. J. Cell Biol., *51*:26, 1971.

Weinstock, M., and C. P. Leblond: Synthesis, migration and release of precursor collagen by odontoblasts as visualized by radioautography after [³H] proline administration. J. Cell. Biol., *60*:92, 1974.

Weston, J.: The migration and differentiation of neural crest cells. Adv. Morph., 8:41, 1970.

Wislocki, G. B., and Sognnaes, R. F.: Histochemical reactions of normal teeth. Am. J. Anat., *87*:239, 1950.

Wolbach, S. B., and Howe, P. R.: The incisor teeth of albino rats and guinea-pigs in vitamin A deficiency and repair. Am. J. Path., 9:275, 1933.

26
The Esophagus and Stomach

ESOPHAGUS

The *esophagus* is a muscular tube 25 cm. (10 inches) in length that conveys food rapidly from the pharynx to the stomach. The greater part of its length is intrathoracic but the terminal 2 to 4 cm. are below the diaphragm. Its wall includes all the layers characteristic of the digestive tube in general (Fig. 26–1). The mucous membrane is 500 to 800 μm. thick. The stratified squamous epithelium (Fig. 26–2) continues from the pharynx into the esophagus. At the junction of the esophagus with the cardia of the stomach, there is an abrupt transition from stratified squamous to simple columnar epithelium (see Fig. 26–5). On macroscopic examination, the boundary line between the smooth, white mucous membrane of the esophagus and the pink surface of the gastric mucosa appears as a jagged line.

In man the flattened cells of the superficial layers of the epithelium contain a small number of keratohyalin granules but do not undergo true cornification. The lamina propria consists of loose connective tissue with relatively thin collagenous fibers and networks of fine elastic fibers. In addition to the usual connective tissue cells, numerous lymphocytes are scattered throughout the tissue.

Small lymphatic nodules are found around the ducts of the esophageal mucous glands.

At the level of the cricoid cartilage the elastic layer of the pharynx is succeeded by the *muscularis mucosae*, which consists of longitudinal smooth muscle fibers and thin elastic networks. Near the stomach the muscularis mucosae attains a thickness of 200 to 400 μm.

The dense connective tissue of the *submucous layer* consists of collagenous and elastic fibers and small infiltrations of lymphocytes about the glands. The submucous layer, together with the muscularis mucosae, forms numerous longitudinal folds, which result in the irregular outline of the lumen in cross section (Fig. 26–1). During the swallowing of food these folds are smoothed out. This is made possible by the elasticity of the connective tissue that forms the submucous layer.

The *muscularis externa* of the human esophagus is 0.5 to 2.2 mm. thick. In the upper quarter of the esophagus both its outer and inner layers consist of striated muscle. In the second quarter, bundles of smooth muscles begin gradually to replace the striated muscle, and in the lower third only smooth muscle is found. The relations between the two types of muscular tissue are subject to individual variations. The two layers of the muscularis externa are not regularly circular and longitudinal, respectively: in the inner layer there are many spiral or oblique bundles.

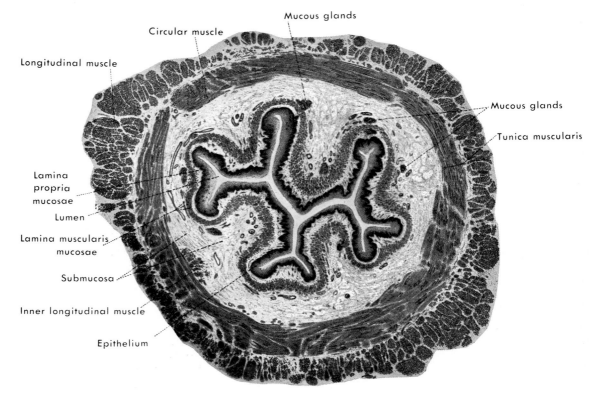

Figure 26–1   Cross section from the middle third of the esophagus of a 28 year old man. × 8. (After Sobotta.)

The longitudinal muscular bundles of the outer layer are also irregularly arranged in many places.

The outer surface of the esophagus is connected with the surrounding parts by a layer of loose connective tissue constituting the *tunica adventitia.*

Glands of the Esophagus

Two kinds of small glands occur in the esophagus: *esophageal glands proper* and *esophageal cardiac glands.* The esophageal glands proper are unevenly distributed, small, compound glands with richly branched tubuloalveolar secretory portions containing only mucous cells (Fig. 26–4). They are located in the submucous layer (Fig. 26–4A) and can just be recognized with the naked eye as elongated white spots. The branches of the smallest ducts are short and fuse into a cystically dilated main duct, which pierces the muscularis mucosae and opens through a small orifice. The epithelium in the smallest ducts is low columnar, whereas in the enlarged main duct stratified squamous epithelium is found. The mucous glands often give rise to cysts of the mucous membrane.

The *esophageal cardiac glands* closely resemble the cardiac glands of the stomach. Two groups of them can be distinguished. One is in the upper part of the esophagus at the level between the cricoid cartilage and the fifth tracheal cartilage; the other is in the lower part of the esophagus near the cardia. They show great individual variation and sometimes are entirely absent.

Unlike the esophageal glands proper, they are always confined to the lamina propria mucosae. Their terminal portions are branched and curled tubules that contain columnar or cuboidal cells with a pale granular cytoplasm, which sometimes gives a staining reaction for mucin. The smallest ducts drain into a large duct that is sometimes cystically dilated and always opens on the tip of a papilla. Its columnar epithelium often gives a distinct reaction for mucin and resembles the mucous epithelium of the gastric foveolae.

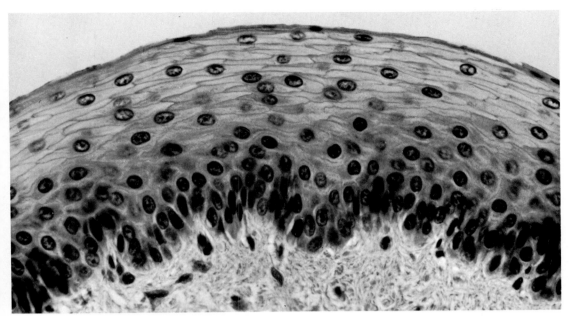

Figure 26-2 Esophageal stratified squamous epithelium of a rhesus monkey. Hematoxylin and eosin. × 500.

In the regions of esophageal mucous membrane that contain the upper and lower groups of cardiac glands, the stratified squamous epithelium may be supplanted in places by a simple columnar epithelium having an appearance similar to that in the gastric pits of the stomach mucosa. Seen with the naked eye, such patches suggest erosions—that is, places denuded of epithelium. Sometimes the patches lined with mucous gastric epithelium are of considerable size and are provided with pitlike invaginations and even with tubular glands like those of the fundus; they may even contain typical zymogenic and parietal cells.

The number and development of the cardiac glands as well as of the islands of gastric mucosa in the esophagus are subject to great individual variation. According to some investigators, the presence of this ectopic gastric epithelium may be of some importance in relation to the origin of diverticula, cysts, ulcers, and carcinomas of the esophagus.

In many mammals, especially those that consume coarse vegetable food (rodents, ruminants, and equids), the stratified squamous epithelium of the esophagus undergoes keratinization. The esophageal glands are present in most of the mammals, but instead of being purely mucous, as in man, they have a mixed character. In some species, no esophageal glands are found (rodents, horse, cat).

Histophysiology of the Esophagus

At the junction of the pharynx and esophagus is a region of higher muscular tone referred to as the pharyngoesophageal "sphincter." Similarly, the terminal few centimeters of the esophagus serve as a gastroesophageal "sphincter" maintaining an intraluminal pressure slightly higher than intragastric pressure. There appears to be no anatomical thickening or local change in orientation of the musculature in these regions. Thus, they seem to be physiological rather than anatomical sphincters. The gastroesophageal sphincter is nevertheless quite efficient in preventing reflux of gastric contents into the esophagus.

In swallowing, the tongue propels the food back into the pharynx. This sets in motion a train of coordinated voluntary and involuntary movements by pharyngeal and esophageal musculature. These involve closure of the glottis, elevation of the larynx, constriction of the pharynx, and reflex relaxation of

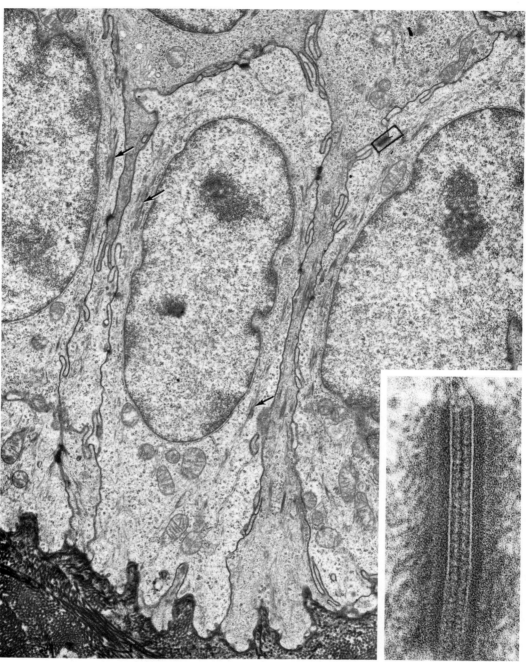

Figure 26–3 Electron micrograph of cells of the basal layer of rodent esophageal epithelium. Division of these cells is responsible for continual renewal of the epithelium. They have abundant free ribosomes and occasional fascicles of cytoplasmic filaments (at arrows). They are attached by well developed desmosomes. One enclosed in rectangle at upper right is shown at high magnification in the inset. Notice the prominent intermediate line in the interspace between the two membranes. (Micrograph courtesy of S. McNutt.)

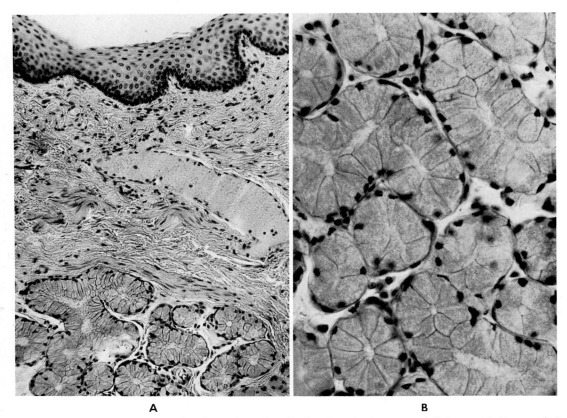

A   **B**

Figure 26-4   *A*, Photomicrograph of esophageal wall, showing the lumen and lining epithelium and the esophageal glands in the submucosa. × 120. *B*, Esophageal glands at higher magnification, illustrating the dark pyknotic appearing nuclei displaced to the base of the cell by the accumulated mucigen in the apical region. × 300.

the pharyngeoesophageal sphincter. When the bolus of food enters the esophagus, the local stimulus of distention initiates a peristaltic wave of contraction which is propagated toward the stomach at a rate of 4 to 6 cm./sec. The gastroesophageal sphincter relaxes transiently in anticipation of the arrival of the peristaltic wave, allowing the food to pass into the stomach.

The nerves to the esophagus are derived from the vagus and the cervical and thoracic sympathetic trunks. They form a plexus of fibers and clusters of cell bodies between the two layers of the muscular coat and a second plexus in the submucosa. They are important for coordination of movements involved in swallowing. Disturbances of the neuromuscular apparatus are fairly common in older persons and individuals of nervous temperament and may result in spasm, difficulty in swallowing, and severe substernal pain.

STOMACH

The stomach is an organ concerned with both storage and digestion of food. In man, storage is a much less important part of its function than in herbivores and particularly in ruminants. In the human stomach the semisolid food resulting from mastication is reduced to a fluid by the contraction of the muscular wall of the organ and the admixture of food with the secretions of the glands of its mucous membrane. The contents of the upper part of the stomach may remain semisolid for some time after a meal, while those of the more distal region are reduced to a pulplike fluid mass, the *chyme*. When the chyme has attained the necessary softness, it is transferred to the duodenum in small portions. Thus, the function of the stomach is in part mechanical and in part chemical.

The cavity of the empty stomach in its

living condition is not of much larger caliber than that of the intestine. The opening from the esophagus into the stomach is called the *cardia*. To the left of the cardia, the wall of the stomach forms a dome-shaped bulge above the level of the gastroesophageal junction, called the *fundus*. The right concave and left convex margins are called the *lesser* and *greater curvatures* of the stomach. The capacious central portion is called the *corpus*, and the region of transition of the stomach into the duodenum is called the *pylorus*. The wall of the stomach consists of the usual layers of the digestive tube: mucosa, submucosa, muscularis, and adventitia.

The mucous membrane of the living stomach is grayish pink, except for paler zones at the pylorus and cardia. The surface of the filled stomach is smooth and evenly stretched. In the empty, contracted stomach the mucosa forms numerous longitudinal folds or *rugae*. This plication of the mucosa is possible because of the loose consistency of the submucosal layer and the contractile action of the muscularis mucosae. Another

much finer and more constant pattern of surface elevations is brought about by shallow furrows that subdivide the surface of the mucous membrane into small, slightly bulging gastric areas 1 to 6 mm. in diameter (Fig. 26–6). With a magnifying lens the surface of each area is seen to be further subdivided by tiny grooves into irregularly convoluted ridges. The pattern of rugae and foveolae is seen most clearly in scanning electron micrographs of the gastric mucosa (Fig. 26–7). In such preparations, the convex apical surfaces of the individual cells can also be identified. In a perpendicular section through the mucous membrane, the transected furrows appear as invaginations, the so-called *gastric pits* or *foveolae gastricae* (Fig. 26–8).

The entire thickness of the mucous membrane in all parts of the stomach is occupied by a multitude of glands, which open into the bottom of the gastric pits (Fig. 26–8). The epithelium that lines the gastric pits and covers the free surface of the mucosa between them is of the same structure throughout. On the basis of differences in the cell pop-

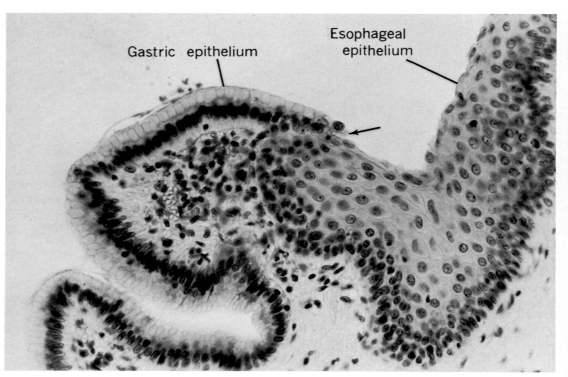

Figure 26–5 Esophagogastric junction. Notice the abrupt transition from stratified squamous to simple columnar epithelium (at arrow). Hematoxylin and eosin. × 375.

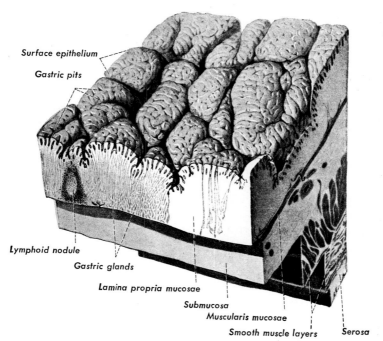

Surface epithelium

Gastric pits

Lymphoid nodule

Gastric glands

Lamina propria mucosae

Submucosa

Muscularis mucosae

Smooth muscle layers

Serosa

Figure 26-6   Surface of gastric mucosa of a man; drawing based on binocular microscope view. The cut surfaces are slightly diagrammatic. At the left, the normal distribution of the gastric glands; to the right, only a few are indicated. Glands, gray; gastric pits, black. × 17. (After Braus.)

ulation in the glands, however, three regions are distinguished in the stomach. The first, which forms a narrow (5 to 30 mm.) ring-shaped area around the cardia, is called the *cardiac area* and contains the *cardiac glands*. The second zone comprises the corpus of the stomach and contains the *gastric glands proper*, or *fundic glands*. The third part, the pyloric region, occupies the distal third of the stomach and extends farther along the lesser curvature than along the greater; it is characterized by the presence of *pyloric glands*. These zones are not sharply delimited, and along the borderline the glands of one region mingle to a certain extent with those of the region adjoining. According to some authors, between the second and third zones is a narrow strip, some millimeters in width, occupied by a fourth type of gland, the *intermediate glands*. In the dog, the animal widely used for physiological experimentation, this intermediate zone is unusually well developed, reaching a width of 1 to 1.8 cm.

In some other mammals, especially the ruminants, the subdivisions of the stomach are much more sharply defined and are marked by deep constrictions that separate the organ into chambers. The stratified squamous epithelium of the esophagus is cornified and may invade a smaller or larger part of the stomach. This esophageal portion, as a rule, has few or no glands. In the ruminants, the lining of the three first chambers of the stomach—the rumen, the reticulum, and the omasum—is of esophageal nature; only in the fourth portion, the abomasum, are gastric glands found, and only here does digestion occur.

Surface Epithelium

The gastric pits and the ridges between them are lined by a tall (20 to 40 μm.) columnar epithelium. At the cardia this epithelium begins abruptly under the overlying edge of the stratified squamous epithelium of the esophagus (Fig. 26–5). At the pylorus it is replaced by the intestinal epithelium. The supranuclear portion of the cells on the free surface is occupied by granules of a peculiar type of mucigen. In sections in which the granules have not been preserved or fail to stain, the supranuclear region of the cell appears clear or highly vacuolated. After proper fixation, the mucigen can be stained with mucicarmine or with the periodic acid–Schiff reaction. With certain other dyes that normally stain mucus, the surface mucous cells are unstained. Upon release, the granules give rise to the layer of mucus that lubricates the surface of the mucosa. The mucus, unlike that secreted by glands of the oral cavity, is not precipitated by acetic acid.

A diplosome can be demonstrated near the free surface and there is a supranuclear or paranuclear Golgi complex. In preparations in which the granules are preserved and stained, it is evident that, in the cells of the foveolae, they become progressively less abundant at deeper levels, and in the bottom of the pits they form only a thin layer immediately beneath the cell surface. Cells of this kind continue into the neck of the gastric glands.

In electron micrographs, the surface mucous cells have short microvilli on their free surfaces and the plasmalemma of these projections has a conspicuous coating of carbohydrate-rich, fine filamentous material. The mucigen granules are spherical, ovoid, or discoid and are, for the most part, dense and homogeneous (Figs. 26–10 and 26–11). However, in some granules of lower density in human surface mucous cells, a characteristic reticular or serpentine pattern is evident within the mucigen. Some may have a dense core and a less dense periphery. The Golgi complex is well developed, the endoplasmic reticulum is sparse, and the mitochondria are in no way unusual. Under physiological conditions, the surface cells are continuously desquamated into the lumen. The population of surface mucous cells is renewed about every three days. Signs of regeneration are

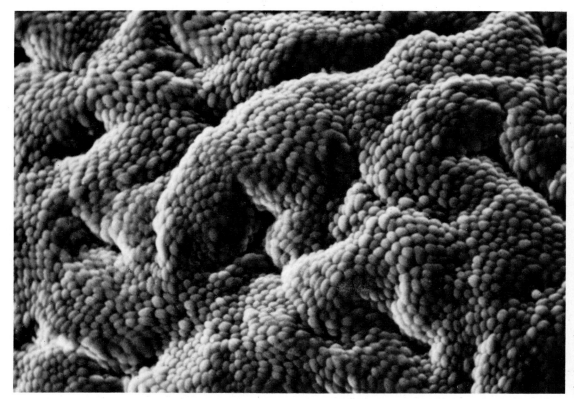

Figure 26–7 Scanning electron micrograph of the luminal surface of the gastric mucosa. The cells are all the same type—surface mucous cells. The convex apical surfaces of the individual epithelial cells are clearly seen. The convoluted pattern of ridges and gastric pits or foveolae is also evident. (Micrograph courtesy of J. Riddell.)

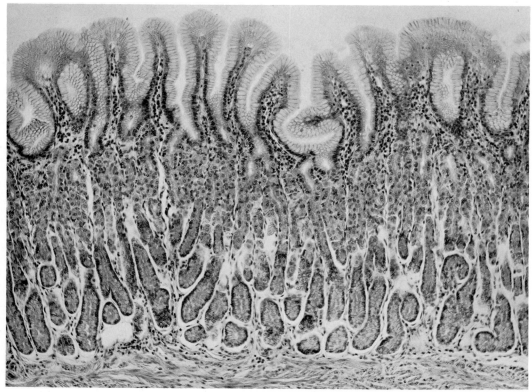

Figure 26-8 Photomicrograph of the gastric mucosa of a macaque, showing the gastric glands opening into the gastric pits, or foveolae. Hematoxylin and eosin. × 120.

seen only in the deeper part of the foveolae and in the necks of the glands, where mitoses are frequent in the less differentiated cells that contain relatively few mucigen granules under their free surface. The newly formed cells are slowly displaced upward and continually replace those lost at the surface.

Gastric Glands

Of the three types of glands found in the gastric mucosa (*cardiac, gastric,* and *pyloric*), the gastric glands are found over the entire corpus and are the most important contributors to the secretion of gastric juice. They are closely packed together and oriented perpendicular to the surface of the mucosa. They extend through its entire thickness of 0.3 to 1.5 mm. From one to several open through a slight constriction or neck into the bottom of each foveola. The overall diameter of the gland is 30 to 50 μm., but the lumen is narrow. The blind ends are slightly expanded

and coiled, and sometimes divide into two or three branches. The number of gastric foveolae is estimated to be 3.5 million and the number of associated glands 15 million.

The gastric glands are composed of four types of cells: (1) *chief* or *zymogenic cells;* (2) *parietal* or *oxyntic cells;* (3) *neck mucous cells;* and (4) *argentaffin cells.* Mitotic activity is largely confined to cells in the necks of the glands, and it is probable that the zymogenic, parietal, and other cell types develop from the relatively undifferentiated cells in this region.

Chief Cells (Zymogenic Cells). The zymogenic cells form a simple cuboidal or low columnar epithelium lining the lumen in the lower half or third of the tubular gastric gland. After death they begin to disintegrate almost immediately, so that adequate preservation is difficult to achieve, but if there is no acid in the stomach, they may remain for some time. When properly fixed, especially after a period of fasting, the cells are full of coarse granules. After intense secretory activity, they are smaller and contain fewer granules, which are located near their surface. The granules are believed to contain *pepsinogen*, the antecedent of the enzyme pepsin. Only certain osmic, sublimate, and formalin mixtures preserve the granules for light microscopy. In most cases they dissolve, and the fixed cytoplasm shows a vacuolated structure. The spherical nucleus does not show any unusual features. In the basal part of the cell, the cytoplasm contains mitochondria and accumulations of basophilic material.

In electron micrographs, the zymogenic cells are found to bear short, irregularly oriented microvilli on their free surfaces (Fig. 26–12). Their fine structure resembles that of other cell types secreting large amounts of protein. The apical cytoplasm contains large round or oval granules of relatively low electron density. A well developed Golgi complex

is located in the supranuclear region. Tubular and cisternal profiles of granular endoplasmic reticulum are found throughout the cytoplasm but are particularly concentrated near the cell base (Fig. 26–12 and 26–13). The abundance of ribosomes, both on the membranes of the reticulum and free in the cytoplasmic matrix, is responsible for the basophilia of these cells in histological sections.

Parietal Cells (Oxyntic Cells). Scattered among the zymogenic cells lining the glands are parietal cells. They are large spheroidal or pyramidal cells with their tapering apical ends wedged between the neighboring zymogenic cells. Sometimes their bases bulge on the outer surfaces of the glands, especially after prolonged secretory activity, when the zymogenic cells are reduced in size.

Each parietal cell usually contains a single large round nucleus, but occasionally two nuclei are present in one cell. The cytoplasm stains deeply with eosin, phloxine, and other acid aniline dyes. The cell contains very numerous rod-shaped or spherical mitochondria, but there are no secretory granules. The most typical feature of a parietal cell is a *secretory canaliculus* that appears to occupy an intracellular position, forming a loose network around the nucleus and opening at the cell apex into the lumen of the gastric gland. The parietal cells do not seem to undergo any marked morphological changes that are visible with the light microscope during the various stages of functional activity.

In electron micrographs the plasma membrane of the free surface appears to lack the filamentous glycocalyx which is conspicuous on other cells of the gastrointestinal mucosa. The apical surface of a parietal cell is invaginated to form the extensive secretory canaliculus that penetrates the cell body and is lined with very numerous, long microvilli that partially occlude the lumen (Figs. 26–14 and 26–15). Although the apex of the pyramidal cell is narrow, the cell has a very large area of free surface exposed to the lumen of the secretory canaliculus. The boundaries between the parietal cells and the adjacent zymogenic or mucous cells are relatively straight and possess typical zonulae occludentes and desmosomes. The cytoplasm is filled with an extraordinary number of plump, closely packed mitochondria having an elaborate internal membrane structure

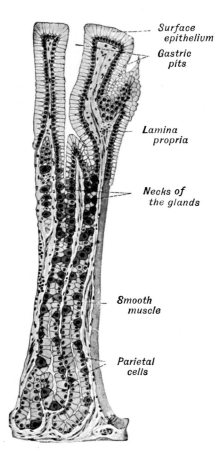

Figure 26-9 Fundic glands of human stomach. Zymogenic cells light gray; parietal cells dark gray. × 130. (After Braus.)

Surface
epithelium

Gastric
pits

Lamina
propria

Necks of
the glands

Smooth
muscle

Parietal
cells

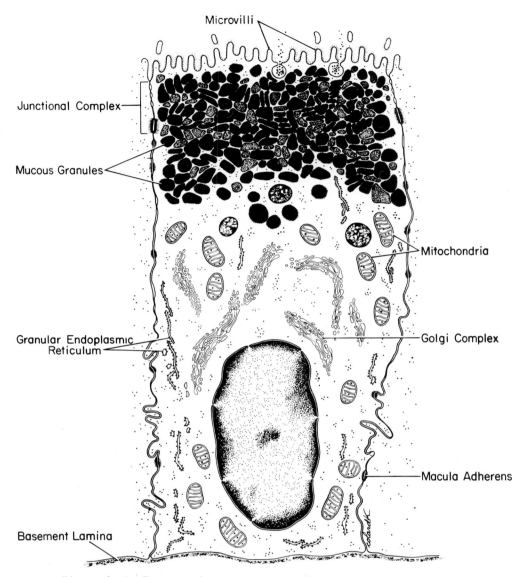

Microvilli

Junctional Complex

Mucous Granules

Mitochondria

Granular Endoplasmic
Reticulum

Golgi Complex

Macula Adherens

Basement Lamina

Figure 26-10   Drawing of a gastric surface mucous cell. (Courtesy of S. Ito.)

and numerous dense granules in the inter-cristal matrix (Figs. 26–14 and 26–15). Cytoplasm near the secretory canaliculus is permeated by an extensive system of minute convoluted tubules. Because of their orientation these were thought by a number of investigators to communicate with the cell surface either permanently or intermittently. However, it has not been possible, by use of electron opaque tracers, to demonstrate continuity. The significance of these tubules in the secretory functions of the cell is still con-

troversial. Profiles of granular reticulum and free ribosomes are relatively few. There are no secretory granules. The Golgi complex is often located between the nucleus and the cell base, in contrast to the supranuclear position that it occupies in most epithelial cells.

Neck Mucous Cells.   These are relatively few in number and are lodged between the parietal cells in the neck of the glands where the latter open into the gastric pits. Deeper in the glands, they are abruptly succeeded by the zymogenic cells. In fresh, unstained preparations they are filled with pale, transparent granules. These cells are easily overlooked or mistaken for zymogenic cells in preparations in which mucus either is not preserved or is unstained. In sections stained with the periodic acid–Schiff reaction, mucicarmine, or mucihematein, the granules that fill the apical cytoplasm are deeply colored, whereas those of the chief cells are unstained. There is evidence that the mucus secreted by these cells is somewhat different from that of the surface mucous cells.

The neck mucous cells appear to be deformed by neighboring cells and therefore tend to be quite irregular in shape; some have a wide base and narrow apex, others a broad apex and narrow base. The nuclei are at the bases of the cells and are often somewhat flattened.

Where the necks of the glands open into the narrow bottoms of the foveolae, the neck mucous cells appear to be connected with the surface epithelium by a series of transitional forms. As mitoses are not found in the neck mucous cells of the adult, it is probable that the new cells arise through a gradual transformation of the undifferentiated epithelium in the bottom of the foveolae and in the neck regions of the glands.

In some gastric glands the neck mucous cells advance far toward the bottom and are sometimes scattered singly between the zymogenic cells. This is especially prominent in the glands near the pyloric region. According to some, the glands of the narrow intermediate zone may contain only neck mucous and parietal cells, and may be devoid of zymogenic cells.

Under the electron microscope the luminal surfaces of the columnar neck mucous cells are studded with short microvilli that have a fuzzy glycocalyx. The lateral surfaces of neighboring cells are attached by small desmosomes and are interdigitated, particularly toward the base of the cell. The apical region of the cell contains numerous dense

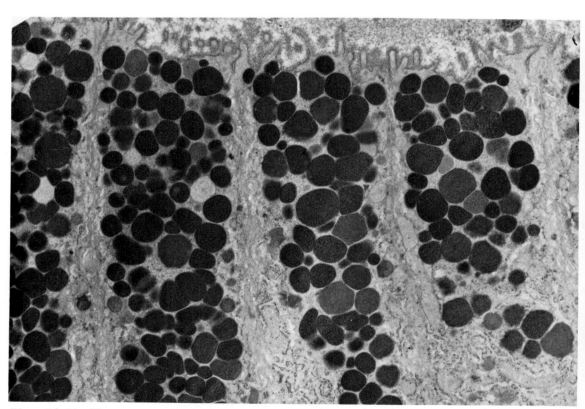

Figure 26-11 Electron micrograph of the apical portion of several surface mucous cells. The short microvilli have a prominent glycocalyx and the surface of the epithelium is covered by a layer of mucus. (Courtesy of S. Ito.)

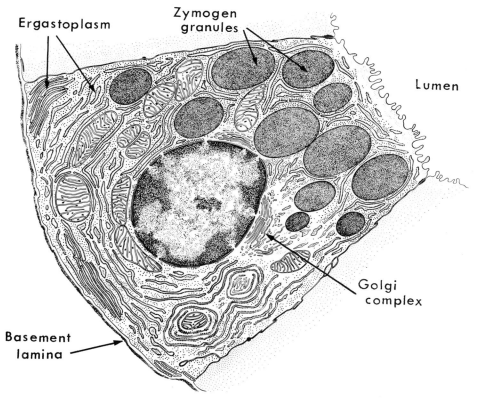

Figure 26-12 Diagram of the chief or zymogenic cell as seen with the electron microscope. (After S. Ito and R. J. Winchester, J. Cell Biol., *16*:541, 1963.)

granules of spheroid, ovoid, or discoid form. Rod-shaped mitochondria of the usual internal structure are scattered through the cytoplasm. There is a sizable supranuclear Golgi complex. Membranous profiles of endoplasmic reticulum are present in small numbers.

Argentaffin Cells. Small granulated cells scattered singly in the epithelium between the bases of the principal cells were observed in the gastric mucosa by Heidenhain in 1870 and later identified throughout the gastrointestinal tract. Their cytoplasmic granules can be stained with silver or chromium salts. These cells were subsequently divided into two categories on the basis of their staining reactions with silver: (1) "argentaffin cells" in which the specific granules reduce silver salts without special pretreatment, and (2) so-called "argyrophilic cells" which require exposure to a reducing substance before their granules will react with silver. The basis for this difference and the relations of the two groups remained poorly understood. It has been the common practice

among light microscopists to refer to all such granulated cells as *enterochromaffin cells.* In recent years, it has been widely accepted that some of these cells are the site of synthesis and storage of *serotonin* (5-hydroxytryptamine).

Electron microscopic studies of the gastrointestinal tract have led to the description of several morphologically distinct types of cells possessing characteristic secretory granules. It is suggested that each may have a different endocrine function. One type, found especially in the pyloric region of the stomach, extends from the basal lamina to the glandular lumen and has spherical membrane limited granules of variable density. Immunocytochemical methods suggest that this cell type produces the hormone *gastrin* (Greider et al.). The predominant category of enterochromaffin cell found throughout the alimentary tract is characterized by electron opaque, polymorphous granules. The cells are pyramidal in shape, with a narrow apical end covered with microvilli. The granules, located near the cell base, have the fluorescence and staining reactions of *serotonin*. A third type of granulated cell bears striking resemblances to the alpha cells of the pancreatic islets and is suspected of being the source of *enteroglucagon* (Orci et al.), but compelling evidence for this is still lacking.

Pyloric Glands

The pyloric glands are found in the distal 4 to 5 cm. of the stomach. In the pyloric region, the foveolae are deeper than elsewhere in the stomach, extending down into the mucous membrane for half its thickness. The glands here are also of the simple, branched tubular type, but they branch more extensively, the lumen is larger, and the tubules are coiled, so that in perpendicular sections they are seldom seen as continuous longitudinal structures (Fig. 26–17). The pyloric glands contain only one type of cell, whose pale cytoplasm shows an indistinct granulation. Secretory capillaries have been described between the cells. The nucleus is often flattened against the base of the cell. In sections

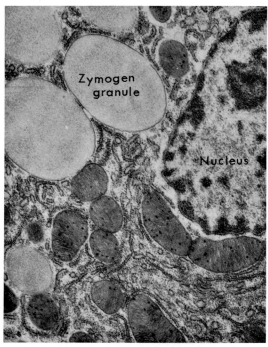

Figure 26–13 Electron micrograph of the apical portion of a gastric zymogenic cell of the bat, showing several pale zymogen granules, numerous mitochondria, and abundant ergastoplasm. Osmic acid fixation. × 17,000. (Courtesy of S. Ito and R. J. Winchester.)

stained with hematoxylin and eosin, they are difficult to distinguish from neck mucous cells or the cells of the glands of Brunner in the duodenum. Some investigators believe that the pyloric glandular cells are identical with the neck mucous cells, for both give similar staining reactions for mucus. Cresyl violet, and the Giemsa mixture of dyes, however, seem to stain them in a specific way. In the human stomach, the pyloric glands in the region of the sphincter may contain parietal cells. Argentaffin cells have also been described in the pyloric glands.

Cardiac Glands

These glands, found in the immediate vicinity of the esophageal orifice, are compound tubular glands that open directly into the gastric pits. They are composed of mucous cells that are histologically quite similar to the mucous cells of the pyloric glands or the neck mucous cells of the gastric glands proper. A few argentaffin cells are found among the mucous cells.

Lamina Propria

Connective tissue of the lamina propria occupies the narrow spaces between the glands and the muscularis mucosae and forms larger accumulations only between the necks of the glands and between the foveolae. It consists of a delicate network of collagenous and reticular fibrils and is almost devoid of elastic elements. In addition to oval pale nuclei, which seem to belong to fibroblasts, the meshes of the fibrous network contain numerous small lymphocytes and some plasma cells, eosinophilic leukocytes, and mast cells. Sometimes, lymphoid cells with coarsely granular acidophilic inclusions, called Russell's bodies, are found between the epithelial cells of the glands. These may develop under physiological conditions but are more common in pathological states. In the lamina propria, especially in the pyloric region, strands of smooth muscle may be found, and small accumulations of lymphatic tissue occur normally.

Other Layers of the Stomach Wall

The muscularis mucosae consists of an inner circular and an outer longitudinal layer of smooth muscle. In some places there is an additional outer circular layer. Strands of

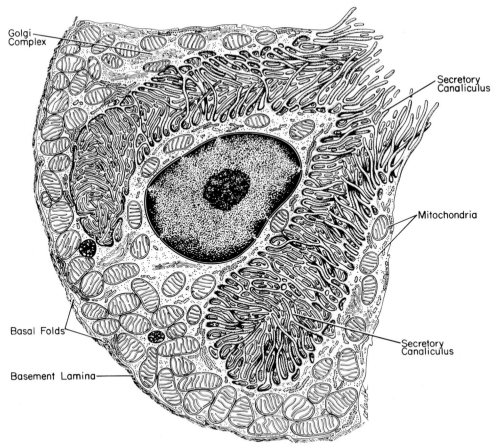

Golgi Complex

Secretory Canaliculus

Mitochondria

Basal Folds

Secretory Canaliculus

Basement Lamina

Figure 26–14 Drawing of the ultrastructure of the gastric parietal cell or oxyntic cell. It is a large cell with very abundant large mitochondria and an intracellular canaliculus lined with microvilli. (Drawing courtesy of S. Ito.)

smooth muscle cells extend from the inner layer between the glands toward the surface. The contraction of these strands compresses the mucous membrane and probably facilitates the emptying of the glands.

The *submucous layer* consists of denser connective tissue that contains some fat cells and is rich in mast cells, lymphoid wandering cells, and eosinophilic leukocytes. This layer contains the large blood and lymph vessels and venous plexuses.

The *muscularis externa* consists of three layers—an outer layer, mainly longitudinal, a middle circular, and an inner oblique. The outermost layer is a continuation of the longitudinal fibers of the esophagus. The muscle fibers maintain their longitudinal course only along the two curvatures, while on the anterior and posterior surfaces of the stomach they gradually become oriented toward the

greater curvature. In the pyloric region, the longitudinal fibers are assembled in a layer that continues into the corresponding layer of the intestinal wall. The middle layer is the most continuous and the most regularly organized of the three. In the pylorus it forms a thick, circular sphincter that helps control the evacuation of the stomach. The emptying of the stomach depends primarily on the contraction of the gastric musculature. The work of all the parts of the muscular coat just described is regulated with marked precision. The wall of the stomach adapts itself to the volume of its contents without alteration in the pressure in its cavity.

The serous membrane, the outermost layer of the stomach wall, is a thin layer of loose connective tissue overlying the muscularis externa and covered on its outer aspect with mesothelium. It is continuous with the serous covering of the large and small omentum.

Histophysiology of the Stomach

The mechanical functions of storage, mixing of stomach contents, and emptying depend upon the muscular apparatus of the stomach. Peristaltic waves originate in the fundus and pass downward over the stomach toward the pyloris. From 5 to 15 ml. of gastric chyme enter the duodenum with each peristaltic wave.

The capacity of the stomach as a reservoir for accumulation of food in intermittent feeders is considerable. Although the luminal volume of the empty stomach is only about 50 ml., nearly 1000 ml. can be swallowed before the intraluminal pressure begins to rise. Distention stimulates peristalsis.

The secretory activity of the stomach is greater than is generally realized. The amount of gastric juice secreted by the human stomach in a fasting subject is from 500 to 1500 ml. After each meal, about 1000 ml. of gastric juice is secreted. This is a clear colorless fluid that contains mucus, water, and electrolytes, as well as the enzyme *pepsin*.

Pepsinogen is synthesized by the chief cells of the gastric glands and is released in response to cholinergic nervous stimulation. The low pH of the gastric contents due to hydrochloric acid secretion by the parietal cells results in severance of a polypeptide fragment from pepsinogen and its conversion to the active enzyme pepsin. The enzyme is optimally active at pH 2 and cleaves peptide bonds. Thus, it is important in the gastric digestion of proteins.

A glycoprotein called *gastric intrinsic factor* is also released into the lumen of the stomach. Formerly attributed to the chief cells, it now is known to be produced by the parietal or oxyntic cells. The intrinsic factor binds to vitamin B_{12} of dietary origin and facilitates its absorption by the intestine. Failure of absorption of vitamin B_{12} leads to impairment of maturation of erythrocytes in the bone marrow and results in *pernicious anemia*. The in-

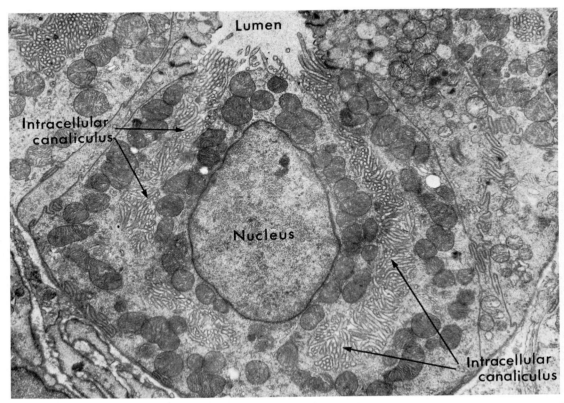

Figure 26–15 Electron micrograph of a parietal cell of bat gastric mucosa. The extensive secretory canaliculus within the limits of the cell is filled by large numbers of irregularly oriented microvilli. × 10,000. (Courtesy of S. Ito.)

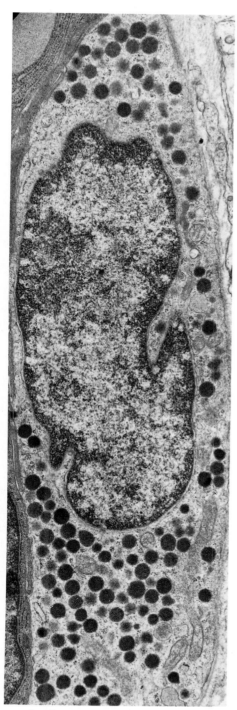

Figure 26-16 Electron micrograph of one of the types of granular argentaffin or endocrine cells. This kind is believed to secrete the hormone gastrin. (Micrograph by S. Ito.)

trinsic factor is sometimes called the *gastric anti-pernicious anemia factor*. Patients with pernicious anemia show atrophy of parietal cells in their gastric glands, which results in defi-

ciency of intrinsic factor and consequent anemia. Surgical resection of most of the stomach may require subsequent administration of vitamin B_{12} to prevent development of severe anemia.

Perhaps the most remarkable aspect of gastric function is its capacity to elaborate a secretion with a pH ranging from 2 to as low as 0.9. Thus the concentration of hydrogen ions may reach a level 10^6 times greater than that of the blood. There no longer seems to be any doubt that acid secretion is a function of the parietal cells, but the intracellular biochemical events involved remain poorly understood. Fractions containing 80 to 95 per cent parietal cells can be separated from dissociated gastric mucosa, and these will secrete chloride directionally in vitro. In keeping with the high energy requirement of the process and the abundance of their mitochondria, they have a much higher oxygen consumption rate than other cell types in the gastric glands (Duncan and Ito).

Despite the very high hydrogen ion concentration in the stomach, there is normally little or no diffusion of acid back across the mucosa. The epithelium thus poses an effective barrier to acid diffusion. However, if the gastric mucosa is exposed to aspirin or to alcohol, the epithelium is extensively damaged, and the efficiency of the barrier is greatly reduced (Fig. 26–18).

The gastrointestinal hormone *gastrin* present in the mucosa of the gastric antrum is a hexadecapeptide produced by one of the several types of argentaffin cell found mainly in the pyloric region and in the duodenum. Gastrin has a number of actions. It binds to receptors on the parietal cells and stimulates acid secretion. It also promotes pepsinogen secretion and stimulates gastric motility. Nearly the entire range of its activities resides in the C-terminal tetrapeptide. This has been synthesized and is used clinically to stimulate acid secretion.

Cell Renewal and Regeneration in the Stomach

The superficial portions of the gastric mucosa have a rapid rate of renewal. Studies on laboratory animals, by means of colchicine blockage of mitosis and autoradiography with tritiated thymidine, indicate that the surface mucous cells are renewed in about three days and the neck mucous cells in about one week (Stevens and Leblond). Although the human

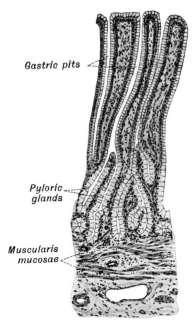

Figure 26-17 Pyloric glands from human stomach. Slightly diagrammatic. × 75. (After Braus.)

gastric mucosa cannot be studied in this way, it is probable that its rate of replacement is also quite rapid. Mitotic activity is largely confined to the surface mucous cells in the depths of the foveolae and the neck mucous cells in the necks of the glands (Fig. 26–19). The epithelial cells exfoliated at the surface are replaced by upward migration from this region of mitotic activity. The neck mucous cells do not appear to migrate, but they may be extruded from time to time directly into the gland lumen.

There is some evidence that parietal cells and zymogenic cells can be replaced by differentiation from neck mucous cells, but most autoradiographic studies have indicated that these cell types are relatively long lived and are renewed only very slowly.

After injury, the gastric mucosa is regenerated in a sequence of events reminiscent of

Figure 26-18 The protective permeability barrier that protects the stomach wall from damage by the acidity of the gastric contents is broken down by aspirin or alcohol. *A*, Normal surface mucous cells of mouse gastric mucosa. *B*, Mucosa 8 minutes after oral administration of a solution of 20 mM aspirin. The superficial cells are pale, their cytoplasm vacuolated, the chromatin marginated. *C*, Mucosa 8 minutes after 20 mM aspirin and 1 mM HCl. Damaged surface cells have exfoliated, exposing blood vessels of the lamina propria. (From R. Hingson and S. Ito, Gastroenterology 61:156, 1971.)

its development in embryonic life. Relatively undifferentiated mucous cells at the margins of the wound proliferate to form an epithelial sheet that migrates over the defect. The epithelium then invaginates to form gastric

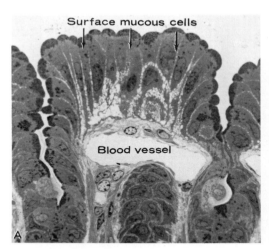

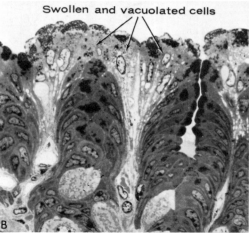

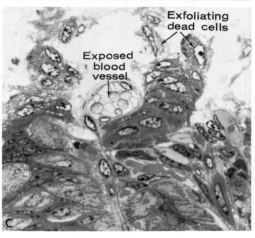

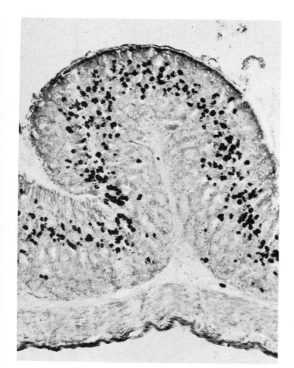

Figure 26–19   Autoradiograph of the gastric mucosa of a mouse given three injections of tritiated thymidine over a 12 hour period preceding fixation of the tissue. The distribution of the black deposits of silver demonstrates that the principal site of mitoses is in the neck region of the gastric glands. × 110. (Courtesy of A. J. Ladman.)

pits and glands. Certain of the cells differentiate into cells resembling neck mucous cells, and these appear to differentiate into parietal and zymogenic cells.

REFERENCES

Baker, B. L.: Cell replacement in the stomach. Gastroenterology, 46:202, 1964.

Bensley, R. R.: The cardiac glands of mammals. Am. J. Anat., 2:105, 1902.

Bertalanffy, F. D.: Cell renewal in the gastrointestinal tract of man. Gastroenterology, 43:472, 1963.

Boas, A., and T. H. Wilson: Cellular localization of gastric intrinsic factor in the rat. Am. J. Physiol., 206:783, 1963.

Davenport, H. W.: Physiology of the Digestive Tract. Chicago, Year Book Medical Publishers, 1971, pp. 85–102.

Dawson, A. B.: Argentophile and argentaffin cells in the gastric mucosa of the rat. Anat. Rec., 100:319, 1948.

Edwards, D. A. W.: The esophagus. Gut, 12:948, 1971.

Erspamer, V., and B. Asero: Identification of enteramine, the specific hormone of the enterochromaffin cell system, as 5-hydroxytryptamine. Nature, 169:800, 1952.

Forssmann, W. G., L. Orci, R. Pictet, A. E. Renold, and C. Rouiller: The endocrine cells in the epithelium of the gastrointestinal mucosa of the rat. J. Cell Biol., 40:692, 1969.

Gershon, M. D., and L. L. Ross: Localization of sites of 5-hydroxytryptamine storage and metabolism by radioautography. J. Physiol. (London), 186:477, 1966.

Greider, M. H., V. Steinberg, and J. E. McGuigan: Electron microscopic identification of the gastrin cell of the human antral mucosa by means of immunocytochemistry. Gastroenterology, 63:572, 1972.

Grossman, M. I.: Gastrin and its activities. Nature, 228:1147, 1970.

Helander, H. F.: Ultrastructure of fundus glands of the mouse gastric mucosa. J. Ultrastruct. Res., (Suppl. 4):1, 1962.

Hingson, D. J., and S. Ito: Effect of aspirin and related compounds on the fine structure of mouse gastric mucosa. Gastroenterology, 61:156, 1971.

Hoedemarker, P. J., J. Abels, J. J. Wachters, A. Arends, and N. O. Nieweg: Investigations about the site of production of Castle's gastrin intrinsic factor. Lab. Invest., 13:1394, 1964.

Holter, H., and K. Linderstrøm-Lang: Beiträge zur enzymatischen Histochemie; die Verteilung des Pepsins in der Schleimhaut des Schweinemagens. Zeitschr. f. physiol. Chem., 226:149, 1934.

Hunt, T. E., and E. A. Hunt: Radioautographic study of proliferation in the stomach of the rat using thymidine-H^3 and compound 48/80. Anat. Rec., 142:505, 1962.

Ito, S.: The endoplasmic reticulum of gastric parietal cells. J. Biophys. Biochem. Cytol., 11:333, 1961.

Ito, S.: Anatomic structure of the gastric mucosa. In Code, C. F., and M. I. Grossman (eds.): Handbook of Physiology, Section 6. Washington, D.C., American Physiological Society, 1967–1968.

Ito, S., and R. J. Winchester: The fine structure of the gastric mucosa in the bat. J. Cell Biol., 16:541, 1963.

Kaye, M. D., and V. P. Showalter: Normal deglutative responses of the human lower esophageal sphincter. Gut, 13:352, 1972.

Landboe-Christensen, E.: Extent of the pylorus zone in the human stomach. Acta Path. Microbiol. Scandinav., Suppl. 54:671, 1944.

Leblond, C. P., and B. E. Walker: Renewal of cell populations. Physiol. Rev., 36:255, 1956.

Lillibridge, C. B.: The fine structure of normal human gastric mucosa. Gastroenterology, 47:269, 1964.

Lipkin, M., P. Sherlock, and B. Bell: Cell proliferation kinetics in the gastrointestinal tract of man. II. Cell renewal in stomach, ileum, colon, and rectum. Gastroenterology, 45:721, 1963.

MacDonald, W. C., J. S. Trier, and N. B. Everett: Cell proliferation and migration in the stomach, duodenum and rectum of man. Gastroenterology, 46:403, 1964.

Orci, L., R. Pictet, W. G. Forssmann, A. F. Renold, and C. Rouiller: Structural evidence for glucagon producing cells in the intestinal mucosa of the rat. Diabetologia, 4:56, 1968.

Samloff, I. M.: Pepsinogens, pepsins, and pepsin inhibitors. Gastroenterology, 60:586, 1971.

Sedar, A. W.: The fine structure of the oxyntic cell in relation to functional activity of the stomach. Ann. N.Y. Acad. Sci., 99:9, 1962.

Stevens, C. E., and C. P. Leblond: Renewal of the mucous cells in the gastric mucosa of the rat. Anat. Rec., 115:231, 1953.

Wolf, S.: The Stomach. New York, Oxford University Press, 1965.

27

Intestines

THE SMALL INTESTINE

The small intestine is the portion of the alimentary tract between the stomach and the large intestine. It is a tubular viscus about 15 to 20 feet long, divisible grossly into three segments, the *duodenum*, the *jejunum*, and the *ileum*. The duodenum is about 10 inches long and largely retroperitoneal, being closely attached to the dorsal wall of the abdomen. The remainder of the small intestine is suspended from the dorsal wall by a mesentery and is freely movable. The proximal part of the freely movable portion of the small intestine is the jejunum, which usually occupies the upper left portion of the abdominal cavity. The distal portion of the small intestine, situated in the lower abdomen, is the ileum. Although there are minor gross and microscopic differences between these three segments, they have the same basic organization, and the transitions between them are gradual. The general description that follows will apply to all. Specific regional differences will be pointed out where they apply.

The principal functions of the small intestine are: to move forward the chyme that it receives from the stomach; to continue its digestion with special juices secreted by its own intrinsic glands and its accessory glands, the liver and pancreas; and to absorb into the blood and lymph vessels in its mucosa the nutrient materials released by digestion.

As in other parts of the gastrointestinal tract, the wall of the small intestine is made up of four concentric layers—the *serosa*, the *muscularis*, the *submucosa*, and the *mucosa*. In relation to the digestive and absorptive function of the intestine, the most important of these is the mucosa.

THE INTESTINAL MUCOSA

To augment the efficiency of this physiologically important layer, there are a number of structural specializations that serve to increase the area of surface exposed to the lumen. The *plicae circulares* (valves of Kerckring) are grossly visible crescentic folds that extend half to two thirds of the way around the lumen (Fig. 27–1). They are permanent structures involving both the mucosa and the submucosa (Fig. 27–2). The larger ones are some 8 to 10 mm. in height, 3 to 4 mm. in thickness, and up to 5 cm. in length. They are absent from the first portion of the duodenum. They begin about 5 cm. distal to the pylorus and reach their greatest development in the last part of the duodenum and proximal portion of the jejunum. From there onward, they gradually diminish in size and number and are seldom found beyond the middle of the ileum.

A second and more effective means of augmenting the surface area of the mucosa is the presence of enormous numbers of *intestinal villi* (Fig. 27–4). These are minute finger-like projections of the mucosa having a length of 0.5 to 1.5 mm., depending upon the degree of distention of the intestinal wall and the state of contraction of smooth muscle fibers in their own interior. They cover the entire surface of the mucosa and give it a characteristic velvety appearance in the fresh condition. Their number varies from 10 to 40 per square millimeter. They are most numerous in the duodenum and proximal jejunum.

The surface of the epithelium is increased not only by elevation of villi, but also by invagination to form tubular glands. Be-

658

tween the bases of the villi are the openings of innumerable *crypts of Lieberkühn* (Fig. 27–5). These are simple tubular glands 320 to 450 μm. long, which extend down into the lamina propria nearly to the thin layer of smooth muscle comprising the *muscularis mucosae*. The spaces between the intestinal glands are occupied by the loose connective tissue of the *lamina propria*.

Epithelium

The epithelium covering the free surface of the mucosa is simple columnar. Three types of cells can be distinguished in the epithelium—*absorptive cells, goblet cells,* and *argentaffin* or *basal granular cells.*

The Intestinal Absorptive Cell. The absorptive cells are columnar in form and 20 to 26 μm. in height, with an ovoid nucleus situated in the lower part of the cell. The free surface has a prominent striated border and beneath this is a clear zone usually devoid of organelles but occupied by the *terminal web* (Fig. 27–8). This may exhibit birefringence when examined with the polarizing microscope and it can be selectively stained by a method which employs tannic acid, phosphomolybdic acid and the dye amido black (Leblond et al.). The cytoplasm below the terminal web is rich in filamentous mitochondria. There is a well developed supranuclear Golgi apparatus.

In electron micrographs, the striated or brush border of the absorptive cells is made up of large numbers of closely packed parallel microvilli which amplify the surface exposed to the lumen about thirty-fold. The microvilli are 1 to 1.4 μm. in length, and about 80 nm. in diameter (Fig. 27–8). The plasmalemma enclosing the microvilli has the usual unit membrane structure but is unusual in having a nap of delicate branching filaments that radiate from its outer leaflet, giving the membrane a fuzzy appearance (Ito). These filaments are longer and more numerous at the tips of the villi than on their sides (Figs. 27–9 and 27–10). The intermingling of the filamentous excrescences of the microvillus tips forms a continuous *surface coat* on the striated border which varies from 0.1 to 0.5 μm. in thickness, depending upon the species (Fig. 27–11). This surface coat is well developed in the human. It is regarded as an integral part of the cell surface. It is glycoprotein in nature and is extremely resistant to both proteolytic and mucolytic agents. It is believed to have a protective role, but it is likely that it also participates actively in the digestive process. Intraluminal digestive enzymes such as pancreatic amylase and proteases are believed to be adsorbed onto the very large surface presented by the glycoprotein filaments of the surface coat. Thus, some of the digestive processes previously thought to occur only in the lumen may also take place

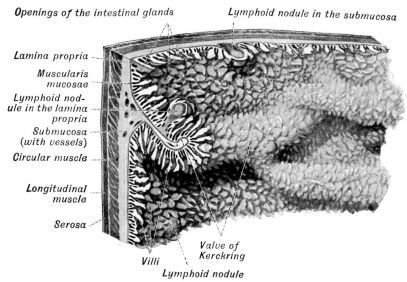

Openings of the intestinal glands   Lymphoid nodule in the submucosa

Lamina propria

Muscularis mucosae

Lymphoid nodule in the lamina propria

Submucosa (with vessels)

Circular muscle

Longitudinal muscle

Serosa

Villi   Valve of Kerckring

Lymphoid nodule

Figure 27–1 Portion of small intestine; drawn from sections using a binocular microscope. $\times$ 17. (After Braus.)

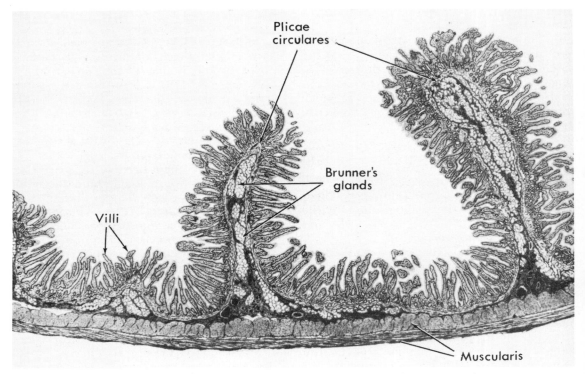

Figure 27-2   Drawing of a longitudinal section through the wall of the duodenum of an adult human, showing the plicae circulares (valves of Kerckring), the villi, and submucosal glands of Brunner. (From W. Bargmann, *Histologie und mikroskopische Anatomie des Menschen,* 6th edition, Stuttgart, Georg Thieme Verlag, 1962.)

on the microvillous surface (Trier). Isolated intestinal striated borders hydrolyze disaccharides and polypeptides to monosaccharides and amino acids. Therefore, the disaccharidases and peptidases involved in the terminal digestion of carbohydrates and proteins are localized in the membrane of the microvilli (Rhodes et al.). In addition to its enzymatic activities, it has been suggested that the surface coat of the jejunum may have specific receptors or binding sites for substances that are selectively absorbed in this portion of the intestine and not in other regions (Trier). Thus, the membrane of the brush border and its surface coat, which were not resolved with the light microscope, have now been shown to be of great physiological importance in the digestive and absorptive function of the small intestine.

In the interior of each microvillus is a bundle of thin straight filaments that run longitudinally in an otherwise homogeneous fine textured cytoplasmic matrix. The filaments extend downward from the microvilli into the terminal web, which is resolved in electron micrographs as a feltwork of exceedingly fine filaments oriented, for the most part, parallel to the brush border. At the sides of the cell, the filaments of the terminal web merge with those of the zonula adherens. The filaments in the core of the microvilli have been shown to form arrowhead complexes with heavy meromyosin and hence are interpreted as actin (see p. 59). It is generally assumed that the filaments of the microvilli and the terminal web are cytoskeletal elements which maintain the stability of the microvillous border. However, the possibility that the microvilli can shorten by virtue of the actin filaments in their core has not been ruled out.

Below the terminal web, the cytoplasm contains numerous elongate mitochondria of orthodox internal structure, and occasional lysosomes. Branching profiles of smooth endoplasmic reticulum are plentiful in this region. The membranes of this organelle contain enzymes essential for synthesis of triglycerides from fatty acids and monoglycerides. This organelle therefore plays an important role in intestinal absorption of fat. Cisternal profiles of granular endoplasmic reticulum are also seen in the supranuclear cytoplasm but these are more abundant toward the base. The Golgi complex has the usual arrays of parallel cisternae and associated vesicles. It shows no morphological evidences of activity except during lipid absorption.

The lateral surfaces of the absorptive cells are in close apposition in the upper part of the epithelium and may have occasional slender interdigitating processes. In phases of active absorption the lateral cell membranes of neighboring cells may diverge toward the base of the epithelium, and *chylomicra* may accumulate in these widened intercellular clefts (Figs. 27–21 and 27–24). A juxtaluminal junctional complex bars access to the intercellular cleft from the lumen. The presence of an occluding junction completely encircling each cell near the lumen insures that material being absorbed from the lumen must traverse the plasma membrane of the brush border, the apical cytoplasm, and the lateral cell membrane to gain access to the intercellular spaces of the epithelium.

The plasma membrane at the cell base is closely applied to a continuous basal lamina which extends across the intercellular spaces at the base of the epithelium. Absorbed material accumulating between cells must traverse this barrier to reach the capillaries and lymphatics of the intestinal villus.

Goblet Cell. The *goblet cells* are irregularly scattered among the absorptive cells (Fig. 27–7). They are described in some detail in Chapter 4, as examples of unicellular glands. Their name derives from their fancied resemblance to a wine glass. Their apical region, called the *theca*, is distended with mucigen droplets, while the base of the cell is relatively free of secretory material and forms a slender stem or stalk. The nucleus tends to be flattened and the surrounding cytoplasm strongly basophilic. The organelles are difficult to study with the light microscope

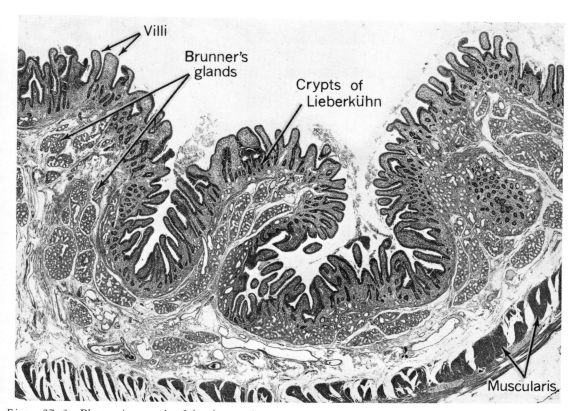

Figure 27–3 Photomicrograph of duodenum from a man who had committed suicide by drinking formalin. The mucosa is unusually well preserved; the muscularis shows considerable shrinkage. × 20. (Courtesy of H. Mizoguchi.)

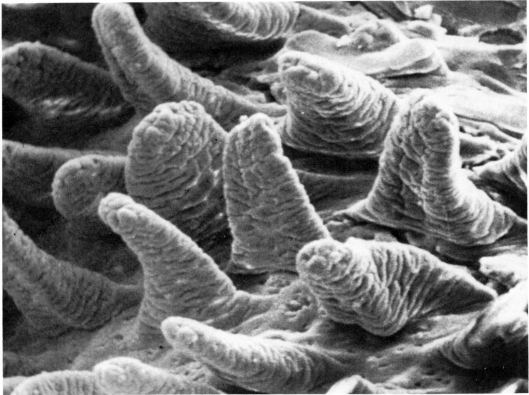

Figure 27-4   Scanning electron micrograph of rat jejunum showing the intestinal villi. (Micrograph courtesy of S. Ito.)

in the mature goblet cell because of their close crowding.

In electron micrographs, cisternae of granular endoplasmic reticulum are arranged more or less parallel to the base and the lateral surfaces of the cell. A few cisternae may continue upward into the thin layer of cytoplasm around the theca (Fig. 4–11). A highly developed Golgi complex is situated between the nucleus and the mucigen droplets in the theca. The individual droplets appear to originate in the Golgi complex and move up into the theca. Each is enveloped by a delicate membrane, which is often disrupted in preparation of the specimen. The basal and lateral plasma membranes are smooth-contoured except for a few lateral interdigitations. The goblet cells are attached to the neighboring absorptive cells by atypical juxtaluminal junctional complexes. Sparse microvilli may be present on the free surface. Their length and number is influenced by the degree of distention of the theca with mucigen. The tend-

ency of mucigen droplets to swell in specimen preparation has made it difficult to study the mechanism of their release, but the membranes of the droplets appear to fuse with each other and with the plasmalemma, permitting the mucus to flow out while maintaining the integrity of the cell surface (Trier).

The secretory product of the goblet cell, *mucus*, is a viscous material with the consistency of raw egg white. It serves to lubricate and protect the surface of the epithelium. Chemical analyses indicate that goblet cell mucus is a very large glycoprotein which is acidic due to presence on the molecule of both sialic acid terminal sugars and sulfate (Forstner et al.). It stains brilliantly with the periodic acid–Schiff reaction for carbohydrates, with Alcian blue, and with thiazine dyes (such as toluidine blue), which stain acidic glycoproteins. There appear to be minor qualitative differences between the mucus in the crypts and that on the villi and also differences along the length of the intestine. The content of acid polysaccharide is generally higher in the goblet cells of the colon than in those of the small intestine.

The synthetic activities of goblet cells include the synthesis of protein from amino acid precursors; the formation of polysaccharides from mono- and disaccharides; the linking of oligo- and polysaccharides to proteins; and the incorporation of sulfate into acid polysaccharides. Autoradiographic studies show that protein synthesis is associated with the abundant granular endoplasmic reticulum at the cell base, whereas synthesis of polysaccharide and its sulfation take place in the Golgi complex.

Basal Granular Cells (Argentaffin or Enterochromaffin Cells). At the base of the epithelium, between the columnar absorptive cells, are scattered small cells that have numerous granules in their cytoplasm. The majority are rounded or pyramidal and confined to the base of the epithelium. An occasional one may be flask-shaped, with a slender process extending to the free surface. Their basal location and the fact that their granules tend to be concentrated between the

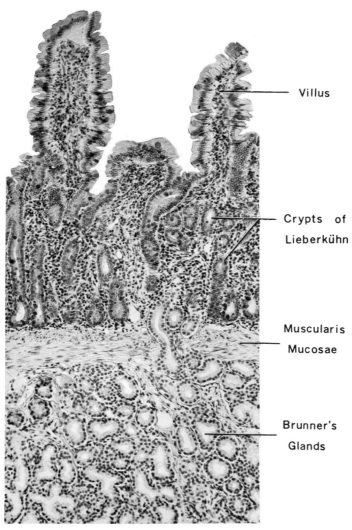

Villus

Crypts of Lieberkühn

Muscularis Mucosae

Brunner's Glands

Figure 27-5 Photomicrograph of a histological section of the duodenum of a macaque. The villi, crypts of Lieberkühn, and Brunner's glands are shown. A duct of Brunner's gland can be seen penetrating the muscularis mucosae to empty into one of the crypts. Hematoxylin and eosin. × 110.

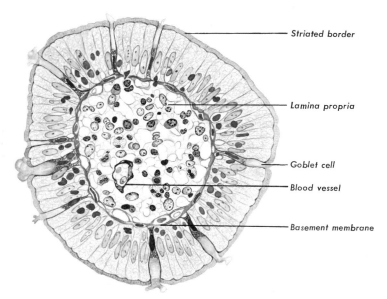

Striated border

Lamina propria

Goblet cell

Blood vessel

Basement membrane

Figure 27–6   Cross section of villus of human jejunum. Iron-hematoxylin-azan. × 350. (Redrawn and slightly modified from V. Patzelt.)

nucleus and the basal lamina suggest that they are *endocrine cells* that liberate their secretion into the lamina propria rather than into the intestinal lumen.

They occur singly and are widely scattered throughout the gastrointestinal epithelium. They are present in moderate numbers in the stomach, and are common in the duodenum, more sparse in the jejunum and ileum, but abundant in the appendix. They have also been demonstrated in the biliary tract and in the ducts of the pancreas. In the intestine, they occur both on the villi and in the crypts.

Many methods were developed by light microscopists for staining the granules of these cells, which have been variously named on the basis of their staining reactions. Cells whose granules reduce ammoniacal silver nitrate solutions and therefore stain brown or black were described as *argentaffin cells*. Cells whose granules turn brown after treatment with bichromate were called *enterochromaffin cells*. These two were formerly believed to constitute a single population of cells, and their widespread occurrence and their cytological characteristics led to the hypothesis that they constituted a diffuse endocrine system—the *enterochromaffin system*.

It was later found that if sections were treated with a reducing substance before being exposed to silver nitrate, a larger number of basal granular cells could be demonstrated. Cells stained after such treatment were described as *argyrophil cells*. The differences in number of argyrophil and argentaffin cells, and the fact that some granulated cells exhibited a yellow fluorescence in ultraviolet light while others did not, gradually led to the realization that not all of the granular cells were identical. In recent years, electron microscopic studies have demonstrated significant differences in the ultrastructure of their organelles and their specific granules. It is now recognized that there are certainly more than one and possibly several distinct cell types.

Cells that fluoresce and exhibit a chromaffin as well as an argentaffin reaction are now known to contain 5-hydroxytryptamine (*serotonin*.) This biologically active substance occurs also in the nervous system and, among other effects, causes vigorous contraction of smooth muscle. It is claimed that as much as two thirds of the serotonin content of the body resides in the gastrointestinal tract, where it is believed to play an important role in generation of the peristaltic movements that propel food and wastes through the gut. Administration of reserpine, which causes release of serotonin, results in a decrease in number of demonstrable basal granular cells. Tumors arising from these cells — *carcinoid tumors* or *argentaffinomas* — are often attended by marked vasomotor, respiratory, and gastrointestinal symptoms caused by their liberation of excessive amounts of serotonin.

The serotonin secreting cell is the predominant gastrointestinal endocrine cell. In electron micrographs, it is characterized by electron-opaque, polymorphous secretion granules, about 200 nm. in diameter. It regularly has a process reaching the lumen and may have a few microvilli like those of the neighboring absorptive cells. The Golgi complex is supranuclear, but the granules preferentially locate in the basal cytoplasm.

A second type of basal granular cell does not reach the lumen. Its granules are almost uniformly round and 500 to 700 nm. in diameter. The position of the Golgi complex is variable, but it is often below the nucleus. The striking ultrastructural resemblance of this cell type to the alpha cells of the pancreatic islets has fostered the speculation that it may be the cell responsible for the synthesis and secretion of the hyperglycemic agent *enteroglucagon* (Orci).

Another cytological type of basal granular cell has been described and held to be responsible for secretion of *gastrin*.

Crypts of Lieberkühn

The epithelium covering the villi continues into the intestinal glands or crypts of Lieberkühn (Fig. 27–5). The upper halves of the walls of the crypts are lined with low columnar epithelium containing absorptive cells, goblet cells, and a few basal granular cells. In the lower halves of the crypts the cells are less clearly differentiated and there are numerous mitoses. It is here that new cells are formed to continually replace those that are exfoliated at the tips of the villi. If tritiated thymidine is given to an animal, it can be shown by biopsies at various later times that the label incorporated into nuclei of dividing cells in the bottom of the crypts of Lieberkühn gradually moves upward onto the villi. About a day after administration of thymidine the labeled cells are on the sides of the villi and by the fifth day they are being exfoliated at the villus tips. Thus billions of cells are being shed every day from the human gastrointestinal tract and are being replaced by upward displacement of cells

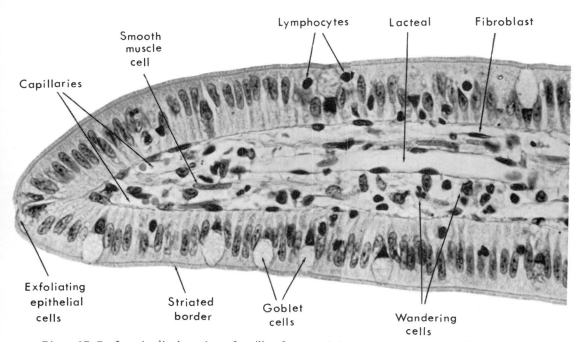

Figure 27-7　Longitudinal section of a villus from cat jejunum. Hematoxylin and eosin. × 600.

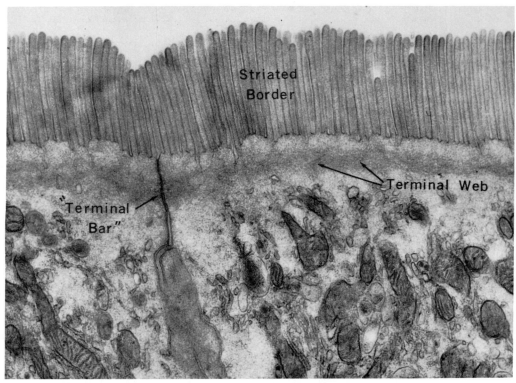

Figure 27-8 Electron micrograph of portions of two intestinal epithelial cells of the hamster, showing the striated border, the terminal web, and the junctional complex, which corresponds to the terminal bar seen with the light microscope. × 25,000. (Courtesy of E. Strauss.)

from localized regions of cell proliferation. In the small intestine, the proliferative activity is confined to the crypts of Lieberkühn.

Discovery of this rapid turnover of cells in the lining of the intestine has altered our interpretations of the physiology of some of the cell types. For example, it was formerly thought that goblet cells might accumulate secretions, discharge and then refill, and that this cycle was repeated many times. It is now realized that the life span of intestinal goblet cells is only 3 or 4 days—the time taken for them to differentiate in the crypts, move up onto the villi and be exfoliated at the tip. Thus, it is probable that goblet cells secrete continuously and normally pass through only one secretory cycle. This consists of an initial phase in the crypts when rate of synthesis of mucus exceeds discharge and mucin accumulates; an intermediate phase when the cells are in the upper part of the crypts and lower half of the villi, synthesis and discharge are approximately in equilibrium, and the cells appear engorged with mucus; and a final

phase when rate of discharge exceeds synthesis as the cells approach the tips of the villi and appear depleted (Moe). Although this is the normal course of events, it can be modified by irritants which cause expulsion of mucus. If mustard oil is administered locally to experimental animals, the goblet cells expel nearly all of their mucus stores. Under these conditions, they then were found to initiate a new cycle of accumulation (Florey).

The discovery of the continual upward migration of epithelial cells immediately posed a number of puzzling morphogenetic problems. Do the cells move with respect to a relatively stationary basal lamina, or does the epithelium as a whole move with respect to the underlying lamina propria? The answers to these questions remain in doubt but valuable new insight into the problem has been gained from autoradiographic studies which reveal that there is also a continuous renewal and upward migration of the pericryptal fibroblasts (Pascal et al.). Much of the relevant experimental work has been carried out on

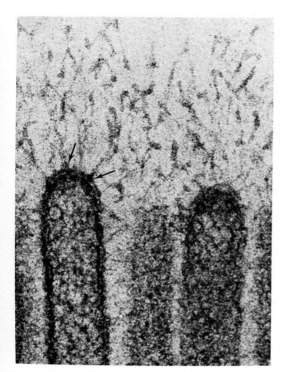

Figure 27–9 Electron micrograph of the tips of several microvilli from cat ileum, showing the branching protein-polysaccharide (mucopolysaccharide) filaments attached at one end to the outer leaflet of the unit membrane (at arrows). × 120,000. (Courtesy of S. Ito, after D. W. Fawcett, J. Histochem. Cytochem., *13*:75, 1965.)

the crypts of the colon but the findings are believed to apply also to those of the small intestine and other parts of the alimentary mucosa.

The crypts are surrounded by a sheath of flattened fibroblasts closely applied to the base of the epithelium and by a highly ordered reticulum laid down with the majority of its small bundles of unit fibers of collagen arranged circumferentially around the crypt. The *pericryptal fibroblasts* are flattened squamous elements that present fusiform profiles in both longitudinal and transverse sections of the glands. At early time intervals after administration of tritiated thymidine, labeled fibroblasts are found in autoradiographs around the lower third of the crypts. At longer time intervals, these labeled cells are localized around the necks of the glands. If the changing distribution of the labeled epithelial cells and labeled pericryptal cells are compared, it is evident that the two cell types migrate in synchrony. Electron micro-

graphs show that that there is a progressive increase in degree of cytological differentiation of the fibroblasts as they move upward. The continuous renewal and upward migration of pericryptal cells constitutes an exception to the generalization that fibroblasts in the adult are a relatively stable population proliferating only in response to injury (Kaye et al.).

Paneth Cell

In addition to the cell types already described, there is a type of cell occurring in small groups only in the depths of the crypts of Lieberkühn—these are the *Paneth cells* (Fig. 27–12). They are pyramidal in form, with a round or oval nucleus situated near the base, and conspicuous secretory granules in the apical cytoplasm. They have the cytological characteristics of cells actively secreting protein. The cytoplasm at the base is basophilic and in electron micrographs contains parallel arrays of cisternae of rough endoplasmic

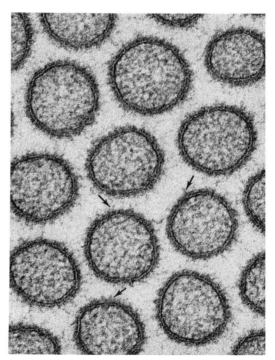

Figure 27–10 Electron micrograph of rat intestinal microvilli in transverse section. The protein-polysaccharide surface coat is present (at arrows), but the filaments are much shorter on the sides of the microvilli than on the tips. × 120,000. (Courtesy of S. L. Palay.)

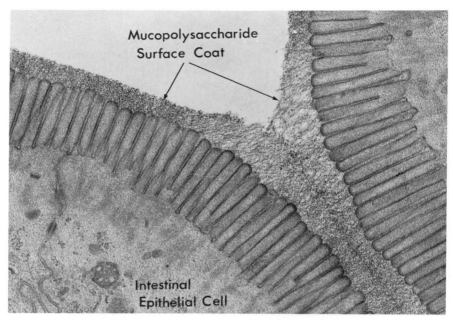

Figure 27–11 Brush borders of epithelial cells in two neighboring villi of cat intestine, illustrating the well-developed mucopolysaccharide surface coat. × 30,000. (Courtesy of S. Ito.)

reticulum. The lumen of the cisternae not infrequently has a dense content and may occasionally be precipitated in crystalline form (Behnke and Moe). The Golgi complex is prominent, as in other active glandular cells, and often contains the formative stages of secretory granules. The granules are homogeneous in density in man and in a number of other species. In the mouse, they have a dense core and lighter peripheral zone (Fig. 27–13). The periphery consists of an acid glycoprotein, whereas the core appears to be a neutral glycoprotein. The granules usually stain with acid dyes such as eosin or orange G.

Paneth cells are a stable population with little or no turnover. They do not incorporate tritiated thymidine and they are not observed in mitosis. They are abundant in humans, monkeys, mice, rats, guinea pigs, and ruminants, but are absent from the intestines of dogs, cats, pigs, and raccoons (Trier).

Paneth cells evidently secrete continuously, but the rate of secretion is enhanced by feeding or administration of pilocarpine. Despite decades of study, the functional role of Paneth cells is still not known. On the basis of microchemical analysis of slices of mucosa at the level of the bottom of the crypts, it was suggested that these cells might secrete a peptidase (Linderström-Lang) but this has not been substantiated in later work. Others have proposed that the granules contain *lysozyme*, an enzyme capable of lysing bacteria. An antibacterial function of Paneth cells has yet to be demonstrated convincingly. Paneth cells are reported to concentrate radioactive zinc, a trace metal that is an essential component of a number of enzymes, but no digestive enzyme has yet been specifically localized to the Paneth cells, and their function remains a mystery.

The Lamina Propria

The lamina propria of the intestinal mucosa fills the spaces between the glands of Lieberkühn and forms the cores of the intestinal villi (Figs. 27–6 and 27–7). It resembles reticular connective tissue in being highly cellular and containing a stroma of argyrophilic fibers not unlike that of lymphoid tissue. Associated with the fibers are cells with oval, pale nuclei comparable to the reticular cells of lymphatic tissue stroma. The reticular fibers are condensed adjacent to the epithelium to support the basal lamina, and in addition there are fine elastic networks surround-

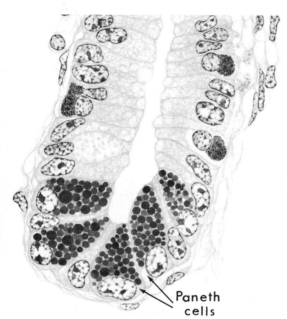

Figure 27–12 Drawing of a crypt of Lieberkühn, illustrating the Paneth cells at the base of the crypt. Higher up in the crypt are four argentaffin cells. Hematoxylin and eosin.

ing the crypts and extending into the villi. Thin strands of smooth muscle extend from the muscularis mucosae into the core of the villi, where they are arranged parallel to the axis of the villus around the central *lacteal*, the minute terminal branch of the lymph vascular plexus that enters each villus and provides an important pathway for the assimilation of absorbed lipid. Periodic contractions of the smooth muscle of the villus core tend to empty the lacteals and propel lymph and absorbed nutrients toward the mesenteric lymphatics and thoracic duct.

Large numbers of lymphocytes, plasma cells, eosinophils, and macrophages are found in the meshes of the lamina propria. These free cells are believed to interact and cooperate in the defenses of the body against bacteria, toxins, and other antigenic substances in the intestinal lumen. The most numerous of the free cells are the lymphocytes, a mobile reserve of immunocompetent cells, some of which are capable of transformation into antibody-producing plasma cells. Many of the lymphocytes penetrate the epithelium on the villi and in the crypts. This phenomenon increases in intensity along the tract and reaches its highest development in the large

intestine. It was formerly thought that lymphocytes by the millions migrated through the gastrointestinal epithelium into the lumen. Autoradiographic studies with tritiated thymidine now cast doubt upon this. Over 95 per cent of the lymphocytes lie in the basal third of the epithelium, and no evidence was found of their entering the lumen. Labeling experiments indicate that the epithelial lymphocyte population has a mean generation time of 15 to 22 days in the mouse (Darlington and Rogers). Their significance is not clear.

Attention has been drawn to the frequent juxtaposition of macrophages, plasma cells, and eosinophils in the lamina propria (Deane). Paradoxically, macrophages, which are known for their ability to digest bacteria and other antigenic materials taken up by phagocytosis, also seem to process antigens in some way that increases their effectiveness. Weak antigens may be hundreds of times more immunogenic when associated with macrophages than they are in the free state. Although the greater part of phagocytosed antigen is destroyed, some appears to persist in or on the macrophages and is liberated gradually and presented to neighboring cells in a manner that facilitates contact between antigen and antigen sensitive lymphocytes. Thus, macrophages seem actively to promote an immune response by priming the host for a secondary reaction to antigen.

The plasma cells produce the protective immunoglobulins called antibodies (see Chapter 14). There are some six different classes of these in man, but the most common and best known are designated IgG, IgM, and IgA. By means of fluorescein labeled antisera specifically reacting with the three types of immunoglobulins, it has been shown that among the plasma cells of the lamina propria, there is a great predominance of cells producing IgA. As IgA passes upward from the lamina propria, it is thought to attach to a protein synthesized in the epithelial cells. The new complex emerging in the secretions is called "secretory IgA" and is thought to protect against viral and bacterial invasions. Quantitative data indicate a mean population density of IgA reactive plasma cells of 180,000 per cu. mm. of lamina propria, as against 18,000 and 30,000 for IgG and IgM reactive cells (Crabbe et al.).

The significance of the large population

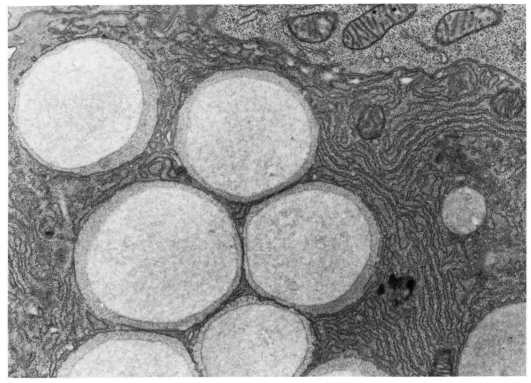

Figure 27-13 Electron micrograph of an area of cytoplasm from a Paneth cell, showing the abundance of granular reticulum and the heterogeneity of the secretory granules. (Micrograph courtesy M. Staley and J. Trier, Am. J. Anat., *117*:365, 1965.)

of eosinophils is not so clear but there is evidence that this cell type accumulates where antigen-antibody complexes have formed and that they phagocytose and destroy these complexes (Litt).

Another peculiar type of wandering cell found in the epithelium of the crypts and in the lamina propria in many animals is the so-called *globular leukocyte*. It has a small, round, dark nucleus and a cell body containing large round granules or droplets that stain brightly with eosin. Their significance and relationships to other leukocytes are not known.

Lymphoid Tissue

The lamina propria of the small intestine contains great numbers of isolated lymphatic nodules varying from 0.6 to 3 mm. in diameter (Fig. 27-14). They are scattered all along the intestine but are more numerous and larger in the distal part. In the ileum they may be found near the surface of the plicae circulares or between them. If they are small, they occupy only the layer of the mucosa above the muscularis mucosae. The larger ones occupy the whole thickness of the mucosa, bulge on its surface (Fig. 27-15), and may even extend through the muscularis mucosae into the submucous layer. They are visible to the naked eye, and their surface is often free of villi and usually also of crypts. Recent studies with the scanning electron microscope reveal, in the flattened epithelium overlying lymphoid nodules, a distinctive cell type not found elsewhere (Owen). These cells scattered randomly in the epithelium have microvilli that are much larger than those of the surrounding intestinal absorptive cells (Figs. 27-15 and 27-16). The functional significance of these cells has yet to be determined.

Groups of many solitary nodules massed together are called *aggregated nodules* or *Peyer's patches*. They occur, as a rule, only in the ileum, but occasionally may be found elsewhere. Their normal number is estimated at 30 to 40. They always occur on the side of the intestinal wall opposite the line of attachment of the mesentery and are recognizable grossly as elongated, oval, slightly thickened areas. Their long diameter varies from 12 to 20 mm.; the short, from 8 to 12 mm. They consist of dense lymphatic tissue with large germinal centers in their interior. The periphery is marked by a thin layer of condensed reticular fibers. The lamina propria and the submucosa in the vicinity of the nodules are always infiltrated with lymphocytes. In old age the solitary follicles and Peyer's patches undergo involution.

A lymphoid organ called the bursa of Fabricius associated with the lower intestinal tract in birds is essential to the development of antibody-producing lymphoid cells (B lymphocytes). The equivalent of the bursa of Fabricius in man and other mammals has not been clearly identified. However, there is evidence that in the rabbit the Peyer's patches and appendix may assume part of this role. The morphological similarity of Peyer's patches to the bursa is not as striking in man, mouse, and some other species as it is in the rabbit, but the possibility remains that those lymphoid nodules associated with the gut are important for development of the capacity for antibody production.

Muscularis Mucosae

This layer averages 38 μm. in thickness and consists of elastic networks and of an inner circular and an outer longitudinal layer of smooth muscle.

Submucosa

The submucous layer consists of rather dense connective tissue with an abundant elastic tissue component and occasional lobules of adipose tissue. In the duodenum it is occupied by a thick layer of *duodenal glands* or *Brunner's glands.*

Duodenal Glands (Submucosal Glands of Brunner)

These submucosal glands, present only in mammals, are usually encountered first in the region of the pyloric sphincter, but in

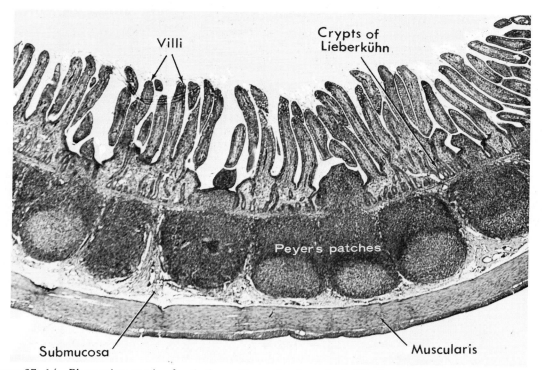

Figure 27–14 Photomicrograph of cat's ileum illustrating intestinal villi. Crypts of Lieberkühn and submucosal lymphoid nodules or Peyer's patches are shown.

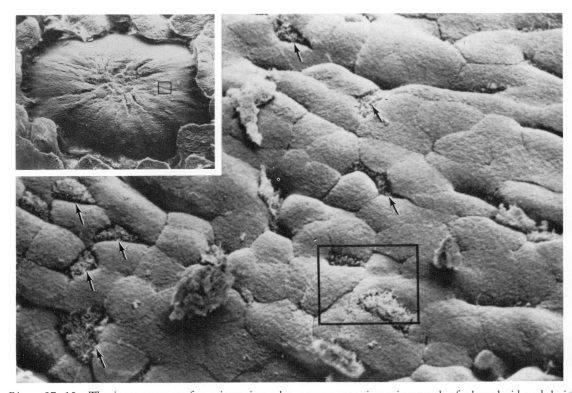

Figure 27-15 The inset presents for orientation a low-power scanning micrograph of a lymphoid nodule in rat intestine covered by an attenuated layer of epithelium and surrounded by villi. The area in the small square is shown at higher magnification in the main figure. The polygonal outlines of the flattened cells is evident and certain of them have a surface texture different from the majority (at arrows). This difference is seen more clearly in Figure 27-16 (a higher magnification of the area enclosed in the rectangle). (Micrograph courtesy of R. Owen and A. Jones, Gastroenterology, 66:189, 1974.)

man they may sometimes extend a few centimeters into the pyloric region of the stomach. In the distal two thirds of the duodenum the glands of Brunner gradually diminish in size and finally disappear. They show a tendency to occupy the cores of the circular folds and are separated by gland-free intervals (Figs. 27-2, 27-3 and 27-5). In some cases they extend into the upper part of the jejunum.

The terminal secretory portions of the glands consist of richly branched and coiled tubules arranged in lobules 0.5 to 1.0 mm. in diameter situated in the submucosa (Fig. 27-5). The ducts penetrate the muscularis mucosae to open into a crypt of Lieberkühn.

Examined with the electron microscope, the secretory cells of the submucosal glands present a combination of the fine structural features of zymogenic and mucus-secreting cells. They have numerous mitochondria and abundant basal granular reticulum. Their dense secretory granules bear a superficial resemblance to those of pancreatic zymogen cells. The Golgi complex is unusually large and is believed to be the site of synthesis of the carbohydrate moiety of the secretory product and of its combination with the protein moiety synthesized in the granular endoplasmic reticulum (Friend).

In the species in which it has been studied, the secretion is a clear, viscous, and distinctly alkaline fluid (pH 8.2 to 9.3). Its principal function is thought to be to protect the duodenal mucosa against the erosive effects of the acid gastric juice. Its mucoid nature, its alkalinity, and possibly the buffering capacity of its bicarbonate content may make it well suited to this role.

Muscularis

The external and internal layers of the muscular coat are well developed in the small intestine. They are usually described as longitudinal and circular layers. Between these layers is the sympathetic *myenteric nerve plexus.* Some strands of smooth muscle cells pass from one layer into the other. The smooth muscle cells have usually been regarded as a static cell population, but autoradiographic studies now demonstrate a slow rate of cell replication distributed throughout the external muscle layer of the colon (Kaye et al.). There are differences in rate of replication in different portions of the alimentary tract.

Serosa

The external serosal coat consists of a layer of mesothelial cells resting on loose connective tissue. At the attachment of the mesentery, the serous layer of the intestines is continuous with the leaves of the mesentery.

THE APPENDIX

The appendix is a blindly ending evagination of the cecum occurring in man and many other animals. Its wall is thickened by an extensive development of lymphoid tissue, which forms an almost continuous layer of large and small lymphatic nodules (Fig. 27–17). The small lumen has an angular outline in cross section and often contains masses of dead cells and acellular detritus. In other cases the lumen is obliterated. It is difficult to draw a distinct line between the normal structure and certain pathological conditions in this organ. Villi are absent. The glands of Lieberkühn radiating from the lumen have an irregular shape and variable length and are largely embedded in the lymphoid tissue.

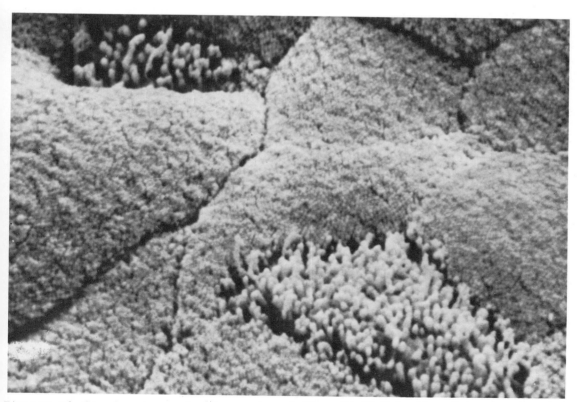

Figure 27–16   Scanning micrograph of the area shown in Figure 27–15. Two of the cells bear loosely packed microvilli that are very much broader than those composing the brush border of the surrounding cells. (Micrograph courtesy of R. Owen and A. Jones, Gastroenterology, 66:189, 1974.)

The epithelium of the surface of the glands contains only a few goblet cells and consists mostly of columnar cells with a striated border. The zone of mitotically active undifferentiated cells in the crypts is shorter than in the small intestine. In addition to occasional Paneth cells, argentaffin cells are regularly present in the depths of the crypts and in smaller numbers in the upper parts of the glands. They are much more plentiful than in the small intestine, and may number 5 to 10 to a gland.

The lymphatic tissue of the appendix is similar to that of the tonsils and often shows chronic inflammatory changes. The muscularis mucosae of the appendix is poorly developed. The submucosa forms a thick layer with blood vessels and nerves and occasional fat lobules. The muscularis externa is reduced in thickness, but the two usual layers are always identifiable. The serous coat is similar to that covering the rest of the intestines.

THE LARGE INTESTINE

The mucosa of the large intestine does not form folds comparable to the plicae circulares except in its last portion, the rectum, and the villi cease, as a rule, above the ileocecal valve. The interior of the large intestine therefore has a smooth surface, which is lined by simple columnar epithelium with a thin striated border.

The glands of Lieberkühn are straight tubules, and they attain a greater length in the large than in the small intestine—up to 0.5 mm., and up to 0.7 mm. in the rectum (Fig. 27–18). They differ from the glands in the small intestine in the greater abundance of their goblet cells (Figs. 27–19 and 27–20). At the bottom of the crypts are the usual proliferating, relatively undifferentiated epithelial cells and occasionally argentaffin cells. As a rule there are no cells of Paneth.

The structure of the lamina propria is es-

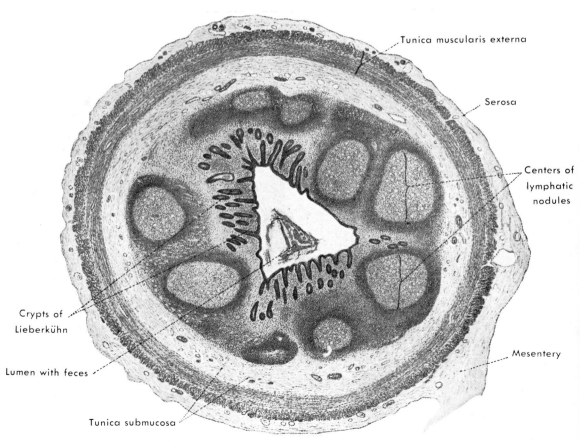

Figure 27–17 Cross section of appendix from a 23 year old man. × 22. (After Sobotta.)

sentially the same as in the small intestine; eosinophilic leukocytes are abundant, often invading the epithelium of the crypts. Scattered nodules of lymphoid tissue are always present in varying numbers and are also found in the rectum. They extend deep into the submucosal layer.

The muscularis mucosae is well developed and consists of longitudinal and circular strands. It may send slender bundles of muscle cells toward the surface of the mucosa. The submucous layer does not present any peculiarities. The muscularis externa differs from the corresponding coat of the small intestine in the arrangement of its outer longitudinal coat, which is not a continuous layer but is localized in three thick, longitudinal bands, the *taeniae coli*. In the rectum the outer component of the muscularis again becomes a continuous layer all around the viscus. The serous coat of the colon in its free portion forms the *appendices epiploicae*, pendulous protuberances consisting of adipose tissue and accumulations of cells similar to those in the omentum.

In the anal region the mucosa is thrown into longitudinal folds, the *rectal columns of Morgagni*. The crypts of Lieberkühn in this region suddenly become short and disappear, and along an irregular line, about 2 cm. above the anal opening, there is an abrupt transition from simple columnar to stratified squamous epithelium. This is the transition zone between the mucosa and skin. At the level of the external muscular sphincter of the anus, the surface layer assumes the histological structure of the skin, and sebaceous glands and large, apocrine, circumanal glands appear. The lamina propria here contains a plexus of large veins, which, when abnormally distended and varicose, present at the anus as hemorrhoids.

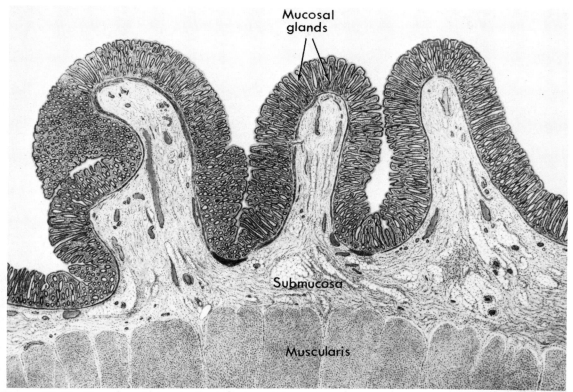

Mucosal glands

Submucosa

Muscularis

Figure 27-18 Drawing of a longitudinal section of the wall of the human colon. (From W. Bargmann, *Histologie und mikroskopische Anatomie des Menschen,* 6th edition, Stuttgart, Georg Thieme Verlag, 1962.)

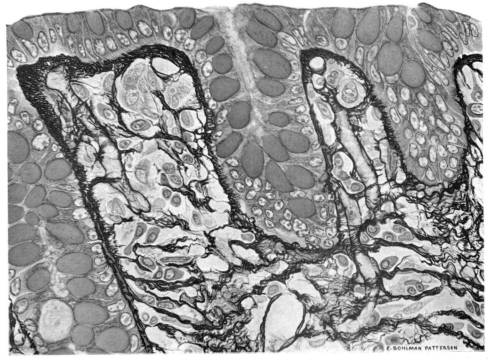

Figure 27-19 Slightly tangential section through mucous membrane of human colon. The reticular fibers are condensed beneath the epithelium and about the blood vessels. The mucigen of the goblet cells is stained blue. Bielschowsky-Foot and Mallory-azan stains. × 600.

THE HISTOPHYSIOLOGY OF INTESTINAL ABSORPTION

Essential to the digestion of the chyme in the small intestine are the secretions of the liver and pancreas, which are delivered into the duodenum at the ampulla of Vater. The bile released from the liver and gallbladder, together with the mechanical mixing action of peristalsis, reduces the ingested lipid to a fine emulsion of triglycerides. The pancreatic juice contributes lipolytic, proteolytic, and carbohydrate splitting enzymes. The mucosa of the intestine itself contributes *intestinal juice* or *succus entericus*, which is mainly a product of the glands of Lieberkühn.

The intestinal secretion was formerly reported to contain several digestive enzymes, but it is now clear from biochemical studies of isolated brush borders that some of the enzymes previously believed to be secreted into the lumen actually reside on the striated border of the intestinal absorptive cells. Among these are *leucine aminopeptidase* and enzymes that hydrolyze disaccharides; *sucrase*, which splits cane sugar into the hexoses glucose and fructose; *lactase*, which splits milk sugar into glucose and galactose; and *maltase*, which hydrolyzes disaccharides derived from glycogen and starch into glucose. As previously stated, these enzymes are not secreted into the lumen but are an integral part of the microvilli of the brush border. They hydrolyze disaccharides in the lumen to hexoses that can be translocated to the blood by hexose pumps residing in the lateral and basal membranes of the absorptive cells. Thus, the brush border not only is a device for increasing the surface area for absorption, but is also the site of the enzymes reponsible for the terminal steps in the digestion of carbohydrates and proteins.

It has recently been recognized that disease can result from genetic defects involving absence of one of the enzymes of the brush border. It has long been known that some babies cannot tolerate milk. Feeding of milk results in bloating and copious diarrhea. The cause of these symptoms has been traced to congenital absence of a single enzyme, *lactase*, from the intestinal epithelium. There is no other enzymatic deficiency in these infants and if lactose is eliminated from the diet they do very well.

The intraluminal digestion of most food reduces it to subunits of molecular size whose path of absorption through the intestinal mucosa cannot be followed by microscopy. However, by labeling certain substances with fluorescent compounds so that they can be visualized by fluorescence microscopy, or with radioactive isotopes for autoradiography, some information has been gained about the absorption of proteins. In the period of suckling, the newborn of many species can absorb intact protein, including antibodies.

This takes place in the jejunum and ileum, but not in the duodenum. Labeled protein and particulate matter introduced into the jejunum appear to be taken into the cells by pinocytosis (Graney). Within a few weeks after birth, this capacity is lost and in adult mammals, including man, no more than trace amounts of intact protein can be assimilated. Ingested protein must first be hydrolyzed to amino acids by intraluminal digestion and these products of hydrolysis are then absorbed.

Of the various classes of nutritive substances, *fat* lends itself best to morphological studies of intestinal absorption because lipid can be fixed in the tissue and intensely stained by osmium tetroxide for study with light or electron microscopes (Fig. 27–21). Dietary fat, consisting mainly of triglycerides, is hydrolyzed by pancreatic lipase in the intestinal lumen to free fatty acids and monogly-

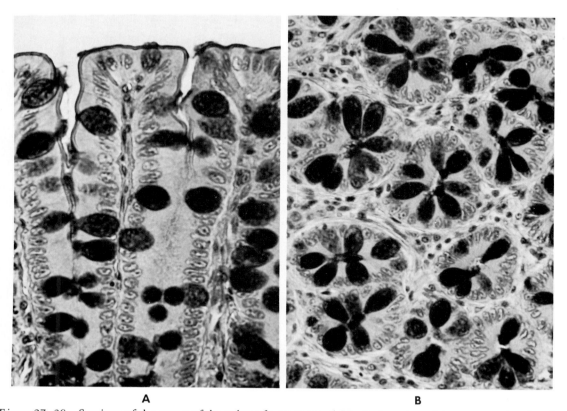

A   **B**

Figure 27–20 Sections of the crypts of the colon of a macaque. *A*, Vertical section of the mucosa, showing the columnar cells and goblet cells. × 550. *B*, Horizontal section of the crypts, showing the radial disposition of goblet cells around the lumen and the cellular lamina propria between crypts. Periodic acid–Schiff reaction and hematoxylin. Photomicrograph. × 425.

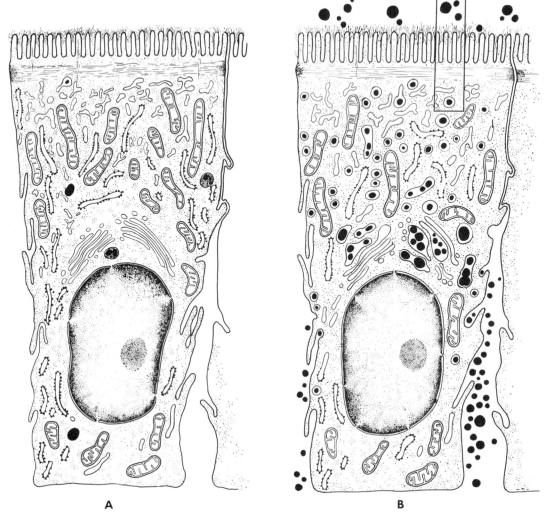

A　　　　　　　　　　　　　　　　**B**

Figure 27–21　Schematic representation of the fine structure of an intestinal absorptive cell (*A*) in the fasting state and (*B*) after a lipid-rich meal. The area in the rectahgle is depicted at higher magnification in Figure 27 – 22. (Redrawn after R. Cardell, S. Badenhausen, and K. R. Porter, J. Cell Biol., *34*:123, 1967.)

cerides. These products combine with bile salts to form minute micelles about 20 Å in diameter (Fig. 27–22). When myriads of these come into contact with the microvilli of the intestinal absorptive cells, the fatty acids and monoglycerides diffuse across the plasma membrane and accumulate in the apical cytoplasm (Strauss). The membranes of the smooth endoplasmic reticulum located there contain the enzymes for resynthesis of triglycerides from fatty acids and monoglycerides. During lipid absorption, the resynthesized triglyceride forms numerous visible droplets

in the lumen of the reticulum in the apical portion of the cell (Cardell et al.). From there the lipid appears to be transported to the Golgi complex for further processing that converts it into *chylomicra*, the complex glycolipoprotein droplets that are transported via the lacteals and intestinal lymphatics to the bloodstream (Fig. 27–21). The precise role of the Golgi complex in lipid absorption has not been established, but it seems likely that the carbohydrate moiety of the chylomicra is added there to the triglyceride synthesized in the smooth reticulum. The chylomicron also

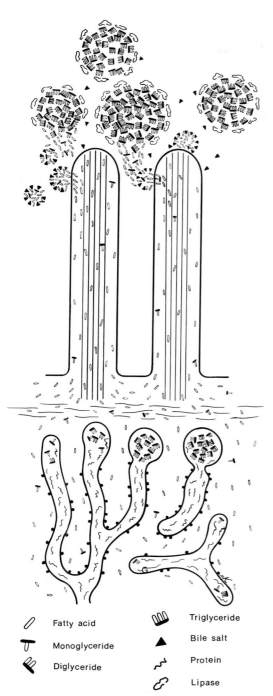

acquires in its passage through the Golgi complex a membranous investment with properties that enable it to coalesce with the lateral plasma membrane of the columnar cell. Vesicles of Golgi origin thus discharge chylomicra into the intercellular cleft between adjacent absorptive cells (Fig. 27-24). From there they move across the basal lamina of the epithelium and into the lymphatic capillaries in the lamina propria of the intestinal villi.

The absorptive cells of the intestine are able to respond rapidly and to modify their internal structure to adapt it to the requirements of lipid absorption (Friedman and Cardell). In the fasting state, there are some profiles of granular endoplasmic reticulum and a limited amount of smooth reticulum in the apical cytoplasm, and a relatively quiescent supranuclear Golgi complex. Ingestion of lipid stimulates the formation of a more extensive smooth reticulum to provide for resynthesis of triglyceride and its transport to the Golgi complex. The rapid turnover of Golgi membranes during lipid absorption and transport also requires accelerated synthesis of new membrane to replace that lost to the cell surface in discharge of chylomicrons. If protein synthesis is blocked by administration of puromycin, membrane replacement in smooth reticulum and Golgi complex is prevented, as is synthesis of protein constituents of the chylomicra. Lipid transport is therefore inhibited and large amounts of lipid accumulate in the cytoplasm of the absorptive cells (Sabesin; Friedman and Cardell).

An important part of the absorptive mechanism is the active movement of the intestinal villi. These can be observed in a living animal if a loop of intestine is split open and the surface of the mucosa is observed with a binocular microscope. A villus is seen to suddenly shorten to about half its length with an appreciable increase in its thickness, and it slowly extends again to its original length. Each villus contracts about six times a minute. During the contraction, its volume is reduced and the contents of the central lacteal are forwarded to the submucous lymphatic plexus. Contraction occurs as a result of shortening of the longitudinally oriented strands of smooth muscle in the core of the villus. The contraction of the villi is believed to be under the nervous control of Meissner's submucous plexus. Direct mechanical stimulation of the base of a villus with a bristle also calls forth

$\mathscr{O}$ Fatty acid	$\underset{\text{lllll}}{\text{llll}}$ Triglyceride
$\top$ Monoglyceride	▲ Bile salt
$\mathscr{R}$ Diglyceride	$\sim$ Protein
	$\mathscr{E}$ Lipase

Figure 27-22 Schematic representation of events occurring in a small area of the apex of an intestinal absorptive cell (see Fig. 27-21). An emulsion of fine droplets of lipid in the lumen is broken down by pancreatic lipase to fatty acids and monoglycerides. These diffuse into the microvilli and apical cytoplasm, where they are esterified to form triglycerides in the smooth endoplasmic reticulum. (Redrawn after R. Cardell, S. Badenhausen, and K. R. Porter, J. Cell Biol., *34*:123, 1967.)

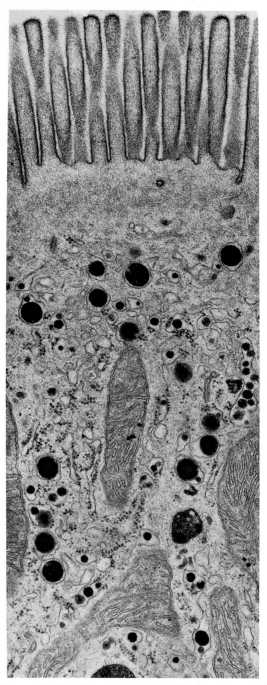

Figure 27–23 Electron micrograph of rat intestinal cell. Lipid accumulates in sizable droplets within the smooth reticulum, but very little is seen in inpocketings of the cell surface or in vesicles traversing the terminal web. Though pinocytosis undoubtedly occurs it is to some extent not the principal mechanism for absorption of lipid. × 32,000. (Courtesy of S. L. Palay and J. P. Revel.)

a contraction, and the stimulus radiates from the affected villus to the surrounding villi.

BLOOD VESSELS OF THE GASTROINTESTINAL TRACT

The arrangements of the blood and lymph vessels in the wall of the stomach and in the wall of the intestine are basically similar. Because the important differences depend mainly on the presence of villi, the small intestine shows significant peculiarities.

In the stomach, the arteries arise from the two arterial arches along the lesser and greater curvatures and are distributed to the ventral and dorsal surfaces. In the intestine, the arteries reach one side in the mesentery. They run in the serosa and break up into large branches that penetrate the muscularis externa and enter the submucosal layer, where they form a large plexus (Fig. 27–26). In the stomach and colon the plexus gives off branches directed toward the surface. Some of these break up into capillaries supplying the muscularis mucosae; others form capillary networks throughout the mucosa and surrounding the glands. The capillary net is especially prominent around the foveolae of the gastric mucosa.

From the superficial, periglandular capillary networks, veins of considerable caliber arise. They form a venous plexus between the bottoms of the glands and the muscularis mucosae. From this plexus, branches run into the submucosa and form a venous plexus. From this submucosal plexus, the large veins follow the arteries and pass through the muscularis externa into the serosa. In the stomach the veins of the submucosal plexus are provided with valves and a relatively thick muscular coat.

In the small intestine, the submucous arterial plexus gives off two kinds of branches that run toward the mucosa. Some of these arteries ramify on the inner surface of the muscularis mucosae and break up into capillary networks that surround the crypts of Lieberkühn in the same way they surround the glands of the stomach. Other arteries are especially destined for the villi, each villus receiving one or sometimes several such small arteries. These vessels enter the base of the villus and form a dense capillary network im-

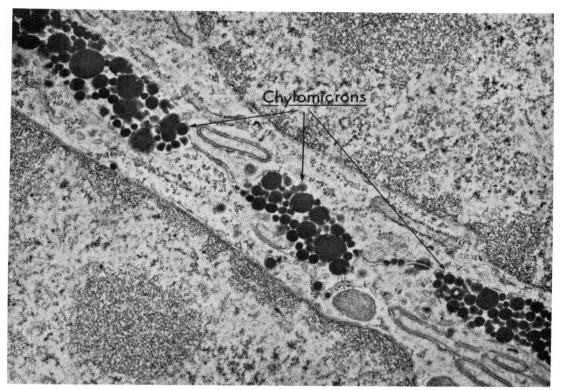

Figure 27-24 Electron micrograph of the boundary between two rat intestinal epithelial cells during lipid absorption. The absorbed lipid has been discharged through the lateral cell surfaces and is seen to have accumulated here as aggregations of chylomicrons in the intercellular spaces. × 30,000. (Courtesy of S. L. Palay and J. P. Revel.)

mediately under its epithelium (Fig. 27–27). Near the tip of the villus one or two small veins arise from the superficial capillary network and run downward, to anastomose with the glandular venous plexus, and then pass on into the submucosa, where they join the veins of the submucosal plexus. These veins in the intestine have no valves. However, their continuations, which pass through the muscularis externa with the arteries, are provided with valves. Valves disappear again in the collecting veins of the mesentery.

LYMPH VESSELS OF THE GASTROINTESTINAL TRACT

In the stomach, the lymphatics begin as an extensive system of large lymphatic capillaries in the superficial layer of the mucosa between the glands. They are always situated more deeply than the blood capillaries. They anastomose everywhere throughout the mucosa. They surround the glandular tubules and take a downward course to the inner surface of the mucosa, where they form a plexus of fine lymphatic vessels. Branches of the plexus pierce the muscularis mucosae and form, in the submucosa, a plexus of lymphatics that is provided with valves. From the submucosal plexus larger lymphatics run through the muscularis externa. Here they receive numerous tributaries from the lymphatic plexus in the muscular coat and then follow the blood vessels into the retroperitoneal tissues. In the wall of the colon the lymphatics show a similar arrangement.

The lymphatic vessels are important in the absorption of fat from the small intestine. During digestion, all their ramifications become filled with milky white lymph—a fine emulsion of neutral fats. This white lymph, drained from the intestine, is called *chyle*, and the lymphatics that carry it away from the epithelium are called *lacteals*.

In the small intestine the most conspicuous parts of the lymphatic system are the central lacteals in the core of the villi. Each conical villus has one lacteal, which occupies an axial position and ends blindly near the tip. The broader villi of the duodenum may contain two or perhaps more lacteals that intercommunicate. The lumen of these lacteals, when distended, is considerably larger than that of the blood capillaries. The wall consists of thin endothelial cells and is everywhere connected with the argyrophilic reticulum and surrounded by thin, longitudinal strands of smooth muscle.

The central lacteals at the base of the villi anastomose with the lymphatic capillaries between the glands. They also form a plexus on the inner surface of the muscularis mucosae. Branches of this plexus, provided with valves, pierce the muscularis mucosae and form, in the submucosa, a loose plexus of larger lymphatics. The latter also receives tributaries from the dense network of large, thin-walled lymphatic capillaries, which closely surround the surface of the solitary and aggregated follicles. The large lymphatics that run from the submucosal plexus through the muscularis externa into the mesentery receive additional branches from a dense, tangential plexus located between the circular and longitudinal layers of the muscularis externa.

NERVES OF THE INTESTINAL TRACT

The nerve supply seems to be similar in its organization in all parts of the intestinal tube and consists of an intrinsic and an extrinsic part. The first of these is composed of nerve cells and their fibers located in the wall of the intestine. The extrinsic nerves are represented by the preganglionic fibers of the vagus nerve and the postganglionic fibers of the sympathetic nerve. The latter run to the intestine from the celiac plexus. They enter the intestinal wall through the mesentery along the branches of the large vessels.

Numerous groups of nerve cells and bundles of nerve fibers are seen between the circular and the longitudinal layers of the muscularis externa. These constitute the *myenteric plexus of Auerbach* (Figs. 27–28 and 27–29). In the submucosa, similar elements form the *submucosal plexus of Meissner*. These plexuses form the intrinsic nervous mechanism of the intestinal wall.

The nerve cells of the enteric ganglia are connected by strands of nonmyelinated nerve fibers of both extrinsic and intrinsic origin. These nerve cells appear in two principal forms, which may present differences in their secondary characteristics. The first type occurs exclusively in the myenteric plexus. It is a multipolar cell with short dendrites that terminate in brushlike arborizations on the bodies of cells of the second type in the same ganglion. The axon can be traced for a considerable distance through neighboring ganglia and is supposed to form connections with cells of the second type in other ganglia. These neurons are associative.

The cells of the second type are far more numerous and show great variations in their forms. Their dendrites vary in number and are often missing. They begin as diffuse receptive endings in relation with nerve cells of

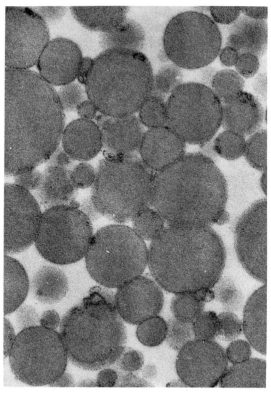

Figure 27–25 Electron micrograph of chylomicrons fixed in osmium tetroxide, embedded and sectioned. They range from 1100 Å to 7000 Å. × 45,000. (From A. Jones and M. Price, J. Histochem. Cytochem., *16*:366, 1968. By permission of the Histochemical Society, Inc.)

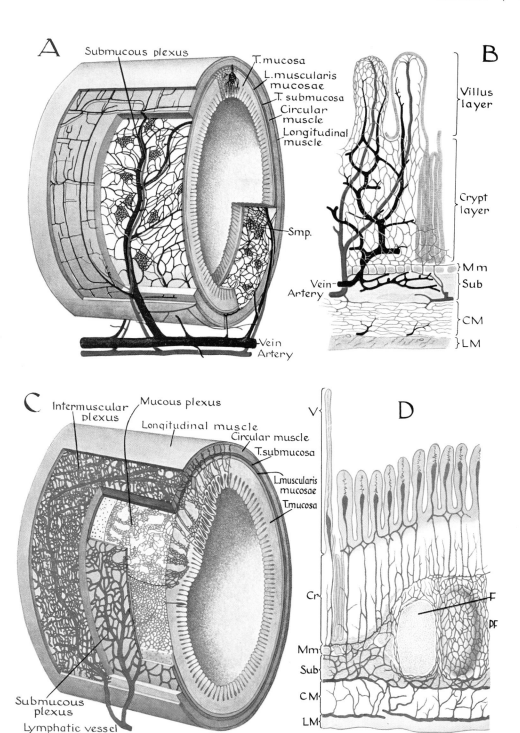

Figure 27-26   Diagrams of distribution of blood vessels (*A* and *B*) and of lymphatics (*C* and *D*) in the small intestine of the dog. *B* and *D* are drawn on a larger scale to show details. *CM*, Circular muscle; *Cr*, crypt; *F*, follicle; *LM*, longitudinal muscle; *Mm*, lamina muscularis mucosae; *PF*, perifollicular plexus; *Smp*, submucous plexus; *Sub*, tunica submucosa; *V*, villus. (Redrawn and slightly modified from Mall.)

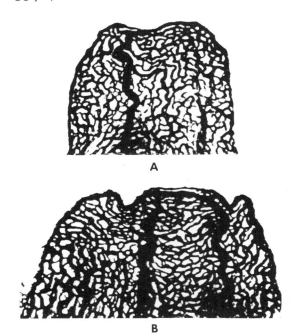

A

B

Figure 27–27 Two villi of rat intestine injected with India ink in gelatin. The villi in this species are thin, leaflike structures whose broad surface is presented in this figure. In the duodenum (*B*) they are larger and more richly vascularized than they are farther along in the jejunum (*A*). The large surface area presented by the villi and their rich network of capillaries favors absorption of nutrients. × 100.

the first and of the same (i.e., second) type in the ganglia of origin or in other ganglia. The axon enters a fiber bundle and divides; its branches terminate in the circular or longitudinal layer of the muscularis externa in connection with smooth muscle cells. Thus, the neurons of the second type are motor. Those in the myenteric plexus supply the muscularis externa; those of the submucosal plexus supply the muscularis mucosae and the muscles of the villi.

Cells of a third type occur in the enteric plexuses and are also scattered in the submucosa and in the interior of the villi. This is the "interstitial cell," with a finely vacuolated protoplasm and short, branching processes that interlace with other processes to form an irregular feltwork. It does not contain obvious neurofibrils and may possibly be of microglial nature.

Most of the nonmyelinated fibers of the bundles that connect the ganglia, and the fibers in the ganglia, are processes of the enteric neurons. The rest are formed by extrinsic fibers, mainly of vagal and to some extent

of sympathetic origin. The vagal fibers terminate as pericellular arborizations on cells of the second type in the enteric ganglia. The sympathetic fibers cannot be distinguished from the axons of the motor cells in the fiber bundles. They do not seem to enter into synaptic relationship with the nerve cells of the ganglia but take part, together with axons of intrinsic neurons, in the formation of the intramuscular plexuses and terminate in connection with the muscular cells. The sympathetic fibers supply the blood vessels, too. Some of them have also been described as forming a plexus in the subserosa and ending freely in the connective tissue.

If the intestine is detached from the mesentery and placed in warm Tyrode solution, it will show normal peristaltic movements if the mucosa is stimulated by objects introduced into the lumen. This shows that the intestine is an autonomous organ whose

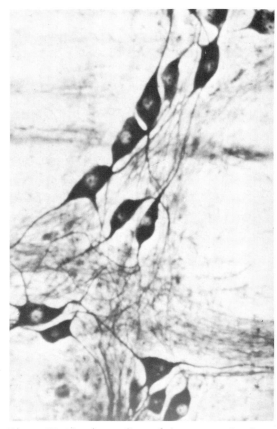

Figure 27–28 A ganglion of the myenteric plexus of cat jejunum containing bipolar and multipolar neurons. Modified Bielschowsky stain. (Photomicrograph courtesy of G. Schofield.)

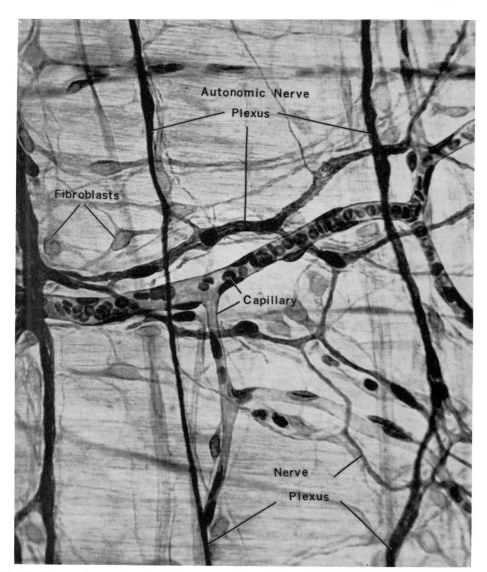

Figure 27-29 Photomicrograph of a whole mount of the longitudinal muscle coat of rabbit intestine impregnated with silver to show the nerve bundles of Auerbach's plexus. × 300. (After K. C. Richardson, J. Anat., 94:451, 1960. Labeling added.)

movements are determined by the local neuromuscular mechanism and that these are only regulated through the extrinsic nerves. Numerous nerve endings of sensory nature have been found under and in the epithelial layers of the villi.

Some investigators believe that the enteric plexuses mediate complete reflex arcs, the sensory component being enteric, a cell of the plexus, with dendritic endings in contact with the epithelium of the villi or the glands of Lieberkühn, whereas the axons transmit the impulse to another enteric neuron whose axon ends in the smooth muscles. Most authors hold, however, that all neurons of the enteric plexuses are of efferent nature and that therefore the sensory nerve endings in the mucous membrane must be of extrinsic nature. The local reflexes in the intestine are explained as "axon reflexes." The axons of the enteric neurons are supposed to divide into two branches, one of which receives stimuli that are transmitted to the other branch without passing through the cell body.

HISTOGENESIS OF INTESTINES

The histogenesis of the mucosa of the intestine resembles that of the stomach. At first the boundary between the epithelium and the connective tissue is even. The development of villi begins in the duodenum in embryos of 20 mm. and gradually extends downward. In the duodenum, jejunum, and the upper part of the ileum, the villi arise as isolated epithelial outgrowths. In the remaining parts of the intestine, longitudinal ridges develop, which later are subdivided by the transverse furrows into single villi. The number of the villi in a given stretch increases through the appearance of new outgrowths in the hollows between the older villi. In a fetus of 100 mm., villi are found all along the intestine, including the colon, although they disappear from the colon in the later stages. This is due either to a fusion of the villi from their bases upward or to their shortening through the stretching of the growing wall. In an embryo of 55 mm., the supranuclear protoplasm of the epithelial cells on the tips of the villi acquires a transparent aspect, while on the free surface a condensed cytoplasmic layer develops. Between these elements, scattered goblet cells appear.

In the fetus of four months, the epithelium of the villi has a manifold appearance. In the lower parts of the small intestine, the common epithelial cells with the clear supranuclear region contain a multitude of coarse yellow granules. These are called *meconium corpuscles* and are similar to those seen in the lumen of the intestine. Their yellowish color is due to adsorption of bile pigment.

Between the common epithelial cells are many typical goblet cells. Beginning with the fourth month, argentaffin cells make their appearance. During the seventh month, the cells of Paneth appear. In the human fetus they seem to occur not only in the crypts but also on the villi.

The development of the glands of Lieberkühn also starts in the duodenum and proceeds downward. In a fetus of the fourth month the excavations between the villi are lined with small, crowded cells with a cytoplasm darker than that of the epithelium on the villi. From these areas, evaginations arise that penetrate the subjacent connective tissue. From the seventh month, in addition to invagination of new glands, dichotomous division of the blind ends of the preexisting glands contributes largely to the continuing increase in the number of glands. Bifurcation of the crypts proceeds in the newborn.

The glands of Brunner make their appearance during the sixth month as massive, epithelial ingrowths from the depths of the duodenal crypts. In a fetus of 290 mm., they are numerous in the upper part of the duodenum and consist of branching tubules. Further downward they are smaller and the intervals between them are larger.

REFERENCES

Behnke, O., and H. Moe: An electron microscopic study of mature and differentiating Paneth cells in the rat. J. Cell Biol., *22*:633, 1964.

Benditt, E. P., and R. L. Wong: On the concentration of 5-hydroxytryptamine in mammalian entero-chromaffin cells and its release by reserpine. J. Exper. Med., *105*:509, 1957.

Bensley, R. R.: The structure of the glands of Brunner. The Decennial Publ., University of Chicago, *10*:279, 1903.

Brown, A. L.: Microvilli of the human jejunal epithelial cell. J. Cell Biol., *12*:623, 1962.

Bulbring, E., and R. C. Y. Lin: The effect of intraluminal application of 5-hydroxy-tryptophan on peristalsis, the local production of 5-HT and its release in relation to intraluminal pressure and propulsive activity. J. Physiol., *140*:381, 1958.

Cardell, R. R., Jr., S. Badenhausen, and K. R. Porter: Intestinal triglyceride absorption in the rat. An electron microscopical study. J. Cell Biol. *34*:123, 1967.

Clarke, S. L., Jr.: The ingestion of proteins and colloidal materials by columnar absorptive cells of the small intestine in suckling rats and mice. J. Biophys. Biochem. Cytol., *5*:41, 1959.

Crane, R. K.: Intestinal absorption of sugars. Physiol. Rev., *40*:789, 1960.

Crane, R. K.: Hypothesis for mechanism of intestinal active transport of sugars. Federation Proc., *21*:891, 1962.

Darlington, D., and A. W. Rogers: Epithelial lymphocytes in the small intestine of the mouse. J. Anat., *100*:813, 1966.

Deane, H. W.: Some electron microscopic observations on the lamina propria of the gut, with comments on the close association of macrophages, plasma cells and eosinophils. Anat. Rec., *149*:453, 1964.

Eicholtz, A., and R. K. Crane: Studies on the organization of the brush border in intestinal epithelial cells. J. Cell Biol., *26*:687, 1965.

Erspamer, V.: Occurrence and distribution of 5-hydroxytryptamine (enteramine) in the living organism. Zeitschr. f. Vit. Hormon Fermentforsch., *9*:74, 1957.

Faulk, W. P.: Peyer's patches: morphologic studies. Cell. Immunol. *1*:500, 1970.

Florey, H. W.: The secretion and function of intestinal mucus. Gastroenterology, *43*:326, 1962.

Florey, H. W., R. D. Wright, and M. A. Jennings: The secretions of the intestine. Physiol. Rev., *21*:141, 1936.

Forstner, J. F., I. Jabbal, and G. G. Forstner: Goblet cell mucin of rat small intestine. Chemical and physical characterization. Can. J. Biochem., *51*:1154–1166, 1973.

Friedman, H. I., and R. D. Cardell, Jr.: Effects of puromycin on the structure of rat intestinal epithelial cells during fat absorption. J. Cell Biol., *52*:15, 1972.

Friend, D. S.: The fine structure of Brunner's glands in the mouse. J. Cell. Biol., *25*:563, 1965.

Garry, R. C.: The movements of the large intestine. Physiol. Rev., *14*:103, 1934.

Gershon, M. D., and L. L. Ross: Studies on the relationship of 5-hydroxytryptamine and the enterochromaffin cell to anaphylactic shock in mice. J. Exper. Med., *115*:367, 1962.

Graney, D. O.: The uptake of ferritin by ileal absorptive cells in suckling rats. Am. J. Anat., *123*:227, 1968.

Grossman, M. I.: The glands of Brunner. Physiol. Rev., *38*:675, 1958.

Hanssen, O., and L. Herman: The presence of an axial structure in the microvillus of the mouse convoluted proximal tubule cell. Lab. Invest., *11*:610, 1962.

Ito, S.: The enteric surface coat on cat intestinal microvilli. J. Cell Biol., *27*:475, 1965.

Jennings, M. A., and H. W. Florey: Autoradiographic observations of the mucous cells of the stomach and intestine. Quart. J. Exper. Pathol., *41*:131, 1956.

Johnston, T. M.: Mechanism of fat absorption. *In* Field, J. (ed.): Handbook of Physiology. Washington, D. C., American Physiology Society, Section 6, Vol. III, 1353, 1968.

Jones, A. L., and R. K. Ockner: An electron microscopic study of endogenous very low density lipoprotein production in the intestine of rat and man. J. Lipid Res., *12*:580, 1971.

Kaye, G. I., N. Lane, and R. Pascal: Colonic pericryptal fibroblast sheath: replication, migration, and cytodifferentiation of a mesenchymal cell system in adult tissue. II. Fine structural aspects of normal rabbit and human colon. Gastroenterology *54*:852, 1968.

Ladman, A. J., H. A. Padykula, and E. W. Strauss: A morphological study of fat transport in the normal human jejunum. Am. J. Anat., *112*:389, 1963.

Landboe-Christensen, E.: The Duodenal Glands of Brunner in Man, Their Distribution and Quantity. An Anatomical Study. Copenhagen, E. Munksgaard; London, Oxford University Press, 1944.

Lane, N., L. Caro, L.R. Otero-Vilardebo, and G. C. Godman: On the site of sulfation in colonic goblet cells. J. Cell Biol., *21*:339, 1964.

Leblond, C. P., and B. Messier: Renewal of chief cells and goblet cells in the small intestine as shown by radioautography after injection of thymidine-3H into mice. Anat. Rec., *132*:247, 1958.

Leblond, C. P., H. Puchtler, and Y. Clermont: Structures corresponding to terminal bars and terminal web in many types of cells. Nature, *186*:784, 1960.

Linderström-Lang, K.: Distribution of enzymes in tissues and cells. Harvey Lectures, *34*:214, 1939.

Lipkin, M.: Cell replication in the gastrointestinal tract of man. Gastroenterology, *48*:616, 1965.

Litt, M.: Studies on experimental eosinophilia. I. Repeated quantitation of peritoneal eosinophilia in guinea pigs. Blood, *16*:1318, 1960.

Miller, D., and R. K. Crane: The digestive function of the epithelium of the small intestine. II. Localization of disaccharidase hydrolysis in the isolated brush border portion of the intestinal epithelial cells. Biochem. Biophys. Acta, *52*:293, 1961.

Moe, H.: The ultrastructure of Brunner's glands of the cat. J. Ultrastruct. Res. *4*:58, 1960.

Moe, H.: The goblet cells, Paneth cells, and basal granular cells of the epithelium of the intestine. Internat. Rev. Gen. and Exper. Zool., *3*:241, 1968.

Monesi, V.: The appearance of enterochromaffin cells in the intestine of the chick embryo. Acta Anat., *41*:97, 1960.

Owen, R. L., and A. L. Jones: Epithelial cell specialization within human Peyer's patches: an ultrastructural study of intestinal lymphoid follicles. Gastroenterology, *66*: 189, 1974.

Palay, S. L., and L. J. Karlin: An electron microscope study of the intestinal villus. I. The fasting animal. II. The pathway of fat absorption. J. Biophys. Biochem. Cytol., *5*:363, 373, 1959.

Palay, S. L., and J. P. Revel: The morphology of fat absorption. *In* Meng, H. C., ed.: Lipid Transport, Springfield, Ill., Charles C Thomas, 1964, pp. 1–11.

Pascal, R., G. Kaye, and N. Lane: Colonic pericryptal fibroblast sheath: replication, migration and cytodifferentiation of a mesenchymal cell system in adult tissue. I. Autoradiographic studies of normal rabbit colon. Gastroenterology, *54*:835, 1968.

Patzelt, V.: Der Darm. *In* von Möllendorff, W., and W. Bargmann, eds.: Handbuch der mikroskopischen Anatomie des Menschen. Berlin, Julius Springer, 1936, Vol. 5, part 3, p. 1.

Ratzenhofer, M., and D. Leb: Über die Feinstruktur der argentaffinen und der anderen Erscheinungsformen der "Hellen Zellen" Feyrter's im Kaninchen-Magen. Zeitschr. f. Zellforsch., *67*:113, 1965.

Richardson, K. C.: Electronmicroscopic observations on Auerbach's plexus in the rabbit with special reference to the problem of smooth muscle innervation. Am. J. Anat., *103*:99, 1958.

Richardson, K. C.: Studies on the structure of the autonomic nerves in the small intestine, correlating the silver-impregnated image in light microscopy with the permanganate-fixed ultrastructure in electronmicroscopy. J. Anat. (London), *94*:457, 1960.

Sabesin, S. M., and K. J. Isselbacher: Protein synthesis inhibition: mechanism for production of impaired fat absorption. Science, *147*:1149, 1965.

Schofield, G. C.: Anatomy of muscular and neural tissues in the alimentary canal. *In* Code, C. F., and M. I. Grossman (eds.): *Handbook of Physiology*. Section 6. Washington, D. C., American Physiological Society, 1967–1968.

Selzman, H. M., and R. A. Liebelt: Paneth cell granules of mouse intestine. J. Cell Biol., *15*:136, 1962.

Senior, J. R.: Intestinal absorption of fats. J. Lipid Res., *5*:495, 1964.

Singh, I.: The prenatal development of enterochromaffin cells in the human gastro-intestinal tract. J. Anat. (London), *97*:377, 1963.

Singh, I.: On argyrophile and argentaffin reactions in individual granules of enterochromaffin cells of the human gastro-intestinal tract. J. Anat. (London), *98*:497, 1964.

Spicer, S. S., M. W. Staley, M. G. Wetzel, and B. K. Wetzel: Acid mucosubstance and basic protein in mouse Paneth cells. J. Histochem. Cytochem., *15*:225, 1967.

Strauss, E. W.: The absorption of fat by intestine of golden hamster *in vitro*. J. Cell Biol., *17*:597, 1963.

Strauss, E. W.: Electron microscopic study of intestinal fat absorption *in vitro* from mixed micelles containing linolenic acid, monoolein, and bile salt. J. Lipid Res., *7*:307, 1966.

Trier, J. S.: Studies on small intestinal crypt epithelium. I. The fine structure of the crypt epithelium of the proximal small intestine of fasting humans. J. Cell Biol., *18*:599, 1963.

Trier, J. S.: Morphology of the epithelium of the small intestine. *In* Handbook of Physiology, Section 6. Washington, D. C., American Physiological Society, 1967–1968.

Zetterqvist, H.: The Ultrastructural Organization of the Columnar Absorbing Cells of the Mouse Jejunum. Stockholm, Aktiebolaget Godvil, 1956.

28

The Liver and Gallbladder

LIVER

The liver is the largest gland in the body, weighing about 1500 gm. in the adult. It functions both as an *exocrine gland*, secreting bile through a system of bile ducts into the duodenum, and as an *endocrine gland*, synthesizing a variety of substances that are released directly into the bloodstream. To appreciate the importance of the liver and to correlate its structure with its functions requires an understanding of its blood supply and its strategic location in the circulation. It receives a large volume of venous blood from the intestinal tract via the *portal vein* and a small volume of arterial blood via the *hepatic artery*. It is drained by the *hepatic veins* into the inferior vena cava near the heart. The liver is thus interposed between the intestinal tract and the general circulation. It therefore receives, in the portal blood, all of the material absorbed from the intestinal tract except the bulk of the lipid, which is transported in the *chyle* via the mesenteric lymphatics to the thoracic duct. The absorbed products of digestion are taken up and metabolized in the liver or are transformed there and returned to the blood for storage or utilization elsewhere. The liver may also receive toxic substances from the intestine or from the general circulation and is capable of degrading them by oxidation or hydroxylation or detoxifying them by conjugation. The products of their degradation or their harmless conjugates are then excreted in the *bile*. The bile is a complex fluid that can be regarded as a secretion in that it plays an important role in digestion, but it can also be regarded as a vehicle for excretion to the extent that it carries detoxified waste and potentially harmful materials to the intestine for ultimate elimination.

The liver also synthesizes several important protein components of the blood plasma, and it exercises an important degree of control over the general metabolism by virtue of its capacity to store carbohydrates as glycogen and to release glucose to maintain the normal concentration of glucose in the blood.

HISTOLOGICAL ORGANIZATION OF THE LIVER

The liver is composed of epithelial cells arranged in plates or laminae that are interconnected to form a continuous tridimensional lattice. The laminae are disposed radially with respect to terminal branches of the hepatic veins, which traditionally have been designated as *central veins* because of their location in the centers of prismatic units of liver parenchyma that constitute the liver *lobules* (Figs. 28–1 and 28–2). The radially disposed plates of liver cells are exposed on either side to the blood flowing in a parallel system of vascular channels, the *hepatic sinusoids*. The radially oriented sinusoids closely conform to the broad surfaces of the cellular laminae and intercommunicate through fenestrations in them to form a labyrinthine system of thin-walled vessels intimately related to a very large surface area of liver parenchyma.

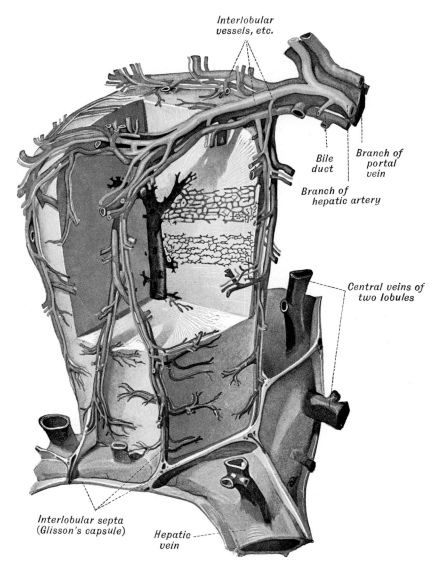

Interlobular
vessels, etc.

Bile
duct

Branch of
portal
vein

Branch of
hepatic artery

Central veins of
two lobules

Interlobular septa
(Glisson's capsule)

Hepatic
vein

Figure 28–1 Wax reconstruction (by A. Vierling) of a lobule of the liver of a pig. A portion of the lobule has been cut away to show the bile capillaries and sinusoids. × 400. (After Braus.)

The Liver Lobule

In the pig and a few other species, a well defined layer of connective tissue clearly demarcates the lobules. However, in most mammals, including the human, there is no boundary between the lobules, the hepatic parenchyma appearing quite continuous. The radial pattern of the cellular plates and sinusoids is such that one can, nevertheless, recognize the units of structure and assign imaginary boundaries to the lobule by relying upon the regularly distributed central veins and portal canals as landmarks (Fig. 28–2).

The lobules in sections are typically hexagonal, with the corners of the polygon each occupied by a *portal canal* (Fig. 28–2 and 28–3). This latter structure consists of a small branch of the portal vein and one of the hepatic artery, as well as a bile ductule, enclosed in a common investment of connective tissue (Fig. 28–4). Blood enters the hepatic sinusoids from small branches of the hepatic artery and portal vein, flows

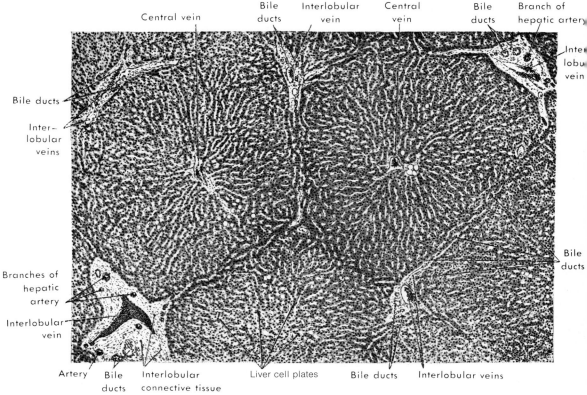

Figure 28–2 Portion of liver from a 22 year old man. Two complete lobules are surrounded by portions of other lobules. × 70. (After Sobotta.)

through the lobule centripetally, and leaves via the central vein (Figs. 28–5 and 28–6).

The traditional lobule as defined above is not comparable with the lobules of most glands, which are centered on the ducts that drain them. The liver lobule as just presented is conceptually convenient, however, for as a result of differential deposition of glycogen or fat, the hepatic tissue of which it is composed, frequently exhibits microscopically distinguishable zones, concentric around the central vein. Moreover, in pathological conditions, necrosis may selectively involve the central or the peripheral zone, depending upon the nature of the disease process.

The lobular pattern appears to develop as a consequence of the hydrodynamics of the blood flow through the liver. From this point of view the liver may be considered as a tough sac filled with fluid, in which is suspended a plastic spongework of liver tissue. In the flow of fluid through the liver, the terminal branches of the portal vein are sources and

the radicles of the hepatic vein are sinks (Figs. 28–3 and 28–5). The flow from the one to the other is thought to determine the radial pattern of the sinusoids characteristic of the lobule. It follows also that the cells nearest the branches of the portal vein receive blood first and therefore have first call upon the nutrient and oxygen content of the portal blood. As the latter diminish in the passage of the blood from the periphery toward the center of the lobule, a gradient of metabolic activity is established, which is expressed in the morphologically detectable zonation of the lobule.

Some histologists have objected to the classical definition of the liver lobule because it is inconsistent with the lobular organization typical of other exocrine glands. In an effort to make the liver conform to the same general plan, Mall proposed an alternative concept of liver lobulation according to which the portal canal was considered to be the center of the lobule, and the branches of the hepatic vein were said to be situated around its periphery. The lobule defined in this way is called a *portal lobule*. In such a lobule, the bile would drain toward a duct located with the vascular supply in the center of the lobule, as is the case in most other glands.

In some respects this is a more satisfactory way of interpreting the architecture of the liver than the *classical lobule*, but it has been argued that the portal lobule is not the smallest unit of functional organization of the liver. A variant of the portal lobule has been proposed by Rappaport and his colleagues, who consider the functional unit to be a mass of parenchymal tissue associated with the fine terminal branches of the portal vein, hepatic artery, and bile duct. These branches leave the portal canals at intervals, coursing perpendicular to the canals and to the central vein, and run along the side of the hexagon that forms the section of the classical lobule. The associated mass of hepatic tissue is smaller than either of the lobules proposed earlier and is composed of parts of two ad-

jacent classical lobules (Fig. 28–7)). It is called a *liver acinus* and is defined as the tissue supplied by a terminal branch of the portal vein and of the hepatic artery and drained by a terminal branch of the bile duct. The limits of the acinus are not defined by any recognizable anatomical landmarks but extend outward to the terminal branches of the hepatic veins and to the imaginary outer limits of acini associated with neighboring portal canals. The parenchyma is continuous from one acinus to the next, and indeed from one classical lobule to the next. Therefore, if the supply and drainage of one unit should fail, it would still be supplied and drained by others. This concept of liver structure, although still not universally accepted, has proved useful in the understanding of some aspects of liver physiology and in accounting for some manifestations of liver pathology, especially that following bile duct occlusion and that found in cirrhosis of the liver.

The *classical lobule*, the *portal lobule*, and the *acinus* should not be considered as con-

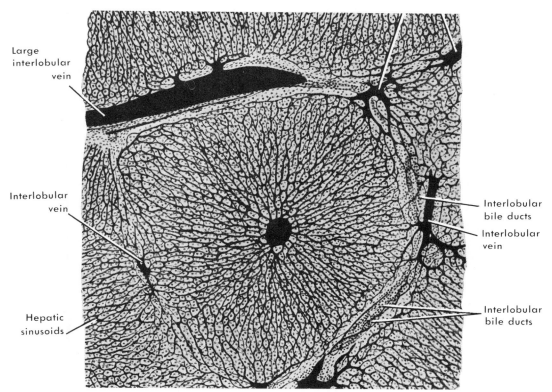

Large interlobular vein

Interlobular vein

Hepatic sinusoids

Interlobular bile ducts

Interlobular vein

Interlobular bile ducts

Figure 28–3 Portion of liver of a rabbit injected through the portal vein with Berlin blue and gelatin. A complex lobule surrounds the central vein. × 54. (After Sobotta.)

flicting concepts of liver structure but as complementary ones. Because of the complexity of the function of the liver, it is sometimes useful to think in terms of one and at other times in terms of another. It is noteworthy that the traditional lobulation is not present in the lower vertebrates nor in the mammalian embryo.

The Blood Supply

The principal afferent blood vessel of the liver is the portal vein, which receives blood from the digestive tract and from the spleen. It enters the liver at the porta, together with the hepatic artery and the bile duct. The hepatic artery, in all mammals, carries much less blood than the portal vein, though the relative amounts vary in different species. These two vessels and the bile duct branch together as they penetrate the liver mass, with fine branches eventually occupying the portal canals at the periphery of the lobules (Figs.

28–1 and 28–4). They are accompanied throughout by a network of lymphatics. It is to be emphasized, however, that none of the vessels of the larger portal canals are in direct communication with the liver parenchyma. The canal is bounded by a continuous plate of hepatic cells, with only occasional fenestrations through which the tiny terminal branches of the artery, vein, and bile duct penetrate the liver parenchyma, running along the boundaries between the classical lobules and occupying the center of the functional units or acini.

These groups of terminal branches are accompanied by very sparse connective tissue and a fine network of lymphatics. The difference in structure and in function between them and typical portal canals needs to be emphasized. It is not via the larger portal canals but through these smaller terminal branches of the vessels that blood enters the sinusoids of the parenchyma. It is here, too, that the terminal ductules of the bile duct,

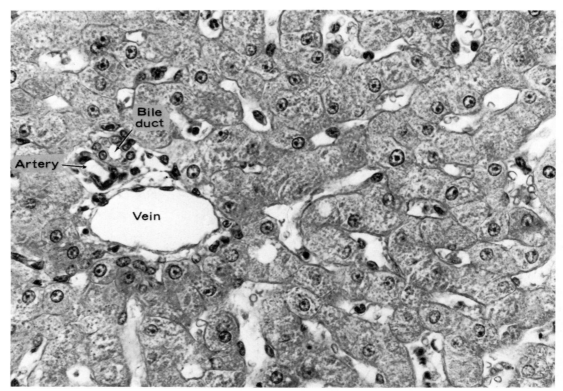

Figure 28–4 Photomicrograph of liver parenchyma at the periphery of a traditional lobule, showing a typical portal triad, consisting of branches of the hepatic artery and portal vein, and a small bile duct.

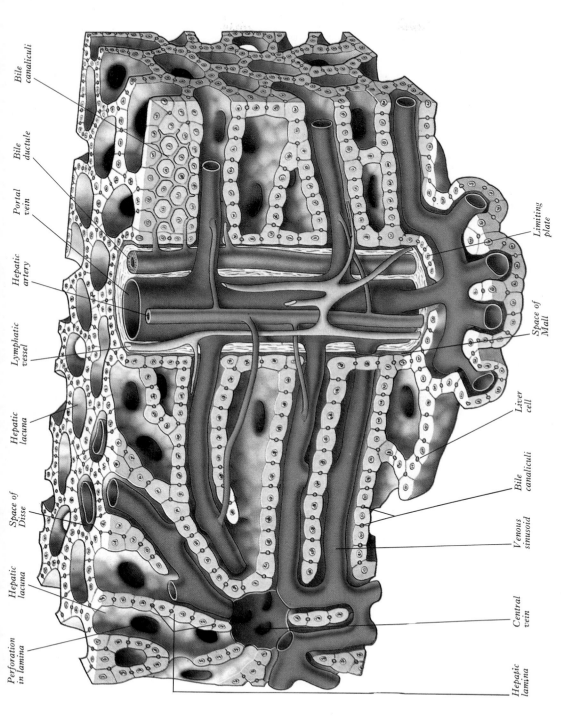

Bile
canaliculi

Bile
ductule

Portal
vein

Hepatic
artery

Lymphatic
vessel

Hepatic
lacuna

Space of
Disse

Hepatic
lacuna

Perforation
in lamina

Limiting
plate

Space of
Mall

Liver
cell

Bile
canaliculi

Venous
sinusoid

Central
vein

Hepatic
lamina

Figure 28–5   Diagram of hepatic structure. (From Gray's Anatomy. London, Longman. After Prof. H. Elias.)

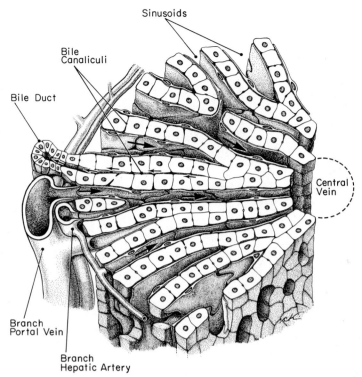

Sinusoids

Bile
Canaliculi

Bile Duct

Central
Vein

Branch
Portal Vein

Branch
Hepatic Artery

Figure 28-6 Diagrammatic representation of the radial disposition of the liver cell plates and sinusoids around the terminal hepatic venule or central vein, showing the centripetal flow of blood from branches of the hepatic artery and portal vein, and the centrifugal flow of bile (small arrows) to the small bile duct in the portal space. (Redrawn and modified from Ham, Textbook of Histology. Philadelphia, J. B. Lippincott Co.)

sometimes called the *canals of Hering,* join the parenchyma to receive the bile from the system of minute canaliculi between the liver cells. Here, too, the lymphatics receive the abundant liver lymph composed of the interstitial fluid and plasma that has drained into the perivascular spaces from the parenchyma and sinusoids. The virtue of the functional unit of Rappaport is that it emphasizes these important relationships.

In the larger portal canals, fine branches of both the portal vein and the hepatic artery supply an elaborate capillary network that is intimately associated with the branches of the bile duct. From this network, collecting venules re-enter the portal vein, so that there is, in a sense, a minute portal system, receiving blood from the hepatic artery, inserted into the greater portal system. From the extent of this capillary plexus it has been suggested that in the normal liver of some species at least, the most important function of the hepatic artery is to supply this plexus in the portal canals. Only a relatively small volume

of arterial blood enters the sinusoids directly from the branches of the hepatic artery in the core of the functional unit.

The details of branching in the core of the functional unit are very difficult to analyze in sections, but they have been studied by injection and corrosion. Throughout its length, the branch of the portal vein gives off distributing venules that send a branch in either direction, and from these arise the final branches that enter the sinusoids. The artery sends off branches that form a more typical arborization and end in the sinusoids. The lymphatic network appears to end blindly in the connective tissue.

Shunt vessels carrying blood directly from the artery to the portal vein have been described, but there is no evidence that they are abundant or functionally important in the normal liver. Also described are fine terminal branches of the artery extending deep into the lobule and entering the sinusoids directly, but these are certainly not common, and it seems possible that their description is the

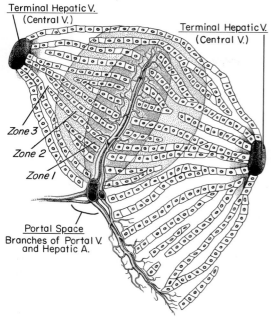

Terminal Hepatic V.
(Central V.)

Terminal Hepatic V.
(Central V.)

Zone 3

Zone 2

Zone 1

Portal Space
Branches of Portal V.
and Hepatic A.

Figure 28-7 Diagram illustrating the functional unit of liver parenchyma (the acinus) according to Rappaport et al. It consists of the parenchyma centered around the terminal branches of the hepatic artery and portal vein. It is to be noted that the cells in Zone 1 nearest these vessels have first call upon the incoming oxygen and nutrients, while the cells of Zone 2 are less favored and those of Zone 3 near the terminal hepatic venules are least favorably situated. (Redrawn after Rappaport, A. M., A. J. Borowy, W. M. Lougheed, and W. N. Lolto, Anat. Rec., *119*:11, 1954.)

result of a misinterpretation of the lobular pattern.

The blood leaves the lobule through a terminal radicle of the hepatic vein, the central vein of the classical lobule. Its wall is penetrated by innumerable pores opening directly into the sinusoidal labyrinth. There is no continuous limiting plate of liver cells around the central vein like that around the portal canal. The central veins are the intralobular branches of the hepatic vein. They join to form an intercalated vein (the sublobular vein of the older literature). Several of these unite to form a collecting vein, and these in turn join to form the hepatic veins, which pursue a course through the liver independent of the portal venous system. There may be two or more hepatic veins that enter the inferior vena cava. The intralobular veins are highly contractile and act as throttle veins to control the flow of blood through the liver lobules

and the entire portal vein bed, which serves as an important blood reservoir.

Experiments involving ligature of the various vessels entering or leaving the liver have often given confusing results because there are other vessels that contribute in a minor way to the circulation of the liver. The most important of these are the arteries and veins of the diaphragm, which sometimes anastomose with vessels in the liver. These anastomoses are variable. They may be rapidly enlarged or new ones may possibly be formed as occasion demands. They are of importance in the interpretation of experiments involving alterations in blood flow after ligation of the main vessels and of changes in the circulation in cirrhosis.

Hepatic Sinusoids

The hepatic sinusoids are larger than capillaries, more irregular in shape, and their lining cells are directly related to the epithelial cells of the parenchyma with essentially no intervening connective tissue. The lining of the sinusoids consists of a thin layer of cells that differ from typical capillary endothelium in two respects: (1) Some of the lining cells are actively phagocytic, and (2) the cell boundaries do not blacken with silver nitrate. This latter property led some early investigators to suggest that the lining was a syncytium. Various cytological and experimental studies that were carried out in the era of light microscopy cast doubt upon this interpretation, and more recent studies with the electron microscope have established beyond doubt that the endothelium is made up of individual cells.

Whether the lining is composed of one or two types of cells has long been a subject of dispute. Those who distinguish two had identified one as a typical endothelial cell and considered the other to be a fixed macrophage called the *cell of Kupffer.* Other investigators observed that, upon repeated injection of colloidal particulate matter into experimental animals, the phagocytic cells of the sinusoids became larger and more numerous; they thought they could recognize forms intermediate between endothelial cells and Kupffer cells. Therefore, it became widely accepted that the endothelial cells could transform into phagocytic cells when the need arose and the different appearance of the lining cells simply

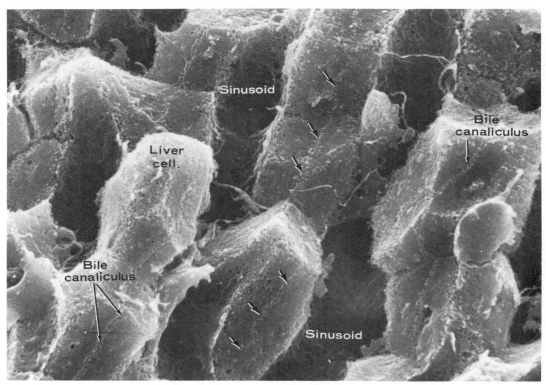

Figure 28-8 Scanning electron micrograph of rat liver fixed by perfusion and then broken open to reveal its internal architecture. The micrograph affords a three dimensional view of the plates of polygonal hepatic cells alternating with sinusoids. Where the liver plates have been broken, the bile canaliculi can be identified on the contact surfaces of the hepatic cells (at arrows). (Micrography courtesy of M. Karnovsky.)

represented different functional states of a single cell type. The application of electron microscopy and histochemical staining reactions seems now to have resolved the controversy in favor of distinct populations having different origins and functions. In electron micrographs of liver fixed by perfusion, it is now possible to identify three cell types associated with the sinusoids—*endothelial cells, Kupffer cells,* and perisinusoidal *fat-storing cells.*

Endothelial Cells. These flattened cells have a large nucleus-to-cytoplasm ratio, and relatively few organelles. They form the greater part of the extremely thin lining layer of the sinusoids. They are not significantly phagocytic to colloidal vital dyes, although some pinocytotic activity is suggested by electron micrographs in which small, coated vesicles are seen associated with both the adluminal and the abluminal surfaces of the cell.

Whether the sinusoidal lining is continuous or discontinuous is an important question that has long been debated. Physiological ob-

servations on rates of clearance of substances from the blood and on the large size of the molecules and colloidal particles that readily pass through the wall of the sinusoid, have made it seem probable that there are openings in it that permit the blood plasma, but not the blood cells, to gain direct access to the surface of the hepatic cells. The electron microscope has provided visual and experimental confirmation. In the common laboratory species the endothelial cells have typical overlapping junctions in some places but in others the attenuated margins of neighboring cells may be separated by intercellular openings 0.1 to 0.5 μm. across. In addition, where the plane of section passes subtangential to the attenuated peripheral part of an endothelial cell it can be seen in electron micrographs to be fenestrated, presenting a sieve-like appearance (Figs. 28–9 and 28–10). These openings are considerably larger and more variable in size than the so called pores in fenestrated capillaries elsewhere in the body.

Thus it appears that in these species there are intracellular fenestrations as well as small discontinuities between adjacent cells. It can be shown that in as short a time as 30 seconds after injection of colloidal thorium dioxide into the portal vein, the dense particles can be found in electron micrographs on both sides of the endothelium and on the surface of the underlying hepatic cells. Since the endothelium of the hepatic sinusoids also lacks a basal lamina in laboratory rodents, the particulate tracer evidently encounters no obstruction to passage through the fenestrations.

Openings in the walls of the blood vessels are rare in the circulatory system of vertebrates. Therefore, when the discontinuities in the hepatic sinusoids were first demonstrated by electron microscopy, there was some concern that they represented artifacts of specimen preparation. The methacrylate embedding material, then in general use, was known to produce discontinuities in some

structures during polymerization. As preparative methods have improved and embedding media have been introduced that are relatively free of such distortions, the lining of the hepatic sinusoids continues to appear interrupted, while the endothelia of capillaries in other organs prepared identically show no such openings. The absence of typical, continuous, cell to cell junctions evidently explains the failure of attempts to impregnate the outlines of the endothelial cells with silver. It is now the consensus that the wall of the sinusoids is discontinuous in most mammals, including man. There are significant species differences in the degree of endothelial discontinuity. The hepatic sinusoids of sheep, goats, and calves have a distinct basal lamina and a continuous endothelium with only rare fenestrae, and these are closed by a thin diaphragm.

In those species with a discontinuous sinusoidal endothelium and no basal lamina,

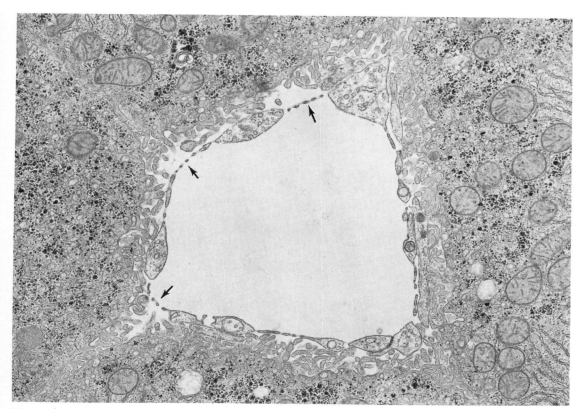

Figure 28–9 Electron micrograph of a sinusoid in rat liver fixed by vascular perfusion. The endothelium is extremely attenuated in some areas where there are fenestrations that give it a sieve-like structure (see arrows). (Micrograph from E. Wisse, J. Ultrastr. Res., *31*:125, 1970.)

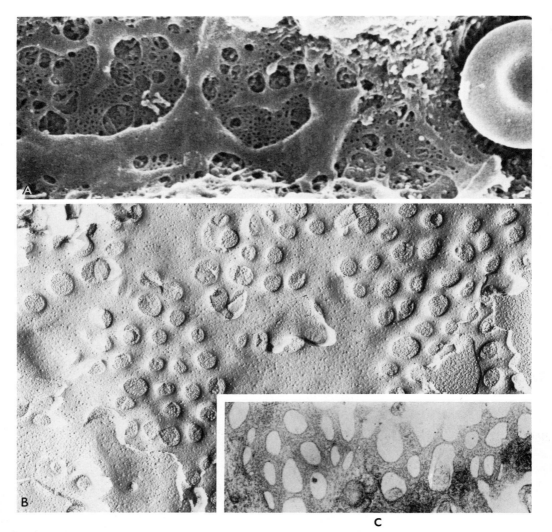

Figure 28-10 *A,* Scanning electron micrograph of a rat liver sinusoid seen from the luminal surface. Fenestrations of the thin areas of the endothelial cells are clearly visible. (Micrograph *A* courtesy of M. Karnovsky.) *B,* Freeze-fracture preparation of the endothelium of an hepatic sinusoid illustrating numerous elevations of varying size representing fenestrations. *C,* A subtangential section of endothelium in a transmission electron micrograph. Fenestrations of varying size and shape correspond to the elevations seen in the replica of the freeze fractured specimen. (Micrographs *B* and *C* as xeroxed copy by E. Wisse, J. Ultrastr. Res., *31*:125, 1970.)

there is evidently no filtration barrier other than for cells. Chylomicra and very low density lipoprotein particles can freely traverse inter- or intracellular fenestrations. The situation is less clear in those species which have a continuous basal lamina and few fenestrations, but low density lipoprotein particles are seen in the space of Disse and in the plasma and are evidently able somehow to traverse the endothelium.

Kupffer Cells. These stellate cells were described by Kupffer in 1898 in liver stained by a gold-chloride impregnation method. They were depicted with their processes traversing the sinusoids. Thus they were thought to lie within the sinusoid but fixed to the endothelium. They frequently contain engulfed erythrocytes in various stages of disintegration, pigment deposits, and granules rich in iron. They actively phagocytize particulate matter injected into the bloodstream and therefore are stained intensely with such vital dyes as lithium carmine or trypan blue. They also take up injected carbon particles or electron opaque particles of thorium dioxide (Fig. 28–11). These cells thus belong to the reticuloendothelial system. They may retain for long periods of time phagocytosed material that cannot be digested by lysosomes.

Electron microscopic studies of Kupffer cells in livers fixed by perfusion have done much to clarify their cytological characteristics and their relations to other cells associated with the sinusoids. They are usually situated on the endothelium with processes extending between the endothelial cells. Their highly variable shape suggests that their form and relations to the endothelium may change continually. They do not form desmosomes or other enduring specializations for attachment to the endothelial cells. The greater part of their irregular cell surface is exposed to the blood in the lumen of the sinusoid. A thin fuzzy coat or glycocalyx can be demonstrated. In addition to surface folds, and slender villous projections there are peculiar sinuous invaginations of the plasma membrane into the peripheral cytoplasm. These have a central dense line between parallel membranes and a faint transverse striation resulting in a highly characteristic appearance in thin sections that has led to their description "worm-like" or "vermiform" structures. These are never seen in endothelial cells but have been reported in macrophages of other organs and in the Langerhans cells of the epidermis.

The cytoplasm of Kupffer cells is richer in organelles and more heterogeneous in appearance than that of endothelial cells. Clear vacuoles of varying size and dense bodies presumed to be lysosomes are usually present. There is a juxtanuclear centrosome and associated Golgi complex. Short cisternal profiles of granular endoplasmic reticulum are scattered throughout the cytoplasm. These are demonstrated with unusual clarity in preparations reacted for peroxidase activity (Fig. 28–12). Peroxidase is present in the perinuclear cisterna, in the lumen of the endoplasmic reticulum, and in the occasional annulate lamellae of Kupffer cells. This reaction serves clearly to distinguish them from endothelial cells which have no peroxidase activity (Wisse; Fahimi).

Until recently it was assumed that increases in the numbers of Kupffer cells after stimulation of the reticuloendothelial system were due either to division of the preexisting cells of this type or to acquisition of phagocytic capacity by endothelial cells transforming into Kupffer cells. This latter source is of course excluded if it be accepted that these are distinct populations. The experimental stimulation of phagocytic cells results in a substantial increase in the number of Kupffer cells incorporating H^3-thymidine. Thus there seems no doubt of their ability to increase by mitosis. There is now also good reason for believing that Kupffer cells can be replaced and augmented by recruitment from extrahepatic sources (Howard). In the relevant experiments, mice were given sufficient whole body x-irradiation to suppress division of their own cells. They then received an intravenous injection of bone marrow cells and lymphocytes from another animal of a compatible strain whose cells carried a chromosomal marker.

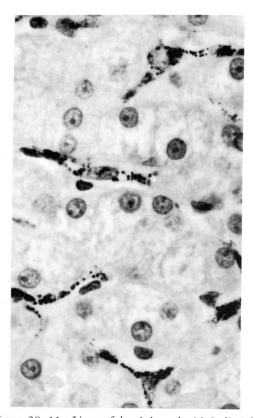

Figure 28–11 Liver of dog injected with India ink, showing uptake of carbon by the lining cells. × 675. (Courtesy of A. J. Ladman.)

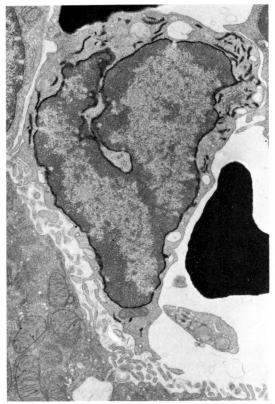

Figure 28–12 Electron micrograph of a Kupffer cell, showing a positive reaction for peroxidase in the nuclear envelope and in cisternae of the endoplasmic reticulum. This reaction serves to distinguish Kupffer cells from endothelial cells. (Micrograph from D. Fahimi, J. Cell Biol., 47:247, 1970.)

When the reticuloendothelial systems of the recipient mice were stimulated, the dividing Kupffer cells could be shown to have originated from the bone marrow of the donor. Similarly, when pairs of unirradiated histocompatible mice were maintained in parabiosis for several months, karyotypic analysis of Kupffer cells revealed limited numbers of partner-derived cells in every instance. These experiments have led to the conclusion that normally many and perhaps all of the Kupffer cells are derived from a precursor in the bone marrow, as are the free mononuclear phagocytes of other organs. They would thus belong to the "mononuclear phagocyte system." However, this view has not yet been accorded general acceptance. Monocytes usually lose all peroxidase activity when they become macrophages. The presence of strong activity in Kupffer cells does not provide support for the view that monocytes are transformed into Kupffer cells.

Fat Storing Cells. The origin of these cells that accumulate lipid is still not clear. They have been described under a variety of names, *interstitial cells* (Satsuki), *lipocytes* (Bronfenmajer), *fat-storing cells* (Ito), and *stellate cells* (Wake). They can be stained with gold chloride (Figs. 28–13 and 28–14), and it is possible that some of the stellate cells described by Kupffer were, in fact, fat-storing cells and not exclusively the phagocytic cells which now bear his name (Wake).

Investigators are agreed that these cells are located in the perisinusoidal spaces. They tend to be more numerous in intermediate and peripheral portions of the hepatic lobule than they are in the central zone. Their functional significance is poorly understood. When exogenous vitamin A is administered it seems to accumulate preferentially in the lipid droplets of the stellate fat-storing cells.

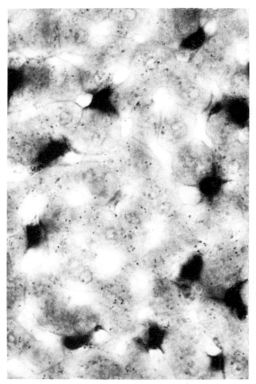

Figure 28–13 Photomicrograph of normal rabbit liver stained by Kupffer's original gold impregnation method. The perisinusoidal stellate or fat-storing cells are stained. × 600. (Photograph by K. Wake, Am. J. Anat., *132*:429, 1971.)

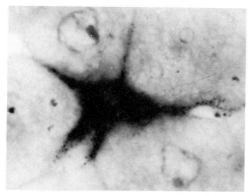

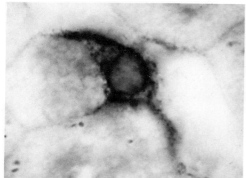

Figure 28-14 Fat-storing cells of rabbit liver after Kupffer's gold impregnation method. × 1800. (Photomicrographs from K. Wake, Am. J. Anat., *132*:429, 1971.)

Perisinusoidal Space (Space of Disse)

The question of the relationship of the sinusoid lining to the underlying liver cells also seems to have been settled by the electron microscope. The controversy stemmed from the fact that in histological sections of human postmortem material, an obvious space, called the *space of Disse,* could be seen between the sinusoid lining and the liver cells. It did not appear in biopsy material nor in the usual sections of livers of laboratory animals used in research. It was therefore regarded by many histologists as a consequence of agonal or postmortem change in the liver. In electron micrographs of well fixed material, the endothelium of the sinusoids is not closely applied to a smooth parenchymal cell surface, as was formerly thought to be the case, but instead rests lightly on the tips of a large number of irregularly oriented microvilli on the surface of the liver cell (Figs. 28–15 and 28–16). There is therefore a true peri-

vascular space in the normal liver into which the microvilli project. The space of Disse described by pathologists was evidently the result of an edematous expansion of this space. The term has now come to be applied freely to the narrow perivascular space revealed by the electron microscope in the normal liver.

Occasional bundles of collagen fibers are encountered in the space of Disse, forming the argyrophilic reticulum described by light microscopists (Fig. 28–28), but the space contains no true ground substance and plasma can apparently move freely through it. Although its content is plasma rather than interstitial fluid, it must be considered an interstitial space and not a lymphatic space, because it is not lined by lymphatic endothelium. The space of Disse may, nevertheless, be important in the formation of the abundant liver lymph.

It is evident that direct access of the plasma to the surface of the liver cell is a structural feature of great functional importance in the active exchange of metabolites between the liver and the bloodstream. The efficiency of this exchange is further promoted by the increase in surface achieved by the microvilli. From measurement of electron micrographs it is estimated that the length of the plasma membrane covering the microvilli and lining the clefts between them is six times greater than the linear extent of cell surface measured across the bases of the microvilli.

The Cytology of the Hepatic Parenchymal Cells

The liver cells are polyhedral, with six or more surfaces. The surfaces are of three sorts: those exposed to the perisinusoidal space; those exposed to the lumen of the bile canaliculus; and those in contact with adjacent liver cells (Fig. 28–17). The nuclei are large and round, with a smooth surface, but may vary in size from cell to cell. The variation in size has been shown to be an expression of polyploidy. Most cells have a single nucleus, but as many as 25 per cent are binucleate; 70 per cent or more of the nuclei are tetraploid, and 1 to 2 per cent are octaploid. The nucleus is typically vesicular, with a few scattered chromatin clumps and one or more prominent nucleoli. In electron micrographs the liver cell nucleus has few features that distinguish it from the nuclei of other cells. The chromatin is repre-

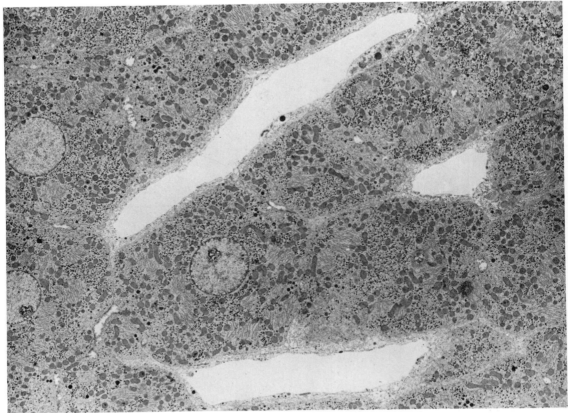

Figure 28-15 Electron micrograph of plates of liver cells and intervening sinusoids. (Micrograph by E. Wisse.)

sented by ill defined masses of fine filaments or granules of moderate density. Somewhat larger granules 300 Å in diameter, called perichromatin granules, are located near the masses of chromatin. These are usually surrounded by a clear zone about 250 Å wide. These granules stain with uranyl acetate and indium and are therefore believed to contain nucleic acids. The nucleoli consist of fine fibrils (60 Å) and dense granules (150 Å), and both of these components are present in the anastomosing strands that constitute the nucleolonema. As in other cell types, the nuclear envelope consists of two parellel membranes bounding a perinuclear cisterna. The outer element of the nuclear envelope bears occasional ribosomes on its cytoplasmic surface and is continuous at certain points with the membranes of the granular endoplasmic reticulum. The cytoplasm of liver cells in well nourished animals contains conspicuous strands or irregular masses of material that are strongly basophilic and can be shown by

histochemical methods to be rich in ribonucleoprotein (Fig. 28–18). After a prolonged fast, these basophilic bodies are reduced in size and number and the cytoplasm is mainly eosinophilic. Owing to such variations in different nutritional conditions, it was formerly thought that the basophilic masses represented a storage form of protein. It is now known that these bodies seen with the light microscope correspond to arrays of cisternae of the granular endoplasmic reticulum in electron micrographs. Therefore they are not stores of protein but sites of protein synthesis. In the normal animal, protein is not stored in cytoplasmic inclusions. The rough reticulum usually occurs in the form of aggregations of from three to 20 cisternae (Fig. 28–19). These are spaced somewhat farther apart and are less precisely parallel than the cisternae in the pancreas and other protein secreting cell types. The cisternae are studded with numerous ribosomes, but the ends of their profiles are apt to be slightly expanded and free of granules. In addition to the ribosomes associated with the cytoplasmic membranes, there are other polysomes in spiral or rosette patterns free in the cytoplasmic matrix.

The liver cell also contains a moderately extensive smooth endoplasmic reticulum that takes the form of a close-meshed plexus of branching and anastomosing tubules, somewhat variable in caliber (Fig. 28–20). Owing to the thinness of the sections, however, the continuity of the system is not always evident, and it may appear as a congeries of separate profiles of irregular outline. Sites of continuity between the rough and smooth surfaced reticulum are frequently observed (Fig. 28–21). Small globules about 300 to 400 Å in diameter are often seen in the lumen of the smooth reticulum (Fig. 28–20). These represent the very low density serum lipoprotein which is synthesized in the liver and released into the blood.

The cytoplasm of the liver cell presents an extremely variable appearance, which reflects to some extent the functional state of the cell. The principal source of variation is in the content of the stored material—glycogen and fat. In the preparation of histological sections, both fat and glycogen have been removed, but the presence of glycogen is indicated by irregular empty spaces, and the presence of lipid is represented by round vacuoles. By appropriate methods of fixation both fat and glycogen can be preserved and stained. The content of these materials in the liver may vary extensively with the diet or the stage of digestion (Fig. 28–22).

When adequately preserved, glycogen appears in electron micrographs of liver cells as dense aggregates or rosettes up to 0.1 μm. in diameter (alpha particles) composed of beta particles 200 to 300 Å in diameter. Glycogen is not uniformly distributed in the cytoplasm but tends to be closely associated with the areas of smooth endoplasmic reticulum (Fig. 28–23).

Lipid occurs in the form of osmiophilic droplets of varying size. These are few in number in the normal liver, but may be dra-

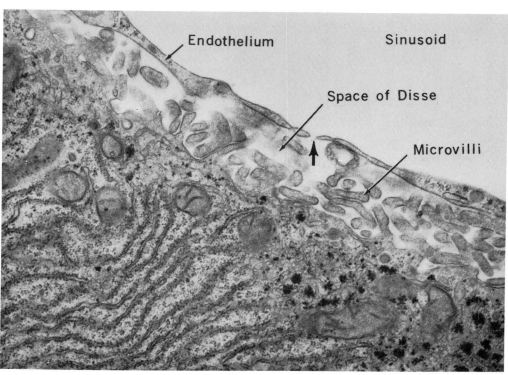

Figure 28–16 Electron micrograph of part of the surface of a rat liver cell bordering on a sinusoid. Numerous irregularly oriented microvilli project into a narrow space between the hepatic cell and the endothelium lining the sinusoid. The perivascular space is often called the space of Disse. Notice the small discontinuity in the lining of the sinusoid (at heavy arrow). × 18,000. (Courtesy of K. R. Porter and G. Millonig; labeling added.)

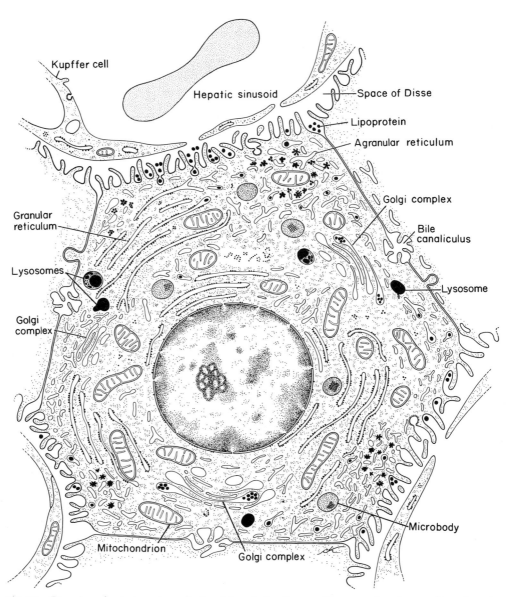

Kupffer cell

Hepatic sinusoid

Space of Disse

Lipoprotein

Agranular reticulum

Golgi complex

Granular reticulum

Bile canaliculus

Lysosomes

Lysosome

Golgi complex

Microbody

Mitochondrion

Golgi complex

Figure 28-17 Drawing depicting the relationship of the liver cells to each other and to the sinusoids and showing the principal components of the hepatic cell as seen in electron micrographs. (Drawing by Sylvia Colard Keene.)

matically increased after consumption of alcohol or other hepatotoxic substances. The lipid droplets are usually not limited by a membrane. They may occur anywhere in the cytoplasm and have no special topographical relation to any of the organelles other than mitochondria which may be closely applied to the surface of the droplet.

Mitochondria cannot be seen in the usual histological preparation, but they can be revealed by special cytological techniques. They are numerous, and for the most part filamentous, but they vary somewhat in size and shape in different parts of the the lobule and in different physiological conditions. The mitochondria are in no way unusual in their fine structure. Lamellar or tubular cristae project into a matrix of relatively low density. A number of matrix granules are usually seen in each mitochondrial profile.

The Golgi system of the cell consists of several parts, each situated near a bile canaliculus. Each complex is made up of three to five flat saccules or cisternae in close parallel array. The ends of the cisternae are often dilated and contain numerous moderately dense granules 300 to 600 Å in diameter. These appear to be identical to the low density lipoprotein particles observed in the smooth reticulum. Associated with each of the Golgi complexes are several membrane limited dense bodies 0.2 to 0.5 μm. in diameter. These peribiliary dense bodies contain histochemically demonstrable acid hydrolases and therefore correspond to the lysosomes isolated from homogenates of liver (de Duve). The lysosomes are believed to be involved in intracellular digestion, but from a consideration of the function of the liver it is not clear what substances would require digestion other than damaged organelles lost to the wear and tear of normal functional activity.

Scattered throughout the cytoplasm of the hepatocyte are related cytoplasmic organelles, the *microbodies* or *peroxisomes* (Figs. 28–24 and 28–25). These are spherical bodies 0.2 to 0.8 μm. in diameter enclosed by a mem-

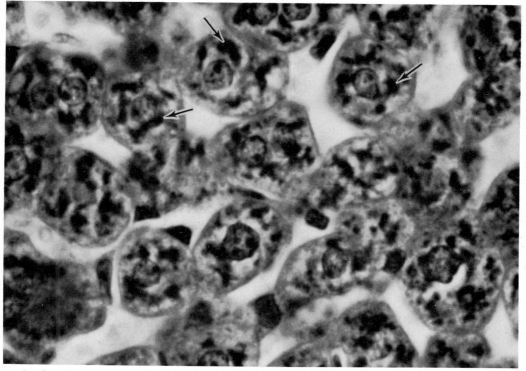

Figure 28–18 Photomicrograph of rat liver stained with eosin and methylene blue. The deeply stained basophilic bodies (at arrows) in the cytoplasm correspond to the aggregations of granular endoplasmic reticulum seen in electron micrographs. × 1250.

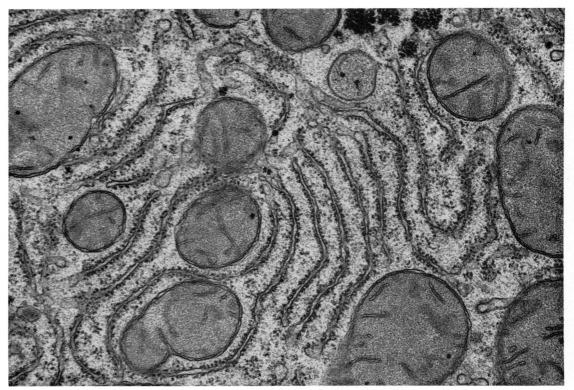

Figure 28–19 Electron micrograph showing an area of granular endoplasmic reticulum from hamster liver, corresponding to one of the basophilic bodies seen with the light microscope. The mitochondria and the granular reticulum are often in close topographical relation to one another. × 34,000. (After Jones, A. L., and D. W. Fawcett, J. Histochem. and Cytochem., *14*:215, 1966.)

brane and containing a crystalline *nucleoid* eccentrically placed in a moderately dense, finely granular matrix. Their crystalline inclusions have been isolated and found to contain *uricase.* The positive staining of peroxisomes with the histochemical reaction for peroxidase activity is attributed to the enzyme *catalase,* which is present in the matrix (Fahimi). It is presumed that microbodies function within the cytoplasm in a manner comparable to the lysosomes, but their actual significance in the economy of the cell remains to be elucidated.

Zonation Within the Liver Lobule

In organs with multiple functions, it is often possible to demonstrate cytological differences between cells performing different functions. In the liver, despite its manifold and quite diverse activities, the cells are all basically very similar in their appearance. All of the parenchymal cells are probably capable of carrying out all of the functions of the liver. However, cytologists have long believed that the degree of their activity under normal conditions depends primarily on their location within the lobule. The classical lobule can be divided into concentric zones on the basis of the cytological evidences of activity of the cells. A zone of varying width around the periphery of the lobule has been designated the "zone of permanent function." Next there is an intermediate "zone of varying activity" and finally a narrow zone around the central vein that is called the "zone of permanent repose" (Noel). These correspond respectively to the portions of the lobule where the liver cells are most favorably situated, are intermediate, and are least favorably situated with respect to the sequence in which oxygen and nutrients reach them in the blood entering the sinusoids from the terminal branches of the hepatic artery and portal vein at the periphery of the lobule (at the center of the functional unit of Rappaport). This zonation is quite striking in the mouse but less obvious in other species.

Typically, after the feeding of a large meal, glycogen is deposited first in the zone of permanent function at the periphery of the lobule. During active digestion, glycogen fills cells progressively farther into the intermediate zone until, in extreme cases, all but the cells immediately adjacent to the central vein may be filled with it. With the conclusion of digestion, carbohydrate is returned to the blood, as needed, by removal of the glycogen, beginning at the most centrally located deposits. If the fast is prolonged, glycogen may ultimately disappear completely at the periphery. Thus, in an animal such as the mouse, which normally feeds at night, there is a diurnal tide of glycogen within the lobule, which may be spectacularly accentuated by restricting the feeding time to one hour, with the animal fasting the rest of the day.

Accompanying this tide is a corresponding change in the mitochondria. Those in the zone of permanent repose are thin, elongated, and sparse, staining so lightly that they are frequently seen only with difficulty in mitochondrial preparations. In the zone of permanent function, however, they are large, deeply staining spheres or short rods that may crowd the cytoplasm. In the intermediate zone, the rods become progressively elongated until, as one approaches the central zone, they are slender filaments. The width of the intermediate zone varies with the state of the diurnal tide of alimentation. In other species including man, such changes are not demonstrable.

Under certain conditions, both pathological and physiological, fat may accumulate in the liver. Usually this appears first in the cells of the central zone as small spherical droplets; these become progressively larger by

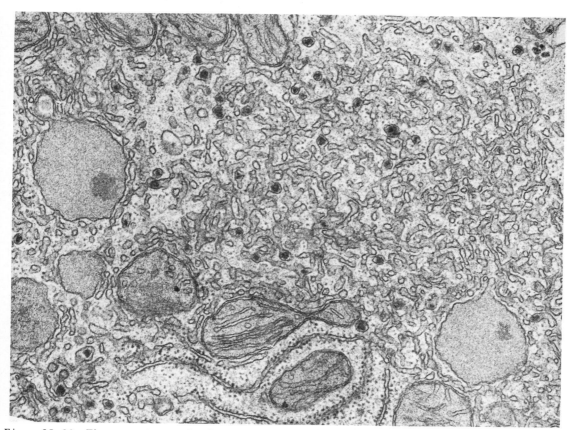

Figure 28–20 Electron micrograph of hepatocyte cytoplasm showing smooth surfaced reticulum containing small, spherical dense particles representing newly synthesized very low density serum lipoprotein. Also present are two microbodies or peroxisomes with eccentrically placed nucleoids. (Micrograph by R. Bolender.)

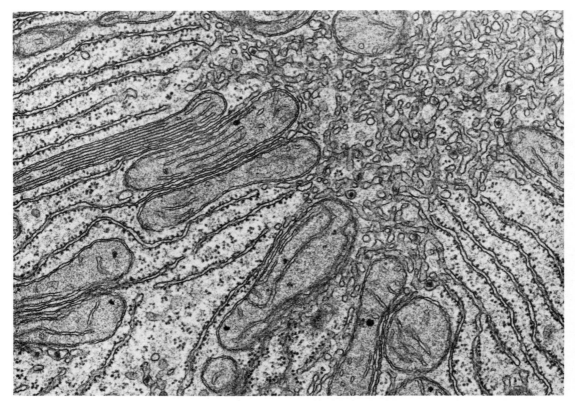

Figure 28–21 Electron micrograph of a small area of hepatocyte cytoplasm including several mitochondria, cisternal profiles of granular endoplasmic reticulum, and, at the upper right, a close meshed plexus of agranular reticulum. (Micrograph by R. Bolender.)

coalescence as well as by further accumulation, until the cell may be distended by a single large drop. In certain conditions, notably some sustained dietary deficiencies, fat is deposited in the peripheral rather than in the central zone. In both cases, fat may disappear when the condition responsible is corrected.

Position in the lobule may not be the only determining factor in the relative activity of liver cells. Application of the fluorescent antibody technique to localize the sites of production of plasma albumin has shown marked differences among liver cells immediately adjacent to one another, and the distribution of active cells in this case appears to bear little relation to the familiar zonation within the lobule.

Bile Canaliculi

These are minute canals that run between liver cells throughout the parenchyma.

As a rule, a single canaliculus runs between each adjacent pair of cells. Thus, in a plate of liver cells that is one cell thick, the bile canaliculi form a network having hexagonal meshes with a single cell in each mesh. However, because the laminae of parenchymal cells branch and anastomose, the canaliculi form a three dimensional net with polyhedral meshes. In amphibians, there are small branches that extend between cells from a core canaliculus and end blindly. It is now generally agreed that there are no such blind branches in the mammalian liver. The canaliculi form a continuous network without a break from lobule to lobule throughout the parenchyma. Intracellular branches have been reported to penetrate the cytoplasm, but these descriptions seem to be a misinterpretation of vacuoles that often occur in the cytoplasm adjacent to the canaliculus and in conjunction with the Golgi complex. These may appear more prominently under conditions of anoxia or during excretion of vital dyes and may, in fact, discharge into the canaliculus, but no permanent intracellular bile canals have been demonstrated. The membrane lining the canaliculi is a site of adenosine triphosphatase activity, and histochemical reactions for this enzyme provide a useful method for selectively staining this system of minute intercellular canals (Fig. 28–26).

From observations with the light microscope, it seemed reasonable to assume that the bile canaliculi were distinct entities having walls of their own. Indeed, it was suggested that their hexagonal network around the hepatic cells contributed significantly to the structural stability of the liver. The electron microscope has now shown that the lumen of the bile canaliculus is merely an expansion of the intercellular space and that its wall is simply a local specialization of the surfaces of adjoining hepatic cells (Fig. 28–27). Over most

of their length, the apposed membranes of the two cells are relatively straight and separated by an intercellular space about 150 Å wide. At the site of the bile canaliculus they diverge to form a canalicular intercellular space 0.5 to 1 μm. in diameter. The portion of the cell membrane bordering on this space bears short microvilli that project into its lumen. Along the margins of the canaliculus the membranes of the opposing cells come into close contact and are fused to form an occluding junction comparable to the zonula occludens of other epithelia. These two bands of tight junction evidently seal the commissures of the canaliculus and prevent its contents from escaping into the narrow intercellular cleft on either side. A narrow zone of cytoplasm immediately adjacent to the canaliculus is free of organelles and has the finely fibrillar structure characteristic of a firmly gelated ectoplasmic layer.

In addition to the zonulae occludentes

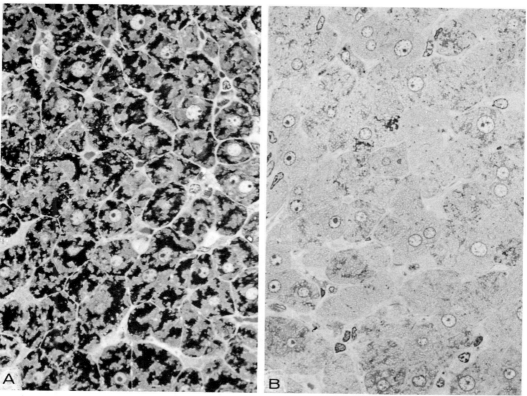

Figure 28–22 Dietary differences in amount of stored glycogen are clearly illustrated by comparison of these photomicrographs of rat liver. *A,* Liver of an animal fasted for 2 hours and containing 8.2 per cent glycogen. *B,* Liver of an animal fasted for 21 hours containing 0.9 per cent glycogen. (From R. Cardell et al., Anat. Rec., *177*:23, 1973.)

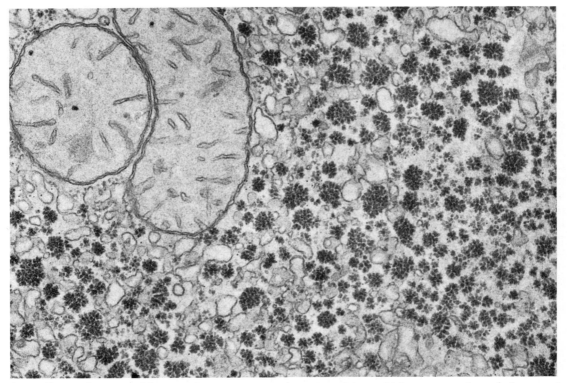

Figure 28-23 An area of hamster hepatocyte cytoplasm containing a high concentration of glycogen in aggregations of varying size (alpha particles). The glycogen is closely associated with profiles of the agranular endoplasmic reticulum.

adjacent to the canaliculus a number of nexuses or gap-junctions are found on the boundaries between adjoining hepatic cells. These are believed to be sites of low electrical resistance that permit communication between cells and provide for coordination of their physiological activities. These junctional specializations are visible in electron micrographs of thin sections, but they are studied to best advantage in freeze-fracture preparations (Fig. 28–28). They have now been isolated for biochemical analysis (Goodenough).

There is probably a matrix material between the microvilli of the bile canaliculi that is not revealed in electron micrographs. That the canaliculi and their junctional complexes form a fairly rigid structure possessing some integrity is demonstrated by the fact that they persist as tubules when the cells are teased apart. Tubular fragments of them may also be found in homogenates of liver tissue.

The bile canaliculi vary in diameter, be-

coming somewhat distended with active secretion and more or less collapsed with decreasing activity. When distended, the microvilli are more widely scattered and appear to be shorter, and when collapsed, the microvilli may pack the lumen so completely that it is virtually occluded. This is possibly the reason why the canaliculi are hard to see with the light microscope.

The junction of the bile canaliculus with the bile duct system is not easily demonstrated. The fine terminal branches of the bile duct leave the portal canal with the terminal branch of the portal vein and penetrate the parenchyma between two lobules—that is, in the core of a functional unit of Rappaport. They are so small and have such thin walls that they are recognized only with difficulty. They appear so different from the smallest bile ducts that they are designated ductules or *cholangioles*. They have small diverticula that expand against the adjacent parenchyma and

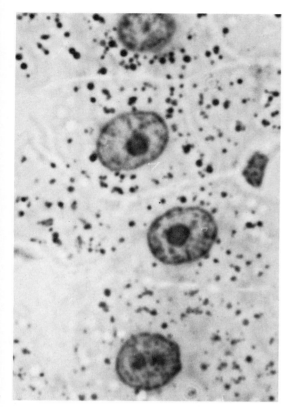

Figure 28-24 Photomicrograph of rat liver stained by a histochemical reaction for demonstration of peroxidase activity. The distribution of reactive granules corresponds to that of the microbodies or peroxisomes identifiable in electron micrographs. (Micrograph from D. Fahimi, J. Cell Biol., *43*:275, 1969.)

are applied tightly to it, cell to cell. The bile capillaries continue between the hepatic cells to empty into the lumen of the diverticulum. The whole arrangement is well demonstrated if the cholangioles and bile canaliculi are distended, as they are following occlusion of the bile duct. The diverticula then appear especially distended and have consequently been designated *ampullae*. The ends of the canaliculi here are the only ends in the continuous polygonal network.

Connective Tissue

For an organ of its size, the liver has remarkably little connective tissue. Underlying the surface capsule, extending into the portal canals, and following them to their finest branches, is a small amount of dense connective tissue. The extent of the connective tissue skeleton of the liver was first clearly revealed by classical histologists after the parenchyma was macerated away in water, leaving the fibrous skeleton floating free. It is called Glisson's capsule. On the surface, it forms the thin connective tissue layer beneath the peritoneal mesothelium. Within the portal canals, it forms a common sheath around the branches of the portal veins, the hepatic artery, and the bile duct, and it contains the network of lymphatics that drains the lymph from the liver. In these sites it is typical connective tissue with dense collagenous fibers and occasional fibroblasts. Within the lobule, the only skeletal structure is a network of reticular fibers between the sinusoid lining and the hepatic cell plates (Fig. 28-29). This is demonstrated by various techniques, but especially well by some of the silver techniques. At the periphery of the lobule, where the portal veins enter the sinusoids, the collagenous fibers of the portal canals become continuous with the network of reticular fibers surrounding the sinusoids. This reticulum is the supporting tissue of the liver parenchyma. It contains no fibroblasts, the fibers apparently being formed by the sinusoid lining cells as they are in other regions of the reticuloendothelial system.

Lymph Spaces

The liver produces a large amount of lymph. The major part of the thoracic duct lymph comes from the liver, less from the intestine via the mesenteric lymphatics, and still less from the other organs of the posterior part of the body. The hepatic lymph differs from the rest of the lymph in that it contains a large amount of plasma protein, with the ratio of albumin to globulin only a little higher than in the plasma. The origin of liver lymph is still a matter of active investigation. The network of lymphatics follows the portal vein to its finest terminal branches. Here it ends in the tenuous connective tissue sheath. No lymphatics have been demonstrated within the lobule. The most probable assumption is that plasma traversing the discontinuities in the sinusoid lining and entering the space of Disse moves along toward the periphery of the lobule, bathing the microvilli and exchanging material with the hepatic cells as

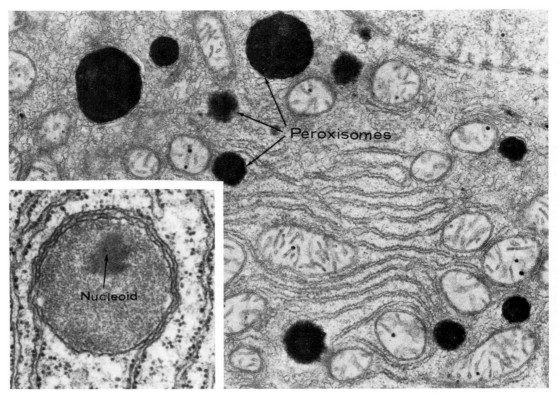

Figure 28–25 Microbodies or peroxisomes of rodent liver are limited by a single membrane and contain a "nucleoid" consisting of a paracrystalline array of tubular subunits. (Micrograph by R. Wood.) When stained for peroxidase activity, the matrix of the microbodies reacts intensely but the nucleoid remains unstained. (From D. Fahimi, J. Cell Biol., *43*:275, 1969.)

it goes. Then it apparently percolates into the tissue space around the interlobular twigs of the bile duct, the portal vein, and their accompanying lymphatics. It thus becomes the tissue fluid of this space, and the liver lymph is drained from it by the lymphatic vessels (Fig. 28–30).

REGENERATION

The liver parenchyma, compared to that of many other organs, is fairly stable in that the cells rarely need to be replaced in a normal adult. It is, nevertheless, capable of spectacular regeneration. In the rat, two thirds of the liver may be removed and in a few days most of the tissue extirpated will be replaced. Similarly, after administration of some hepatotoxic agents, notably the chlorinated hydrocarbons, a substantial part of each lobule may

be destroyed, and in this case too, the lost tissue is rapidly replaced.

Regeneration after partial hepatectomy consists of growth and cell division throughout the remaining liver mass. Hence, the division into lobes is not restored. Most of the research on regeneration has been done on the rat and the mouse, in which the amount restored is usually as great as the amount removed, although in old rats it may be somewhat less. In other animals, the amount regenerated may be considerably less, in inverse ratio to the size of the animal.

Central necrosis after a toxic dose of carbon tetrachloride may involve as much as one third to one half of each lobule and is remarkably uniform throughout the liver in the rat or mouse. In an uncomplicated case, only the parenchymal cells are killed, leaving the sinusoid linings intact, so that the circulation through the lobule is maintained. The necrotic cells are removed by autolysis, while the

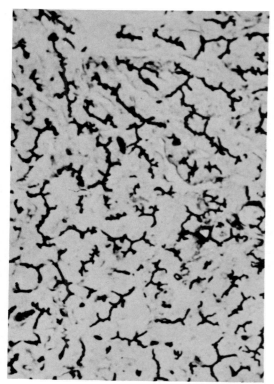

Figure 28-26 Photomicrograph of rat liver, showing the branching pattern of bile canaliculi, which are demonstrated here by their positive histochemical staining reaction for adenosine triphosphatase. × 200. (Courtesy of A. Novikoff.)

cells in the remaining part of the lobule divide rapidly by mitosis. The mass of normal liver tissue increases until in five or six days the original pattern of the liver is completely restored. If the dose of carbon tetrachloride is repeated at regular intervals when regeneration is still in progress, thus repeatedly producing new injury before the old has been repaired, fibrosis appears, and if it is continued long enough, cirrhosis of the liver ensues.

If the cellular injury is at the periphery of the lobule, as after bile duct occlusion or after treatment with certain hepatotoxic agents, there may be cell division throughout the remaining tissue, but there is also considerable mitotic activity in the epithelium of the bile ductules and smaller bile ducts, with a corresponding increase in the number of ductules and small ducts. The ductules penetrate into the injured peripheral part of the lobule, apparently to re-establish a pathway

for bile drainage that has been interrupted by the death of the peripheral cells and dissolution of their bile canaliculi. If the injury continues, the increase in ductules and ducts may develop into a spectacular proliferation of the bile ducts. If it does not continue, the normal architecture of the liver is rapidly restored, with the disappearance of the new ducts and ductules. It is not clear whether the duct cells atrophy and disappear or transform into parenchymal cells. In repair after severe injury, the occurrence of intermediate cells gives credence to the latter possibility.

The problem of the initiation of mitosis in a normally quiescent tissue and of its cessation when the lost tissue has been replaced has been extensively investigated, and partial hepatectomy with the ensuing regeneration is an important system in which to study a great variety of biological problems.

HISTOPHYSIOLOGY

Because of the remarkable range of its biochemical functions in intermediary metabolism and its strategic location in the circulation, the liver acts as a vital organ for processing nutrients absorbed from the gastrointestinal tract and for transforming them into materials needed by the other specialized tissues of the body.

One of its most important functions is the maintenance of the normal blood glucose concentration. Liver cells take up glucose from the blood and by means of a series of enzymatic reactions polymerize it to form glycogen, the storage form of carbohydrate. Simpler compounds, such as lactic acid, glycerol, and pyruvic acid, can be converted in the liver into glucose and thence to glycogen. As the need arises, glycogen is broken down to glucose again by a process of phosphorylation, catalyzed by the enzyme phosphorylase. This enzyme usually occurs in an inactive form but is specifically activated by the hormones epinephrine and glucagon, which act upon the liver and cause it to release glucose into the blood.

Many of the enzymes involved in glycogenesis and glycogenolysis are free in the cytoplasmic matrix. These functions, therefore, cannot be attributed to any particular cell organelle. However, in electron micrographs, the glycogen is usually localized in

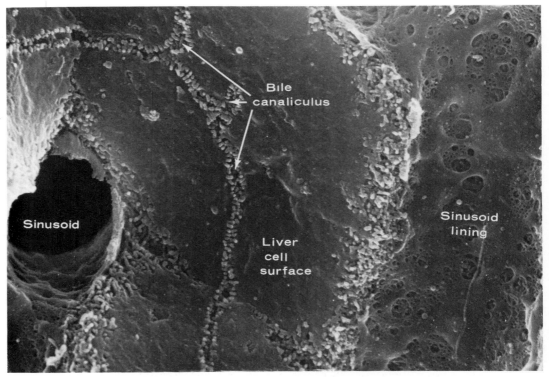

Figure 28-27 A scanning electron micrograph of rat liver in which a plate of liver cells between two sinusoids has been broken across, revealing the bile canaliculus as a groove lined with short microvilli. The other half of the canaliculus would be on the surface of the liver cell broken away from cells shown here. (Micrograph courtesy of M. Karnovsky.)

areas of cytoplasm rich in smooth surfaced endoplasmic reticulum. The exact significance of this close topographical relationship is not yet clear, but the enzyme glucose-6-phosphatase, which is known to reside in these membranes, may participate in some way in the release of glucose to the blood.

The liver also plays a decisive role in the metabolism and transport of lipids and in the maintenance of lipid levels in the circulating blood. The lipids in the blood plasma are derived from ingested food, from mobilization of fat reserves in adipose tissue, or from synthesis from carbohydrate or protein in the liver. The main vehicle for the transport of lipids from all of these sources is the plasma *lipoprotein*, and it is in the liver that the transformation of lipids into serum lipoprotein takes place. Small spherical particles 300 to 1000 Å in diameter are seen in electron micrographs of the livers of fed animals in agranular terminal expansions of the granular reticulum, in tubular elements of the smooth reticulum, in exocytotic vesicles at the cell

surface, and in the space of Disse. These particles are thought to contain a triglyceride lipid core surrounded by a more water soluble, polar surface coat of protein, phospholipid, and cholesterol.

In the isolated perfused liver, the number of these particles is strikingly increased when fatty acids are added to the perfusate. These particles represent very low density lipoproteins being formed in the liver and released into the space of Disse. Triglycerides are formed from fatty acids in the smooth reticulum, and these are combined there with protein synthesized in the granular reticulum to form lipoprotein particles (Fig. 28-31). There is also good evidence that the reticulum, particularly the agranular form, plays an important part in the synthesis of cholesterol in the liver. An experimentally induced increase in the abundance of smooth reticulum is accompanied by an enhanced capacity to synthesize cholesterol from acetate (Jones).

The liver is the site of synthesis of *plasma*

proteins, and the rate of their production is quite substantial. Studies on the isolated perfused organ indicate that the liver of an adult rat synthesizes in excess of 13 mg. of albumin per day. It is likely that the organelle principally involved is the granular endoplasmic reticulum. A fine flocculent or filamentous substance is sometimes observed in the lumen of the cisternae, and protein with the properties of albumin has been identified in liver microsomes, but the entire secretory pathway has not been worked out.

In addition to serum albumin, the liver produces alpha and beta globulins, the enzymes of the blood plasma, glycoproteins, and lipoproteins. The concentrations of these substances in the blood can be used clinically as a measure of liver cell function. Because

prothrombin and a number of other protein factors involved in blood clotting are formed by the hepatocytes, liver disease may result in a tendency to bleed excessively from minor injuries.

The liver is responsible for the metabolism of a large variety of lipid soluble drugs, including the barbiturates commonly used as sedatives. The enzymes responsible for the degradation of these compounds are localized mainly in the smooth surfaced microsome fraction of liver homogenates and hence reside in the agranular reticulum of the intact liver cell. Moreover, it has recently been found that administration of such drugs induces a marked increase in the smooth surfaced membranes of the cytoplasm and that this morphological change is accompanied by

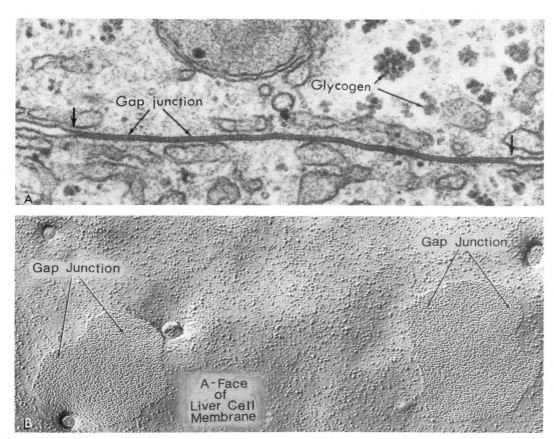

Figure 28–28 *A,* An electron micrograph of a portion of the boundary between two liver cells in thin section, showing the cell membranes converging at the arrows and coming into close apposition to form a nexus or gap junction between the arrows. (Micrograph courtesy of R. Wood.) *B,* A surface replica of an area of liver cell membrane freeze-fractured to expose its A-face. In addition to the population of randomly distributed intramembranous particles, there are two gap junctions exhibiting closely packed particles of uniform diameter. (Micrograph courtesy of A. Yee.)

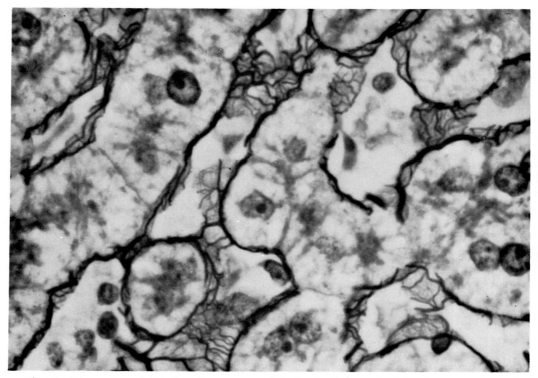

Figure 28-29 Photomicrograph of rat liver prepared by Pap's silver method for demonstrating reticulum. A fine meshwork of argyrophilic fibers is situated between the hepatic cells and the cells lining the sinusoids. × 1250.

a concomitant increase in the drug metabolizing enzymes (Figs. 28–19, 28–20, and 28–21). These changes evidently do not represent toxic effects of the drug but rather an adaptive response of the liver cell, which enhances its efficiency in eliminating the inducing drug. These morphological and biochemical changes thus appear to be the basis of *drug tolerance* — the progressive loss of effectiveness of a drug with continued use. Certain of the steps in the metabolism of steroid hormones in the liver take place also in the endoplasmic reticulum and probably depend upon some of the same hydroxylating enzymes that are involved in the metabolism of exogenous drugs.

An important excretory function of the liver is the uptake and excretion of the pigment *bilirubin*, which originates from the breakdown of aged red blood cells being eliminated from the circulation by Kupffer cells and other phagocytes of the reticuloendothelial system. This substance, carried in the blood, is normally conjugated with glucuronide in the liver by enzymes in the endoplasmic reticulum. The conjugate, bilirubin glucuronide, is excreted into the bile. In the intestine, it is reduced by the action of bacteria into a group of compounds collectively referred to as *urobilinogens*. While most of this is eliminated in the feces, some is reabsorbed and re-excreted in the bile. When bilirubin accumulates in the blood (hyperbilirubinemia), a person becomes jaundiced. This may result from (1) increased production of bilirubin beyond the capacity of the liver to excrete it—e.g., in hemolytic jaundice; (2) decreased uptake of bilirubin by the liver; (3) disturbance in conjugation of bilirubin in the liver—e.g., in jaundice of the newborn; (4) interference with excretion due to obstruction of the bile duct system. Determination of the relative amounts of conjugated and unconjugated bilirubin in the blood is therefore an important means of evaluating liver function and of distinguishing among the several causes of jaundice in patients.

BILE DUCTS

The constituents of the bile are emptied into the bile canaliculi, which communicate with the interlobular bile ducts by the canals of Hering. The finest radicles of the bile ducts are 15 to 20 μm. in diameter and have a small lumen surrounded by cuboidal epithelial cells. They do not have a striated border, and their cytoplasm rarely contains fat droplets. The cells show occasional mitoses. These small ducts lie on a basal lamina immediately surrounded by dense collagenous bundles.

The interlobular bile ducts form a richly anastomosing network that closely surrounds the branches of the portal vein. Closer to the porta, the lumen of the ducts gradually be-comes larger, while the epithelium becomes taller (the ducts of the second order) and has a layer of mitochondria at the base of its cells and another near the free border. These cells commonly contain fat droplets and, when these are numerous, cholesterol crystals. Although a faint thickening of the periphery of these cells may be seen in some animals, it is not found in man. Lymphocytes are frequently seen migrating through the epithelium into the lumen. As the ducts become larger, the surrounding layers of collagenous connective tissue become thicker and contain many elastic fibers. At the transverse fossa of the liver, the main ducts from the different lobes of the liver fuse to form the *hepatic duct*, which, after receiving the *cystic duct*, continues from the gallbladder to the duodenum as the *common bile duct (ductus choledochus)*.

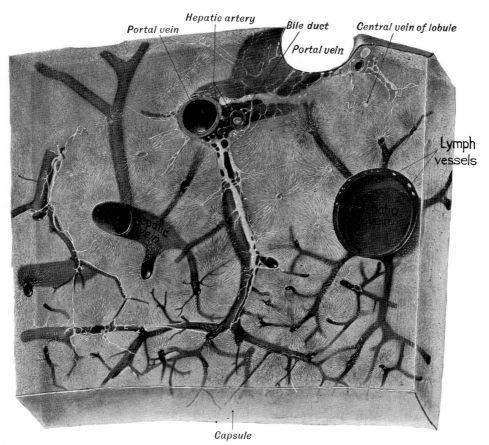

Figure 28–30 Thick section of liver of adult cat, cleared in oil of wintergreen. The lymphatic network appears pale and the blood vessels dark. The lymphatic vessels are confined to the interlobular connective tissue, where they surround the branches of the larger blood vessels and bile ducts. × 16. (After F. C. Lee.)

The epithelium of the extrahepatic ducts is tall columnar. The mucosa is thrown into many folds and is said to yield an atypical variety of mucus. The scanty subepithelial connective tissue contains large numbers of elastic fibers, some lymphoid cells and occasional leukocytes; many of these penetrate the epithelium and pass into the lumen. Scattered bundles of smooth muscles first appear in the common bile duct; they run in the longitudinal and oblique directions, and form an incomplete layer around the wall of the duct. As it nears the duodenum, the smooth muscle layer of the ductus choledochus becomes more prominent, and its intramural portions function as a sort of sphincter in regulating the flow of bile.

THE GALLBLADDER AND CHOLEDOCHODUODENAL JUNCTION

The gallbladder is a pear-shaped, hollow viscus closely attached to the posterior surface of the liver. It consists of a blindly ending fundus, a body, and a neck, which continues into the cystic duct. Normally it measures ap- proximately 10 by 4 cm. in adult man, and in most animals it has a capacity of 1 to 2 ml. per kg. of body weight. It shows marked variations in shape and size and is frequently the seat of pathological processes that change its size and the thickness of its wall. The mucosa is easily destroyed, so that in most specimens removed even a short time after death, large areas of epithelium are found to be desquamated or disintegrating.

Histology of the Gallbladder

The choledochoduodenal junction comprises the portion of the duodenal wall that is traversed by the common bile duct (ductus choledochus) the pancreatic duct (ductus pancreaticus) and the short ampulla into which they empty. For most of its length it consists of an oblique passage through the tela submucosa; it is guarded proximally by a contractile "window" in the muscle of the duodenum and distally by the valvules of the ampulla of Vater. From fenestra to ostium, the associated bile and pancreatic passages are invested by a common musculus proprius, the *sphincter of Oddi.*

In man this may consist of four parts: the *sphincter choledochus,* a strong annular sheath which invests the common bile duct from just outside the fenestra to its junction with the pancreatic duct; the *fasciculi longitudinales,* longitudinal bundles which span the interval between the two ducts and extend from the margins of the fenestra to the ampulla; the *sphincter ampullae,* a meshwork of fibers about the ampulla of Vater (if present), which is strongly developed in only one sixth of adults; and the *sphincter pancreaticus,* present in variable form, either alone or combined with the sphincter choledochus in a figure-eight configuration. The sphincter choledochus is so placed that its contraction stops the flow of bile. The longitudinal fasciculi tend to shorten the intramural portion of the ducts, thus facilitating the flow of bile into the duodenum. The sphincter ampullae, when strongly developed, can create abnormally a continuous channel between bile and pancreatic ducts. An undesirable consequence of this is to permit reflux of bile into the pancreatic duct.

The wall consists of the following layers: a mucosa consisting of a surface epithelium and a lamina propria, a layer of smooth muscles, a perimuscular connective tissue

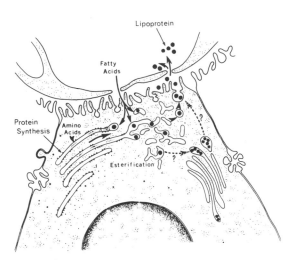

Figure 28–31 Diagram illustrating intracellular pathway of synthesis and release of very low density serum lipoprotein (VLDL). Fatty acids from the blood are esterified in the smooth reticulum to form triglycerides. These are combined with protein synthesized on ribosomes associated with the rough reticulum. The particles are released into the space of Disse and enter the blood in the sinusoids.

layer (Fig. 28–32), and a serous layer, covering a part of the organ. The mucosa is thrown into frequent folds or rugae. The major folds are subdivided into many smaller folds; they are easily seen in the contracted or even the partially distended organ. But when the viscus is greatly distended its wall becomes much thinner and most of the folds disappear, although some of them can always be seen.

The epithelium consists of a single layer of tall columnar cells, with oval nuclei (Fig. 28–32). The cytoplasm stains faintly with eosin. An inconspicuous striated border is present in histological sections, but with the electron microscope the apical surface of the tall columnar cells is found to bear a large number of microvilli (Fig. 28–34). These are somewhat shorter and less regular in their orientation than are those of the striated border of the intestinal epithelium. At the tips of the microvilli the membrane bears minute filiform appendages similar to the filamentous surface coat found on intestinal mucosa and on various other epithelia.

From a study of thin sections with the transmission electron microscope one gains the erroneous impression that the microvilli are not especially numerous (Fig. 28–34). However, when this epithelium is viewed with the scanning microscope, the surface has a velvety appearance due to the presence of very large numbers of short microvilli (Figs. 28–35 and 28–36).

The lateral cell boundaries are relatively straight at the apical portion of the epithelium, but from the level of the nucleus to the basal lamina there is a complex plication and interdigitation of the cell surface. The intercellular space in the upper portion of the epithelium is 150 to 200 Å wide and is sealed near the lumen by a typical zonula occludens. Toward the base, the intercellular space may be narrow or greatly widened. The degree of distention of the intercellular clefts at the base appears to depend upon the functional state of the gallbladder epithelium.

In the lamina propria and in the perimuscular layer near the neck of the gallbladder are simple tubuloalveolar glands. Their epithelium is cuboidal and clear, and the dark nuclei are compressed at the base of the cell. They thus stand out sharply against the darker, tall columnar epithelium of the gallbladder. These glands are said to secrete mucus.

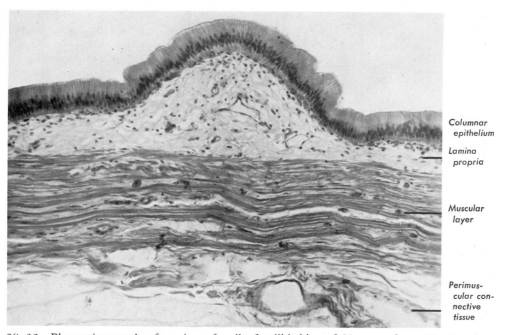

Columnar
epithelium

Lamina
propria

Muscular
layer

Perimus-
cular con-
nective
tissue

Figure 28–32 Photomicrograph of section of wall of gallbladder of *Macacus rhesus*. Fixation by vascular perfusion. × 142.

Outpouchings of the mucosa have sometimes been confused with glands. These are lined by and are continuous with the surface epithelium and extend through the lamina propria and the muscular layer. They are called *Rokitansky-Aschoff sinuses* and probably are indicators of a pathological change in the wall of the organ that permits an evagination of the mucosa through the enlarged meshes of the submucosal muscular network. They are not found in embryonic gallbladders and should not be confused with the "true" ducts of Luschka (vide infra), for the latter never communicate with the lumen of the gallbladder.

Beneath the epithelium is an irregular network of longitudinal, transverse, and oblique smooth muscle fibers, accompanied by a network of elastic fibers. The spaces between the bundles of muscles are occupied by collagenous, reticular, and some elastic fibers, with a sprinkling of fibroblasts. The blood vessels and lymphatics contained in the peri-

muscular layer send branches into and through the muscular layer to the mucosa.

External to the muscular layer is a fairly dense connective tissue layer which completely surrounds the gallbladder and is in places continuous with the interlobular connective tissue of the liver. It contains many collagenous and a few elastic fibers and scattered fibroblasts, with a few macrophages and lymphoid wandering cells, small lobules of fat cells, and the blood vessels, nerves, and lymphatics supplying the organ.

Not infrequently, particularly in the hepatic surface and near the neck, peculiar ductlike structures may be seen. They can be traced for considerable distances in this connective tissue layer, and some of them connect with the bile ducts. They never connect with the lumen of the gallbladder and are probably aberrant bile ducts laid down during the embryonic development of the biliary system. They have been called "true" *Luschka ducts*, to distinguish them from epithelial outpouchings of the mucosa.

The portion of the gallbladder not attached to the liver is covered with the peritoneum. Through it the ramifying arteries, veins, and lymphatics can be seen with the unaided eye. This serosal layer is continuous with that covering the liver.

The gallbladder continues at its neck into the cystic duct. The wall of the latter is thrown into prominent folds which constitute the *spiral valve of Heister.* These folds are said to contain smooth muscle bundles and are thought to prevent distention or collapse of the cystic duct when the latter is subjected to sudden changes of pressure.

Blood Vessels

The gallbladder is supplied with blood by the cystic artery. The venous blood is collected by veins that empty primarily into capillaries of the liver and only secondarily into the cystic branch of the portal vein. A prominent feature of the gallbladder is its rich supply of lymphatic vessels, of which there are two main plexuses, one in the lamina propria (but not within the rugae) and the other in the connective tissue layer. The latter plexus receives tributaries from the liver, thus affording an explanation for hepatogenous cholecystitis. These plexuses are collected into larger lymphatics, which pass through the lymph node or nodes at the neck

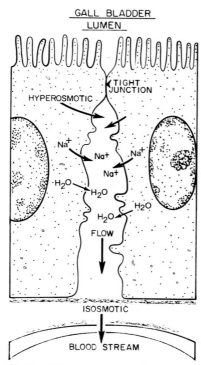

GALL BLADDER
LUMEN

HYPEROSMOTIC

TIGHT JUNCTION

Na+   Na+   Na+

Na+

H₂O   H₂O   H₂O

H₂O

FLOW

ISOSMOTIC

BLOOD STREAM

Figure 28-33 Diagram illustrating the probable mechanism of concentration of the bile. Sodium is actively pumped into the intercellular cleft below the occluding junction, creating a standing gradient that moves water from the lumen to the blood vessels in the wall of the gallbladder.

of the bladder and then accompany the cystic and common bile ducts. They pass through several lymph nodes near the duodenum and finally communicate with the cisterna chyli.

Nerves

The nerves are branches of the splanchnic sympathetic and the vagus nerves. Study of the effects of stimulation of these nerves has given rise to contradictory reports by different investigators. It is probable that both excitatory and inhibitory fibers are contained in each of them. Of greater clinical importance are the sensory nerve endings, because overdistention or spasms of the extrahepatic biliary tract inhibit respiration and set up reflex disturbances in the gut.

Histophysiology of the Gallbladder

The gallbladder serves as a site of concentration and storage of bile, which is secreted continuously by the liver. The bile does not normally enter the intestine until a specific stimulus causes the gallbladder to contract. The stimulus is usually the presence of lipid in the small intestine. Ingestion of fat automatically causes discharge of the contents of the gallbladder. After a test meal of egg yolks or cream, three fourths of its content are expelled within 40 minutes.

When fat enters the small intestine, it causes release of a hormone, *cholecystokinin*, from the mucosa. This is carried via the blood to the gallbladder, inducing rhythmic contractions. In the peristalsis of the duodenum, as waves of relaxation of its smooth muscle pass by the ampulla of Vater, the tonic contraction of the sphincter of Oddi (vide infra) relaxes, permitting intermittent outflow of bile. Thus the emptying of the gallbladder results from the combined action of cholecystokinin on the musculature of the gallbladder and peristalsis in the duodenum.

Of special clinical importance is the concentrating function of the gallbladder. Its mucosa withdraws water and inorganic ions

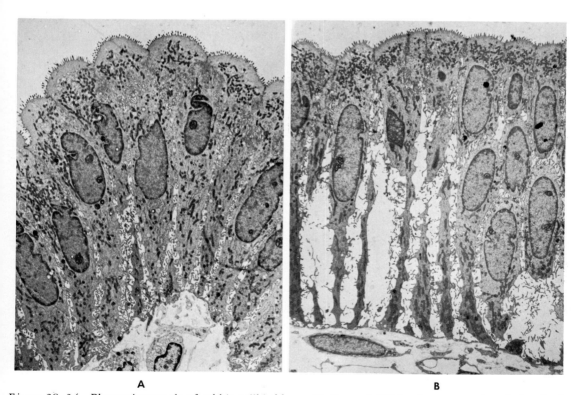

A **B**

Figure 28-34 Photomicrograph of rabbit gallbladder epithelium. *A,* With a hyperosmotic solution in the lumen the net water flux is very low and the intercellular spaces at the base of the epithelium are relatively inconspicuous. *B,* In a gallbladder actively transporting fluid in vitro, the intercellular spaces are greatly distended. × 1400. (Courtesy of G. Kaye, J. Cell Biol., 30:237, 1966.)

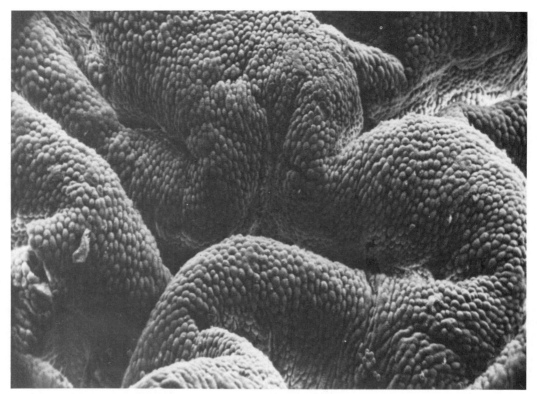

Figure 28–35 A scanning electron micrograph of mucosal folds of the guinea pig gallbladder. The convex apical ends of the individual epithelial cells are clearly identifiable. (Micrograph from Mueller, Jones, and Long, Gastroenterology, *63*:856, 1972. © 1972 The Williams & Wilkins Co., Baltimore.)

from the bile. Recent experimental studies suggest the mechanism. In gallbladders known to be transporting fluid in vivo, the intercellular spaces at the base of the epithelium are always distended and the subepithelial capillaries are dilated. In experiments carried out in vitro, if either sodium or calcium is omitted from the medium, there is no fluid transport and the intercellular spaces are narrow. If either ion is replaced, fluid transport is restored and the intercellular spaces again appear distended. It is believed that during concentration of bile, active transport of solute across the lateral cell membrane increases the concentration of solute in the intercellular space (Figs. 28–33 and 28–34). Because of the resulting osmotic gradient, water moves into and through the cell to the intercellular space, causing its distention. Development of hydrostatic pressure in this space drives the solution across the basal lamina into the submucosa (Kaye et al.).

The functional capacity of the gallbladder is assessed clinically by observing its capacity to concentrate halogen salts of phenolphthalein which are opaque to x-rays (Graham-Cole test). Failure to visualize the gallbladder after this test indicates that the organ is diseased or occluded. If the mucosa is damaged, it may lose its concentrating power. Undoubtedly, absorption of bile salts under such conditions is an important factor in the precipitation of gallstones. After obstruction of the cystic duct the bile may be resorbed in toto or replaced by a colorless fluid consisting largely of exudate and mucus.

There is little evidence in favor of a secretory function of the gallbladder. In the pathological gallbladder two or three types of granular inclusions are found in the epithelial cells. Their chemical nature is not known, but it is likely that they are lysosomal rather than secretory. They probably represent abnormal deposits of material absorbed from

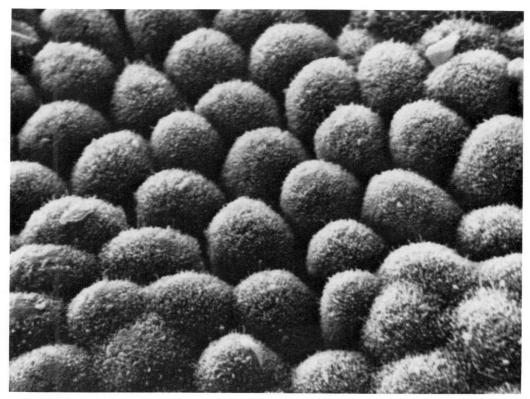

Figure 28-36 Scanning electron micrograph of the luminal surface of gallbladder epithelium. The convex apical ends of the cells are covered with short microvilli. (Micrograph from Mueller, Jones, and Long, Gastroenterology, *63*:856, 1972. © 1972 The Williams & Wilkins Co., Baltimore.)

the bile. Some mucus is added to the bile as it passes down the larger bile ducts, and mucus secreting glands are fairly numerous in the neck. In some mammalian species no gallbladder is present. Its surgical removal in man is often followed by a marked dilatation of the biliary passages.

REFERENCES

Liver

Arey, L. B.: On the presence of so-called portal lobules in the seal's liver. Anat. Rec., *51*:315, 1932.

Ashworth, C. T., and E. Sanders: Anatomic pathway of bile formation. Am. J. Path., *37*:343, 1960.

Ashworth, C. T., V. A. Stembridge, and E. Sanders: Lipid absorption, transport and hepatic assimilation studied with electron microscope. Am. J. Physiol., *198*:1326, 1960.

Biava, C. G.: Studies on cholestasis: A re-evaluation of the fine structure of normal human bile canaliculi. Lab. Invest., *13*:840, 1964.

Boak, J. L., G. H. Christie, W. L. Ford, and J. G. Howard: Pathways in the development of liver macrophages; alternative precursors contained in populations of lymphocytes and bone-marrow cells. Proc. Roy. Soc. B., *169*:307, 1968.

Brauer, R. W.: Liver circulation and function. Physiol. Rev., *43*:115, 1963.

Bronfenmajer, S., F. Schaffer, and H. Popper: Fat-storing cells (lipocytes) in human liver. Arch. Path., *82*:447, 1966.

Bruni, C., and K. R. Porter: The fine structure of the parenchymal cell of the normal rat liver. I. General observations. Am. J. Path., *46*:691, 1965.

Bucher, N. L. R.: Experimental aspects of hepatic cell regeneration. New Eng. J. Med., *277*:686, 1967.

Cardell, R. R., Jr., J. Larner, and M. B. Babcock: Correlation between structure and glycogen content of livers from rats on a controlled feeding schedule. Anat. Rec., *177*:23, 1973.

Daems, W. Th.: The micro-anatomy of the smallest biliary pathways in mouse liver tissue. Acta Anat., *46*:1, 1961.

Deane, H. W.: The basophilic bodies in hepatic cells. Am. J. Anat., *78*:227, 1946.

Elias, H.: A re-examination of the structure of the mammalian liver. I. Parenchymal architecture. II. The hepatic lobule and its relation to the vascular and biliary systems. Am. J. Anat., *84*:311 and *85*:379, 1949.

Fahimi, H. D.: Cytochemical localization of peroxidatic activity of catalase in rat hepatic microbodies (peroxisomes). J. Cell Biol., *43*:275, 1969.

Fahimi, H. D.: The fine structural localization of endogenous and exogenous peroxidase activity in Kupffer cells of rat liver. J. Cell Biol., *47*:247, 1970.

Fawcett, D. W.: Observations on the cytology and electron microscopy of hepatic cells. J. Nat. Cancer Inst., *15* (Suppl.):1475, 1955.

Fouts, J. R.: Factors influencing the metabolism of drugs in liver microsomes. Ann. N. Y. Acad. Sci., *104*:875, 1963.

Goodenough, D. A.: Isolation and characterization of gap junctions from mouse liver. Proc. 1972 ICN–UCLA Symposium on Molecular Biology (C. F. Fox, ed.). New York, Academic Press, 1972.

Goodenough, D. A., and J. P. Revel: The permeability of isolated and in situ mouse hepatic gap junctions studied by enzymatic tracers. J. Cell Biol., *50*:81, 1971.

Greenway, C. V., and R. D. Stark: Hepatic vascular bed. Physiol. Rev., *51*:23, 1971.

Grubb, D. J., and A. L. Jones: Ultrastructure of hepatic sinusoids in sheep. Anat. Rec., *170*:75, 1971.

Hamashima, Y., J. G. Harter, and A. H. Coons: The localization of albumin and fibrinogen in human liver cells. J. Cell Biol., *20*:271, 1964.

Hampton, J. C.: Liver. *In* Kurtz, S. M. (ed.): Electron Microscopic Anatomy. New York, Academic Press, 1964, p. 41.

Hanzon, V.: Liver cell secretion under normal and pathologic conditions studied by fluorescence microscopy on living rats. Acta Physiol. Scandinav., Suppl. 101, 28:1, 1952.

Harkness, R. D.: Regeneration of liver. Brit. Med. Bull., *13*:87, 1957.

Helweg-Larsen, J. F.: Nuclear class series; studies on frequency distribution of nuclear sizes and quantitative significance of formation of nuclear class series for growth of organs in mice with special reference to influence of pituitary growth hormone. Acta Path. Microbiol. Scandinav., Suppl. 92, p. 3, 1952.

Howard, J. G.: The origin and immunological significance of Kupffer cells. *In* van Furth, R. (ed.): Mononuclear Phagocytes. Oxford, Blackwell Scientific Publications, 1970, pp. 178–199.

Ito, T.: Cytological studies on stellate cells of Kupffer and fat-storing cells in the capillary wall of the human liver. Acta Anat. Nippon., *26*:2, 1951.

Ito, T., and S. Shibasaki: Electron microscopic study on the hepatic sinusoidal wall and the fat-storing cells in the normal human liver. Arch. Histol. Jap. *29*:137, 1968.

Jefferson, N. C., M. I. Hassan, H. L. Popper, and H. Necheles: Formation of effective collateral circulation following excision of hepatic artery. Am. J. Physiol., *184*:589, 1956.

Jezequel, A., K. Arakawa, and J. W. Steiner: The fine structure of the normal neonatal mouse liver. Lab. Invest., *14*:1894, 1965.

Johnson, F. P.: The isolation, shape, size, and number of the lobules of the pig's liver. Am. J. Anat., *23*:273, 1918.

Jones, A. L., and D. T. Armstrong: Increased cholesterol biosynthesis following phenobarbital induced hypertrophy of agranular endoplasmic reticulum. Proc. Soc. Exper. Biol. Med., *119*:1136, 1965.

Jones, A. L., and D. W. Fawcett: Hypertrophy of the agranular endoplasmic reticulum in hamster liver induced by phenobarbital (with a review of the functions of this organelle in liver.) J. Histochem. Cytochem., *14*:215, 1966.

Jones, A. L., N. B. Ruderman, and M. G. Herrera: Electron microscopic and biochemical study of lipoprotein synthesis in the isolated perfused rat liver. J. Lipid Res., *8*:429, 1967.

Knisely, M. H.: The structure and mechanical functioning of the living liver lobules of frogs and Rhesus monkeys. Proc. Inst. Med. Chicago, *16*:286, 1947.

Kuhn, N. O., and M. L. Olivier: Ultrastructure of the hepatic sinusoid of the goat *Capra hircus.* J. Cell Biol., *26*:977, 1965.

von Kupffer, C.: Über Sternzellen der Leber. Arch. Mikr. Anat., *12*:353, 1876.

von Kupffer, C.: Über die sogenannten Sternzellen der Saugthierleber. Arch. f. Mikr. Anat., *54*:254, 1899.

Laschi, R., and S. Casanova: Fenestrae closed by a diaphragm in the endothelium of liver sinusoids. J. Microscopie, *8*:1037, 1969.

Lee, F. C.: On the lymph-vessels of the liver. Carnegie Contributions to Embryol., *15*:63, 1923.

Luck, D. J. L.: Glycogen synthesis from uridine diphosphate glucose; the distribution of the enzyme in liver cell fractions. J. Biophys. Biochem. Cytol., *10*:195, 1961.

Mahley, R. W., R. L. Hamilton, and V. S. LeQuire: Characterization of lipoprotein particles isolated from the Golgi apparatus of rat liver. J. Lipid Res., *10*:433, 1969.

Matter, A., L. Orci, and C. Rouiller: A study of the permeability barriers between Disse's space and the bile canaliculus. J. Ultrastr. Res., *11* (Suppl.), 1969.

Noel, R.: Recherches histo-physiologiques sur la cellule hépatique des mammifères. Arch. Anat. Micr., *19*:1, 1923.

Novikoff, A. B., and E. Essner: The liver cell; some new approaches to its study. Am. J. Med., *29*:102, 1960.

Orrenius, S., J. L. E. Ericksson, and L. Ernster: Phenobarbital induced synthesis of microsomal drug metabolizing enzyme system and its relationship to the proliferation of endoplasmic membranes. J. Cell Biol., *25*:627, 1965.

Palade, G. E., and P. Siekevitz: Liver microsomes; an integrated morphological and biochemical study. J. Biophys. Biochem. Cytol., *2*:171, 1956.

Peters, T., B. Fleischer, and S. Fleischer: The biosynthesis of rat serum albumin. IV. Apparent passage of albumin through the Golgi apparatus during secretion. J. Biol. Chem., *246*:240, 1971.

Porter, K. R., and C. Bruni: An electron microscope study of the early effects of 3′-Me-DAB on rat liver cells. Cancer Res., *19*:997, 1959.

Rappaport, A. M., Z. J. Borowy, W. M. Lougheed, and W. N. Lotto: Subdivision of hexagonal liver lobules into a structural and functional unit; role in hepatic physiology and pathology. Anat. Rec., *119*:11, 1954.

Remmer, H., and H. J. Merker: Effect of drugs on the formation of smooth endoplasmic reticulum and drug metabolizing enzymes. Ann. N. Y. Acad. Sci., *123*:79, 1965.

Wake, K.: "Sternzellen" in the liver; perisinusoidal cells with special reference to storage of vitamin A. Am J. Anat., *132*:429, 1971.

Wakim, K. G., and F. C. Mann: The intrahepatic circulation of blood. Anat. Rec., *82*:233, 1942.

Wilson, J. W.: Liver. Ann. Rev. Physiol., *13*:133, 1951.

Wilson, J. W.: Hepatic structure in relation to function. *In* Brauer, R. W., ed.: Liver Function: A Symposium on Approaches to the Quantitative Description of Liver Function. Washington, American Institute of Biological Sciences, Publ. No. 4, 1958, p. 175.

Wilson, J. W., and E. H. Leduc: Role of cholangioles in restoration of the liver of the mouse after dietary injury. J. Path. Bact., *76*:441, 1958.

Wisse, E.: An electron microscopic study of the fenestrated endothelial lining of rat liver sinusoids. J. Ultrastr. Res., *31*:125, 1970.

Wisse, E., and W. Th. Daems: Fine structural study on the sinusoidal lining cells of rat liver. *In* van Furth, R. (ed.):

Mononuclear Phagocytes. Oxford, Blackwell Scientific Publications, pp. 200–211, 1970.

Gallbladder and Bile Ducts

Bergh, G. S., and J. A. Layne: A demonstration of the independent contraction of the sphincter of the common bile duct in human subjects. Am. J. Physiol., *128*:690, 1940.

Boyden, E. A.: An analysis of the reaction of the human gall bladder to food. Anat. Rec., *40*:147, 1928.

Boyden, E. A.: The anatomy of the choledochoduodenal junction in man. Surg., Gynec. Obstet., *104*:641, 1957.

Chapman, G. B., A. J. Chiardo, R. J. Coffey, and K. Weineke: The fine structure of the human gall bladder. Anat. Rec., *154*:579, 1966.

Diamond, J. M.: Transport of salt and water in rabbit and guinea pig gall bladder. J. Gen. Physiol., *48*:1, 1964.

Elfving, G.: Crypts and ducts in the gall-bladder wall. Acta Path. Microbiol. Scand., *49* (Suppl. 135), 1960.

Evett, R. D., J. A. Higgins, and A. L. Brown, Jr.: The fine structure of normal mucosa in the human gall bladder. Gastroenterology, *47*:49, 1964.

Halpert, B.: Morphological studies on the gall bladder. II. The "true Luschka ducts" and "Rokitansky-Aschoff sinuses" of the human gall bladder. Bull. Johns Hopkins Hosp., *41*:77, 1927.

Hayward, A. F.: Aspects of the fine structure of gall bladder epithelium of the mouse. J. Anat., *96*:227, 1962.

Hayward, A. F.: Electron microscopic observations on absorption in the epithelium of the guinea-pig gall bladder. Zeitschr. f. Zellforsch., *56*:197, 1962.

Hayward, A. F.: The structure of gall-bladder epithelium. Int. Rev. Gen. Exp. Zool., *3*:205, 1968.

Jorpes, J. E., and V. Mutt: Secretin, pancreozymin and cholecystokinin; their preparation and properties. Gastroenterology, *36*:377, 1959.

Kaye, G. I., H. O. Wheeler, R. T. Whitlock, and N. Lane: Fluid transport in rabbit gall bladder. A combined physiological and electron microscope study. J. Cell Biol., *30*:237, 1966.

Mueller, J. C., A. L. Jones, and J. A. Long: Topographical and subcellular anatomy of the guinea-pig gall bladder. Gastroenterology, *63*:856, 1972.

Petrén, T.: Die Venen der Gallenblase und der extrahepatischen Gallenwege beim Menschen und bei den Wirbeltieren. Stockholm. Idun, 1933.

Pfuhl, W.: Die Leber und die Gallenblase und die extrahepatischen Gallengänge, *In* von Möllendorff, W., and W. Bargmann (eds.): Handbuch der mikroskopischen Anatomie des Menschen. Berlin, Julius Springer, 1932, Vol. 5, Part 2, pp. 235, 426.

Satsuki, S., K. Tsunoda, and K. Shindo: Uber das Verhalten der Leberzellen, Sternzellen, und Feltspeicherungszellen der Meerschwickenleber gegenüber der intravenös verbreichten. Feltemulsion. Arch. Histol. Jap., *9*:514, 1956.

Schwegler, R. A., Jr., and E. A. Boyden: The development of the pars intestinalis of the common bile duct in the human fetus, with special reference to the origin of the ampulla of Vater and the sphincter of Oddi. I. The involution of the ampulla. II. The early development of the musculus proprius. III. The composition of the musculus proprius. Anat. Rec., *67*:441, *68*:17, and *68*:193, 1937.

Torsoli, A., M. L. Ramorino, L. Palagi, C. Colagrande, I. Baschieri, S. Ribotta, and M. Marinosci: Observations roentgencinématographiques et electromanométriques sur la motilité des vôies biliaries. Sem. Hôp. Paris, *37*:790, 1961.

Whitlock, R. T., and H. O. Wheeler: Coupled transport of solute and water across rabbit gall bladder epithelium. J. Clin. Invest., *43*:2249, 1964.

Yamada, E.: The fine structure of the gall bladder epithelium of the mouse. J. Biophys. Biochem. Cytol., *1*:445, 1955.

29
Pancreas

The pancreas is a pinkish white organ lying retroperitoneally at about the level of the second and third lumbar vertebrae (Fig. 29–1). On the right its head is adherent to the middle portion of the duodenum, and its body and tail extend transversely across the back wall of the abdomen to the spleen. In the adult it measures from 20 to 25 cm. in length and varies in weight from 65 to 160 gm. It is covered by a thin layer of connective tissue which does not, however, form a definite fibrous capsule. It is finely lobulated, and the outlines of the larger lobules can be seen with the naked eye.

Next to the liver, the pancreas is the largest gland connected with the alimentary tract. It consists of an *exocrine portion*, which elaborates about 1200 ml. of digestive juice a day, and an *endocrine portion*, whose secretion plays an important part in the control of the carbohydrate metabolism of the body. Unlike the liver, in which the exocrine and endocrine functions are both carried on by the same cells, the pancreas has exocrine and endocrine functions that are carried on by different groups of cells.

THE EXOCRINE PANCREAS

Acinar Tissue

The pancreas is a compound acinous gland whose lobules are bound together by loose connective tissue through which run blood vessels, nerves, lymphatics, and excretory ducts. The acini that produce the exocrine secretory product vary from rounded structures to short tubules (Fig. 29–2). They consist of a single row of pyramidal epithelial cells converging toward a central lumen and resting upon a basal lamina supported by delicate reticular fibers. The size of the lumen varies with the functional condition of the organ, being small when the organ is at rest but becoming distended during active secretion. Between the acinar cells are fine secretory capillaries connected with the central lumen.

The acinar cells show rather striking differences in the various stages of secretion. In general, the basal part of the cell, when seen in the living condition, is homogeneous or may show a faint striation, owing to the presence of filamentous mitochondria in it. The apical portion of the cell is filled with highly refractile secretion granules or droplets, which vary greatly in number, depending on the degree of secretory activity.

In sections stained with hematoxylin and eosin after Zenker-formol fixation, the basal region of the acinar cells stains a dark purple, while the secretory granules are a bright orange-red. In sections stained with the basic dye methylene blue, the basal cytoplasm stains intensely, owing to the presence of a high concentration of ribonucleoprotein in this part of the cell. The basophilic material, formerly called *ergastoplasm*, may have a lamellar or filamentous appearance after some fixatives (Fig. 29–3). The Golgi apparatus is located in the supranuclear region and varies in its size and location in different physiological conditions. The *zymogen* granules or droplets arise in the Golgi region; they are particularly numerous in fasting animals and relatively few after a large meal or after injection of pilocarpine, which causes a massive release of secretion. After discharge of the zymogen droplets, the Golgi apparatus enlarges as new secretory droplets are formed.

The fine structure of the pancreatic acinar cell has probably been studied more

726

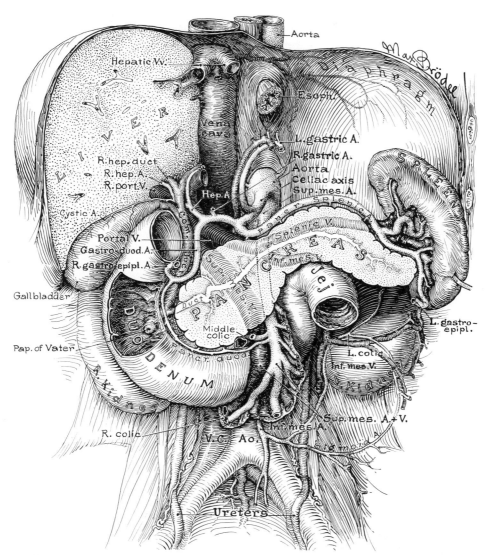

Figure 29–1 Drawing of the upper abdominal viscera with the stomach, transverse colon and most of the liver cut away to show the location and relationships of the pancreas. (Drawing by M. Brödel, from Trimble, Parsons, and Sherman, Surg. Gynec. Obstet., 73:711, 1941. By permission of Surgery, Gynecology & Obstetrics.)

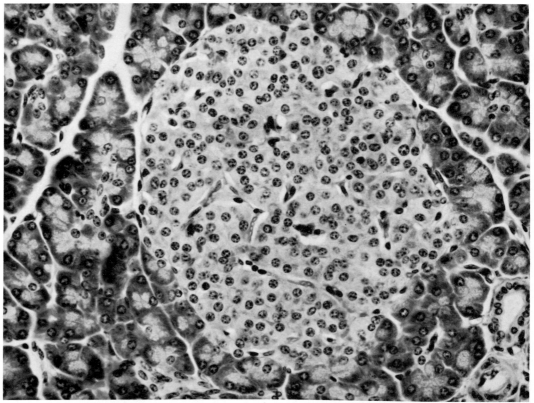

Figure 29–2 Photomicrograph of an islet of Langerhans and surrounding acinar tissue in guinea pig pancreas. Hematoxylin and eosin. × 500.

intensively than any other glandular cell. The intracellular synthetic pathway and the mechanism of discharge of its granules were described in considerable detail in Chapter 4 (see pp. 109–114) and will only be reviewed here.

The basal half is occupied by tubular elements of granular endoplasmic reticulum and extensive parallel arrays of cisternae (Fig. 29–4). Free ribosomes are abundant in the cytoplasmic matrix. The long mitochondria have well developed cristae and numerous matrix granules. The Golgi complex consists of stacks of parallel cisternae, numerous small vesicles, and condensing vacuoles containing secretory material of relatively low density. Mature zymogen "granules" or droplets with very dense contents are also found in close topographical relation to the Golgi complex. Occasional lipid droplets and lysosomes are commonly found in this region.

The free surfaces of the acinar cells usually bear a few short, irregularly oriented microvilli. The apical cytoplasm is crowded with zymogen granules (Fig. 29–5), and some are found in the process of discharging their contents into the lumen of the acinus (Figs. 29–6 and 29–7). It is evident from such images that at the time of release the zymogen is not in the form of a granule but is fluid and flows out through an opening created by fusion of its limiting membrane with the cell surface membrane. The lumen of the acinus is usually filled with moderately dense homogeneous material representing zymogen already secreted. Normally the zymogen droplets in the apex of the cell remain discrete even though closely crowded together. In cells that are very actively secreting, however, a zymogen droplet whose membrane has become continuous with the plasma membrane may be joined in similar fashion by a second and this one in turn by a third. In this way, a series of interconnected zymogen droplets may come to extend for some distance downward into the apical cytoplasm (Fig. 29–7).

The digestive enzymes of the pancreas are believed to be synthesized in the basal cytoplasm of the acinar cells, where they accumulate in the lumen of the endoplasmic reticulum. Through it, they are channeled into the Golgi region, where they are segregated in vesicular elements of the Golgi complex and concentrated into typical zymogen granules. In most species it is only after the product has undergone this concentration that it is sufficiently insoluble to resist extraction during specimen preparation. Consequently, zymogen granules are visible in the Golgi region and apex of the cell, but their precursors in the endoplasmic reticulum are extracted, and its lumen usually appears empty. Nevertheless, the presence of the digestive enzymes within the reticulum has been established in biochemical studies of the microsome fraction. In the guinea pig, and occasionally in the bat and the dog, electron micrographs of stimulated glands reveal, in the lumen of the reticulum, dense spherical bodies that resemble small zymogen granules. In these species, at least, segregation of the product evidently can occur in the reticulum as well as in the Golgi apparatus.

THE ENDOCRINE PANCREAS

Islets of Langerhans

Scattered throughout the exocrine portion of the pancreas are richly vascularized small masses of endocrine cells composing the *islets of Langerhans* (Fig. 29–2). These can be stained differentially by perfusion of the gland with a dilute solution of neutral red. When this is done, the islets can be identified with the naked eye and counted. In the adult human their number is estimated to range

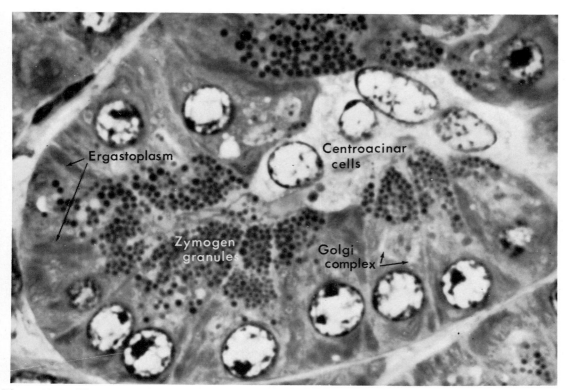

Figure 29–3 Photomicrograph of human pancreas, showing an acinus and its centoacinar cells. The ergastoplasm, Golgi complex, and zymogen granules of the acinar cells are clearly identifiable. The fixation of the nuclei is less than ideal, but adequate preservation of this organ from postmortem material is difficult. Formalin, osmium fixation, Epon section, stained with toluidine blue. × 3200. (Courtesy of S. Ito.)

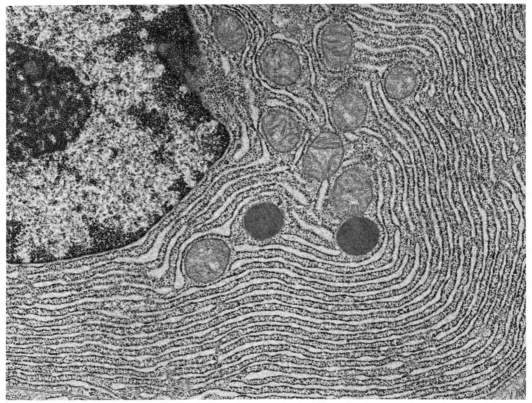

Figure 29-4 Electron micrograph of the basal region of a human pancreatic acinar cell, showing a portion of the nucleus and the extensive development of cisternae of granular endoplasmic reticulum. (Micrograph courtesy of A. Like and S. Ito.)

from 200,000 to 1,800,000. They are somewhat more numerous in the tail of the pancreas than in its body or head.

The islets are more or less completely demarcated from the surrounding acinar tissue by a thin layer of reticular fibers, but there is normally very little reticulum within the islet other than that associated with the capillaries. Isolated islet cells or groups of a few cells may occasionally be found among the acinar cells or closely associated with the small ducts. The islet cells are arranged in irregular cords and are paler staining than the surrounding acinar cells (Fig. 29-8). No secretory granules can be seen within them in routine hematoxylin and eosin preparations, but with special stains such as Mallory-azan at least three types of granular cells can be distinguished. One of these, called the *alpha cell* (A cell), contains granules that are insoluble in alcohol, while the granules of the other

principal type, the *beta cell* (B cell), are soluble in alcohol. The alpha cells are less numerous and in man tend to be situated around the periphery of the islet with the beta cells in the interior.

The mitochondria of the islet cells resemble those of the ducts in being slender filaments compared to the coarser filamentous mitochondria of the acinar cells. The Golgi apparatus of the beta cell is distinctly larger than that of the alpha cell but in neither cell type is this organelle as conspicuous as it is in the acinar tissue.

In a number of animal species, if the pancreas is freshly fixed in Zenker-formol and stained with Mallory-azan, three types of granular cells can be identified in the islets (Fig. 29-8). The granules of the alpha cells are relatively large and are colored a brilliant red, and those of the beta cells are smaller and stain brownish orange. A third type, called the *delta cell* (Bloom; Thomas), is filled with small blue-staining granules. In the dog the alpha, beta, and delta cells are estimated to constitute 20, 75, and 5 per cent, respectively, of the total. In addition to the granular cell types, the islets of the guinea pig pancreas also contain a nongranular cell designated the *C cell*.

The presence of the four cell types just described has now been verified in electron microscopic studies. The alpha cells are the most striking, owing to their large numbers of very dense spherical granules (Fig. 29–9). These are enclosed in a membrane, which, in osmium fixed material, is separated from the granule by a narrow clear zone. In tissue preserved with aldehyde fixatives, the very dense granule appears to have a less dense outer zone to which the membrane is closely applied. It is believed that this less dense outer component is extracted in the usual preparative procedure, leaving a clear space between the dense core of the granule and the limiting membrane.

In ultrathin sections, favorably oriented mitochondria are seen as long slender rods having the usual internal membrane structure, but shorter profiles are more common. There are a few cisternal profiles of the granular endoplasmic reticulum and a juxtanuclear Golgi complex that may contain developing secretory granules.

The beta cells have somewhat larger mitochondria and a more prominent Golgi complex. The endoplasmic reticulum is usually somewhat less extensive than that of the alpha cell. The beta cells show marked species variations in the character of their granules. In some species, the granules are homogeneous and moderately dense and are therefore distinguishable from alpha cell granules only by their slightly different size and density. In man, bat, dog, and certain other species, the beta granules have a very distinctive appear-

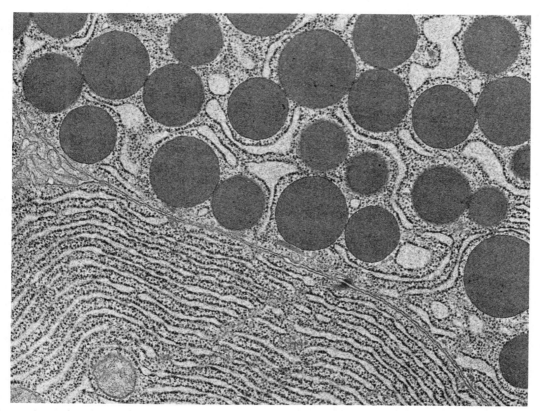

Figure 29–5 A portion of two neighboring human pancreatic acinar cells. Below is the endoplasmic reticulum of the paranuclear region of one cell, and above is the apical region of the adjacent cell filled with zymogen granules and tubular elements of reticulum. (Micrograph courtesy of A. Like and S. Ito.)

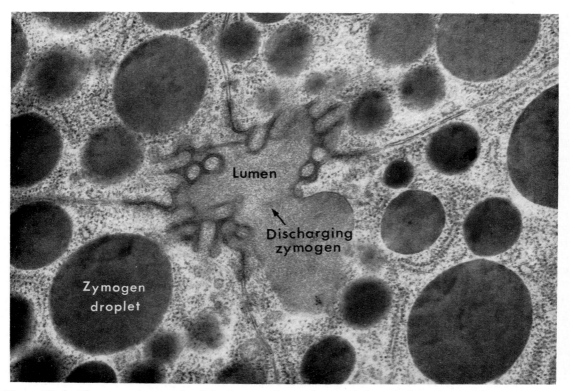

Figure 29-6 Electron micrograph of the lumen of an acinus and the apical portions of four acinar cells. Large dense zymogen droplets or granules are found in the cell apex. The limiting membrane of one of these has fused with the cell membrane and its zymogen is being discharged into the lumen. The free surface of the acinar cells bears short microvilli. × 38,000.

ance because they contain one or more small dense crystals (Fig. 29–10). In the human these are rectangular or polygonal and at high magnification show periodic internal stucture (Like). The crystals are surrounded by a matrix that appears to be easily extracted in specimen preparation, for in electron micrographs, the dense crystals, enclosed in a loose fitting membrane, stand out against an almost clear background (Fig. 29–10).

The existence of the delta cell as a type morphologically distinguishable from alpha and beta cells was long a subject of controversy. The existence of such cells in many, if not all, mammalian species can no longer be questioned, but whether they are a physiologically distinct cell type or merely a stage in the secretory cycle of one of the other cell types remains an open question. Their granules tend to be slightly larger and considerably less dense than the alpha granules (Fig 29–11). Some authors consider their separate

identity well established (Munger). However, the fact that in man, forms intermediate between typical alpha granules and delta granules can be found, and the fact that both types of granule may be present in the same cell, has led others to consider the delta cells to be altered alpha cells (Like). This possibility was considered by Bloom in the original description of these cells. In electron micrographs, the transition from alpha to delta type granules is often accompanied by a gradual loss of the morphological integrity of the mitochondria, Golgi complex, and other membranous components of the cytoplasm. The nucleus, however, remains nearly normal in appearance and the cell is evidently viable. If the delta cells are the result of some regressive change in alpha cells, the physiological significance of this change and its regular occurrence in a number of species remain to be explained.

The cells of the islets tend to be polarized

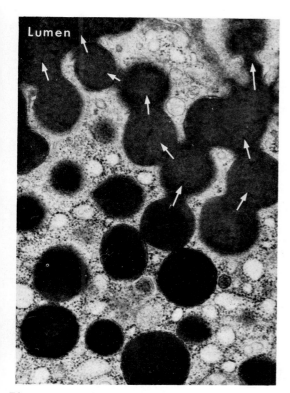

Figure 29-7 Electron micrograph of the apical portion of an acinar cell from a dog pancreas. A zymogen granule or droplet opening onto the lumen may be joined to a second and this to a third, so that zymogen may be discharged through several intercommunicating membrane limited vacuoles. × 24,500. (After A. Ichikawa, J. Cell Biol., 24:369, 1965.)

toward the capillaries. Granules are seen in very close association with the cell membrane at the vascular pole of the cell.

The cytoplasmic matrix of the endocrine cells contains small numbers of microtubules. The observation that administration of colchicine, which suppresses formation of microtubules, also prevents release of insulin from beta cells suggests that the microtubules may be involved in movement of the granules to the cell surface prior to their release (Lacy). However, recent work indicates that colchicine also affects other components of the cell and its action on the release of secretory products may be more complex than was initially believed. The granules seem to be discharged by exocytosis, but they must disintegrate almost immediately in the extra-cellular environment, for they are rarely seen outside the cell.

The capillaries of the islets of Langerhans are of the type in which areas of endothelium of appreciable thickness alternate with extremely attenuated areas penetrated by numerous pores or fenestrations. The capillaries of the acinar tissue are usually not fenestrated.

THE DUCT SYSTEM

The lumen of each acinus is continuous with the lumen of a small duct bounded by the *centroacinar cells,* so named because they are surrounded by and appear to extend into the center of the acinus (Fig. 29–12). The centroacinar cells are easily distinguished by their pale staining in histological sections and by the very low density of their cytoplasm and the paucity of their organelles in electron micrographs. Near the termination of the duct system part of the wall may be made up of centroacinar cells and part by acinar cells (Fig. 29–13). The terminal portion of the duct system drains proximally into the *intralobular* or *intercalated ducts.* These are lined by cells similar to the centroacinar cells that form a low columnar epithelium. These ducts are tributaries of larger *interlobular ducts* (Fig. 29–14) lined by a columnar epithelium in which goblet cells and occasional argentaffin cells are interspersed. Small mucous glands may bulge slightly from the ductal epithelium. The interlobular ducts join the main pancreatic ducts, of which there are two. The larger or *duct of Wirsung* begins in the tail and runs through the substance of the gland, receiving throughout its course numerous branches, so that it gradually increases in size as it nears the duodenum. In the head of the pancreas, it runs parallel with the ductus choledochus, with which it may have a common opening, or it may open independently in the ampulla of Vater. The opening and closing of these ducts are controlled by the sphincter of Oddi (p. 718). The accessory *duct of Santorini* is about 6 cm. long. It is nearly always present and lies cranial to the duct of Wirsung. These larger ducts have around the epithelium a moderately thick layer of dense connective tissue containing some elastic fibers.

In addition to the system of ducts just described, the pancreas is said to contain a

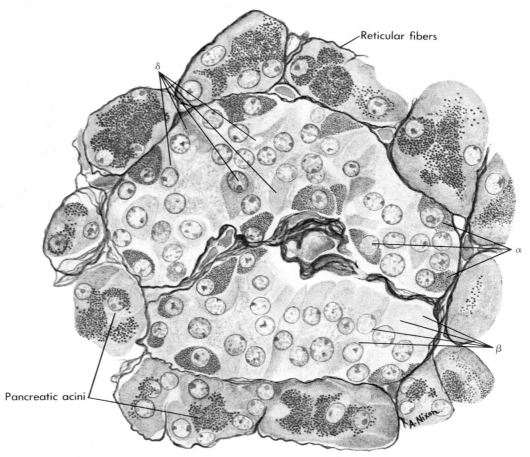

Reticular fibers

δ

α

β

Pancreatic acini

Figure 29–8   Section of human pancreas. The central part of the figure is an islet of Langerhans with granular cells of types alpha, beta, and delta. Mallory-azan stain. × 960. (After Bloom, 1931.)

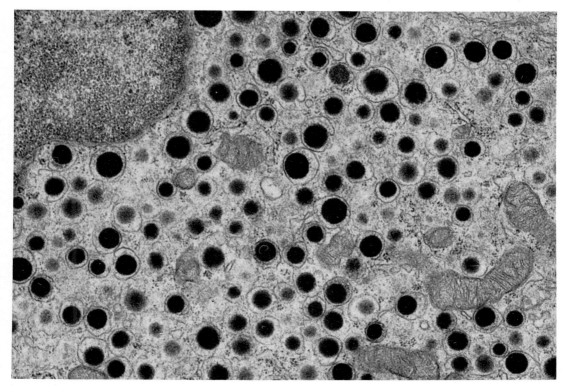

Figure 29–9 Electron micrograph of a juxtanuclear area of an alpha cell in a human islet of Langerhans. The alpha granules have a very dense spherical core and a less dense outer region bounded by a membrane. × 24,000. (Courtesy of A. Like.)

system of anastomosing small tubules which arise from the large ducts and run in the connective tissue surrounding them. These tubes have a diameter of 12 to 27 μm.; they are connected with the islets of Langerhans and only occasionally with the acini. These structures, although studied most extensively in the guinea pig, are also said to be present in man. Their epithelium is of a low, irregularly cuboidal type. They show occasional mitoses. Occasional goblet cells and a few cells with true mucous granules may be found within them. Some of the projections from these tubules consist of islet cells, singly or in groups, but the most striking feature of the tubules is their connection, by one or more short stalks, with large islets of Langerhans. It has long been thought that these ductules are composed of undifferentiated epithelium from which new islets can arise after destruction of the endocrine pancreas by disease or injury. This interpretation is now less widely accepted, for it has been shown that the islet cells themselves can divide mitotically and have considerable regenerative capacity.

BLOOD VESSELS, LYMPHATICS, AND NERVES

The arterial supply of the pancreas is from branches of the celiac and superior mesenteric arteries. From the celiac it receives branches through the pancreaticoduodenal and splenic arteries; it also receives small branches from the hepatic artery. The inferior pancreaticoduodenal artery is a branch of the superior mesenteric. The vessels run in the interlobular connective tissue and give off fine branches that enter the lobules. Veins accompany the arteries throughout and lead the blood either directly into the portal vein or indirectly through the splenic vein.

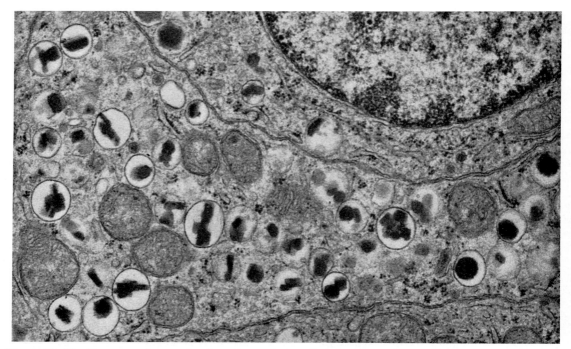

Figure 29–10 Electron micrograph of portions of two adjoining beta cells. The beta granules in man and several other species are membrane bounded spherical vesicles containing dense crystals of varying configuration. × 26,000. (Courtesy of A. Like.)

The lymphatic supply of the gland has not been worked out in detail. The lymphatic drainage is principally into the celiac nodes about the celiac artery.

The nerve supply is mainly by unmyelinated fibers arising from the celiac plexus. These fibers accompany the arteries into the gland and end about the acini. There are also many sympathetic ganglion cells in the interlobular connective tissues. The organ also receives myelinated fibers from the vagus nerves.

In electron micrographs axons are seen penetrating the basal lamina to end in intimate contact with the base of the acinar cells (Fig. 29–15). These nerve terminals often contain numerous synaptic vesicles. The source of these nerves is not clear, but it is likely that they are the terminations of branches from the vagus and may be involved somehow in regulation of secretion.

The presence of unmyelinated nerves in the islets of Langerhans has also been reported, and some of these end on the endocrine cells (Legg; Esterhuizen et al.). The axons are lodged between islet cells or in deep recesses in their bases inside the basal lamina (Fig. 29–16). Two types of endings are distinguishable. Those presumed to be cholinergic contain small, empty appearing synaptic vesicles, whereas in those endings believed to be adrenergic, many of the vesicles contain dense cores or granules of irregular shape. Both kinds of endings have been found in intimate relation to both alpha and beta cells.

It is generally believed that the regulation of secretion in both the exocrine and endocrine pancreas depends largely upon gastrointestinal hormones. There is strong evidence for this in the observation that grafted or denervated pancreas secretes zymogen in response to the hormones *secretin* and *pancreozymin* and releases insulin in response to elevated blood sugar. The physiological evidence concerning the role of nerves is contradictory, but the morphological evidence for innervation of the cells is indisputable. If the nerves to the pancreatic islets and acinar cells do not directly activate the secretory mechanism, it is possible that they may modulate the permeability of the cell membranes or the sensitivity of the cells to hormones.

REGENERATION

If the bulk of the pancreas is removed experimentally, the organ regenerates only slightly. If a portion of the tissue is injured by a wound, mitotic figures appear in the ductal epithelium and many new islets are formed, but few, if any, new acini develop as a result of the injury. If the main pancreatic ducts are ligated, there is at first a rapid disintegration of the pancreatic acini, followed by a much slower disintegration of the islets. This process extends over a period of months and even years. One week after the ligation, in the guinea pig and rabbit, most of the acini have degenerated; after one month, there is considerable generation of new islets and some acini. After nearly three years, it is said that only the main duct is present as a blindly ending structure, there are no acini left, but a few islets persist.

HISTOPHYSIOLOGY OF THE EXOCRINE PANCREAS

The external secretory function of the pancreas follows a rhythmical cycle, with a low level of continuous secretion accentuated periodically by nervous and hormonal stimulation associated with eating. The relative importance of hormonal and nervous control of pancreatic function is still a subject of debate. The presence of food in the antrum of the stomach and passage of the acid products of gastric digestion into the duodenum result in release into the blood of two different hormones, *secretin* and *pancreozymin*. Secretin, a polypeptide hormone consisting of 27 amino acid residues, causes the pancreas to secrete a large volume of fluid containing a high concentration of bicarbonate but very little enzymatic activity. This alkaline juice serves to neutralize the acid chyme entering the intestine from the stomach and provides the neutral or alkaline pH required for optimal activity of the pancreatic enzymes. Pancreozymin, carried by the blood to the pancreas,

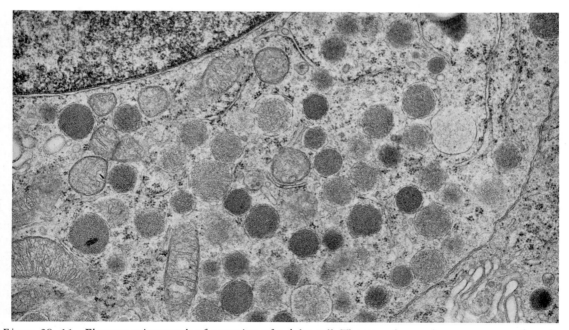

Figure 29–11   Electron micrograph of a portion of a delta cell. The granules are homogeneous and tend to fill their limiting membrane, but they vary considerably in density. It is not clear whether these cells represent a distinct type or are altered alpha cells. × 21,000. (Courtesy of A. Like.)

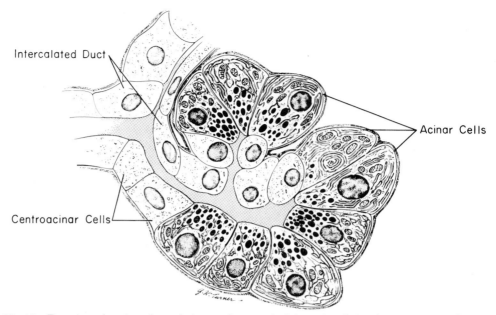

Intercalated Duct

Acinar Cells

Centroacinar Cells

Figure 29-12 Drawing showing the relations of a terminal branch of the duct system and centroacinar cells to the acinus.

causes secretion of large amounts of digestive enzymes. Acting alone, it does not significantly increase the volume of outflow from the pancreatic duct, but the coordinated action of secretin and pancreozymin results in a copious secretion of enzyme-rich pancreatic juice. Pancreozymin, a polypeptide hormone possessing 33 amino acid residues, is now known to be the same hormone as *cholecystokinin*, produced in the intestinal mucosa and released in response to the presence of amino acids and fats in the intestinal lumen. Its primary function is to activate contraction of the gallbladder, adding bile to the duodenal contents, but it also stimulates digestive enzyme secretion by the pancreas.

Because of the similarity in structure of its terminal tetrapeptide, *gastrin*, a hormone released from the antral mucosa, has an effect on pancreatic secretion similar to cholecystokinin but quantitatively less important.

Stimulation of the vagus nerve has an effect similar to that of pancreozymin, increasing enzyme secretion but not greatly influencing the volume of pancreatic juice. Because food in the intestine can stimulate pancreatic flow and enzyme secretion when all nervous connections between the in-

testine and the pancreas have been severed, some physiologists have been inclined to discount the importance of the nervous system in pancreatic secretion. However, atropine, which blocks the action of the parasympathetic nervous system, causes a marked inhibition of enzyme secretion from the intact pancreas. This fact suggests that cholinergic nervous stimulation is important.

The pancreas secretes *proteases, nucleases, amylases,* and *lipases*—enzymes for digestion of the three major classes of nutrients (proteins, carbohydrates, and fats). Proteolytic enzymes account for 70 per cent of the enzymes of the pancreatic juice and include *endopeptidases (trypsin, chymotrypsins,* and *elastases)* that split central peptide bonds and *exopeptidases (carboxypeptidase A* and *B)* that cleave terminal bonds of peptides or proteins. Thus the combined effect of the pancreatic proteolytic enzymes is to hydrolyze proteins to peptide fragments and then to reduce these to amino acids. The nucleases *ribonuclease* and *deoxyribonuclease* degrade ribonucleoprotein and deoxyribonucleoprotein. Pancreatic amylase hydrolyzes starch and glycogen to yield disaccharides, and pancreatic lipase splits triglycerides into fatty acids and glycerol.

The proteolytic enzymes are secreted as inactive precursors. In the intestine the enzyme *enterokinase* from the intestinal mucosa converts inactive trypsinogen to trypsin, the active enzyme. Trypsin in turn can activate all of the other precursors of proteolytic enzymes. Lipase and amylase appear to be secreted in the active form.

When these enzymes are within the acinar cells, they are enclosed in membranes and are present as inactive precursors. Thus, they do not injure the pancreas, but in the pathological condition *acute pancreatitis,* the proenzymes may be converted into active enzymes that destroy the pancreas itself.

HISTOPHYSIOLOGY OF THE ENDOCRINE PANCREAS

The principal product of the endocrine pancreas is *insulin,* a polypeptide composed of 51 amino acid residues in two chains, designated A and B, which are linked by two disulfide bonds. It is a very important hormone, directly or indirectly affecting the function of nearly every organ in the body. One of its most general effects is on the movement of glucose through the membranes of various cell types, especially muscle, adipose cells, and liver. The insulin binds to the cell membrane but the exact mechanism by which it accomplishes its augmentation of glucose entry is still poorly understood. Because brain, muscles, and many other organs are heavily dependent upon glucose as an energy source, the facilitation by insulin of entry of this sugar into the cells is extremely important for normal metabolism. Within the cell, glucose is rapidly phosphorylated, and in this form cannot diffuse out. The result then is a trapping of glucose in the cells and a lowering of the glucose in the circulating blood. There is a corresponding increase in intracellular hexose phosphates, which may be metabolized to yield energy or converted

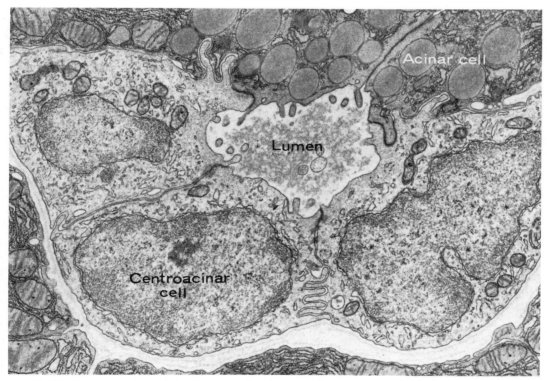

Figure 29-13 Electron micrograph of a terminal segment of the duct system of guinea pig pancreas showing the lumen bounded on one side by acinar cells and on the other by centroacinar cells. (From R. P. Bolender, J. Cell Biology, *61*:269, 1974.)

to glycogen, the storage form of carbohydrate in animals. In addition to its action on transport, insulin also has intracellular effects on glucose utilization by enhancing the activity of enzymes such as glucokinase and glycogen synthetase. In adipose cells, insulin causes accumulation of fat by facilitating entry of glucose and its conversion to fatty acids and triglycerides, and by inhibiting release of fatty acid from the adipose cells to the blood.

A deficiency of insulin production results in the serious metabolic disease, *diabetes mellitus*. Impairment of glucose utilization results in elevation of blood sugar, and excretion of sugar in the urine. The involvement of the pancreas in this disease was discovered in the late 1800's by Minkowski who pancreatectomized dogs. An attendant was observant enough to note that flies were attracted to the urine of these animals in greater number than to that of normal animals and this led to clinical demonstration of sugar in the urine. It was later shown that ligation of the pancreatic ducts was followed by degeneration of

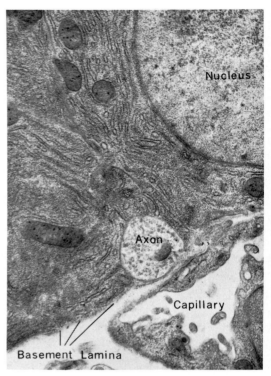

Figure 29-15 Electron micrograph of a nerve axon between the bases of two neighboring pancreatic acinar cells from bat. The axon contains "synaptic vesicles" and lies within the basal lamina of the acini. × 10,000.

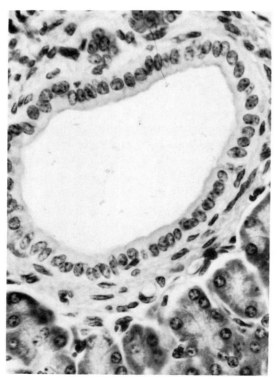

Figure 29-14 Photomicrograph of a small interlobular pancreatic duct.

the acinar tissue, but such animals did not develop signs of diabetes, thus suggesting that the disease was not due to interference with the exocrine secretory product, but that a blood-borne endocrine secretion was involved. This was corroborated by the finding that symptoms of diabetes could be prevented in pancreatectomized dogs by transplanting pancreatic tissue subcutaneously. Proof of the presence of pancreatic hormone controlling carbohydrate metabolism came in 1922 when Banting and Best extracted from pancreas some time after ligation of the ducts, a protein capable of alleviating the symptoms of diabetes. It subsequently became possible to inactivate the proteolytic enzymes of fresh bovine pancreas from the slaughter house and to isolate the hormone. This led directly to one of the great achievements of modern therapeutics, the treatment of diabetes with insulin. Crystallization of insulin was accomplished in 1926 by Abel, and its structure and amino acid sequence were determined in 1956 by Sanger — the first naturally occurring protein of biological importance for which the precise structure was shown. By combining insulin with protamine, a preparation was obtained that was effective over a longer period of time after injection.

Insulin is synthesized in the beta cells of the islets of Langerhans in the form of *proinsulin*, a precursor consisting of a single polypeptide chain of about 73 amino acid residues. Some type of specific proteolytic cleavage is believed to result in removal of a segment of 22 amino acid residues, with formation of insulin, in which the A and B chains are linked by two sulfide bonds.

In the pancreas of diabetic humans, there is a hyalinization or fibrosis of the islets of Langerhans, with a striking deficiency of the beta cells. Diabetes can be produced and the pathological changes in the pancreas simulated in experimental animals by administration of *alloxan*, which causes a more or less selective destruction of the beta cells.

Tumors of the beta cells may occasionally occur in man. These may produce excessive amounts of insulin resulting in low blood sugar, bizarre behavior, and episodes of unconsciousness.

The alpha cells of the islets produce *glucagon*, a 29 amino acid peptide. Administration of cobalt chloride to experimental animals causes varying degrees of destruction of the alpha cells, and the amount of extractable glucagon is then diminished. In comparative studies on different species, the amount of glucagon extractable from the pancreas has been found to correlate with the relative abundance of alpha cells.

Glucagon is secreted in response to cholecystokinin or insulin, and has an action opposite to that of insulin; namely, it causes an elevation of the blood sugar level. It appears to exert its effect by activating the enzyme phosphorylase in the liver, promoting glycogenolysis and release of glucose into the blood.

Recent studies using fluorescent antibod-

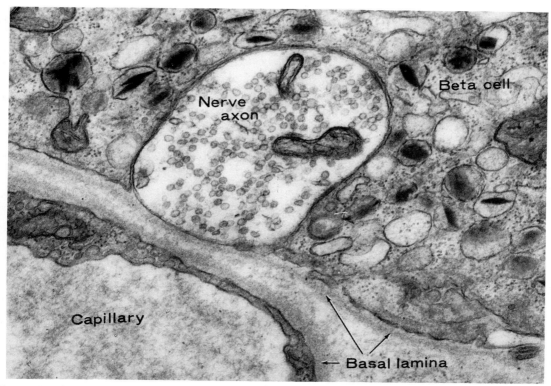

Figure 29-16 Electron micrograph of the vascular pole of a beta cell of the cat pancreas, and a portion of an adjacent capillary. An unmyelinated axon containing numerous "synaptic vesicles" occupies a deep recess in the cell base inside the basal lamina. (Micrograph from P. G. Legg Zeitschr. Zellforsch., *80*:307, 1967.)

ies seem to localize gastrin in the pancreatic islets, possibly in the alpha cells. Its physiological significance there is unknown. Rare islet cell tumors of man produce considerable amounts of gastrin and result in gastric hypersecretion and severe gastric ulcers.

REFERENCES

Banting, F. G., and C. H. Best: The internal secretion of the pancreas. J. Lab. Clin. Med., 7:251, 1922.

Baum, J., B. E. Simmons, R. H. Unger, and L. L. Madison: Localization of glucagon in the alpha cells in the pancreatic islet by immunofluorescent techniques. Diabetes, 11:371, 1962.

Benscome, S. A., and D. C. Pease: Electron microscopy of the pancreatic islets. Endocrinology, 63:1, 1958.

Bensley, R. R.: Studies on the pancreas of the guinea pig. Am. J. Anat., 12:297, 1911.

Björkman, N., C. Hellerström, B. Hellman, and B. Petersson: The cell types in the endocrine pancreas of the human fetus. Zeitschr. f. Zellforsch., 72:425, 1966.

Bloom, W.: A new type of granular cell in the islets of Langerhans of man. Anat. Rec., 49:363, 1931.

Caramia, G., B. L. Munger, and P. E. Lacy: The ultrastructural basis for the identification of cell types in the pancreatic islets. I. Guinea pig. Zeitschr. f. Zellforsch., 67:533, 1965.

Caro, L. G., and G. E. Palade: Protein synthesis, storage and discharge in the pancreatic exocrine cell: An autoradiographic study. J. Cell Biol., 20:4, 1964.

de Duve, C.: Glucagon; the hyperglycaemic glycogenolytic factor of the pancreas. Lancet, 2:99, 1953.

Dunn, S. J., H. L. Sheehan, and N. G. B. McLetchie: Necrosis of islets of Langerhans produced experimentally. Lancet, 1:484, 1943.

Gomori, G.: Observations with differential stains on human islets of Langerhans. Am. J. Path., 17:395, 1941.

Gomori, G.: Pathology of the pancreatic islets. Arch. Path., 36:217, 1943.

Grossman, M. I.: Nervous and hormonal regulation of pancreatic secretion. In de Reuck, A. V. S., and M. P. Cameron (eds): The Exocrine Pancreas. Ciba Foundation Symposium. Boston, Little, Brown & Co., 1961, p. 220.

Ichikawa, A.: Fine structural changes in response to hormonal stimulation of the perfused canine pancreas. J. Cell Biol., 24:369, 1965.

Janowitz, H. D.: Pancreatic secretion of fluid and electrolytes. In Code, C. F., and M. I. Grossman (eds.): Handbook of Physiology. Section 6. Washington, D. C., American Physiological Society, 1967–1968.

Lacy, P. E.: Electron microscopy of the islets of Langerhans. Diabetes, 11:509, 1962.

Lacy, P. E.: The pancreatic beta cell: structure and function. New Eng. J. Med., 276:187, 1967.

Lacy, P. E., and J. R. Williamson: Quantitative histochemistry of the islets of Langerhans. II. Insulin content of dissected beta cells. Diabetes, 11:101, 1962.

Latta, J. S., and H. T. Harvey: Changes in the islets of Langerhans of the albino rat induced by insulin administration. Anat. Rec., 82:281, 1942.

Lazarow, A.: Protection against alloxan diabetes. Anat. Rec., 97:37, 1947.

Lazarow, A.: Cell types of the islets of Langerhans and the hormones they produce. Diabetes, 6:22, 1957.

Legg, P. G.: The fine structure and innervation of the beta and delta cells in the islets of Langerhans of the rat. Zeitschr. f. Zellforsch., 80:307, 1967.

Like, A. A.: The ultrastructure of the islets of Langerhans in man. Lab. Invest., 16:937, 1967.

Like, A. A., and W. L. Chick: Mitotic division in pancreatic beta cells. Science, 163:941, 1969.

Like, A. A., and L. Orci: The embryogenesis of the human pancreatic islets, a light microscopic and electron microscopic study. Diabetes, 21(Suppl. 2):511, 1972.

Mayhew, D. A., P. H. Wright, and J. Ashmore: Regulation of insulin secretion. Pharmacol. Rev., 21:183, 1969.

Munger, B. L., F. Caramia, and P. E. Lacy: The ultrastructural basis for the identification of cell types in the pancreatic islets. II. Rabbit, dog, and opossum. Zeitschr. f. Zellforsch., 67:776, 1965.

Palade, G. E., P. Siekewitz, and L. G. Caro: Structure, chemistry and function of the pancreatic exocrine cell. In de Reuck, A. V. S., and M. P. Cameron (eds.): The Exocrine Pancreas. Ciba Foundation Symposium. Boston, Little, Brown & Co., 1961.

Renold, A. E.: Insulin biosynthesis and secretion—a still unsettled topic. New Eng. J. Med., 282:173, 1970.

Robb, P.: The development of the islets of Langerhans in the human fetus. Quart. J. Exper. Physiol., 46:335, 1953.

Sanger, F., and E. O. P. Thompson: Amino-acid sequence in the glycyl chain of insulin. Biochem. J., 53:353, 1953.

Sanger, F., and H. Tuppy: Amino-acid sequence in the phenylalanyl chain of insulin. Biochem. J., 49:481, 1951.

Soskin, S., and R. Levine: Carbohydrate Metabolism. 2nd ed. Chicago, University of Chicago Press, 1952.

Staub, A., L. Sinn, and O. K. Behrens: Purification and crystallization of glucagon. J. Biol. Chem., 214:619, 1955.

Thomas, T. B.: Cellular components of the mammalian islets of Langerhans. Am. J. Anat., 62:31, 1937.

Thompson, E. O. P.: The insulin molecule. Sci. Amer., 192:36, 1955.

Warren, S., and P. M. LeCompte: The Pathology of Diabetes Mellitus. 3rd. ed. Philadelphia, Lea & Febiger, 1952.

Warshawsky, H., C. P. Leblond, and B. Droz: Synthesis and migration of proteins in the cells of the exocrine pancreas as revealed by specific activity determinations from electron micrographs. J. Cell Biol., 16:1, 1963.

30
Respiratory System

To maintain their metabolic processes, higher animals require molecular oxygen. The respiratory system provides for the intake of oxygen and the elimination of carbon dioxide, which are transported to and from the tissues of the body by the circulatory system. The respiratory tract may be divided into the *conducting* and the *respiratory portions*. The former comprises the air-conducting tubes that connect the exterior of the body with that portion of the lungs where the exchange of gases between blood and the air takes place. These tubes are the passages of the *nose*, the *pharynx*, the *larynx*, the *trachea*, and the *bronchi* of various sizes. At the ends of the smallest branches of the air conducting passages is the respiratory portion of the lungs, formed by many small air filled vesicles called *alveolar sacs* and *alveoli*. In addition to its function in respiration, the pharynx serves as part of the alimentary tract connecting the mouth with the esophagus. The larynx also contains the organ of phonation.

THE NOSE

The nose is a hollow organ composed of bone, cartilage, muscles, and connective tissue. Its skin is provided with unusually large sebaceous glands and small hairs. The integument continues through the anterior nares into the vestibule of the nose. The epithelium here is stratified squamous, and there are stiff hairs that are believed to help in excluding particles of dust from the inspired air. The remainder of the nasal cavity is lined with mucus-secreting, pseudostratified ciliated epithelium and with a highly specialized form of ciliated epithelium in the olfactory sensory area.

The ciliated columnar epithelium is like that of the larynx and trachea in having goblet cells richly interspersed among the ciliated cells. A basal lamina separates the epithelium from the underlying connective tissue layer, which contains mixed mucous glands. The mucus from these glands keeps the lining of the nasal cavity moist. Beneath the epithelium of the lower nasal conchae are rich venous plexuses, which serve to warm the air passing through the nose. The tissue containing these plexuses is capable of considerable engorgement but differs from erectile tissue by the absence of septa containing smooth muscle.

Lymphocytes and other leukocytes migrating through the epithelium, and collections of lymphatic tissue beneath it, are characteristic features of the respiratory epithelium of the nose, especially near the nasopharynx.

The inspired air passes from the nasal cavity by way of the nasopharynx and pharynx to the larynx. The nasal part of the pharynx is lined by ciliated columnar epithelium. In its oral part it is lined by stratified squamous epithelium, which is continuous with that of the mouth above and the esophagus below. The structure of the pharynx is described on page 617.

The Organ of Olfaction

The receptors for the sense of smell are located in the *olfactory epithelium*. In fresh condition this epithelium is yellowish brown in contrast to the surrounding pink mucous

743

membrane. The olfactory area extends from the middle of the roof of the nasal cavity some 8 to 10 mm. downward on each side of the septum and onto the surface of the upper nasal conchae. The total surface of these areas on both sides is about 500 sq. mm. The outlines of the olfactory area are irregular.

The olfactory epithelium is a tall pseudostratified columnar epithelium about 60 μm. thick. It consists of three kinds of cells: supporting cells, basal cells, and olfactory cells.

The *supporting cells* were traditionally described as tall, slender elements with an axial bundle of tonofibrils and a prominent "cuticular plate" immediately beneath the free surface, inserting at either side into a prominent "terminal bar." In electron micrographs these specializations are found to be a typical terminal web associated with the zonula adherens of a well developed junctional complex that attaches the supporting cells to the adjacent sensory cells. The free surface of the cell bears numerous long slender microvilli that project into the overlying blanket of mucus. There is a small Golgi complex in the apical cytoplasm, and pigment granules that are responsible for the brown color of the olfactory area. In some species the supporting cells are secretory and contain numerous mucigen granules in the apical cytoplasm.

Between the bases of the supporting cells, the *basal cells* form a single layer of small conical elements with dark nuclei and branching processes.

The *olfactory cells*, evenly distributed between the supporting cells, are bipolar nerve cells. Their round nuclei occupy a zone between the nuclei of the supporting cells and the connective tissue. The apical portion of the cell, a modified dendrite, extends as a cylindrical process from the nucleus to the surface of the epithelium. The proximal end tapers into a thin, smooth process about 1 μm. thick. This is an axon—a fiber of the olfactory nerve. It passes into the subepithelial connective tissue and, with similar fibers, forms small nerve bundles. These are collected into about 20 macroscopically visible *fila olfactoria*.

The cytoplasm of the olfactory cell contains a network of neurofibrils, which are especially distinct around the nucleus. The cell may be slightly constricted at the level of its junctional complexes with the neighboring supporting cells. Distal to this, the bulbous head of the olfactory cell dendrite projects above the general surface of the epithelium (Fig. 30-4). This protruding portion is sometimes inappropriately called the *olfactory vesicle*. Radiating from its surface are six to eight *olfactory cilia* originating from basal bodies set

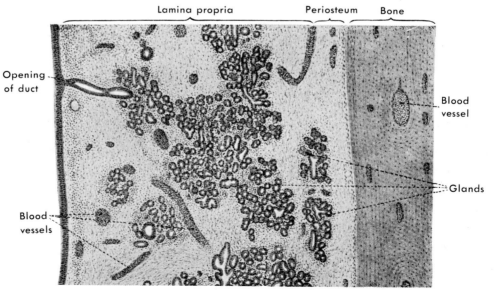

Figure 30-1 Section of respiratory mucosa of osseous portion of nose of a 22 year old man. × 45. (After Sobotta.)

nerve are enmeshed in a delicate connective tissue rich in macrophages. The fila olfactoria pass through openings of the cribriform plate of the ethmoid bone and enter the olfactory bulb of the brain, where the primary olfactory center is located. The olfactory mucosa is also provided with myelinated nerve fibers originating from the trigeminal nerve. After losing their myelin sheaths, the fibers enter the epithelium and end with fine arborizations below its free surface between the supporting cells. These endings are receptors for stimuli other than odors.

The lamina propria of the olfactory mucosa is continuous with the dense connective tissue of the underlying periosteum. In it are numerous pigment cells and some lymphoid cells.

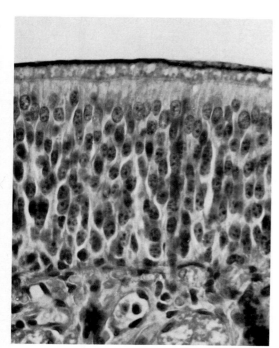

Figure 30-2 Photomicrograph of a celloidin embedded section of mammalian olfactory epithelium. Masson stain. × 475.

in a superficial ectoplasmic layer of cytoplasm having the character of a terminal web. These olfactory cilia are for the most part nonmotile and extremely long. In the frog, in which they have been studied in some detail with the electron microscope, they attain lengths of 150 to 200 μm. They have an atypical structure. The proximal segment of the ciliary shaft is about 250 nm. in diameter and contains the usual $9 + 2$ arrangement of longitudinal microtubules. A few micrometers from their base there is an abrupt narrowing of the shaft to about 150 nm. This slender portion of the shaft continues to the tip of the cilium, constituting some 80 per cent of its overall length. In this segment, the axoneme consists of 11 singlets instead of the usual two singlets and nine doublets. The slender distal segments of the olfactory cilia course parallel to the surface of the epithelium embedded within a thick layer of mucus, but with their tips near its surface. On the basis of the anatomical and physiological evidence now available, these specialized cilia appear to be the component of the sense organ that is excited by contact with odorous substances.

The unmyelinated fibers of the olfactory

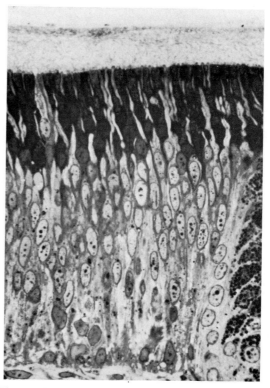

Figure 30-3 Photomicrograph of an araldite embedded section of olfactory epithelium from a frog. The slender, lighter-staining cells that extend to the surface of the epithelium are the olfactory rods of the bipolar receptor cells. The darker cells making up the bulk of the upper third of the pseudostratified epithelium are sustentacular cells. At the lower right is a portion of a gland of Bowman. Toluidine blue stain. × 600. (After T. Reese, J. Cell Biol., 25:209, 1965.)

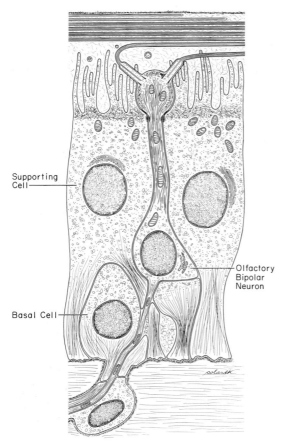

Supporting
Cell

Olfactory
Bipolar
Neuron

Basal Cell

Figure 30-4 Diagrammatic representation of the essential features of the olfactory epithelium based upon electron microscopic studies. The height of the epithelium has been foreshortened. The vertical lines in the rod or dendrite of the olfactory bipolar neuron represent microtubules.

Beneath the epithelium the lamina propria contains a rich plexus of blood capillaries. In its deeper layers it includes a plexus of large veins and dense networks of lymphatic capillaries. The latter continue into large lymphatics, which course toward the lymph nodes on either side of the head. If a colored material is injected into the subarachnoid spaces of the brain it can penetrate into the lymph capillaries of the olfactory region as well as into the sheaths of the fila olfactoria. This indicates a possible pathway for infections to spread from the nasal mucosa to the meninges.

The lamina propria in the olfactory area also contains the branched, tubuloalveolar *ol-*

factory glands of Bowman. The secretory portions are oriented mainly parallel to the surface, whereas the narrow ducts assume a perpendicular course and open onto the surface. Immediately under the epithelium the duct is often considerably enlarged. The low pyramidal cells of the secretory portions are serous and contain obvious secretory granules.

Histophysiology. The olfactory stimuli are of chemical nature. The secretion of the glands of Bowman keeps the surface of the olfactory epithelium moist and furnishes the necessary solvent. As most odoriferous substances are much more soluble in lipids than in water, and as the membranes and other constituents of olfactory cells and their cilia contain a considerable amount of lipids, odoriferous substances, even if present in extreme dilution, may presumably become concentrated in these structures. The continuous stream of the secretion of the olfactory glands, by removing the remains of the stimulating substances, keeps the receptors ready for new stimuli. In this respect the olfactory glands doubtless have a function similar to that of the glands associated with the taste buds.

The olfactory epithelium in man is easily affected by inflammation of the nasal mucosa and may be altered or replaced by atypical epithelium.

Paranasal Sinuses

Connected with the nasal cavity, and forming cavities in the respective bones, are the frontal, ethmoidal, sphenoidal, and maxillary sinuses—the *accessory sinuses of the nose.* These are lined with ciliated epithelium similar to that of the nasal cavity but containing fewer and smaller glands. The cilia beat so as to move a blanket of mucus toward the nasal cavity. The mucosa of all the sinuses is thin and the lamina propria cannot be differentiated as a separate layer from the periosteum of the bones, to which it is tightly adherent.

THE LARYNX

The larynx is an elongated structure of irregular shape, whose walls contain hyaline and elastic cartilage, connective tissue, striated muscles, and a mucosa with associated glands. It serves to connect the pharynx with the trachea. As a result of changes resulting from the contraction of its muscles, it produces variations in the width of the opening between the vocal cords. The size of this opening and the degree of muscular tension exerted upon the cords determine the pitch of the sounds made by the passage of air through the larynx.

The framework of the larynx is made up of several cartilages. Of these, the thyroid and cricoid cartilages and the epiglottis are unpaired, whereas the arytenoid, corniculate, and cuneiform cartilages are paired. The thyroid and cricoid and the lower parts of the arytenoids are hyaline cartilage. The *extrinsic muscles* of the larynx support and connect it with surrounding muscles and ligaments and their contraction raises it during deglutition. The *intrinsic muscles* join together the carti-

lages of the larynx. By their contraction they give different shapes to the laryngeal cavity and thus play a role in phonation.

The anterior surface of the *epiglottis*, the upper half of its posterior surface (the *aryepiglottic folds*), and the *vocal cords* are all covered with stratified squamous epithelium. In the adult, ciliated epithelium usually begins at the base of the epiglottis and extends down the larynx, trachea, and bronchi.

The cilia, which are 3.5 to 5 μm. long, beat toward the mouth, and thus move foreign particles, bacteria, and mucus from the lungs toward the exterior of the body.

Goblet cells are scattered among the cylindrical cells of the laryngeal epithelium in varying numbers. The glands of the larynx are of the tubuloacinous, mixed mucous variety. The alveoli secrete mucus and may have serous crescents. A few taste buds are scattered on the undersurface of the epiglottis.

The *true vocal cords* contain the vocal or inferior thyroarytenoid ligaments. Each of these (one on each side of the midline) consists of a band of elastic tissue bordered on its lateral side by the thyroarytenoid muscle and covered medially by a thin mucous membrane consisting of stratified squamous epithelium. The anteroposterior dimension of the space between the vocal cords is said to be about 23 mm. in men and 18 mm. in women. The shape of this opening between the vocal cords undergoes great variations in the different phases of respiration and in the production of various sounds in talking and singing. Contraction of the thyroarytenoid muscle approximates the arytenoid and thyroid cartilages, and this relaxes the vocal cords.

Blood Vessels, Lymphatics, and Nerves

The larynx is supplied by the upper, middle, and lower laryngeal arteries, which, in turn, arise from the superior and inferior thyroid arteries. The veins from the larynx empty into the thyroid veins. The larynx contains several rich plexuses of lymphatics, which lead into the upper cervical lymph nodes and to those about the trachea. The superior laryngeal nerve carries sensory nerves to the mucous membrane, and the inferior laryngeal nerve sends motor nerves to the muscles of the larynx.

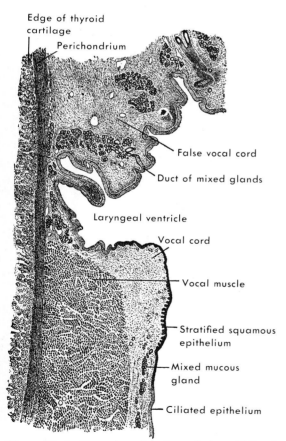

Edge of thyroid cartilage
Perichondrium
False vocal cord
Duct of mixed glands
Laryngeal ventricle
Vocal cord
Vocal muscle
Stratified squamous epithelium
Mixed mucous gland
Ciliated epithelium

Figure 30–5 Frontal section through the middle of the glottis of a 9 year old boy. × 15. (After von Ebner.)

THE TRACHEA

The trachea is a thin walled, flexible tube about 11 cm. long and 2 to 2.5 cm. in diameter. It is continuous with the larynx above and ends below by dividing into the two main bronchi.

The lining of the trachea is ciliated pseudostratified columnar epithelium and rests on an unusually thick basal lamina. Numerous goblet cells are scattered throughout the epithelium. The lamina propria contains an abundance of elastic fibers and numerous small glands similar to those of the larynx. These glands, most of which are external to the layer of elastic fibers, open by short ducts onto the free surface of the epithelium. In the posterior portion of the trachea, the glands extend through the muscular layer. Stimulation of the recurrent laryngeal nerve activates secretion in these glands. The lamina propria also contains occasional accumulations of lymphoid tissue.

The most characteristic feature of the trachea is its supporting framework of 16 to 20 C-shaped hyaline cartilages that encircle it on its ventral and lateral aspects. Because the successive incomplete cartilaginous rings are separated by interspaces bridged by fibroelastic tissue, the tube has much more pliability and extensibility than if they formed a continuous sheet. Some of the cartilages branch obliquely around the trachea. With advancing age they become fibrous, but they do not ossify, as the thyroid cartilage of the larynx often does. They are surrounded by dense connective tissue that contains many elastic and reticular fibers.

The posterior wall of the trachea, adjacent to the esophagus, is devoid of cartilages (Fig. 30–6). In their place is a thick layer of smooth muscle bundles, which, in the main, run transversely. They are inserted into the dense elastic fiber bundles surrounding the tracheal cartilages and are joined to the mucosa by a layer of loose connective tissue.

Blood Vessels, Lymphatics, and Nerves

A delicate network of lymphatics is found in the mucosa, and a much coarser plexus occurs in the submucosa. These lead into the lymph nodes, which accompany the trachea along its entire length. The arteries

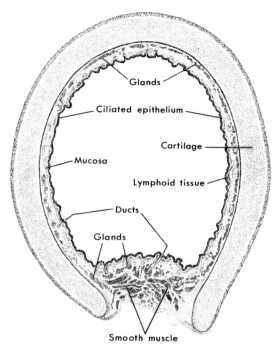

Figure 30-6 Cross section through the trachea of a 9 year old boy. × 6. (Redrawn and modified from Kölliker-von Ebner.)

for the trachea are mainly from the inferior thyroid. The nerves supplying the trachea arise from the recurrent branch of the vagus nerve and from the sympathetic chain. The sympathetic nerves of the trachea contain small ganglia, from which fibers lead to the smooth muscle in its posterior wall. Myelinated sensory nerves are also found.

THE LUNGS

The lungs are paired organs occupying a great part of the thoracic cavity and constantly changing in form and size in the different phases of respiration. The right lung consists of three lobes and the left lung of two, with each lobe receiving a branch of the primary bronchus of the same side. The outer surface of the lungs is closely invested by a serous membrane, the *visceral pleura.*

In children the lungs are a pale pink because of their rich blood supply. With advancing age they become gray, owing to accumulation of inhaled carbon particles in phagocytic cells in the connective tissue septa. This darkening of the lung is especially marked in city dwellers, who are chronically exposed to smoke and atmospheric pollution.

Each of the five lobes of the lungs is divided by thin connective tissue septa into great numbers of roughly pyramidal portions of pulmonary tissue, the *lobules*. These are so arranged that the apex of each points toward the hilus, and the base is oriented toward the surface of the lung. These gross lobules are not seen as easily in the adult lung as in the embryonic lung, except at the surface. The progressive deposition of carbon under the pleura from the inspired air marks the outlines of these lobules distinctly. Each lobule is supplied by a small bronchiole.

Bronchial Tubes

The trachea divides into two main branches called the *primary bronchi*. These enter the substance of the lungs at the hilus, one on each side, and, coursing downward and outward, divide into two smaller bronchi on the left side and three on the right. These give rise to smaller *secondary bronchi*, from which several orders of *bronchioles* originate. With the development of lung surgery, knowledge of the segmental distribution of the secondary bronchi in the lobes has become important. According to Boyden, the right lung is made up of 10 principal bronchopulmonary segments, while the left lung can be divided into eight segments. The basic pattern of the secondary bronchi appears, however, to be subject to considerable variation. It has been estimated that there are from 50 to 80 terminal bronchioles in each lobule. Each *terminal bronchiole* continues into one, two, or more *respiratory bronchioles*. These break up into 2 to 11 *alveolar ducts*, from which arise the *alveolar sacs* and *alveoli*. Thus, the main successive divisions of the bronchial tree are primary bronchi, secondary bronchi, bronchioles, alveolar ducts, alveolar sacs, and alveoli. An *atrium* has been described as connecting the alveolar sacs and the alveolar ducts (see p. 752).

Before the bronchi enter the lungs, their

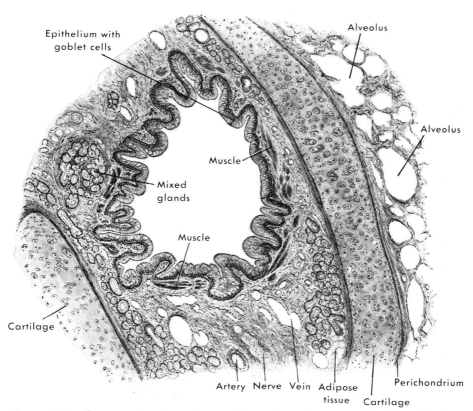

Figure 30-7 Cross section through a small bronchus of a man. × 30. (After Schaffer.)

structure is practically identical with that of the trachea. But as soon as they enter the lungs, the *cartilage rings* disappear and are replaced by irregularly shaped *cartilage plates*, which completely surround the bronchi. As a result, the intrapulmonary bronchi and their branches are cylindrical and not flattened on one side, as are the trachea and the extrapulmonary portions of the bronchi. As one follows the air passages peripherally, the cartilage plates become smaller and irregularly distributed around the tube, while the muscular layer completely surrounds the bronchus. The cartilage disappears from the wall when the diameter of the bronchiole reaches about 1 mm.

The bronchus is lined by a mucous membrane continuous with that of the trachea and having the same type of epithelium. The epithelium is ciliated columnar in the larger branches and nonciliated cuboidal in the terminal branches.

The lamina propria consists of a small amount of reticular and collagenous connective tissue and many elastic fibers. It contains a few lymphoid cells and is set off from the epithelium by a prominent basal lamina. The mucosa of the bronchus, in histologic sections, shows a marked longitudinal folding due to the contraction of the smooth muscle in the wall. It is claimed that these folds disappear when the lung is distended.

Nerves enter the epithelium from the lamina propria and terminate in close relationship to specialized cells characterized by the presence of dense-cored granules in their basal cytoplasm. These cells, occurring singly or in small clusters, have a small area of their apical surface exposed to the lumen of the bronchiole. A single cilium often projects from their lateral surface near the lumen. This complex, consisting of mitochondria-rich intraepithelial nerve endings and associated granular cells, is interpreted as a sensory receptor unit in the bronchioles (Hung et al.). These probably correspond to the receptors shown by physiological studies to be stimulated in bronchial and bronchiolar epithelium by cigarette smoke, ammonia, and other noxious vapors. Beneath the mucosa is a layer of smooth muscle fiber bundles that run around the tube but never form a closed ring, as they do in the blood vessels and intestines. Instead, the muscles form an interlacing feltwork, the meshes of which become larger in the smaller bronchioles. Numerous elastic fibers are intimately associated with the smooth muscle cells. As will be discussed later, the elastic fibers and smooth muscles throughout the lung play an important part in the changes in its volume that occur during respiration. A dense network of small blood vessels accompanies this myoelastic layer.

The outermost layer of the bronchial wall consists of dense connective tissue, which contains many elastic fibers. It surrounds the plates of cartilage and is continuous with the connective tissue of the surrounding pulmonary tissue and with that accompanying the large vessels.

Mucous and mucoserous glands are found as far out in the bronchial tree as the cartilage extends. The glands are usually situated deep to the muscular layer, through which their ducts penetrate to open on the free surface.

Diffuse lymphatic tissue occurs regularly in the mucosa and in the fibrous tissue around the cartilage, especially where the bronchi branch.

With the progressive decrease in the size of the bronchi and bronchioles toward the periphery, the layers of their walls become thinner, and in some of them the various elements intermingle to form a single layer. The smooth muscle, however, is distinct up to the end of the respiratory bronchioles, and a few strands even continue into the walls of the alveolar ducts.

RESPIRATORY STRUCTURES OF THE LUNGS

The functional unit of the lung, often called the *primary lobule*, is composed of all the structures beginning with a respiratory bronchiole, and including alveolar duct, atria, alveolar sac, and alveoli, together with all the associated blood vessels, lymphatics, nerves, and connective tissue. In the newborn, the pulmonary lobule is small. The respiratory bronchiole has not yet developed, and the alveoli are represented as shallow diverticula on the walls of the alveolar ducts (see Fig. 30–12A).

In a thin section of lung the respiratory portion of the organ appears as a lacework of large spaces separated by thin septa (see Fig. 30–12B). Here and there this lacework is traversed by the thick walled bronchi and ar-

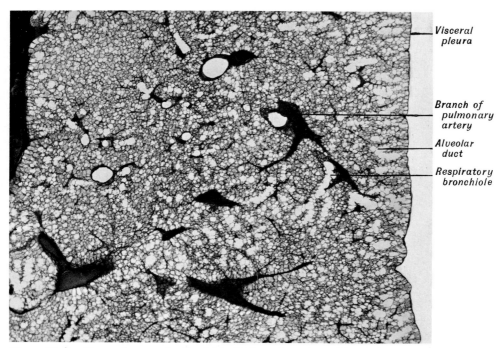

Visceral
pleura

Branch of
pulmonary
artery

Alveolar
duct

Respiratory
bronchiole

Figure 30–8   Photomicrograph of a thick (120 μm.) section of lung of *Macacus rhesus.* × 10.

teries and veins of various sizes. A different picture is seen if a thick section is examined with the binocular microscope. Then the lung has the appearance of an irregular honeycomb in which the polyhedral alveoli and alveolar sacs form the "cells" (Figs. 30–8 and 30–9). This honeycomb is traversed by the system of bronchioles and the alveolar ducts, which are continuous with the atria, alveoli, and alveolar sacs.

For histological purposes, the lungs should ideally be fixed by introducing the solutions through the trachea or by perfusion through the pulmonary artery, with the lungs still in the body to prevent overdistention. The more common method of dropping a bit of lung into fixing fluid gives a highly distorted picture, for the lung shrinks greatly under these conditions, and the air in the organ prevents the penetration of the fixative. Some aspects of the structure of the lung may be understood best by examination of sections of 60 to 120 μm. thickness. Hematoxylin and eosin staining gives but a poor idea of the architecture of the lung. Special staining and injection methods are necessary for a more complete demonstration of its organization. Furthermore, it should be borne

in mind that the internal configuration of the lung changes continuously with every inspiration and expiration.

Respiratory Bronchioles

In the adult, the respiratory bronchioles begin with a diameter of about 0.5 mm. They are short tubes, lined in their first part with a ciliated columnar epithelium devoid of goblet cells. A short distance down the bronchiole, the ciliated columnar epithelium loses its cilia and becomes low cuboidal. These bronchioles have walls composed of collagenous connective tissue containing bundles of interlacing smooth muscles and elastic fibers. They lack cartilage. A few alveoli bud from the respiratory bronchiole on the side opposite that along which runs the branch of the pulmonary artery. A thinner continuation of the cuboidal epithelium of the bronchiole extends onto the alveolar wall. These alveoli are the first of the respiratory structures of the lung and are responsible for the term "respiratory bronchiole." These bronchioles soon branch into 2 to 11 radiating *alveolar ducts.* They are surrounded by alveoli that have risen from adjacent ducts.

Alveolar Ducts

The structure of the alveolar ducts is difficult to visualize in ordinary histological sections of the distended lung. However, in thick sections studied with the binocular microscope, the alveolar ducts are seen as thin tubes with highly discontinuous walls. They usually follow a long, tortuous course and give off several branches, which in turn may branch again. They are closely beset with thin walled outpouchings, the alveolar sacs. These blind polyhedral sacs open only into the alveolar duct. Because the alveolar sacs are closely packed against one another, their openings occupy the greater part of the wall of the alveolar duct, so that in sections of usual thickness its tubular nature is not apparent. The wall of the alveolar duct between the mouths of the alveolar sacs is supported by strands of elastic and collagenous fibers and a few smooth muscle cells. In thin sections of the lung, only small portions of these fibers and muscle are seen. They appear as slight enlargements coursing parallel to the long axis of the alveolar duct. In thicker sections it becomes evident that these are merely transversely or

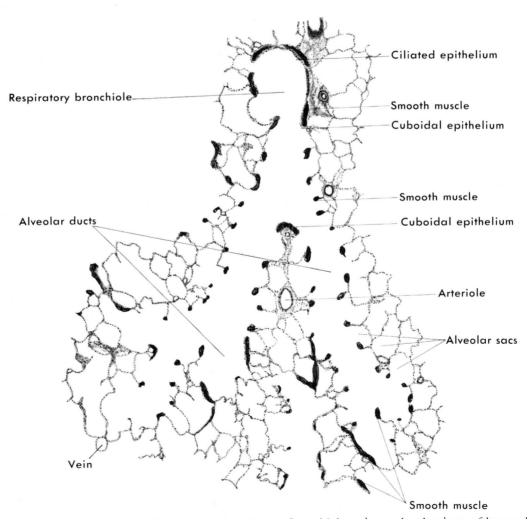

Figure 30-9 Drawing of a section through a respiratory bronchiole and two alveolar ducts of human lung. Note the smooth muscle in the walls of the alveolar ducts. (Slightly modified from Baltisberger.)

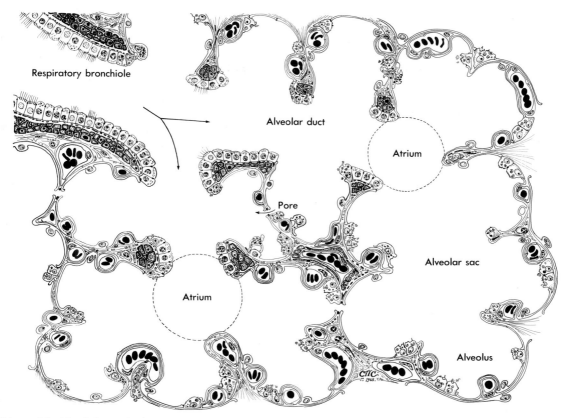

Respiratory bronchiole

Alveolar duct

Atrium

Pore

Alveolar sac

Atrium

Alveolus

Figure 30-10 Schematic representation of the respiratory unit of the lung: respiratory bronchiole, alveolar ducts, alevolar sacs, and alveoli. The atria indicated by the circles are spaces bounded on one side by the termination of the alveolar duct and on the other by the openings of the alveolar sacs. (Slightly modified after S. Sorokin, *in* R. O. Greep, ed.: Histology. 2nd ed. New York, McGraw-Hill Book Co., 1966.)

tangentially cut small portions of the long connective tissue fibers and muscle bundles, which are interwoven around the mouths of the alveolar sacs.

Alveolar Sacs and Alveoli

From the alveolar ducts arise both single alveoli and alveolar sacs comprising two to four or more alveoli. It has been suggested that the space between the ends of the alveolar duct and the alveolar sacs be termed the *atrium*. The structures described under this term have not been generally accepted as forming a distinct entity, and some authors consider them simply parts of the alveolar ducts.

The alveoli are thin walled polyhedral sacs, open on one side. Air may thus diffuse freely from the alveolar ducts into the alveo-

lar sacs and into the cavities of the alveoli. The most conspicuous feature of the alveolar wall is a dense network of capillaries that anastomose so freely that many of the spaces between them are smaller than the diameters of the vessel lumina (Fig. 30–13). The alveolar walls also contain a closely woven network of branching reticular fibers. These, along with less numerous elastic fibers, form the tenuous supporting framework for the thin walled air sacs and their numerous capillaries. The capillaries are thick relative to the rest of the alveolar wall, so that they bulge into the alveoli, and thus the greater portion of their surface is presented to the alveolar air. The larger reticular and elastic fibers occupy a central position in the interalveolar septa, with the anastomosing capillaries weaving back and forth through the meshes of the fibers to jut first into one and then into the

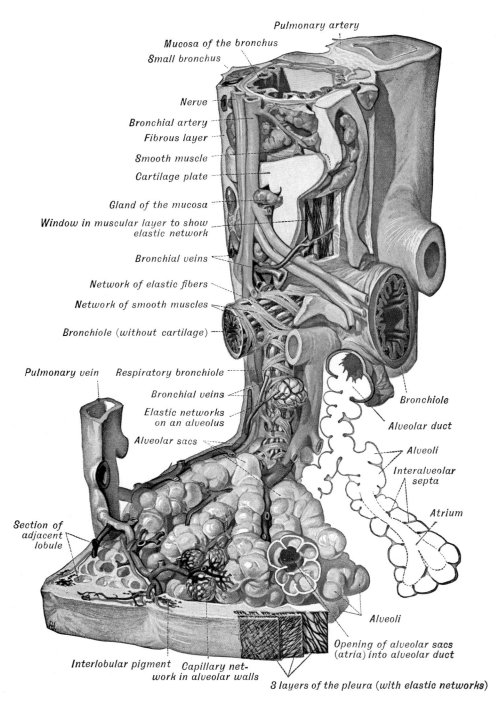

Pulmonary artery

Mucosa of the bronchus

Small bronchus

Nerve

Bronchial artery

Fibrous layer

Smooth muscle

Cartilage plate

Gland of the mucosa

Window in muscular layer to show elastic network

Bronchial veins

Network of elastic fibers

Network of smooth muscles

Bronchiole (without cartilage)

Pulmonary vein *Respiratory bronchiole*

Bronchial veins

Elastic networks on an alveolus

Alveolar sacs

Bronchiole

Alveolar duct

Alveoli

Interalveolar septa

Atrium

Section of adjacent lobule

Alveoli

Interlobular pigment *Capillary net-work in alveolar walls*

Opening of alveolar sacs (atria) into alveolar duct

3 layers of the pleura (with elastic networks)

Figure 30–11   Portion of a pulmonary lobule from the lung of a young man. Free reconstruction by Vierling, somewhat foreshortened. Mucosa and glands, green; cartilage, light blue; muscles and bronchial artery, orange; elastic fibers, blue-black; pulmonary artery, red; pulmonary and bronchial veins, dark blue. × 32. (After Braus.)

other of the adjacent alveolar spaces. This relationship of supporting fibers to capillaries is best seen in the lung of the newborn, in which the interalveolar septa have a thick, cellular central stroma that becomes more and more attenuated with advancing age, as a result of thinning and stretching of the alveolar walls.

Small openings called *alveolar pores* are found in the thin wall separating adjacent alveoli. Their presence was first detected in sections of lung from a patient with fibrinous pneumonia, in which strands of fibrin could be seen passing through from one alveolus to the other. Their existence in normal lungs has since been confirmed. These minute apertures measure only about 7 to 9 μm. in diameter and are found in the openings between capillaries (Fig. 30–13). From one to six may be found in an alveolar septum, and larger numbers have been reported. There is no longer any doubt of their occurrence, but their significance is problematical. They may conceivably provide a collateral air circulation that tends to prevent atelectasis when second-

ary bronchi become obstructed. They may also have the disadvantage of providing pathways that permit the spread of bacteria from one alveolus to its neighbors in pneumonia.

The mouths of the alveolar sacs are completely surrounded by a wavy wreath of collagenous fibers. These fibers continue from one sac to the next and help to give some substance to the wall of the alveolar duct. These wavy wreaths probably straighten out with deep inspiration. The collagenous fibers are accompanied by elastic fibers. The dense networks of reticular fibers within the walls of the alveoli and alveolar sacs are continuations of these collagenous fibers, which, in turn, merge with the collagenous fibers in the walls of the arteries, veins, and bronchioles. The elastic fibers are likewise continuations of those of the bronchioles.

Lining of the Alveoli

Throughout several decades of study of the lungs with the light microscope, one of

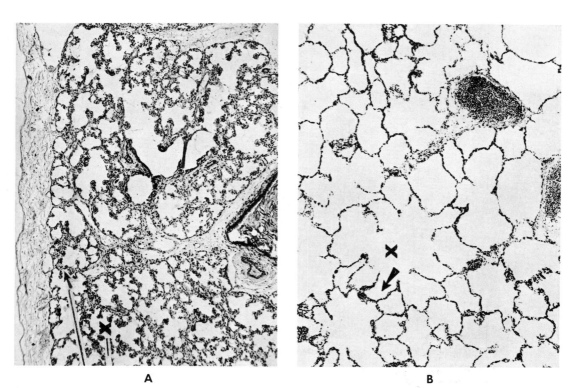

A   **B**

Figure 30–12   Photomicrographs of section of lung. *A,* Human newborn. *B,* 12 year old girl. Both specimens fixed immediately after death by the intratracheal injection of Zenker-formol solution. Note increase in size of alveolar ducts (*x*) and alveoli (arrow). Mallory-azan stain. × 82. (Courtesy of C. G. Loosli.)

the most controversial problems in histology was that of the lining of the alveolar wall. All agreed that the entire respiratory tract in the embryo was lined with continuous epithelium of endodermal origin. According to some histologists, the epithelial lining present in the fetus persisted postnatally throughout life, but the growth of alveoli in late fetal life and their expansion after birth resulted in an extreme attenuation of those portions of the epithelial cells overlying the capillaries, while the thicker portions of the cells containing the nuclei remained grouped in the meshes of the capillary net. However, the thin film of epithelium presumed to extend over the capillaries usually was not visible with the light microscope, and other histologists insisted that the alveolar lining was discontinuous, with only isolated groups of epithelial cells present between the capillaries, whose walls were believed to be exposed directly to the alveolar air. Still others regarded the alveolar ducts and alveoli as connective tissue spaces entirely devoid of a lining of endodermal origin.

This controversy was finally settled by electron microscopic studies (Low; Karrer) which clearly demonstrated that there is a thin continuous cellular covering of the al-

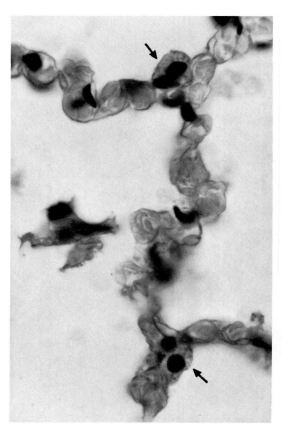

Figure 30-14 Photomicrograph of alveolar wall of lung of 18 year old man. Note the thin membrane between the lumina of the capillaries and the air spaces. Arrows point to "septal cells" or "alveolar cells" in their characteristic location on the alveolar walls. Hematoxylin-eosin-azure II stain. × 1000. (Courtesy of C. G. Loosli.)

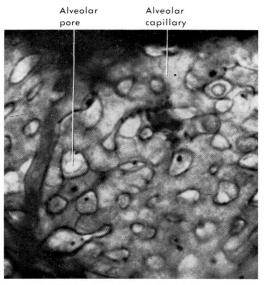

Alveolar pore Alveolar capillary

Figure 30-13 Photomicrograph of lung, showing a surface view of an alveolar septum with its close meshed capillary plexus. An alveolar pore is shown in one of the meshes of the capillary net. (After E. R. Weibel, Zeitschr. f. Zellforsch., 57:648, 1962.)

veoli which is at or just below the limit of visibility with the light microscope (Fig. 30–16). In many places it is as thin as the most attenuated areas of capillary endothelium. The alveolar epithelium is separated from the endothelium by a continuous basal lamina. In addition to the squamous *pulmonary epithelial cells* (small alveolar cells, pneumonocytes type I), there are numerous rounded or cuboidal cells in the lining that are called *septal cells* or *alveolar cells* (great alveolar cells, pneumonocytes type II).

The extremely thin pulmonary epithelial cells form a continuous lining layer in the alveolar wall, interrupted only by occasional alveolar cells that protrude into the air space. The nuclei are flattened and resemble those of endothelial or mesothelial cells. The shapes and thickness of the cells are, of course, related to the degree of inflation of the lung and the tension on the interalveolar septa at the time of fixation.

The alveolar cells (pneumonocytes type II) are cuboidal or rounded elements of the alveolar epithelium readily visualized with the light microscope. They may occupy niches in the alveolar wall and lie mainly deep to the squamous epithelial cells, or they may be so situated in the epithelium that they bulge some distance into the alveolar lumen. They occur singly or in groups of two or three. In electron micrographs, they are found to rest on the basal lamina of the epithelium. They possess short microvilli on their free surface and form junctional complexes with neighboring squamous alveolar epithelial cells (Fig. 30–17). They are therefore considered to be part of the epithelium and not merely cells of mesenchymal origin wandering through the epithelium (Sorokin). Their Golgi complex is extensive, and vesicular and cisternal profiles of granular endoplasmic reticulum are common. There are abundant free ribosomes in the cytoplasmic matrix. The cell thus has some of the fine structural characteristics of a secretory cell.

The most distinctive cytological feature of the alveolar cell is the presence of numerous dense, osmiophilic bodies 0.2 to 1.0 μm. in diameter that have an internal structure consisting of thin parallel or concentric lamellae (Fig. 30–18). These *multilamellar bodies* or *cytosomes* seen in electron micrographs correspond in number and location to the vacuoles observed in these cells in histological sections of paraffin embedded lung tissue. They are limited by a membrane, and their histochemical reactions and solubilities suggest that they are rich in lipid, particularly phospholipid. These bodies are occasionally seen at the free surface of the cell, where they appear to discharge their contents in much the same manner as described for the release of secretory products by various glandular cells. These bodies have recently been the subject of intensive investigation because of the suggestion that they represent intracellular stores of a surface active material which,

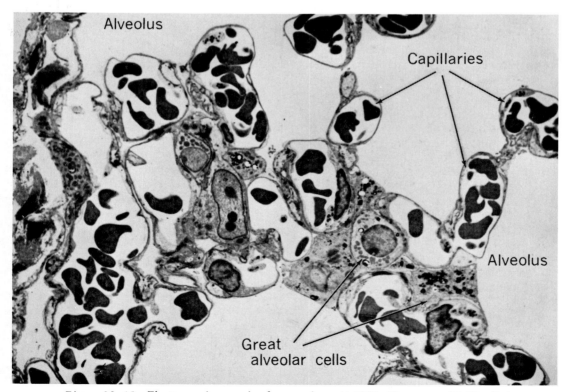

Figure 30–15 Electron micrograph of mouse lung. × 1800. (Courtesy of J. Rhodin.)

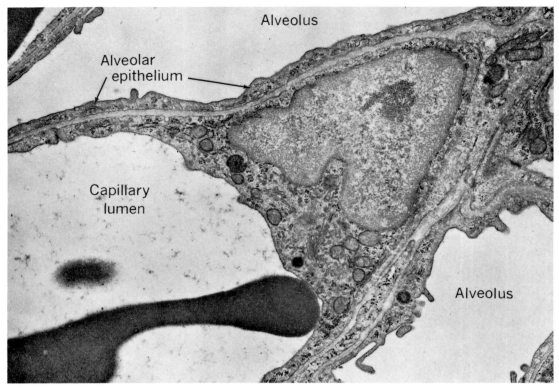

Figure 30-16 Electron micrograph of part of a capillary and adjacent alveoli, illustrating (*upper left*) the nature of the alveolocapillary membrane or blood-air barrier, which consists of three layers: the alveolar epithelium, an interstitial space occupied by a basal lamina, and the capillary endothelium. × 20,500. (Courtesy of E. R. Weibel.)

upon release, spreads upon the surface of the epithelium, lowering surface tension and tending to stabilize alveolar diameter. Inadequate surfactant production is considered to be responsible for the *respiratory distress syndrome* of the human newborn, a disease which frequently accompanies premature birth.

Nerve endings have been described in the alveolar walls of some species (Hung et al.; Meyrick and Reid). Some of these are rich in mitochondria and are believed to be sensory; other endings, near alveolar cells, contain dense-cored vesicles and may be involved in neural control of surfactant secretion.

Alveolar Phagocytes (Dust Cells)

In practically every section of lung, free phagocytic cells are encountered in the alveoli. Because they contain particles of in-

haled dust they are sometimes called "dust cells." In certain cardiac diseases attended by pulmonary vascular congestion, they become filled with granules of *hemosiderin* resulting from phagocytosis and degradation of blood pigment. There is no general agreement as to the origin of the alveolar phagocytes. Some investigators claim that they arise by exfoliation of the alveolar or septal cells; others consider them indistinguishable from macrophages in other parts of the body and trace their origin to hematogenous monocytes that emigrate from the capillaries. The bulk of the evidence now favors this interpretation. Although it may be that the fixed alveolar cells possess a limited capacity for phagocytosis, there is a marked difference between their activity and that of the free alveolar phagocytes. There are also marked differences in cytochemical reactions of the septal cells and free macrophages that suggest that they are functionally distinct (Sorokin).

In tissue cultures of the lungs and in certain in vivo experiments, inconspicuous cells in the septa mobilize in a few hours and assume the appearance and function of typical macrophages. Whether these arise from the alveolar cells in the epithelium or from interstitial histiocytes is not clear. In acute pneumococcal infections of the lung of dogs and monkeys, the principal reaction of the "septal cells" appears to be one of enlargement without detachment from the alveolar walls. No phagocytic properties are observed in them. Under these conditions the chief source of macrophages appears to be hematogenous monocytes that transform into macrophages after they enter the alveoli early in the disease. Whatever the origin of the alveolar phagocyte, it acts as a typical macrophage in defense of the lung, including the continual removal of dust particles. The number of these cells and their burden of phagocytosis is much greater in smokers than in nonsmokers (Figs. 30–20 and 30–21).

Blood Vessels

The lungs receive most of their blood from the pulmonary arteries. These are of large caliber and of elastic type. The branches of these arteries in general accompany the bronchi and their branches as far as the respiratory bronchioles. The arterial paths in the lung, however, are subject to considerable variation. From the respiratory bronchioles they divide, and a branch passes to each alveolar duct and is distributed in a capillary network over all the alveoli that communicate with this duct. The venules arise from the capillaries of the pleura and from the capillaries of the alveolar septa and portions of the alveolar ducts. They run in the intersegmental connective tissue, independently of the arteries, and join to form the pulmonary veins. In passing through the lung, the pulmonary artery is usually above and behind its accompanying bronchial tube, whereas the vein is below and in front of it.

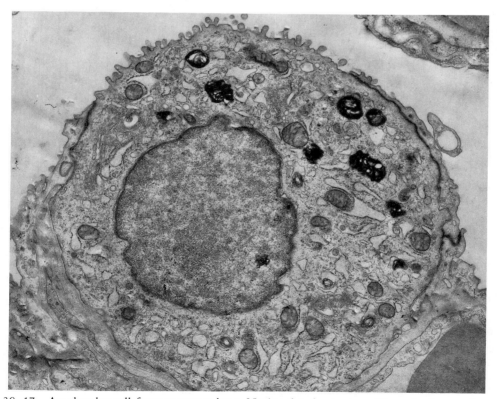

Figure 30–17 An alveolar cell from opossum lung. Notice the short microvilli on its free surface and its junctional complexes with the thin alveolar epithelial cells that partially cover its sides. A Golgi complex and numerous dilated cisternae of granular endoplasmic reticulum can be seen in its cytoplasm. (After S. Sorokin, J. Histochem. Cytochem., *14*:834, 1966.)

The bronchial arteries and veins are much smaller than the pulmonary vessels. These arteries arise from the aorta or the intercostal arteries and follow the bronchi. They are distributed to the walls of the bronchi, their glands, and the interlobular connective tissue beneath the pleura. Most of the blood carried by the bronchial arteries is brought back by the pulmonary veins. In the alveoli that arise from the respiratory bronchioles, there are capillary anastomoses between the terminations of the pulmonary and the bronchial arteries.

Lymphatics

There are two main divisions of the lymphatics of the lungs. One set is in the pleura and the other in the pulmonary tissue. They communicate infrequently. Both drain into the lymph nodes at the hilus of the lung. The lymphatics of the pleura form a dense network with large and small polygonal meshes. The large meshes are formed by large vessels

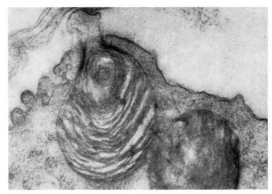

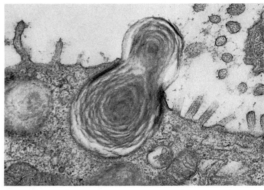

Figure 30-19 Lamellar bodies in mouse alveolar cells apparently in the process of being secreted in much the same manner as that described for merocrine secretions in the¹ pancreas and other glands. × 37,500. (After K. Hatasa and T. Nakamura, Zeitschr. f. Zellforsch., *68:*266, 1965.)

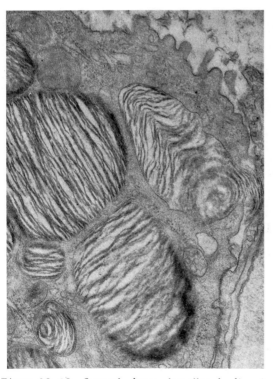

Figure 30-18 Several dense lamellar bodies in an alveolar cell of mouse lung. One at the right is apparently releasing some of its content into the lumen. × 37,500. (After K. Hatasa and T. Nakamura, Zeitschr. f. Zellforsch., *68:*266, 1965.)

and demarcate the lobules; the small meshwork is formed of smaller vessels that mark out the anatomical units. There are many valves in these lymphatics that control the flow of lymph so that it passes toward the hilus and not into the pulmonary tissue. These pleural lymphatics join to form several main trunks, which drain into the lymph nodes at the hilus.

The pulmonary lymphatics may be divided into several groups, which include those of the bronchi, of the pulmonary artery, and of the pulmonary vein. The lymphatics in the bronchi extend peripherally as far as the alveolar ducts, and their end branches join the lymphatic radicles of the plexuses about the pulmonary artery and vein. There are no lymphatic vessels beyond the alveolar ducts. The pulmonary artery is accompanied and drained by two or three main lymphatic trunks. The lymphatics associated with the pulmonary vein begin with its radicles in the alveolar ducts and in the pleura. All the lymphatics of the pulmonary tissue drain toward the hilar nodes. Efferent trunks from the hilar nodes anastomose to form the right lymphatic duct, which is the principal channel of lymph drainage from both the right and left lungs. There are no valves in the intrapulmonic lymphatics except in a few vessels, in the interlobular connective tissue near the pleura, which accompany the branches of the pulmonary veins. These lymphatic vessels connect the pulmonary and pleural lymphatic plexuses. As their valves point only toward the pleura, they provide a mechanism whereby lymph can flow from the pulmonary tissue into the pleural lymphatics if the normal flow of lymph from the pulmonary tissue toward the hilus is interrupted.

As has been mentioned, the mucosa of the bronchi is infiltrated with lymphocytes and often contains germinal centers. There are other accumulations of lymphatic tissue in the adventitia of the pulmonary arteries and veins.

Nerves

The pulmonary plexuses at the root of the lung are formed by branches of the vagus and of the thoracic sympathetic ganglia. The bronchoconstrictor fibers are from the vagus nerve, whereas the bronchodilator fibers are from the sympathetic nerve and arise mainly from the inferior cervical and first thoracic ganglia. The pulmonary vessels are supplied with both sympathetic and parasympathetic nerve fibers. The effect of these fibers on the vessels is not understood, as the experimental evidence is contradictory. The sympathetic fibers act as vasoconstrictors for the bronchial arteries.

The Pleura

The cavities containing the lungs are lined by a serous membrane, the *pleura*, which consists of a thin layer of collagenous tissue containing some fibroblasts and macrophages and several prominent layers of elastic fibers running at various angles to the

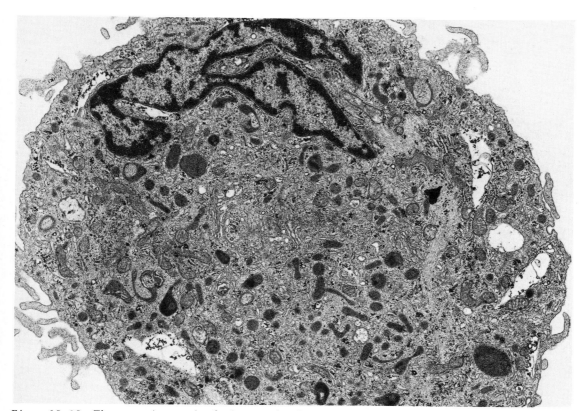

Figure 30–20   Electron micrograph of a human alveolar macrophage from a nonsmoker. Numerous small lysosomes are present but relatively few heterophagic vacuoles are seen. (Micrograph courtesy of S. Pratt and A. J. Ladman.)

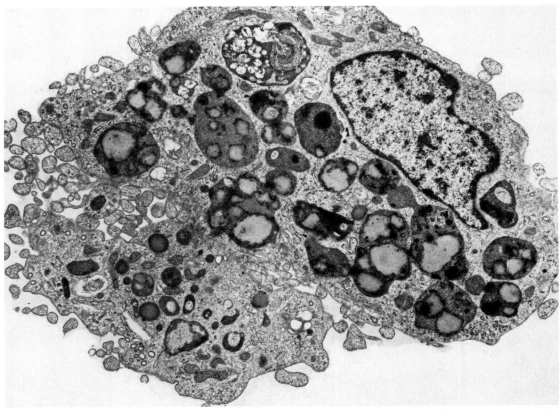

Figure 30-21. Electron micrograph of an alveolar macrophage from an 18 year old cigarette smoker. The cytoplasm is crowded with pigment masses representing undigestible residues of material phagocytized from the alveoli. (Micrograph courtesy of S. Pratt and A. J. Ladman.)

outer surface. It is covered by a layer of mesothelial cells like those of the peritoneum. The layer lining the wall of the thoracic cavity is called the *parietal pleura;* that reflected over the surface of the lungs is known as the *visceral pleura.* A prominent feature of the pleura is the great number of blood capillaries and lymphatic vessels distributed in it. The few nerves of the parietal pleura are connected with the phrenic and intercostal nerves. The nerves to the visceral pleura are believed to be branches of the vagus and of the sympathetic nerves supplying the bronchi.

Histogenesis

The lung arises in the embryo as a median diverticulum of the foregut caudal to the branchial clefts. Its prenatal growth can be divided into three periods: glandular, canalicular, and alveolar (Loosli and Potter). The diverticulum growing caudally is the primordium of the trachea, and it divides into right and left branches representing the primary bronchi. These rapidly elongate and branch dichotomously during the second to sixth week of gestation to produce several successive generations of hollow tubules lined with columnar epithelial cells. These tubules grow into a highly cellular mesenchyme in such a way as to resemble a glandular organ. From 16 to 23 generations of bronchial branches are formed during fetal life, and no new terminal bronchioles are formed after birth. Thus the air conducting portion of the respiratory tract completes its branching phase of growth quite early in intrauterine life. The branching of the pulmonary arteries that accompany the bronchial tree also appears to occur in this same period.

During the canalicular period of development, from the fourth to the seventh month, there is a more rapid growth of the mesenchymal tissue associated with the peripheral portions of the bronchial tree. Connective tissue cells and fibrils become prominent and an extensive system of capillaries develops. The capillaries are closely associated with air channels in a manner not unlike their relation to the respiratory membrane in the adult. No alveoli are present at this stage.

The alveolar stage of development occupies the period from 6½ months to full term. The lung loses its glandular character and becomes increasingly vascular. The bulbous expansions at the ends of the bronchial tree branch further, and alveoli arise as shallow evaginations from the sides of the channel walls. The connective tissue fibers become distributed around the alveolar openings. The epithelium becomes attenuated, and the capillaries establish a close relation to the future respiratory surface.

The majority of investigators consider the initial respiratory air spaces to be alveoli similar in size to those seen in the adult lung. In man it would seem that these saccular spaces correspond more correctly to alveolar ducts and that definitive alveoli are absent. At the end of gestation, the alveoli are shallow indentations on the respiratory channels. According to Dubreuil and co-workers, the adult type of respiratory unit does not become apparent until several years after birth. One has only to compare (in Fig. 30–12) the inflated lung of the newborn with the expanded lung of a 12 year old to note the marked increase in size of the alveolar ducts and the alveoli. Whether growth of the lung takes place only by an increase in size and distention of existing ducts and alveoli, or also by some other process, needs further study.

Results on postnatal growth of the human lung are conflicting; some workers report that no new pulmonary acini develop after birth, whereas others conclude that

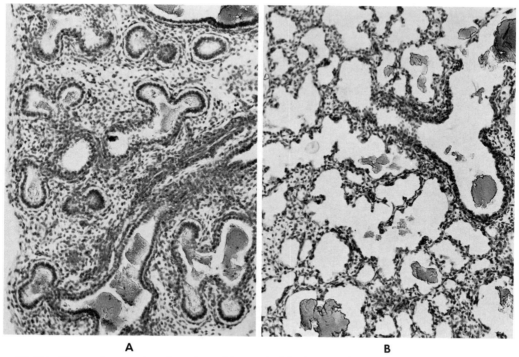

A   **B**

Figure 30–22 Photomicrographs of section of lung. *A,* Of 147 gm. (4 month) fetus. *B,* Of a 440 gm. (6½ month) fetus. Both specimens show Thorotrast aspirated by intrauterine respirations. Although fetal respiration is considered by some to be normal, the majority now believe it occurs only in fetal distress. The lung of the 6½ month fetus was expanded by extrauterine respiration. Note change in character of lung structure from glandular type (previable) to respiratory type (viable). Respiratory portion of lung of older fetus consists essentially of alveolar ducts; alveoli are absent or are represented only by shallow indentations on duct walls. Hematoxylin and eosin. × 45. (After Davis and Potter.)

there is a rapid and steady increase in the number of alveoli in early childhood. It seems likely that the respiratory portion of the lung grows mainly by enlargement in length and width of respiratory bronchioles, alveolar ducts, alveolar sacs, and alveoli, rather than by increased numbers of these structures (Loosli and Potter).

Repair of the Lung

The lung is frequently the seat of inflammatory conditions that leave it unimpaired on healing. In certain infections, however—notably tuberculosis—large masses of pulmonary tissues are destroyed. In such cases, healing is always attended by connective tissue scar formation. There is no evidence to show that the pulmonary tissue can regenerate after destruction.

Histophysiology

The primary function of the lungs is to serve as a means for the assimilation of oxygen from the air and for the removal of carbon dioxide from the body. The network of blood capillaries in the wall of the air sacs is separated from the air by a thin, moist membrane, which permits the ready diffusion of oxygen into the blood and carbon dioxide out of it. The exchange of gases between blood and inspired air takes place across a barrier consisting of three layers: the thin epithelium, the basal lamina, and the capillary endothelium. The movement of the gases is considered to be by a process of passive diffusion, except that the liberation of carbon dioxide from carbonic acid is now known to be greatly accelerated by *carbonic anhydrase*.

The capillaries in the respiratory portions of the human lung are estimated to have a surface area of 140 square meters. The lung also eliminates approximately 800 ml. of water a day in the expired air. Under abnormal conditions it may also remove certain other substances from the blood, such as alcohol.

The lung has a large margin of reserve; that is, the body at rest uses but a small portion—about one twentieth—of the pulmonary aerating surface.

The alveoli probably change but little during inspiration, and the flow of blood is actually faster then. It appears more and more likely that the great increase in the volume of the lungs in inspiration takes place mainly through a great distention of the alveolar ducts, but the smaller bronchi and bronchioles also distend with inspiration.

The pressure within the lung is equal to that of the atmosphere. The lungs are maintained in a partially distended condition by the reduced pressure of the potential space between the two layers of the pleura. An increase in the size of the thorax, such as occurs with every inspiration, decreases pressure in the pleural cavity; consequently the lung sucks in more air and becomes larger, and its elastic and reticular fibers are put under greater tension. This is a purely passive activity on the part of the lung. In expiration, as the thoracic cavity becomes smaller, the pressure in the pleural cavity rises slightly (although it is still below atmospheric pressure). This decreases the tension on the elastic and reticular fibers, and they recoil, pulling the lung into a more contracted state and thus forcing some of the air out of it. It is probable that the smooth muscles of the alveolar ducts and the bronchioles also help force the air out of the lung by their contraction.

When the pleural cavity on one side is connected with the outside air, either by accident or by surgical intervention, the pressure in the lungs and in the pleural cavity becomes equalized at that of the atmosphere. The lung then collapses immediately, because the force that normally opposes the contraction of its elastic elements has been removed. This condition is known as *pneumothorax*. Such a lung remains collapsed until pressure in the pleural cavity is reduced by absorption of the air contained in it.

With each inspiration the descent of the diaphragm enables the bronchi in the lower lobes of the lungs to extend. Because the main bronchi are not fixed in the thorax but descend on inspiration, a mechanism is provided whereby the bronchi of the upper lobes of the lungs extend at the same time.

REFERENCES

Adams, F. H.: Fetal and neonatal cardiovascular and pulmonary function. Annual Rev. Physiol., 27:257, 1965.

Adams, F. H.: Functional development of the fetal lung. J. Pediat., 68:794, 1966.

Avery, M. E.: The alveolar lining layer. A review of studies on its role in pulmonary mechanics and in pathogenesis of atelectasis. Pediatrics, 30:324, 1962.

Avery, M. E., and J. Mead: Surface properties in relation to atelectasis and hyaline membrane disease. Am. J. Dis. Child., 97:517, 1959.

Bargmann, W.: Die Lungenalveole. *In* von Möllendorff, W., and W. Bargmann, eds.: Handbuch der mikroskopischen Anatomie des Menschen. Berlin, Julius Springer, 1936, Vol. 5, part 3, p. 799.

Bertalanffy, F. D.: Respiratory tissue: Structure, histophysiology and cytodynamics. Int. Rev. Cytol., 16:233, 1964.

Beusch, L., K. Schaefer, and M. E. Avery: Granular pneumonocytes: Electron microscopic evidence of their exocrine function. Science, 145:1318, 1964.

Bloom, G.: Studies on the olfactory epithelium of the frog and the toad with the aid of light and electron microscopy. Zeitschr. f. Zellforsch., 41:89, 1954.

Boyden, E. A.: Segmental Anatomy of the Lungs; A Study of the Patterns of the Segmental Bronchi and Related Pulmonary Vessels. New York, Blakiston Division, McGraw-Hill Book Co., 1955.

Boyden, E. A.: The terminal air sacs and their blood supply in a 37-day infant lung. Am. J. Anat., 116:413, 1965.

Boyden, E. A., and D. H. Tompsett: The changing patterns in the developing lungs of infants. Acta Anat., 61:164, 1965.

Bremer, J. L.: Postnatal development of alveoli in the mammalian lung in relation to the problem of the alveolar phagocyte. Carnegie Contributions to Embryol., 25:83, 1935.

Buckingham, S.: Studies on the identification of an antiatelectasis factor in normal sheep lung. Am. J. Dis. Child., 105:521, 1961.

Buckingham, S., and M. E. Avery: Time of appearance of lung surfactant in the foetal mouse. Nature, 193:688, 1962.

Campiche, M.: Les inclusions lamellaires des cellules alvéolaires dans le poumon du raton. Relations entre l'ultrastructure et la fixation. J. Ultrastruct. Res., 3:302, 1960.

Campiche, M., A. Gautier, E. I. Hernandez, and A. Raymond: An electron microscopic study of the fetal development of the human lung. Pediatrics, 32:976, 1963.

Clements, L. P.: Embryonic development of the respiratory portion of the pig's lung. Anat. Rec., 70:575, 1938.

de Lorenzo, A. J.: Electron microscopic observations of the olfactory mucosa and olfactory nerve. J. Biophys. Biochem. Cytol., 3:839, 1957.

Dubreuil, G., A. Lacoste, and R. Raymond: Observations sur le développement du poumon humain. Bul. d'Histol. Appliq. à la Physiol., 13:235, 1936.

Hatasa, K., and T. Nakamura: Electron microscopic observations of lung alveolar epithelial cells of normal young mice with special reference to formation and secretion of osmiophilic lamellar bodies. Zeitschr. f. Zellforsch., 68:266, 1965.

Hung, K. S., M. S. Hertweck, J. D. Hardy, and C. G. Loosli: Ultrastructure of nerves and associated cells in bronchial epithelium of mouse lung. J. Ultrastr. Res., 43:426, 1973.

Hung, K. S., M. S. Hertweck, J. D. Hardy, and C. G. Loosli: Electron microscopic observations on nerve endings in the alveolar walls of mouse lungs. Am. Rev. Resp. Dis., 108:328, 1973.

Karrer, H. E.: The ultrastructure of mouse lung; general architecture of capillary and alveolar walls. J. Biophys. Biochem. Cytol., 2:241, 1956.

Karrer, H. E.: The ultrastructure of mouse lung: The alveolar macrophage. J. Biophys. Biochem. Cytol., 4:693, 1958.

Krahl, V. E.: Anatomy of the mammalian lung. *In*: American Physiological Society: Handbook of Physiology. Baltimore, Williams & Wilkins Co., 1964, Section 3, Vol. I, p. 213.

Ladman, A. J., and T. N. Finley: Electron microscopic observations of pulmonary surfactant and the cells which produce it. Anat. Rec., 154:372, 1966.

Le Gros Clark, W.: Inquiries into the anatomical basis of olfactory discrimination. Proc. Roy. Soc. B, 146:299, 1957.

Loosli, C. G.: Interalveolar communications in normal and in pathologic mammalian lungs. Arch. Path., 24:743, 1937.

Loosli, C. G.: The pathogenesis and pathology of experimental type I pneumococcic pneumonia in the monkey. J. Exper. Med., 76:79, 1942.

Loosli, C. G., and R. F. Baker: The human lung: microscopic structure and diffusion. Ciba Foundation Symposium on Pulmonary Structure and Function, 1962, p. 194.

Loosli, C. G., and E. L. Potter: Pre- and postnatal development of the respiratory portion of the human lung, with special reference to the elastic fibers. Am. Rev. Resp. Dis., 80:5, 1959.

Low, F. N.: The pulmonary alveolar epithelium of laboratory mammals and man. Anat. Rec., 117:241, 1953.

Low, F. N., and M. M. Sampaio: The pulmonary alveolar epithelium as an entodermal derivative. Anat. Rec., 127:51, 1957.

Macklin, C. C.: The musculature of the bronchi and lungs. Physiol. Rev., 9:1, 1929.

Macklin, C. C.: Residual epithelial cells on the pulmonary alveolar walls of mammals. Tr. Roy. Soc. Canada, 3rd ser., Sec. V, 40:93, 1946.

Meyrick, B., and L. Reid: Nerves in the rat intraacinar alveoli: an electron microscopic study. Resp. Physiol., 11:367, 1971.

Miller, W. S.: The Lung. 2nd ed. Springfield, Ill., Charles C Thomas, 1947.

Pattle, R. E.: Properties, function, and origin of the alveolar lining layer. Proc. Roy. Soc. B., 148:217, 1958.

Pratt, S. A., M. H. Smith, A. J. Ladman, and T. N. Finley: The ultrastructure of alveolar macrophages from human cigarette smokers and non-smokers. Lab. Invest., 24:331, 1971.

Pump, K. K.: The circulation of the primary lobule of the lung. Dis. Chest., 39:614, 1961.

Pump, K. K.: The bronchial arteries and their anastomoses in the human lung. Dis. Chest., 43:245, 1963.

Pump, K. K.: The morphology of the finger branches of the bronchial tree of the human lung. Dis. Chest., 46:379, 1964.

Reese, T. S.: Olfactory cilia in the frog. J. Cell Biol., 25:209, 1965.

Robertson, O. H.: Phagocytosis of foreign material in the lung. Physiol. Rev., 21:112, 1941.

Sorokin, S. P.: A morphologic and cytochemical study on the great alveolar cell. J. Histochem. Cytochem., 14:884, 1967.

Spencer, H., and D. Leof: The innervation of the human lung. J. Anat. (London), 98:599, 1964.

Tobin, C. E.: Human pulmonic lymphatics. Anat. Rec., 127:611, 1957.

Weibel, E. R.: Morphometrische Analyse von Zahl, Volumen und Oberfläche der Alveolen und Kapillaren der menschlichen Lunge. Zeitschr. f. Zellforsch., 57:648, 1962.

Weibel, E. R.: Morphometrics of the lung. *In* American Physiological Society: Handbook of Physiology. Baltimore, Williams & Wilkins Co., 1964, Section 3, Vol. I, p. 285.

31

The Urinary System

The urinary system consists of the kidneys, ureters, urinary bladder, and urethra. The system functions to clear the blood of the waste products of metabolism and to regulate the concentrations of many constituents of the body fluids. In addition to their excretory function, the kidneys have an endocrine function—producing and releasing into the bloodstream a humoral agent that affects blood formation (erythropoietin) and another that influences blood pressure (renin). In the male, the urethra not only conveys the urine to the outside but also serves the reproductive system as the pathway for the discharge of semen.

KIDNEYS

The human kidneys are paired organs situated retroperitoneally on the posterior wall of the abdominal cavity on either side of the vertebral column. They are roughly bean-shaped, 10 to 12 cm. in length, 5 to 6 cm. in width, and 3 to 4 cm. in thickness. A concavity, the *hilus,* is found on the medial border. The large excretory duct, the *ureter,* emerges from the hilus and courses downward to the urinary bladder, which is situated in the pelvis directly behind the pubis. The kidney is closely invested by a thin but strong capsule of dense collagenous fibers. The glandular part of the kidney surrounds a large cavity, the *renal sinus,* that extends inward from the hilus and contains the *renal*

pelvis. The remainder of the sinus around the renal pelvis is occupied by loose connective tissue and adipose tissue, through which the blood vessels and nerves pass into the renal tissue.

The renal pelvis is a funnel-shaped expansion of the upper end of the ureter, which sends into the substance of the kidney two or three sizable outpocketings called *major calyces.* These in turn have a number of smaller branches called *minor calyces* (Fig. 31–1).

When the cut surface of the hemisected kidney is viewed with the naked eye, a darker reddish brown *cortex* is readily distinguishable from a lighter *medulla.* The medulla is made up of 8 to 18 conical subdivisions called *renal pyramids,* each having its base toward the cortex and its apex or *papilla* projecting into the lumen of a minor calyx. The lateral boundaries of each pyramid are defined by inward extensions of the darker cortical tissue forming the *renal columns* (of Bertin). A renal pyramid together with the cortical tissue overlying its base and covering its sides constitutes a *renal lobe.* Each lobe of the human kidney corresponds to the entire unipyramidal kidney of common laboratory rodents. During embryonic development, each lobe arises in association with a different minor calyx, and during fetal life the several lobes are recognizable as distinct convexities on the surface of the organ, but later in development they fuse into a continuous smooth-contoured cortex.

The gray substance of each pyramid is radially striated with brownish lines that con-

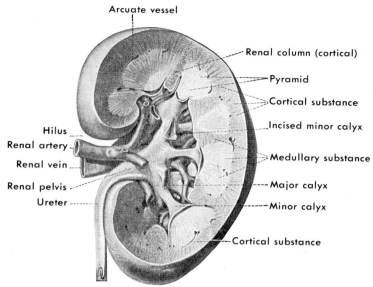

Arcuate vessel

Renal column (cortical)

Pyramid

Cortical substance

Incised minor calyx

Medullary substance

Major calyx

Minor calyx

Cortical substance

Hilus

Renal artery

Renal vein

Renal pelvis

Ureter

Figure 31–1 Human kidney, seen from behind, after removal of part of the organ. Three fifths natural size. (After Braus.)

verge toward the apex of the papilla. These striations are a reflection of the orientation of the straight portions of the microscopic uriniferous tubules and of the blood vessels that course parallel to them. The tip of each papilla, called the *area cribrosa*, is perforated by 10 to 25 small openings, where the terminal segments of the uriniferous tubules open into a minor calyx.

The myriad renal tubules that constitute the parenchyma of the kidney are specialized along their length for different functions, and each of the specialized segments tends to be located at a particular level. This consistency in distribution of corresponding segments is reflected in grossly distinguishable zones in the medulla, which differ slightly in color or pattern. There is an *inner* and *outer zone* of the medulla and the outer zone is sometimes further subdivided into a darker and thicker *inner band* or *stripe* and a lighter and thinner *outer band*.

From the bases of the medullary pyramids thin, radially directed striations extend into the cortical substance. These bear some resemblance to the striations in the pyramid but do not extend through the entire thickness of the cortex. These markings are called the *medullary rays* (of Ferrein) and represent continuations of bundles of tubules from the pyramid into the cortex (Figs. 31–2

and 31–3). Each medullary ray and its immediately associated cortical tissue are considered to be a *renal lobule*, although they are not separated from one another by connective tissue septa as is often the case of lobules of other glands. The structural basis of the patterns that are visible on the cut surface of the normal kidney will be better understood after the description of the uriniferous tubules. It is sufficient here to note that recognition of these gross markings is not only an aid to comprehension of the complex microscopic organization of this organ, but it is also of practical value to the pathologist to the extent that loss or distortion of the normal pattern is associated with particular disease entities.

URINIFEROUS TUBULES

The tubules composing the kidney have two principal portions. The first portion, the *nephron*, corresponding to the secretory elements of other glands, is concerned with the formation of urine, and the second portion, the *collecting tubule*, carries out a final concentration of urinary solute to form a hypertonic urine, and serves as the excretory duct conveying the urine to the renal pelvis. These two components arise in the embryo from separate primordia which become connected secondarily. This is in contrast to the development of other glands, in which the ducts and secretory portions arise from a single primordium that branches dichotomously and becomes secretory in the distal part of its arborescent pattern.

The Nephron

The nephron is the tubular functional unit of this organ. There is estimated to be about two million in each kidney, and the output of urine represents a summation of the functions of this very large number of units. Along the length of the nephron are several morphologically distinct segments, each having a characteristic configuration and occupying a definite position in the cortex or medulla. Each segment is lined with a specific type of epithelium specialized for a particular role in the formation of urine.

At the proximal end of each is a thin-walled expansion called *Bowman's capsule,*

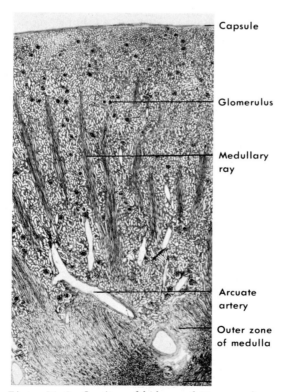

Figure 31-2 Section of kidney of *Macacus rhesus.* Fixation by vascular perfusion—hence the empty blood vessels. Photomicrograph (slightly retouched). × 13.

which is deeply indented by a globular tuft of capillaries, the *glomerulus.* This mass of capillaries and its surrounding chalice-shaped epithelial capsule together constitute the *renal corpuscle.* It has a vascular pole where the afferent and efferent vessels enter and leave the glomerulus, and a *urinary pole* where the slit-like cavity within the capsule of Bowman is continuous with the lumen of the next segment of the nephron, the *proximal tubule* (Fig. 31–4). This consists of a convoluted and a straight portion. The latter is followed by a *thin segment* and this in turn by the straight and convoluted portions of the *distal tubule.* The convoluted portion of the proximal tubule (*proximal convoluted tubule*) and the convoluted portion of the distal tubule (*distal convoluted tubule*) are both located in the cortex close to the renal corpuscle. The portion of nephron between the two convoluted segments (namely, the straight portion of the proximal tubule, the thin segment, and the straight portion of the distal tubule) forms a loop, the *loop of Henle,* extending from the cortex for a variable distance into the medulla. The radially oriented descending and ascending limbs of the loop run parallel to each other and are connected by a sharp bend (Fig. 31–4). The same segments are represented in the same sequence in all nephrons, but the length of the loop and the proportions of the segments of which it is formed vary with the position of the glomerulus in the cortex. Nephrons whose glomeruli are in the outer or subcapsular portion of the cortex have short loops of Henle with abbreviated thin segments, and these loops extend only a very short distance into the outer zone of the medulla. Nephrons whose glomeruli are situated in the deep or juxtamedullary region of the cortex form a loop with long descending and ascending limbs and an extensive thin segment, which penetrates deep into the inner zone of the medulla. Nephrons with glomeruli midway in the cortex have intermediate characteristics. In addition, there are significant differences in the vascular supply to these three categories of nephrons. These will be described later. The distal convoluted tubules are joined to the collecting duct system by a short connecting segment often referred to as the *arched collecting tubule* to distinguish it from the radially oriented *straight collecting tubules.* The latter are continuous with the *papillary ducts* which deliver urine to the minor calyces.

Figure labels: Capsule, Glomerulus, Medullary ray, Arcuate artery, Outer zone of medulla

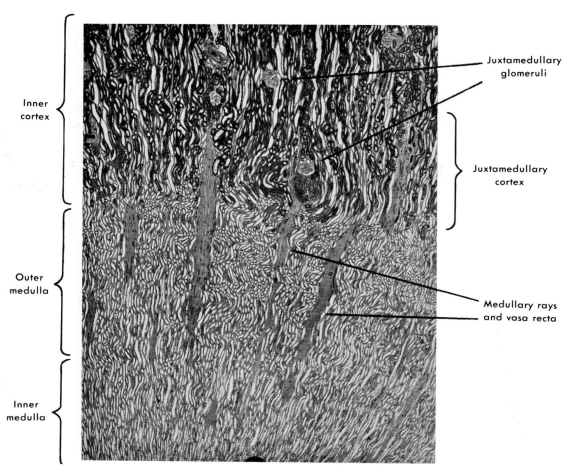

Inner cortex

Juxtamedullary glomeruli

Juxtamedullary cortex

Outer medulla

Medullary rays and vasa recta

Inner medulla

Figure 31–3 Section of dog kidney, showing medullary rays and vasa recta extending from juxtamedullary glomeruli to the border of the inner medulla. Mallory stain. × 30. (After Thorburn et al., Circulation Res., 13:290, 1963.)

The tortuous convoluted tubules of neighboring nephrons in the cortex intermingle so extensively that the identity and shape of the individual units cannot be ascertained from study of histological sections. What is known of their three-dimensional configuration has been established by their reconstruction from serial sections (Grafflin) or by maceration of the tissue and teasing out the individual nephrons by time-consuming micromanipulation (Oliver). It has also been possible by micropuncture to penetrate individual glomerular capsules and to observe directly the progress of injected contrast media through the lumen of a single nephron (Beuckes).

The renal corpuscles have evolved as efficient ultrafiltering devices for clearing the blood of wastes. About 1200 ml. of blood flows through the kidneys per minute and about a fifth of the plasma volume is filtered off in the renal corpuscles. Thus, about 120 ml. of a fluid, called the *glomerular filtrate,* enters the renal tubules each minute. As this fluid passes through the various segments of the nephron, its composition is modified by secretion of certain substances into it and reabsorption of water and other constituents from it. The final product, *urine,* is drained through the collecting ducts into the renal pelvis.

Renal Corpuscle. The capsule of Bowman around the tuft of glomerular capillaries is a double walled cup composed of squamous epithelium. Although not strictly true, it is conceptually useful to consider that in the embryonic development of the renal corpuscle, the glomerulus is pushed into, and deeply indents, a blind terminal expansion of the uriniferous tubule. From this mode of development it would follow that there is a *visceral layer* of epithelium (the glomerular epithelium) applied to the capillaries, as well as a *parietal layer* (the capsular epithelium). Between these is a narrow chalice-shaped cavity, the *capsular space* (Bowman's space). At the vascular pole of the renal corpuscle, the visceral layer is reflected off the afferent and efferent glomerular vessels to become continuous with the squamous epithelium of the parietal layer. At the urinary pole, the capsular epithelium is continuous with the cuboidal epithelium in the neck of the proximal convoluted tubule (Fig. 31–5).

In the development of the renal corpuscle, the parietal layer remains a typical squamous epithelium of flat polygonal cells, but the cells of the visceral layer become so extensively modified that, in the adult, they bear little resemblance to any other epithelial cells.

These cells, called *podocytes*, are closely applied to the capillaries and are basically stellate, with several radiating *primary processes* that embrace the vessels in a manner reminiscent of the pericytes of ordinary capillaries (Fig. 31–6). The primary processes give rise to very numerous *secondary processes*, also called *foot processes* or *pedicels*. These interdigitate with corresponding elements of neighboring podocytes to create an extraordinarily elaborate system of intercellular clefts, called *slit pores* (Figs. 31–8 and 31–9).

In thin sections examined with the electron microscope, the cell bodies of the podocytes are rarely found in extensive contact with the basal lamina. Instead, they stand off 1 or 2 μm. and are attached to it via their primary processes, which then ramify over its surface. The cell body and major processes of one podocyte may arch over, undermining

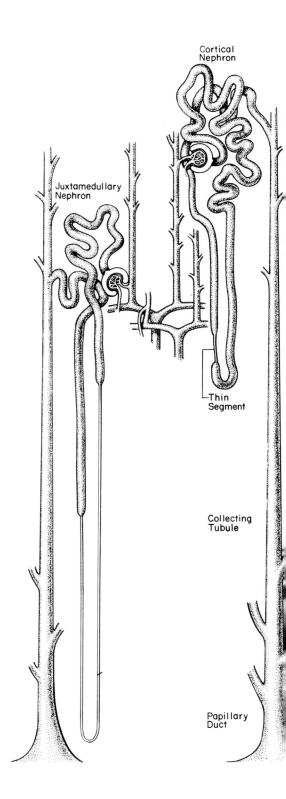

Figure 31–4 Highly schematic drawing of a cortical nephron and a juxtamedullary nephron, comparing the renal corpuscles, proximal convoluted tubules, straight descending portions of proximal tubule, thin segments, straight ascending portions of the distal tubule, distal convoluted tubules and collecting tubules. The cortical nephrons have a short loop of Henle with a very short thin segment, whereas these structures are long and extend deep into the medulla in juxtamedullary nephrons.

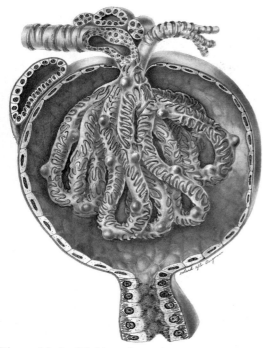

Figure 31–5 Highly schematic representation of the renal corpuscle. The parietal layer of Bowman's capsule is depicted considerably thicker than it actually is, and the visceral layer overlying the capillaries of the glomerulus is greatly simplified, with only the major processes of the podocytes depicted. Although earlier described as a cluster of simple loops, the capillaries are now believed to branch and anastomose to form a network. (Redrawn and modified after Bargmann.)

podocytes and the finer details of the filtration barrier requires the higher resolution available in transmission electron micrographs. The podocytes have nuclei of complex form, often deeply infolded. Their cytoplasm contains a well developed Golgi complex, cisternal profiles of granular endoplasmic reticulum and abundant free ribosomes. Cytoplasmic filaments and microtubules are plentiful, both in the cell body and in the primary and secondary processes. The foot processes are aligned upon the outer surface of a continuous basal lamina, which they share with the endothelium of the underlying glomerular capillary (Fig. 31–11). Adjacent pedicels are not in intimate contact but are separated by slits about 250 Å wide. In micrographs of good resolution, these gaps are seen to be bridged by a thin dense line 60 Å or less in thickness (Fig. 31–12). This thin line is interpreted as a section of an exceedingly thin *slit membrane* extending between the outer leaflets of the plasma membranes of adjacent foot processes at the level of the basal lamina. This structure is considered to be similar to the tenuous diaphragm that closes the pores of fenestrated capillaries.

The basal lamina beneath the foot processes is 0.1 to 0.15 μm. in thickness and consists of a feltwork of fine filaments embedded in a glycoprotein matrix. It contains

primary processes of neighboring podocytes (Fig. 31–9). As a consequence of these relationships, the greater part of the capsular surface of the glomerular capillaries is carpeted by interdigitating pedicels thus providing a maximal area of slit pores for filtration. By laborious study of thin sections with the transmission electron microscope and imaginative reconstruction, students of renal cytology ventured to depict the three dimensional configuration of the podocytes, as shown in Figures 31–5 and 31–6. With the recent introduction of scanning electron microscopy, it is now possible to obtain three dimensional images of the cellular topography of this remarkably specialized epithelium. Its actual complexity (Figs. 31–7 and 31–8) far exceeds the most daring earlier interpretations of its structure based upon conventional light and electron microscopy.

Demonstration of the cytology of the

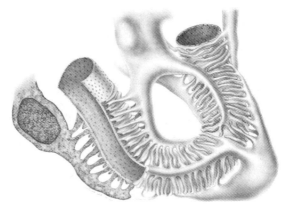

Figure 31–6 Highly schematic representation of the interdigitating pattern of secondary processes (foot processes or pedicels) of the podocytes on the outer surface of a glomerular capillary loop. This arrangement provides a very large area of slender filtration slits or slit pores between adjacent processes. (Redrawn and modified after Gordon, *in* A. W. Ham: Histology. 5th ed. Philadelphia, J. B. Lippincott Co., 1965.)

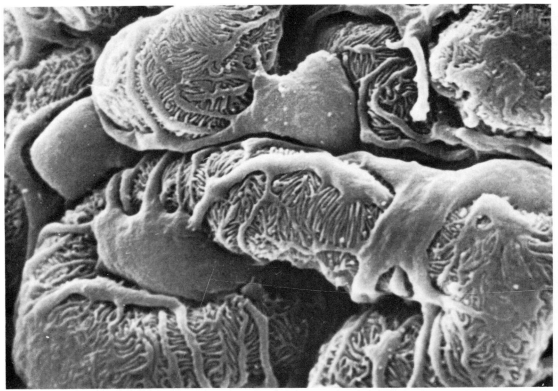

Figure 31-7 Scanning electron micrograph of a small area of the glomerulus, showing the visceral epithelium, consisting of podocytes with their interdigitating processes forming an elaborate filigree around the cylindrical capillaries. (Micrograph courtesy of F. Spinelli, Ciba-Geigy Ltd. Research Laboratories, Basle, Switzerland.)

collagen, but this appears to be in macromolecular form rather than in cross striated fibrils. The basal lamina becomes markedly thickened in diabetes and in certain other diseases affecting the kidney.

On the other side of the basal lamina, the endothelium lining the glomerular capillary is extremely attenuated and is perforated by circular pores or fenestrae 700 to 900 Å in diameter. These pores are said to differ from those of fenestrated capillaries elsewhere in the body in that they seem to lack the thin pore diaphragm. The abundance and distribution of the endothelial pores are best seen in the extended surface views offered by the freeze-cleaving technique of specimen preparation (Fig. 31-13). The thicker portions of the endothelial cells containing the nucleus are usually on the side of the capillary away from the capsular space. Also associated with this deep surface of the capillaries are the *mesangial cells.* These are stellate in form and

have a number of characteristics in common with the pericytes of capillaries elsewhere.

The filtration barrier between the blood circulating in the glomerular capillaries and the capsular space consists of the fenestrated endothelium, the basal lamina, and the slit pores between the interdigitating podocyte foot processes of the visceral epithelium. The endothelial pores appear to hold back only the cellular elements of blood and large particulate components of the plasma. The basal lamina is the only continuous layer in the wall of the glomerular capillary and is an important filtering component holding back large molecules. Evidence for this is derived from use of particulate tracers, such as ferritin (molecular weight, 400,000). When this large electron dense protein is administered intravenously to experimental animals, electron micrographs of their kidneys show that it easily traverses the endothelial pores of the glomerulus but tends to accumulate against

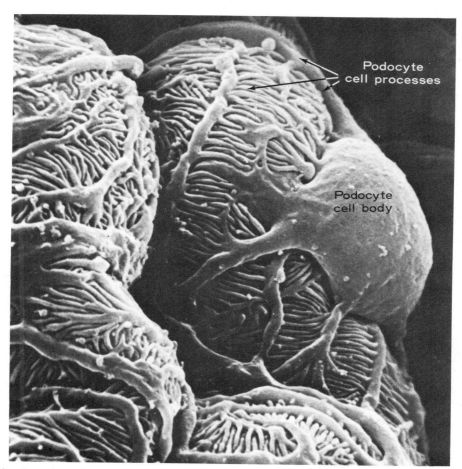

Podocyte cell processes

Podocyte cell body

Figure 31-8 Scanning micrograph of two adjacent capillary loops of rat glomerulus, illustrating the remarkable complexity of the primary and secondary processes of the podocytes, whose ramification and interdigitation leaves an enormous area of filtration slits through which the glomerular filtrate passes into the capsular space. (Micrograph courtesy of F. Spinelli, Ciba-Geigy Ltd. Research Laboratories, Basle, Switzerland.)

the inner aspect of the basal lamina. Ferritin molecules gradually infiltrate this layer and some may ultimately pass through it, but it is evident that the basal lamina is capable of significantly retarding ferritin and of preventing the passage of larger molecules. The impedance of ferritin, however, cannot be taken as evidence that this is the site of filtration of smaller protein molecules. Similar experiments have been carried out using horse-radish peroxidase (molecular weight, 40,000) and myeloperoxidase (molecular weight, 160,000) as protein tracers that are detectable by ultrastructural cytochemistry. The smaller peroxidase is found to pass rapidly through the endothelial pores, across the basal lamina, and through the slit pores into Bowman's space. The larger myeloperoxidase, on the other hand, readily traverses the basal lamina but is held up at the level of the slit membranes. These findings are interpreted to mean that the epithelial slit pores permit passage of molecules of 40,000 but retain molecules of 160,000 molecular weight (Graham and Karnovsky).

It has been shown that the basal lamina is not a static structural component but is constantly being renewed. The fact that the visceral epithelial cells exhibit some of the cytological characteristics of synthetically active cells has led to the suggestion that they play a role in the formation and continual renewal of the basal lamina. Experimental substantiation of this belief has been provided by adding silver nitrate to the drinking water of rats for a period of time sufficient to mark the glomerular basal lamina with a black line of deposited silver. In the weeks following cessation of silver nitrate ingestion, it can be shown that new, unlabeled basal lamina has been deposited on the epithelial side (Kurtz and Feldman). It is also speculated that the mesangial cells may be involved in the maintenance and reconditioning of the basal lamina by removal of residues of filtration. They probably participate in the turnover of this layer by removal of the older, deep portions of the filter as it is renewed at the epithelial surface (Farquhar).

The Proximal Tubule. At the urinary pole of the renal corpuscle, the squamous parietal epithelium of Bowman's capsule is continuous with the cuboidal epithelium of the proximal tubule (Fig. 31–5). This seg-

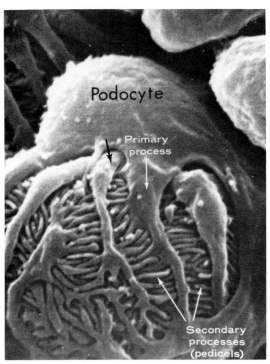

Figure 31-9 Scanning micrograph showing the relationship of primary processes and small secondary processes of the podocytes, called pedicels. Notice that the cell body of the podocyte may be elevated from the capillary surface and processes of a neighboring podocyte may extend under it (at arrow) to interdigitate with its own pedicels. (Micrograph courtesy of F. Spinelli, Ciba-Geigy Ltd. Research Laboratories, Basle, Switzerland.)

ment of the nephron is about 14 mm. long, 60 μm. in diameter, and makes up the bulk of the renal cortex. It is composed of a convoluted portion (*pars convoluta*) and a straight portion (*pars recta*). In addition to many small loops, the convoluted portion rather consistently forms a large loop directed toward the kidney capsule. The recurrent limb of this loop returns to the vicinity of the renal corpuscle and then courses toward the nearest medullary ray, where it straightens out to become the pars recta, running inward toward the medulla.

The epithelium of the proximal convoluted tubule consists of a single layer of cells with a conspicuous brush border on their luminal surface. In kidney tissue fixed by routine methods, the lumen of the proximal tubule is often occluded by the apposition of the brush borders of the surrounding cells. It was formerly thought that this was the normal condition, and that the glomerular filtrate might percolate through the interstices among the microvilli of the brush borders. It is now known that this constriction of the tubules and obliteration of the lumen is an artifact. If the fixative is dripped onto the surface of the living kidney, or if the organ is perfused under conditions that involve no agonal fall of blood pressure, all of the proximal tubules will have a wide open lumen (Figs. 31–14 and 31–15). Each proximal tubule cell contains a single spherical nucleus in an eosinophilic cytoplasm. In cytological preparations, the Golgi apparatus forms a crown around the upper pole of the nucleus, and long rodlike mitochondria in the basal half of the cell tend to be oriented parallel to the cell axis. In well preserved tissues, this orientation of the mitochondria may result in a faint vertical striation of the cell base, even without special staining of the mitochondria. The lateral limits of the cells are rarely resolved with the light microscope because their sides are elaborately fluted and deeply interdigitated with complementary ridges and grooves on the neighboring cells. In favorable preparations, affording surface views of the epithelium, some of the major interdigitations of the cell surfaces can be seen, but the true complexity of the shape of these cells can only be appreciated by careful study of electron micrographs. There are columnar lateral ridges that extend the full height of the cell. An even greater number of slender lateral processes near the cell base extend under adjacent cells (Fig. 31–16). The resulting compartmentation of the base of the epithelium seen in micrographs of thin sections was originally attributed to a simple infolding of the basal plasma membrane. However, most of the membrane bounded basal compartments are not open at any point to the cytoplasm of the overlying cell. It is clear, therefore, that many of them are, in fact, sections of undermining basal processes of neighboring cells. In addition to the basal processes, there are smaller lateral processes that are confined to the juxtaluminal region of the epithelium (Bulger).

In electron micrographs, the microvilli of the brush border appear long, regularly oriented, and closely packed. Arising from the clefts between the microvilli and extending downward into the apical cytoplasm are numerous tubular invaginations called *apical canaliculi* (Fig. 31–15). The membrane lining them has a filamentous outer surface coat and short projections from the cytoplasmic

face of the membrane. In this respect, the tubules closely resemble the so-called coated vesicles seen in many other cell types. Also found in the apical cytoplasm are clear vacuoles of varying size and others with a content of appreciable density. The apical canaliculi and the associated vacuoles appear to be involved in the cellular mechanism for absorption and concentration of protein from the glomerular filtrate. Evidence for this was obtained at the light microscope level by intravenous injection of peroxidase and subsequent demonstration of a peroxidase reaction in the apical vacuoles of the proximal convoluted tubule (Straus). In a recent application of the sensitive new peroxidase method for ultrastructural cytochemistry, it has been reported that the exogenous enzyme can be demonstrated in the brush border and apical canaliculi as early as 90 seconds after its intravenous injection (Fig. 31–17). Later it is found in the vacuoles, where it undergoes progressive concentration. Whether the apical canaliculi open directly

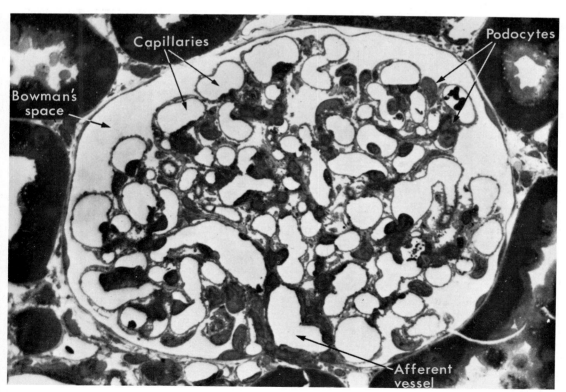

Figure 31–10 A thin plastic section of a renal corpuscle from a rat kidney fixed by perfusion and showing the open lumens of the capillaries. The irregularity of their outer surface is due to the sections of podocyte processes on their exterior. × 700. (Courtesy of A. Aoki.)

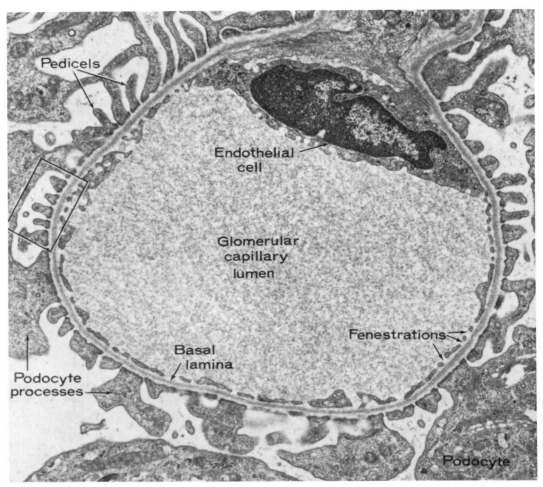

Figure 31–11 Transmission electron micrograph of a transverse section of a glomerular capillary, showing its basal lamina interposed between the fenestrated capillary endothelium on the inside and the slit pores between pedicels of the visceral epithelium on the outside. An area comparable to that in the rectangle is shown at higher magnification in Figure 31–12. (Micrograph from G. Tyson and R. Bulger, Anat. Rec., *172*:669, 1972).

into the vacuoles or whether vesicles bud off from their ends and transport quanta of the absorbed material to the vacuoles has not been settled. Many of the protein absorption vacuoles give histochemical reactions for acid photophatase and are evidently secondary lysosomes, i.e., sites of intracellular digestion of the absorbed protein by lysosomal enzymes.

Although the entire length of the proximal tubule seems to have much the same structure in ordinary histological preparations electron micrographs show that in the straight portion the brush border and lateral interdigitations are less highly developed,

and the mitochondria are somewhat shorter and less numerous. Certain experiments (vital staining; poisoning with uranium, chromium, or bichloride of mercury; and others) allow subdivision of the proximal tubule into three or four successive segments, which show specific reactions to the different noxious agents. Similar conclusions on functional differentiation within this segment of the nephron have been drawn from histochemical studies.

The Thin Segment. The *loop of Henle* consists of the straight portion of the proximal tubule, the thin segment, and the ascending or straight portion of the distal tubule. In the outer zone of the medulla, the descending portion of the proximal tubule abruptly narrows from a width of about 60 μm. to continue as the thin segment, about 15 μm. in diameter (Fig. 31–18). The epithelium changes from cuboidal to squamous with a height of only 0.5 to 2 μm. There is a sudden termination of the brush border, which gives way to very sparse, irregularly oriented, short microvilli on the luminal surface of the thin segment. The nuclei cause the central portions of the cells to bulge into the lumen. Owing to the small caliber of the tubule, its thin wall, and the bulging of the perikaryon into the lumen, the thin segment of Henle's loop in cross section bears a superficial resemblance to a capillary (Fig. 31–19).

In electron micrographs, typical cellular units containing a nucleus make up only a small portion of the wall. Most of the epithelium is composed of small membrane bounded units 1 to 3 μm. across, separated from one another by intermembranous clefts extending from basal lamina to lumen. These short segments of the epithelium are too small to contain a nucleus and often enclose only one or two mitchondria. They are attached to one another by juxtaluminal junctional complexes. This unusual appearance of the epithelium is attributed to the fact that its cells, like those of the proximal convolution, have extraordinarily complex shapes, with elaborately interdigitated outlines. The short anucleate segments seen in micrographs of the thin limb thus represent sections through the deeply intercrescent processes of the cells. These do not commonly extend under the adjacent cells to form basal compartments, as do those seen in sections of the thicker epithelia of the proximal and distal tubules. Instead, the processes take up the full thickness of the epithelium, and interdigitate with those of neighboring cells like the teeth of gears. The epithelium rests upon

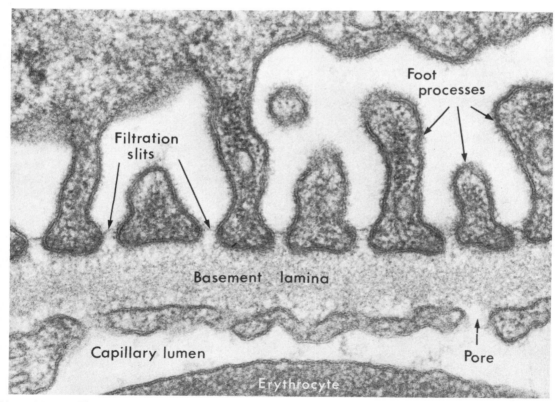

Figure 31–12 Electron micrograph of a portion of the wall of a glomerular capillary, showing pores in the extremely attenuated endothelium. On the outer surface of the basal (basement) lamina are the foot processes of the podocytes, with the narrow filtration slits between them. × 70,000. (Courtesy of D. Friend.)

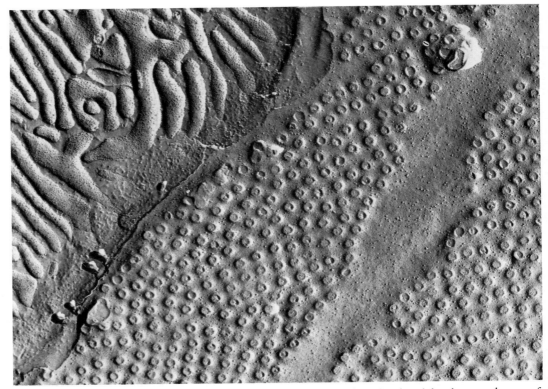

Figure 31–13 Freeze-cleaving preparation of rat kidney glomerulus. At the right the membrane of the endothelium of a capillary has been cleaved, showing the very uniform size and regular distribution of the endothelial pores. At the upper left, the membranes of a number of pedicels on the outer aspect of the capillary have been cleaved. (Micrograph courtesy of D. Goodenough.)

a moderately thick basal lamina and the cytoplasm contains relatively few organelles. The cells of the thin segment of the nephron show a gradual simplification of their structure as the loop descends deeper into the pyramid. The interdigitating processes become fewer and the microvilli shorter and less abundant.

In the human kidney, the epithelium is appreciably higher, and the shape of the cells in the thin limb is less complex than in the rat and mouse. The interdigitating lateral cell processes are relatively few or entirely lacking. The basal cell membrane is, for the most part, smooth contoured and rests upon a basal lamina that is distinctly thicker than that in laboratory rodents. The luminal surface has a few short microvilli coated with radiating fine filaments, and each cell bears a single flagellum (Bulger et al.).

In rats and certain other species whose kidneys have a single pyramid, the corresponding segments of the loops tend to be in register. As mentioned earlier, this regularity of arrangement is reflected in a zonation within the medulla that is detectable on naked eye inspection of the cut surface. An *outer* and *inner zone of the medulla* can be recognized, and an *inner* and *outer band* or *stripe* are distinguishable within the outer zone of the medulla. In these species, the boundary between the outer and inner band of the outer medulla is at the junctions of the straight portion of the proximal tubules with the descending thin limbs of Henle's loops. The transition between the inner and outer medulla is at the junctions of the ascending thin limbs with the ascending straight portion of the distal tubule. The inner medulla therefore contains collecting tubules, thin limbs of the loop of Henle, and blood vessels (Fig. 31–20B).

In the human, a similar zonation of the medulla is detectable, though less easily, because the loops of Henle are of different lengths depending upon the position of their renal corpuscle in the cortex and the length of their thin segment (Fig. 31–4). The short loops are associated with the renal corpuscles located nearer the surface of the kidney. Loops of this type are about seven times as numerous as the long ones. Their bend which is distal to the thin segment is located in the outer part of the medulla and is formed by the thick ascending limb. The thin segment is in the descending limb of the loop and may be very short or in some instances may even be absent. In the latter event, the straight descending portion of the proximal tubule continues directly into the thick ascending limb. In the longer loops, which are associated with the deeper lying juxtamedullary renal corpuscles, the bend is formed by the thin limb. These long loops may extend nearly to the apex of the papilla. In this event, the length of the thin limb may be 10 mm. or even more.

The junction of the outer and inner zones of the medulla is marked by the transition of the thin limb to the ascending thick limb of the long loops of Henle (Fig. 31–20*A*). The boundary between the outer and inner bands of the outer medulla in the human kidney is somewhat obscured by the prevalence in this region of short loops having the junctions between their successive segments at different levels.

The Distal Tubule. The distal tubule is shorter and somewhat thinner than the proximal tubule and is composed of three parts: the straight portion (*pars recta*); the portion adjacent to the renal corpuscle, containing the macula densa (*pars maculata*); and the convoluted portion (*pars convoluta*). The

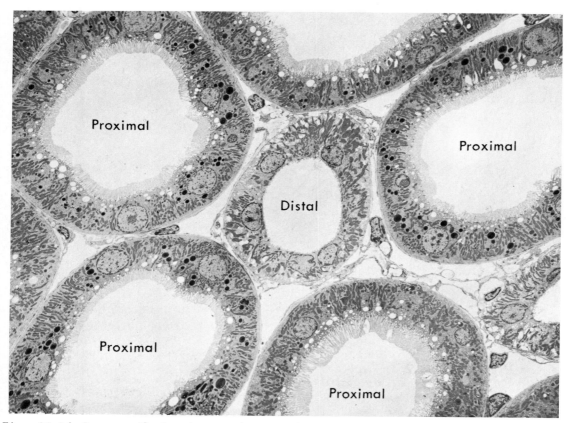

Figure 31–14 Low magnification electron micrograph from the cortex of rat kidney fixed by vascular perfusion. The field includes five proximal convoluted tubules in transverse section, showing their open lumen and prominent brush border. Two distinct segments of the proximal convolution can be recognized. The first portion has a deeper brush border (section at *lower right*). The second portion has a thinner brush border and prominent dense bodies in the cytoplasm (other three labeled sections). × 2000. (After A. Maunsbach, J. Ultrastr. Res., *15*:252, 1966.)

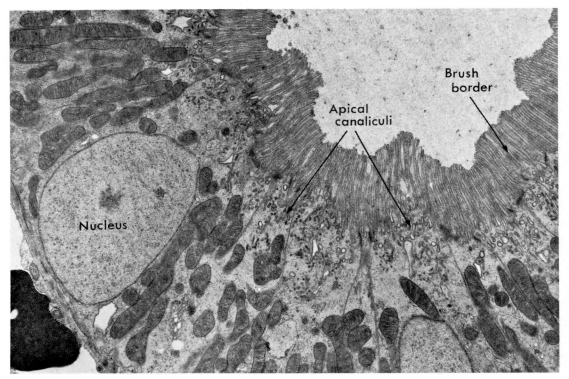

Figure 31-15 Electron micrograph of a sector of the wall of a proximal tubule of rat kidney. × 6000. (Courtesy of R. Bulger.)

straight portion begins in the inner band of the outer zone of the medulla and constitutes the ascending thick limb of the loop of Henle. The transition from the thin segment (15 μm.) to the ascending limb of the distal tubule (35 μm.) is usually fairly abrupt. The height of the epithelium increases, but the lumen is generally wider than that of the proximal tubule. A brush border and apical canaliculi are lacking, and the lateral borders of the cells are somewhat more easily distinguished than in the proximal tubule. In electron micrographs, the base of the epithelium is elaborately compartmentalized by infoldings of the basal membrane that make deep incursions into the cell (Fig. 31-21). In addition, there are undermining basal processes of neighboring cells comparable to those described for the proximal tubule. Long mitochondria are lodged in these basal compartments and their orientation parallel to the axis of the cell results in a prominent striation of the basal cytoplasm. The mitochondria have a complex internal membrane structure and numerous matrix granules. The Golgi complex is small and forms a crown around the upper pole of the nucleus. There are a few cisternal profiles of granular endoplasmic reticulum and a moderate number of free ribosomes. A pair of centrioles is located in the apical cytoplasm, and from one of these a single flagellum may project into the lumen. The distal tubule cells of carnivores may contain numerous lipid droplets, but this is not a normal feature of the primate kidney.

The thick ascending limb of Henle's loop or straight portion of the distal tubule has on the average a length of 9 mm. It enters the cortical tissue, returns to its renal corpuscle and attaches to its vascular pole, particularly to the afferent arteriole. That side of the tubule in contact with the afferent arteriole forms an elliptical disk of taller cells measuring 40 by 70 μm. in man. This area, called the *macula densa*, has been reported to have some significance in the hemodynamics of the kidney, but its precise role has not been defined (Fig. 31-22). From here the straight portion passes into the distal convoluted portion of the tubule. This portion of the tubule has many short loops and irregular contortions. It usually courses toward the surface above the corresponding renal corpuscle. Its length is estimated at 4.6 to 5.2 mm., its diameter at 20 to 50 μm.

Collecting Tubules

The connections of the nephrons with the collecting tubules are located in the cortex of the kidney along medullary rays. The distal tubules are continuous with *arched collecting tubules,* which are tributaries of straight collecting tubules located in the medullary rays. In the medullary ray, the collecting tubules pass inward through the outer zone of the medulla without further fusions. When they reach the inner zone, they join at acute angles with other, similar tubules. There are about seven such convergences in the medulla near the pelvis, and they result in the formation of large, straight tubules called *papillary ducts* (of Bellini). These have a lumen measuring 100 to 200 μm. in diam-

eter and open on the area cribrosa at the apex of each papilla.

The system of the intrarenal excretory ducts has an epithelium typically quite different from that of the various parts of the nephron. In the smallest collecting tubules, the cells are cuboidal and very distinctly outlined; they contain a darkly staining round nucleus and have a clear cytoplasm (Fig. 31–23). The latter contains a few fine mitochondria and, at the surface, a pair of centrioles with a central single flagellum.

As the collecting tubules grow larger, the cells become higher, and finally, in the papillary ducts, they acquire a columnar form. They are always arranged in a single layer, with all the nuclei at one level and with the free surfaces bulging slightly into the lumen of the tubule. The cytoplasm keeps its pale appearance. The centrioles remain at the bulging free surface. In the area cribrosa, the simple columnar epithelium of the ducts continues onto the surface of the papilla.

The length of the collecting tubules is estimated at 20 to 22 mm. and the length of the nephron at 30 to 38 mm.

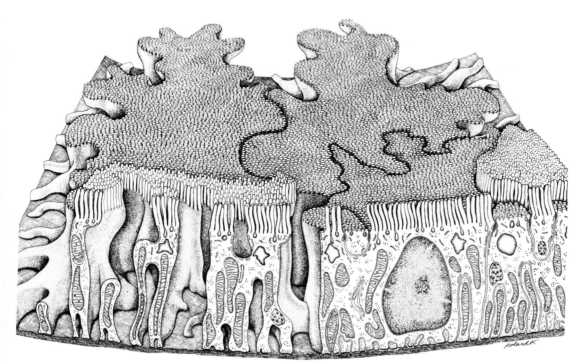

Figure 31–16   Drawing of the shapes and interrelations of the cells of the proximal convoluted tubule. As in fluted columns, some of the interdigitated lateral processes extend the full height of the cell; others are confined to the base and extend beneath adjacent cells. (After R. Bulger, Am. J. Anat., *116:*237, 1965.)

JUXTAGLOMERULAR COMPLEX

In addition to their function in excretion, the kidneys have a role in the regulation of blood pressure. There is a clear association between certain types of kidney disease and high blood pressure (hypertension). The kidney produces and may release into the blood a substance called *renin*. This has no vasomotor effect itself but is an enzyme that acts upon a plasma globulin, *angiotensinogen*, to split off a decapeptide, *angiotensin I*. A converting enzyme in the blood plasma then acts upon this to split off two more amino acids, converting it to *angiotensin II*—the most potent vasoconstrictor known. Renin is synthesized in the juxtaglomerular region of the nephron where the ascending straight portion of the distal tubule returns to the renal corpuscle and comes into intimate relation with its vascular pole.

Among the smooth muscle cells in the wall of the afferent arteriole just proximal to its entrance into the glomerulus are cells that contain conspicuous cytoplasmic granules. These granular *juxtaglomerular cells* are in contact with the intima of the arteriole on the one side, and on the other side they are intimately related to the base of the epithelial cells comprising the *macula densa* in the wall of the distal tubule (Fig. 31–24). Also associated with the granular cells are a few nongranular ones and a group of pale staining extraglomerular mesangial cells (also called lacis cells, polkissen, or polar cushion) located in the angle between the afferent and efferent arterioles at the vascular pole of the glomerulus. The interrelations of the granular juxtaglomerular cells, the macula densa, and the extraglomerular mesangial cells are poorly understood. They are believed to have related functions, however, and together they comprise the *juxtaglomerular apparatus* or *complex*. The juxtaglomerular cells are described as "myoepithelioid" because they appear to be highly modified smooth muscle cells. They have a slightly basophilic cytoplasm and their specific granules are most clearly demonstrated by the Bowie stain, the PAS reaction, or by the fluorchrome dye thioflavine T. In electron micrographs they have a moderately abundant granular endoplasmic reticulum and a well developed Golgi complex. The granules appear to arise in the cisternae of the Golgi complex, as in other glandular cells. When first formed the granules are of variable shape, and have a crystalline internal structure with a periodicity of 50 to 100 Å. Coalescence of these elements gives rise to mature granules, which are irregularly shaped conglomerates that may retain evidences of crystalline order but more often appear homogeneous.

The secretory nature of these granules was established in experimental studies that demonstrated changes in granule content of the juxtaglomerular cells in renal ischemia (Goormaghtigh), in variations in salt intake, and in adrenalectomy (Hartroft; Dunihue and Boldosser). These studies led to the hypothesis that these cells are the site of production of renin. Support for this thesis has come from the finding that the solubility characteristics of renin and of the granules of the juxtaglomerular cells are similar and

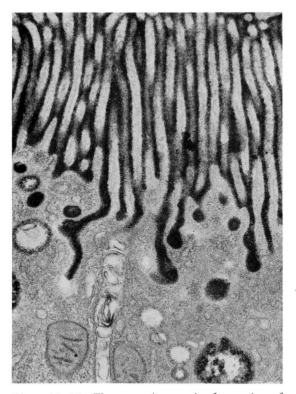

Figure 31–17 Electron micrograph of a portion of the brush border of the proximal convoluted tubule a few seconds after intravenous injection of myoglobin. The myoglobin has passed into the glomerular filtrate and appears between the microvilli and in the apical canaliculi. It is also present in vacuoles in the apical cytoplasm. (Micrograph courtesy of W. Anderson.)

that there is a direct correlation between the level of renin determined by bioassay and the degree of granulation of the juxtaglomerular cells. Microdissection methods have localized the renin to the immediate vicinity of the renal corpuscle, and recently, by application of the fluorescent antibody technique, renin has been shown to reside in the granules of the juxtaglomerular cells (Edelman and Hartroft). Other investigators using similar methods, have found the fluorescence both in the juxtaglomerular cells and in the macula densa (Warren et al.).

The bases of the cells of the macula densa are in very close relation to the juxtaglomerular cells, and the basal lamina between them is exceedingly thin. This close topographical relationship has been interpreted as suggesting some interchange of substances between the macula densa and the juxtaglomerular cells. Consistent with such a relationship is the report that

the polarity of the Golgi complex in the cells of the macula densa is toward the juxtaglomerular cells, whereas in the remainder of the circumference of the distal tubule, it is toward the lumen (McManus).

The finding that the cells of the macula densa show changes in their histochemically demonstrable enzymatic activities when the rate of secretion of the juxtaglomerular cells is altered provides further indication that the two structures are functionally related. The juxtaglomerular complex also has an important function in regulation of tissue hydration and blood volume. Any condition that reduces blood or extracellular fluid volume seems to be sensed by the afferent arteriole acting as a baroreceptor or by the macula densa as a sensor of sodium concentration. The juxtaglomerular cells are stimulated to synthesize and release renin. The resulting angiotensin II in the blood directly stimulates the zona glomerulosa of the adrenal cortex to

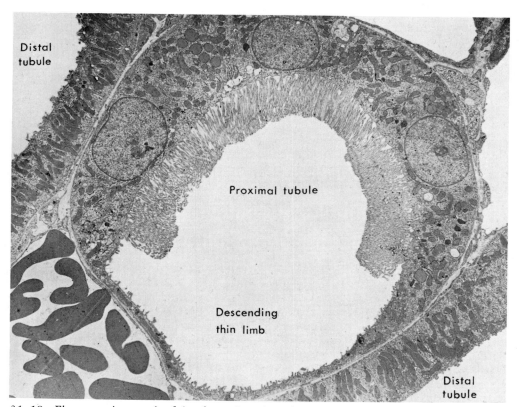

Figure 31–18 Electron micrograph of the abrupt junction of the straight portion of the proximal tubule with the thin limb of the loop of Henle. Slightly oblique section through the junction. The brush border stops suddenly and the epithelium becomes very thin. × 4200. (After Osvaldo and Latta, J. Ultrastr. Res., *15*:144, 1966.)

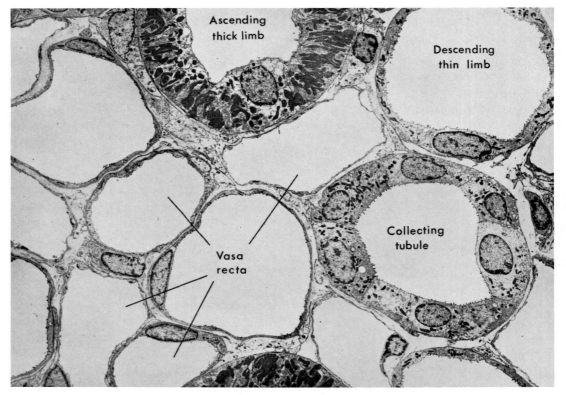

Figure 31-19 Electron micrograph of the inner band of the outer zone of rat kidney medulla, showing ascending thick limb, descending thin limb, collecting tubule, and the vasa recta. × 3000. (After A. Maunsbach, J. Ultrastr. Res., *15*:242, 1966.)

release *aldosterone,* which acts in turn upon the collecting ducts of the kidney to induce sodium and water retention, which tends to correct the reduction of plasma and interstitial tissue fluid volume.

BLOOD SUPPLY

Because the kidneys serve to clear the blood of accumulated waste products of metabolism, they have a very large blood flow, averaging about 1200 ml./min. through both kidneys. A knowledge of the blood supply of the kidney is essential to an understanding of its function.

The *renal artery* enters the hilus of the kidney and divides into two main sets of branches directed toward the dorsal and ventral aspects of the organ. In the adipose tissue surrounding the pelvis, these branches in turn divide into smaller *interlobar arteries* that enter the substance of the kidney and course peripherally in the renal columns between the pyramids or lobes of the kidney. At the level of the base of the medullary pyramids the interlobar arteries arch over to run parallel to the surface of the organ as the *arcuate arteries* at the corticomedullary junction. Small *interlobular arteries,* given off from the arcuate arteries at regular intervals, course radially toward the kidney surface (Fig. 31-26).

The interlobular arteries running radially in the cortex give off numerous *afferent arterioles* to the glomeruli (Fig. 31-27). The blood is carried from the glomeruli via *efferent arterioles.* The efferent vessels of glomeruli situated in the outer part of the cortex are of small diameter and break up to form the cortical intertubular capillary network. The efferent vessels of the more deeply situated juxtamedullary glomeruli are of larger caliber and pass downward into the medulla, breaking up into bundles of thin-walled vessels somewhat larger than ordinary capillaries, called *vasa recta* (Fig. 31–28). The efferent vessels of the juxtamedullary glomeruli and the vasa recta both contribute branches to an intertubular capillary network in the medulla.

The vasa recta form hairpin loops at various levels in the medulla, turning back toward the cortex and running close to and parallel with the vessels from which they recur. The descending vessels penetrate the outer medulla to different depths before turning back. The descending and ascending limbs of these loops form a countercurrent system of vessels called a *vascular bundle* or *rete mirabile*. As more vessels turn back, the vascular bundles taper down as they approach the inner medulla. The descending vessels forming the arterial limbs of the vascular bundle or rete are slightly smaller than the recurrent vessels that constitute the venous limbs (Fig. 31–29). The fine structure of the

vessel walls also differs, the arterial component having a continuous endothelium, whereas the venous component has a thin fenestrated endothelium. The proximity of the vessels in the vascular bundles and the large surface they present to one another facilitate rapid movement of diffusible substances between the ascending and descending limbs of the loops. The vasa recta thus serve as efficient countercurrent exchangers for diffusible substances.

The capillaries of the outermost layers of the cortex are drained toward the surface by radially arranged branches, the *superficial cortical veins*, which join veins of characteristic configuration on the surface of the kidney, called *stellate veins*. This outer mantle of venous channels is drained by a relatively small number of *interlobular veins* into the *arcuate veins* that accompany the arteries of the same name. The capillaries in the deeper part of the cortex empty into radially oriented *deep*

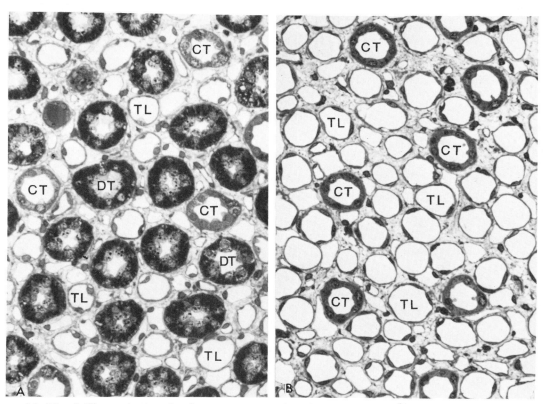

Figure 31–20 *A*, Photomicrograph of a transverse section through the outer medulla, which is composed of thin segments (TL) ascending straight portions of distal tubules (DT), and collecting tubules (CT). *B*, Transverse section through the inner medulla, composed of thin limb (TL) of the loop of Henle and collecting tubules (CT).

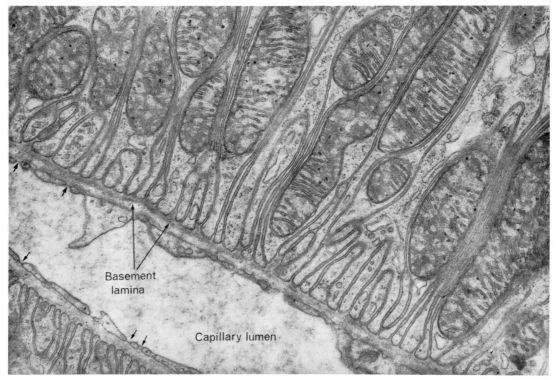

Figure 31-21 Electron micrograph of a portion of the base of a distal convoluted tubule of guinea pig kidney, illustrating the small and large basal compartments. The latter contain long mitochondria oriented perpendicular to the cell base. Notice that the peritubular capillary is of the fenestrated type with several of its pores indicated by arrows. × 20,000. (Courtesy of A. Ichikawa.)

cortical veins, of which there are some 400 per square centimeter running parallel to a corresponding number of interlobular arteries. The blood in these flows inward to the arcuate veins and thence to the *interlobar* veins, which finally become confluent in the hilus to form the *renal vein*.

The hemodynamics of the renal circulation are such that the flows to various zones of the kidney are very different. Measurements of blood flow distribution in the unanesthetized dog give values of 472 ml./100 gm./min. in the cortex; 132 ml./100 gm./min. in the outer medulla, and 17 ml./100 gm./min. in the inner medulla (Thorburn et al.). Although the cortical flow is normally very rapid, strong stimulation of sympathetic nerves may diminish it almost to zero. Under various stressful circumstances, the cortex of the kidney becomes pale, and red blood may appear in the renal vein. Evidently under these conditions the renal cortex is relatively

ischemic and the bulk of the blood that would normally pass through the cortical glomeruli for filtration is bypassed through the juxtamedullary glomeruli and the vasa recta into the interlobular veins and thence to the renal vein.

LYMPHATICS

Networks of lymphatic capillaries are found both in the capsule of the kidney and in the parenchyma. Both groups are connected by occasional anastomoses. The lymphatics of the capsule join the lymph vessels of the neighboring organs. The lymph capillaries in the parenchyma form dense networks between the uriniferous tubules, especially in the cortex. They pass into lymphatics that accompany the larger blood vessels and leave the kidney at the hilus. They are not present in the glomeruli or medullary rays.

NERVES

Macroscopic dissection shows that the sympathetic celiac plexus sends many nerve fibers into the kidney. Their distribution inside the organ has not been worked out satisfactorily. It is relatively easy to follow non-myelinated and myelinated fibers along the course of the larger blood vessels. They provide the adventitia with sensory nerve endings and the muscular coat with motor endings. Along with the afferent arterioles, nerve fibers may reach the renal corpuscles, and some of them seem to end on their surfaces. A nerve supply of the uriniferous tubules, however, has not been convincingly demonstrated. Some investigators describe plexuses of fine nerve fibers that surround and seem to penetrate the basal lamina. On its inner surface they are said to form another plexus, from which terminal branches arise to end between the epithelial cells. There is a good possibility that the silver stains on which these descriptions are based were impregnating reticulum and not axons. The finer innervation of the kidneys has not been systematically studied at the electron microscope level, where the fine nerve fibers can be identified with greater certainty.

HISTOPHYSIOLOGY OF THE KIDNEYS

In forming urine, the kidneys do not produce new material in significant amounts but eliminate water and some of the waste products of metabolism that are carried in solution in the blood. In addition to their *excretory function*, in which they dispose of waste and foreign substances, the kidneys have equally important *conservative functions*, by which they retain the amounts of water, electrolytes, and other substances needed by the body, while eliminating excesses of these substances. They therefore play an important role in the maintenance of the constancy of the internal environment of the organism. The kidney carries out its functions by a combination of filtration, passive diffusion, active secretion, and

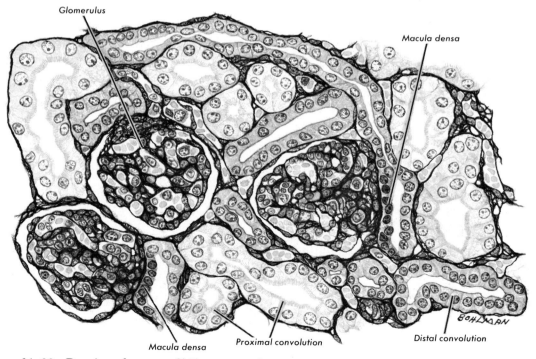

Figure 31-22   Drawing of an area of kidney cortex from a six month old infant, showing the macula densa, a specialized area of the distal tubule adjacent to the renal corpuscle and its afferent arteriole. Mallory-azan stain. × 200.

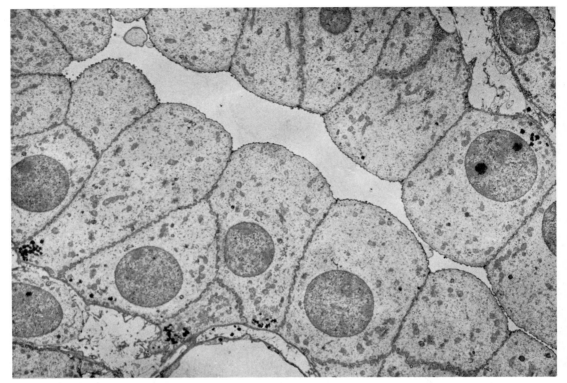

Figure 31-23 Electron micrograph of large collecting tubule or duct of Bellini. The cell surface is smoothly contoured and convex; the cytoplasm contains relatively few organelles and does not give the appearance of being metabolically active. × 2000. (Courtesy of J. Rhodin.)

selective absorption. The form, topographical relations, and microscopic organization of its components represent structural adaptations favoring these processes.

The Glomerulus

The blood circulates through the glomerular capillaries with a *hydrostatic pressure* of about 70 mm./Hg. This tends to press the fluid constituents of the blood through the pores and intercellular spaces of the endothelium, across the basal lamina, through the filtration slits between foot processes of the podocytes, and into Bowman's capsule. The hydrostatic pressure in the capillaries is opposed by an average *colloid osmotic pressure* of about 32 mm. Hg and a *capsular pressure* of about 20 mm. Hg. The net *filtration pressure* is thus about 18 mm. Hg. With some 1300 ml. of blood flowing through the glomeruli of both kidneys each minute, approximately 125 ml. of glomerular filtrate is produced. Analy-

sis of fluid aspirated from Bowman's capsule by micropuncture has established that it is an ultrafiltrate of blood plasma with nearly the same composition as the interstitial fluid. It contains small molecules such as phosphates, creatinine, uric acid, and urea, and small amounts of albumin, but is free of larger protein molecules and substances combined with them. As stated earlier, the site of the barrier to large molecules is still debated, but the most recent evidence indicates that molecules of molecular weight 100,000 and larger are arrested at the slit pores rather than in the basal lamina.

Of the 125 ml. of filtrate formed per minute in the glomeruli, 124 ml. are reabsorbed as the fluid passes through the various segments of the nephrons and the collecting ducts, leaving a volume of only 1 ml. to be excreted as urine. This small remainder is not simply derived by absorption of water; its contents are modified in its passage along the tubules by (1) diffusion of some substances

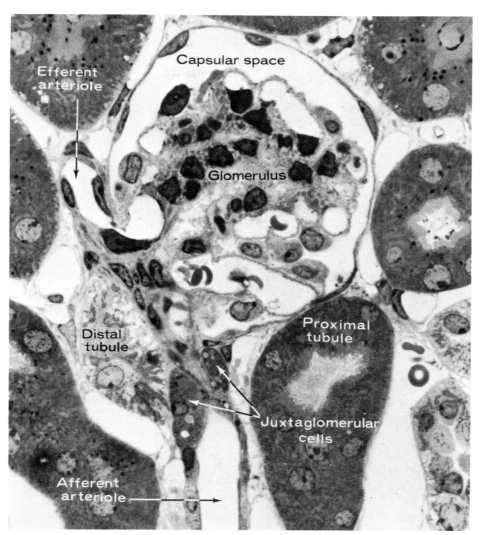

Figure 31-24 Photomicrograph of a thin plastic section of rat kidney, showing a glomerulus and clusters of juxtaglomerular cells in the wall of its afferent arteriole. (Micrograph by courtesy of R. Bolender.)

back into the blood, (2) absorption by osmotic work, and (3) excretion of other substances into the lumen.

The transport of certain substances into and out of the nephron can be rather precisely measured in healthy humans and is the basis of a variety of clinical measurements of their kidney function. *Inulin* is a nonmetabolized carbohydrate which, when injected intravenously, rapidly appears in the glomerular filtrate but is not secreted or absorbed by the tubules. It can be used, therefore, as a means of measuring the amount of plasma filtered by all of the glomeruli of both kidneys. This calculation is based upon the concentrations of inulin in the urine and in the plasma during the experiment. The volume of plasma containing the same amount of inulin as that found in the urine is the amount of plasma which has been "cleared" of this substance by filtration during the period of the test. The *inulin clearance* furnishes a standard from which it is possible to estimate what proportions of other substances are reabsorbed or excreted by cells in various parts of the tubule.

Proximal Convolution

Much of our knowledge of the functions of renal tubules has been derived from studies on amphibian species, in which it is possible to puncture the glomerular capsule and the tubules at different levels in living animals and carry out microchemical analyses on the fluid aspirated. The change in the composition of the filtrate as it passes along the nephron can thus be studied directly. Similarly, fluid of known composition can be perfused through a segment of tubule between two pipettes and the substances added to or subtracted from it can be determined. By these and other methods, it has been shown that 85 per cent or more of the sodium chloride and water of the glomerular filtrate is reabsorbed in the proximal tubule. In this process, the cells actively transport sodium from the lumen, and the water and chloride passively follow it to maintain osmotic equilibrium.

Normally all of the glucose in the filtrate

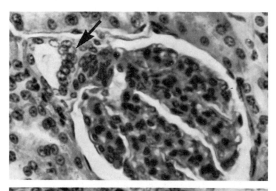

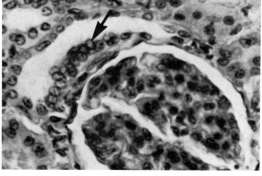

Figure 31–25 Photomicrograph of two renal corpuscles from macaque kidney, showing (at arrows) two typical examples of the macula densa, an area of the wall of the distal tubule where the cells are thicker and the nuclei are crowded together and superimposed. × 175.

is also reabsorbed in the proximal convoluted tubule, and it is calculated that nearly half a pound of glucose and more than three pounds of sodium chloride are recovered per day from the glomerular filtrate of man. If the level of glucose in the blood is raised experimentally above a certain level, the glucose is not completely absorbed and appears in the urine. This *tubular maximum for reabsorption of glucose* (glucose Tm) is a useful index of the reabsorptive capacity of the kidney tubules.

Other metabolically important substances that are reabsorbed in the proximal tubule are amino acids, protein, acetoacetic acid, and ascorbic acid. On leaving the proximal tubules, the fluid contains essentially none of these substances. The absorption of proteins in the proximal tubule has been followed morphologically by intravenous administration of peroxidase and its subsequent detection by a histochemical method (Graham and Karnovsky). Similar studies have been carried out by administration of ferritin and ^{125}I labeled albumin by micropuncture, followed by direct or autoradiographic visualization of the tracer substance (Maunsbach). The results of these studies are in close agreement, all showing uptake in the apical invaginations and apical vacuoles of the proximal tubule within a very few minutes. In 30 to 60 minutes, the label is localized in dense granules containing acid phosphatase, interpreted as lysosomes. It is assumed that absorbed albumin is degraded by the lysosomes and is not returned to the bloodstream.

Thus, some useful substances are conserved by reabsorption. On the other hand, the end products of metabolism, *urea, uric acid,* and *creatinine,* which are of little or no use to the body, are not avidly reabsorbed but are allowed to remain in the urine and are eliminated from the body. While some 99 per cent of the water of the glomerular filtrate is conserved, only 40 per cent of the urea and none of the creatinine is reabsorbed.

In addition to its capacity for active reabsorption, the proximal tubule has the capacity to secrete creatinine, para-aminohippuric acid, the organic iodine compound Diodrast, and sulfonic dyes such as phenol red. The secretory capacity of the proximal tubule does not have the physiological importance in man that it does in some lower animals, particularly those fish that have aglomerular kidneys. However, the substances that are secreted are useful in the clinical evaluation of kidney function and renal blood flow. When

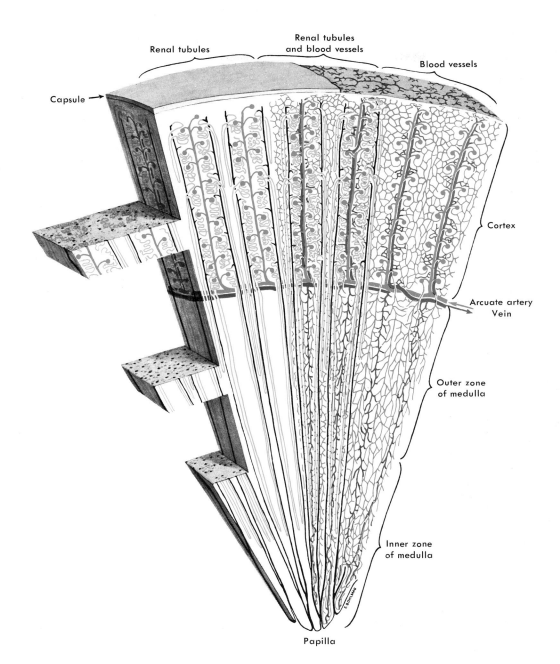

Figure 31-26 Diagram of relations of blood vessels, nephrons, and collecting ducts in kidney. The actual structures are much more complicated than those indicated here. Arteries, red; veins, blue; glomeruli, red dots; nephrons, green; collecting ducts, black. Six interlobular arteries and attached glomeruli are shown. The right-hand pair shows their relation to the veins, the left-hand pair their relation to nephrons, and the central pair their relations to both nephrons and veins. The intertubular capillaries of the cortex and medulla are shown, but the descending bundles of vasa recta running downward from the juxtamedullary glomeruli are not clearly illustrated. (Extensively modified from the diagrams of Peter, Braus, and von Möllendorff.)

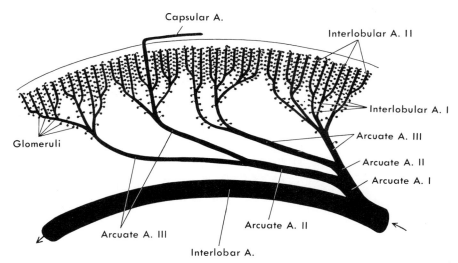

Figure 31-27 Schematic representation of the finer arterial branching in the dog kidney. (After A. Kügelgen and K. J. Otto, *in* Zwanglose Abhandlungen aus dem Gebiet der normalen und pathologischen Anatomie. Vol. 5. Stuttgart, Georg Thieme, 1959.)

introduced into the blood in moderate concentrations, Diodrast and para-aminohippuric acid are entirely removed during a single passage of blood through the kidneys. Since it is impossible to remove by filtration all the substances dissolved in the blood and have any fluid plasma left, the complete removal of a substance in one passage of blood through the kidney must occur in part by filtration and in part by excretory work. Knowing the concentration of such a substance in the blood and the amount found in the urine produced in a given period of time, one can calculate the blood flow through the kidney. The blood flow is equal to the plasma flow plus the cell volume found by hematocrit. From the values for Diodrast clearance and for inulin clearance, one can determine the fraction of renal plasma flow which is filtered by the glomeruli.

If one then raises the concentration of Diodrast in the blood, a point is reached at which the kidney fails to remove all the material from the blood. The maximum concentration that is completely cleared is taken as a measure of the *excretory capacity of the tubule* (*Tm*, or *tubular maximum*). If the values are known for renal plasma flow and inulin clearance, the measurement of other substances (such as urea, uric acid, and phosphate and bicarbonate buffers) in the blood and urine can be related to the activities of the total number of nephrons with regard to these substances. In this way it has been deter-

mined which substances are secreted, which are reabsorbed, and which diffuse passively from the glomerular filtrate. The localizations of these specific events in various portions of the tubule are less well known.

Loop of Henle and Distal Tubule

The loop of Henle is an essential element in the production of hypertonic urine. Only those birds and mammals which have a thin segment in the loop produce a urine that is hypertonic to the blood plasma. The fluids in the renal cortex are isosmotic with plasma, but there is a continuous increase in osmotic pressure from the corticomedullary junction to the tip of the papilla. This is attributed to the arrangement of the loop of Henle and the properties of the different segments of its wall. In the descending limb, the wall is freely permeable to sodium and to water, whereas the ascending limb is believed to be impermeable to water; its cells are the site of a "sodium pump" that moves sodium from the urine into the interstitial spaces of the medulla, increasing the osmotic concentration there. Water therefore leaves the descending limb of the loop by passive diffusion and the urine becomes increasingly concentrated as it passes deeper into the medulla toward the turn of the loop. A constantly increasing proximodistal osmotic gradient is therefore maintained. The descending and ascending

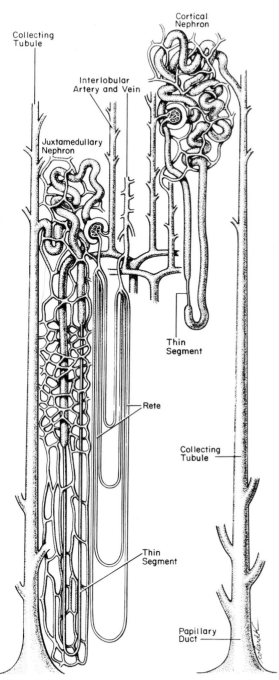

Collecting Tubule

Cortical Nephron

Interlobular Artery and Vein

Juxtamedullary Nephron

Thin Segment

Rete

Collecting Tubule

Thin Segment

Papillary Duct

Figure 31–28 Schematic drawing of the blood supply associated with cortical and juxtamedullary nephrons. In the latter, the efferent arteriole runs downward into the medulla, where it gives rise to a bundle of vasa recta. These together with their recurrent venules form long bundles of parallel vessels called retia mirabilia. Here the arterial and venous elements have been separated to illustrate their continuity in long loops. In life, the arterial and venous limbs of the loops intermingle, as shown in Figure 31–29.

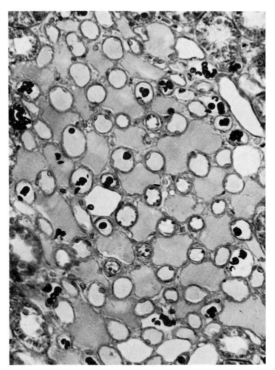

Figure 31–29 Photomicrograph of a rete mirabile from a dog kidney. Notice that the vessels are of two morphological types: the descending arterial limbs are capillaries with a round cross section and walls of appreciable thickness; the ascending venous limbs are larger, more irregular in outline, and have exceedingly thin walls. The latter are filled here with gray precipitate of plasma, while the former appear empty or contain a few erythrocytes. × 250.

limbs of the vessels in the bundles of vasa recta are arranged very close to one another (Figs. 31–28 and 31–29), and thus constitute a countercurrent exchange system. This permits the concentration of the blood in the descending and ascending limbs to equilibrate, an arrangement which is thought to keep these vessels from disturbing the osmotic gradient in the medulla, which is necessary for concentration of the urine.

The active pumping of sodium out of the ascending limb of the loop of Henle renders the urine hypertonic by the time it reaches the distal convoluted tubule. The pumping of sodium continues in the distal convolution, but some of the sodium is replaced by other cations, such as potassium and hydrogen, or by ammonia derived from glutamine by oxidative deamination. The distal tubule is therefore the principal site of acidification of the urine.

In the *absence* of the antidiuretic hormone of the posterior lobe of the hypophysis, the distal tubule and collecting ducts are impermeable to water. Under these conditions the urine passing through the medulla would remain dilute in spite of the concentration gradient in the surrounding interstitium. In the *presence* of antidiuretic hormone, the collecting ducts become highly permeable to water, and thus exposure to the high osmolarity maintained in the peritubular spaces of the medulla results in removal of water and secretion of concentrated urine. By hormonal regulation of the permeability of the distal tubule and collecting ducts, the concentration of the urine can be varied over a wide range.

The efficiency of reabsorption of sodium is under hormonal control. Aldosterone secreted by the zona glomerulosa of the adrenal cortex acts specifically on the renal tubules to increase their rate of sodium absorption. In the absence of aldosterone, there is a serious loss of sodium in the urine; when this hormone is present in normal amounts, some 1200 gm. of sodium are reabsorbed each day and only a few hundred milligrams escape in the urine.

PASSAGES FOR THE EXCRETION OF URINE

The excretory passages convey the urine from the parenchyma of the kidney to the outside. Their walls are provided with a well developed coat of smooth muscle. Its contractions move the urine forward.

The calyces, the pelvis, the ureter, and the bladder all have a similar structure, but the thickness of the wall gradually increases from the upper to the lower part of the urinary tract. The inner surface is lined with a mucous membrane. There is no distinct submucosa, and the lamina propria of the mucosa blends with the smooth muscle coat, which in turn is covered by an adventitial layer of connective tissue.

All the excretory passages of the urinary tract are lined with transitional epithelium. In the calyces, it is two or three cells thick and in the ureter four or five. When the wall of the bladder is contracted, the epithelium is six to eight cells thick and its superficial cells are rounded or even club shaped. When the bladder is distended, the epithelium is thin and the cells are greatly flattened and stretched (Figs. 31–30 and 31–31).

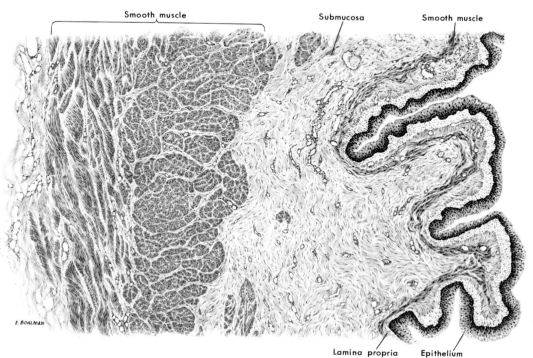

Figure 31–30 Low power view of section of wall of contracted urinary bladder of *Macacus rhesus.*

Electron micrographs of transitional epithelium reveal fine structural features peculiar to this tissue. The free surface of the cells at the lumen has a characteristic scalloped appearance. Segments of membrane of varying length are quite straight and seemingly stiff (Fig. 31–32). Neighboring straight segments may be so oriented as to produce angular surface contours not seen on other cells. There is a superficial ectoplasmic layer of cytoplasm rich in fine filaments, and bundles of filaments course through the deeper cytoplasm as well. Flattened, elliptical, or lenticular vesicles are present in the superficial cytoplasm, and these are bounded by thick membranes of the same character as that on the luminal surface. Vesicles of this kind are peculiar to the cells of transitional epithelium. It is speculated that they may be formed within the cell and may be added to the surface membrane, providing for its replacement or for its rapid expansion in distention of the bladder (Porter and Bonneville).

The luminal plasma membrane of the superficial cells of bladder epithelium has a unique ultrastructure and unusual physiological properties. It is thicker (120 Å) than most cell membranes and asymmetric in sections, with the outer dense line of the unit membrane significantly thicker than the inner dense line. When this membrane is isolated and examined by negative staining and optical diffraction (Warren and Hicks), it is found to have a highly ordered substructure consisting of hexagonally arranged subunits. Each subunit seems to be a hexamer composed of twelve smaller subunits arranged in a stellate configuration (Fig. 31–33). The significance of this lattice structure in relation to the function of the bladder epithelium is by no means clear. It is known, however, that in man the tonicity of the bladder urine may be 2 to 4 times higher than that of the plasma in the capillaries of the lamina propria. If the transitional epithelium were to act as a semipermeable membrane, water would pass

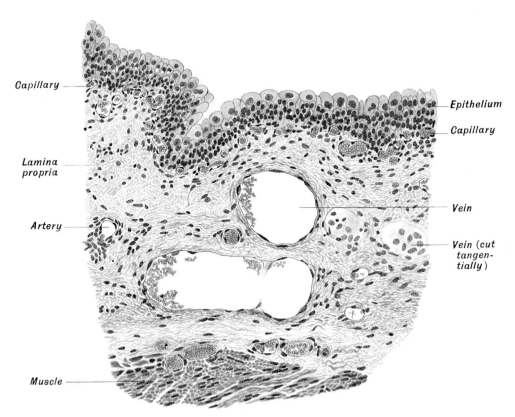

Figure 31–31 Section of wall of human urinary bladder in contracted condition; capillaries penetrate the epithelium. × 150. (After A. A. Maximow.)

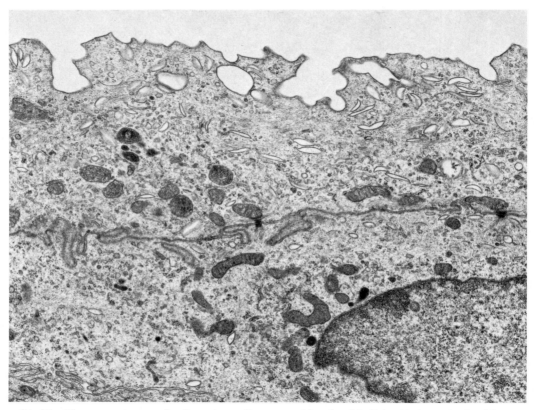

Figure 31-32 Electron micrograph of portions of two transitional epithelial cells from the bladder. Notice the flattened elliptical vesicles in the cytoplasm of the upper cell and the peculiar angular appearance of the luminal surface. This apparently results from insertion of relatively stiff segments of membrane into the surface when the lenticular vesicles fuse with the plasma membrane. (Micrograph courtesy of M. Hicks and B. Ketterer, J. Cell Biol., 45:542, 1970.)

from blood to urine, and the latter would become diluted. This does not occur, and it seems evident therefore that the epithelium possesses an effective barrier preventing water loss. The barrier function is diminished or lost if the thick surface membrane is chemically altered or mechanically damaged. The barrier is believed to reside in occluding junctions between the superficial cells that close the intercellular spaces, and in the special properties of their thick luminal membrane (Hicks).

No true glands are present in the calyces, the pelvis, or the ureter, but glands may be simulated here by small, solid nests of epithelial cells within the thickness of the epithelial sheet. In the urinary bladder, however, and in the vicinity of the internal urethral orifice, small invaginations of the epithelium into the subjacent connective tissue can be found. They contain numerous clear, mucus-secreting cells and are similar to the glands of Littre in the urethra.

There is a thin basal lamina between the epithelium and the lamina propria. The connective tissue of the latter forms thin folds that may penetrate deep into the epithelium.

The connective tissue underlying the mucosa is abundant and contains elastic fiber networks and sometimes small lymphatic nodules. Its deeper layers have a loose arrangement. The mucous membrane in the empty ureter, therefore, is thrown into several longitudinal folds, which in cross section give a festooned appearance to the margin of the lumen (Fig. 31–32). In the bladder, the deep, looser layer of connective tissue is especially abundant so that in the contracted condition of the organ, the mucous membrane forms numerous thick folds.

The muscular coat of the urinary passages, in contrast to that of the intestine, does not form clearly defined separable layers. Instead, it occurs as loose anastomosing strands of smooth muscle separated by abundant collagenous connective tissue. In general, the muscular coat consists of an inner longitudinal and an outer circular layer, but their limits are ill defined. Beginning in the lower third of the ureter, a third external longitudinal layer is added. This is especially prominent in the bladder.

In the small calyces capping the papillae of the pyramids, the strands of the inner

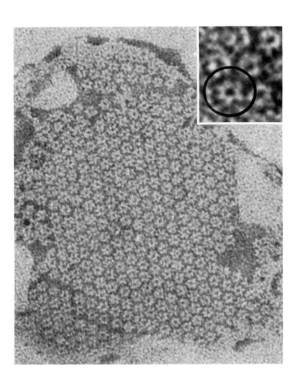

Figure 31–33 Electron micrograph of a negatively stained portion of the cell membrane at the free surface of transitional epithelium. This membrane has a unique substructure (see inset) consisting of hexagonally arranged subunits. This structure may be related to the unusual permeability properties of the bladder epithelium. (Micrograph courtesy of M. Hicks and B. Ketterer, J. Cell Biol., 45:542, 1970.)

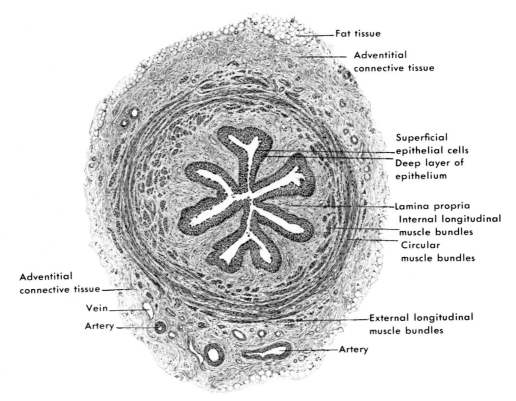

Figure 31-34 Cross section of markedly contracted human ureter. × 30. (After Schaffer.)

longitudinal muscle layer end at the attachment of the calyx to the papilla. The outer circular strands reach higher up and form a muscular ring around the papilla. The calyces show periodic contractions. This muscular activity is believed to assist in moving the urine out of the papillary ducts into the calyces. The muscular coat of the ureter also performs slow peristaltic movements. The waves of contraction proceed from the pelvis toward the bladder.

Because the ureters pierce the wall of the bladder obliquely, their openings are usually closed by the pressure of the contents of the bladder and are open only when the urine is forced through them. A fold of the mucous membrane of the bladder extending over the ureteral orifice and acting as a valve usually prevents the backflow of the urine. In the intramural part of the ureters, the circular muscular strands of their wall disappear, and the connective tissue of the mucous membrane contains longitudinal muscular strands whose contraction opens the lumen of the ureter.

The muscular coat of the bladder is very strong. Its thick strands of smooth muscle cells form three layers, which intermingle at their margins and cannot be separated from one another. The outer longitudinal layer is developed best on the dorsal and ventral surfaces of the viscus, while in other places its strands may be wide apart. The middle circular or spiral layer is the thickest of all. The inner layer in the body of the bladder consists of relatively sparse, longitudinal or oblique strands. In the region of the trigone, thin, dense bundles of smooth muscle form a circular mass around the internal opening of the urethra, forming the *internal sphincter* of the bladder.

Blood Vessels, Lymphatics, and Nerves

The blood vessels of the excretory passages penetrate first through the muscular coat and provide it with capillaries. Then they form a plexus in the deeper layers of the mucous membrane. From here small arteries pass toward the surface and form a rich capillary plexus immediately under the epithelium.

The deeper layers of the mucosa and the muscularis in the renal pelvis and the ureters also contain a well-developed network of lymph capillaries. In the bladder lymph vessels are said to be present only in the muscularis.

Nerve plexuses, small ganglia, and scattered nerve cells can be found in the adventitial and muscular coats of the ureter. Most of the fibers supply the muscle, but some fibers apparently of efferent nature have been traced into the mucosa and the epithelium.

A sympathetic nerve plexus in the adventitial coat of the bladder, the *plexus vesicalis*, is formed in part by the pelvic nerves, which originate from the sacral nerves, and in part by the branches of the hypogastric plexus. The vesical plexus sends numerous nerves into the muscular coat. A continuation of the nerve plexus, but seemingly without nerve

cells, is found in the connective tissue of the mucosa. Here the sensory nerve endings are located. Many fibers penetrate into the epithelium between the cells, forming varicose free endings.

URETHRA

Male Urethra

The male urethra has a length of 18 to 20 cm. Three parts can be distinguished. The short proximal segment surrounded by the prostate is the *pars prostatica (prostatic urethra)*. Here the posterior wall of the urethra forms an elevation, the *colliculus seminalis (verumontanum)*. On its surface in the midline is the opening of the *utriculus prostaticus*, the rudimentary homologue of the uterus in the male. Located to the right and to the left of this are the two slit-like openings of the *ductus ejaculatorius (ejaculatory ducts)* and the numerous openings of the ducts of the prostate gland. The second, very short segment of the urethra (18 mm. long), the

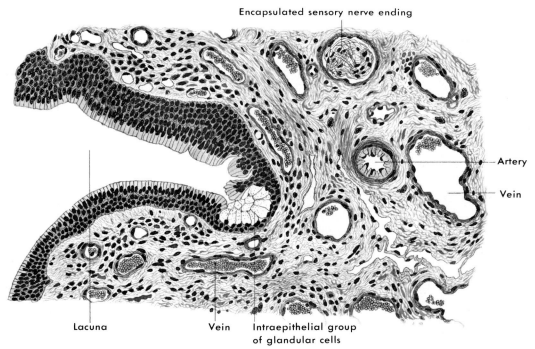

Encapsulated sensory nerve ending

Artery

Vein

Lacuna   Vein   Intraepithelial group
                          of glandular cells

Figure 31-35   Section of cavernous part of male human urethra. × 165. (After A. A. Maximow.)

pars membranacea (membranous urethra), extends from the lower pole of the prostate to the bulb of the corpus spongiosum of the penis. The third portion, *pars spongiosa (penile urethra)*, which is about 15 cm. long, passes longitudinally through the corpus spongiosum of the penis.

The prostatic part is lined with the same transitional type of epithelium as the bladder. The pars membranacea and the pars spongiosa are lined with a stratified or pseudostratified columnar epithelium (Figs. 31–35 and 31–36). Patches of stratified squamous epithelium are common in the pars spongiosa. In the terminal enlarged part of the canal, the *fossa navicularis*, stratified squamous epithelium occurs as a rule. In the surface epithelium, occasional mucous goblet cells may be found. Intraepithelial cysts containing a colloid-like substance are common.

The lamina propria of the mucosa is a loose connective tissue with abundant elastic networks. No separate submucous layer can be distinguished. This connective tissue contains numerous scattered bundles of smooth muscle, mainly oriented longitudinally. In the outer layers, however, circular bundles are also present. The lamina propria has no distinct papillae extending into the epithelium; these appear only in the fossa navicularis. The membranous portion of the urethra is surrounded by a mass of striated muscle, a part of the urogenital diaphragm.

The surface of the mucous membrane of the urethra shows many recesses, the *lacunae of Morgagni*. These outpocketings continue into deeper, branching tubules, the *glands of Littre* (Fig. 31–37). The larger ones among them are found especially on the dorsal surface of the pars spongiosa of the urethra. They run obliquely in the lamina propria and are directed with their blind end toward the root of the penis. They sometimes penetrate far into the corpus spongiosum. The glands of Littre are lined with the same epithelium as the surface of the mucous membrane, but in many places this epithelium is transformed into compact intraepithelial nests of clear cells, which have the staining reactions of mucus. In old age some of the recesses of the urethral mucosa may contain concretions similar to those of the prostate.

Female Urethra

The female urethra is 25 to 30 mm. long. Its mucosa forms longitudinal folds and is lined with stratified squamous epithelium. In many cases, however, pseudostratified columnar epithelium can be found. Numerous invaginations are formed by the epithelium (Fig. 31–38). The outpocketings in their wall are lined in many places with clear mucous cells, as in the glands of Littre of the male urethra. The glands may accumulate colloid material in their cavities or may even contain concretions. The lamina propria, devoid of papillae, is a loose connective tissue with abundant elastic fibers. It is provided with a highly developed system of venous plexuses and has, therefore, a character resembling the corpus spongiosum of the male. The mucous membrane with its veins is surrounded by a thick mass of smooth muscles; the inner layers of the latter have a longitudinal, the outer layers a circular, arrangement. Distally, the smooth muscles are strengthened by a sphincter of striated muscle.

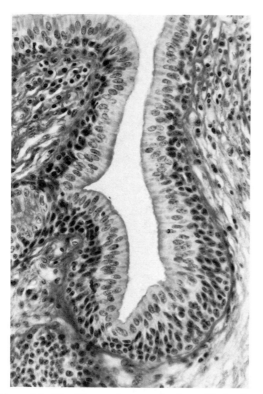

Figure 31–36 Photomicrograph of stratified columnar epithelium of human urethra.

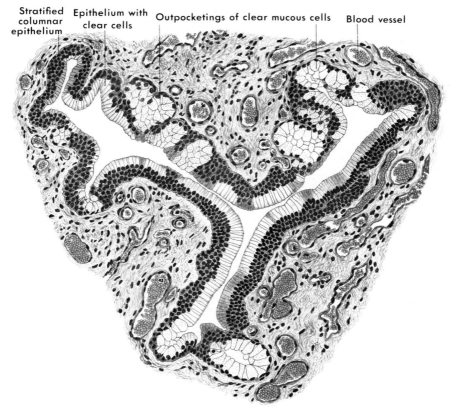

Stratified columnar epithelium   Epithelium with clear cells   Outpocketings of clear mucous cells   Blood vessel

Figure 31–37   Section of urethral gland (gland of Littre) from cavernous part of male human urethra. × 165. (After A. A. Maximow.)

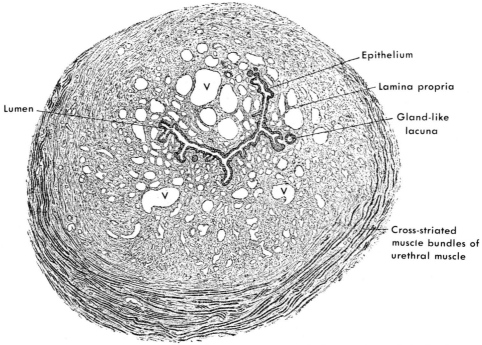

Figure 31–38 Cross section through urethra of a woman. The darker portions of the lamina propria are smooth muscle bundles. × 10. (After von Ebner.)

REFERENCES

Arakawa, M.: A scanning electron microscopy of the glomerulus of normal and nephrotic rats. Lab. Invest., 23:489, 1970.

Barajas, L.: The development and ultrastructure of the juxtaglomerular cell granule. J. Ultrastr. Res., 15:400, 1966.

Beeuwkes, R.: Efferent vascular patterns and early vascular-tubular relations in the dog kidney. Am. J. Physiol., 227:1361, 1974.

Bulger, R. E.: The shape of rat kidney tubular cells. Am. J. Anat., 116:237, 1965.

Bulger, R. E., C. C. Tisher, C. H. Myers, and B. F. Trump: Human renal ultrastructure. II. The thin limb of Henle's loop and the interstitium in healthy individuals. Lab. Invest., 16:124, 1967.

Bulger, R. E., and B. F. Trump: Fine structure of the rat renal papilla. Am. J. Anat., 118:685, 1966.

Buss, H.: Die morphologische Differenzierung des visceralen Blattes der Bowmanschen Kapsel. Raster-und durstrahlungselektronenmikroskopische Untersuchungen. Z. Zellforsch., 111:346, 1970.

Chambers, R., and R. T. Kempton: Indications of function of the chick mesonephros in tissue culture with phenol red. J. Cell Comp. Physiol., 3:131, 1933.

Chandra, S., J. C. Hubbard, F. R. Skelton, L. L. Bernardis, and S. Kamura: Genesis of juxtaglomerular cell granules. A physiologic, light and electron microscopic study concerning experimental renal hypertension. Lab. Invest., 14:1834, 1965.

Dunihue, F. W., and W. G. Boldosser: Observations on the

similarity of mesangial to juxtaglomerular cells. Lab. Invest., 12:1228, 1963.

Edelman, R., and P. M. Hartroft: Localization of renin in the juxtaglomerular cells of the rabbit and dog through the use of the fluorescent antibody technique. Circulation Res., 9:1069, 1961.

Ericsson, J. L. E.: Transport and digestion of hemoglobin in the proximal tubule. I. Light microscopy and cytochemistry of acid phosphatase. Lab. Invest., 14:1, 1965.

Ericsson, J. L.: Transport and digestion of hemoglobin in the proximal tubule. II. Electron microscope. Lab. Invest., 14:16, 1965.

Ericsson, J. L. E., A. Bergstrand, G. Andres, H. Bucht, and G. Cinotti: Morphology of the renal tubular epithelium in young, healthy humans. Acta Pathol. Microbiol. Scand., 63:361, 1965.

Farquhar, M. G.: Glomerular permeability investigated by electron microscopy. In Small Blood Vessel Involvement. In Diabetes, p. 31, American Institute of Biological Sciences, 1964.

Farquhar, M. G., and G. E. Palade: Functional evidence for the existence of a third cell type in the renal glomerulus. Phagocytosis of filtration residues by a distinctive "third" cell. J. Cell Biol., 13:55, 1962.

Farquhar, M. G., S. L. Wissig, and G. E. Palade: Glomerular permeability. I. Ferritin transfer across the normal glomerular capillary wall. J. Exper. Med., 113:47, 1961.

Forster, R. P.: Kidney cells. In Brachet, J., and A. E. Mirsky (eds.): The Cell; Biochemistry, Physiology, Morphology. New York, Academic Press. 1961, Vol. 5, p. 89.

Goormaghtigh, N.: Existence of an endocrine gland in the

media of the renal arterioles. Proc. Soc. Exper. Biol. Med., *42*:688, 1939.

Gottschalk, C. W.: Micropuncture studies of tubular function in the mammalian kidney. Fifth Bowditch Lecture. Physiologist, *4*:35, 1961.

Grafflin, A. L.: The normal, acromegalic and the hyperplastic human nephron. Arch. Path., *27*:691, 1939.

Graham, R. C., and M. J. Karnovsky: The early stages of absorption of injected horseradish peroxidase in the proximal tubules of mouse kidney: Ultrastructural cytochemistry by a new technique. J. Histochem. Cytochem., *14*:291, 1966.

Graham, R. C.: Glomerular permeability. Ultrastructural cytochemical studies using peroxidases as protein tracers. J. Exper. Med., *124*:1123, 1966.

Hartroft, P. M.: Juxtaglomerular cells. Circulation Res., *12*:525, 1963.

Hicks, R. M.: The fine structure of transitional epithelium of the rat ureter. J. Cell Biol., *26*:25, 1965.

Hicks, R. M.: The permeability of rat transitional epithelium keratinization and the barrier to water. J. Cell Biol., *28*:21, 1966.

Hicks, R. M., and B. Ketterer: Isolation of the plasma membrane of the luminal surface of rat bladder epithelium, and the occurrence of a hexagonal lattice of subunits both in negatively stained whole mounts and in sectional membranes. J. Cell Biol., *45*:542, 1970.

Koss, L. G.: The asymmetric unit membranes of the epithelium of the urinary bladder of the rat. Lab. Invest., *21*:154, 1969.

von Kugelgen, A., B. Kuhlo, M. Kuhlo, and K. J. Otto: Die Gefassarchitectur der Niere. Stuttgart, Georg Thieme Verlag, 1959.

Kurtz, S. M., and J. D. Feldman: Experimental studies on the formation of the glomerular basement membrane. J. Ultrastr. Res., *6*:19, 1962.

Lassen, N. A., and J. B. Longley: Countercurrent exchange in vessels in the renal medulla. Proc. Soc. Exper. Biol. Med., *106*:743, 1961.

Latta, H., A. B. Maunsbach, and L. Osvaldo: The fine structure of renal tubules in cortex and medulla. *In* Dalton, A. J., and F. Haguenau (eds.): Ultrastructure of the Kidney. New York, Academic Press, 1967, pp. 1–56.

Longley, J. B., and E. R. Fisher: Alkaline phosphatase and the periodic acid-Schiff reaction in the proximal tubule of the vertebrate kidney; a study in segmental differentiation. Anat. Rec., *120*:1, 1954.

Maunsbach, A. B.: The influence of different fixatives and fixation methods on the ultrastructure of rat kidney proximal tubule cells. I. Comparison of different perfusion fixation methods and of glutaraldehyde, formaldehyde and osmium tetroxide fixatives. J. Ultrastr. Res., *15*:242, 1966.

Maunsbach, A. B.: Absorption of I^{125} labeled homologous albumin by rat kidney proximal tubule cells. J. Ultrastr. Res., *15*:197, 1966.

Maunsbach, A. B.: Isolation and purification of acid phosphatase containing autofluorescent granules from homogenates of rat kidney cortex. J. Ultrastr. Res., *16*:13, 1966.

Miller, F.: Hemoglobin absorption by the cells of the proximal convoluted tubule in mouse kidney. J. Biophys. Biochem. Cytol., *8*:689, 1960.

Miller, F., and G. Palade: Lytic activities in renal protein absorption droplets. An electron microscopical cytochemical study. J. Cell Biol., *23*:519, 1964.

Miyoshi, M., T. Fujita, and J. Tokunuga: The differentiation of renal podocytes. A combined scanning and transmission electron microscope study in the rat. Arch. Histol. Jap., *33*:161, 1971.

von Möllendorff, W.: Der Exkretionsapparat. *In* von Möllendorff, W., and W. Bargmann (eds.): Handbuch der mikroskopischen Anatomie des Menschen. Berlin, Julius Springer, 1930, Vol. 7, Part 1, p. 1.

Neustein, H. B., and A. B. Maunsbach: Hemoglobin absorption by proximal tubule cells of the rabbit kidney. A study by electron microscopic autoradiography. J. Ultrastr. Res., *16*:141, 1966.

Oliver, J.: New directions in renal morphology; A method, its results and its future. The Harvey Lectures, *40*:102, 1944–45.

Osvaldo, L., and H. Latta: The thin limb of the loop of Henle. J. Ultrastr. Res., *15*:144, 1966.

Osvaldo, L., and H. Latta: Interstitial cells of the renal medulla. J. Ultrastr. Res., *15*:589, 1966.

Peter, K.: Untersuchungen über Bau und Entwicklung der Niere. Jena, G. Fischer, 1927.

Pierce, E. C.: Renal lymphatics. Anat. Rec., *90*:315, 1944.

Policard, A.: Le tube urinaire des mammifères. Rev. Gén. d'histol., *3*:fasc. 10, 1905.

Porter, K. R., and M. Bonneville: An Introduction to the Fine Structure of Cells and Tissues. Philadelphia, Lea & Febiger, 1964.

Rhodin, J.: Correlation of ultrastructural organization and function in normal and experimentally changed proximal convoluted tubule cells of the mouse kidney. Stockholm, Aktiebolaget Godvil, 1954.

Rhodin, J.: Anatomy of kidney tubules. Int. Rev. Cytol., *7*:485, 1958.

Rhodin, J.: Electron microscopy of the kidney. Am. J. Med., *24*:661, 1958.

Richards, A. N., and A. M. Walker: Methods of collecting fluid from known regions of the renal tubules of amphibia and of perfusing the lumen of a single tubule. Am. J. Physiol., *118*:111, 1937.

Richards, A. N.: Processes of urine formation. Proc. Roy. Soc. B., *126*:398, 1938.

Richter, W. R., and S. M. Moize: Electron microscopic observations on the collapsed and distended mammalian urinary bladder. J. Ultrastr. Res., *9*:1, 1963.

Schloss, G.: The juxtaglomerular E-cells of rat kidneys in diuresis and antidiuresis, after adrenalectomy and hypophysectomy, and in avitaminosis A, D and E, Acta Anat., *6*:80, 1948.

Schmidt-Nielsen, B.: Urea excretion in mammals. Physiol. Rev., *38*:139, 1958.

Sjöstrand, F. S., and J. Rhodin: The ultrastructure of the proximal convoluted tubules of the mouse kidney as revealed by high resolution electron microscopy. Exper. Cell Res., *4*:426, 1953.

Smith, H. W.: The Kidney. New York, Oxford University Press, 1951.

Smith, H. W.: Principles of Renal Physiology. New York, Oxford University Press, 1956.

Spargo, B.: Kidney changes in hypokalemic alkalosis in the rat. J. Lab. Clin. Med., *43*:802, 1954.

Spargo, B., F. Straus, and F. Fitch: Zonal renal papillary droplet change with potassium depletion. Arch. Path., *70*:599, 1960.

Sternberg, W. H., E. Farber, and C. E. Dunlap: Histochemical localization of specific oxidative enzymes. II. Localization of diphosphopyridine nucleotide and triphosphopyridine nucleotide diaphorase and the succindehydrogenase system in the kidney. J. Histochem., *4*:266, 1956.

Straus, W.: Localization of intravenously injected horseradish peroxidase in the cells of the convoluted tubules of rat kidney. Exper. Cell Res., *20*:600, 1960.

Suzuki, Y.: An electron microscopy of the renal differentiation. II. Glomerulus. Keio J. Med., *8*:129, 1959.

Thorburn, G. D., H. H. Kopald, J. A. Herd, M. Hollenberg, C. C. C. O'Morchoe, and A. C. Barger: Intrarenal distribution of nutrient blood flow determined with krypton[85] in the unanaesthetized dog. Circulation Res., *13*:290, 1963.

Tisher, C. C., R. E. Bulger, and B. F. Trump: Human renal ultrastructure. I. Proximal tubule of healthy individuals. Lab. Invest., *15*:1357, 1966.

Tisher, C. C., R. E. Bulger, and B. F. Trump: Human renal ultrastructure. III. The distal tubule in healthy individuals. Lab. Invest., *18*:655, 1968.

Tobian, L.: Relationship of juxtaglomerular apparatus to renin and angiotensin. Circulation, *25*:189, 1962.

Trueta, J., A. E. Barclay, P. M. Daniel, K. J. Franklin, and M. M. L. Prichard: Studies of the Renal Circulation. Springfield, Ill., Charles C Thomas, 1947.

Trump, B. F., and R. E. Bulger: New ultrastructural characteristics of cells fixed in glutaraldehyde-osmium tetroxide mixture. Lab. Invest., *15*:368, 1966.

Tyson, G., and R. Bulgar: Endothelial detachment sites in glomerular capillaries of vinblastin-treated rats. Anat. Rec., *172*:669, 1972.

Ullrich, K. J., K. Kramer, and J. W. Boylan: Present knowledge of the countercurrent system in the mammalian kidney. Progr. Cardiovas. Dis., *3*:395, 1961.

Walker, A. M., P. A. Bott, J. Oliver, and M. C. MacDowell: The collection and analysis of fluid from single nephrons of the mammalian kidney. Am. J. Physiol. *134*:580, 1941.

Warren, R. C., and R. M. Hicks: Structure of the subunits in the thick luminal membrane of rat urinary bladder. Nature, *227*:280, 1970.

Wirz, H., B. Hargitay, and W. Kuhn: Lokalisation des Konzentrierungsprozesses in der Niere durch direkte Kryoskopie. Helvet. Physiol. Pharmacol. Acta, 9:196, 1951.

Yamada, E.: The fine structure of the renal glomerulus of the mouse. J. Biophys. Biochem. Cytol., *1*:551, 1955.

Zimmerman, K. W.: Über den Bau des Glomerulus der Säugetiere, Weitere Mitteilungen. Zeitschr. f. mikr.-anat. Forsch., *32*:176, 1933.

32

Male Reproductive System

TESTIS

The testis is a compound tubular gland enclosed in a thick fibrous capsule, the *tunica albuginea.* On the posterior aspect of the organ, a thickening of the connective tissue capsule projects into the gland as the *mediastinum testis.* Thin fibrous septa, called the *septula testis,* extend radially from the mediastinum to the tunica albuginea, dividing the organ into about 250 pyramidal compartments, the *lobuli testis.* The septula may be incomplete toward the periphery, so that the lobules intercommunicate, but where their apices converge upon the mediastinum they are more completely separated.

Each lobule is composed of one to four highly convoluted *seminiferous tubules.* These are 150 to 250 μm. in diameter, 30 to 70 cm. long and extremely tortuous (Fig. 32–3).

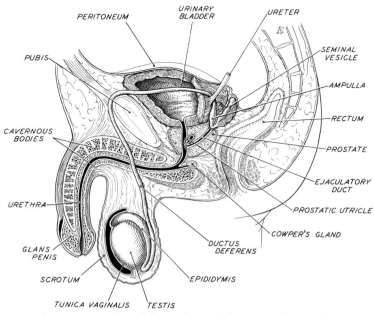

Figure 32–1 Diagrammatic representation of the male genital system. The midline structures are shown in sagittal section; bilateral structures, such as testis, epididymis, vas deferens, and seminal vesicle, are depicted intact. (After C. D. Turner.)

805

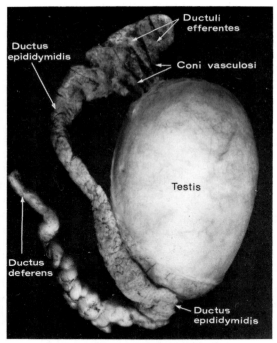

Figure 32-2 Photomicrograph of human testis, epididymis, and ductus deferens. The epididymis has been dissected free and drawn away from the testis to reveal more clearly the coni vasculosi. (Photograph courtesy of A. F. Holstein.)

Each testis is suspended in the scrotum at the end of a long vascular pedicle, *the spermatic cord*, which consists of the excretory duct of the testis, the *ductus deferens*, and the blood vessels and nerves supplying the testis on that side. The *epididymis*, an organ closely applied to the posterior surface of the testis, is made up of the convoluted proximal part of the excretory duct system (Figs. 32-2 and 32-3). Each testis and epididymis is surrounded on its anterior and lateral surfaces by a cleftlike serous cavity that arises late in embryonic development as a detached portion of the peritoneal cavity.

The testes develop early in embryonic life in the dorsal wall of the abdominal cavity and later descend into the scrotum, each carrying with it an outpocketing of the periton-

The seminiferous tubules constitute the exocrine portion of the testis, which is in essence a cytogenous gland whose holocrine secretory product is whole cells, the *spermatozoa*. The tubules are usually highly convoluted loops, but they may also branch or end blindly. At the apex of each lobule its seminiferous tubules pass abruptly into the *tubuli recti*, the first segment of the system of excretory ducts. They in turn are confluent with the *rete testis*, a plexiform system of epithelium lined spaces in the connective tissue of the mediastinum.

On the inner aspect of the tunica albuginea, dense connective tissue gives way to a looser layer provided with numerous blood vessels, the *tunica vasculosa testis*. A loose connective tissue of similar character extends inward from this layer to fill all of the interstices among the seminiferous tubules. It contains fibroblasts, macrophages, mast cells, and perivascular mesenchymal cells. In addition, there are clusters of epithelioid *interstitial cells*, also called *Leydig cells*. These constitute the endocrine tissue of the testis.

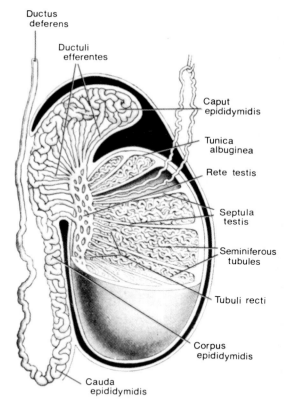

Figure 32-3 Cutaway diagram of the architecture of the testis and excurrent duct system. The septula divide the organ into a number of compartments occupied by highly convoluted seminiferous tubules. One has been unravelled and drawn out to show its length and the fact that it is a loop terminating in the rete testis. (Drawing modified from W. J. Hamilton, Textbook of Human Anatomy. London, Macmillan & Co., 1957.)

eum, the *tunica vaginalis propria testis*, which forms the serous cavity around the testis. It consists of an outer parietal and an inner visceral layer that is closely applied to the tunica albuginea of the testis on its anterior and lateral surfaces. On the posterior aspect of the testis, where the blood vessels and nerves enter the organ, the visceral layer is reflected from its surface and is continuous with the parietal layer. After removal of the parietal layer, the visceral coat covering the testis appears as a glistening, smooth surface covered with mesothelium, which is the remnant of the coelomic or germinal epithelium that covered the primordium of the gonad in the embryo. The tunica vaginalis enables the testis, which is sensitive to pressure, to glide freely in its envelopes.

SEMINIFEROUS TUBULES

The Lamina Propria or Boundary Tissue

The seminiferous tubules are enclosed by one or more layers of adventitial cells derived from primitive connective tissue elements of the interstitium. The organization of this boundary tissue varies from species to species. In the common laboratory rodents, there is a single layer of flattened polygonal cells that meet edge to edge to form a continuous epithelioid sheet surrounding the tubule. In their ultrastructure, these cells have all of the cytological characteristics of smooth muscle and are presumed to be contractile. They cannot be called true smooth muscle cells because of their atypical shape and epithelioid organization. Therefore, they are referred to as *myoid cells* or *peritubular contractile cells*. They are believed to be responsible for the rhythmic shallow contractions that can be observed in the seminiferous tubules of these species. The contractions seem to be intrinsically generated, since no nerves have been observed in or near this layer.

In larger species, such as ram, boar and bull, there are multiple layers of adventitial cells. In these, only the innermost layer is muscle-like, the next layer has some of the characteristics of smooth muscle, and outer layers appear to be fibroblasts. In monkey and man, there are also multiple layers of cells but these are not epithelioid, and the cells do not resemble smooth muscle as much as in other species. Contractility of seminif-

erous tubules has not been observed in primates. In many cases of human male infertility, the boundary tissue becomes greatly thickened.

The Seminiferous Epithelium

In the adult, the seminiferous tubules are lined by a complex stratified epithelium composed of two major categories of cells: *supporting cells* and *spermatogenic cells*. The supporting elements are of a single kind, the *Sertoli cells*, whereas the spermatogenic cells include several morphologically distinguishable types: *spermatogonia, primary spermatocytes, secondary spermatocytes, spermatids,* and *spermatozoa* (Figs. 32–6 and 32–7). These germ cells are not ontogenetically distinct cell types but are successive stages in a continuous process of differentiation of the male germ cells.

The three dimensional configuration of the Sertoli cell is extraordinarily complex, but it can be thought of as basically columnar, resting upon the basal lamina and extending upward through the full thickness of the epithelium to its free surface. From the columnar portion of these cells an elaborate system of thin processes radiate laterally to surround the spermatogenic cells and occupy all of the interstices among them. The earliest of the germ cells, the spermatogonia, also rest upon the basal lamina, while the more advanced stages of the germ cell line are found at successively higher levels in the epithelium (Figs. 32–7 and 32–8). The proliferative activity in the epithelium is confined to the spermatogonia and spermatocytes near the base. The continual formation of new generations of cells in this region displaces the more advanced cells to higher levels until, as mature sperm, they come to border directly upon the lumen. To understand spermatogenesis, it is important to bear in mind that the seminiferous epithelium consists of (1) a fixed population of nonproliferating supporting cells, and (2) a proliferating and differentiating population of germ cells that move slowly upward along the sides of the Sertoli cells to the free surface. This dynamic relationship of the cells makes the lining of the seminiferous tubules unique among epithelia.

Owing to the elaborate shape of the Sertoli cells and the limitations of resolution of the light microscope, their outlines cannot be seen distinctly. Earlier, this gave rise to the widespread belief that they constituted a syncytium, but this interpretation is now known to be erroneous. In sections parallel to the basal lamina of the epithelium, the bases of the Sertoli cells can be seen with the light microscope as distinctly outlined polygonal areas. Electron micrographs clearly show pairs of apposed membranes at the boundary between adjacent Sertoli cells and between the latter and the germ cells. Therefore, the spermatogenic cells are not embedded in a "Sertolian syncytium," but instead occupy deep recesses of conforming shape in the lateral and apical surfaces of the sustentacular cells. The elaborate shape of the Sertoli cells (Fig. 32–9) is probably attributable to their close coaptation to the highly irregular and changing contours of the differentiating germ cells that they surround.

The nucleus of the Sertoli cell is generally ovoid in outline but may have one or more deep infoldings of its surface. It is about 9 by 12 μm. in average size, with a relatively homogeneous nucleoplasm, except for a large and highly characteristic nucleolus, consisting of a round or oval central body flanked by two rounded basophilic masses. In electron micrographs, the tripartite structure of this complex is confirmed. The central element consists of a typical nucleolonema organized around a homogeneous central area of relatively low density. The two adjacent darker masses of finely granular material appear to be nucleolus associated chromatin.

The cytoplasm contains numerous slender elongated mitochondria often oriented parallel to the long axis of the cell. Numerous lipid droplets and occasional lipofuscin pigment granules are found near the cell base.

The granular endoplasmic reticulum is sparse but the agranular reticulum is well developed, especially near the cell base. It usually occurs in the form of a network of

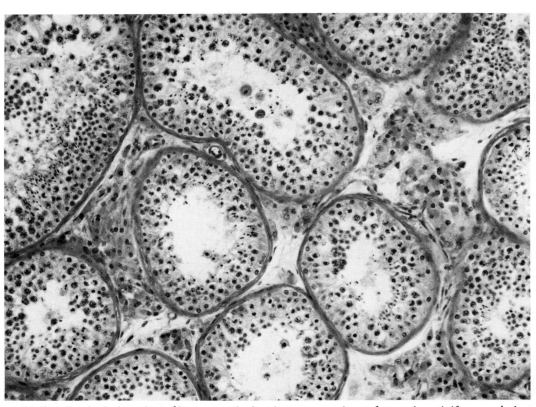

Figure 32-4 Histological section of human testis showing cross sections of several seminiferous tubules and clusters of Leydig cells in the angular interstices among them.

smooth surfaced tubules, but in some species it may form concentric systems of membranes around lipid droplets. The presence of a well developed smooth endoplasmic reticulum at the cell base has been interpreted by some as evidence for secretion of steroid hormones, but such a function has yet to be clearly established for the Sertoli cell. In certain stages of the spermatogenic cycle, close aggregations of smooth reticulum are found in the cytoplasm immediately adjacent to the developing acrosomal cap of each associated spermatid (Fig. 32–9). The significance of this striking localization remains unexplained,

but may be an expression of the "nurse cell" function of Sertoli cells.

The Golgi complex is extensive but relatively simple in its organization and shows no sign of involvement in secretory activity. The slender mitochondria have the usual foliate internal membrane structure and are remarkable only for their length. The lysosomal system of the cell exhibits a diversity of components, ranging from membrane-limited, spherical primary lysosomes to pleomorphic, dense, secondary lysosomes, to large irregular conglomerates of lipochrome pigment with a very heterogeneous content

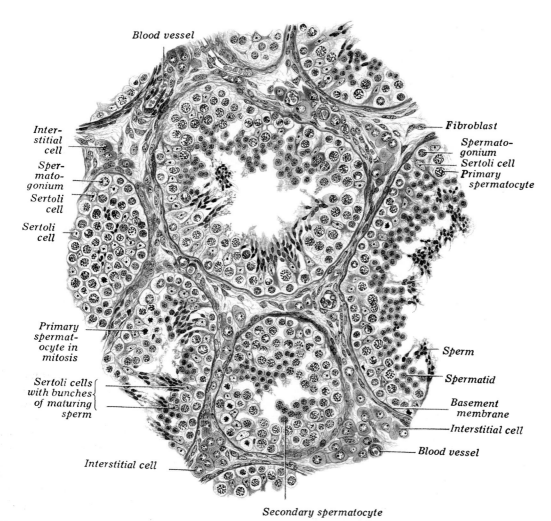

Figure 32–5 Section of human testis (obtained at operation). The transected tubules show various stages of spermatogenesis. × 170. (After A. A. Maximow.)

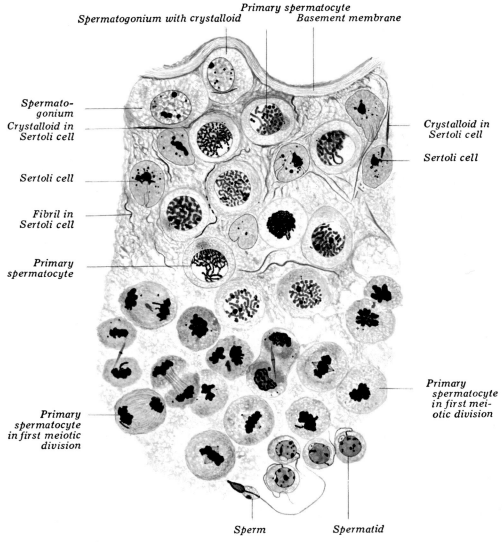

Figure 32–6 Section of same testis as in Figure 32–5; seminiferous epithelium with primary spermatocytes in first meiotic division. Iron-hematoxylin stain. × 750. (After A. A. Maximow.)

of globular and granular components of varying density. Although the lysosomal digestive system of these cells is well developed, the amount of accumulated pigment is not large when one considers that they are responsible for degradation and disposal of the residual cytoplasm of generation after generation of spermatozoa.

The filamentous component of the cytoplasmic matrix of Sertoli cells is more abundant than in many other cell types. A feltwork of 70 to 90 Å filaments excludes organelles and inclusions and results in a thin clear

zone surrounding the nucleus. Filaments in lower concentrations are randomly dispersed in the cytoplasm. Occasionally they associate laterally to form fascicles parallel to the long axis of the cell. At certain stages of the spermatogenic cycle, microtubules are also abundant in the supranuclear columnar portion of the Sertoli cell. They are very uniformly spaced and oriented parallel to the cell axis. The escalation of the germ cells in the epithelium and the release of spermatozoa probably depend upon active changes in shape of the supporting cells. The filaments and microtubules of the Sertoli cells are very probably the agents of these cytoplasmic movements.

Inclusions peculiar to the human Sertoli cell are the crystalloids of Charcot-Böttcher. These are slender, fusiform structures 10 to 25 μm. long, often visible with the light microscope. In electron micrographs, they consist of dense straight filaments 150 Å in diameter. These subunits are generally parallel or converge toward the ends of the crystalloid. They are often rather poorly ordered and there may be irregular defects in the interior of these crystalloids, occupied by cytoplasmic matrix. Their chemical nature and physiological significance are unknown.

The Sertoli cells provide mechanical support and protection for the developing germ cells, and they probably participate in their nutrition. They also seem to play an active role in the release of the mature spermatozoa. The Sertoli cells are never observed in division in the mature testis. They are resistant to heat, ionizing radiation, and various toxic agents that destroy the more sensitive spermatogenic cells.

It will facilitate the student's understanding of the complex cytological changes that take place in the germ cells of the seminiferous epithelium if the structure of the end product—the spermatozoon—is described first.

THE SPERMATOZOON

The mature spermatozoon is an actively motile, free swimming cell consisting of a *head*, which contains a nucleus with all of the genetic traits a father can transmit to his offspring, and a *tail* or flagellum, which provides the motility that assists in transport of the sperm to the site of fertilization and insures that it is appropriately oriented for penetration of the coatings of the ovum (Figs. 32–10 and 32–11).

The human sperm head is ovoid in outline in frontal view and pyriform when seen on edge, being thicker near the neck and tapering toward the tip. The head is 4 to 5 μm. in length and 2.5 to 3.5 μm. in width. The greater part of its bulk consists of the

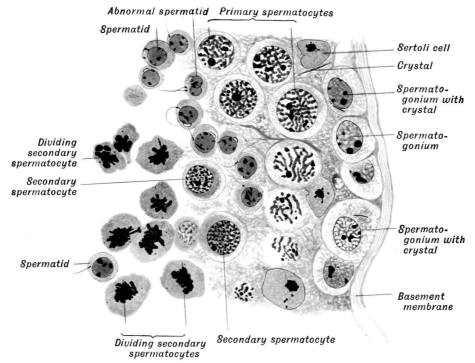

Figure 32–7 Section of same testis as in Figure 32–5; seminiferous epithelium with mitoses of secondary spermatocytes—second meiotic division. The loosening of the spermatocytes and spermatids from their normal attachment to the Sertoli cells is an artifact of specimen preparation. × 750. (After A. A. Maximow.)

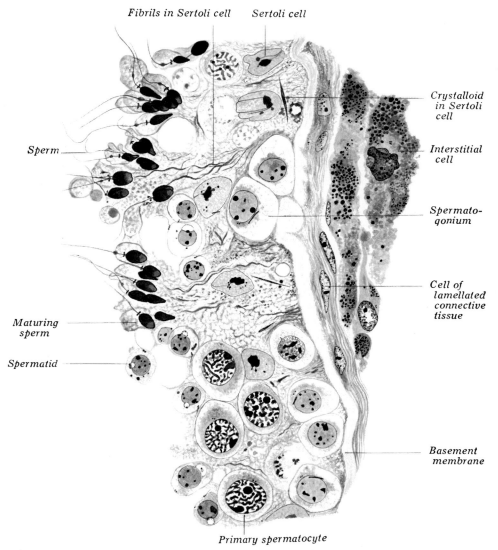

Fibrils in Sertoli cell   *Sertoli cell*

Crystalloid in Sertoli cell

Interstitial cell

Sperm

Spermatogonium

Cell of lamellated connective tissue

Maturing sperm

Spermatid

Basement membrane

Primary spermatocyte

Figure 32–8 Section of same testis as in Figure 32–5; seminiferous epithelium with clusters of maturing sperm, connected with Sertoli cells. Iron-hematoxylin stain. × 750. (After A. A. Maximow.)

nucleus, whose chromatin has become greatly condensed to diminish its volume for greater mobility and to protect its genome from damage in transit to the egg. The anterior two thirds of the nucleus is covered by the *acrosomal cap*—an organelle containing enzymes that are believed to have an important role in sperm penetration during fertilization (Figs. 32–11 and 32–12). The mammalian sperm head varies greatly in size and shape from species to species.

The sperm tail is about 55 μm. long and varies in thickness from about 1 μm. near the base to 0.1 μm. near its tip. It presents four segments along its length recognizable with the light microscope by slight differences in thickness and in the nature of their sheaths. From proximal to distal, these regions are the *neck*, the *middle piece*, the *principal piece*, and the *end piece* (Fig. 32–11). There are significant differences in the internal structure of these segments. These cannot be clearly resolved in fresh preparations but require special cytological techniques, or preferably electron microscopy, for their demonstration. The more detailed description of

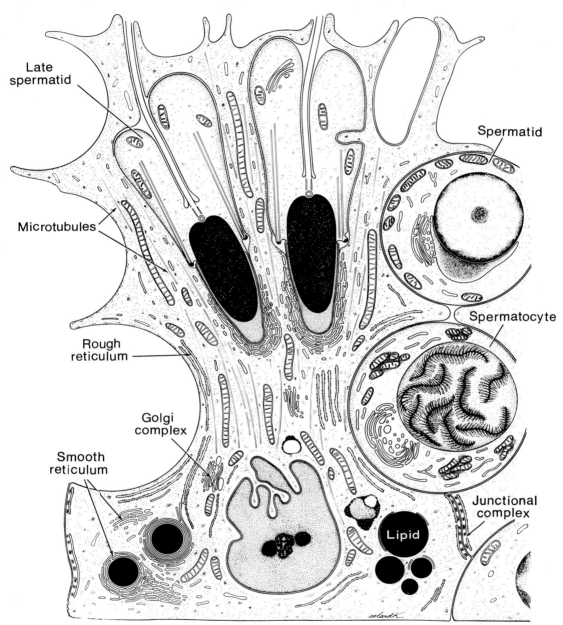

Figure 32-9 Drawing illustrating the ultrastructure of the Sertoli cell and its relationship to the germ cells. The spermatocytes and early spermatids occupy niches in the sides of the columnar supporting cell, while late spermatids reside in deep recesses in its apex. (After D. W. Fawcett, in *Male Fertility and Sterility*. Serono Symposium, 1973.)

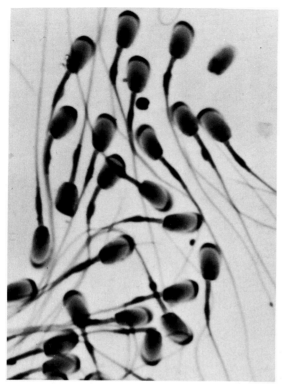

Figure 32-10 Photomicrograph of chinchilla sperm stained by the Feulgen reaction and counterstained with light green. The crescentic apical segment of the acrosome can be seen at the leading edge of the sperm head. × 3000.

spermatozoon structure that follows is based largely upon electron microscopic studies.

The Acrosome. The acrosome is a membrane limited organelle that closely conforms to the contours of the tapering anterior portion of the sperm nucleus. The inner acrosomal membrane, which is adherent to the nuclear envelope, is continuous at the posterior margin of the cap with the outer acrosomal membrane. The two membranes run parallel throughout most of their course and enclose a narrow cavity occupied by a homogeneous amorphous material—the acrosomal contents. In the human spermatozoon, the acrosome is relatively small and does not extend anteriorly much beyond the leading edge of the nucleus. In many other mammalian species, however, there is a conspicuous thickening of the cap that extends well beyond the nucleus and may exhibit a highly specific shape. It is useful to designate this region as the *apical segment* of the acrosomal cap. The main portion of the acrosome is

then called the *principal segment.* In addition, in all mammalian species, there is a specialized caudal region where there is an abrupt narrowing of the cap and a slight condensation of its contents. With special staining techniques, this region was visible to light microscopists as a band around the middle of the head and was therefore called the *equatorial segment* (Fig. 32–12). The functional significance of this specialization has yet to be discovered.

The acrosome of mammalian spermato-

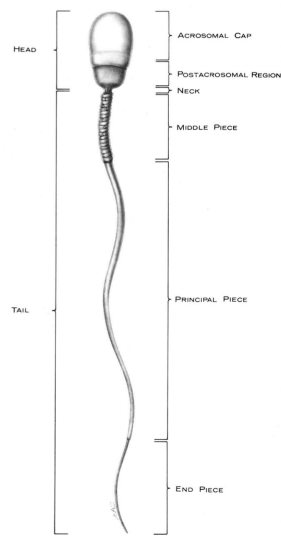

Figure 32-11 Drawing of a mammalian spermatozoon as seen with the light microscope, presenting the terms used in describing its various regions.

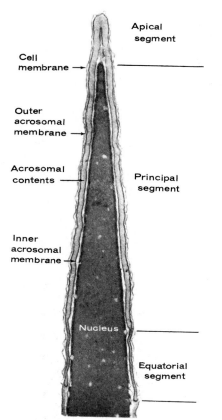

Apical segment

Cell membrane →

Outer acrosomal membrane →

Acrosomal contents →

Principal segment

Inner acrosomal membrane →

Nucleus

Equatorial segment

Figure 32-12 Electron micrograph of a monkey spermatozoon, illustrating the relationship of the acrosomal cap to the condensed nucleus and to the cell membrane.

zoa stains with the periodic acid–Schiff reaction and hence contains appreciable amounts of carbohydrate. In addition, it is known to contain several enzymes of lysosomal nature. Among those identified to date are hyaluronidase, neuraminidase, acid phosphatase, β-N-acetylglucosamidase, and aryl sulfatase. There is also a proteolytic enzyme remarkably similar to trypsin in its substrate specificity, pH optimum, and range of inhibitors. The precise role of these enzymes in fertilization is still unclear, but extracts of sperm acrosomes will disperse the adhering cells of the corona radiata and will digest the zona pellucida from recently ovulated eggs of some species. Sperm in the vicinity of ova in the oviduct undergo a sequence of structural changes called the *acrosome reaction:* The outer membrane of the acrosome fuses at multiple points with the overlying plasma membrane of the sperm head to create numerous openings through which the enzyme-rich contents of the acrosome are liberated in a process not unlike the release of secretory products from a glandular cell. The release of the enzymes is believed to facilitate sperm entry.

Nucleus. The nucleus of the mature mammalian spermatozoon is usually dense and homogeneous in electron micrographs (Figs. 32–12 and 32–13). Human spermatozoa are subject to considerably more variation in size, shape, and texture of the chromatin than are those of other species. In ejaculates of fertile men the chromatin in a certain proportion of the sperm nuclei is not homogeneous but is a dense conglomerate of closely packed coarse granular subunits. In these, the process of chromatin condensation during spermiogenesis does not seem to have progressed to completion. Another peculiarity of human sperm nuclei is the frequent occurrence of irregularly shaped clear spaces of varying size in the chromatin. These are commonly referred to as nuclear vacuoles, although they are not membrane bounded. They seem to result from randomly occurring defects in condensation of the chromatin, and there is no evidence at present that they interfere with fertilizing capacity. Despite the absence of resolvable order in the fine structure of the nucleoplasm, there are indications that the chromosomes retain their identity and have a consistent arrangement within the nucleus. For example, quinacrine mustards have been found to stain the Y chromosome of man more or less selectively. When this method is applied to human sperm, a yellow fluorescent spot is located in approximately the same position in the heads of half of the sperm population.

Caudal to the acrosome a specialized dense layer is found between the plasma membrane and the nuclear envelope which exhibits a characteristic pattern of fine structure that differs from species to species (Fig. 32–13). It seems more closely adherent to the inner aspect of the cell membrane than to the underlying nucleus. This component corresponds to the "postnuclear cap" of classical light microscopy. However, inasmuch as it is not continuous over the posterior surface of the nucleus but is simply a broad band encircling the postacrosomal region, the term postacrosomal cap is no longer appropriate. Although the chemical nature and functional

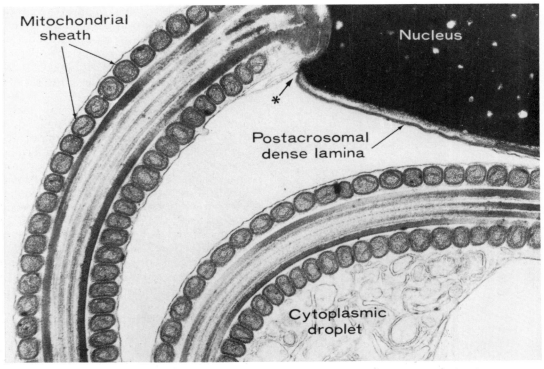

Figure 32–13 Electron micrograph of portions of two spermatozoa of the dormouse (*Glis glis*). In the post-acrosomal region, the membrane is reinforced by a dense lamina. This specialization may be important for fertilization, for it is this region that first fuses with the egg membrane. The asterisk indicates the site of the posterior ring, a circumferential line of fusion of the plasmalemma and the outer and inner membranes of the nuclear envelope. (Micrograph by D. Phillips, from D. W. Fawcett, Biol. Reprod., *2* (Suppl. 2, 1970.)

significance of this layer are not known, it is thought to be an important structure, for it is specifically in this region that the membrane of the sperm first fuses with that of the egg during fertilization.

The plasma membrane is firmly adherent to the nuclear envelope along a line, called the *posterior ring*, which encircles the sperm head at the caudal edge of the post-acrosomal dense layer (Fig. 32–13). Behind this line or groove the membrane diverges somewhat from the underlying structures of the nucleus. The nuclear envelope which is generally closely applied to the condensed chromatin diverges from it caudal to this line of membrane adherence and forms a fold of variable size extending back into the neck region. Pores and annuli which are absent from the nuclear envelope over the condensed nucleus are abundant in the fold or scroll that extends back into the neck. This portion of the envelope is interpreted as an excess resulting from the diminution in vol-

ume of the nucleus associated with nuclear condensation during spermiogenesis. The nuclear envelope over the caudal surface of the head is again devoid of pores, and its membranes are in close apposition. The nuclear envelope lines the shallow *implantation fossa* where the tail attaches to the head. In this area there are regular periodic densities bridging the 100 Å interspace between the leaves of the nuclear envelope. These may help strengthen this region of attachment of tail to head.

The Neck. Immediately behind the head is a *connecting piece* which has a dense *capitulum* conforming in shape to the implantation fossa to which it attaches (Fig. 32–26). Extending backward from this capitulum are nine segmented columns 1 to 1.5 μm. long that are continuous at their caudal ends with nine *outer dense fibers* of the sperm flagellum. In the interior of the connecting piece immediately subjacent to the articular surface of the capitulum is a transversely oriented juxtanuclear or *proximal centriole* (Fig. 32–26). The triplet microtubules of the centriole wall are embedded to varying degrees in the dense material composing the articular surface and segmented columns of the connecting piece. A *distal centriole* oriented in the axis of the sperm flagellum is usually absent from the mature spermatozoon, but vestiges of its nine triplets may be associated with the inner aspect of the segmented columns. The central pair of microtubules of the flagellar axoneme may extend anteriorly in the interior of the connecting piece as far as the proximal centriole.

One or two longitudinally oriented mitochondria may be found in the neck region outside the connecting piece, and these may have processes that extend between the segmented columns into its interior. In the human sperm, a sizeable mass of residual cytoplasm may surround the neck, but in most mammals this *cytoplasmic droplet* is either absent from mature sperm or located at the caudal end of the middle piece.

The Middle Piece. In the core of the sperm flagellum is the *axoneme* consisting of two central singlet microtubules surrounded by nine evenly spaced doublets, frequently written as (9 + 2). These extend without significant change in structure throughout the length of the tail from the neck to near the tip of the end piece. The sperm flagellum differs from other flagella in that the axoneme is surrounded by nine outer dense fibers (9 + 9 + 2). Each dense fiber is continuous anteriorly with one of the segmented columns of the connecting piece, and each courses longitudinally in close relation to one of the nine doublets of the axoneme. The axoneme and its associated outer dense fibers are considered to be the motor elements of the tail.

Three regions of the sperm tail are defined by the nature and extent of the sheaths that surround the 9 + 9 + 2 core complex (Fig. 32–19). The middle piece is characterized by a sheath of circumferentially oriented mitochondria arranged end to end in a tight helix (Fig. 32–14). These mitochondria are believed to generate the energy for sperm motility. The structural organization of the middle piece is basically similar in all mammalian spermatozoa but the length of the mitochondrial helix varies from about 15 gyres in primates to over 300 in some rodents. In the human, the middle piece is from 5 to 7 μm. long and somewhat more than 1 μm. thick.

Immediately caudal to the last turn of the mitochondrial sheath is the *annulus*, a ring of dense material to which the flagellar membrane is firmly adherent (Fig. 32–15). The annulus and its attachment to the membrane are presumed to prevent caudal displacement of the mitochondria during the tail movements.

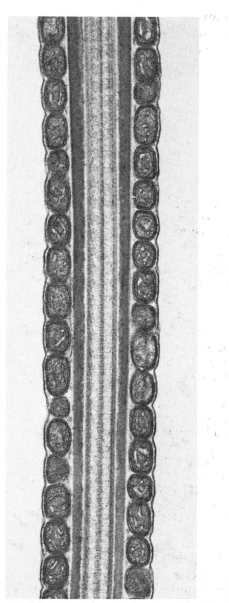

Figure 32–14 Electron micrograph of the midpiece of a spermatozoon in longitudinal section, showing the close apposition of the mitochondrial sheath to the outer dense fibers of the flagellum.

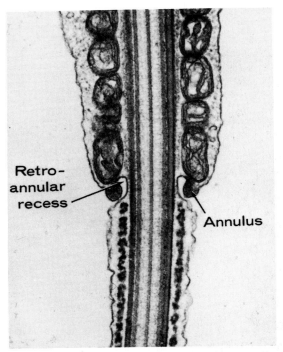

Figure 32–15 Electron micrograph of the junction of the midpiece and principal piece of a rodent spermatozoon. This is the site of the annulus, a dense ring fused to the plasma membrane. In some species the cell membrane forms a deep groove or recess immediately behind the annulus. In others, the membrane is relatively smooth.

The Principal Piece. The principal piece of the spermatozoon is about 45 μm. long and about 0.5 μm. thick at the base, gradually tapering toward the end piece. It has a highly characteristic *fibrous sheath* (Fig. 32–19). Studied by electron microscopy, it is seen to consist of continuous dorsal and ventral longitudinal columns connected by regularly spaced circumferential ribs that extend halfway around the sheath and are continuous at their ends with the longitudinal columns (Fig. 32–16). In cross sections of the principal piece, it is apparent that outer dense fibers 3 and 8 terminate a short distance beyond the annulus (Fig. 32–17). Distal to their termination, the tapering inner edges of the dorsal and ventral columns of the sheath extend into the position of these fibers and are attached to a short flange projecting radially from doublets 3 and 8 of the axoneme. A plane through the longitudinal columns of the fibrous sheath coincides approximately with the plane

through the centers of the central pair of microtubules of the axoneme. This plane divides the cross section of the tail asymmetrically (Fig. 32–17). On one side is a *minor compartment* containing three outer dense fibers and on the other is a *major compartment* containing four. The asymmetry in the distribution of these fibers in the cross section is believed to be reflected in the movements of the sperm tail. The principal plane of bending appears to be perpendicular to the dorsoventral axis of the tail, and the more rapid "power stroke" observed in the proximal portion of the tail is assumed to be toward the side having four outer dense fibers, two of which (numbers 5 and 6) are especially large. The details of the mechanism of sperm tail movement have yet to be worked out. It is now believed that the microtubules of the axoneme produce bending by a

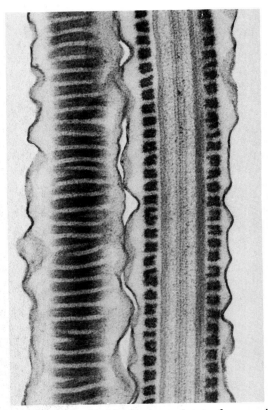

Figure 32–16 Longitudinal sections of two adjacent sperm tails. One has been cut tangentially to the fibrous sheath and shows some of its ribs in surface view; the other is a midline section and therefore shows the circumferential ribs of the sheath in cross section.

sliding mechanism comparable to that of skeletal muscle.

The End Piece. The fibrous sheath ends abruptly 5 to 7 μm. from the tip of the flagellum. The terminal portion, distal to this point, consisting of the axoneme covered only by the flagellar membrane, is called the *end piece* (Fig. 32–19). Its structure is essentially identical to that of a simple flagellum or cilium. The manner in which the axoneme ends varies somewhat from species to species. In some, the doublets terminate at different levels in the tapering tip, but in primates, the nine doublets dissociate into 18 single microtubules. Thus, including the central pair, cross sections through the terminal half micrometer may show 20 closely spaced single microtubules.

SPERMATOGENESIS

Spermatogenesis comprises the entire sequence of events by which spermatogonia are transformed into spermatozoa. For convenience of description it may be divided into three principal phases. In the first, called *spermatocytogenesis,* the most primitive spermatogonia proliferate by mitotic division to replace themselves and to give rise to several successive generations of spermatogonia, each somewhat more differentiated than the preceding. Division of the last generation of spermatogonia (Type B) yields preleptotene spermatocytes. In the second phase, *meiosis,* the spermatocytes undergo two maturation divisions, which reduce the chromosome number by half and produce a cluster of

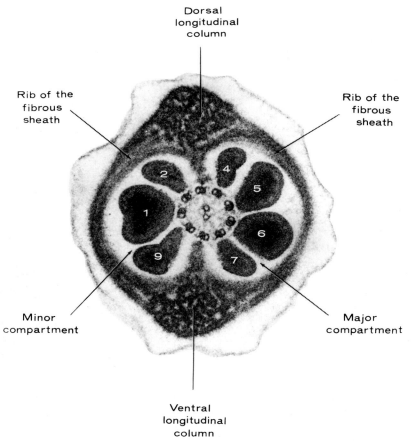

Figure 32–17 Transverse section through the principal piece of a hamster spermatozoon. Outer fibers 3 and 8 have terminated and their place is filled by inward extensions of the dorsal and ventral longitudinal columns of the fibrous sheath. The cross section is asymmetrical, with a major compartment containing four dense fibers and a minor compartment containing three.

spermatids. In the third phase, called *spermiogenesis*, the spermatids undergo a remarkable series of cytological transformations leading to the formation of spermatozoa.

For spermatogenesis to continue without exhausting the supply of stem cells, the spermatogonia must perpetuate themselves

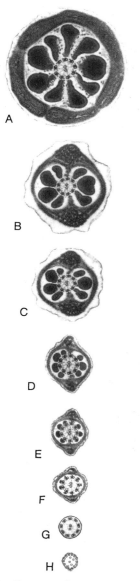

Figure 32–18 Cross sections at successive intervals along the length of the Chinese hamster sperm tail, illustrating the reduction in diameter of the outer dense fibers and the tapering of the tail as a whole. *A* is a section at the level of the midpiece. *B–F,* Successive levels in the principal piece. *G* and *H* are through the end piece. (Micrographs courtesy of D. Phillips.)

and also produce generation after generation of spermatocytes. In human testicular tissue preserved in Zenker-formol fixative, at least two types of spermatogonia (*A* and *B*) can be distinguished with little difficulty. The *type A spermatogonium* has a spherical or ellipsoid nucleus with very fine chromatin granules and one or two irregularly shaped nucleoli attached to the inner aspect of the nuclear envelope. The cytoplasm is homogeneous and pale-staining. In some spermatogonia of this type, the nucleoplasm is dark, and a large pale-staining nuclear vacuole is present. These cells in the human and monkey are designated as dark type A spermatogonia, to distinguish them from the others with paler nucleoplasm and no nuclear vacuole. The *type B spermatogonium* has a spherical nucleus containing chromatin granules of varying size, many of which are distributed along the nuclear envelope. The single nucleolus is centrally located and often has granules of chromatin associated with it. The cytoplasm is not significantly different from that of the type A spermatogonium.

The type A spermatogonium undergoes a series of divisions that give rise to other type A spermatogonia. Of these progeny, certain ones serve as stem cells for future cycles of spermatogonial renewal and spermatocytogenesis. Others proceed to differentiate through recognizable intermediates into type B spermatogonia. The division of type B spermatogonia then gives rise to primary spermatocytes.

In somatic cells, chromosomes are present in pairs. These cells are conventionally described as *diploid* in chromosome number, while the gametes which contain only one chromosome of each pair are *haploid*. The reduction in chromosome number of the gametes to half the somatic number is part of an orderly process which maintains a constant number of chromosomes for each species. At fertilization the spermatozoon and ovum each contribute a haploid set of chromosomes to the zygote, reestablishing the diploid chromosome number. The special type of nuclear division that results in the formation of the haploid gametes is called *meiosis* (see p. 74). In spermatogenesis it occurs in the spermatocytes.

The primary spermatocytes at first resemble in size and cytological characteristics the spermatogonia from which they arise, but as they move away from the basal lamina of the germinal epithelium, they accumulate more cytoplasm and become distinctly larger. Almost immediately after their formation, the spermatocytes enter prophase of the first maturation division. Their chromatin becomes reorganized into thin threadlike chromosomes characteristic of the *leptotene* stage of meiosis. The homologous chromosomes, which have duplicated themselves during the preceding interphase, undergo intimate pairing during the *zygotene* stage through the formation of the *synaptonemal complex*. Because of the greater thickness and deeper staining of the paired chromosomes at this stage they show up more clearly than those of the leptotene stage. When the pairing of the chromosomes to form bivalents or *tetrads* is complete they continue the process of coiling and shortening to form the much

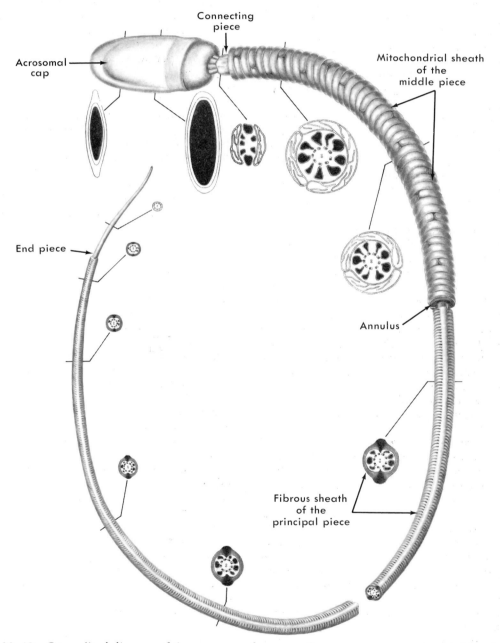

Connecting piece

Acrosomal cap

Mitochondrial sheath of the middle piece

End piece

Annulus

Fibrous sheath of the principal piece

Figure 32–19   Generalized diagram of the structure of a mammalian spermatozoon as revealed by electron microscopy.

coarser and more obvious chromosomal strands typical of the *pachytene* stage. At this stage, the duplicated chromosomes can be identified as *dyads* or *sister chromatids* held together by *centromeres*. Each pachytene element consists of four chromatids. It is also at this period that *crossing over* occurs, in which corresponding regions of the chromatids of the paired chromosomes are exchanged. During *diplotene* and *diakinesis* the chromosomes complete their process of shortening and the synaptonemal complexes disappear.

These stages of meiotic prophase are extremely prolonged, extending over about 22 days. For this reason, a great many spermatocytes in different stages of prophase can be seen in cross sections of seminiferous tubules.

At the end of prophase, the nuclear membrane disappears. The tetrads, or bivalents, arrange themselves at the equatorial plate in *metaphase I*. At *anaphase I* the centromeres of each homologous pair move to opposite poles of the spermatocyte, taking both chromatids (dyads) along with them. This is in contrast to mitosis, during which the duplicated chromosomes line up on the equatorial plate and the centromeres divide, sending copies of each chromosome to the opposite poles. The chromosomes that separate in meiosis are also unique in that they may differ from both maternal and paternal chromosomes because of exchanges that have taken place during crossing over. Anaphase I and *telophase I* are quickly completed, resulting in the formation of secondary spermatocytes carrying only half the number of chromosomes originally present. Since the chromosomes have already been duplicated, the secondary spermatocytes remain in interphase only briefly and they are therefore encountered only infrequently in sections of seminiferous tubules. The secondary spermatocytes quickly complete the second phase of the meiotic division with a brief *prophase II* followed by *metaphase II* with the chromosomes aligned on the equatorial plate. *Anaphase II* differs from anaphase I in that the centromeres divide, permitting the sister chromatids to move to opposite poles. Upon completion of meiosis at *telophase II*, spermatids are formed which have a haploid set of chromosomes.

In the human spermatogonium there are 46 chromosomes, consisting of 22 pairs of *autosomes* and one pair of *sex chromosomes* (XX or XY). The different pairs of autosomes vary in size and in the location of the kinetochore,

but the two members of any given pair of autosomes are morphologically identical. The sex chromosomes in the female (XX) are also identical, but those of the male (XY) differ markedly in size (Fig. 2–34). At the end of the first maturation division in spermatogenesis, each bivalent, including the XY pair, separates into its two constituent chromosomes along the line of their previous conjugation. Therefore of any two secondary spermatocytes resulting from the first maturation division, one will contain 22 autosomes and an X chromosome, while the other will contain 22 autosomes and a Y chromosome. Since all of the eggs produced by the female are the same, containing 22 autosomes plus X, those sperm developing from spermatocytes containing X will be *female determining*, because fertilization will result in a zygote containing 44 + XX (female), whereas sperm developing from secondary spermatocytes containing a Y chromosome will be *male determining*, for the zygote will contain 44 + XY (male).

Electron microscopic studies have shown that the division of all male germ cells, except the most undifferentiated spermatogonia, differ from somatic cell divisions in another important respect. Following division of the nucleus (*karyokinesis*), division of the cell body (*cytokinesis*) is incomplete, and the daughter cells remain connected by protoplasmic bridges at the site where the constricting cleavage furrow encounters the spindle remnant. Such spindle bridges occur as transient structures in mitosis of somatic cells, but in the seminiferous epithelium they remain, after resorption of the spindle, as sizable communications between the daughter cells (Fig. 32–20). They persist to a late stage in the differentiation of the spermatids into spermatozoa. It has been the traditional view that each spermatogonium divided and the daughter cells each developed into a primary spermatocyte; this ultimately divided into two secondaries, and these in turn divided to form four individual spermatids. This interpretation is now known to be incorrect. In all but the earliest spermatogonial division cytokinesis is incomplete, resulting in groups of conjoined spermatogonia and larger syncytial clusters of primary spermatocytes. These produce double the number of interconnected secondary spermatocytes. Their division in turn produces very large numbers of conjoined spermatids (Figs. 32–20 and 32–21). The progeny of a single spermatogonium thus form a cluster of germ cells that remain in protoplasmic continuity throughout their differentiation. This arrangement is probably responsible for the synchrony of development of large numbers of germ cells in any one area of the seminiferous tubule. Individual sperm are separated from the syncytia at the moment of their release from the epithelium. Partial failures of this process may account for the frequency of abnormal double spermatozoa in the ejaculate.

The term *spermiogenesis* describes the sequence of developmental events by which spermatids are transformed into spermatozoa. Each of the relatively small spherical or polygonal spermatids resulting from division of the secondary spermatocytes has a nucleus 5 to 6 μm. in diameter with pale-staining finely granular chromatin. A small Golgi apparatus can be seen in the juxtanuclear cytoplasm. The first sign of differentiation of a specific component of the spermatozoon is the appearance of several small granules within the Golgi apparatus (Fig. 32–22*A, B*). In some species these are first observed in the spermatocytes; in others they are not seen until

the spermatid stage. These *proacrosomal granules* are rich in carbohydrate and are most clearly demonstrated in specimens stained by the periodic acid–Schiff reaction. In electron micrographs, each is found to be enclosed within a membrane limited vesicle of the Golgi apparatus. Although the general features of spermiogenesis can be followed with the light microscope, the finer details described here can be visualized only with the electron microscope. As development progresses, the several separate granules in the Golgi region coalesce into a single large globule, the *acrosomal granule*, contained within a membrane bounded *acrosomal vesicle* or vacuole (Fig. 32–22*C, D*). This becomes adherent to the outer aspect of the nuclear envelope. The point of its adherence marks the future anterior tip of the sperm nucleus. The Golgi apparatus remains closely associated with the surface of the acrosomal vesicle, and it continues to form smaller vesicles that coalesce with the membrane of the acrosomal vesicle, contributing their contents to its enlargement (Fig. 32–22*E, F, G*).

It is convenient to divide spermiogenesis

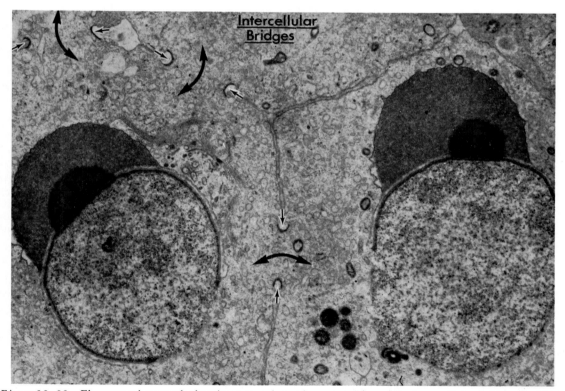

Figure 32–20 Electron micrograph showing two guinea pig spermatids and the intercellular bridges by which they are joined to each other and to two other spermatids of the same cluster. The small arrows indicate the local thickening of the cell membrane encircling the bridges. The large arrows passing through the bridges indicate the sites of continuity of the cytoplasm from cell to cell. × 9000.

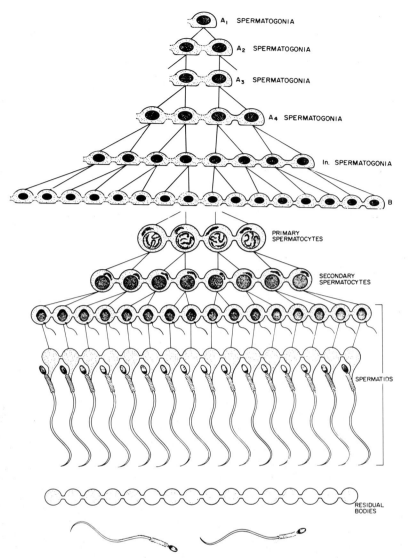

Figure 32–21 Diagram illustrating the clonal nature of the male germ cells. Only the most primitive spermatogonia, dividing to replace the stem cell population, complete cytoplasmic division and give rise to separate daughter cells. Once committed to differentiation, the daughter cells of all subsequent spermatogonial divisions and the two meiotic divisions remain connected by intercellular bridges. Individual sperm are ultimately separated from syncytial chains of residual bodies still connected by bridges. The numbers of interconnected cells are considerably larger than depicted in this figure.

into four phases. That period from the appearance of the proacrosomal granules to the development of a hemispherical acrosomal granule fixed to the nuclear envelope is referred to as the *Golgi phase*. In the second or *cap phase*, the limiting membrane of the acrosomal vesicle increases its area of adherence to the nuclear envelope, forming a thin fold that spreads over the pole of the nucleus, ultimately to cover its entire anterior hemisphere as a membranous *head cap*. The acro-

some meanwhile remains localized at the pole of the nucleus (Fig. 32–22F, G).

In the third or *acrosomal phase* of spermiogenesis, there is redistribution of the acrosomal substance, a condensation of the nucleoplasm, and an elongation of the spermatid. The bulk of the acrosome remains localized at the anterior pole of the nucleus, but during this phase of spermiogenesis its substance gradually spreads in a thin layer into the fold of membrane composing the

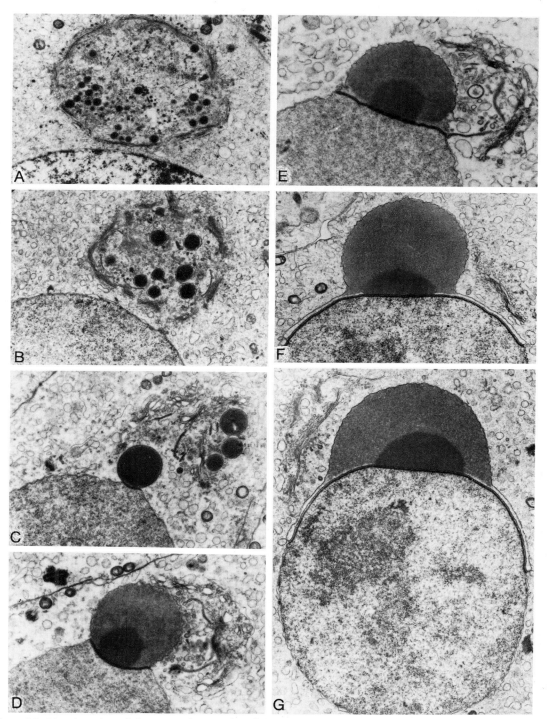

Figure 32–22 A series of electron micrographs of the juxtanuclear region of a guinea pig spermatocyte (*A*) and spermatids (*B–G*), showing the successive stages of formation of the acrosomal vesicle (*C–E*) and its conversion to an acrosomal cap (*F, G*). The guinea pig is selected because the large size of its acrosome makes it favorable material for study of the process of differentiation, which is qualitatively similar in all mammals.

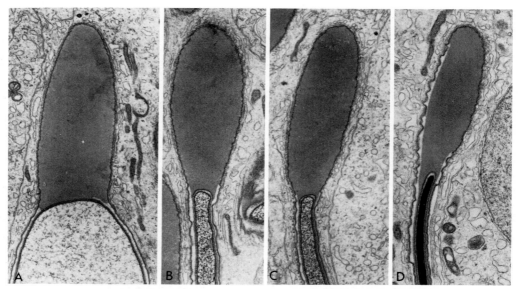

Figure 32–23 Further development of the acrosome of guinea pig spermatozoon. When the acrosome has attained its full size, the Golgi migrates into the postnuclear cytoplasm and the subsequent changes consist of a progressive modification of its shape taking place concurrently with a condensation of the chromatin and flattening of the nucleus. (From D. W. Fawcett and D. M. Phillips, J. Reprod. Fertil., Suppl. 6, pp. 405–418, 1969.)

head cap until the acrosome and head cap are coextensive and constitute the *acrosomal cap* (often simply called the *acrosome*). In its definitive form it is a caplike structure, limited by a membrane and containing a substance rich in carbohydrate and hydrolytic enzymes. It varies in its size and shape in different species but is present on the sperm of all mammals. The spermatid nucleus becomes elongated and flattened during this period. Its uniformly dispersed finely granular nucleoplasm becomes transformed into thin strands or filaments that subsequently shorten and thicken into coarse dense granules.

During the fourth or *maturation phase* of spermiogenesis, there is little further change in the simple acrosome of the human sperm, but in other species it continues to undergo further alterations and gradually takes on the shape characteristic of the species (Fig. 32–23).

The dense granules in the condensing nucleus become coarser, increasing in size at the expense of the intervening spaces until they finally coalesce and the nucleus is transformed into a homogeneous dense mass devoid of visible substructure. By the time this condition has been reached, the nucleus has attained the flattened pyriform shape characteristic of the human sperm head. Defects in

the condensation of the nucleoplasm often leave one or more clear areas of variable shape and size, recognized with the light microscope as nuclear "vacuoles." These are large and of frequent occurrence in the human sperm but are small and relatively uncommon in the spermatozoa of other species.

While the early stages of acrosome formation are in progress at the anterior pole of the nucleus, the centrioles migrate to the opposite end of the spermatid. There the distal centriole becomes oriented perpendicular to the cell surface and gives rise to a slender flagellum that grows out into the narrow extracellular cleft between the spermatid and the surrounding Sertoli cell (Fig. 32–24). As the nucleus begins to elongate and condense, the pair of centrioles and the base of the flagellum recede from the surface and take up a position at the caudal pole of the nucleus (Fig. 32–25). At about the same time, cytoplasmic microtubules arise and become laterally associated to form a roughly cylindrical structure, called the *manchette*, which extends caudally from a ringlike specialization of the cell membrane located at the posterior margin of the acrosomal cap. Concurrently with the appearance of the manchette, there is a marked elongation of the

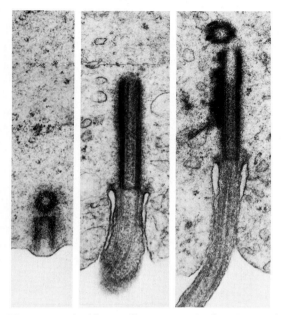

Figure 32–24 The earliest events in formation of the tail consist of migration of the centrioles to cell surface in the postnuclear region, and polymerization of microtubule protein on the template provided by the distal centriole. A typical 9 + 2 axoneme is formed and the simple flagellum elongates by accretion of microtubule subunits to its distal end.

spermatid, so that the bulk of the cytoplasm is displaced well behind the caudal pole of the nucleus, where it surrounds the proximal part of the flagellum (Fig. 32–27*B*, *C*).

The flagellum at this time consists only of the axial filament complex or *axoneme*, with two central fibrils and nine peripheral doublets. The latter are continuous with the wall of the distal centriole. The centriole is encircled by a ring of moderately dense filamentous or granular material. This annular structure was called the "ring centriole" by classical cytologists in the belief that it arose by unequal division of one of the centrioles. Electron microscopic studies provide no evidence in support of this interpretation. Instead, the ring appears to be a derivative of the *chromatoid body* (Fig. 32–26*A*). This loose ring is intimately associated with another small, dense ring that arises as a local specialization on the inner aspect of the plasma membrane, where the latter is reflected from the cell body onto the flagellum.

In the further differentiation of the tail, nine longitudinally oriented segmented columns arise around the centrioles. These are

joined to each other proximally and to the base of the nucleus to constitute the connecting piece. Distally the nine structural elements forming the connecting piece are joined to nine longitudinal dense fibers that develop just peripheral to the doublets of the axoneme. The distal centriole and the large ring that earlier encircled it gradually disappear as the connecting piece and outer fibers of the tail develop. The smaller, dense ring fixed to the flagellar membrane persists, and in the further elongation of the tail, it is carried distally several micrometers. As it moves back, the manchette disappears and mitochondria gather around the segment of flagellum between the annulus and the nucleus and become disposed helically around it, to complete the differentiation of the middle piece (Fig. 32–27*C*, *D*, *E*).

While these developmental events are in progress, a succession of circumferentially oriented ribs or hoops are deposited around the tail distal to the annulus to form the fibrous sheath of the principal piece.

With the completion of differentiation of the tail, the spermatozoon is separated from

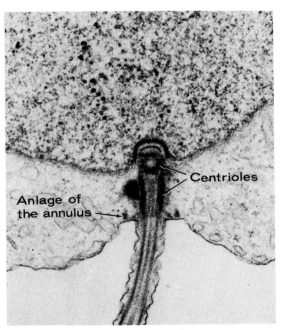

Centrioles

Anlage of the annulus

Figure 32–25 The proximal member of the pair of centrioles comes to occupy a shallow groove, the implantation fossa, in the caudal pole of the nucleus. The anlage of the future annulus then appears as a ring-like density adjacent to the membrane at its site of reflection onto the flagellum.

the excess cytoplasm, which remains in the epithelium (Fig. 32–28) as a membrane limited anucleate mass called the *residual body (of Regnaud)*, consisting of fine granules, lipid droplets, and degenerating excess organelles.

The Cycle of the Seminiferous Epithelium

Spermatogenesis has been most thoroughly studied in the common laboratory rodents, where it displays a degree of order and regularity that facilitates a systematic analysis of the process. As stated earlier, several steps of germ cell development are found at different levels in the germinal epithelium, with the stem cells found at the base and the more differentiated cells located at successively higher levels (Fig. 32–29). The development of any one generation of germ cells goes on concurrently with the development of earlier and later generations at other levels in the epithelium. The cells in different phases of development are not randomly distributed within the epithelium but occur in a number of well defined and easily recognized combinations or associations. The number of distinguishable cell associations varies with the species. In the guinea pig, for example, 12 such cellular associations or *stages* are identified. These are illustrated in the 12 vertical columns of Figure 32–32 and are designated by the Roman numerals at the bottom of each column. In any histological section of guinea pig testis, the cross sections of neighboring seminiferous tubules will vary in their appearance because of the different cell associations they contain (compare Figs. 32–30 and 32–31). If enough tubules are examined, all 12 cell associations or stages will be found, corresponding to the vertical columns in Figure 32–32. In studying this figure, it should be realized that a spermatogonium, in the course of its differentiation into a spermatozoon, passes though all of the cell types encountered by starting at the bottom of column I in this figure and reading from left to right along the horizontal rows from the bottom to the top row.

Spermatids at different phases of differentiation are always associated with spermatocytes and spermatogonia at their specific phases of development. The particular association of cells found at any point

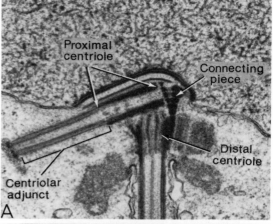
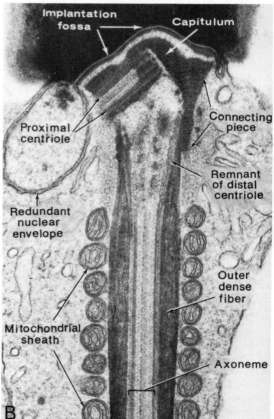

Figure 32–26 A, After establishing contact with the implantation fossa, the proximal or juxtanuclear centriole forms, at its distal end, the centriolar extension or adjunct. The segmented connecting piece begins to form around the distal centriole. *B,* Later in development, the centriolar adjunct disappears and the distal centriole disintegrates, leaving the proximal centriole in a vault or niche in the connecting piece that joins the nucleus to the outer dense fibers of the tail.

along the length of a seminiferous tubule changes with time, passing successively through all 12 stages and then repeating the sequence. The *cycle of the seminiferous epithelium* is defined as the series of changes occurring in a given area of the epithelium between two successive appearances of the same cellular association. The duration of the cycle has not been determined for the guinea pig, but it is about 12 days in the rat, and a spermatogonium takes about four cycles or 48 days to complete its differentiation and be released as a mature spermatozoon (Clermont and Leblond).

The various cell associations also occur in a numerically orderly sequence along the length of the seminiferous tubule. Thus, instead of considering the changes at a given point in the tubule, one can look at it from a different point of view, namely, as a series of successive cell associations found along the length of the same tubule. The *wave of the seminiferous epithelium* is then the distance between two successive identical cell associations. That portion of the length of a wave occupied by one cell association is referred to as a *segment.*

The sequence of pictures along a wave is similar to the sequence of events taking place in one given area during a cycle of the seminiferous epithelium. In the rat there are said to be about 12 waves along the length of each tubule. The length of each segment in the wave corresponds roughly to the relative duration of that particular cell association or stage of the cycle.

In contrast to the very regular ordering of germinal elements in rodents, the appearance of the seminiferous epithelium in histological sections of the human testis at first suggests a haphazard arrangement of its cell types. Because of this apparent disorder, it was believed until recently that no synchronicity of germ cell development comparable to

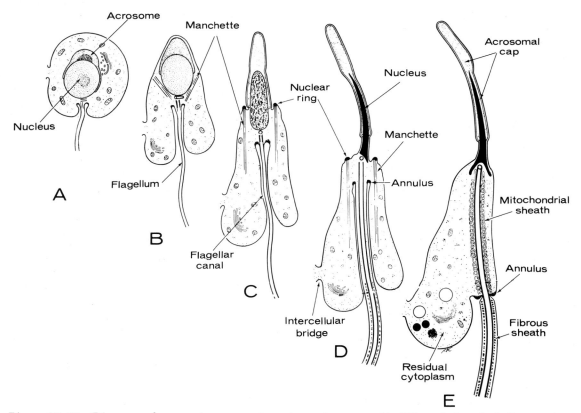

Figure 32-27 Diagram of successive stages in guinea pig spermatid differentiation, including nuclear condensation, appearance of the manchette, elongation of the cell, appearance of the fibrous sheath, caudal migration of the annulus, and formation of the mitochondrial sheath. (From D. W. Fawcett, W. A. Anderson, and D. M. Phillips, Develop. Biol., *26*:220, 1971.)

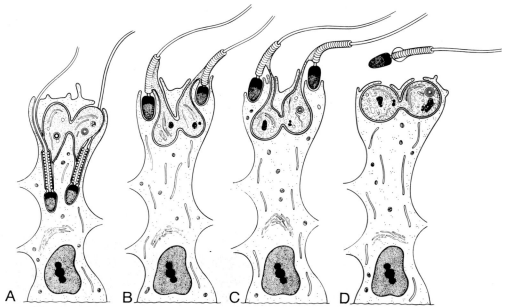

Figure 32–28 Diagrammatic representation of successive stages in sperm release. The axial components of the sperm are gradually extruded while the syncytial mass of spermatid cell bodies is retained in the epithelium. The attenuated stalk connecting the sperm to the residual cytoplasm finally gives way, freeing the spermatozoon. (From D. W. Fawcett, *in* S. J. Segal et al. (eds.): The Regulation of Mammalian Reproduction. Springfield, Ill., Charles C Thomas, 1973.)

that found in rodents existed in man, and that no "cycle of the seminiferous epithelium" could be defined.

This has now been found to be erroneous. Six well defined stages can be recognized, but instead of each occupying the entire cross section of the seminiferous tubule, as in rodents, the recognizable stages or cell associations in man occupy small wedge-shaped areas in the tubular epithelium (Fig. 32–33).

The human germinal epithelium is therefore a mosaic of irregularly shaped areas made up of the six different cell associations. Three or more stages of the cycle may be seen in a single cross section of a tubule. The situation is further complicated by the fact that the cells at the borders of these areas may intermingle to give atypical or heterogeneous associations of cells. The six typical associations are depicted in Figure 32–34.

The duration of the cycle of the human seminiferous epithelium has recently been determined by autoradiographic analyses of testicular biopsies of volunteers. Within one hour of local injection of tritiated thymidine the label was found in nuclei of preleptotene spermatocytes in stage III, but not in the pachytene spermatocytes of that stage or in

any other cells more advanced in their development. With the passage of time these labeled cells would be expected to pass through leptotene, zygotene, and early pachytene stages of meiotic prophase and reappear at the end of the cycle in a stage III cell association as mid-pachytene spermatocytes. Serial biopsies revealed that the mid-pachytene spermatocytes of stage III first showed the label 16 days after the initial injection of thymidine. It was thus established that the duration of one cycle is 16 days. As expected, labeled spermatids in stage III were found at 32 days (two cycles). Assuming one cycle for the cells to develop from spermatogonia to preleptotene spermatocytes, and one to advance from spermatids to release of spermatozoa, the total duration of spermatogenesis in man is estimated to be four consecutive cycles or 64 days (Clermont).

Degenerative and Regenerative Phenomena

In seasonally breeding mammals, active spermatogenesis, beginning at puberty, is discontinued and reinitiated periodically for the rest of the life of the animal. Each time, it continues only during the period of rut, at the end of which the majority of the spermatogenic cells are eliminated by degeneration or maturation depletion. Concomitantly, the seminiferous tubules shrink and gradually come to contain only Sertoli cells and some spermatogonia. In this condition, they resemble the tubules of a prepubertal testis. At the beginning of a new period of sexual activity, spermatogonia multiply and rapidly replace the various generations of spermatogenic cells. In the lower vertebrates, these seasonal changes of the testis are even more prominent.

In man and other mammals that are not seasonal breeders, spermatogenesis is continuous. Nevertheless, in an active human testis the tubules contain scattered degenerating spermatogenic cells in the seminiferous epithelium. This is not pathologic unless it exceeds certain limits. The degenerating cells are seen in segments of the tubule in which the seminiferous epithelium is active and normal spermatogenesis is in full progress. The significance of the normal degeneration of a certain number of germ cells is not known.

Abnormal spermatogenic cells can often be found. In spermatogonia and spermatocytes, giant forms, as well as cells with two nuclei, are not uncommon. Multinucleated giant spermatids likewise are not infrequent. These abnormalities appear to be a consequence of the peculiar mode of cytokinesis in the dividing germinal cells, which normally leaves them connected by intercellular bridges. Failure of initial constriction between the daughter cells or a subsequent opening up of the bridges between two or more cells may lead to the formation of multinucleated spermatocytes or spermatids. Spermatids with two nuclei may continue to develop; thus, monstrous sperm with two tails, or with one tail and two heads, may arise. These abnormal sperm are carried with the normal mature sperm into the

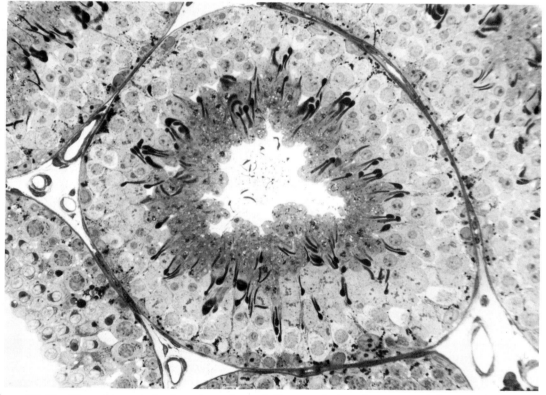

Figure 32--29 Photomicrograph of a guinea pig seminiferous tubule and portions of adjacent tubules. Notice that the epithelium in these four tubules exhibits different associations of cell types, representing different stages of spermatogenesis.

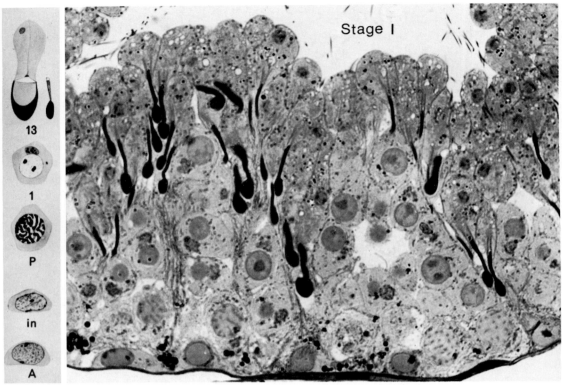

Figure 32–30 Photomicrograph of Stage I of guinea pig spermatogenesis, which includes type A spermatogonia (*A*), intermediate spermatogonia (*in*), pachytene spermatocytes (*P*), spermatids at the beginning of acrosome formation (*1*); and a more advanced generation of elongated spermatids with flattened, condensed nuclei (*13*). (Inset from Y. Clermont, Fertil. Steril., 6:563, 1960.)

epididymis, where some degenerate, but others persist and are also found in ejaculated semen.

The germ cells of the seminiferous epithelium are sensitive to noxious agents. In pathological conditions of general (infectious diseases, alcoholism, dietary deficiencies) or local (inflammation) character, degenerative changes, especially the formation of multinucleated giant cells by the coalescing spermatids, may become prominent. Exposure of the testis to a sufficient dose of x-rays causes an extensive degeneration of spermatogenic cells and may result in sterility. These cells are also sensitive to high temperature. Even the normal internal temperature of the body is incompatible with spermatogenesis. In the majority of adult mammals, the testes are therefore lodged in a scrotum, which has a temperature a few degrees lower than the rest of the body. Testes that fail to descend into the scrotum during development and remain in the abdomen never produce mature sperm. They show atrophic tubules containing only Sertoli cells and scattered spermatogonia. Failure of descent of the testis is called *cryptorchidism*. In experimentally produced cryptorchidism the testis soon decreases in size and comes to contain only Sertoli cells and a few spermatogonia. The seminiferous tubules atrophy in experimental animals fed a diet lacking vitamin E; they also undergo regression in vitamin A deficiency.

In all such cases, the Sertoli cells are more resistant than spermatogenic cells. Some spermatogonia frequently remain. Thus, under favorable conditions, when the noxious factor is removed, a more or less complete regeneration of the seminiferous epithelium may take place. In mammals with a short life span, spermatogenesis continues undiminished until death. Although spermatogenesis continues far into senility in man, the seminiferous tubules do undergo gradual involution with advancing age. A testis of a man older than 35 usually shows scattered atrophic tubules; in the remainder of the organ, however, spermatogenesis may continue without visible alterations. In very old men, all the tubules may be depleted of spermatogenic cells.

INTERSTITIAL TISSUE

The endocrine component of the testis, the Leydig cells, are located in the angular interstices between the convoluted seminiferous tubules (Fig. 32–35). The blood vessels and lymphatics form peritubular plexuses in the intertubular spaces. The extravascular interstitial tissue is a loose areolar connective tissue exceptionally rich in extracellular fluid. In addition to fibroblasts and small bundles of collagen fibers, there are a few macrophages, occasional mast cells and relatively

undifferentiated cells of mesenchymal origin that are capable of developing into Leydig cells in response to gonadotropic stimulation.

The interstitial cells of Leydig occur in clusters of varying size, sometimes closely associated with blood vessels. They are usually irregularly polyhedral, 14 to 20 μm. across, where they are closely packed, but at the periphery of the clusters or when occurring individually they may be elongated or spindle shaped. The large spherical nucleus contains a small amount of peripherally disposed heterochromatin and one or two prominent nucleoli. Binucleate cells are common. Adjacent to the nucleus is a large clear area which is found in electron micrographs to be occupied by a well developed Golgi apparatus. Although the Golgi complex is prominent and responds to gonadotropic stimulation by enlargement, the role of this organelle in the biosynthetic and secretory processes of this cell type is not known. There is no visual evi-

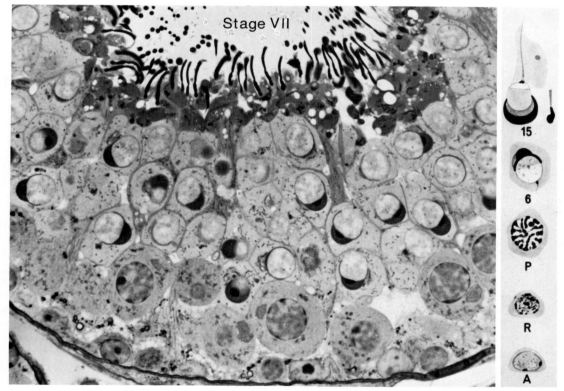

Figure 32–31 Photomicrograph of Stage VII of guinea pig spermatogenesis, characterized by the presence of spermatogonia (*A*); large pachytene spermatocytes (*P*); spermatids in the cap phase of acrosome formation (*6*); nearly mature spermatids projecting into the lumen (*15*); and residual bodies with dense cytoplasm forming a layer adjacent to the lumen.

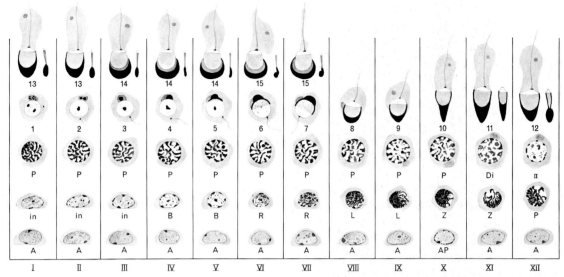

Figure 32–32 In these vertical columns, all 12 different cell associations or stages found in guinea pig seminiferous tubules have been assembled in their correct temporal sequence. Reading from the lower left to the right and from bottom to top, one follows the morphogenetic events from spermatogonium to release of spermatozoa. The time from the appearance of any one of these cell associations at a given point along the tubule until the reappearance of the same cell association is defined as one cycle of the seminiferous epithelium. For photomicrographs of Stages I and VII, see Figures 33–30 and 33–31. (From Y. Clermont, Fertil. Steril., 6:563, 1960.)

dence of accumulation of a product in secretory granules in the Golgi region and at present we have no clues as to the mechanism of release of steroid hormones by these cells. Mitochondria are abundant and quite variable in size and shape. In electron micrographs, their cristae tend to be tubular instead of lamellar, but this is not true in all mammalian species. The cytoplasm is acidophilic in routine preparations and may contain a number of vacuoles where lipid droplets have been extracted. In common with other steroid secreting endocrine cells, the most striking ultrastructural feature of the interstitial cell is its extensive smooth surfaced endoplasmic reticulum (Fig. 32–36). Cisternal profiles of granular reticulum are also present, but the bulk of the cytoplasm is filled with a branching and anastomosing system of smooth surfaced tubules. These membranes contain the enzymes necessary for several of the steps in the biosynthesis of androgenic steroids. Peroxisomes and lysosomes are found in abundance, but their function in the economy of these cells is not understood. Golden brown deposits of lipochrome pigment occur in the Leydig cells in men of all ages, but they become increasingly prominent with advancing age (Fig. 32–38).

A feature peculiar to the human Leydig cell is the presence of conspicuous cytoplasmic crystals 3 μm. or more in thickness and up to 20 μm. in length. These *crystals of Reinke* are highly variable in size and shape; they may be rounded or pointed at the ends (Fig. 32–38). They have little affinity for the common histological stains and appear nearly colorless in routine preparations. They can, nevertheless, be recognized in negative image in ordinary preparations and, if desired, they can be stained by azocarmine. They are isotropic in polarized light and have the solubility properties of protein. In electron micrographs they present a highly ordered structure differing in its pattern depending upon the plane of section. The crystal consists of filamentous molecules about 50 Å thick (Fig. 32–39). In x-ray diffraction its pattern bears some resemblance to catalase, but the spacing is different (Nagano). The crystals occur in the testes of most men from puberty to senility, but their abundance is subject to considerable variation. They are found in no other mammalian species and their significance is unknown.

The interstitial tissue of the testis exhibits rather remarkable species differences in the relative volume of the Leydig cells (compare

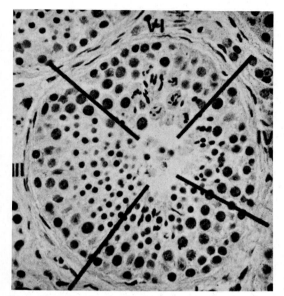

Figure 32-33 In the human, the stages of spermatogenesis do not occupy the whole circumference of a tubule as in other species. In this photomicrograph, for example, four different associations of cells are found in the same cross section. (From Y. Clermont, Am. J. Anat., *112*:50, 1963.)

Figs. 32–29 and 32–35). In the human they are said to make up 12 per cent of the volume of the testis, whereas in the boar they may account for 35 to 40 per cent. In some species the cells contain large amounts of lipid; others contain very little. The physiological correlates of these differences are not yet clear.

BLOOD VESSELS AND LYMPHATICS OF THE TESTIS

The blood supply of the human testis is from a branch of the abdominal aorta called the *internal spermatic* or *testicular artery*. It divides either before reaching the testis or on its surface, giving rise to several main branches that penetrate the organ. These in turn give rise to *centripetal branches* that course toward the rete testis. Major branches of these vessels run in the opposite direction as *centrifugal branches*. The branching of the centripetal and centrifugal arteries gives rise to many *intertubular arterioles* located in the angular columns of interstitial tissue between the seminiferous tubules. The *intertubular capillaries* derived from these form networks in the interstitial tissue. The capillaries in neighboring interstitial columns are connected by ladder-like circumferentially oriented *peritubular capillaries* (Kormano and Suoranta).

Postcapillary venules join to form collecting venules, and the confluence of these in turn forms veins that course toward the tunica albuginea (*centrifugal veins*) or toward the rete testis (*centripetal veins*). The former drain into veins of the tunica; the latter, running in the septula testis, converge upon a venous plexus associated with the rete testis. Upon reaching the surface, these veins join those of the tunica in forming the *pampiniform plexus* of veins in the spermatic cord. The right pampiniform plexus drains directly into the inferior vena cava via the *internal spermatic vein*. The corresponding vein on the left joins the left renal vein. This evidently results in some slight impairment of venous return, so that the left pampiniform plexus is often more distended than the right, and the left testis is generally lower. The veins of the left pampiniform plexus are sometimes varicose, a condition described as *varicocoele*.

In many animal species and possibly in man, the arrangement of blood vessels in the spermatic cord (the internal spermatic artery surrounded by the pampiniform plexus) constitutes a countercurrent heat exchange system that allows the arterial blood to lose heat to the cooler venous blood in the pampiniform plexus. This precooling of the arterial blood helps maintain the temperature of the testis a few degrees below deep body temperature. This lower temperature is essential for continued spermatogenesis.

The intertubular areas of the human testis also contain thin walled lymphatic vessels (Fig. 32–40) that drain into larger lymphatics in the septula testis and tunica albuginea and thence upward in lymph vessels of the cord to para-aortic lymph nodes and nodes associated with the renal blood vessels.

The lymphatics show considerable variation in pattern from species to species. In the common laboratory rodents, they form very extensive peritubular sinusoids. The aggregations of Leydig cells in these species are centrally located and closely associated with the walls of the blood vessels. They are surrounded by sinusoidal lymphatics. The steroid secreting cells are thus interposed between the blood vascular elements on the one side and the lymphatic sinusoids on the other and release their hormone into both. In larger species—ram, bull, and man—the lym-

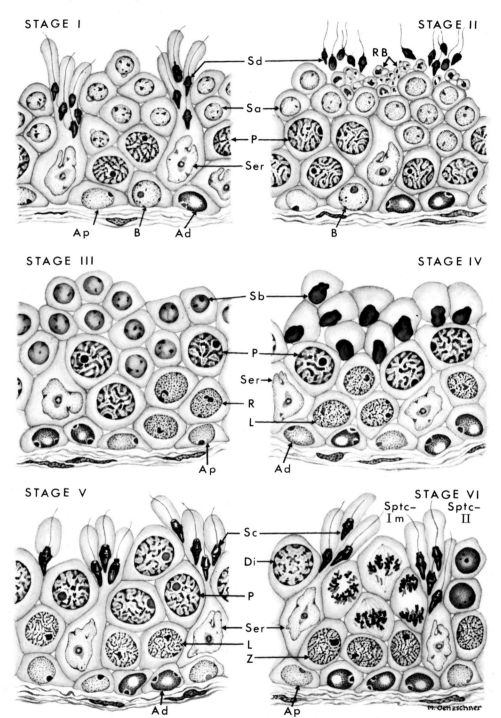

Figure 32–34 Diagram of the six recognizable cell associations or stages of the cycle of the human seminiferous epithelium. *Ser*, Sertoli cell; *Ad* and *Ap*, dark and pale type A spermatogonia; *B*, type B spermatogonia;
R, resting primary spermatocyte; *L*, leptotene spermatocyte; *Z*, zygotene spermatocyte; *P*, pachytene sperma-
tocyte; *Di*, diplotene spermatocyte; *Sptc-Im*, primary spermatocyte in division; *Sptc-II*, secondary spermatocyte
in interphase; *Sa, Sb, Sc, Sd*, spermatids in various stages of differentiation; *RB*, residual bodies of Regnaud.
(From Y. Clermont, Am. J. Anat., *112*:35, 1963.)

phatics are not sinusoidal but form thin-walled vessels more or less centrally located in the intertubular areas. The Leydig cells are not intimately related to either the blood vessels or the lymphatics, but evidently they release androgen into the abundant extracellular fluid of the interstitial tissue, whence it diffuses to the tubules for its local effect on spermatogenesis, and to the vessels for its effect on distant target organs.

HISTOPHYSIOLOGY OF THE TESTIS

Endocrine Function of the Testis

The function of the testis as an endocrine gland resides mainly in the Leydig cells, which elaborate androgenic steroid hormones, principally *testosterone*. This hormone has both local actions on the seminiferous tubules and distant actions on the accessory glands of the male reproductive tract and on many other tissues and organs. The seminiferous epithelium is dependent upon the continual presence of high concentrations of androgen to enable the germ cells to proliferate and differentiate. An adequate production of testosterone is also necessary for maintenance of the normal size and secretory activity of the seminal vesicles, prostate, and bulbourethral glands. After castration, these glands undergo a striking diminution in size, but this regression can be prevented by administration of exogenous testosterone. Testosterone is also responsible for the development and maintenance of secondary sex characteristics, such as the male pattern of pubic hair, growth of beard, male distribution of subcutaneous fat, low pitch of voice, and muscular build. Castration of boys in the prepubertal period results in failure of these characteristics to develop normally.

Unlike the germinal cells of the testis, the endocrine cells are not especially temperature sensitive. Therefore, individuals whose testes have failed to descend into the scrotum

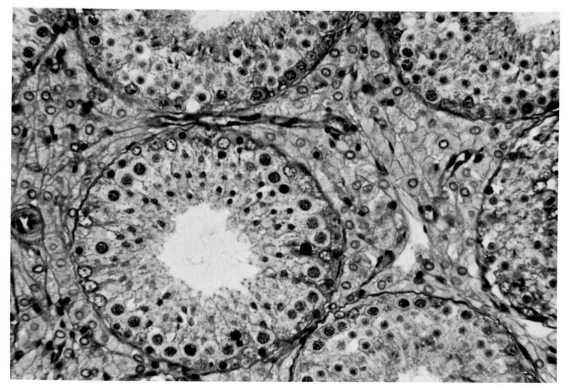

Figure 32–35 The amount of interstitial tissue varies greatly with the species. In the opossum testis shown in this photomicrograph it is exceptionally abundant. In the human it is relatively sparse. × 450.

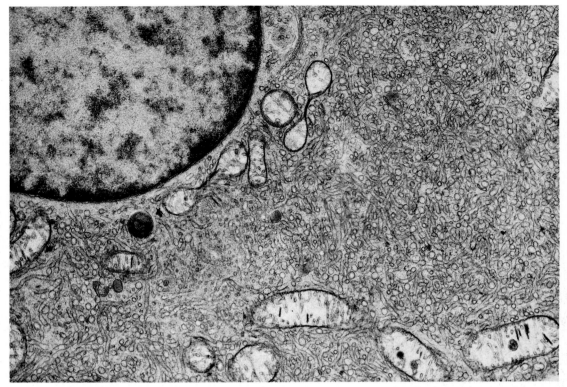

Figure 32–36 Interstitial cells in some species contain abundant droplets of lipid, whereas others are virtually devoid of lipid. The electron micrograph of opossum interstitial cell shown here is free of lipid. The cytoplasm is occupied by a very extensive agranular endoplasmic reticulum. × 10,000. (After A. Christensen and D. W. Fawcett, J. Biophys. Biochem. Cytol., 9:653, 1961.)

may have normal secondary sex characteristics, but they will be sterile because the higher intraabdominal temperature will have caused atrophy of their seminiferous tubules.

The dependence of the prostate upon testosterone secreted by the testis is the rationale for castration in the treatment of men with prostatic cancer. The tumor often undergoes marked shrinkage after removal of the testis or administration of female sex hormone (estrogens), and the survival of the patient can be considerably prolonged.

The secretory activity of the Leydig cells is under control of one of the gonadotropic hormones of the hypophysis, luteinizing hormone (LH), also called *interstitial cell stimulating hormone* (ICSH) in the male. Hypophysectomy leads to testicular atrophy, which can be reversed by injection of gonadotropins. The testes and the hypophysis are reciprocally related in that variations in levels of circulating testosterone affect the release of LH by the pituitary. Administration of androgen decreases gonadotropin release, and conversely castration causes accumulation of gonadotropin in the pars distalis of the hypophysis. The basophils responsible for gonadotropin production show characteristic changes that permit their identification as "castration cells."

Exocrine Function of the Testis

The spermatozoa may be considered a holocrine secretory product of the seminiferous tubules. The numbers of sperm produced are astronomical. Accurate estimates of the daily production are not available, but considering that there are 200 to 300 million sperm per ejaculate, it is probably considerably more than this number. The ram is more prodigal, with some 2 billion per ejaculate; it can sire up to 40 lambs in a single day. In all mammals, the males produce a great excess of gametes; a single ejaculate of the bull, for

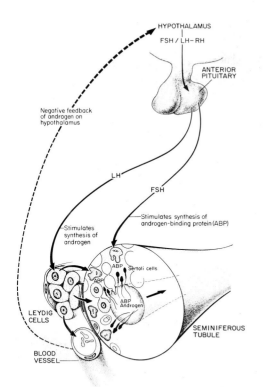

HYPOTHALAMUS

FSH / LH–RH

ANTERIOR PITUITARY

Negative feedback of androgen on hypothalamus

LH

FSH

Stimulates synthesis of androgen-binding protein (ABP)

Stimulates synthesis of androgen

ABP

ABP

Sertoli cells

ABP Androgen

LEYDIG CELLS

SEMINIFEROUS TUBULE

BLOOD VESSEL

Figure 32–37 Diagram of the hypophyseal control of male reproduction in which luteinizing hormone (LH) acts upon the Leydig cells and follicle stimulating hormone acts upon the seminiferous tubules.

example, is sufficient for fecundation of 40 cows by artificial insemination. It is thus theoretically possible for a single bull to father 30,000 calves in a decade. The production of such enormous numbers of sperm in man as well is attributable to the fact that there are in the two testes 800 to 1200 seminiferous tubules, each 30 to 70 cm. long, thus totaling about one third of a mile of continuously proliferating seminiferous epithelium.

The role of gonadotropin in control of spermatogenesis has long been controversial. The importance of LH is quite clear (Fig. 32–37). It causes production of androgen necessary for sperm maturation. The fact that FSH administered to immature or to hypophysectomized adult rats causes some increase in weight of the testes without any obvious stimulation of Leydig cells suggests a direct effect of this hormone on the seminiferous tubules. On the other hand, the observation that spermatogenesis can be maintained in hypophysectomized mature

males with testosterone alone seemed to indicate that FSH is unnecessary in the adult or at best plays only a minor role. However, it has now been shown that FSH administered to immature or to hypophysectomized adult rats is rapidly bound to cell membranes in the tubules; and this is followed within 15 minutes by an acceleration of nuclear transcription of DNA, and within an hour stimulation of protein synthesis is demonstrable (Means). Since this protein synthesis is induced in immature animals in which spermatids have not yet appeared, it must be attributed to Sertoli cells, or early germ cells, or both. This effect of FSH persists after destruction of the germ cells by radiation and hence is believed to represent a stimulation of the Sertoli cells. Consistent with this conclusion is autoradiographic evidence that radioactive precursors of nucleic acid localize very rapidly in Sertoli cell nucleoli but disappear from these cells long before they disappear from spermatocytes—suggesting a rapid turnover of RNA in the supporting cells (Kierszenbaum). The formation of androgen-binding protein (ABP) in the seminiferous tubules is also stimulated by FSH, suggesting that one of the principal functions of this hormone in the male is to promote the synthesis by the Sertoli cells of a binding protein which enables the tubules to accumulate androgens in the high local concentrations required for completion of spermatogenesis (Hansson et al.).

The exocrine secretory function of the seminiferous epithelium thus includes production and release of androgen-binding protein, and the elaboration of a considerable volume of fluid that serves as a vehicle in which the sperm are transported to the rete testis and into the epididymis. This fluid is rich in ions, especially potassium, and also in glutamate and inositol. These are presumed to be secreted by the seminiferous epithelium and may be important for survival of the spermatozoa.

Blood-Testis Permeability Barrier

It has been known for several decades that vital dyes and many other substances introduced into the bloodstream readily leave the vessels and enter the extracellular spaces of most of the tissues and organs except the brain. This vital organ seems to be protected by a *blood-brain barrier* that resides in the en-

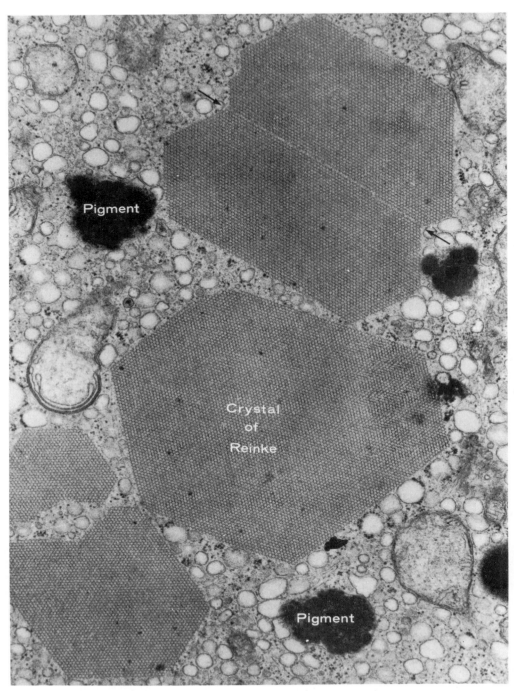

Figure 32-38   Electron micrograph of Leydig cell cytoplasm from human testis showing lipochrome pigment deposits, vesicular elements of smooth reticulum and several crystals of Reinke. (Micrograph from T. Nagano and I. Ohtsuki, J. Cell Biol., *51*:148, 1971.)

dothelial junctions of the brain capillaries. More recently a *blood-testis barrier* has been described. The permeability barrier in this case does not reside in the walls of the blood vessels, which are in fact unusually permeable in the interstitial tissue. Instead, the exclusion of dyes and other large molecules from the seminiferous tubules depends upon the presence of special junctional complexes between adjacent Sertoli cells near the base of the seminiferous epithelium. They consist of many parallel lines of fusion of the apposed membranes, thus effectively preventing entry of substances into the system of intercellular clefts in the upper parts of the epithelium. These occluding junctions are situated at the interface between overarching Sertoli cell processes just above the spermatogonia (Fig. 32–41). Thus, they divide the epithelium into a *basal compartment,* containing the spermatogonia, and an *adluminal compartment,* containing the more advanced stages of germ cell differentiation. Substances in the extracellular spaces of the interstitium have relatively unimpeded access to the basal compartment but are barred from deeper penetration into the epithelium by the Sertoli cell junctional specializations. At certain stages of the spermatogenic cycle, these must become locally dissociated in order to allow the spermatocytes of the next germ cell generation to move upward into the adluminal compartment. After this event they evidently re-form, restoring the barrier.

The full significance of this arrangement is still being studied, but it seems likely that a barrier near the base of the epithelium may be necessary for fluid secretion. It may also enable the Sertoli cells to maintain in the adluminal compartment a microenvironment especially favorable for germ cell differentiation. Finally, it must be recalled that the postmeiotic germ cells are genetically different from the parent cells. The blood-testis barrier may be needed to prevent foreign protein from these cells from reaching the blood and inducing the formation of antibodies.

EXCRETORY DUCTS OF THE TESTIS

The Tubuli Recti and Rete Testis

The seminiferous tubules occupy lobules or compartments within the testis that are demarcated by connective tissue septula extending inward from the tunica albuginea (Fig. 32–3). The several tubules in each lobule form convoluted loops, the ends of which converge toward a posteriorly situated region of highly vascular connective tissue described as the *mediastinum of the testis.* Within its substance is a labyrinthine plexus of epithelium lined channels called the *rete testis* (Figs. 32–3 and 32–42).

Near the ends of the seminiferous tubules, the germ cells disappear from the epithelium, leaving a short terminal segment lined by Sertoli cells only. An abrupt narrowing then occurs where the seminiferous tubule is continuous with the *tubulus rectus,* a short, narrow channel connecting the seminiferous tubule to the rete testis. The tubuli recti and rete testis are lined by a simple cuboidal epithelium. The cells are relatively

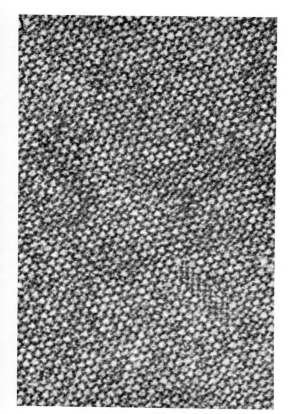

Figure 32–39 High-magnification electron micrograph of the lattice of a crystal of Reinke. (Courtesy of H. Fahrenbach.)

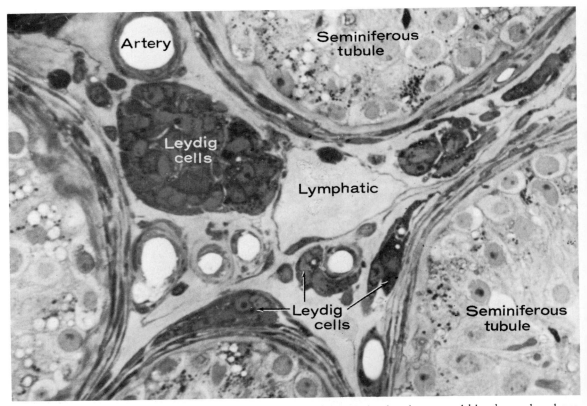

Figure 32-40 Photomicrograph of interstitial tissue of human testis, showing several blood vessels, a large thin walled lymphatic vessel, and clumps of Leydig cells not closely associated with blood vessels. (Micrograph from K. Christensen, *in* E. Rosemberg and C. A. Paulsen (eds.): The Human Testis. Advances in Experimental Medicine and Biology, Vol. 10. New York, Plenum Press, 1970.)

simple in their fine structure and do not give the appearance of being highly active cells. Their free surface bears a sparse covering of microvilli. Many—perhaps all—of the lining cells have a single flagellum projecting into the lumen. This is presumed to be motile, although it is not obvious what function it could serve other than some degree of agitation of the fluid contents of the rete.

In the guinea pig, the cells of the tubuli recti and the proximal portion of the rete testis store a remarkable amount of glycogen, which displaces the nucleus toward the lumen and all other organelles toward the cell periphery. This has not been reported in other species.

Ductuli Efferentes

From the posterosuperior aspect of the testis, 12 or more *ductuli efferentes* arise from the rete and emerge on the surface of the testis. Through numerous spiral windings and convolutions they form 5 to 10 conical bodies about 10 mm. in length called the *coni vasculosi*. These have their bases toward the free surface of the head of the epididymis and their apices toward the mediastinum testis (Fig. 32-2 and 32-3). They are held together by connective tissue and constitute part of the head of the epididymis.

The ductuli efferentes have a characteristic epithelium. The lumen has a festooned outline because it is lined by alternating groups of tall and low cells. The shorter cells may form small, cuplike excavations in the thickness of the epithelium. The cells of these excavations may contain granules. These were formerly interpreted as secretory material, but ultrastructural and histochemical studies now indicate that they are lysosomes. There is no evidence that the epithelium of the ductuli efferentes is secretory. Two cell types are recognized—one ciliated and the other bearing sparse microvilli. The nonciliated cells have canalicular invaginations of the free surface and other evidences of endocytosis. In animals injected with vital dyes, the cells contain dye inclusions, as a result of absorption from the lumen. The tall ciliated cells usually have a conical form, with the broad end toward the lumen. The cilia on the free surface beat toward the epididymis and move the nonmotile sperm in this direction.

Outside the basal lamina of the epithelium is a thin layer of circularly arranged smooth muscle cells. In the distal portion of the ductuli forming the coni vasculosi, the muscular layer becomes more prominent.

Ductus Epididymidis

The convoluted tubules of the coni vasculosi gradually fuse with one another to

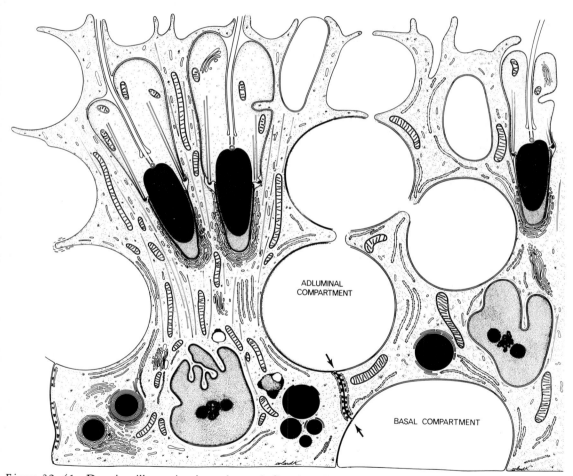

ADLUMINAL COMPARTMENT

BASAL COMPARTMENT

Figure 32-41 Drawing illustrating how the occluding junction (at arrows) between overarching processes of adjacent Sertoli cells divides the epithelium into basal and adluminal compartments. Substances diffusing from the interstitium have direct access to the spermatogonia in the basal compartment but are excluded from the adluminal compartment by membrane fusion in the junction complexes. These then constitute the main structural basis of the blood-testis permeability barrier. (From D. W. Fawcett, *in* Handbook of Physiology. Vol. 3. Baltimore, Williams and Wilkins, 1975.)

form the single *ductus epididymidis.* Though it forms a compact organ less than 7.6 cm. long, if the duct were uncoiled and straightened out, it would be over 6 m. long. The epididymis is the site of accumulation and storage of spermatozoa. In addition, there is evidence from work on experimental animals that the spermatozoa are not physiologically mature when they leave the testis but gradually acquire the ability to fertilize and the capacity for normal motility as they slowly move through the long epididymal duct. The epithelium lining this organ may play an important role in creating a fluid environment favorable for continued maturation of the spermatozoa. The epididymis is customarily subdivided into three regions for descriptive convenience: the *caput* (head), *corpus* (body), and *cauda* (tail) (Fig. 32–3). At the distal end of the cauda the duct gradually straightens out and continues as the *ductus deferens.*

The epididymis is lined with a pseudostratified columnar epithelium in which at least two cell types are distinguishable. The *principal cells* in the initial segment of the caput are very tall but gradually become lower in successive segments and are low columnar or cuboidal in the cauda epididymidis. The free surface of each principal cell bears a tuft of very long, nonmotile stereocilia (Fig. 32–44). These have no basal bodies and in electron micrographs appear to be enormous microvilli. They have a bundle of fine filaments in their core that extends downward for some distance into the apical cytoplasm. The cell surface between stereocilia is irregular in contour, exhibiting numerous invaginations suggestive of active pinocytosis. Large numbers of coated vesicles and large multivesicular bodies are present in the apical cytoplasm. These structural elements are believed to participate in the absorptive functions of the epididymal epithelium. Over ninety per cent of the fluid leaving the testis is absorbed in the ductuli efferentes and ductus epididymidis. If horseradish peroxidase or an electron opaque particulate marker is injected into the rete testis, it can be shown to be taken into vacuoles and ultimately into multivesicular bodies of the principal cells. Lysosomes are also found in these cells, and in certain segments of the epididymis of some species they are so large and numerous as to be easily visualized with the light microscope. They were interpreted as secretory granules by a number of early investigators, but this view has now been abandoned.

The principal cells have a number of cytological characteristics typical of actively synthesizing secretory cells. Their basal cytoplasm is filled with cisternae of granular endoplasmic reticulum, and the apical portion of the cell contains many profiles of smooth or sparsely granulated reticulum that are distended with a homogeneous content of low density. The supranuclear Golgi complex is remarkably large, but there is no indication that it is involved in segregation of a secretory product. There are no secretory granules and no indication of exocytosis. The functional significance of the high degree of differentiation of the principal cells still eludes us. The epididymal epithelium is known to produce glycerophosphorylcholine, and there is evidence that it has the capacity to synthesize steroids, but neither of these functions adequately explains the prevalence of granular reticulum, which is usually associated with protein synthesis.

Cells of the second type, the *basal cells,*

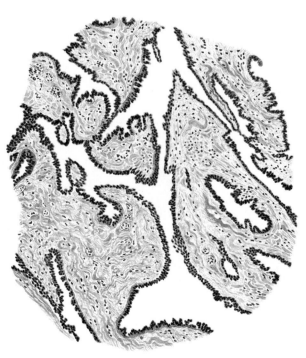

Figure 32–42 Section of human rete testis. × 140. (After A. A. Maximow.)

are small round or pyramidal elements lodged between the bases of the columnar cells (Fig. 32–44). Their cytoplasm has little affinity for stains and is of low density in electron micrographs. The organelles are few and relatively simple in their structure. Lipid droplets are common in the basal cells of some species. The basal cell surface may interdigitate extensively with the neighboring principal cells. The function of the basal cells is even more obscure than that of the principal cells.

Scattered among the columnar cells at various levels in the epithelium are small cells with pale cytoplasm and dark heterochromatic nuclei. These have been termed "halo cells" by some authors, but recent electron microscopic studies identify them as intraepithelial lymphocytes.

External to the epithelium of the ductus epididymidis is its smooth musculature, which exhibits a gradual proximodistal increase in thickness. In the caput, the contractile cells are very slender, and the bundles they form are, for the most part, oriented circumfer-

entially. In the corpus, sparse strands of longitudinally and obliquely oriented cells form an incomplete outer layer. At the transition from the corpus to the cauda, typical large smooth muscle cells are added to the smaller contractile cells characteristic of more proximal portions of the epididymis (Fig. 32–45). These progressively increase in number. In the distal portion of the cauda, the two-layered muscle coat is transformed into a three-layered coat, which continues into the ductus deferens.

The regional differences in the cytology of the musculature are associated with differences in the motility of the ductus epididymidis. In the caput and upper corpus, where slender muscle cells predominate, the duct undergoes spontaneous rhythmic peristaltic contractions that serve to transport the spermatozoa slowly along the tract. These contractions are independent of nervous stimulation and continue when the duct is excised and maintained in vitro. Contractions of this character are much reduced in the cauda, the principal site of sperm storage. The larger

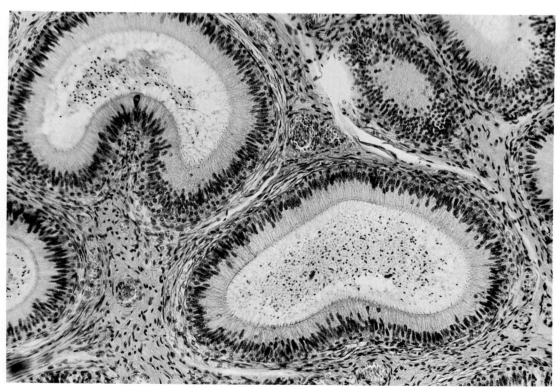

Figure 32–43   Section of ductus epididymidis from an adult man. Spermatozoa are seen in the lumen. × 180.

smooth muscle fibers that predominate in this region evidently require adrenergic sympathetic nervous stimulation. The sympathetic nerve net increases in density along the cauda and reaches a maximum in the intraabdominal portion of the ductus deferens, which is principally involved in the powerful contractions that expel sperm during the ejaculatory reflex.

Ductus Deferens

On passing into the ductus deferens, the excretory pathway acquires a larger lumen and a thicker wall. The epithelium and the lamina propria mucosae form longitudinal folds, which result in the highly irregular outline of the lumen seen in cross section (Figs. 32–46 and 32–47). The pseudostratified columnar epithelium is lower than in the epididymis, and the cells usually have stereocilia. The connective tissue of the mucous membrane contains extensive elastic networks. The highly developed muscular coat forms a layer 1 mm. thick. It consists of inner and outer longitudinal layers, and a powerful intermediate layer of circular muscle. Outside the muscle there is an adventitial coat of connective tissue. The firm duct is easily palpable through the thin skin of the scrotum.

The *spermatic cord* consists of the ductus deferens and its accompanying spermatic artery, pampiniform plexus of veins, and nerves of the spermatic plexus. The cord is enclosed

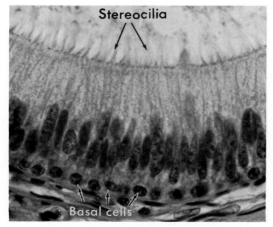

Figure 32–44 Photomicrograph of human epididymal epithelium, showing the characteristic row of basal cells and the stereocilia on the free surface.

by the *cremaster muscle*, a discontinuous layer of loose longitudinal strands of striated muscle. This layer extends downward to similarly invest the testes and serves to raise them in response to cold, fear, and other stimuli.

The ductus deferens, after crossing the ureter in the abdominal cavity, forms a fusiform enlargement, the *ampulla*. At the distal end of the ampulla it receives the duct of a large, glandular evagination, the *seminal vesicle*. Then, as the short (19 mm.) straight *ejaculatory duct* (0.3 mm. in diameter), it pierces the body of the *prostate gland*, at the base of the urinary bladder, and finally it opens by a small slit into the prostatic part of the urethra, on a small thickening of its posterior wall, the *colliculus seminalis* or *verumontanum* (Figs. 32–48 and 32–50). The openings of the ejaculatory ducts are located to the right and to the left of a blind invagination on the summit of the colliculus, the *utriculus masculinus*, which represents in the male the vestigial homologue of the uterus.

In the ampulla of the ductus deferens, the mucosa is thrown into numerous thin, irregularly branching folds, which in many places fuse to give the appearance in sections of a netlike system of partitions with angular meshes. The epithelium shows evidence of secretion. From the excavations between the folds, numerous tortuous branched outpocketings reach far into the surrounding muscular layer and are lined with a single layer of columnar, clear cells of glandular nature containing secretion granules. The musculature is much less regularly arranged here than in the other parts of the ductus deferens.

Ejaculatory Ducts

The epithelium lining the ejaculatory ducts is a simple or pseudostratified columnar epithelium, probably endowed with glandular functions. Its cells contain a large quantity of yellow pigment granules. Near the openings of the ducts the epithelium often assumes the structure of "transitional" epithelium. The mucosa of the ducts forms many thin folds reaching far into the lumen; its connective tissue is provided with abundant elastic networks. The dorsomedial walls of the ducts contain a series of glandular outpocketings, which may be accessory seminal vesicles. The ducts proper are surrounded only by connective tissue.

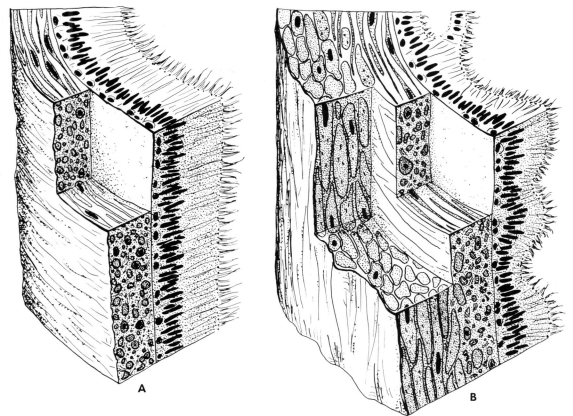

Figure 32-45 *A,* Drawing showing circumferentially oriented thin contractile cells underlying the epithelium of the initial portion of the ductus epididymidis. *B,* Corresponding illustration of the transitional zone between the corpus and the cauda. Slender contractile cells are found immediately subjacent to the epithelium and several layers of typical large smooth muscle cells are found peripheral to these. (From H. Baumgarten, A. Holstein, and E. Rosengren, Z. Zellforsch., *120:*37, 1971.)

ACCESSORY GLANDS OF THE MALE REPRODUCTIVE TRACT

Seminal Vesicles

The seminal vesicles are elongated saccular organs with numerous lateral outpocketings from an irregularly branching lumen. They arise as evaginations of the ductus deferens and are basically similar to it in structure. The wall consists of an external connective tissue layer rich in elastic fibers, a middle layer of smooth muscle thinner than in the duct, and an epithelium resting upon a thin layer of loose connective tissue. The mucosa forms an intricate system of thin, primary folds, which branch into secondary and tertiary folds. These project far into the lumen and anastomose frequently. In this way, numerous cavities in different sizes are formed, separated by thin, branching partitions (Fig. 32–49). All of these cavities open into the larger central cavity, but in sections many of them may seem to be isolated.

The epithelium shows great individual variations, which probably depend on age and physiological conditions. As a rule, it is pseudostratified and consists of rounded basal cells lodged between larger cuboidal or low columnar cells. All basal cells have a supranuclear pair of centrioles, whereas in the superficial cells the centrioles are located just beneath the surface and give rise to a central flagellum. The cells contain numerous

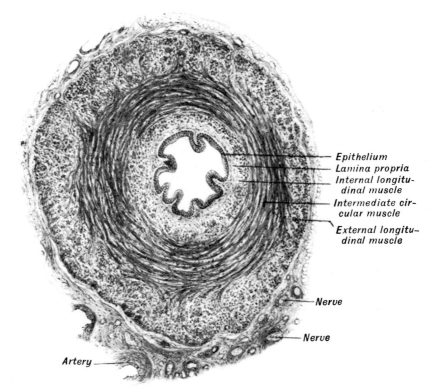

Epithelium
Lamina propria
Internal longitu-
  dinal muscle
Intermediate cir-
  cular muscle
External longitu-
  dinal muscle

Nerve

Nerve

Artery

Figure 32-46   Cross section of human ductus deferens. × 30. (After Schaffer.)

granules and clumps of yellow lipochrome pigment that first appears at the time of puberty. Similar pigment may also be found in the smooth muscles and in the connective tissue of the seminal vesicles. The epithelial cells contain secretion granules. The secretion of the seminal vesicles is a slightly yellowish, viscid liquid. In sections it appears as coagulated, netlike, deeply staining masses in the lumen. After castration, the epithelium atrophies, but it can be restored by injections of testosterone.

The muscular wall of the seminal vesicles is provided with a plexus of nerve fibers and contains small sympathetic ganglia.

Prostate Gland

The prostate is the largest of the accessory glands of the male reproductive tract. Its secretion, together with that of the seminal vesicles, serves as a diluent and vehicle for transport of sperm from the male to the female. The prostate is about the size of a horse chestnut and surrounds the urethra at

its origin from the urinary bladder. It is a conglomerate of 30 to 50 small, compound tubuloalveolar or tubulosaccular glands, from which 16 to 32 excretory ducts open independently into the urethra on the right and left sides of the colliculus seminalis (Fig. 32-50). The form of the glands is irregular. Large cavities, sometimes cystic, alternate with narrow, branching tubules. The blind ends of the secreting portions are sometimes narrower than the excretory ducts. In many places, branching papillae and folds with a thin core of connective tissue project far into the lumen. In sections they may appear as isolated, epithelium lined islands in the cavities. The basal lamina is indistinct, and the glandular epithelium rests upon a layer of connective tissue with dense elastic networks and numerous blood capillaries. In the larger alveolar cavities the epithelium may be low cuboidal or even squamous, but in most places it is simple or pseudostratified columnar. The cytoplasm of the cells contains numerous secretory granules. The epithelial cells become smaller and lose their secretion

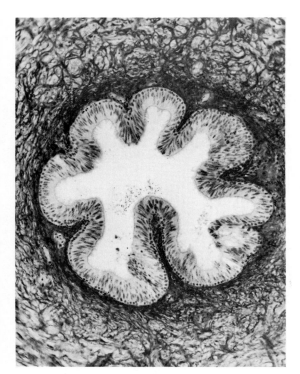

Figure 32-47 Histological section of the human ductus deferens, showing its irregular lumen, pseudostratified epithelium, lamina propria, and surrounding bundles of longitudinal smooth muscle. (Micrograph courtesy of A. Hoffer.)

granules after castration. Injections of testosterone restore the cells quickly to their normal appearance and activity.

The abundant stroma of the prostate consists of dense connective tissue with collagenous fibers, elastic networks, and many smooth muscle fibers arranged in strands of varying thickness. The connective tissue also forms a capsule at the periphery of the organ. Together with the smooth muscle fibers, it is arranged in thick, broad septa, widely separating the glands and radiating from the region of the colliculus seminalis to the periphery. Around the urethra, smooth muscle forms a thick ring—the internal sphincter of the bladder.

The secretion of the prostate is a thin, opalescent liquid with a slightly acid (pH 6.5) reaction. It has a rather low protein content but contains diastase, beta glucuronidase, several proteolytic enzymes, and a potent fibrinolysin. It is the main source of the citric acid and acid phosphatase of the semen. In sections, the secretion in the glandular cavities

appears granular. It contains occasional desquamated cells and spherical or ellipsoid concentrically lamellated bodies—the *prostatic concretions* (Fig. 32-51). These are believed to originate through condensation of the secretions. They may become calcified, and may exceed 1 mm. in diameter. The concretions are added to the semen and can be found in the ejaculate. The larger ones are unable to pass out through the ducts and may remain in the gland lodged in cysts. Their number increases with age.

The prostate is abundantly provided with plexuses of nonmyelinated nerve fibers connected with small sympathetic ganglia. Sensory nerve endings of various kinds (end bulbs, genital corpuscles, and so on) are scattered in the interstitial connective tissue. Free nerve endings have been described in the epithelium.

The *utriculus prostaticus*, situated deep in the interior of the prostate gland and opening on the colliculus seminalis, according to some recent observations, is not merely a functionless vestigial organ but may be an accessory gland of the male sexual apparatus. It is a blind vesicle of considerable size lined with an epithelium with many folds and glandlike invaginations. The epithelium is similar to that of the prostate. Sometimes patches of ciliated columnar epithelium can also be found.

The prostate is of great medical interest because *benign nodular hyperplasia of the prostate* is the most common tumor in the aging male. The disease begins at about 45 years of age and by the time the age of 80 years is reached, 80 per cent of the male population is affected with varying degrees of obstruction of the bladder neck and urinary retention. Cancer of the prostate is also the most common malignant tumor in the male.

Unfortunately, the physiology of the gland is not well understood, and even its morphology has been a subject of controversy and terminological confusion. On the basis of embryological studies, the prostate has traditionally been subdivided into middle, lateral and posterior lobes, all pyramidal in form and situated respectively anterior, lateral, and posterior to the axis determined by the course of the ejaculatory ducts through the gland (Lowsley). These lobes merge at their boundaries as development progresses and in the adult they have no reality. There is now a tendency to abandon these regional designa-

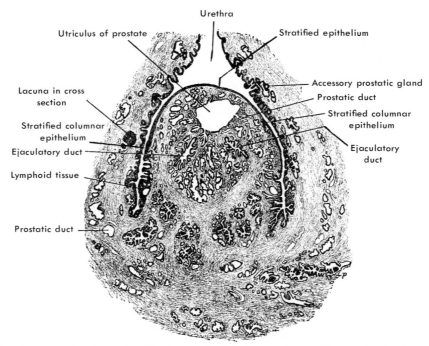

Figure 32–48 Cross section through colliculus seminalis of a young man. The urethra has been incised above. The utriculus of the prostate has prostatic ducts emptying into it. × 10. (After von Ebner, from Schaffer.)

tions. Some authors do, however, distinguish *central* and *peripheral zones* on the basis of histological criteria. In the central zone, the stroma is denser, the branching of the duct system is more elaborate, the epithelium is more exuberant, and the sacculations are larger, with prominent intraluminal partitions. In the peripheral zone, the stroma is looser, the duct system simpler, and the sacculations smaller and less partitioned. This histological heterogeneity may well be reflected in functional differences.

For the interpretation of prostatic disease, it is probably more important to realize that in addition to the glandular tissue of the prostate proper, there are smaller glands that originate as diverticula of the urethra above the verumontanum. These extend radially into the periurethral connective tissue and the smooth muscle of the surrounding sphincter. Although surrounded by the prostate and formerly considered a part of it, these urethral glands are ontogenetically and functionally distinct. It is now widely accepted that these are the site of origin of benign "prostatic" hyperplasia (BPH). On the other hand, the prostate proper is the site of predilection for the development of cancer.

Bulbourethral Glands

The bulbourethral glands (Cowper's glands), each the size of a pea, are of the compound tubuloalveolar variety. In some respects they resemble mucous glands. Their ducts enter the membranous urethra or the posterior portion of the cavernous urethra. The ducts as well as the secreting portions are of irregular size and form, and in many places they show cystlike enlargements. The terminal portions end blindly. The connective tissue partitions between the glandular lobules measure 1 to 3 mm. across and contain elastic nets and thick strands of striated and smooth muscles. The latter may penetrate with the connective tissue into the interior of the lobules.

The structure of the epithelium in the secreting portions and in the ducts is subject to great functional variations. In the enlarged alveoli, the cells are usually flattened; in the other glandular spaces they are cuboidal or columnar, with the nuclei at the base (Fig.

32–52). The cytoplasm contains small mucoid droplets and spindle-shaped inclusions staining with acid dyes. It has been suggested that they leave the cell body as such and then dissolve and mix with the mucin. The cells also contain droplets of various sizes. The excretory ducts are lined with a pseudostratified epithelium resembling that of the urethra and may contain large patches of secreting cells. They are also provided with small accessory glandular outpocketings having the structure of the glands of Littre of the urethra.

After fixation, the secretion appears in the lumen of the glandular spaces and ducts as angular precipitates that stain brightly with eosin. In life the secretion is a clear, viscid, mucuslike lubricant, which can be drawn out into long, thin threads. Unlike true mucus, it does not form a precipitate with acetic acid. In the boar, the secretion is extremely viscous and rubbery and plays an important role in the gelation of the seminal plasma that takes place soon after ejaculation in this species. The secretion is rich in sialoprotein.

THE PENIS

The penis is formed of three cylindrical bodies of cavernous or erectile tissue, the two *corpora cavernosa penis* and the unpaired *corpus cavernosum urethrae*. Arising from the ascending rami of the pubis on either side, the corpora cavernosa converge and join at the pubic angle. From there they run distally side by side to their conical distal ends, forming the dorsal two thirds of the shaft of the penis. On the upper surface of the penis, along the line of their junction, is a shallow longitudinal groove occupied by the dorsal artery and vein. On their lower surface the corpora cavernosa form a deep groove occupied by the corpus cavernosum urethrae (corpus spongiosum) (Fig. 32–53). The latter is traversed throughout its length by the *urethra* and ends with an acorn-shaped enlargement, the *glans penis*, bearing on its posterior aspect a pair of concavities which cap the conical ends of both corpora cavernosa penis.

The erectile tissue of the corpora cavernosa is a vast spongelike system of irregular

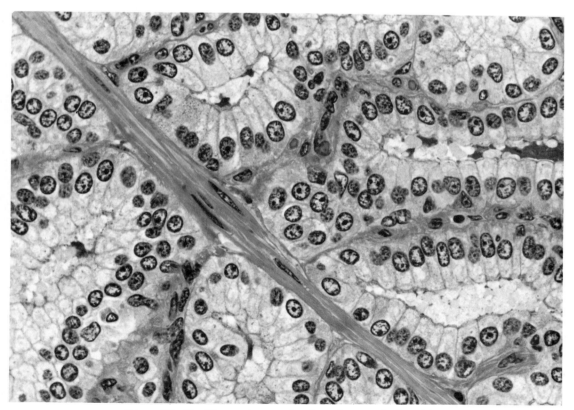

Figure 32-49 Photomicrograph of monkey seminal vesicle.

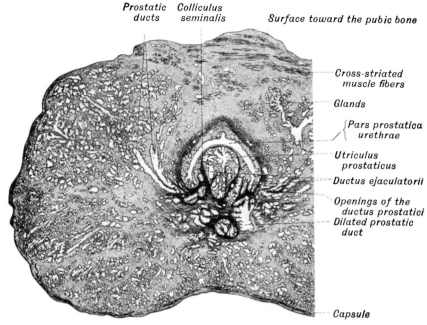

Prostatic ducts   Colliculus seminalis   Surface toward the pubic bone

Cross-striated muscle fibers
Glands
{Pars prostatica urethrae
Utriculus prostaticus
Ductus ejaculatorii
Openings of the ductus prostatici
Dilated prostatic duct
Capsule

Figure 32-50   Cross section of human prostate. × 4. (After Braus.)

vascular spaces fed by the afferent arteries and drained by the efferent veins. In the flaccid condition of the organ, the cavernous spaces contain but little blood and appear as collapsed irregular clefts. In erection they become large cavities engorged with blood under pressure. This increased inflow of blood and relative restriction of outflow causes the enlargement and the rigidity of the erect penis.

Each of the *cavernous bodies* is surrounded by a thick (1 mm.), resistant fibrous capsule, the *tunica albuginea.* Its collagenous fibers are arranged in an outer, mainly longitudinal, and an inner, circular layer, and are accompanied by elastic networks. Between the two cavernous bodies the tunica albuginea forms a fibrous partition, which is pieced by numerous clefts through which the cavernous spaces of both sides communicate. On the inner surface of the albuginea, especially in the posterior part of the corpora, there is a layer of dense connective tissue containing a multitude of small veins draining the cavernous spaces.

The cavernous spaces are largest in the central zone of the cavernous bodies. In the collapsed condition, they may have a diameter of 1 mm. Toward the periphery, they gradually diminish in size. The partitions between them, the *trabeculae,* consist of dense fibrous tissue and contain thick collagenous bundles, elastic fibers, fibroblasts, and strands of smooth muscle fibers. Their surface is lined with endothelium, which is continuous with that of the incurrent arteries and of the excurrent veins.

The tunica albuginea of the corpus cavernosum urethrae is much thinner than that of the corpora cavernosa penis and contains circularly arranged smooth muscle fibers in its inner layer. It also is provided with abundant elastic networks. The blood lacunae here, unlike those of the corpora cavernosa, are everywhere the same in size. The trabeculae between them contain more numerous elastic fibers, whereas smooth muscle fibers are relatively scarce. The cavernous spaces occupying the axis of the corpus cavernosum urethrae gradually pass into the venous plexus of the urethral mucosa.

The *glans penis* consists of dense connective tissue containing a plexus of large anastomosing veins, with circular and longitudinal smooth muscles in their thick walls. The longitudinal muscle strands often bulge into the lumen of the veins.

The skin covering the penis is thin and is provided with an abundant subcutaneous layer containing smooth muscles, but is devoid of adipose tissue. The skin on the distal part of the shaft of the penis is devoid of hair and has only sweat glands in limited numbers. The glans is covered by an encircling fold of skin, the *prepuce*. Its inner surface, adjacent to the glans, is moist and has the character of a mucous membrane. The dermis of the glans penis is fused with the deeper connective tissue of the glans. In this region there are peculiar sebaceous glands (*glands of Tyson*), which are not associated with hairs. They show great individual variations in number and distribution.

Blood Vessels

The erectile tissue of the penis is supplied with blood from the *arteria penis*. It breaks up into several large branches (*arteria profunda penis* and *dorsalis penis*, among them), which run to different parts of the organ, but all anastomose. In all these branches, even before they enter the erectile tissue, the intima forms long ridgelike thickenings which project into the lumen. These consist of loosely arranged collagenous and elastic fibers and contain strands of smooth muscle fibers, mostly arranged longitudinally.

Wherever the arterial branches enter into the corpora cavernosa through the tunica albuginea, they assume a longitudinal, forward course and give off many new branches. In the flaccid condition of the penis, they have a convoluted or curled course—*helicine arteries*. They have a thick media. When they reach 65 to 80 μm. in diameter (precavernous arteries), they run in the longitudinal trabeculae of the corpora cavernosa and open directly into the cavernous spaces.

The intima of the helicine arteries is also provided with longitudinal ridges of connective tissue and smooth muscle fibers, as in the branches of the arteria penis before they enter the erectile tissue. The ridges are more

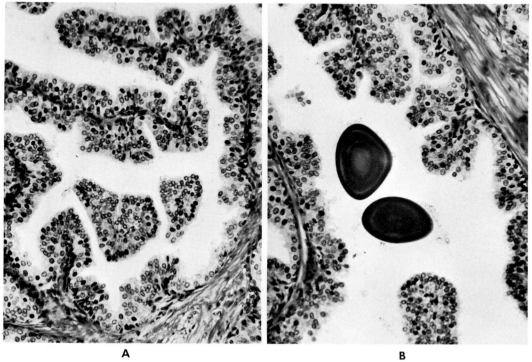

A   **B**

Figure 32–51 Photomicrographs of human prostate. *A,* The character of the epithelium. *B,* Typical concretions. Hematoxylin and eosin. × 150.

frequent at the sites of division of the vessels. The arterial supply of the corpus cavernosum urethrae is similar to that of the corpora cavernosa penis.

The major part of the blood leaves the corpora cavernosa penis through the vena profunda penis. Its radicles have a thick muscular wall. They arise under the albuginea, especially in the posterior regions of the erectile bodies, through confluence of a multitude of branched "postcavernous" venules. The latter run parallel to the surface under the tunica albuginea, have a length of 300 to 400 μm. or more, and have no muscle in their thin walls. They originate from the peripheral cavernous spaces, which are in direct or indirect communication with the largest axial blood spaces. The blood from the corpus spongiosum is drained mainly through the vena dorsalis penis. Unlike those of the corpora cavernosa penis, the first radicles of this vein start from the lacunae with large openings and leave the corpus by the shortest route, by piercing the albuginea.

The arrangement and structure of the afferent and efferent blood vessels in the cor-

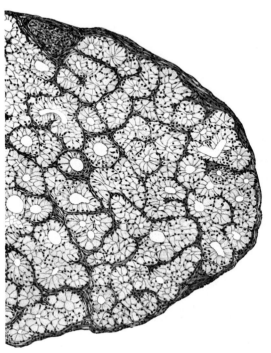

Figure 32–52 Part of the lobule of the bulbourethral gland of a 23 year old man. Zenker. × 120. (Slightly modified from Stieve.)

pora cavernosa penis helps to explain the mechanism of erection. The arteries play the active, and the veins the passive, role. The erection begins with the relaxation of the tonus of all smooth muscles in the arteries and in the erectile bodies. The blood pressure overpowers the elastic resistance of the tissue and stretches the media in the arteries. The presence of longitudinal ridges in the intima is believed to enable the lumen in such places to enlarge greatly and quickly. The lacunae of the cavernous bodies are filled with arterial blood. As the helicine arteries open, especially into the large axial spaces, these spaces compress the peripheral, smaller spaces and the thin-walled veins under the tunica albuginea that drain them. In this way, the outflow of the blood is throttled down. The blood accumulates in the corpora cavernosa under increasing pressure, and the erectile tissue therefore becomes rigid. The helicine arteries during erection are passively stretched, and their convolutions are straightened out. Since in the corpus spongiosum there is no difference between axial and peripheral lacunae and the draining veins are not compressed, there is relatively little retention of blood, and the circulation continues freely. Consequently, the corpus spongiosum never attains great rigidity during erection.

After ejaculation, the arterial musculature regains its tonus. The afflux of the arterial blood is reduced to the usual amount. The excess blood that has accumulated in the corpora cavernosa penis is slowly pressed out into the veins through the contraction of the smooth muscles of the trabeculae and the recoil of the elastic networks. Owing to the compression of the peripheral small veins and to the presence of the valves, the return of the penis to the flaccid condition is accomplished only gradually.

Lymphatics

Dense, superficial networks of lymphatic capillaries are found in the skin of the penis, of the prepuce, and of the shaft. They form a dorsal superficial lymph vessel, which runs toward the medial inguinal lymph nodes. Deep nets of lymphatic capillaries collect the lymph from the glans; they form a plexus on each side of the frenulum and continue into a dorsal subfascial lymph vessel.

Nerves

The nerves of the penis come both from the sacral plexus, via the pudendal nerve, and from the pelvic sympathetic system. The former supply the striated muscles of the penis (such as the bulbocavernosus) and also furnish the sensory nerve endings in the skin and the mucosa of the urethra. Among these sensory endings, free nerve endings can be demonstrated in the epithelium of the glans, the prepuce, and the urethra. In addition, there are free nerve endings in the subepithelial connective tissue of the skin and the urethra. Finally, numerous encapsulated corpuscles of various types are present: *corpuscles of Meissner* in the papillae of the skin of the prepuce and the glans, *genital corpuscles* in the deeper layers of the stratum papillare of the dermis of the glans and in the mucosa of the ure-

thra, and *corpuscles of Vater-Pacini*, which occur along the dorsal vein in the subcutaneous fascia, in the deeper connective tissue of the glans, and under the albuginea in the corpora cavernosa. The sympathetic nervous plexuses are connected with the smooth muscles of the vessels and form extensive, nonmyelinated networks among the smooth muscles of the trabeculae in the corpora cavernosa.

SEMEN

As the sperm pass along the excretory ducts, the secretions of the ducts and accessory glands are added to them. The final product is the *semen*. The sperm in the seminiferous tubules are nonmotile. They are slowly forwarded into the tubuli recti and the rete testis by the fluid secreted into the tu-

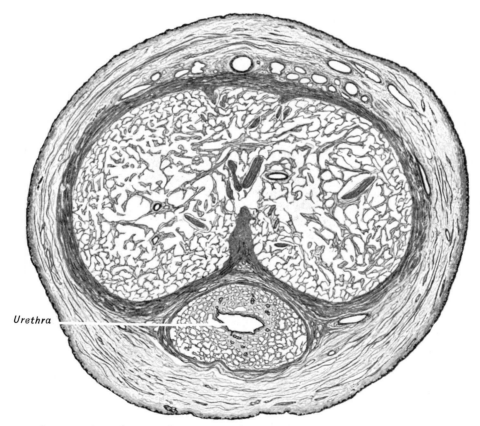

Figure 32-53   Cross section of penis of a 21 year old man. The septum in the corpus cavernosum penis is incomplete, because the section is from the distal part of the organ. The penis was fixed by injection of formalin into the corpus cavernosum. × 3½. (Slightly modified from Stieve.)

bules. The seminiferous tubules may also actively move the quiescent sperm by executing peristaltic movements. The flattened cells investing the seminiferous tubules have been shown to have many of the fine structural characteristics of smooth muscle cells (Clermont; Ross). In some species slow contractile movements of the excised seminiferous tubules have been observed. In the ductuli efferentes, the epithelium with its cilia beating toward the epididymis contributes to the transport of the sperm.

The long, winding duct of the epididymis is slowly traversed by the sperm propelled by peristaltic contractions of smooth muscle in the duct wall. They are kept here, especially in the tail, for a long time, sometimes for several weeks. In some species, the sperm acrosome undergoes continuing morphological differentiation during the passage through the epididymis, and the fertilizing capacity of the spermatozoa is known to increase progressively. As previously noted, the ductus epididymidis has an outer layer of smooth muscle that is responsible for rhythmic peristaltic movements that move the sperm along the duct. During ejaculation contraction of the ductus deferens is of primary importance in expulsion of stored sperm.

The epididymis is the site of storage of spermatozoa. The sperm do not accumulate to any great extent in the ductus deferens. This part of the excretory system, with its heavy muscular coat, is adapted for their speedy transportation during sexual activity.

The function of the seminal vesicles is primarily glandular. Their thick secretion contributes substantially to the volume of the ejaculate. It is rich in fructose, which is the principal sugar of the semen and provides the carbohydrate substrate utilized as an energy source by motile spermatozoa of the ejaculate. The secretion contains small amounts of yellowish pigment, mainly flavins, which give the semen a strong fluorescence in ultraviolet light—a property of some medicolegal importance in the detection of semen stains.

In the process of ejaculation, the muscular tissue of the prostate also contracts and discharges its abundant liquid secretion. The semen, entering the urethra and mixing with the secretion of the glands of Cowper and Littre, is expelled by the contraction of the bulbocavernosus muscle compressing the bulbus urethrae.

The average volume of the ejaculate in man is about 3.5 ml., and of this the sperm account for less than 10 per cent, the rest being *seminal plasma.* The sperm density varies from 50 to 150 million per ml. Each ejaculate therefore contains 200 to 300 million sperm.

Under suitable conditions the sperm may remain alive outside the body for several days. They also survive for some time in the excretory ducts after death. In the uterus and the fallopian tube, living sperm have been found some days after coitus. They can now be stored in the frozen state for months or years and retain their fertilizing capacity upon thawing.

Besides the sperm, the semen contains degenerated cells, probably cast off from the epithelium of the excretory ducts and the urethra. Occasionally, columnar epithelial cells and wandering cells of connective tissue origin may also occur. There are, furthermore, round, hyaline bodies of unknown origin, lipid granules, concretions from the prostate, and a multitude of fat, protein, and pigment granules. When the semen cools and begins to dry, peculiar crystals of various forms develop—the *crystals of Böttcher.* They are believed to consist of phosphate of spermine, a polyamine compound present in considerable amounts in human semen and contributed mainly by the prostate.

It has been claimed that the different components of the semen are discharged from the urethra in a certain sequence. With the development of the erection the slippery secretion of the glands of Cowper and Littre lubricates the urethra. At the beginning of the ejaculation, the prostatic secretion is discharged first. Then the masses of sperm accumulated in the ductus deferens and distal portion of the ductus epididymidis are expelled. The final portion of the ejaculate is mainly the thick secretion of the seminal vesicles. In some animals (e.g., mouse) the abundant secretion of the seminal vesicles is coagulated in the vagina by an enzyme contained in the prostatic juice, and thus a solid plug is formed in the vagina which temporarily occludes its lumen and prevents the escape of the semen.

REFERENCES

Anberg, A.: The ultrastructure of the human spermatozoon. Acta Obstet. Gynec. Scandinav., *36*(Suppl. 2):1, 1957.
Baumgarten, H. G., A. F. Holstein, and E. Rosengren: Arrangement, ultrastructure and adrenergic innervation

of smooth musculature of the ductuli efferentes, ductus epididymidis and ductus deferens of man. Zeitschr. f. Zellforsch., *120*:37, 1971.

Bishop, M. W. H., and A. Walton: Spermatogenesis and the structure of mammalian spermatozoa. *In* Marshall's Physiology of Reproduction. 3rd ed. London, Longmans, Green & Co., 1960, Vol. 1, Part 2, p.1.

Bishop, D.: Sperm motility. Physiol. Rev., *42*:1, 1962.

Brockelman, J.: Fine structure of germ cells and Sertoli cells during the cycle of the seminiferous epithelium in the rat. Zeitschr. f. Zellforsch., *59*:820, 1963.

Christensen, A. K.: The fine structure of testicular interstitial cells in guinea pig. J. Cell Biol., *26*:911, 1965.

Christensen, A. K., and D. W. Fawcett: The normal fine structure of opossum testicular interstitial cells. J. Biophys. Biochem. Cytol., *9*:653, 1961.

Clermont, Y.: Contractile elements in the limiting membrane of the seminiferous tubules of the rat. Exper. Cell Res., *15*:438, 1958.

Clermont, Y.: The cycle of the seminiferous epithelium of man. Am. J. Anat., *112*:35, 1963.

Crabo, B.: Fine structure of the interstitial cells of the rabbit testes. Zeitschr. f. Zellforsch., *61*:587, 1963.

Dym, M., and D. W. Fawcett: Further observations on the numbers of spermatogonia, spermatocytes, and spermatids joined by intercellular bridges in mammalian spermatogenesis. Biol. Reprod., *4*:195, 1971.

Dym, M., and D. W. Fawcett: Observations on the blood-testis barrier and on physiological compartmentation of the seminiferous epithelium. Biol. Reprod., *3*:308, 1970.

Fawcett, D. W.: Intercellular bridges. Exper. Cell Res., Suppl. *8*:174, 1961.

Fawcett, D. W.: A comparative view of sperm ultrastructure. Biol. Reprod., *2*(Suppl. 2):90, 1970.

Fawcett, D. W.: Ultrastructure and functions of the Sertoli cell. Handbook of Physiology. Washington, D.C., American Physiological Society (in press).

Fawcett, D. W.: The anatomy of the mammalian spermatozoon with particular reference to the guinea pig. Zeitschr. f. Zellforsch., *67*:279, 1965.

Fawcett, D. W., W. B. Neaves, and M. N. Flores: Comparative observations on intertubular lymphatics and the organization of interstitial tissue of the mammalian testes. Biol. Reprod. (in press).

Glover, T. D.: Some aspects of function in the epididymis. Int. J. Fertil., *14*:216, 1969.

Hamilton, D. W.: The mammalian epididymis. *In* Balin, H., and S. Glasser (eds.): Reproductive Biology. Amsterdam, Excerpta Medica, 1972.

Hoffer, A., D. W. Hamilton, and D. W. Fawcett: The ultrastructure of the principal cells and intraepithelial leucocytes in the initial segment of rat epididymis. Anat. Rec., *175*:169, 1973.

Horstmann, E.: Die Kerneinschlüsse im Nebenhodenepithel des Hundes. Zeitschr. f. Zellforsch., *65*:770, 1965.

Horstmann, E., R. Richter, and E. Roosen-Runge: Zur elektronenmikroskopie der Kerneinschlüsse im menschlichen Nebenhodenepithel. Zeitschr. f. Zellforsch., *69*:69, 1966.

Huckins, C.: Spermatogonial stem cell population in the rat. I. Their morphology, proliferation, and maturation. Anat. Rec., *169*:533, 1971.

Huggins, C.: The physiology of the prostate gland. Physiol. Rev., *25*:281, 1945.

Kormano, M., and H. Suoranta: Microvascular organization of the adult human testis. Anat. Rec., *170*:31, 1971.

Ladman, A. J., and W. C. Young: An electron microscopic study of the ductuli efferentes and rete testis of the guinea pig. J. Biophys., Biochem. Cytol., *4*:219, 1958.

Leblond, C. P., and Y. Clermont: Definition of the stages of the cycle of the seminiferous epithelium of the rat. Ann. N.Y. Acad. Sci., *55*:548, 1952.

Lowsley, O. S.: Development of the human prostate with reference to the development of other structures at the neck of the bladder. Am. J. Anat., *13*:299, 1912.

Lowsley, O. S.: Embryology, anatomy and surgery of the prostate gland. Am J. Surg., *8*:526, 1930.

Macklin, C. C., and M. T. Macklin: The seminal vesicles, prostate and bulbo-urethral glands. *In* Cowdry, E. V. (ed.): Special Cytology. 2nd ed. New York, Paul B. Hoeber, Inc., 1932, Vol. III, p. 1771.

Mann, T.: Biochemistry of Semen and of the Male Reproductive Tract. London, Methuen & Co., 1964.

McNeal, J. E.: The prostate and prostatic urethra: a morphologic synthesis. J. Urol., *107*:1008, 1972.

Means, A. R.: Concerning the testicular actions of FSH on cells of the seminiferous epithelium. *In* Velardo, J. T., and B. T. Kasprow (eds.): Biology of Reproduction. Pan American Congress of Anatomy 1972, pp. 385–388.

Orgebin-Crist, M. C.: Studies on the function of the epididymis. Biol. Reprod., (Suppl.) *1*:155, 1969.

Price, D.: Normal development of the prostate and seminal vesicles of the rat, with a study of experimental postnatal modifications. Am. J. Anat., *60*:79, 1936.

Rasmussen, A. T.: Interstitial cells of the testis. *In*: Cowdry, E. V. (ed.): Special Cytology. 2nd ed. New York, Paul B. Hoeber, Inc., 1932, Vol. III, p. 1973.

Roosen-Runge, E. C.: The process of spermatogenesis in mammals. Biol. Rev., *37*:343, 1962.

Roosen-Runge, E. C., and L. O. Giesel, Jr.: Quantitative studies on spermatogenesis in the albino rat. Am. J. Anat., *87*:1, 1950.

Setchell, B. P.: Testicular blood supply, lymphatic drainage, and secretion of fluid. *In* Johnson, A. D., et al. (eds.): The Testis. Vol. 1, pp. 101–218. New York, Academic Press, 1970.

Steinberger, A., and E. Steinberger: Hormonal control of mammalian spermatogenesis. *In* S. Segal et al. (eds): Regulation of Mammalian Reproduction. Springfield, Ill., Charles C Thomas, 1973, pp. 139–150.

Stieve, H.: Männliche Genitalorgane, *In* von Möllendorff, W., and W. Bargmann, eds.: Handbuch der mikroskopischen Anatomie des Menschen. Berlin, Julius Springer, 1930, Vol. 7, part 2, p. 1.

Waites, G. M. H., and B. P. Setchell: Physiology of the testis, epididymis and scrotum. *In* Advances in Reproductive Physiology, *4*:1. London, Logos Press, 1969.

Yamada, E.: Some observations on the fine structure of the interstitial cell in the human testis as revealed by electron microscopy. Gunma Symp. on Endocr., Vol. 2, p. l. Maebashi, Japan, Gunma University Institute of Endocrinology, 1965.

Young, W. C.: Die Resorption in den Ductuli efferentes der Maus und ihre Bedeutung fur das Problem der Unterbindung im Hoden-Nebenhodensystem. Zeitschr. f. Zellforsch., *17*:729, 1933.

33
Female Reproductive System

The female genital system consists of the ovaries, oviducts, uterus, vagina, and external genitalia (Fig. 33–1). In the sexually mature female the ovaries, oviducts, and uterus undergo marked changes in their structure and functional activity in relation to the menstrual cycle and pregnancy. These changes are regulated by complex neural and hormonal mechanisms.

OVARY

The human ovaries are slightly flattened paired organs, each measuring 2.5 to 5 cm. in length, 1.5 to 3 cm. in width, and 0.6 to 1.5 cm. in thickness. One of the edges, the *hilus,* is attached by the *mesovarium* to the broad ligament, which extends from the uterus laterally to the wall of the pelvic cavity.

The ovary has a thick peripheral zone or *cortex,* which surrounds the *medulla* or *zona vasculosa.* Embedded in the connective tissue of the cortex are *follicles* containing the female sex cells, *oocytes.* The follicles are present in a wide range of sizes representing various stages of their development. When a follicle reaches maturity it ruptures at the surface of the ovary to release the ovum, which then

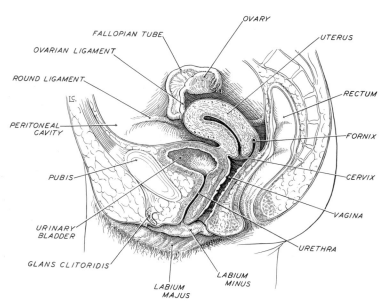

Figure 33-1   A diagrammatic sagittal section of the female pelvis, showing the genital organs and their relations to the bladder, urethra, and rectum. (After C. D. Turner.)

858

gains access to the open end of the neighboring oviduct. The boundary between the ovarian cortex and medulla is poorly defined. The medulla consists mainly of loose connective tissue and a mass of contorted blood vessels that are large in proportion to the size of the ovary.

The ovary is covered by a continuous sheet of squamous or cuboidal epithelium, which was named the *germinal epithelium* in the mistaken belief that the primordial oocytes originated from it (Fig. 33–4). The term persists although the evidence now overwhelmingly favors the extragonadal origin of the primordial germ cells. Beneath the germinal epithelium is a layer of dense connective tissue, the *tunica albuginea* (Fig. 33–5).

Ovarian Follicles

Embedded in the stroma of the cortex deep to the tunica albuginea are the follicles. The younger the person, the more numerous they are. In a normal young adult over 400,000 have been counted in serial sections of both ovaries. Of this large number, fewer than 1000 are released by the process of ovulation during a woman's reproductive life. The others degenerate and become atretic.

Their number decreases progressively throughout life and at menopause follicles are hard to find, although a few may persist into old age. The vast majority are *primordial* or *unilaminar follicles.* They are found mainly in the periphery of the cortex, immediately beneath the tunica albuginea (Figs. 33–5 and 33–6). Each consists of a large round *oocyte* surrounded by a single layer of flattened *follicular cells.* Owing to the large size of the oocyte, there may be several follicular cells around its circumference in sections. Primordial follicles may rarely contain more than one oocyte, but such polyovular follicles are quite uncommon.

Primordial Follicles (Unilaminar Follicles). The oocyte has a large, eccentrically placed, vesicular nucleus with a large nucleolus. In favorable thin sections the meiotic chromosomes can be seen (Fig. 33–6). Associated with the juxtanuclear cell center is a well developed Golgi apparatus surrounded by numerous small mitochondria. The primordial oocyte is enveloped by a single layer of flattened follicular cells. The surfaces of the oocyte and the enveloping follicular cells at this stage are smooth and in close apposition.

In electron micrographs the prominent juxtanuclear Golgi complex exhibits short

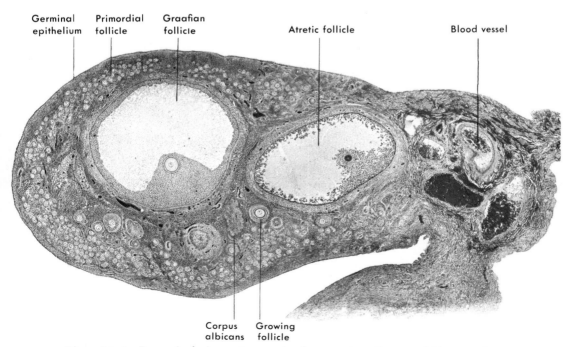

Figure 33–2 Retouched photomicrograph of transection of ovary of *Macacus rhesus.*

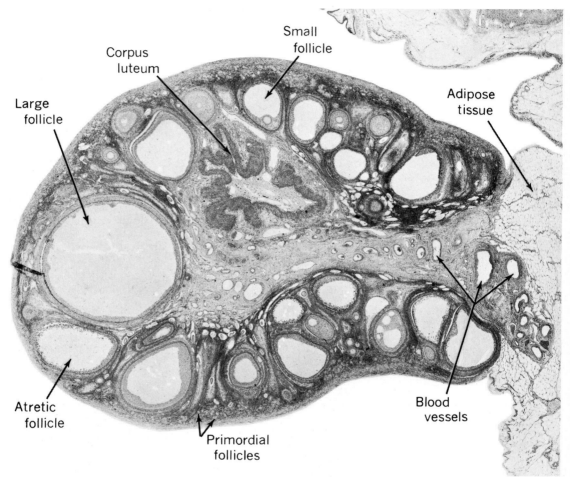

Figure 33-3 Unretouched photomicrograph of an ovary of *Macacus rhesus*. ×8. (Courtesy of H. Mizoguchi.)

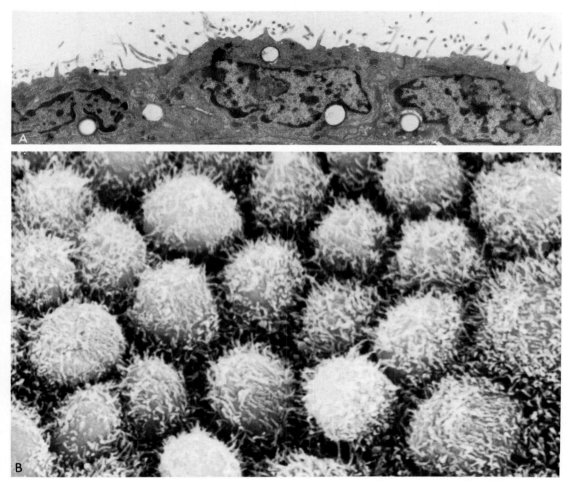

Figure 33-4 *A*, Cells of the germinal epithelium of the ovary as seen with the transmission electron microscope in a thin section. The surface bears irregularly oriented microvilli. *B*, Scanning electron micrograph of the germinal epithelium of the ovary. The bulging free surfaces have many more microvilli than one would infer from study of thin sections of this epithelium. The germinal epithelium resembles the peritoneal mesothelium covering other abdominal and pelvic organs. (Micrographs courtesy of E. Anderson.)

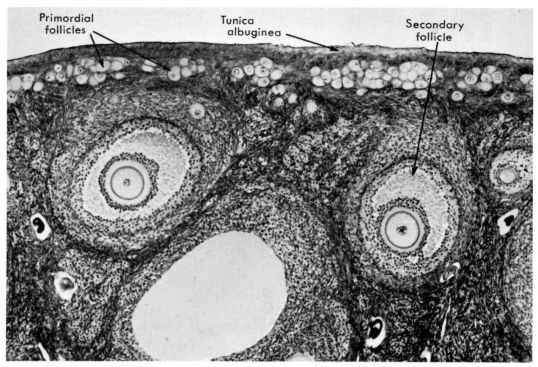

Figure 33–5 Photomicrograph of cat ovary, showing numerous primordial follicles and two secondary follicles with a well developed antrum. ×100.

parallel arrays of cisternal profiles and large numbers of small vesicles. Similar vesicular profiles are distributed in smaller numbers throughout the ooplasm, and it is believed that these may originate in the Golgi apparatus. Annulate lamellae are often found adjacent to the nucleus or free in the neighboring ooplasm. The spherical or short plump mitochondria tend to congregate in the vicinity of the cell center. Later, when the oocyte begins to grow, they become dispersed throughout the ooplasm. The endoplasmic reticulum in the early stages of oocyte development takes the form of vesicles or slightly elongated profiles bearing a few ribosomes. Longer cisternal profiles subsequently arise in limited numbers and finally become associated in parallel arrays. Multivesicular bodies are a common component of the ooplasm but are more numerous in later stages of development.

Primary Follicles. The transition from an inactive primordial follicle to a developing primary follicle involves cytological changes in the oocyte, the follicular cells, and the ad-

jacent connective tissue. As the oocyte enlarges, the single layer of flattened follicular cells first becomes cuboidal or low columnar (Fig. 33–7), and then through mitotic proliferation gives rise to *granulosa cells* that form a stratified epithelium (Figs. 33–8 and 33–9).

As the oocyte grows, there is a noticeable change in the distribution of its organelles. The Golgi complex, which initially was single and located in the juxtanuclear region of the early oocyte, gives rise to multiple Golgi complexes widely dispersed in the ooplasm. In the full grown oocyte these are located mainly at the periphery near the cell membrane or *oolemma*. Although granular endoplasmic reticulum is not a prominent organelle in the oocyte, it gradually becomes more extensive, and the number of free ribosomes in the ooplasm increases. The number of small vesicles and multivesicular bodies also increases markedly. There are a few lipid droplets and occasional heterogeneous masses identified as lipochrome pigment. Dense granules rich in lipid, believed to correspond to the yolk platelets of eggs in lower animals, are found in mammalian oocytes, but these are smaller and less numerous in primates than in other species.

In electron micrographs of advanced primary follicles, irregular microvilli on the surface of the oocyte project into discontinuous spaces that develop between the oocyte and the surrounding granulosa cells. Amorphous material deposited around the microvilli in these clefts represents the onset of formation of the *zona pellucida* which later becomes a refractile, deeply staining layer of uniform thickness. It becomes visible with the light microscope, around oocytes 50 to 80 μm. in diameter, in multilaminar primary follicles. The zona pellucida is a gel-like neutral glycoprotein. Its secretion is usually attributed to the granulosa cells, but there is some evidence that the oocyte may also participate in its formation.

In the granulosa cells of the growing primary follicle, the mitochondria, the granular reticulum, and free ribosomes gradually increase in abundance and the Golgi apparatus becomes more prominent. In some species, lipid droplets are common in the cytoplasm. Slender processes from those cells nearest the oocyte penetrate into the zona pellucida, where they mingle with microvillous projections from the oocyte (Fig. 33–11). Some of these may make contact with the oolemma, but protoplasmic continuity between the granulosa cells and the oocyte has not been demonstrated.

As the growing follicles increase in size, they gradually move deeper into the cortex (Figs. 33–2 and 33–3). Concurrently with the proliferation of the granulosa cell layer, a sheath of stromal cells develops around the follicle to form the *theca folliculi*. This layer subsequently differentiates into a highly vascular, inner layer of secretory cells, the *theca interna*, and an outer layer, the *theca externa*, composed mainly of connective tissue. Numerous small vessels penetrate the theca externa to supply a rich capillary plexus in the

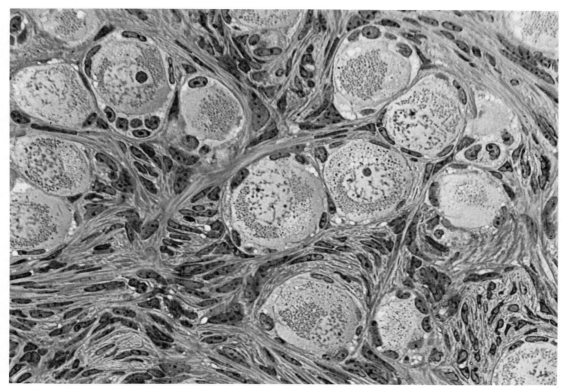

Figure 33-6 Photomicrograph of a number of primordial follicles in the cortex of a monkey ovary. The chromosomes of the dictyate stage of meiosis are visible in the oocyte nuclei. The oocytes are surrounded by a single layer of flattened follicular cells.

Nucleus of ovum

Nucleolus of ovum

Cytoplasm of ovum

Perinuclear mitochondria

Follicular cell with mitochondria

Basal lamina

Interstitial connective tissue

Blood vessel

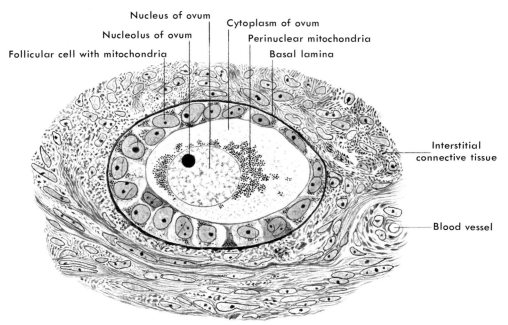

Figure 33-7 Follicle in first stages of growth from ovary of adult woman. Aniline-acid fuchsin stain. ×780. From a preparation of C. M. Bensley. (After A. A. Maximow.)

theca interna, but the granulosa cell layer remains avascular throughout the growth of the follicle.

Secondary Follicles (Antral Follicle). In the course of the continuing proliferation of the follicular cells, the enlarging follicle becomes oval in shape and the oocyte eccentric in position. When the follicle reaches a diameter of about 0.2 mm. and has 6 to 12 layers of cells, irregular spaces filled with clear fluid appear among the granulosa cells. This fluid, called *liquor folliculi*, increases in amount as the follicle enlarges and the irregular spaces among the granulosa cells become confluent to form a single crescentic cavity, the *antrum*. Thenceforth the follicle is described as a *secondary follicle*, or *antral follicle* (Fig. 33-12). By the time the formation of the antrum begins, the oocyte has usually attained its full size. The ovum grows no more thereafter, but the follicle as a whole continues to enlarge until it reaches a diameter of 10 mm. or more.

The typical small antral follicle is lined with a stratified epithelium of granulosa cells, which displays a local thickening on one side called the *cumulus oophorus*. This thicker region protruding into the fluid filled cavity

has the oocyte in its center (Figs. 33-12 and 33-13). Although the lining of the follicle is described as a stratified epithelium, its granulosa cells are less compact in their organization than the cells of most epithelia. They may be columnar immediately surrounding the zona pellucida, but elsewhere liquor folliculi accumulates between them and they become angular or stellate in form and are connected with one another by short processes. In growing follicles, small accumulations of densely staining material may appear among the granulosa cells. These are the *Call-Exner bodies* (Figs. 33-8 and 33-9). Whether they are intra- or extracellular was formerly a subject of dispute, but electron micrographs clearly show that they are extracellular (Fig. 33-10). They stain positively with the PAS reaction.

Mature Follicle (Graafian Follicle). In the human, follicles require 10 to 14 days from the beginning of the cycle to reach maturity. As they approach their maximum size they are large vesicles that occupy the full thickness of the ovarian cortex and bulge from the free surface of the organ. The follicles appear tense, as though the liquid in the follicular cavity were under considerable pressure, but actual measurements have not borne out this impression. The protein and polysaccharide of the follicular fluid are precipitated by fixatives and appear finely granular in sections.

The epithelium around the follicular cavity is limited on the outside by a prominent basal lamina that separates it from the theca. In late stages of follicular growth, mitotic figures gradually decrease in number among the granulosa cells. Intercellular spaces among the cells of the inner layers of the epithelium become more prominent. The connection of the ovum and the immediately associated granulosa cells of the cumulus oophorus with the rest of the epithelium is gradually loosened by the development of new liquid filled intercellular spaces. In the loosening up of the cumulus, one or more layers of radially disposed, columnar granu-

losa cells remain attached to the ovum, forming the *corona radiata*, a loose cellular investment which persists around the ovum even after ovulation.

The theca folliculi reaches its greatest development in the mature follicle. The theca interna is composed of large spindle-shaped or polyhedral cells with oval or elliptical nuclei and fine lipid droplets in their cytoplasm (Figs. 33–14 and 33–15). They are enmeshed in a network of reticular fibers that are continuous with those of the theca externa and the rest of the ovarian stroma. Although they are modified stromal cells and superficially resemble fibroblasts, the cells of the theca interna in electron micrographs have cytological characteristics similar to those of cells in other steroid secreting endocrine glands. They are principally responsible for elaboration of the female sex hormones,

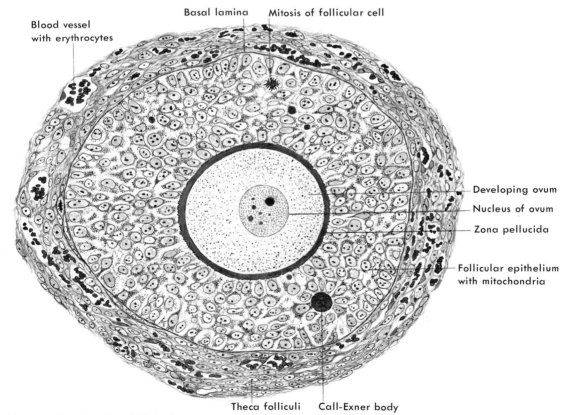

Figure 33–8 Growing follicle from same ovary as Figure 33–7, with developing ovum already five sixths its full size. ×375. (After A. A. Maximow.)

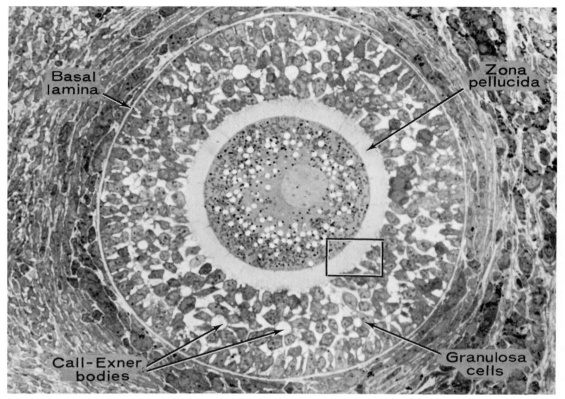

Figure 33–9 Photomicrograph of a primary follicle in a plastic section of ovary, showing the prominent basal lamina of the stratified epithelium of granulosa cells, and the thick zona pellucida around the oocyte. Spherical clear areas among the granulosa cells are the Call-Exner bodies (see Figure 33–10). An area similar to that in the rectangle is seen at higher magnification in Figure 33–11. (Micrograph courtesy of E. Anderson.)

estrogens. Consistent with the presumed endocrine function of the theca interna is its rich capillary plexus.

The theca externa consists of concentrically arranged fibers and fusiform cells that do not appear to have any secretory function. Electron microscopic studies have shown that some of the fusiform cells of the theca externa háve the ultrastructural characteristics of smooth muscle cells (O'Shea). Their role in ovulation remains problematic. Contraction of circumferentially oriented cells in the theca externa would be expected to compress the follicular contents and raise intrafollicular pressure. However, pressure recordings have failed to demonstrate a rise in intrafollicular pressure immediately preceding follicular rupture (Blandau). Therefore, the smooth muscle cells of the theca probably do not play a major role in this process. They may, however, play a significant role in the postovulatory collapse of the follicle.

The number of follicles that begin to develop in each cycle is considerably greater than the number that reach maturity. They may degenerate at any stage of development from primordial follicles onward (see page 873). Of the few that reach maturity, some involute, but, as a rule, one ruptures and releases an ovum.

Ovulation

The process by which the follicle ruptures and sets free the ovum is called *ovulation.* A follicle ripens at intervals of about 28 days in the human female, although variations of a week or more are not uncommon. Normally ovulation occurs on or about the fourteenth day of an ideal 28 day cycle. Usually only one ovum is released, but occasionally two, and rarely more, may be discharged. Cycles of typical duration may occur without associated ovulation. These are called

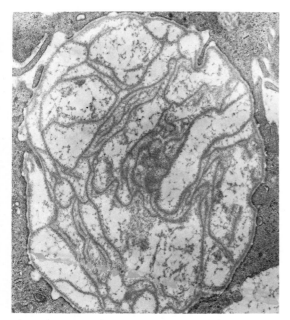

Figure 33–10 Electron micrograph of Call-Exner body. It appears to consist of a cavity lined with a distinct basal lamina and with a filigree of excess basal lamina in the interior. There is also a sparse flocculent precipitate of proteinaceous material. (Micrograph courtesy of E. Anderson.)

anovulatory cycles. The stages preparatory to rupture of the follicle have been extensively studied in histological sections of ovaries, and the actual process of ovulation has been directly observed and photographed in living rats (Blandau) and in humans (Decker; Doyle).

The ovum and the granulosa cells immediately surrounding it are loosened from the cumulus oophorus in the last stages of follicular maturation and float free in the liquor folliculi. During this period, the follicular fluid seems to accumulate faster than the follicle grows, and the part of the follicular wall that bulges on the surface of the ovary becomes progressively thinner. The follicular fluid that forms just before ovulation is more watery than the rest and appears to be secreted at a rapid rate. The first indication of impending ovulation is the appearance on the outer surface of the follicle of a small oval area, the *macula pellucida* or *stigma*. In this area the flow of blood slows and then ceases, resulting in a local change in color and translucency of the follicular wall. The germinal epithelium overlying this area becomes discontinuous and the intervening stroma greatly thinned out. The stigma then bulges outward as a clear vesicle or cone. In the rat, in which these events have been observed in greatest detail, the formation of the stigma takes place in 5 minutes or less. The cone then ruptures and in a minute or two the ovum and its adherent mass of cumulus cells are pushed through the orifice, followed by a gush of follicular fluid (Fig. 33–16). The fluid immediately associated with the ovum appears viscous, while that which follows is quite thin.

The turgid fronds or fimbriae of the oviduct or fallopian tube are closely applied to the surface of the ovary at the time of ovulation. Their active movements, and the currents created in the surface film by the cilia on their epithelial cells, are responsible for drawing the ovum into the open ostium of the oviduct.

Hormonal Control of Ovulation

Ovulation depends upon a complex relationship between the hypothalamus, the hypophysis, and the ovary. Gonadotropin releasing hormone (FSH/LH-RH) carried in the hypophyseoportal vessels to the anterior lobe of the hypophysis stimulates synthesis and release of follicle stimulating hormone (FSH) and luteinizing hormone (LH) into the general circulation. These result in follicular growth and maturation in the ovary. At about mid-cycle there is an additional surge of LH release, which appears to cause the FSH-primed follicle to rupture and discharge its ovum. The ruptured follicle is then transformed into a corpus luteum, which synthesizes progesterone and small amounts of estrogen. These steroid hormones of the ovary then inhibit the hypothalamus and hypophysis, thereby decreasing ovarian stimulation by gonadotropins. If fertilization does not occur, the corpus luteum is transient. When it involutes, ovarian hormones are no longer produced in appreciable quantity; menstruation then follows; the hypothalamus and hypophysis resume their function; and the cycle repeats itself.

Infertility due to failure to ovulate can sometimes be corrected by administering human gonadotropic hormones or clomiphene citrate, a drug that stimulates the hypothalamus and hypophysis.

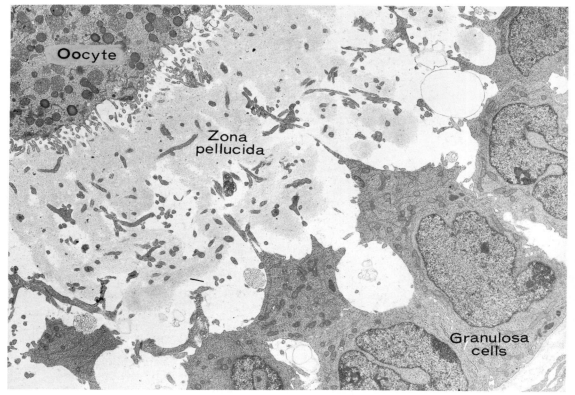

Figure 33–11 Electron micrograph of a field including portions of the zona pellucida, oocyte, and follicular cells. There are many small microvilli on the oocyte, some of which extend into the amorphous substance of the zona pellucida. Many larger processes also extend from the granulosa cells into the zona. (Micrograph courtesy of E. Anderson.)

Maturation of the Ovum

In very early embryos the primordial germ cells are located in the endoderm of the yolk sac, and they subsequently migrate along the root of the mesentery and laterally into the germinal ridges which give rise to the ovaries. During their migration they proliferate by mitosis, greatly increasing their number. Mitosis continues for some time after the primordial germ cells have taken up residence in the developing ovaries. The resulting *primary oocytes* then enter prophase of the first meiotic division and proceed to the so-called dictyate stage. Meiosis is then arrested, and the oocytes remain in this condition throughout the remainder of gestation, childhood, and puberty. Then, in the adult, one oocyte, as a rule, undergoes maturation and completes meiosis shortly before ovulation each month throughout the woman's reproductive life. This long interruption in the continuity of the meiotic process,

lasting from 12 to 40 years is one of the most remarkable phenomena in reproductive biology. We know little or nothing about how meiosis is suppressed during this period, but there has been some progress in our understanding of the factors involved in resumption of meiosis. Although each month a number of oocytes enlarge as their follicles are stimulated to grow, only the oocyte residing in the one follicle that progresses to large size can be stimulated to undergo maturation. A surge in the release of luteinizing hormone (LH) occurring near the middle of the cycle seems to be the trigger for resumption of meiosis. When enlarged follicles are removed from rat ovaries and placed in organ culture before the LH surge has occurred, the oocytes remain in the dictyate stage. However, addition of LH to the culture medium or microinjection of dibutyryl cyclic AMP into the antrum will induce resumption of meiosis and completion of maturation in vitro (Tsafriri et al.). Thus, the LH surge seems to activate the prepared oocyte, and the action of the hormone is mediated by the adenyl cyclase/cyclic AMP system.

In the resulting division of the primary oocyte, the chromatin is equally divided between the daughter cells but one of them, the *secondary oocyte*, receives nearly all the cytoplasm. The other daughter cell becomes the *first polar body*, a minute cell containing a nucleus and a minimal amount of cytoplasm. The first meiotic division, begun in fetal life, is completed within the follicle of the adult ovary a short time before ovulation (Figs. 33–17 and 33–18).

Immediately after the expulsion of the first polar body, the nucleus of the secondary oocyte enters the second meiotic division, but it progresses only to metaphase, where it is arrested, and proceeds no further unless the ovulated oocyte is fertilized. The chromatin is then divided equally, but again the bulk of the cytoplasm is retained by one daughter cell—the mature *ovum*. The other daughter cell is the small *second polar body*. In the human, observations on the formation of the polar bodies are incomplete. The first polar body undergoes rapid fragmentation and disappears. The second, which is formed after fertilization of the ovum, persists only through the first few cleavages of the fertilized ovum and then disappears. As in spermatogenesis, the consequence of the meiotic divisions is the production of a mature gamete with the haploid number of chromosomes.

Fertilization

The newly ovulated tubal ovum in most mammalian species is surrounded by a corona radiata of adhering granulosa cells. With the invasion of this mass of cells by spermatozoa, their attachments to one another are loosened. The gradual dispersion of the cells of the corona radiata is attributed to a depolymerization of the intercellular substance by enzymes released from the acrosomes of the spermatozoa. Increased

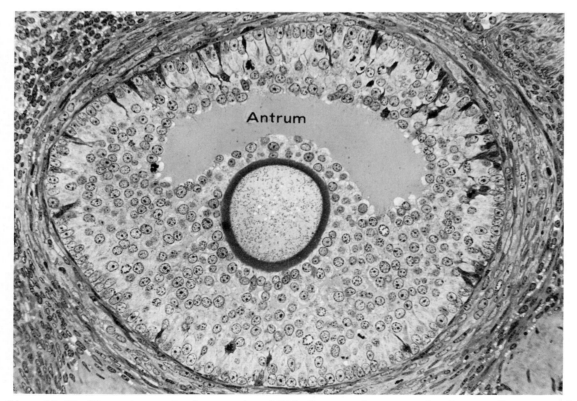

Figure 33–12 Photomicrograph of a secondary follicle from monkey ovary, showing a small antrum and cumulus oophorus. A well developed theca is seen around the periphery of the follicle.

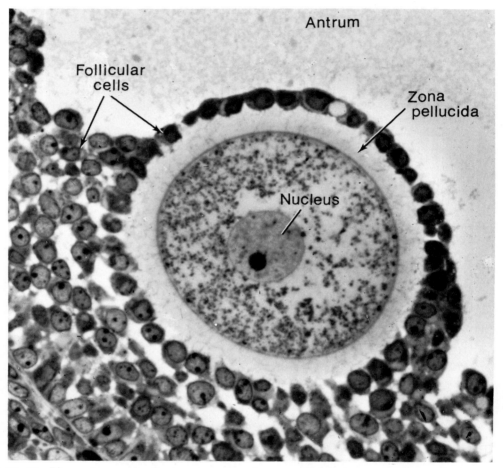

Figure 33-13 Photomicrograph of a human oocyte in an antral follicle. (Photomicrograph courtesy of L. Zamboni.)

surface activity of the cells themselves may also be involved.

Upon reaching the zona pellucida, the sperm head gradually penetrates this layer. The details of this process are still not completely understood. The spermatozoon remains actively motile during its penetration. This movement may contribute to the process, but local lysis of the zona by enzymes of the sperm acrosome is also believed to play an important role in sperm penetration. Once within the vitelline space, the movements of the sperm cease. The membrane overlying the postacrosomal region of the sperm head fuses with the oolemma, and the sperm sinks into the ooplasm. *Fertilization* proper consists of the entry of the spermatozoon into the ovum. This event somehow stimulates the ovum to complete the second meiotic division and cast off the second polar body. This is followed by fusion of the egg and sperm nuclei to restore the diploid chromosome number, and cleavage of the zygote ensues.

If the ovum is not fertilized it gradually fragments and is absorbed or phagocytized. The length of the period during which the human ovum remains fertilizable is not precisely known, but it is probably less than 24 hours.

Formation of the Corpus Luteum

Following ovulation and discharge of the liquor folliculi, the wall of the follicle collapses, and its granulosa cell lining is thrown into folds (Fig. 33–19). There may be some associated bleeding from the capillaries of the theca interna, resulting in the formation of a central clot. The cells of the plicated granulosa layer and those of the theca interna then undergo striking cytological alterations. They enlarge, accumulate lipid, and are transformed into plump, pale-staining polygonal cells—the *lutein cells*. After these postovulatory changes have taken place, the follicle is called the *corpus luteum*. Two kinds of lutein cells are distinguishable within it. Those derived from the granulosa cells make up the bulk of the lutein tissue and are called *granulosa lutein cells*. Those at the periphery, originating from the cells of the theca interna, are smaller and more deeply staining and are called the *theca lutein cells* (Figs. 33–20 and 33–21). The lipid in the lutein cells is dis-

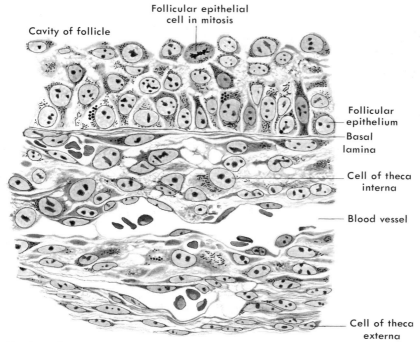

Follicular epithelial cell in mitosis

Cavity of follicle

Follicular epithelium

Basal lamina

Cell of theca interna

Blood vessel

Cell of theca externa

Figure 33-14   Section of part of wall of large follicle under high magnification. ×780. (After A. A. Maximow.)

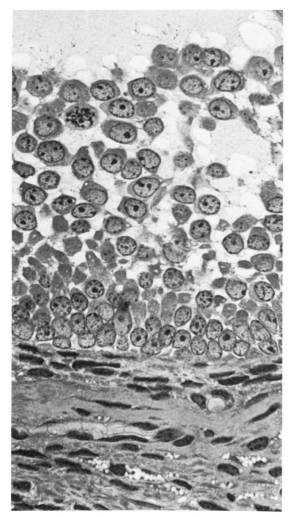

Figure 33-15 Photomicrograph of a portion of the wall of an antral follicle, illustrating the loose organization of the follicular epithelium (above) and the fusiform thecal cells (below), with multiple lipid droplets in their cytoplasm, appearing here as clear vacuoles.

the lutein tissue. Connective tissue elements also penetrate the developing corpus luteum from its periphery, forming a delicate reticulum around the lutein cells and gradually converting the resolving blood clot in the central cavity into a fibrous core.

If the ovum is not fertilized, the ruptured follicle gives rise to a *corpus luteum of menstruation*, which lasts for only about 14 days. Its rate of secretion of progesterone then drops as it undergoes histological involution. The lutein cells become loaded with lipid and ultimately degenerate. In the succeeding months the connective tissue cells become pyknotic, hyaline intercellular material accumulates, and the former corpus luteum is reduced to a white scar, the *corpus albicans* (Fig. 33-24). This slowly sinks deeper into the interior of the ovary and gradually disappears over a period of many months or years.

If ovulation is followed by fertilization, the corpus luteum enlarges further and becomes a *corpus luteum of pregnancy*, which persists for about 6 months and then gradually declines up to full term. After delivery its involution is accelerated and it undergoes changes leading to the formation of a scar similar to that left behind by the corpus luteum of menstruation.

The development of the corpora lutea of pregnancy and of the menstrual cycle has now been studied by electron microscopy in the human and in the rhesus monkey. In addition to vascular and connective tissue in-

solved in routine histological preparations, leaving numerous vacuoles. Their vacuolated cytoplasm gives them an appearance reminiscent of the cells of the adrenal cortex. In electron micrographs they have mitochondria with tubular cristae and the abundant smooth endoplasmic reticulum characteristic of steroid secreting cells (Fig. 33-22). The corpus luteum secretes the hormone *progesterone*.

While the cells of the collapsed follicular wall are undergoing luteinization, the capillaries of the theca interna sprout and invade

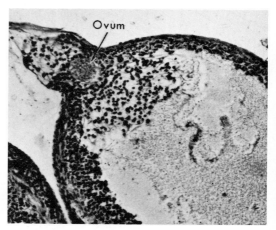

Figure 33-16 Photomicrograph of an ovulating ovarian follicle from the rat. The cumulus with the enclosed egg (at arrow) can be seen passing through the stigma. (Courtesy of R. J. Blandau.)

A

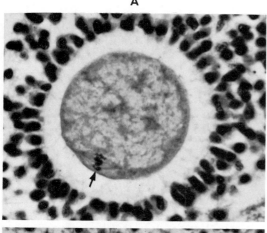

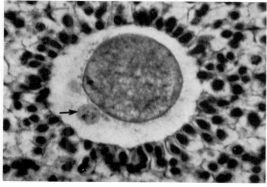

B

Figure 33–17 Photomicrographs of two stages in the maturation of the rat ovum. *A*, Section of a rat egg shortly before ovulation, showing the first polar spindle with diploid chromosomes on the metaphase plate (arrow). (Courtesy of R. J. Blandau.) *B*, Ovulated egg recovered from the ampulla of the oviduct but before sperm penetration. The first polar body lies in the perivitelline space (arrow). The second maturation spindle can be seen just above it. (Courtesy of R. J. Blandau.)

vasion of the ruptured follicular epithelium, there is an hyperplasia and hypertrophy of the cells. Two distinct populations of lutein cells are morphologically distinguishable, especially in corpora lutea of pregnancy (Fig. 33–21). The lighter appearing granulosa lutein cells are very large, measuring up to 30 μm. in diameter, in contrast to darker theca lutein cells, which are only about 15 μm. in diameter. In the luteinization of granulosa cells there is (1) a transformation of a dense heterochromatic pattern in the nucleus to a more homogeneous nucleoplasm with a single prominent nucleolus, (2) a change in form

of the mitochondria from elongate organelles with lamelliform cristae to highly pleomorphic mitochondria with a dense matrix, tubular cristae, and often with osmiophilic inclusions, (3) an increase in lipid droplets and in the smooth membranes of the agranular reticulum, which take the form of networks of anastomosing tubules or concentric systems of cisternae, (4) evolution of the single Golgi complex of the granulosa cells to multiple small stacks of cisternae widely dispersed in the cytoplasm of the lutein cells, (5) an increase in lysosomes and lipofuscin pigment deposits, (6) development of many microvilli on the surface of granulosa lutein cells, that project into intercellular clefts and invaginations of the cell surface which are reminiscent of the intracellular canaliculi of gastric parietal cells. This surface amplification is less apparent on the theca lutein cells, which remain smaller and generally have a somewhat less extensive smooth endoplasmic reticulum, and more numerous lipid droplets.

The cytological changes described for luteinization *in vivo* have also been observed in tissue cultures of granulosa cells from preovulatory follicles. The acquisition of the ultrastructural characteristics of lutein cells is correlated with the synthesis of increased amounts of progesterone (Crisp and Channing).

Late in pregnancy, a new population of small dense granules appears in the cytoplasm of the lutein cells. These do not contain lysosomal enzymes. They are believed to represent sites of storage of the polypeptide hormone *relaxin* which has been localized to the corpus luteum by fluorescent antibody methods (Belt et al.; Long; Zarrow and O'Connor). The exact physiological role of this hormone is still poorly understood, but it is known to inhibit contractions of the myometrium in pregnancy. It also promotes dilatation of the cervix, and in some species loosens the symphysis pubis, thus facilitating parturition.

Atresia of Follicles

In the human female, during the early part of each cycle, a group of follicles starts to grow. Usually only one of these goes on to develop into a mature follicle, and all the others undergo a degenerative process called *follicular atresia*. Some 99 per cent of the oocytes present in the ovary at birth are des-

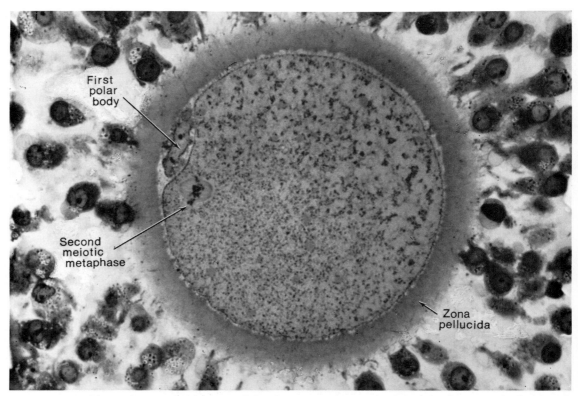

First
polar
body

Second
meiotic
metaphase

Zona
pellucida

Figure 33-18 Photomicrograph of human follicular oocyte at completion of the first meiotic division. A first polar body has been extruded and the chromosomes and spindle of the second meiotic metaphase are visible. (Photomicrograph courtesy of L. Zamboni.)

tined to degenerate. This depletion of the stock of oocytes begins in intrauterine life, becomes prominent at birth and before puberty, and continues on a smaller scale throughout reproductive life. Every normal ovary, therefore, contains degenerating follicles. Why only a few follicles reach maturity and rupture, while the great majority degenerate at various stages of development, is not known. The mechanism by which a single follicle is selected to complete its development is also unknown. Nor do we have any clear idea of the biological significance of this wastage of oocytes.

Atresia may begin at any stage of development of the follicle, even in ones that are apparently mature. In a primary follicle doomed to destruction, the ovum shrinks and degenerates, a process followed by the dissolution of the granulosa cells. The resulting small cavity in the stroma is closed rapidly without leaving a trace. In small secondary follicles, the earliest sign of abnormality is often the eccentric location of the egg nucleus, which goes on to develop a coarse granularity and finally becomes pyknotic. In follicles of larger size the histological changes in atresia become somewhat more complex and variable. In the cyclic atresia of follicles in the adult human ovary the process appears to be initiated in the follicle wall, with secondary effects upon the oocyte. One of the earliest indications of this atretic process is the invasion of the granulosa layer and cumulus oophorus by strands of vascularized connective tissue. This is followed by a loosening and shedding of the granulosa cells into the follicular cavity and a hypertrophy of the theca interna. In follicles exhibiting these changes, the oocyte may still appear normal in routine histological preparations. As the degeneration of the granulosa cells advances, the follicle collapses, its outlines become wavy, and the cavity is filled by a large number of fibroblasts and wandering cells. The remnants of the degenerated follicular epithelium are rapidly resorbed. The folded and collapsed zona pellucida may remain alone amid the connective tissue elements.

The theca interna also undergoes important changes. The basal lamina that separates it from the epithelium often increases in thickness and is transformed into a thick layer of hyaline substance, the "glassy membrane," which is characteristic of follicles in advanced atresia. The large cells of the theca interna increase further in size and are usually arranged in radial groups or strands, separated from one another by partitions of collagenous fibers and smaller fusiform cells. The cells acquire a typical epithelioid character and are filled with lipid droplets. They are very similar in appearance to the theca lutein cells but reach a higher degree of

development in the atretic follicle. The cavity of the atretic follicle, containing the collapsed zona pellucida and connective tissue, is now surrounded by a broad, festooned layer of epithelioid, lipid-containing theca interna cells, arranged in radial cords and provided with a rich capillary network. The microscopic appearance of such an atretic follicle is rather similar to that of an old corpus luteum. Such structures have therefore been given the misleading name *corpora lutea atretica.* The main differences are, of course, the presence of the glassy membrane, degenerated granulosa cells, and sometimes a zona pellucida in the center.

Strands of fibrous connective tissue and blood vessels ultimately penetrate the glassy membrane, and the remains of the degenerated elements in the interior are destroyed. The resulting scar with its hyaline streaks

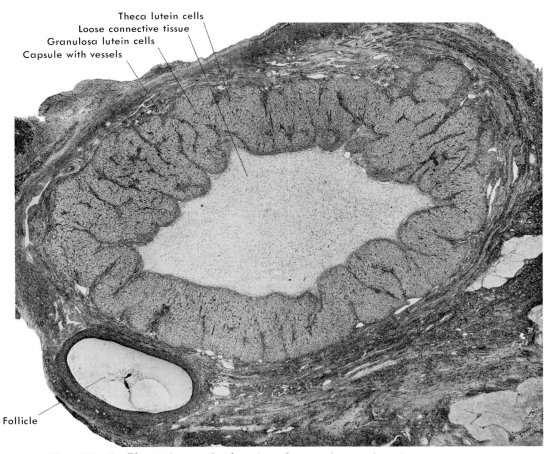

Figure 33-19 Photomicrograph of section of corpus luteum from human ovary. ×11.

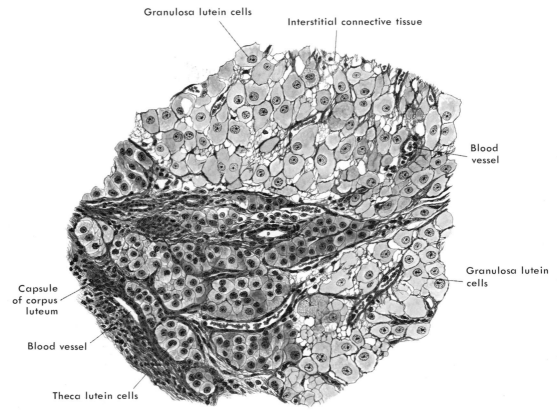

Granulosa lutein cells

Interstitial connective tissue

Blood vessel

Granulosa lutein cells

Capsule of corpus luteum

Blood vessel

Theca lutein cells

Figure 33-20 Drawing of a peripheral area of human corpus luteum of pregnancy, stained for reticular fibers by the Bielschowsky method. The smaller darker cells at the lower left are theca lutein cells, the larger paler cells above are granulosa lutein cells. (After A. A. Maximow.)

sometimes resembles a corpus albicans derived from old corpora lutea but is usually much smaller, and sooner or later it disappears in the stroma of the ovary. The layer of hypertrophic theca interna cells surrounding the atretic follicle is broken up by the invading strands of fibrous tissue into separate cell islands of various shapes and sizes. These islands are irregularly scattered in the stroma and may persist for a time. They contribute to the so-called "interstitial gland" of the ovary.

The Interstitial Tissue of the Ovary

The stroma of the human ovarian cortex consists of spindle-shaped cells and networks of reticular fibers. Elastic fibers occur only in the walls of blood vessels. The cells bear a superficial resemblance to smooth muscle but do not have myofilaments in their cytoplasm. The stromal cells can differentiate into ovarian *interstitial cells* and, in ovarian pregnancy, they are capable of transformation to *decidual cells*.

The endocrine function and developmental potentialities of the layer of specialized interstitial tissue composing the theca folliculi have already been described. Thus the interstitial tissue of the ovarian cortex comprises reticular fibers and spindle-shaped cells with potentialities distinct from those of ordinary fibroblasts. The medulla, on the other hand, is made up of more typical loose connective tissue with fibroblasts, many elastic fibers, and strands of smooth muscle cells accompanying the blood vessels.

In many mammals the ovarian stroma contains conspicuous clusters and cords of large epithelioid interstitial cells. They are rich

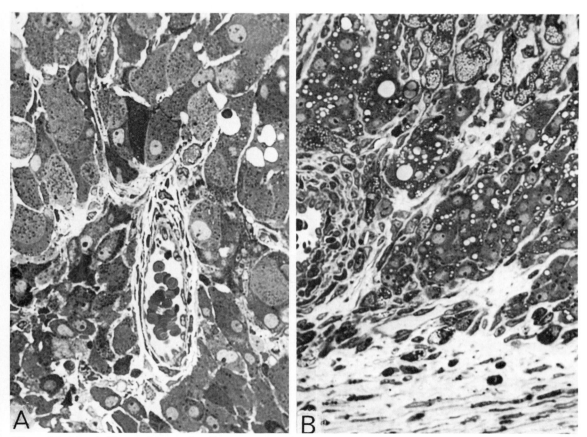

Figure 33–21 *A*, Photomicrograph of human corpus luteum at 9 weeks' gestation. The larger cells above are granulosa lutein cells, and the smaller ones below are theca lutein cells derived from the theca interna. *B*, Corpus luteum of the human menstrual cycle about one day after ovulation. Cells of the theca interna have luteinized and are migrating into the developing corpus luteum. (Photomicrographs from T. M. Crisp et al., Am. J. Anat., *127*:37, 1970.)

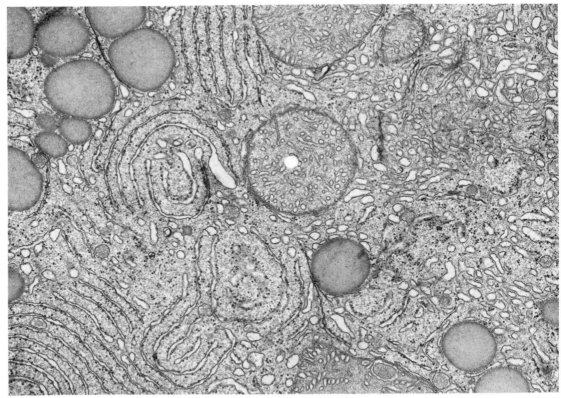

Figure 33-22 Electron micrograph of a portion of a theca lutein cell of a human corpus luteum at 9 weeks' gestation. The granular and agranular endoplasmic reticulum are well developed and lipid droplets are abundant. The mitochondria are highly variable in size and have tubular cristae. (From T. M. Crisp et al., Am. J. Anat., *127*:37, 1970.)

in lipid and resemble lutein cells. In some species they have been shown to secrete ovarian hormones. Because of their epithelioid appearance and presumed secretory function, these cells, dispersed in the stroma, are referred to collectively as the *interstitial gland*. In animal species that have large litters, particularly among the rodents, the development of the interstitial gland may be very extensive. Cell foci originating from the breaking up of the hypertrophied theca interna of atretic follicles persist, enlarge, and fuse. Through the continuous addition of new cells, a large part of the organ is ultimately transformed into a diffuse mass of large, closely packed, lipid-containing interstitial cells that are almost identical in appearance to granulosa lutein cells. The follicles and the corpora lutea are embedded in this cell mass, and only a thin tunica albuginea separates it from the germinal epithelium on the surface.

The interstitial gland is poorly developed in the human ovary. Interstitial cells are found in the greatest numbers during the first year of life, when atretic follicles are most numerous, and they are believed to arise from the hypertrophied theca interna of regressing follicles. The interstitial gland involutes at puberty with the onset of menstruation and the cyclic development of corpora lutea. In the adult human ovary, cells of this kind either are absent or are present only in small numbers widely scattered in the stroma.

In the hilus of the ovary and in the adjacent mesovarium, groups of another kind of large epithelioid cell may be found closely associated with vascular spaces and unmyelinated nerve fibers. These cell clusters, now simply called *hilus cells*, were originally named the *sympathicotropic hilus gland* and were considered to be chromaffin cells. This view is now less widely accepted, since they do not always stain with chromates. More-over, convincing evidence has been pre-sented that they are similar to the Leydig cells of the testis. They are rich in lipid, contain cholesterol esters and lipochrome pigment, and may even have cytoplasmic crystals apparently identical to the crystals of Reinke (see Chapter 32). They have the histochemical and cytologic characteristics of actively secreting endocrine cells. They are prominent during pregnancy and at the menopause. Tumor or hyperplasia of the ovarian hilus cells is accompanied by mascu-linization. This clinical observation and their cytological and cytochemical resemblances to Leydig cells suggest that they secrete androgens.

In the broad ligament and in the meso-varium, the occurrence of small accumula-tions of "interrenal tissue" corresponding to adrenal cortical tissue has also been de-scribed.

Vestigial Organs Associated with the Ovary

Certain vestigial organs are found in connection with the ovary. The most obvious of these is the *epoöphoron*. It consists of several parallel or divergent tubules, running in the mesovarium from the hilus of the ovary toward the oviduct and fusing with a longitudinal canal parallel to the oviduct. All of these tubules end blindly. They are lined with low cuboidal or columnar epithelium, which is sometimes ciliated, and are sur-rounded by a condensed connective tissue layer containing smooth muscle. The upper end of the longitudinal duct sometimes ends in a cyst-like enlargement, the *hydatid of Morgagni*, while its other end may extend far toward the uterus as the so-called *duct of Gartner*. The transverse tubules and the longi-tudinal duct of Gartner together comprise the *epoöphoron*. Between the epoöphoron and

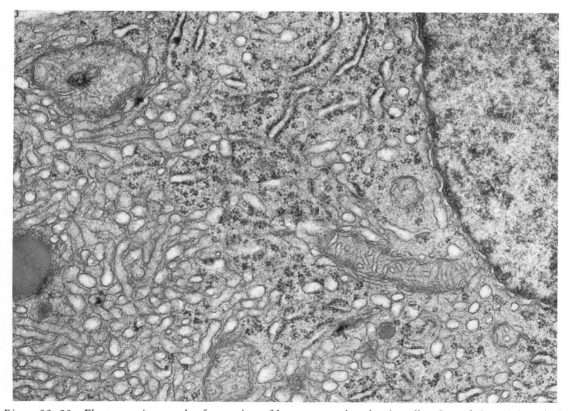

Figure 33–23 Electron micrograph of a portion of human granulosa lutein cell at 9 weeks' gestation. As in other steroid producing endocrine glands, there is an extensive development of tubular smooth reticulum, and lesser amounts of the granular form. (From T. M. Crisp et al., Am. J. Anat., *127*:37, 1970.)

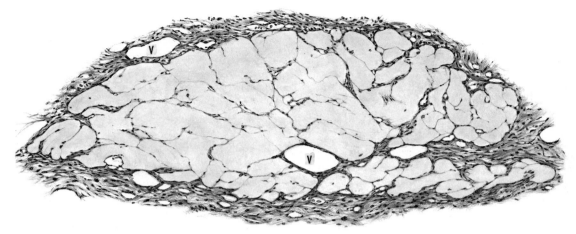

Figure 33-24 Corpus albicans of human ovary. Fixation by perfusion—hence the empty vessels (*V*). Dense hyaline material separates the residual cells of the corpus luteum. The whole structure is surrounded by the stroma of the ovary. ×135.

the uterus in the tissue of the broad ligament is another group of irregular fragments of epithelial tubules, the *paroöphoron.* The epoöphoron is a rudiment of the embryonic mesonephros and is the homologue of the ductuli efferentes and epididymis of the male. The paroöphoron is the remnant of the caudal part of the mesonephros and corresponds to the vestigial paradidymis of the male.

Vessels and Nerves

The principal arterial supply to the ovary is from the ovarian artery, which arises from the aorta below the level of the renal vessels and reaches the ovary through the infundibulopelvic ligament. Along the mesovarial border of the ovary this vessel anastomoses with the uterine artery, which courses upward along the lateral aspect of the uterus from the region of the cervix. Relatively large vessels from the region of anastomosis of the uterine and ovarian arteries enter the hilus of the ovary and branch profusely as they course through the medulla. Because of their tortuous course, they are called *arteriae helicinae,* or helicine arteries. These vessels, like those in the corpora cavernosa penis, may show longitudinal ridges on their intima. In the periphery of the medulla they form a plexus, from which smaller twigs penetrate radially, passing between the follicles to enter the cortex, where they break up into loose networks of capillaries. These are continuous with dense networks in the theca of the larger follicles. The veins accompany the arteries. In the medulla they are large and tortuous and form a plexus in the hilus.

Networks of lymph capillaries arise in the cortex, especially in the theca externa of the large follicles. Lymph vessels with valves are found only outside the hilus.

The nerves of the ovary are derived from the ovarian plexus and from the uterine nerves. They enter the organ through the hilus, together with the blood vessels. They consist, for the most part, of nonmyelinated fibers, but thin myelinated fibers are also present. The presence of sympathetic nerve cells in the ovary has not been confirmed. The majority of the nerves supply the muscular coat of blood vessels. Many fibers penetrate into the cortex and form plexuses around the follicles and under the germinal epithelium. It seems doubtful that they penetrate through the basal lamina into the epithelium of the follicles. Sensory fibers ending in corpuscles of Pacini have been described in the ovarian stroma.

THE OVIDUCT OR FALLOPIAN TUBE

The *oviduct* or *fallopian tube* is the part of the female reproductive tract that receives the ovum, provides the appropriate environment for its fertilization, and transports it to the uterus. It is a muscular tube about 12 cm. long situated in the edge of the mesosalpinx, which is the upper free margin of the broad ligament of the uterus. Its lumen communicates with the uterine cavity at one end and is open to the peritoneal cavity at the other. Several segments along its length are identified by different descriptive terms. The part of the tube traversing the wall of the uterus is called the *pars interstitialis*. The narrow medial third near the uterine wall is the *isthmus*. The expanded intermediate segment is the *ampulla*, and the funnel-shaped abdominal opening is the *infundibulum*. The margins of the latter are drawn out into numerous tapering, fringe-like processes, the *fimbriae*.

Histological Organization

The wall of the oviduct consists of a mucosa, a muscular layer, and an external serous coat. The mucosa in the ampulla is thick and forms numerous elaborately branched folds. The lumen in cross section, therefore, is a labyrinthine system of narrow spaces between profusely branching folia covered by epithelium (Fig. 33–26C). In the

isthmus the longitudinal folds are much shorter and less highly branched (Fig. 33–26B), and in the interstitial part they are reduced to low ridges (Fig. 33–26A).

The epithelium is of the simple columnar variety (Fig. 33–27) but may sometimes appear pseudostratified when cut obliquely. It is highest in the ampulla and diminishes in height toward the uterus. It consists of two kinds of cells. One of these, especially numerous on the fimbriae and in the ampulla, is provided with cilia that beat toward the uterus. The other cell type is devoid of cilia and is commonly considered to be secretory. The secretion may provide the ovum with nutritive material, and in some species, notably the rabbit, it adds to the ovum an outer albuminous envelope. In the monotremes and some marsupials, a shell, as well as an albuminous coat, is formed around the ova. The two types of epithelial cells are probably different functional states of a single cell type. In women the epithelium of the oviduct undergoes cyclic changes along with those of the uterine mucosa. True glands are absent in the oviduct.

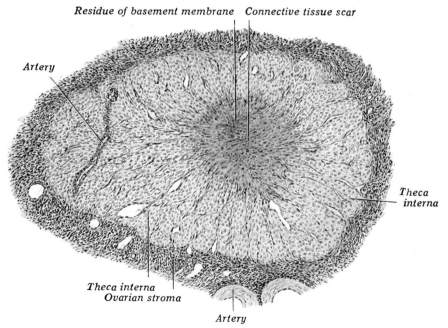

Figure 33–25 An atretic follicle from the ovary of a 39 year old woman. The conspicuous layer of theca cells results from their aggregation after collapse of the follicle. In the majority of atretic follicles this layer is less prominent than depicted here. (After Schaffer.)

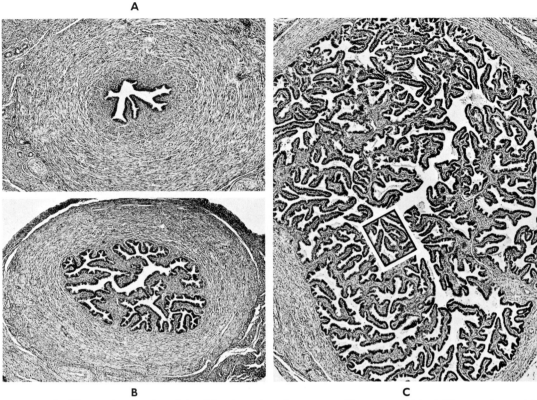

Figure 33–26 Photomicrographs of the fallopian tube of a 23 year old woman. ×30. *A*, The pars interstitialis; *B*, the isthmus; *C*, the outer portion of the ampulla. The area enclosed in the rectangle is shown at higher magnification in Figure 33–27.

The relative proportions of ciliated and nonciliated cells is under endocrine control. Ciliated cells are said to increase in height in the human oviduct during the follicular phase of the cycle and to decrease during the luteal phase, but they do not seem to lose their cilia completely. The cyclic changes have been most thoroughly studied in the rhesus monkey. The changes are most marked in the fimbria and upper ampulla and diminish toward the isthmus. On the fimbria, the epithelium becomes devoid of cilia and non-secretory in the late luteal phase of the cycle. In the early follicular phase, the cells hypertrophy, divide, and begin active ciliogenesis. There is also cytological evidence of secretory activity. These changes reach their peak at mid-cycle. Dedifferentiation is so complete on the fimbriae in the late luteal phase that one cannot distinguish deciliated cells from atrophic secretory cells. The degree of dedifferentiation is less marked toward the isthmus, suggesting that this segment of the oviduct is less estrogen dependent.

After castration the oviductal epithelium rapidly atrophies and dedifferentiates. Within a few weeks the fimbriae are almost completely deciliated and all of the cells are structurally indistinguishable (Fig. 33–28). In the ampulla some cells retain their cilia, and in the isthmus regression is still less marked. Similar dedifferentiation after ovariectomy is observed in the rabbit and in other species (Fig. 33–30). Within a week after administration of estradiol, there is a remarkable hypertrophy, with restoration of cilia and secretory activity. Ciliated epithelia in other parts of the body are completely indifferent to circulating estrogens.

Steroid hormones also appear to affect the rate of ciliary beat. A significant increase has been reported 48 hours after copulation in the rabbit and after progesterone treatment of the estrogen-primed monkey ovi-

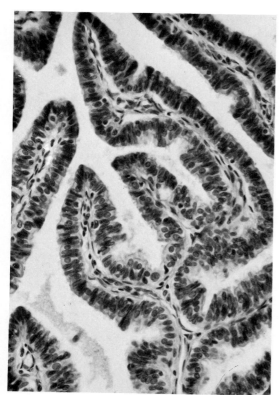

Figure 33-27 Photomicrograph of the branching folds of the mucous membrane of the human fallopian tube. ×280. For orientation, see rectangle in Figure 33–26.

duct. Thus, estrogen seems to prepare the ciliated surface destined to transport the ovum, and progesterone accelerates the ciliary beat at the time an ovum is available to be transported. Later in the cycle, progesterone favors the loss of cilia (Brenner).

The lamina propria of the mucosa in the oviduct consists of a network of reticular fibers and of numerous fusiform cells. Wandering cells and mast cells also occur in limited numbers. The fixed cells here seem to have the same developmental potentialities as those in the uterus. In cases of tubal pregnancy, some of them are transformed into typical decidual cells.

No true muscularis mucosae can be distinguished in the oviduct. The mucosa is surrounded directly by the muscularis, which consists of two layers of smooth muscle bundles. The inner layer is circular or spiral; the outer is principally longitudinal, but there is no distinct boundary between the two. Toward the periphery, longitudinal bundles

gradually appear in increasing numbers among the circular bundles. The smooth muscle bundles are embedded in an abundant, loose connective tissue, and they extend into the broad ligament. Toward the uterus the muscularis increases in thickness. The peritoneal coat of the fallopian tube has the usual serosal structure.

At the time of ovulation the oviduct exhibits active movements. The abdominal opening of the oviduct contains large blood vessels in its mucosa, especially veins, and these extend into the fimbriae. Smooth muscle bundles form a network between the blood vessels. This results, in effect, in a sort of erectile tissue. At the time of ovulation the vessels are engorged with blood, and the resulting enlargement and turgescence of the fimbriae, together with the contraction of their intrinsic muscle, brings the opening of the tubal infundibulum into contact with the surface of the ovary.

The rhythmic contractions of the oviduct are probably of primary importance in the transport of the ovum. Contraction waves pass from the infundibulum to the uterus, and the beat of the cilia on the mucosa is in the same direction.

Blood Vessels, Lymphatics, and Nerves

The mucous membrane and its folds, as well as the serous coat, contain abundant blood and lymph vessels. The lymph channels within the folds of the mucous membrane are extensive and appear in sections as long clefts that are often mistaken for artifactitious splits in the tissue, but careful inspection reveals their smooth endothelial lining. In periods of vascular engorgement, when these lymphatics are also distended with lymph, they no doubt contribute to the increased turgor of the tissue and stiffen the mucosal folds.

Larger nerve bundles are found accompanying the vessels in the serous layer and in the peripheral parts of the longitudinal muscle. The circular muscle layer contains a dense plexus of thin nerve bundles supplying the muscle fibers and penetrating into the mucous membrane.

UTERUS

The uterus is the portion of the reproductive tract that receives the fertilized ovum from the oviduct, provides its attachment, and establishes the vascular relations necessary for sustenance of the embryo throughout its development. In the human it is a single pear-shaped organ with a thick muscular wall (Fig. 33–31). It is slightly flattened dorsoventrally and contains a correspondingly flattened uterine cavity. In the

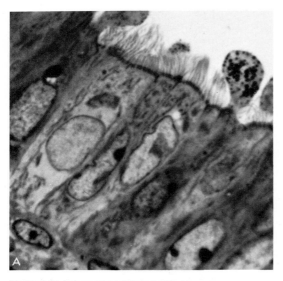

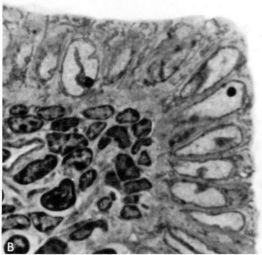

Figure 33–28 A, Photomicrograph of oviductal epithelium from a normal macaque in the follicular phase of the cycle. Ciliated and nonciliated cells are distinguishable. *B*, Oviductal epithelium of a macaque six weeks after ovariectomy. The cells are shorter, nonciliated, and two types of cells are no longer distinguishable. (From R. Brenner, *In* Hafez, E. S., and R. J. Blandau [eds.]: *The Mammalian Oviduct.* Chicago, University of Chicago Press, 1969.)

nonpregnant condition, the uterus is about 6.5 cm. long, 3.5 cm. wide, and 2.5 cm. thick. Several regions are distinguished. The expanded upper portion, constituting the bulk of the organ, is called the *body* or *corpus uteri.* The rounded upper end of the body, where the oviducts join the uterus, is often referred to as the *fundus.* The slightly constricted portion below the corpus is the *isthmus,* and the cylindrical lower part is the *cervix.* The portion of the cervix that protrudes into the vagina is the *portio vaginalis.* The slender cervical canal that passes from the uterine cavity down through the cervix opens into the vagina at the *external os.*

A serous membrane, the peritoneum, covers the fundus and much of the posterior aspect of the uterus. The peritoneum is reflected onto the bladder anteriorly and onto the rectum posteriorly, so that this layer is found only on part of the surface of the organ. The greater part of the thickness of the uterine wall is a mass of smooth muscle, the *myometrium.* The uterus is lined by a glandular mucosa called the *endometrium.*

Myometrium

The smooth muscle fibers of the muscular layer are arranged in cylindrical or flat bundles separated by thin septa of connective tissue. Several layers can be distinguished in the myometrium according to the direction and disposition of the bundles. The layers are not sharply demarcated, however, because fiber bundles frequently cross over from one layer into another.

Immediately beneath the mucosa is a thin layer called the *stratum submucosum.* Its fibers are predominantly longitudinal, but some oblique and circular bundles may be found. This layer forms distinct muscular rings around the intramural portions of the oviducts. The next layer is the thickest and is called the *stratum vasculare,* because it contains many large blood vessels that give it a spongy appearance. Circular and oblique muscle bundles are predominant. In the succeeding *stratum supravascular,* the fibers are mainly circular and longitudinal. Finally, the outermost *stratum subserosum* is a thin longitudinal muscle layer. The two most superficial layers send muscular bundles out into the wall of the oviduct, the broad ligament, and the round ligament.

The smooth muscle cells of the myometrium ordinarily have a length of about 50 μm. In pregnancy, when the mass of the uterus increases about 24 times, they hypertrophy to a length of more than 500 μm. Although smooth muscle hypertrophy accounts for much of the enlargement of the gravid uterus, there also appears to be an increase in the number of the muscle fibers through division (Fischer-Wasels) and possibly through transformation of persisting embryonic connective tissue cells into new muscular elements, especially in the innermost layers of the myometrium (Stieve). There is also a marked increase in the amount of connective tissue as indicated by a five-fold increase in the amount of collagen. There is evidence that smooth muscle cells can synthesize collagen in response to estrogen stimulation (Ross and Klebanoff).

During return of the uterus to normal size after delivery, the muscle cells rapidly diminish in size. It is possible that some of them degenerate.

The connective tissue between the muscular bundles consists of collagenous fibers, fibroblasts, primitive connective tissue cells, macrophages, and mast cells. A typical argyrophilic reticulum surrounds the smooth muscle cells and is continuous with the intermuscular collagenous tissue. Elastic networks are especially prominent in the peripheral layers of the uterine wall. From there they extend inward between the muscle bundles. The innermost layers of the myometrium do not contain elastic fibers, except those found in the walls of the blood vessels.

The cervix is composed mainly of dense collagenous and elastic fibers, among which are distributed fibroblasts and a variable number of smooth muscle cells. The dense fibrous nature of the cervix accounts for the very firm consistency of this part of the uterus.

Histophysiology of the Myometrium. Contractions of the myometrium are very largely responsible for expulsion of the fetus

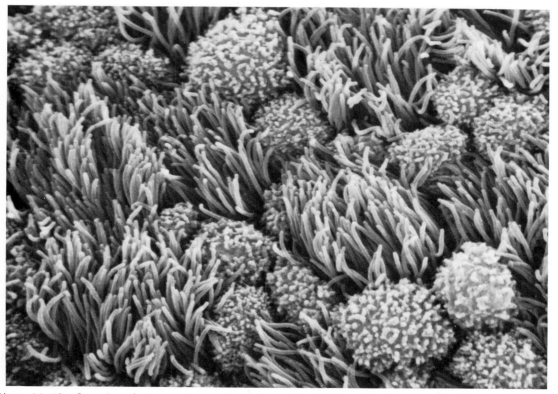

Figure 33–29 Scanning electron micrograph of the surface of the epithelium on the fimbria of the rabbit oviduct in the postovulatory period, showing the dense ciliation and the convex apices of the secretory cells covered with microvilli. (From R. E. Rumery and E. M. Eddy, Anat. Rec., *178*:83, 1974.)

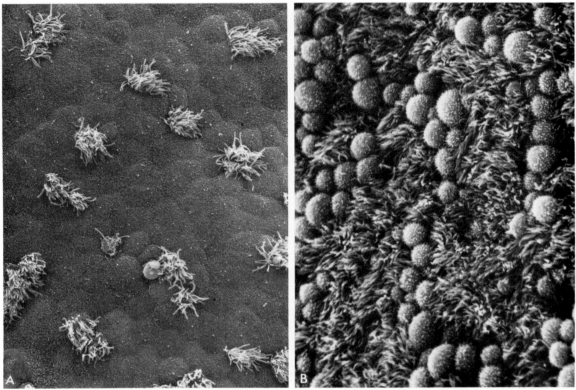

Figure 33-30   Scanning micrographs illustrating the dependence of cytological differentiation of the oviductal epithelium upon hormones. *A*, From the fimbria of a rabbit oviduct 16 months after ovariectomy. The epithelium is flat and smooth, with only occasional ciliated cells. *B*, The other oviduct of the same rabbit after receiving estrogen replacement for 10 days. (From R. E. Rumery and E. M. Eddy, Anat. Rec., *178*:83, 1974.)

at parturition. In the normal nonpregnant uterus, the musculature is continually undergoing shallow, intermittent myogenic contractions that are not attended by any subjective sensation. These may become exaggerated in sexual stimulation or during menstruation, resulting in cramp-like pain. The factors regulating this activity are poorly understood.

When pregnancy ensues, the activity of the myometrium is greatly reduced. Experiments on animals have led to a widely held belief that the elevated level of progesterone produced by the corpus luteum of pregnancy inhibits myometrial contractility, and that withdrawal of this inhibition at the end of gestation initiates labor. This theory is now seriously challenged. An unequivocal demonstration of an effect of progesterone on the human uterine muscle is lacking, and in several animal species, progesterone has been shown to have no effect. Cross circulation ex-

periments between pregnant and nonpregnant animals clearly show that another blood-borne substance plays a more important role than progesterone (Porter). There is some reason to believe that it may be the hormone *relaxin.*

Uterine contractility is increased by *oxytocin,* a hormone of the neurohypophysis. This substance is sometimes used by the obstetrician to initiate labor or to increase the effectiveness of the uterine contractions. Another class of compounds that affect the uterine musculature is the *prostaglandins.* These stimulate smooth muscle in general and, although their mechanism of action is not well understood, they are now widely used as abortifacients.

The maintenance of the normal size and degree of cytological differentiation of the uterine smooth muscle depends upon estrogens produced by the ovary and carried to the uterus in the blood. In the absence of estrogen, uterine smooth muscle atrophies and loses its capacity to generate action potentials.

Endometrium

The primary functions of the endometrium are preparation for implantation of a fertilized ovum, participation in implantation, and formation of the maternal portion of the placenta. The structural and functional changes of the endometrium are dependent upon the endocrine secretory activity of the ovaries. Upon removal of the ovaries, the endometrium atrophies. Upon administration of estrogen, there is a rapid increase in the blood flow to the uterus, the endometrium becomes edematous, its cells begin to proliferate and hypertrophy, and there is a marked increase in its metabolic activity.

Beginning with puberty at 11 to 15 years of age and continuing until *menopause* at age 45 to 50, the uterine mucosa undergoes monthly cyclic changes in its structure in response to rhythmic variations in the secretion of ovarian hormones. At the end of each cycle there is a partial degeneration and sloughing of the endometrium, accompanied by a more or less abundant extravasation of blood. The products of these destructive changes appear as a bloody vaginal discharge, the *menstrual flow*, which normally continues for 3 to 5 days.

The endometrium is approximately 5 mm. in thickness at the height of its development in an ordinary menstrual cycle. It consists of a surface epithelium invaginated to form numerous tubular *uterine glands* that extend down into a very thick lamina propria, usually referred to as the *endometrial stroma*.

The surface epithelium is simple columnar and is composed of a mixture of ciliated and secretory cells. The epithelium of the uterine glands is similar, but the ciliated cells are fewer. The direction of ciliary beat is said to be upward in the glands and toward the vagina on the endometrial surface. The glands are, for the most part, simple tubules, but they may show some bifurcation in the zone adjacent to the myometrium. They occasionally penetrate a short distance among the muscle bundles. Under pathological conditions the myometrium may be extensively invaded in this manner, a change described

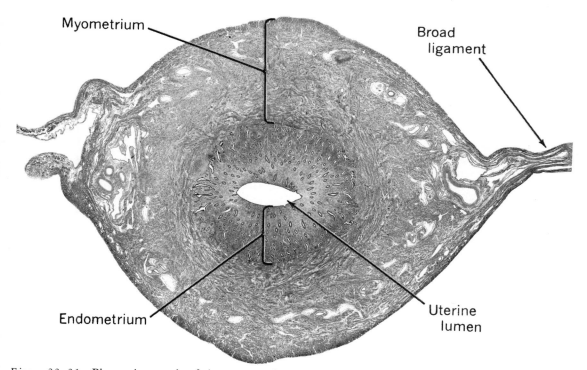

Figure 33–31 Photomicrograph of the uterus of a macaque in transverse section, illustrating the relative thickness of the myometrium and the late proliferative endometrium. ×9. (Courtesy of H. Mizoguchi.)

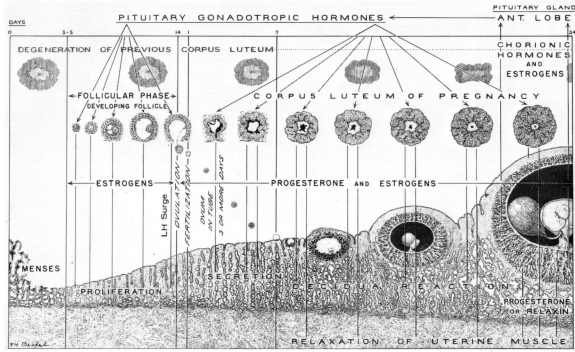

Figure 33–32 Drawing depicting the morphological changes in the ovary and the endometrium in the course of the menstrual cycle and the hormones controlling these changes. (From Eastman, N. J., Williams Obstetrics, 11th ed., 1956. Courtesy of Appleton-Century-Crofts, Publishing Division of Prentice-Hall, Inc., Englewood Cliffs, N.J.)

by the term *adenomyosis.* In old age, the endometrium atrophies and becomes thin. The openings of the glands may become partly obliterated and they then become distended to form small cysts.

The endometrial stroma strongly resembles mesenchyme. Its irregularly stellate cells have large, ovoid nuclei. The cell processes appear to be in contact throughout the tissue and adhere to a delicate framework of reticular fibers. Elastic fibers are absent except in the walls of the arterioles. There is a ground substance, which at times is rich in metachromatic glycoprotein. In the interstices of the reticulum of stellate cells are lymphoid wandering cells and granular leukocytes. Macrophages are not uncommon, but, for some unknown reason, they are not mobilized to phagocytize the blood extravasated in menstruation.

A knowledge of the blood supply of the endometrium is of special importance for an understanding of the mechanisms of menstruation and of placentation. From the uterine arteries that course in the broad liga-

ments along the sides of the uterus, branches penetrate to the stratum vasculare of the myometrium. In this layer, circumferentially oriented *arcuate arteries* run toward the midline, where they anastomose with corresponding vessels from the other side. Branches from the arcuate arteries pass through the deeper layers of the myometrium to reach the endometrium. Where they cross the myometrial-endometrial junction, they give off small *basal arteries* supplying the deepest portion of the endometrium, the *basalis* or *stratum basale* (the portion which is not sloughed off during menstruation). Continuing upward into the thicker layer commonly called the *functionalis,* the arteries are unbranched but highly contorted. These "coiled arteries" ramify into arterioles that supply a rich capillary bed in the superficial portion of the endometrium. The thin walled veins form an irregular anastomosing net with sinusoidal enlargements at all levels of the endometrium. During most of the cycle, the coiled arteries constrict and dilate rhythmically, so that the surface is alternately blanched or suffused with blood. These vessels play an important role in menstruation.

Cyclic Changes in the Endometrium

In the course of a normal menstrual cycle, the endometrium passes through a continuous sequence of morphological and functional changes, but for convenience of description the cycle is divided into three recognizable stages that are correlated with the functional activities of the ovary. These are the *proliferative*, the *secretory*, and the *menstrual* phases. The proliferative phase coincides with the growth of the ovarian follicles and their secretion of estrogenic hormone. The secretory phase is the period when the corpus luteum is functionally active and secreting progesterone, and the menstrual phase ensues when the hormonal stimulation of the endometrium by the ovary declines (Fig. 33–32).

The Proliferative or Follicular Phase. During this phase, which begins at the end of the menstrual flow, there is a two- to threefold increase in thickness of the endometrium. Mitoses are numerous in the epithelium and in the stroma. The straight tubular glands increase in number and in length (Fig.

33–33). Their epithelium is columnar, and the lumen narrow. The ground substance of the stroma is abundant and metachromatic. The coiled arteries are elongating but are only moderately convoluted and do not extend into the superficial third of the endometrium. Toward the end of this phase, the glands become somewhat sinuous and their cells begin to accumulate glycogen (Fig. 33–33B).

The proliferative growth of the endometrium may continue for a day after ovulation, on about day 14 of an ideal 28 day cycle. There may be some diapedesis of erythrocytes into the stroma beneath the surface epithelium, and rarely a little blood may enter the uterine lumen and reach the vagina. Such *intermenstrual bleeding* is rare in the human, but estrous bleeding is common in the dog.

When the endometrium has been prepared by the normal sequential action of estrogen and progesterone, it is capable of undergoing *decidualization* — a change in which its stromal cells transform into large, pale *decidual cells* rich in glycogen. The normal stimulus for this transformation is an implanting blastocyst, but electrical stimulation, intraluminal injection of oil, or simple me-

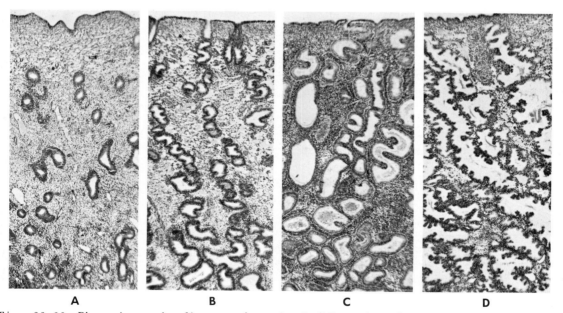

| A | B | C | D |

Figure 33–33 Photomicrographs of human endometrium in different days of the cycle. *A*, Proliferative endometrium of the ninth day. *B*, Early secretory endometrium, fifteenth day. *C*, Secretory endometrium, nineteenth day. *D*, Gestational hyperplasia, twelfth day of pregnancy. (Courtesy of A. T. Hertig.)

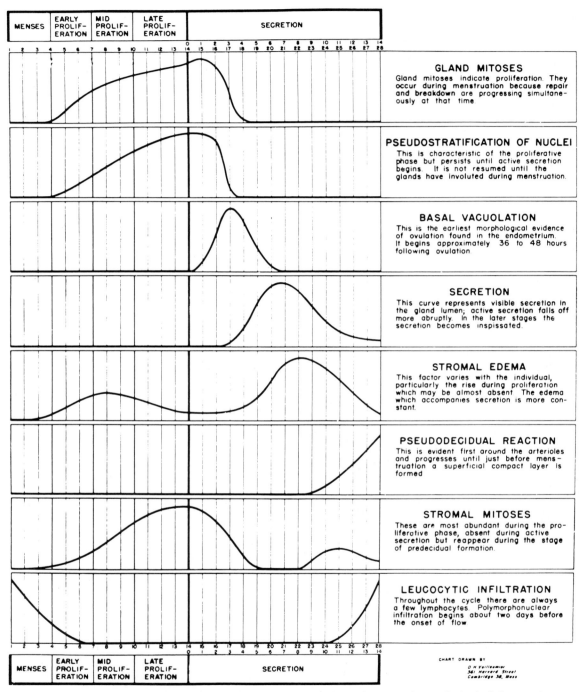

Figure 33–34 Schematic representation of the cyclic changes in the several morphological factors that are useful in dating the endometrium. (From R. W. Noyes, A. T. Hertig, and J. Rock, Fertil. Steril., *1*:3, 1950. The Williams & Wilkins Company.)

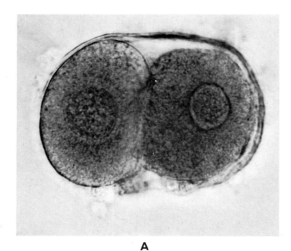

A

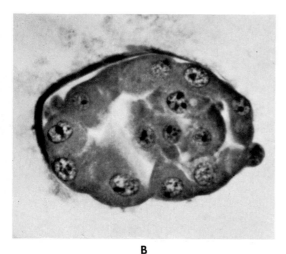

B

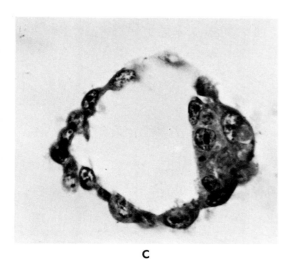

C

chanical traumatization of the endometrium will induce the same changes and result in formation of a mass of decidual cells, called a deciduoma. The exact function of the decidual tissue is still a subject of debate, but there is agreement that it provides a favorable milieu for nourishment of the conceptus and creates a specialized layer facilitating dehiscence of the placenta at the termination of pregnancy.

The Secretory or Luteal Phase. Some further thickening of the endometrium occurs in this phase, but this is largely attributable to edema of the stroma and to the accumulation of secretion in the uterine glands. The glandular epithelium early in the secretory phase of the endometrium shows a characteristic displacement of the nuclei toward the free surface, owing to the accumulation of a large amount of glycogen in the basal cytoplasm. This appearance is transient and is no longer seen after active secretion is established. The glands continue to grow, becoming quite tortuous and ultimately developing a marked sacculation, resulting in a relatively wide lumen of irregular outline, containing a carbohydrate-rich secretion (Fig. 33–33C).

The elongation and convolution of the coiled arteries continues in this phase. They extend into the superficial portion of the endometrium and become more prominent in sections because of the enlargement of the periarterial stromal cells.

The Menstrual Phase. About two weeks after ovulation, in a cycle in which fertilization fails to occur, the stimulation of the endometrium by ovarian hormones declines and marked vascular changes take place. The coiled arteries constrict, so that the superficial zone of the endometrium is blanched for hours at a time. The glands cease secreting, and there is a loss of interstitial fluid, so that

Figure 33–35 Photomicrographs of early human ova. *A,* Segmenting human ovum. Two-cell stage recovered from the fallopian tube. Ovulation age 1½ to 2½ days. Notice polar body between the two blastomeres. ×500. *B,* Free human blastocyst. Section of a 58 cell intrauterine blastocyst. Segmentation cavity is just beginning to form. Zona pellucida is disappearing. Ovulation age 4 days. ×600. *C,* Free human blastocyst. Section of a 107 cell blastocyst recovered from the uterine cavity. The inner cell mass is at the right. Ovulation age 4½ days. ×600. (All three micrographs after A. Hertig, J. Rock, and E. Adams, Am. J. Anat., 98:435, 1956.)

the height of the endometrium shrinks some-what, while the stroma appears more cellular and stains more deeply. Many leukocytes are found in the stroma at this time. After about two days of intermittent ischemia, the coiled arteries close down, making the superficial zone ischemic, while blood continues to circu-late in the basal zone. After a variable

number of hours, the constricted arteries open up for a short time; the walls of the damaged vessels near the surface burst, and blood pours into the stroma and soon breaks out into the uterine lumen. Normally such blood does not clot. Subsequently, patches of blood-soaked tissue separate off, leaving the torn ends of glands, arteries, and veins open

A

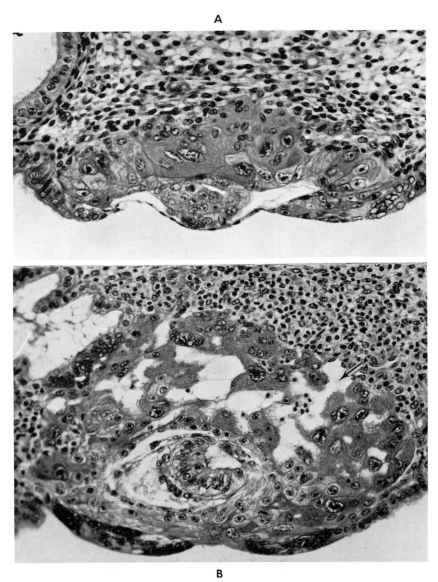

B

Figure 33–36 Photomicrographs of early human implantation sites. *A,* Human 7 day implantation. The embryo is a simple bilaminar disk. Development of an amniotic cavity is beginning. There is a solid plaque of syncytio- and cytotrophoblast. ×300. (After Hertig and Rock, 1941. Courtesy of the Carnegie Institution of Washington.) *B,* Human 9 day implantation. The embryo is a bilaminar disk. The syncytiotrophoblast now shows prominent lacunae. Notice at arrow a maternal blood space communicating with lacuna. ×25. (After Hertig and Rock. Courtesy of the Carnegie Institution of Washington.)

to the surface. Blood may ooze from such veins, refluxing from the intact basal circulation. The menstrual discharge thus contains (1) altered arterial and venous blood, with normal, hemolyzed, and sometimes agglutinated erythrocytes; (2) partially disintegrated or autolyzed epithelial and stroma cells; and (3) the secretions of the uterine and cervical glands. Sometimes there are tissue fragments in the menstrual discharge, but blood clots are considered abnormal. The average loss of blood is 35 ml. By the third or fourth day of the flow, the entire lining of the uterus presents a raw appearing surface.

The endometrium deep to the zone of extravasation remains intact during menstruation, although it does shrink down. The deep ends of glands typical of the secretory phase may be recognizable as such until the end of menstruation. Before the vaginal discharge has ceased, epithelial cells glide out from the torn ends of the glands, and the surface epithelium is quickly restored. The superficial circulation is then resumed, the stroma again becomes rich in ground substance, and the follicular phase of the new cycle begins.

The typical condition illustrated in Figure 33–32 is not always realized. In some cycles, the ovary may not produce a ripe follicle. In such *anovulatory cycles* the endometrial changes are minimal. The proliferative endometrium develops as usual, but since there is no ovulation and no corpus luteum is formed, the endometrium does not progress to the secretory phase but continues to be of the proliferative type until menstruation begins.

The various events of the normal menstrual cycle are so characteristic and reproducible that an experienced pathologist can establish the date of the cycle with surprising accuracy from examination of endometrial curettings or biopsies (Fig. 33–34). It is also possible from examination of biopsies in the second half of the cycle to determine whether a woman is having an ovulatory or an anovulatory cycle. Such examinations are essential in the clinical investigation of the causes of infertility, or the nature of disease of the ovaries, or disorders of menstruation. It is therefore of practical value to be able to recognize the principal phases of the endometrial cycle. The criteria, in brief, are as follows. (1) *Proliferative or follicular phase:* endometrium 1 to 5 mm. thick; straight, narrow

glands becoming wavy; the epithelium tall, becoming vacuolated; many mitoses in all tissues; and no coiled arteries in the superficial third. (2) *Secretory or luteal phase:* endometrium 3 to 6 mm. thick; glands wavy or sacculated, with wide lumina; epithelial cells tall, with surface blebs; stroma edematous superficially; mitoses confined to coiled arteries, which are present near the surface. (3) *Premenstrual phase:* endometrium 3 to 4 mm. thick, greatly contorted glands and arteries; dense stroma with leukocytosis. (4) *Menstrual phase:* endometrium 0.5 to 3 mm. thick; superficially extravasated blood; the glands and arteries appear collapsed; the stroma is dense; and the surface is denuded.

Isthmus and Cervix

The mucosa of the corpus uteri passes over abruptly into that of the isthmus, which

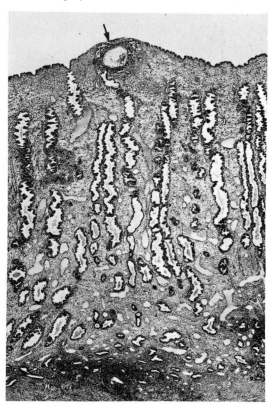

Figure 33–37 Human gestational endometrium with an 11 day implantation site (arrow). The entire thickness of the endometrium is shown. The glands are secretory, the stroma edematous, and the superficial veins are dilated. ×18. (After Hertig and Rock, 1941. Courtesy of Carnegie Institution of Washington.)

remains thin and shows few morphological signs of cyclic changes. It lacks coiled arteries and usually does not bleed during menstruation.

The cervical mucosa has a thickness of 2 to 3 mm. and a structure quite different from that of the corpus uteri. There are branching folds on its surface called the *plicae palmatae*. Its stroma is dense and the glands, which are relatively sparse, are oblique to the surface.

The cervical canal is lined by a tall columnar epithelium whose nuclei are located near the base of the cells, and the greater part of whose cytoplasm is filled with mucus. The mucosa of the cervical canal contains numerous large glands, which differ from those of the corpus and isthmus in that they are ex-

tensively branched and are lined with tall, mucus secreting columnar cells similar to those of the surface epithelium. Occasional cells are ciliated. The cervical canal is usually filled with mucus. Not infrequently in the human, the ducts of some of the glands become occluded and accumulation of secretion then transforms the glands into cysts that may reach 5 to 6 mm. in diameter. These are the so-called *Nabothian cysts*.

The outer surface of the portio vaginalis is smooth and covered with a stratified squamous epithelium similar to that of the vagina. The cells of this epithelium are rich in glycogen. The transition between the columnar mucus-secreting epithelium of the cervical canal and the stratified squamous epithelium

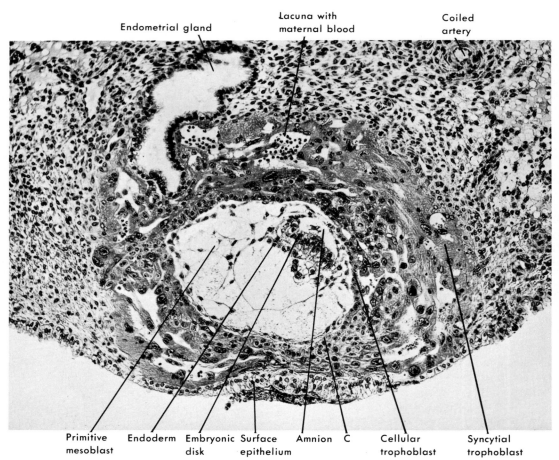

Figure 33–38 Photomicrograph from the same section as Figure 33–36, magnified 160 diameters. The bulk of the ovum consists of masses of trophoblast (syncytium) invading the endometrium. Within the syncytial trophoblast is the cellular trophoblast with obvious cell boundaries. The cells are arranged as a simple epithelium except for the clump at *C*. The cellular trophoblast immediately surrounds the primitive chorionic mesoblast in which the embryo is suspended. (After Hertig and Rock, 1941. Courtesy of the Carnegie Institution of Washington.)

of the portio vaginalis is abrupt. As a rule, the borderline is just inside the external os of the cervix. In some individuals, however, particularly after childbearing, patches of the columnar epithelium of the endocervix may extend for varying distances out onto the portio vaginalis. These are commonly called cervical "erosions." They are especially susceptible to inflammatory reactions and are a common cause of increased vaginal discharge, *leukorrhea*. Virtually all multiparous women have some degree of cervical inflammation. If untreated, cervical erosions and their attendant chronic inflammation may predispose to cancer of the cervix, which accounts for 10 per cent of all cancer deaths in women.

The superficial cells of the cervical epithelium are constantly being exfoliated into the vaginal fluid. These can be examined in stained "vaginal smears," and the discovery of abnormal cells may provide a very early diagnosis of cancer (Papanicolaou).

Histophysiology of the Cervix

The mucosa of the cervix does not take part in the menstrual changes that are characteristic of the endometrium. There are, however, cyclic changes in the secretory activity of its mucous glands. The gland cells are affected by the circulating levels of ovarian hormones so that the amount and properties of the mucus secreted vary at different times in the menstrual cycle. There are normally about a hundred crypts or aggregations of glands in the cervix, and they secrete up to 60 mg. of mucus a day throughout much of the cycle. At mid-cycle, there is a ten-fold increase in secretion rate, probably as a result of increasing estrogenic stimulation. There is also a change in the consistency of the mucus, from the highly viscous state that prevails during most of the cycle, to a less viscous, more highly hydrated condition at mid-cycle. These changes have significance for fertility in that the cervical mucus appears to be a hostile environment and a serious impediment to progress of spermatozoa throughout much of the cycle. The changes occurring at mid-cycle seem to favor sperm migration. Some efforts are now being directed to development of endocrinological means of altering the properties of the cervical mucus as a means of contraception.

In pregnancy, the cervical glands enlarge, proliferate, and accumulate large quantities of mucus. The connective tissue between them is reduced to thin partitions.

ENDOCRINE REGULATION OF THE FEMALE REPRODUCTIVE SYSTEM

The histology of the female reproductive system cannot be fully understood without some overview of the interactions of the brain, the hypophysis, the ovaries, and the uterus in the regulation of the cyclic changes involved in reproduction. Although some of these relations have already been presented in Chapter 18, a brief recapitulation may promote understanding of the cyclic changes described in this chapter.

The cyclic activities of the ovary are under the control of the anterior lobe of the hypophysis. The secretion of follicle stimulating hormone (FSH) is responsible for the

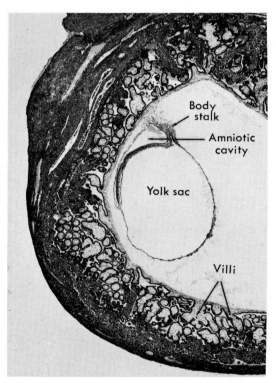

Figure 33–39 Human embryo of ovulation age 18 to 19 days. The curved embryonic disc lies between a large yolk sac and a smaller crescentic amniotic cavity. The body stalk bends back and blends with the chorionic mesoblast. Many secondary villi project into an extensive intervillous space. ×15. (Courtesy of A. T. Hertig.)

growth of the follicle up to the point of ovulation. Luteinizing hormone (LH), together with FSH, is required for ovulation and for the early development of the corpus luteum. The endometrium of the uterus exhibits two phases of functional activity that are correlated with the events in the ovary—a *follicular* (or *proliferative*) *phase* of endometrial growth, coinciding with maturation of the follicles and their ovulation, and a *luteal (or secretory) phase,* correlated with the development of a corpus luteum and during which the endometrium is prepared for reception of a fertilized egg.

At the end of the follicular phase in most mammals, morphological and neural changes occur that make the female receptive to the male at or near the time of ovulation. This is the period of heat or *estrus.* Although the menstrual cycle in the human female is basically similar to the estrus cycle of other species, receptivity to the male is not limited to

the end of the follicular phase and there is no behavioral indication that ovulation has occurred or is imminent.

During the ensuing luteal phase of the cycle the preparation of the endometrium for reception of a fertilized ovum is more extensive in the primates than in many other animals. If no egg reaches the uterus, the bulk of the endometrium breaks down after about two weeks. Its discharge is attended by uterine bleeding—menstruation.

In a cycle in which the ovum is fertilized, the secretion of gonadotropins by the trophoblast of the implanting ovum helps to maintain the corpus luteum beyond its usual lifespan, and it becomes the corpus luteum of pregnancy. The continuing function of this corpus luteum prevents the regressive and ischemic changes that lead to menstruation in an infertile cycle. Instead of regressing, the secretory endometrium persists and undergoes further hyperplasia (Fig. 33–33*D*),

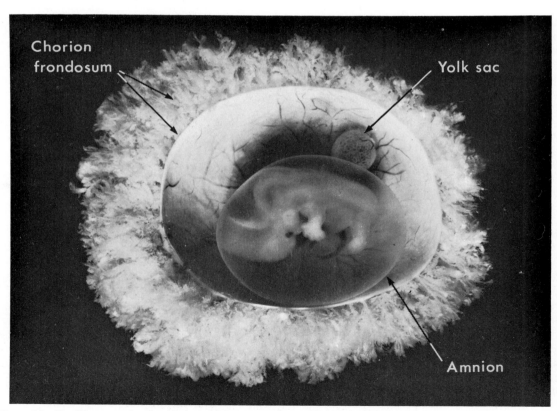

Figure 33–40 Photograph of a 40 day old human embryo (Carnegie No. 8537), showing placental villi projecting from the entire surface of the chorion. (After D. G. McKay, C. C. Roby, A. T. Hertig and M. V. Richardson. Am. J. Obst. Gynec., 69:735, 1955. Courtesy of the Carnegie Institution of Washington.)

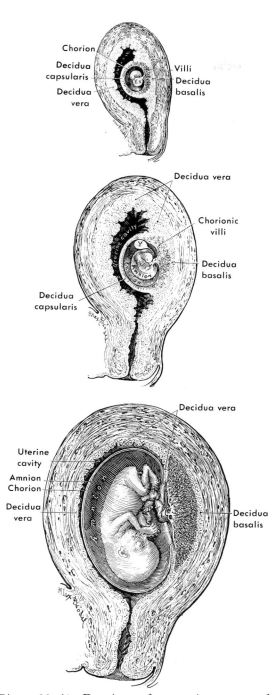

and menstruation is suppressed for the duration of pregnancy.

The temporal correlation of the events in the endometrium with those of the ovary is mediated by ovarian hormones. The developing follicle, particularly its theca interna, secretes the steroid hormones *estradiol* and *estrone,* collectively described as *estrogens.* These stimulate growth of the uterine endometrium. In species exhibiting estrus, the estrogens also act upon the central nervous system to bring about sexual receptivity and its associated behavioral manifestations. After ovulation, the collapsed follicle is reorganized and transformed into a corpus luteum that secretes *progesterone.* This hormone is responsible for the secretory changes in the endometrium that are characteristic of the luteal phase of the cycle.

The secretion of gonadotropins by the hypophysis is influenced by various factors. The rhythm of hypothalamic stimuli carried by the neurohumoral pathway to the anterior hypophysis appears to be determined by some internal clock, but it can also be influenced by psychic factors and various external stimuli. Production of excess ovarian hormones also acts back upon the hypothalamus to diminish gonadotropin secretion. This feedback mechanism is not only operative in the regulation of the normal cycle but is also the basis for the successes in conception control, wherein orally administered analogues of ovarian steroids act upon the hypothalamus and hypophysis to suppress release of the gonadotropins essential for ovulation.

IMPLANTATION

After fertilization takes place in the upper part of the oviduct, segmentation of the ovum proceeds as it passes down the tube (Fig. 33–35*A* and *B*). When it reaches the uterus on about the fourth day, it consists of many cells arranged in a hollow sphere called the *blastocyst* (Fig. 33–35*C*). The blastocyst remains free in the lumen of the uterus for a day or so and then attaches to the surface of the secretory endometrium. The blastocyst by this time has differentiated into (1) an assemblage of cells at one pole called the *inner cell mass,* which is destined to form the embryo proper, and (2) a layer of primitive *trophoblast cells* making up the rest of the wall of the blastocyst. The trophoblast cells are concerned

Figure 33–41 Drawings of successive stages of human pregnancy, showing the gradual obliteration of the uterine lumen, the disappearance of the decidua capsularis, and the establishment of the definitive discoid placenta. (Drawings by M. Brödel, from J. Williams, *Am. J. Obst. Gynec., 13*:1, 1927.)

with the attachment and implantation of the ovum and with the subsequent establishment of the *placenta*, the organ in which the physiological exchange of nutrients and waste products takes place between the embryonic and the maternal circulations. When the trophoblast makes contact with the surface of the endometrium, its cells proliferate rapidly, forming, at the interface between the ovum and the maternal tissue, a multinucleate mass of protoplasm in which no cell boundaries are discernible. This is called the *syncytial trophoblast*. This actively erosive syncytium destroys the surface epithelium and permits the blastocyst to invade the underlying stroma (Fig. 33–36*A*). By the eleventh day the blastocyst is entirely within the endometrium, the trophoblast has formed a broad layer completely surrounding the inner cell mass, and the uterine epithelium has repaired the breach made in it by the implanting ovum (Figs. 33–37 and 33–38). This form of implantation, in which the embryo and its associated membranes become embedded in and completely encapsulated by the endometrium, is called *interstitial implantation* and is characteristic of the human.

From the ninth to the eleventh day, the expanding trophoblastic shell becomes permeated by a labyrinthine system of intercommunicating lacunae containing blood liberated by erosion of maternal blood vessels (Fig. 33–38). This extravasated blood evidently serves as a source of nourishment for the embryo and represents the first step toward the establishment of the uteroplacental circulation upon which the growth of the embryo will later depend. Two forms of trophoblast are recognizable, an inner layer of *cytotrophoblast*, composed of individual cells, and a thicker outer layer of *syncytiotrophoblast*. The cytotrophoblast is mitotically active and contributes to the increasing mass of the syncytiotrophoblast by forming new cells that fuse with and become part of the syncytium.

At the 11-day stage, the embryo proper consists of a bilaminar disk of epithelial cells — a thick plate of ectoderm and a thinner layer of primitive endoderm. The ectodermal plate is continuous at its margins with a thin layer of squamous cells of cytotrophoblastic origin that enclose a small *amniotic cavity*. The endoderm is similarly continuous with a thin sheet of cells forming the *yolk sac*. Surrounding these structures are large spaces traversed by tenuous strands of extraembryonic mesen-

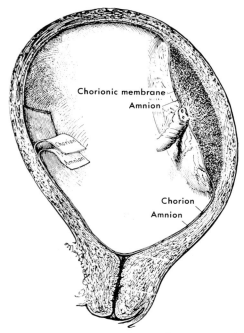

Figure 33–42 Drawing of the disposition of the fetal membranes in the later months of pregnancy. The amnion and chorion have come into contact and have become adherent to each other and to the decidua vera. (Drawings by M. Brödel, from J. Williams, Am. J. Obst. Gynec., *13*:1, 1927.)

chyme (mesoblast). These spaces constitute the *exocoelom*. The surrounding broad zone of trophoblast is called the *chorion*.

PLACENTA

Formation and Structure

From the eleventh to the sixteenth day of pregnancy the trophoblast continues to proliferate rapidly, and the implantation cavity is progressively enlarged at the expense of the surrounding maternal tissue. Invasion of the maternal blood vascular system by syncytiotrophoblast becomes increasingly extensive. The large lacunae in the syncytial labyrinth communicate at many places with venous sinuses in the endometrium. From the fifteenth day onward, solid cords of trophoblast grow outward from the surface of the chorion to form the *primary chorionic villi*. These are soon invaded at their base by chorionic mesenchyme, which advances toward their growing tips, converting the primary villi into

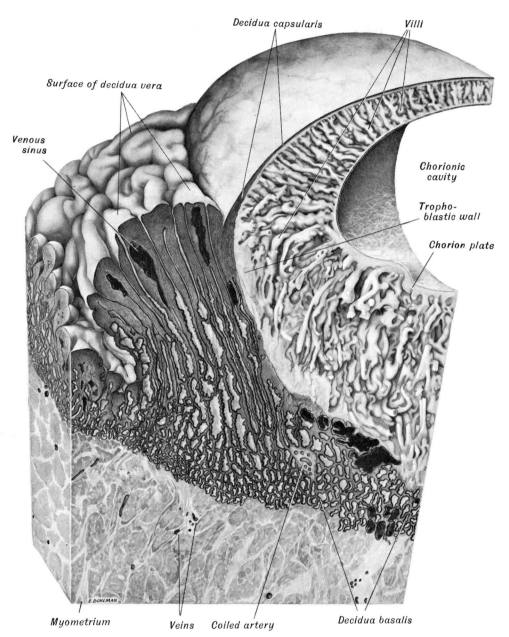

Figure 33-43 Margin of implantation site from a 4 week pregnancy. The ovum is enclosed in the maternal decidua. The villi adjacent to the decidua basalis are long, have many secondary and a few tertiary branches, and are anchored to the decidua by a wall of cytotrophoblast. The decidua vera exhibits three zones: (1) a superficial compact zone with decidual cells; (2) a spongy zone of dilated and sacculated glands; (3) a basal zone of narrow glands, which may be entirely absent. In the implantation site the compact zone has been obliterated by the developing ovum except for the attenuated decidua capsularis. The embryo and the amnion surrounding it are not shown. ×17. (Courtesy of G. W. Bartelmez.)

secondary villi (Fig. 33–39). The secondary villi then consist of an outer layer of syncytial trophoblast, an inner layer of cytotrophoblast, and a mesenchymal core. They are bathed in maternal blood that flows sluggishly through a labyrinthine system of intercommunicating channels collectively making up the *intervillous space.*

From the ends of the secondary chorionic villi, solid cords of trophoblast, the *cytotrophoblastic cell columns,* extend across the intervillous space and, upon reaching the opposite wall, spread along it, coalescing with similar outgrowths from neighboring villi to form a more or less continuous *trophoblastic shell,* interrupted only at sites of communication of maternal vessels with the intervillous space. It consists mainly of cytotrophoblast, but some areas of syncytiotrophoblast can be found. Through its interstitial growth the trophoblastic shell provides a mechanism for rapid circumferential expansion of the entire implantation site and for enlargement of the intervillous space. From the time of its formation throughout the remainder of pregnancy, the intervillous space is lined by trophoblast and traversed by anchoring villi that are attached to the maternal tissue via the trophoblastic shell. The villi absorb nutriments from the maternal blood in the intervillous space and excrete wastes into it. The efficiency of this process is greatly enhanced by the development of a functioning vascular system in the embryo.

Fetal blood vessels differentiate in the mesenchymal cores of the secondary villi as discontinuous endothelial-lined spaces, which later fuse to form continuous vascular channels. These become connected with the embryonic heart via vessels that differentiate in the mesenchyme of the inner surface of the chorion and in the body stalk of the umbilical cord. By the twenty-first to the twenty-third day, fetal blood begins to circulate through the capillaries of the villi. With their vascularization, the secondary villi become *tertiary* or *definitive placental villi* (Fig. 33–44). These radiate from the entire periphery of the chorion (Fig. 33–40). In the subsequent growth of the placenta, the anchoring or stem villi, which extend across to the trophoblastic shell, develop numerous lateral branches whose unattached tips float free in the blood of the intervillous space.

The products of conception occupy only

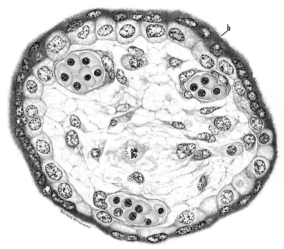

Figure 33–44 Section through placental villus from a 2 cm. human embryo. The brush border (*b*) on the syncytial trophoblast is barely visible. Beneath it is the continuous layer of cellular trophoblast. The vessels in the mesenchyme are filled with primitive erythrocytes. One mesenchymal cell in mitosis. ×450.

a portion of the entire endometrium of pregnancy (*decidua*). Different regions are identified by separate terms descriptive of their topographical relation to the implantation site. The portion that underlies the implantation site and forms the maternal component of the placenta is the *decidua basalis.* The thin superficial portion between the implantation site and the lumen is the *decidua capsularis,* and that lining the remainder of the uterus down to the internal os is the *decidua vera* (Figs. 33–41, 33–42 and 33–43).

Up to about the eighth week, the villi are equally numerous around the entire surface of the chorion (Fig. 33–40), but as pregnancy advances the villi adjacent to the decidua basalis enlarge and rapidly increase in number, while those facing the decidua capsularis degenerate, leaving this surface of the chorion smooth and relatively avascular after the third month. This region is thenceforth called the *chorion laeve,* while the villous portion toward the base is called the *chorion frondosum.* This latter becomes confined to a circular area that goes on to form the definitive discoid placenta.

As the volume of the conceptus increases and it bulges further into the lumen, the decidua capsularis becomes greatly attenuated. Its vascularity is jeopardized, and it

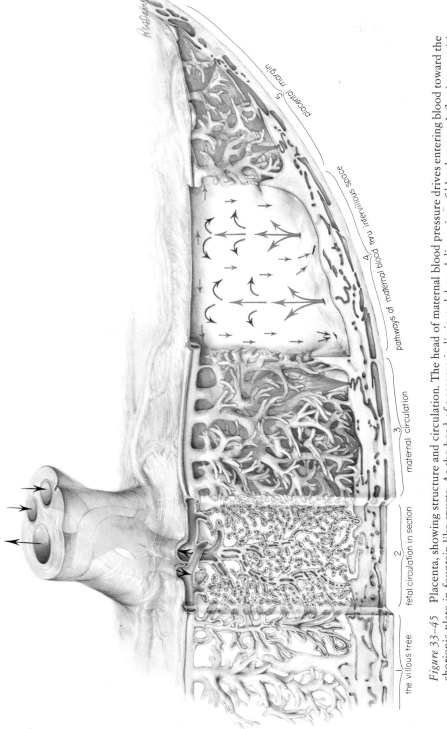

Figure 33–45 Placenta, showing structure and circulation. The head of maternal blood pressure drives entering blood toward the chorionic plate in fountain-like spurts. As the head of pressure is dissipated, lateral dispersion of blood occurs. Inflowing arterial blood pushes venous blood out into the endometrial veins. (After E. M. Ramsey and J. W. Harris, Contributions to Embryology, No. 261, Vol. 38, 1966. Courtesy of the Carnegie Institution of Washington. Drawing by RaniceDavis Crosby.)

degenerates. By four and a half months, the decidua capsularis has disappeared, and the chorion laeve has fused with the decidua vera of the opposite wall, largely obliterating the uterine lumen (Fig. 33–42). The later development of the placenta involves a steady growth in size and length of the villi of the chorion frondosum and a concomitant expansion of the intervillous space. During the fourth and fifth months the placental disk is partitioned into 15 to 20 *cotyledons* by the formation of incomplete septa that project from the decidual plate into the intervillous space. There are also changes during this period in the histological organization of the villi.

Early in gestation the syncytiotrophoblast of the villi is underlain by a more or less continuous layer of cytotrophoblast. Autoradiographic studies have established that the cytotrophoblast constitutes a rapidly dividing germinal layer that provides cells which coalesce with the syncytium. In the placenta from the fourth month onward, the proliferation of cytotrophoblast cells in the villi declines, and they continue to fuse with the syncytium until they have virtually all disappeared. Cytotrophoblast persists, however, in the basal plate in the placental septa, and in isolated islands on the stem villi. Until recently, histochemical evidence tended to implicate cytotrophoblast of these sites in the elaboration of placental hormones. Immunohistochemical studies have now localized human chorionic gonadotropin in the syncytiotrophoblast. The cytotrophoblast is therefore regarded by many as a rapidly proliferating, relatively undifferentiated tissue, while the syncytiotrophoblast is considered to be the synthetically active, differentiated form of trophoblast.

Placental Circulation

Blood poor in oxygen is carried from the fetus to the placenta in the *umbilical arteries* of the umbilical cord. At the junction of the cord with the placenta, the umbilical arteries divide into a number of radially disposed placental arteries that branch freely in the chorionic plate. Numerous branches from these pass downward into the stem villi and ramify in the arborescent pattern of subsidiary villi down to the capillary networks of the terminal villi. The oxygen-rich venous blood is collected into thin walled veins, which return the blood through vessels of increasing caliber that follow the course of the arteries to the chorionic plate. There they join veins that converge upon the single *umbilical vein*, which carries the blood through the umbilical cord to the ductus venosus, whence it enters the inferior vena cava near its point of confluence with the right atrium.

On the maternal side, blood from the arcuate branches of the uterine arteries is carried by the coiled arteries through openings in the basal plate of the placenta into the intervillous space. The flow from the maternal arterioles is pulsatile and is delivered at a pressure considerably higher than that prevailing in the intervillous space. It therefore spurts from the basal plate deep into the intervillous space in jets (Fig. 33–45). As its pressure is dissipated, it flows back around and over the surface of the placental villi, permitting exchange of metabolites with the fetal blood (Ramsey). Since the human has a *hemochorial placenta*, the trophoblast of the villi is exposed directly to maternal blood, and the diffusion barrier in the mature placenta consists only of the thin layer of syncytiotrophoblast, its basal lamina, and the wall of the subjacent fetal capillaries.

The pressure of the incoming blood and its fountain-like distribution tends to force the blood back toward the basal plate, where it is drained away through numerous communications between the intervillous space and dilated veins in the decidua basalis.

VAGINA

The vagina is a distensible muscular tube extending from the vestibule of the female external genitalia to the cervix of the uterus. The lower end of the vagina in the virgin is marked by a transverse semicircular fold or fenestrated membrane, the *hymen*. The wall of the vagina consists of three layers: the mucosa, the muscular coat, and the adventitial connective tissue.

The adventitial coat is a thin layer of dense connective tissue, which merges into the loose connective tissue joining the vagina to the surrounding structures. In this connective tissue there is an extensive venous plexus, nerve bundles, and small groups of nerve cells.

The interlacing smooth muscle bundles of the muscular layer are arranged circularly and longitudinally. The longitudinal bundles are far more numerous, especially in the outer half of the layer. Striated fibers of the bulbocavernosus muscles form a kind of sphincter around the ostium of the vagina.

The mucosa consists of a surface epithelium and an underlying lamina propria. The epithelium is of the stratified squamous variety and has a thickness of 150 to 200 μm. Under normal conditions the superficial cell layers in primates do not show cornification. The nuclei usually remain stainable and the cells become loaded with glycogen. In a prolapsed vagina, when the mucosa is exposed to air, the superficial cells do keratinize like those in the epidermis.

The lamina propria is a moderately dense connective tissue. Toward the muscular layer it becomes looser, and this layer may

be considered a submucosa. In the anterior wall of the vagina, papillae associated with the deep surface of the epithelium are few and small, but in the posterior wall the lamina propria sends numerous papillae far into the covering epithelium. Immediately under the epithelium there is a dense network of fine elastic fibers. From there fine fibers run downward to the muscular layer. Accumulations of lymphocytes are numerous, and sometimes lymph nodules are present. Lymphocytes are always found migrating into the epithelium. The deeper layers of the lamina propria contain a dense plexus of small veins.

There are no glands in the vagina. The mucus lubricating it originates from the glands of the cervix and is made acid by the fermentative action of bacteria on the glycogen from the vaginal epithelium.

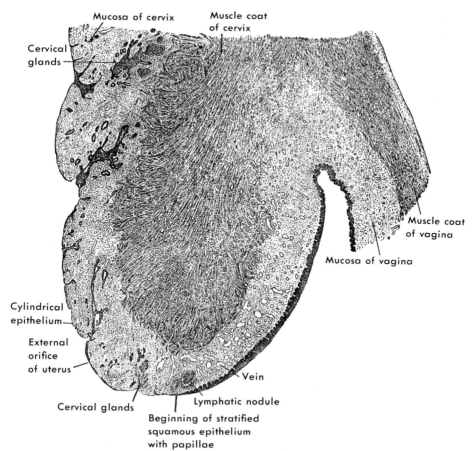

Figure 33-46 Sagittal section through posterior half of the portio vaginalis uteri and the fornix vaginae of a young woman. ×10. (After von Ebner.)

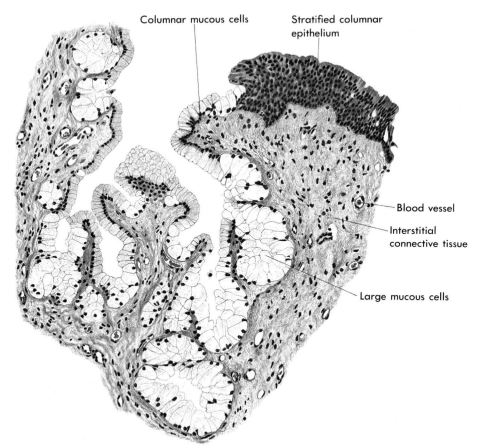

Columnar mucous cells

Stratified columnar epithelium

Blood vessel

Interstitial connective tissue

Large mucous cells

Figure 33–47 Section of gland of Bartholin. A large duct with patches of stratified columnar epithelium gives off smaller branches lined with columnar mucous cells and continuing into tubuloalveolar terminal portions, which are lined with large mucous cells. ×185. (After A. A. Maximow.)

EXTERNAL GENITALIA

The external genital organs of the female comprise the *clitoris*, the *labia majora* and *minora*, and certain glands that open into the *vestibule*, the space flanked by the labia minora.

The *clitoris* corresponds embryologically to the dorsal part of the penis. It consists of two small, erectile, corpora cavernosa ending in a rudimentary *glans clitoridis*. The vagina and the urethra open into the vestibule which is lined with stratified squamous epithelium. Around the opening of the urethra and on the clitoris are several small *vestibular glands* (*glandulae vestibulares minores*). They resemble the glands of Littré in the male urethra and contain mucous cells.

Two larger glands, the *glands of Bartholin* (*glandulae vestibulares majores*), each about a centimeter in diameter, are located in the

lateral walls of the vestibule and open on the inner surface of the labia minora. They are of the tubuloalveolar type, closely corresponding structurally to the bulbourethral glands of the male and secreting a similar lubricating mucus (Fig. 33–47). After the thirtieth year they begin to undergo gradual involution.

The *labia minora* are covered with stratified squamous epithelium and have a core of spongy connective tissue permeated by fine elastic networks. Blood vessels are very numerous. The epithelium contains pigment in its deeper layer and has a thin keratinized layer on the surface. Numerous large sebaceous glands are found on both surfaces. There are no associated hairs (Fig. 33–48).

The *labia majora* are folds of skin containing a large amount of subcutaneous adipose tissue and a thin layer of smooth muscle, corresponding to the tunica dartos of the scro-

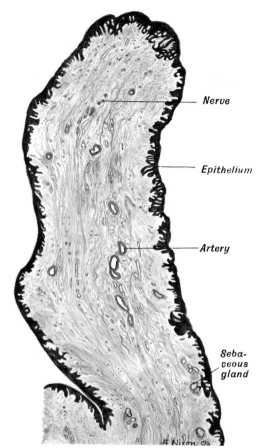

Figure 33–48 Cross section of labium minus of a 34 year old woman.

tum. The outer surface is covered with hair; the inner is smooth and hairless. Sebaceous and sweat glands are numerous on both surfaces.

The outer genital organs are richly supplied with sensory nerve endings. Meissner corpuscles are scattered in the papillae of the epithelium, and genital corpuscles are present in the subpapillary layer. Pacinian corpuscles have been found in the deeper parts of the connective tissue of the labia majora and in the cavernous bodies of the clitoris.

REFERENCES

Adams, E. C., and A. T. Hertig: Studies on guinea pig oocytes. I. Electron microscopic observations on the development of cytoplasmic organelles in oocytes of primordial and primary follicles. J. Cell Biol., *21*:397, 1964.

Adams, E. C., A. T. Hertig, and S. Foster: Studies on guinea pig oocytes. II. Histochemical observations on some phosphatases and lipid in developing and atretic oocytes and follicles. Am. J. Anat., *119*:303, 1966.

Amoroso, E. C.: Placentation. *In* Parkes, A. S. (ed.): Marshall's Physiology of Reproduction. 3rd ed. London, Longmans, Green & Co., Ltd., 1952, Vol. 2, p. 127.

Amoroso, E. C., and C. A. Finn: Ovarian activity during gestation, ovum transport, and implantation. *In* Zukerman, S. (ed.): The Ovary, New York, Academic Press, 1962, p. 451.

Amoroso, E. C.: Histology of the placenta. Brit. Med. Bull., *17*:81, 1961.

Anderson, E., and H. W. Beams: Cytological observations on the fine structure of the guinea pig ovary with special reference to the oogonium, primary oocyte and associated follicle cells. J. Ultrastr. Res., *3*:432, 1960.

Austin, C. R.: The Mammalian Egg. Oxford, Blackwell Scientific Publications, 1961.

Baker, T. G.: A quantitative and cytological study of oogenesis in the rhesus monkey. J. Anat., *100*:761, 1966.

Baker, T. G.: A quantitative and cytological study of germ cells in human ovaries. Proc. Roy. Soc. B. *158*:417, 1963.

Björkman, N.: A study of the ultrastructure of the granulosa cells of the rat ovary. Acta Anat., *51*:125, 1962.

Blanchette, E. J.: A study of the fine structure of the rabbit primary oocyte. J. Ultrastr. Res., *5*:349, 1961.

Blandau, R. J.: Ovulation in the living albino rat. Fertil. Steril., *6*:391, 1955.

Blandau, R. J.: Biology of eggs and implantation. *In* Young, W. C. (ed.): Sex and Internal Secretions. 3rd ed. Baltimore, Williams & Wilkins, 1961, Vol. 2, p. 797.

Blandau, R. J., and K. Moghissi: The Biology of the Cervix. Chicago, University of Chicago Press, 1973.

Brenner, R. M.: Electron microscopy of estrogen effects on ciliogenesis and secretory cell growth in rhesus monkey oviduct. Anat. Rec., *157*:218, 1967.

Brenner, R. M.: The biology of oviductal cilia. *In* Hafez, E. S. E., and R. J. Blandau (eds.): The Mammalian Oviduct. Chicago, University of Chicago Press, 1969, p. 203.

Chiquoine, A. D.: The identification, origin and migration of the primordial germ cells in the mouse embryo. Anat. Rec., *118*:135, 1954.

Corner, G. W.: Ourselves Unborn. New Haven, Yale University Press, 1945.

Crisp, T. M., D. A. Dersouky, and F. R. Denys: The fine structure of the human corpus luteum of early pregnancy and during the progestational phase of the menstrual cycle. Am. J. Anat., *127*:37, 1970.

Crisp, T. M., and C. Channing: Fine structural events correlated with progestin secretion during luteinization of rhesus monkey granulosa cells in culture. Biol. Reprod., *7*:55, 1972.

Danforth, D. N.: The fibrous nature of the human cervix, and its relations to the isthmic segment in gravid and non-gravid uteri. Am. J. Obstet. Gynec., *53*:541, 1947.

Daron, G. H.: The arterial pattern of the tunica mucosa of the uterus in *Macacus rhesus.* Am. J. Anat., *58*:349, 1936.

Decker, A.: Culdoscopic observations on the tubo-ovarian mechanism of ovum reception. Fertil. Steril., *2*:253, 1951.

Doyle, J. B.: Exploratory culdotomy for observation of tubo-ovarian physiology at ovulation time. Fertil. Steril., *2*:474, 1951.

Enders, A. C.: Observations on the fine structures of lutein cells. J. Cell Biol., *12*:101, 1962.

Enders, A. C.: A comparative study of the fine structure of trophoblast in several hemochorial placentas. Am. J. Anat., *116*:29, 1965.

Enders, A. C. and W. R. Lyon: Observations on the fine structure of lutein cells. II. The effects of hypophysectomy and mammotrophic hormones in the rat. J. Cell Biol., *22*:127, 1964.

Everett, J. W.: The mammalian female reproductive cycle and its controlling mechanisms. *In* Young, W. C. (ed.): Sex and Internal Secretions. 3rd ed. Baltimore, Williams & Wilkins, 1961, Vol. 1, p. 497.

Finn, C. A., and D. G. Porter: The Uterus. Handbooks of Reproductive Biology. London, Paul Elek Ltd., 1974.

Gay, V. L., A. R. Midgley, and G. D. Niswender: Patterns of gonadotropin secretion associated with ovulation. Fed. Proc. *29*:1880, 1970.

Gillim, S. W., A. K. Christensen, and C. E. McLennan: Fine structure of human granulosa and theca lutein cells at the stage of maximum progesterone secretion during the menstrual cycle. Anat. Rec., *163*:189, 1969.

Greep, R. O.: Histology, histochemistry and ultrastructure of adult ovary. *In* Smith, D. E. (ed.): The Ovary. Baltimore, Williams & Wilkins, 1962.

Hafez, E. S. E., and R. J. Blandau: The Mammalian Oviduct. Chicago, University of Chicago Press, 1969.

Hertig, A. T.: Gestational hyperplasia of the endometrium. Lab. Invest., *13*:1153, 1964.

Hertig, A. T., and J. Rock: Two human ova of the previllous stage, having an ovulation age of about eleven and twelve days respectively. Carnegie Contributions to Embryol., *29*:127, 1941.

Hertig, A. T., and J. Rock: Two human ova of the previllous stage, having a development age of about seven and nine days respectively. Carnegie Contributions to Embryol., *31*:67, 1945.

Hertig, A. T., J. Rock, E. C. Adams, and W. J. Mulligan: On the preimplantation stages of the human ovum; a description of four normal and four abnormal specimens ranging from the second to the fifth day of development. Carnegie Contributions to Embryol., *35*:199, 1954.

Jost, A.: The role of fetal hormones in prenatal development. The Harvey Lectures, Series 55, 1959–60, p. 201. New York, Academic Press, 1961.

Long, J. A.: Corpus luteum of pregnancy in the rat—ultrastructural and cytochemical observations. Biol. Reprod., *8*:87, 1973.

Markee, J. E.: Menstruation in intraocular endometrial transplants in the Rhesus monkey. Carnegie Contributions to Embryol., *28*:219, 1940.

Moghissi, K. S.: The function of the cervix in fertility. Fertil. Steril., *23*:295, 1972.

Odor, D. L.: Electron microscopic studies on ovarian oocytes and unfertilized tubal ova in the rat. J. Biophys. Biochem. Cytol., *7*:567, 1960.

Odor, D. L.: The ultrastructure of unilaminar follicles of the hamster ovary. Am. J. Anat., *116*:493, 1965.

O'Shea, J. D.: An ultrastructural study of smooth muscle-like cells in the theca externa of ovarian follicles in the rat. Anat. Rec., *167*:127, 1970.

Pinkerton, J. H. M., D. G. McKay, E. C. Adams, and A. T. Hertig: Development of the human ovary—a study using histochemical techniques. Obstet. Gynec. N. Y. *18*:152, 1961.

Price, D.: An analysis of the factors influencing growth and development of the mammalian reproductive tract. Physiol. Zool., *20*:213, 1947.

Ramsey, E. M.: Circulation in the intervillous space of the primate placenta. Am. J. Obstet. Gynec., *84*:1649, 1962.

Ramsey, E. M., and J. W. S. Harris: Comparison of uteroplacental vasculature and circulation in Rhesus monkey and man. Carnegie Contributions to Embryol., *38*:61, 1966.

Rock, J., and A. T. Hertig: Information regarding the time of human ovulation derived from a study of three unfertilized and eleven fertilized ova. Am. J. Obstet. Gynec., *47*:343, 1944.

Snyder, F. F.: Changes in the human oviduct during the menstrual cycle and pregnancy. Bull. Johns Hopkins Hosp., *35*:141, 1924.

Tersakis, J.: The ultrastructure of normal human first trimester placenta. J. Ultrastr. Res., *9*:268, 1963.

Tsafriri, A., H. R. Lindner, V. Zor, S. A. Lamprecht: In-vitro introduction of meiotic division in follicle enclosed oocytes by *LH,* cyclic *AMP,* and prostaglandin E_2. J. Reprod. Fertil., *31*:39, 1972.

Wislocki, G. B., and H. S. Bennett: The histology and cytology of the human and monkey placenta, with special reference to the trophoblast. Am. J. Anat., *73*:335, 1943.

Wislocki, G. B., and G. L. Streeter: On the placentation of the macaque (*Macaca mulatta*) from the time of implantation until the formation of the definitive placenta. Carnegie Contributions to Embryol., *27*:1, 1938.

Witschi, E.: Migration of the germ cells of human embryos from the yolk sac to the primitive gonadal folds. Carnegie Contributions to Embryol., *32*:67, 1948.

Young, W. C. (ed.): Sex and Internal Secretions. 2 vols. 3rd ed. Baltimore, Williams & Wilkins Co., 1961.

Zarrow, M. X., and W. B. O'Connor: Localization of relaxin in the corpus luteum of the rabbit. Proc. Soc. Exp. Biol. Med., *121*:612, 1966.

34
Mammary Gland

The mammary glands are specialized accessory glands of the skin that have evolved in mammals to provide for the nourishment of their offspring, which are born in a relatively immature and dependent state. They are paired glands that are laid down in the embryo along two lines called the *mammary lines*, extending from the axilla to the groin on either side of the midline on the ventral aspect of the thorax and abdomen. Mammary glands may arise anywhere along these lines. The number formed and their location vary with the species. In man only two normally develop, but additional accessory nipples or glandular masses are not uncommon.

In their structure and mode of development, mammary glands somewhat resemble sweat glands. Their differentiation during embryonic life is similar in the two sexes. In the male, however, little additional development occurs in postnatal life, whereas in the female the glands undergo extensive structural changes correlated with age and with the functional condition of the reproductive system. The greatest development of the female breast is reached in about the twentieth year, with atrophic changes setting in by the age of 40 and becoming marked after the menopause. In addition to these gradual changes there are variations in the size of the breasts correlated with the menstrual cycle and striking changes in the amount and functional activity of the glandular tissue during pregnancy and lactation.

Resting Mammary Gland

The mammary gland is a compound tubuloalveolar gland consisting of 15 to 25 irregular lobes radiating from the *mammary papilla* or *nipple*. The lobes are separated by layers of dense connective tissue and surrounded by abundant adipose tissue. Each lobe is provided with a *lactiferous duct* 2 to 4.5 mm. in diameter and lined by stratified squamous epithelium. The duct opens on the nipple and has an irregular angular outline in cross section. Beneath the *areola* (the circular pigmented area around the nipple) each of the ducts has a local dilatation, the *sinus lactiferus*. Distal to this the duct becomes constricted again and emerges at the end of the nipple as a separate opening 0.4 to 0.7 mm. in diameter.

Each lobe is subdivided into lobules of various orders, of which the smallest consist of elongated tubules, the *alveolar ducts*, covered by small saccular evaginations, the *alveoli*. The interlobular connective tissue is dense; the intralobular connective tissue is more cellular and contains fewer collagenous fibers and almost no fat. This intralobular loose connective tissue surrounding the system of ducts is believed to permit greater distensibility when the epithelial portions of the organ hypertrophy during pregnancy and lactation. The secretory portions of the gland, the alveolar ducts and alveoli, consist of cuboidal or low columnar secretory cells resting on a basal lamina and a discontinuous layer of processes of *myoepithelial cells*. The highly branched myoepithelial cells enclose the glandular alveoli in a loosely meshed, basket-like network. They usually lie between the secretory cells and the basal lamina. The presence of myoepithelial cells is interpreted as further evidence that mammary glands are morphogenetically related to sweat glands.

907

There has been much discussion about the presence of alveoli in the nonlactating breast. According to most descriptions of the resting phase, the epithelial structures consist only of ducts and their branches. Some authors, however, believe that the resting breast always has a few alveoli budded off from the ends of the duct system and that these are arranged into small lobules. Part of the difficulty in resolving this question naturally arises from the rarity of the opportunity to obtain normal human breast tissue at known phases of the menstrual cycle. It is clear, however, that early in the cycle the cytoplasmic mass of the epithelial elements is greatly reduced, and there is little or no lumen. In this condition, in which the cells seem to form more or less solid strands, it is not easy to distinguish alveoli from primary ducts. Late in the cycle, the epithelial cells are cuboidal or low columnar, the lumen is evident and contains some secretion, and the surrounding connective tissue stroma is highly vascular. To determine whether these elements are alveolar ducts or alveoli, or both, would require study of serial sections. Because both are potentially secretory, the distinction does not seem an important one. There are microscopically detectable cyclic changes in the terminal ductular and possibly in the alveolar portions of the mammary glands, but these are relatively slight. The gross changes of size, and the sense of engorgement experienced by women at certain times in the cycle, are attributable mainly to hyperemia and some edema of the connective tissue of the breast.

It is to be noted that the mammary gland does not have a single duct. Each lobe is an independent compound alveolar gland whose primary ducts join into larger and larger ducts. These drain into a lactiferous duct, and each of these opens separately at the tip of the nipple. The mammary gland is therefore a conglomeration of a variable number of such independent glands.

Nipple and Areola

The epidermis of the nipple and areola is invaded by unusually long dermal papillae, whose capillaries bring blood close to the surface, imparting a pinkish color to this region in immature and blonde individuals. The skin becomes pigmented at puberty, and the degree of pigmentation increases during pregnancy. An elaborate pattern of bundles of smooth muscle disposed longitudinally along the lactiferous ducts and circumferentially both within the nipple and around its base make it possible for the nipple to become erect in response to certain stimuli. At other times it is flat. In the areola are the accessory *areolar glands of Montgomery*, which are intermediate in their structure between sweat glands and true mammary glands. Along the margin of the areola are large sweat glands and sebaceous glands, which usually lack associated hairs (Fig. 34–1).

The skin at the tip of the nipple is richly innervated with free nerve endings and Meissner's corpuscles in the dermal papillae. There are only very few superficial nerves or nerve end organs on the sides of the nipple or on the areola. This is in contradiction to the widespread notion that nipples and areolae are erogenous areas, highly sensitive to tactile stimulation (Montagna). The skin beyond the areola has neural plexuses around hair follicles, as well as nerve endings resembling Merkel's disks and Krause's end-bulbs. Pacinian corpuscles may also be found deep in the dermis and in the glandular tissue. The innervation of the nipple area is of functional importance, because the stimulus of suckling is required for maintenance of normal lactation.

The Active Mammary Glands

Pregnancy brings about changes in the levels of circulating hormones that result in profound changes in the mammary glands. During the first half of gestation, there is a rapid growth and branching from the terminal portion of the duct system of the resting gland. The growth of epithelial structure takes place, at least in part, at the expense of the interstitial adipose tissue of the breast, which regresses concurrently with the growth of the glandular tissue. There is also, in this period of growth, an increasing infiltration of the interstitial tissue with lymphocytes, plasma cells, and eosinophils. In the later months of pregnancy, the actual hyperplasia of the glandular tissue slows down, and the subsequent enlargement of the breasts is largely a consequence of enlargement of the parenchymal cells and distention of the alveoli with an eosinophilic secretion rich in lactoproteins but relatively poor in lipid. This constitutes the *colostrum*, the first milk that

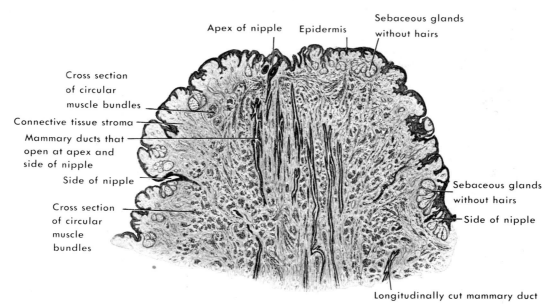

Cross section of circular muscle bundles

Connective tissue stroma

Mammary ducts that open at apex and side of nipple

Side of nipple

Cross section of circular muscle bundles

Apex of nipple

Epidermis

Sebaceous glands without hairs

Sebaceous glands without hairs

Side of nipple

Longitudinally cut mammary duct

Figure 34-1   Nipple of female breast in perpendicular section. × 6. (After Schaffer.)

comes from the breasts after birth. It has special laxative properties and is believed to contain antibodies that provide the newborn with some measure of passive immunity. During the first few days after delivery the degree of infiltration of the stroma of the gland by lymphoid elements becomes less intense, and the colostrum gives way to a copious secretion of milk rich in lipid.

The histological appearance of different parts of the active mammary gland varies considerably (Figs. 34–3 and 34–4). Apparently different areas are not all in the same functional state at the same time. In some places, the secretory portions are filled with milk: their lumen is wide and the walls are dilated and thin. In other areas, the lumen is narrow and the epithelium relatively thick.

The shape of the epithelial cells varies from flat to low columnar. The boundary between them is usually indistinct. If the cells are tall, their distal ends, as in sweat glands, are often definitely separated and project into the lumen of the alveoli as rounded or dome-shaped protrusions. The nucleus may be round or oval and is at about the middle of the cell. If the cells are short, their free surface is usually more or less smooth.

In the cytoplasm are short, rod-shaped mitochondria, few in number in the flattened cells but more plentiful in the taller ones. The cells are generally acidophilic but some basophilic substance may be found at the base of the cells. Droplets of fat, often of large size, accumulate near the free surface and often project into the lumen. After the extraction of fat in preparing histological sections, large clear vacuoles remain in place of the lipid droplets. In addition to the accumulations of lipid, small proteinaceous secretory granules can also be seen in the apical region of the cell. Cyclic changes in the Golgi apparatus during the different phases of secretion have been described. The lumen of the alveoli is crowded with fine granular material and lipid droplets similar to those that protrude from the cells.

The mammary gland was formerly believed to have a mode of release of its product that was intermediate between *merocrine* secretion, in which the secretory materials pass out through the cell apex without appreciable loss of cytoplasm, and *holocrine* secretion, in which the entire cell is given up in contributing its contents to the secretion. The cells of the mammary gland were believed to undergo a partial disintegration in which the fat-filled apical portion of the cell, projecting into the lumen, was described as constricting off from the base of the cell, which remained in place. It was believed that the remainder of

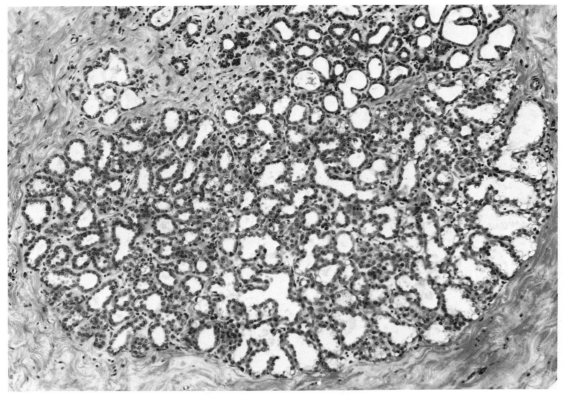

Figure 34–2 Photomicrograph of human mammary gland at eight months of pregnancy.

the cell did not die but rapidly replaced the lost protoplasm and reaccumulated secretion. This mode of release was called *apocrine secretion.* Studies with the electron microscope have now radically changed our views as to the various mechanisms of release of cell products, and it is now doubtful whether the traditional concept of apocrine secretion is still applicable to the mammary gland.

In electron micrographs the main cytological features of the glandular cells are in accord with descriptions resulting from use of the light microscope. The chromophilic areas of the cytoplasm contain cisternal profiles of the granular endoplasmic reticulum. There are a moderate number of mitochondria, a supranuclear Golgi complex, and a number of dense lysosomes. It is evident that the cell has two distinct secretory products, formed and released by different mechanisms. The protein constituents of the milk, like other protein secretions, are elaborated on the ribosome-studded membranes of the

endoplasmic reticulum; they first become visible in the form of moderately dense spherical granules about 400 nm. in diameter in vesicles associated with the Golgi complex. They are transported to the cell surface in these membranous vesicles, which fuse with the plasmalemma and discharge their contained granules into the lumen of the acinus. The mode of formation and release of this particulate component of the milk is therefore identical to that of other protein secreting glands that are generally classified as *merocrine.* The fatty components of the milk do not appear to develop in association with the Golgi apparatus but arise as lipid droplets free in the cytoplasmic matrix. These increase in size and move into the apical region, where they come to project into the lumen covered by a thin layer of cytoplasm. These droplets are ultimately cast off, enveloped by a detached portion of the cell membrane and a thin rim of the subjacent cytoplasm (Fig. 34–8). This mode of release could be considered *apocrine* in the sense that it involves loss of some cytoplasm, but the amount lost is certainly far less than envisioned by the classical cytologists responsible for the term.

Lymphocytes are sometimes encountered among the alveolar epithelial cells. Between these cells and the basal lamina are occasional cells with pale cytoplasm rich in lipid droplets and vacuoles with highly heterogeneous granular and membranous contents. These have been interpreted by some as degenerating epithelial cells, but it seems more likely that they are macrophages.

The myoepithelial cells lie on the epithelial side of the basal lamina. Their processes are filled with parallel arrays of myofilaments 50 Å in diameter. There are spindle-shaped densities among the myofilaments like those found in smooth muscle cells. The cell organelles are concentrated in the perinuclear region of the cell body, but occasional mitochondria and profiles of the endoplasmic reticulum extend into the cell processes. Con-

sidering that myoepithelial cells are derived from the embryonic ectoderm, whereas smooth muscle cells have a mesodermal origin, the cytological characteristics of the two are remarkably similar.

Endocrine Control of Mammary Gland Function

The functioning of the mammary glands is dependent upon the interplay of multiple and complex nervous and endocrine factors. Some are involved in development of the mammary glands to a functional state (mammogenesis), others in the establishment of milk secretion (lactogenesis), and still others are responsible for maintenance of lactation (galactopoiesis).

The primary and secondary ducts that develop during embryonic and fetal life continue to grow in both sexes only in proportion to the growth of the body as a whole, until shortly before puberty, when, in the female, a

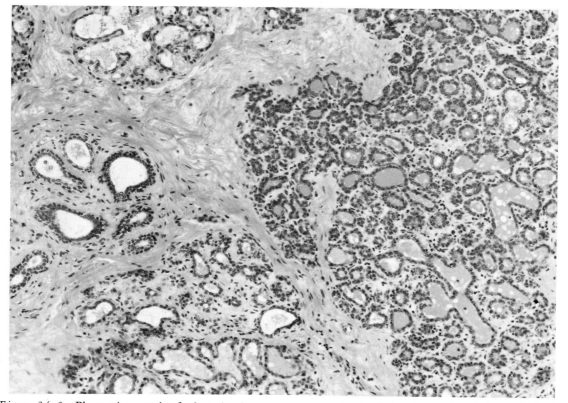

Figure 34–3 Photomicrograph of a lactating human mammary gland. Notice the local variations within the gland. Alveoli in some areas have a large lumen and abundant secretion, whereas in other areas the lumen is very small.

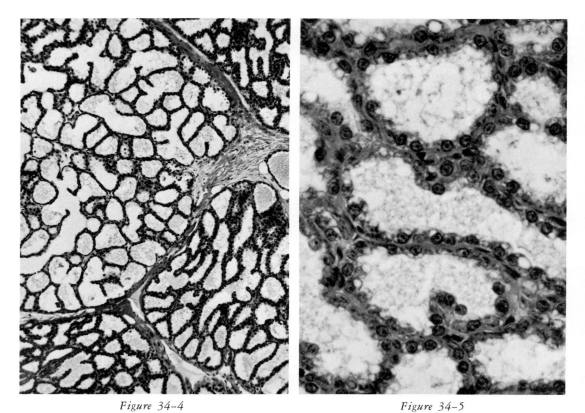

Figure 34-4   *Figure 34-5*

Figure 34-4 Photomicrograph of mammary gland from a lactating cat. Notice the variation from lobule to lobule in the degree of distention of the alveolar ducts and alveoli. × 110.

Figure 34-5 Photomicrograph of lactating cat mammary gland at higher magnification. Large vacuoles can be seen in some of the cells. These represent lipid droplets extracted in specimen preparation. The precipitate in the gland lumen is principally lactoproteins. × 560.

more rapid extension of the duct system begins. This does not take place in the absence of the ovaries. The growth of the duct system thus appears to depend primarily upon estrogen, but for complete development of the alveoli, both estrogen and progesterone are probably required. However, estrogen and progesterone alone fail to produce full mammary development in hypophysectomized animals, and there is now ample evidence that the hypophysis also has a direct effect upon mammary growth by reason of its secretion of *prolactin* and *somatotropin* (STH). Minor effects upon mammary growth have also been traced to indirect effects of *adrenocorticotropic hormone* (ACTH) and *thyrotropic hormone* (TSH), acting upon the adrenal cortex and thyroid. It is now believed that to obtain full morphological development of the gland comparable to that

normally attained in late pregnancy, prolactin, progesterone, estrogen, somatotropin, and adrenal corticoids are all needed (Turner; Cowie and Folley). It should be recalled that the placenta also secretes estrogen, progesterone, and a potent prolactin-like hormone, and no doubt it contributes importantly to the growth stimulus for the mammary glands.

Even in the presence of fully developed prolactational mammary glands, the initiation of milk secretion will not take place in hypophysectomized animals, and in a number of animal species adrenal cortical hormone has also been shown to be essential. Therefore, it is now thought that when the inhibiting levels of circulating estrogen and progesterone fall abruptly at the end of pregnancy, the increased output of prolactin by the hypophysis and the secretion of adrenal cortical steroids bring about milk secretion from the fully developed mammary gland.

Insulin also appears to be involved. Mammary gland explants in organ culture undergo cellular differentiation only if insulin, hydrocortisone, and prolactin are added to the chemically defined culture medium. The alveolar epithelial cells may be induced to divide by insulin in the medium. Addition of hydrocortisone stimulates development of an extensive granular endoplasmic reticulum and enlargement of the Golgi complex. When these changes have taken place, addition of prolactin can then bring about complete differentiation of the cells and can induce synthesis of the specific proteins casein and lactose synthetase (Mills and Topper; Turkington et al.). The regulation of gene expression in mammary epithelial cells in vitro seems to depend upon the sequential action of these hormones. In the absence of any one of them, secretory ultrastructure is not achieved, and there is no augmentation in synthesis of milk proteins.

The continued secretion of prolactin by the hypophysis appears to be necessary for maintenance of lactation, for hypophysectomy results in abrupt cessation of milk pro-

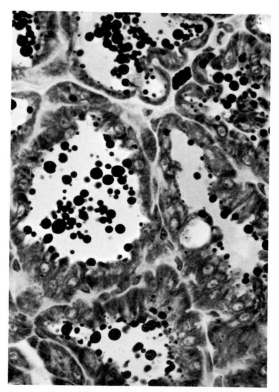

Figure 34-7 Photomicrograph of lactating mammary gland from a mouse, fixed in osmium tetroxide. The large droplets of lipid are preserved both in the apex of the cells and in the lumen of the acini. The smaller protein granules are not visible. × 560. (Preparation by N. Feder.)

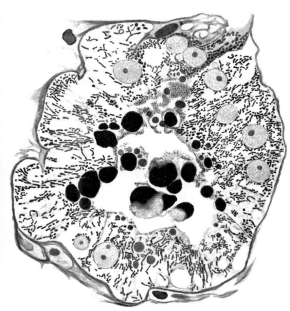

Figure 34-6 Alveolus of lactating mammary gland of a rabbit. The cells contain mitochondria and droplets of fat (stained black with osmic acid). The latter, with the adjacent protoplasm, are extruded into the lumen. × 1000. (After A. A. Maximow.)

duction. The secretion of normal levels of prolactin by intact animals is dependent upon a neurohormonal reflex, in which the periodic sensory stimulus of suckling acts upon supraoptic and paraventricular nuclei in the hypothalamus of the brain to promote the release of prolactin. Interruption of this reflex by denervation of nipples results in failure of lactation.

The discussion until now has been concerned with endocrine stimulated growth of the gland and the initiation and maintenance of secretion. We turn now to the mechanisms for removal of milk from the glands. The milk secreted in the intervals between suckling remains for the most part within the alveoli and alveolar ducts. Only a small proportion passes into the larger ducts and lactiferous sinuses. This small amount can be expressed or withdrawn passively by cannulation of the ducts, but the great bulk of the milk can only be obtained by active participa-

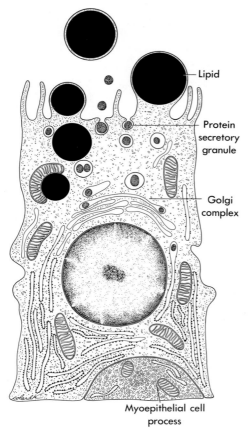

Lipid

Protein secretory granule

Golgi complex

Myoepithelial cell process

Figure 34-8 Diagrammatic representation of a cell from a lactating mammary gland, showing large lipid droplets being cast off enclosed in a layer of cytoplasm, and small granules of protein secretion being concentrated in the Golgi apparatus and released by coalescence of their small vesicles with the plasma membrane. A myoepithelial cell process is depicted in cross section between the epithelial cell and the basal lamina. (Drawing based upon observations of W. Bargmann and A. Knoop, Zeitschr. f. Zellforsch., 49:344, 1959.)

tion of the mother and baby and depends upon the stimulus of suckling, which acts via the hypothalamus to cause release of the hormone *oxytocin* from the neurohypophysis. This in turn stimulates the myoepithelial cells of the gland to contract, ejecting the accumulated milk from the alveoli and fine ducts into the larger ducts and sinuses of the gland.

Regression of the Mammary Gland

If regular suckling is permitted, lactation can be maintained for many months or even for several years. However, if milk is not removed, the glands become greatly distended and milk production quickly ceases. This is in part due to interruption of the neurohormonal reflex mechanism for maintenance of prolactin secretion, but the engorgement of the breasts may also compress the blood vessels, resulting in diminished access of oxytocin to the myoepithelial cells. After a few days the secretion remaining in the alveolar spaces and ducts is absorbed, and the glandular elements gradually return to the resting state. The gland, however, does not return completely to its original state, because many of the alveoli that had formed during the period of pregnancy do not disappear entirely, and the remains of the secretion may sometimes be retained in the mammary ducts for a considerable time. The gland remains in such a resting condition until the following pregnancy, when the same cycle of changes is repeated.

The process of mammary gland regression has been studied mainly in laboratory animals, but the changes are undoubtedly very similar in the human. A few days after weaning, the alveoli are greatly distended with secretory products, and the epithelium is correspondingly flattened. Later there is a gradual collapse of the alveoli and an associated increase in perialveolar connective tissue and adipose tissue. There is an increase in macrophages in the interstitial tissue but no true inflammatory reaction. By 10 days after weaning, the glandular tissue is largely replaced by connective and adipose tissue, and the remaining alveoli appear as scattered solid cords of epithelial cells.

Examined in electron micrographs, the alveolar cells show an early accumulation of intracellular secretory protein in large vacuoles. There is also a marked progressive increase in the number of intraepithelial macrophages. Whereas autophagic vacuoles are rare in the alveolar epithelium of the lactating gland, they rapidly increase in number and size in the first few days after weaning. Their contents include mitochondria, granular reticulum, and secretory granules. There is a concomitant increase in the heterophagic activity of the intraepithelial macrophages. Since they may contain ingested secretory granules, it is concluded that they take up organelles and inclusions from regressing or degenerating epithelial cells. Some of the latter clearly slough in later stages of regression, and these are disposed of by macrophages (Helminen et al.).

Concomitant with the electron microscopic appearance of increases in autophagic and heterophagic vacuoles in the first few days after weaning, there is also a marked increase in activity of the lysosomal enzymes aryl sulfatase, cathepsin D, and acid phosphatase despite the fact that the activity of other nonlysosomal enzymes is declining. Thus, there is apparently a synthesis of new lysosomal enzymes during the early phases of regression.

Involution of the Mammary Gland

In old age, the mammary gland gradually undergoes involution. The epithelium of the secretory portions, and partly also of the excretory ducts, atrophy, and the gland tends, in a general way, to return to the prepubertal condition, in which there are only a few scattered ducts.

On the other hand, the epithelium not

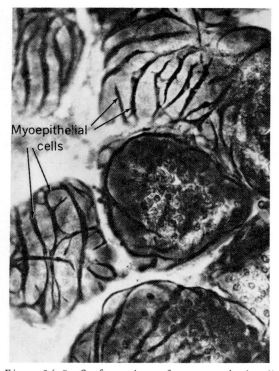

Figure 34-9 Surface view of contracted alveoli from the goat mammary gland, showing silver stained, basket-like processes of the myoepithelial cells. (After K. C. Richardson, Proc. Roy. Soc. B., *136*:30, 1949.)

infrequently is the site of pathological changes. The disorder known as chronic cystic disease is very common in women between 30 and 50 years of age. The terminal ducts and acini may lose their continuity with the remainder of the duct system and form fluid-filled cysts of varying size. The breast is the most common site of cancer among women. About one in every 17 newborn girls (6 per cent) may be expected to develop breast cancer at some time during her life—an incidence 3 times that of cancer of the colon, the second most common type.

Equally striking changes occur in the interstitial connective tissue. This becomes decidedly less cellular; the number of collagenous fibrils decreases, and the whole mass becomes more homogeneous and stains much less intensely with eosin.

Blood and Lymphatic Vessels

The blood supply of a functioning mammary gland is much greater than that of a resting gland. The arteries arise from the anterior thoracic (internal mammary) artery, the thoracic branches of the axillary artery, and the intercostal arteries. They pass mainly along the larger ducts and break up into dense capillary networks on the external surface of the basal lamina of the secretory portions. The veins drain into the axillary and anterior thoracic veins.

The lymphatic vessels begin with capillary networks located in the connective tissue layers surrounding separate alveoli. They collect along the course of the mammary ducts into a subpapillary lymphatic network. From here several large vessels lead the lymph mainly into the lymph nodes in the axilla and subclavicular area, but they also have connections with the lymphatics that penetrate the intercostal spaces to reach parasternal lymph nodes.

Innervation

Noradrenalin-containing nerve fibers are abundant among the smooth muscle cells of the nipple and at the interface between media and adventitia of the arteries of the breast. This is in accord with physiological observations indicating that the efferent nerves to these structures are sympathetic adrenergic. There seems to be no evidence that cholinergic fibers supply any part of the gland.

The majority of mammary nerves follow the arteries and arterioles and supply these structures. A few fibers leave the perivascular networks and lie near the walls of the ducts. They may correspond to sensory fibers for sensing milk pressure, postulated on the basis of behavioral and electrophysiological studies. There is no morphological evidence of a nerve supply to the secretory cells or myoepithelial cells (Hebb and Linzell).

REFERENCES

Bargmann, W., and A. Knoop: Über die Morphologie der Milchsekretion. Licht- und elektronenmikroskopische Studien an der Milchdrüse der Ratte. Zeitschr. f. Zellforsch., 49:344, 1959.

Cowie, A. T., and S. J. Folley: The mammary gland and lactation. *In* Young, W. C. (ed.): Sex and Internal Secretions. 3rd ed. Baltimore, Williams & Wilkins Co., 1961, p. 590.

Dempsey, E. W., H. Bunting, and G. B. Wislocki: Observations on the chemical cytology of the mammary gland. Am. J. Anat., 81:309, 1947.

Foote, F. W., and F. W. Stewart: Comparative studies of cancerous versus non-cancerous breasts. I. Basic morphological characteristics. Ann. Surg., 121:6, 1945.

Gardner, W. U., and G. van Wagenen: Experimental development of the mammary gland in the monkey. Endocrinology, 22:164, 1938.

Hebb, C., and J. L. Linzell: Innervation of the mammary gland. A histochemical study in the rabbit. Histochem. J., 2:491, 1970.

Helminen, H. J., and J. L. E. Ericsson: Studies on mammary gland involution. I. On the ultrastructure of the lactating mammary gland. J. Ultrastr. Res., 25:193, 1968.

Helminen, H. J., and J. L. E. Ericsson: Studies on mammary gland involution. II. Ultrastructural evidence for auto- and heterophagocytosis. J. Ultrastr. Res., 25:214, 1968.

Helminen, H. J., J. L. E. Ericsson, and S. Orrenius: Studies on mammary gland involution. IV. Histochemical and biochemical observations on alterations in lysosomes and lysosomal enzymes. J. Ultrastr. Res., 25:240, 1968.

Hollmann, K. H.: Sur des aspects particuliers des protéines élaboriés dans la glande mammaire. Étude au microscope électronique chez la lapine en lactation. Zeitschr. f. Zellforsch., 69:395, 1966.

Jeffers, K. R.: Cytology of the mammary gland of albino rat. I. Pregnancy, lactation and involution. II. Experimentally induced conditions. Am. J. Anat., 56:257, 179, 1935.

Kon, S. K., and A. T. Cowie: Milk; The Mammary Gland and Its Secretion. New York, Academic Press, 1961.

Miller, M. R., and M. Kasahara: Cutaneous innervation of the human female breast. Anat. Rec., 135:153, 1959.

Mills, E. S., and Y. J. Topper: Some ultrastructural effects of insulin, hydrocortisone and prolactin on mammary gland explants. J. Cell Biol., 44:310, 1970.

Montagna, W.: Histology and cytochemistry of human skin. XXXV. The nipple and areola. Brit. J. Dermat., 83(Suppl.):2, 1970.

Richardson, K. C.: Contractile tissues in the mammary gland, with special reference to myoepithelium in the goat. Proc. Roy. Soc. B, 136:30, 1949.

Turkington, R. W., G. C. Majumder, and M. Riddle: Inhibition of mammary gland differentiation in vitro by 5-bromo-2'-deoxyuridine. J. Biol. Chem., 246:1814, 1971.

Turner, C. D.: General Endocrinology. 4th ed. Philadelphia, W. B. Saunders Co., 1966.

Verley, J. M., and K. H. Hollmann: Synthese et réabsorption des protéines, dans las glande mammaire en stase: Étude autoradiographique au microscope électronique. Zeitschr. f. Zellforsch. 75:605, 1966.

Weatherford, H. L.: A cytological study of the mammary gland: Golgi apparatus, trophospongium and other cytoplasmic canaliculi, mitochondria. Am. J. Anat., 44:199, 1929.

Wellings, S. R., K. B. DeOme, and D. R. Pitelka: Electron microscopy of milk secretion in the mammary gland of the C3H/Crgl mouse. I. Cytomorphology of the prelactating and the lactating gland. J. Nat. Cancer Inst., 25:393, 1960.

Wellings, S. R., B. W. Grunbaum, and K. B. DeOme: Electron microscopy of milk secretion in the mammary gland of the C3H/Crgl mouse. II. Identification of fat and protein particles in milk and in tissue. J. Nat. Cancer Inst., 25:423, 1960.

Wellings, S. R., and J. R. Phelp: The function of the Golgi apparatus in lactating cells of the BALB/cCrgl mouse: An electron microscopic and autoradiographic study. Zeitschr. f. Zellforsch., 61:871, 1964.

35
The Eye

The ability to react to light is a widespread property of living matter, but in complex animals, certain cells are specifically adapted to respond to light. Scattered photoreceptive cells in lower animals probably distinguish only varying intensities of light and only crudely perceive the direction of the light stimuli. Vertebrates have evolved a more efficient organ. A distortion-free image of the visual world is focused on the retina, which not only reacts to various intensities and colors of light, but also encodes spatial and temporal parameters of images for transmission to the brain.

STRUCTURE OF THE EYE IN GENERAL

The anterior segment of the eye, the *cornea*, is transparent, permitting the rays of light to enter. The rest of the wall of the eye is opaque and possesses a darkly pigmented inner surface, which absorbs light rays. The posterior segment of the eye is to a great extent lined with photosensitive nervous tissue, the *retina*, which develops as an outgrowth from the brain. The cavity of the eyeball is filled with transparent media arranged in separate bodies, which, together with the cornea, act as a system of convex lenses. These produce an inverted, reduced image of the objects in the outside world on the photoreceptive layer of the retina.

The wall of the eyeball is composed of three layers: the tough, fibrous, *corneoscleral coat;* the middle, vascular coat, or *uvea;* and the innermost layer, the photosensitive retina. The thick fibrous layer protects the delicate inner structures of the eye and, together with the intraocular fluid pressure, serves to maintain the shape and turgor of the eyeball. It is divided into a large opaque posterior segment, the *sclera,* and a smaller transparent anterior segment, the cornea. The uvea is concerned with the nutrition of the ocular tissues and also provides mechanisms for visual accommodation and control of the amount of light entering the eye. Its three regional differentiations are the *choroid,* the *ciliary body,* and the *iris.* The choroid is the highly vascular portion of the uvea that underlies the photosensitive retina. Extending forward, from the *ora serrata* (the scalloped anterior margin of the photosensitive retina) to the corneoscleral junction, is the *ciliary body.* It forms a belt 5 to 6 mm. wide around the interior of the eyeball and contains the smooth muscle that makes this the instrument of accommodation, acting upon the lens to bring light rays from different distances to focus upon the retina. The iris is a thin continuation of the ciliary body projecting over the anterior surface of the lens, with its free edge outlining the pupil. The diameter of the iris is approximately 12 mm. Its opening, the *pupil,* can be reduced or expanded through the contraction or relaxation of the *constrictor* and *dilator muscles* of the pupil. In this way, the iris functions as an adjustable *optic diaphragm* regulating the amount of light entering the eye (Figs. 35–1 and 35–2).

The innermost tunic, the retina, contains in its sensory part the receptors for light and complex neural networks which elaborate the visual information and send impulses through the *optic nerve* to the brain. The spot where the nerve enters the eyeball, the *papilla* of the optic nerve, is a pink disk approximately 1.4 mm. in dia-

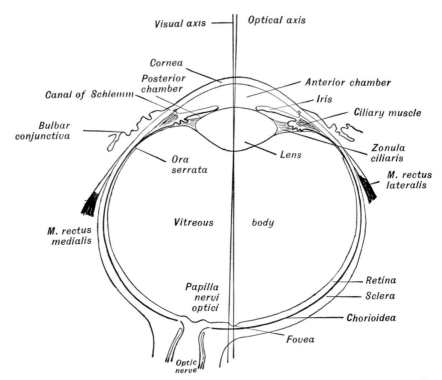

Figure 35–1   Diagram of horizontal meridional section through the right eye of man.

meter and about 3 mm. medial to the posterior pole of the eye. The portion of the retina anterior to the ora serrata and lining the inner surface of the ciliary muscle (*ciliary portion* of the retina) and that lining the posterior surface of the iris (*iridial portion* of the retina) are not photosensitive; these will be discussed with uvea and iris.

The transparent *dioptric media* include the cornea and the contents of the cavity enclosed by the tunics of the eye. Because of the considerable difference between the index of refraction of the cornea (1.376) and of the surrounding air (1.0), the cornea is the chief refractive element of the eye. Of the enclosed transparent media, the most anterior is the *aqueous humor*. It is contained in the *anterior chamber*, a small cavity bounded in front by the cornea and behind by the iris and the central portion of the anterior surface of the lens. The *posterior chamber*, also filled with aqueous humor, is a narrow, annular space enclosed by the lens, the iris, and the ciliary and vitreous bodies (Figs. 35–1 and 35–2).

The next of the transparent media is the *crystalline lens*. This is an elastic biconvex body suspended from the inner surface of the ciliary body by a circular ligament, the *ciliary zonule*. It is placed directly behind the pupil, between the aqueous humor of the anterior chamber anteriorly and the vitreous body posteriorly. The lens is second in importance to the cornea as a refractive element of the eye, and is the dioptric organ of accommodation.

The greater portion of the cavity of the eye, situated between posterior surface of the lens, ciliary body, and retina is the *vitreal cavity*, filled with a viscous transparent substance, the *vitreous humor* or *vitreous body*. It permits light to pass freely from the lens to the photoreceptors.

The retina is transparent during life. Only its outermost layer, the pigment epithelium, is opaque and forms the first barrier to the rays of light.

DIMENSIONS, AXES, PLANES OF REFERENCE

The adult human eyeball is a roughly spherical body about 24 mm. in diameter and

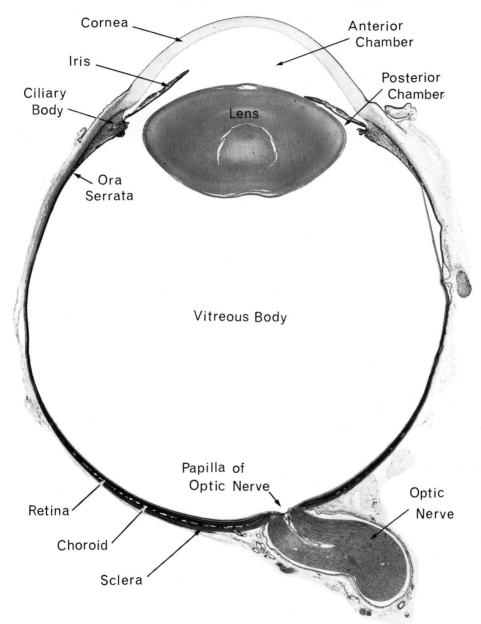

Figure 35-2 Photomicrograph of a meridional section of the eye of a Rhesus monkey. × 10. (Courtesy of H. Mizoguchi.)

weighing 6 to 8 gm. The center of the cornea is the *anterior pole;* the *posterior pole* is located between the *fovea* (the spot of most distinct vision) and the optic papilla. The line connecting the two poles is the *anatomical axis.* The *visual axis* is the line drawn from the center of the fovea to the apparent center of the pupil (Fig. 35–1). The *equatorial plane* is vertical and perpendicular to the visual axis, passing through the greatest expansion of the eyeball, the *equator.* Other planes passing through the axis determine the *meridians* of the eye. The two most important are the vertical and the horizontal meridians. The first passes through the fovea and divides the eyeball, including the retina, into nasal and temporal halves. The plane of the horizontal meridian divides the eyeball and retina into an upper and a lower half. These two planes divide the eyeball and the retina into four quadrants, an upper nasal and an upper temporal, a lower nasal and a lower temporal.

The *anteroposterior diameter* along the axis of the eye is 24 mm., or a little more. The *inner axis,* the distance between the inner surface of the cornea and the inner surface of the retina at the posterior pole, measures a little less than 22 mm. The *optical axis* passes through the optical centers of the refractive media, and is almost identical with the anatomical axis. The visual axis, where it touches the retina, is from 4 to 7 degrees lateral and 3.5 degrees below the optical axis.

The *radius of the curvature* of the large posterior segment around the fundus measures somewhat less than 13 mm., and gradually decreases toward the corneoscleral junction. The cornea has the smallest radius of curvature, approximately 7.8 mm. (outer corneal surface).

The eyeball is lodged in a soft tissue cushion filling the bony orbit of the skull and made up of loose connective and fatty tissue, muscles, fasciae, blood and lymphatic vessels, nerves and a gland. This permits the eye to move freely around its *center of rotation.* The eye is connected to the general integument by the conjunctiva. The lids are a mechanical protection against external noxious agents.

FIBROUS TUNIC

Sclera

The sclera is 1 mm. thick at the posterior pole, 0.4 to 0.3 mm. at the equator, and 0.6 mm. toward the edge of the cornea. It consists of flat collagenous bundles that run in various directions parallel to the surface. Between these bundles are networks of elastic fibers. The cells of the sclera are flat, elongated fibroblasts. Melanocytes also can be found in the deeper layers, especially in the vicinity of the entrance of the optic nerve.

The tendons of the eye muscles are attached to the outer surface of the sclera, which, in turn, is connected with a dense layer of connective tissue—the *capsule of Tenon*—by an exceedingly loose system of thin collagenous membranes separated by clefts—the *space of Tenon.* The eyeball and the capsule of Tenon rotate together in all directions on a bed of orbital fat.

Between the sclera and the choroid is a layer of loose connective tissue with elastic networks and numerous melanocytes and fibroblasts. When these two tunics are separated, part of this loose tissue adheres to the choroid and part to the sclera as its *suprachoroid lamina.*

Cornea

The cornea is slightly thicker than the sclera, measuring 0.8 to 0.9 mm. in the center and 1.1 mm. at the periphery. In man the refractive power of the cornea, which is a function of the index of refraction of its tissue (1.376) and of the radius of curvature of its surface (7.8 mm.), is twice as high as that of the lens.

In a cross section through the cornea, the following layers can be seen: (1) the epithelium, (2) the membrane of Bowman, (3) the stroma, or substantia propria, (4) the membrane of Descemet, and (5) the endothelium or mesenchymal epithelium (Fig. 35–3).

Epithelium. The epithelium is stratified squamous, with an average thickness of 50 μm. It consists, as a rule, of five layers of cells. The outer surface is quite smooth and is composed of large squamous cells. As in other types of stratified squamous epithelium, the cells are connected with one another by many short interdigitating processes that adhere at desmosomes. The cytoplasm contains numerous mitochondria and scattered profiles of granular endoplasmic reticulum in a cytoplasmic matrix filled with randomly oriented fine filaments.

The epithelium of the cornea is extremely sensitive and contains numerous free nerve endings. It is endowed with a remark-

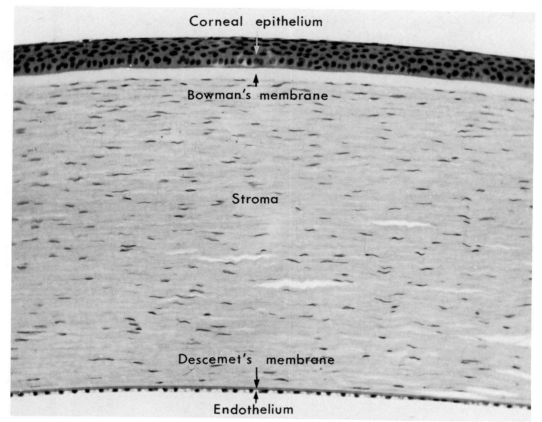

Figure 35–3 Photomicrograph of a section of human cornea. × 160. (After T. Kuwabara, *in* R. O. Greep, ed.: Histology. 2nd ed. New York, McGraw-Hill Book Co., 1966.)

able capacity for regeneration. Minor injuries heal rapidly by a gliding movement of the adjacent epithelial cells to fill the defect. Mitoses in the basal epithelial cells appear later and may be found at considerable distances from the wound. A few mitoses can be found in the basal cell layer under normal conditions.

Bowman's Membrane. The corneal epithelium rests upon a faintly fibrillar membrane of Bowman, 6 to 9 μm. thick. This structure is not actually a membrane but the outer layer of the substantia propria, from which it cannot be separated, but it is nevertheless distinguishable with the optical microscope because its fibers are not so well ordered. With the electron microscope it is seen to consist of a feltwork of randomly arranged collagen fibrils, about 180 Å in diameter, which may show a periodic banding. The membrane does not contain elastin and ends abruptly at the margin of the cornea. Bow-

man's membrane is not present in all mammals; in rabbits the corneal epithelium rests upon a simple basal lamina.

Stroma or Substantia Propria. This layer forms about 90 per cent of the cornea (Fig. 35–3). It is a transparent, regular connective tissue whose bundles form thin lamellae arranged in many layers. In each layer the direction of the bundles changes and those in successive layers cross at various angles (Figs. 35–3 and 35–4). The lamellae everywhere interchange fibers and thus are kept tightly together. The collagen fibrils are somewhat thicker than those in Bowman's membrane, measuring about 230 Å on the average. Between the fibrils, the bundles, and the lamellae, there is a metachromatic glycoprotein ground substance. The substances responsible for its metachromasia are chondroitin sulfate and keratosulfate. The cells of the stroma are long slender fibroblasts (kerato-

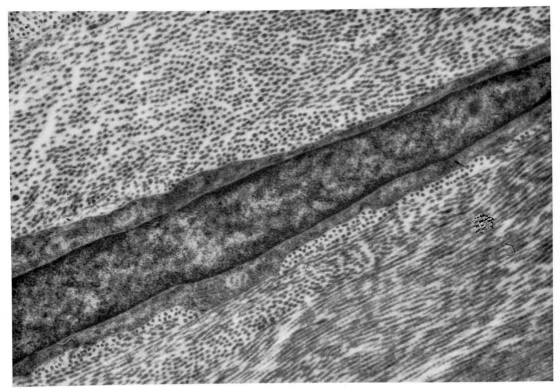

Figure 35–4 Electron micrograph of part of a fibroblast or keratocyte from the cornea and the surrounding layers of collagen fibers at right angles to one another. (Courtesy of M. Jakus.)

cytes) lodged in narrow clefts among the parallel bundles of collagen fibrils. In addition, the stroma always contains a number of lymphoid wandering cells, which migrate from the blood vessels of the corneal limbus. In inflammation, enormous numbers of neutrophilic leukocytes and lymphocytes penetrate between the lamellae.

Membrane of Descemet and Corneal Endothelium. This homogeneous appearing lamella, 5 to 10 μm. thick, can be isolated from the posterior surface of the substantia propria. At the periphery of the cornea, Descemet's membrane continues as a thin layer on the surface of the trabeculae of the limbus. In its structure it is essentially a very thick basal lamina, and it is probably elaborated by the corneal endothelium, which rests upon it (Figs. 35–3 and 35–5). Although it may appear homogeneous under the light microscope, when examined with the electron microscope Descemet's membrane of older individuals may show an apparent cross striation, with bands about 1070 Å apart, con-

nected by filaments less than 100 Å in width and about 270 Å apart (Fig. 35–6A). Tangential sections of such corneas reveal a two dimensional array of nodes, about 1070 Å apart and connected by filaments to form hexagonal figures (Fig. 35–6B). The diagram in Figure 35–7 shows the relationship between the images seen in the two planes. Histochemical data, chemical analyses, and x-ray diffraction studies support the conclusion that the filaments forming this hexagonal array are an atypical form of collagen. In young individuals Descemet's membrane is more homogeneous in appearance. It is suggested that the hexagonal pattern of fibers forms with advancing age by aggregation of collagen that is normally dispersed in the amorphous ground substance as tropocollagen. This and other atypical forms of collagen occur in the membrane at the periphery of the cornea, where randomly oriented fibrous bands with a 1000 Å periodicity are frequently encountered. These are particularly common in *Hassall-Henle bodies* or warts, the dome-shaped protrusions from the periphery of Descemet's membrane into the anterior chamber, which occur with increasing frequency in human eyes after the age of 20.

The inner surface of the membrane of Descemet is covered by a layer of large squamous cells (Fig. 35–5).

Histophysiology of the Cornea

The transparency of the cornea is great, though it is less than that of the aqueous humor. It is due, at least in part, to the uniform diameter and regular spacing of its collagen fibrils, so that scattered rays cancel each other by destructive interference. Glycoproteins of the ground substance may be responsible for the orderly arrangement of the fibrils, since increase in the amount of the interfibrillar fluid, such as occurs in swelling, causes cloudiness of the cornea.

The cornea is avascular, and its central region depends on the aqueous humor for its nourishment. The blood vessels of the limbus supply the peripheral cornea by diffusion and account for the presence, in the corneal stroma, of leukocytes and substances which are excluded from the aqueous humor. Oxygen for the corneal epithelium comes directly from the atmosphere. The contribution of tears to corneal nourishment seems to be negligible.

The cornea is one of the few organs which can be successfully transplanted into allogeneic recipients. One possible explanation for this phenomenon is that the lack of blood vessels protects the transplanted cornea from the host's immune system.

The Limbus

The limbus or sclerocorneal junction is an important region of the eye because it represents a valuable landmark for the ophthalmologist and contains the apparatus for the outflow of the aqueous humor (Figs. 35–8 and 35–9). About 1.5 to 2 mm. wide, its outer surface displays a shallow depression called the *external scleral sulcus*, where the gently curving

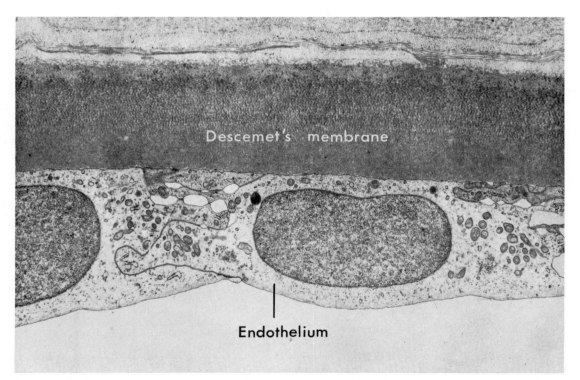

Figure 35–5 Electron micrograph of the endothelium and underlying Descemet's membrane from a human eye. (Courtesy of T. Kuwabara.)

A

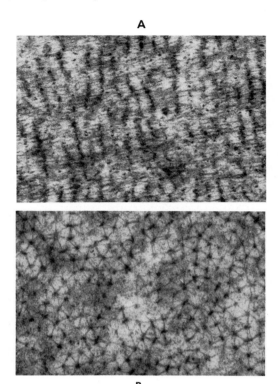

B

Figure 35-6 Electron micrographs of Descemet's membrane, showing the unusual configuration of collagen, characteristic of this layer. *A,* Cross section with its striated appearance. *B,* Tangential section, illustrating hexagonal arrangement of nodes connected by filaments. (Courtesy of M. Jakus.)

sclera is continuous with the more convex cornea. On its inner aspect, the sclerocorneal stroma is marked by a circular depression, the *internal scleral sulcus,* which is filled in by the trabecular meshwork and the canal of Schlemm, specialized tissues constituting the outflow system for the aqueous humor. On the posterior lip of the internal scleral sulcus, the scleral stroma projects toward the interior of the eye, forming a small circular ridge, the *scleral spur;* this affords attachment to the trabecular meshwork anteriorly and to the ciliary muscle posteriorly.

At the limbus, there is a gradual transition of the corneal epithelium into that of the conjunctiva of the bulb (Fig. 35–10). The membrane of Bowman terminates and is replaced by the conjunctival stroma and the anterior margin of the capsule of Tenon. In the connective tissue underlying the epithelium,

the conjunctival vessels form arcades which extend radially into the cornea for about 0.5 mm. beyond the limbal edge. These vessels nourish the periphery of the cornea and supply the corneal stroma with the wandering leukocytes mentioned earlier. The blood vessels that invade the corneal stroma in chronic inflammation arise from these loops. When the limbus is examined in a living subject with the slit-lamp microscope, veins containing aqueous humor instead of blood, also called *aqueous veins,* may be seen emerging from the limbal stroma and emptying into the episcleral veins. At the limbus, the collagenous sclera gradually continues into the corneal stroma and its collagenous bundles progressively acquire the uniform small diameter and orderly arrangement typical of the cornea. Deep to the stroma of the limbus, Descemet's membrane ends and gives way to the spongy tissue of the *trabecular meshwork,* situated between the anterior chamber, the root of the iris, the limbal stroma, and the scleral spur (Fig. 35–11). The trabecular meshwork is composed of a large number of flattened, fenestrated connective tissue sheets or branching and anastomosing beams or trabeculae. These are completely invested by an attenuated endothelium, continuous with the corneal endothelium (Fig. 35–12). They bound a labyrinthine system of minute passages, the intertrabecular spaces, which communicate with the anterior chamber and are filled with aqueous humor.

Interposed between the trabecular meshwork and the limbal stroma is the *canal of Schlemm,* a flattened vessel which extends around the entire circumference of the limbus. The canal of Schlemm has a varicose outline and in places breaks up into irregular branches that coalesce again. The wall of the

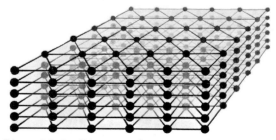

Figure 35-7 Diagram of structure of Descemet's membrane based on electron micrographs. See text for explanation. (Courtesy of M. Jakus.)

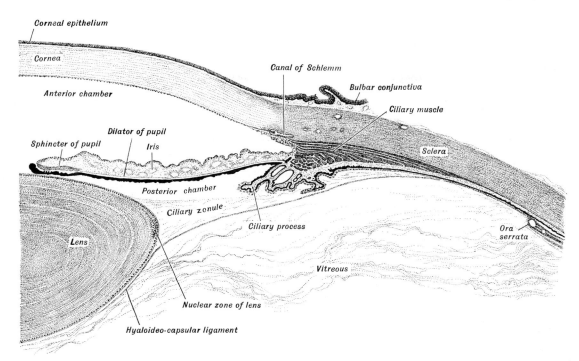

Figure 35–8 Part of meridional section of human eye. × 14. (Modified from Schaffer.)

canal consists of endothelium, a discontinuous basal lamina, and a thin layer of connective tissue. On the outer wall of the canal—that is, toward the limbal stroma—the endothelium is extremely attenuated (Fig. 35–13); on the inner wall of the canal—toward the trabecular meshwork—the endothelium varies greatly in thickness with different techniques of specimen preparation and may display large intra- or intercellular vacuoles. Great importance has been attributed in the past to these "giant vacuoles," for it was believed that they were involved in the process of aqueous humor reabsorption from the anterior chamber. More recent studies, however, seem to suggest that they represent a postmortem artifact.

The lumen of the canal does not communicate directly with the spaces of the trabecular meshwork but is separated from them by the following layers: (1) the endothelium that invests the internal wall of the canal; (2) the connective tissue adventitia of the canal, which here becomes especially rich in stromal cells and is usually referred to as juxtacanali-

cular connective tissue; and (3) the endothelial lining of the trabecular spaces.

From the outer wall of the canal, 25 to 35 channels arise, which join the deep veins of the limbus or pass as aqueous veins to the surface of the limbal stroma and empty into the episcleral veins.

The aqueous humor contained in the anterior chamber permeates the maze of minute intercommunicating passages of the trabecular meshwork; thence, it reaches the lumen of the canal of Schlemm and is finally drained by the episcleral veins. The precise pathway followed by the aqueous humor from the intertrabecular spaces to the lumen of the Schlemm canal is poorly understood. The Schlemm canal usually contains aqueous humor, but it may rarely fill with blood when there is stasis and back pressure in the venous system. Obstruction to the filtration of aqueous humor through the intertrabecular spaces or to its drainage via the canal of Schlemm results in the rise in intraocular pressure characteristic of the serious eye disease *glaucoma*.

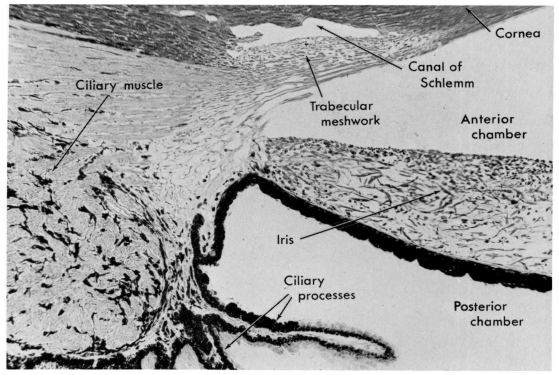

Figure 35-9 Photomicrograph of the sclerocorneal angle of a normal human eye. (Courtesy of T. Kuwabara.)

THE UVEA (THE VASCULAR TUNIC)

Choroid Membrane

The choroid is a thin, soft, brown membrane adjacent to the inner surface of the sclera. Between the sclera and the choroid is a potential cleft, the perichoroidal space; it is traversed by thin lamellae which run obliquely from the choroid to the sclera and form a loose, pigmented tissue layer—the suprachoroid lamina. This is composed of fine, transparent sheets, with fibroblasts on their surface and with a rich network of elastic fibers. Everywhere between and in the connective tissue lamellae, large, flat melanocytes are scattered. In the suprachoroid, as in the rest of the uvea, there are also scattered macrophages. The lamellae of the suprachoroid pass without a distinct boundary into the substance of the choroid proper. This tunic can be subdivided into three main layers. From outside inward, they are: (1) the

vessel layer, (2) the capillary layer, and (3) the glassy membrane or Bruch's membrane (Fig. 35–14).

Vessel Layer. This layer consists of a multitude of large and medium-sized arteries and veins. The spaces between the vessels are filled with loose connective tissue rich in melanocytes. The lamellar arrangement here is much less distinct than in the suprachoroid. According to some, the vessel layer contains strands of smooth muscle independent of the arteries.

Choriocapillary Layer. This is formed by a capillary network arranged in one plane. In places this layer is connected with the vascular layer. The individual capillaries have a large and somewhat irregular caliber; toward Bruch's membrane their endothelium is fenestrated. The net is especially dense and the capillary layer much thicker in the region underlying the fovea. Anteriorly it ends near the ora serrata.

Bruch's Membrane (Glassy Membrane). This is a refractile hyaline layer 1 to

4 μm. thick, between the choroid and the pigment epithelium. The electron microscope has demonstrated that Bruch's membrane is not a homogeneous structure but consists of five different layers: (1) the basal lamina of the endothelium of the capillaries of the choriocapillary layer; (2) a first layer of collagen fibers; (3) a network of elastic fibers; (4) a second layer of collagen fibers; and (5) the basal lamina of the pigment epithelium of the retina.

Ciliary Body

If the eyeball is cut across along its equator, and its anterior half, after removal of the vitreous, is inspected from within, a sharply outlined, dentate border is seen running around the inner surface of the wall in front of the equator (Fig. 35–15). This is the ora serrata or *ora terminalis* of the retina. The zone between the ora and the edge of the lens is

the ciliary body, a thickening of the vascular tunic. Its surface is covered by the darkly pigmented ciliary portion of the retina, which is not photosensitive. In a meridional section through the eye bulb, the ciliary body appears as a thin triangle with its small base facing the anterior chamber of the eye and attached by its outer angle to the scleral spur. The long, narrow angle of its triangular section extends backward and merges with the choroid (Fig. 35–8). The inner surface of the ciliary body is divided into a narrow anterior zone, the *ciliary crown*, and a broader posterior zone, the *ciliary ring*. Seen in surface view, the inner surface of the ring has shallow grooves, *ciliary striae*, which run foward from the teeth of the ora serrata. On its inner surface, the ciliary crown has 70 radially arranged ridges, the *ciliary processes* (Figs. 35–8, 35–9, and 35–15).

The main mass of the ciliary body, exclusive of the ciliary processes, consists of the

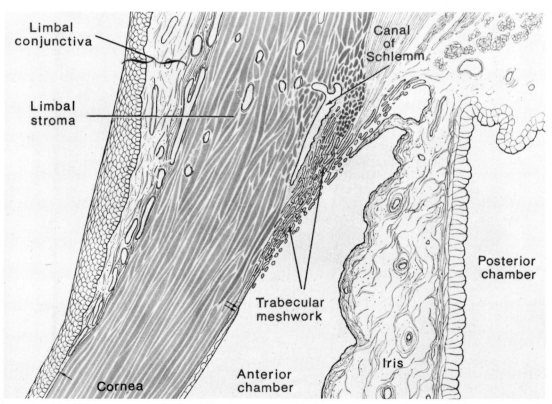

Figure 35–10 Diagram of the limbus. Single arrow, end of Bowman's membrane; double arrow, end of Descemet's membrane. (After Hogan, M. Y., et al., Histology of the Human Eye. Philadelphia, W. B. Saunders Co., 1971.)

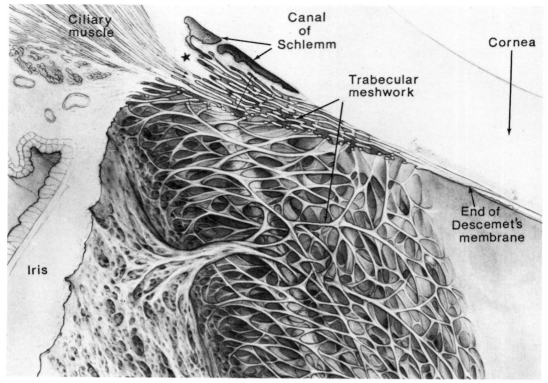

Figure 35-11 Diagram of the outflow system of the aqueous humor. Star indicates scleral spur. (After Hogan, M. Y., et al., Histology of the Human Eye. Philadelphia, W. B. Saunders Co., 1971.)

muscle of accommodation, or *ciliary muscle*. It is smooth muscle and is composed of three portions. Closest to the sclera is the *muscle of Brücke*, whose bundles are deployed chiefly in the meridional direction. This outer part of the ciliary muscle stretches the choroid and is also called the *tensor muscle of the choroid*. In the next inward portion of the ciliary muscle, the bundles of muscle cells radiate fanlike from the region of the scleral spur toward the cavity of the eyeball. This is the *radial or reticular portion* of the ciliary muscle. The third or *circular portion* of the ciliary muscle (*Müller's muscle*) is usually absent in the newborn, appearing in the course of the second or third year. The contraction of this portion relaxes the tension on the lens and thus is important in accommodation for near vision. More recently, the classical subdivision of the ciliary muscle into three portions has been challenged as too schematic; the muscle fibers seem to be interwoven in a tridimensional network, with regions of prevailing meridion-al, radial, and circular orientation. The interstices between the muscular bundles are filled with a small amount of connective tissue containing abundant elastic fibers and melanocytes (Fig. 35-9). The latter become especially numerous toward the sclera, where the connective tissue gradually passes into the lamellae of the suprachoroid.

The inner, *vascular layer of the ciliary body* consists of connective tissue with numerous blood vessels. In the ciliary ring it is the direct continuation of the same layer of the choroid. In the region of the ciliary crown it covers the inner surface of the ciliary muscle and forms the core of the ciliary processes. The vessels are almost exclusively capillaries and veins of varying caliber. The corresponding arteries ramify in the peripheral layers of the ciliary body. The capillary endothelium is fenestrated and freely permeable to plasma proteins. The connective tissue is dense, especially near the root of the iris, and contains abundant elastic fibers. In old age it often shows hyaline degeneration. Melanocytes are usually found only near the surface of the muscle.

The ciliary portion of the retina continues forward beyond the ora serrata and as the *ciliary epithelium* invests the inner surface of the ciliary body; its function is the production of the aqueous humor. The ciliary epithelium consists of two layers of cells, an inner layer of nonpigmented elements bounding the posterior chamber, and an outer pigmented layer, which rests on the stroma of the ciliary body (Fig. 35–16). Toward the root of the iris, the cells of the inner epithelial layer gradually accumulate pigment granules. Because of the embryonal origin of the ciliary epithelium from the edge of the doubled walled optic cup, the pole of the nonpigmented cells directed toward the interior of the eye is usually referred to as the cell base, whereas the base of the pigmented cells corresponds to the pole which adjoins the stroma of the ciliary body; thus, the apices of the pig-

mented and nonpigmented epithelial cells face each other.

A basal lamina invests both surfaces of the ciliary epithelium; that toward the stroma of the ciliary body is continuous with the basal lamina of the pigment epithelium of the retina; the other lamina is continuous with the inner limiting membrane of the retina.

The basal and lateral regions of the nonpigmented cells are occupied by a labyrinth of interdigitating processes formerly called "membrane infoldings" (Fig. 35–17). In this respect, the nonpigmented cells resemble other epithelial elements actively engaged in transport of ions and water. Between the central nucleus and the cell apex is the cell center, consisting of a well developed Golgi apparatus, a centriole, and occasionally a cilium, which protrudes from the cell surface in a channel bounded by the plasma membrane. The cytoplasm is permeated by flat cisternae of the granular endoplasmic reticulum, tubules of the agranular reticulum, and

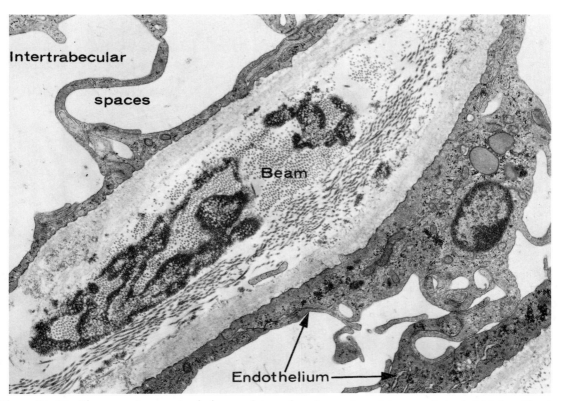

Figure 35–12 Electron micrograph of a beam of the trabecular meshwork in a monkey. A thick basal lamina separates the connective tissue core of the beam from the investing endothelium. The intertrabecular spaces are criss-crossed by processes of the endothelial cells. × 8600. (From Raviola, G., Invest. Ophthalm., *13*:828, 1974.)

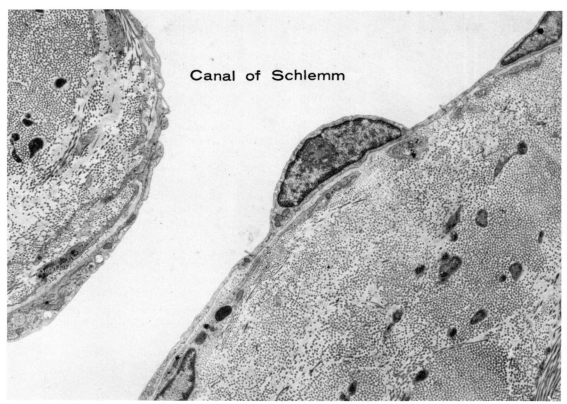

Figure 35-13 Canal of Schlemm in a monkey. The external wall of the canal consists of an attenuated endothelium, a discontinuous basal lamina, and an adventitial layer of flattened fibroblasts. The collagen fibrils of the limbal stroma are seen in cross section. × 6200. (From Raviola, G., Invest. Ophthalm., *13*:828, 1974.)

bundles of filaments radiating from the desmosomes which join adjacent cells. The mitochondria are not especially numerous, nor do they appear to be arranged in an orderly manner with respect to the plasmalemmal invaginations, as is the case for the convoluted tubules of the kidney or the striated ducts of the salivary glands. Especially prominent in the pigmented epithelial cells are the melanin granules, which completely fill the cytoplasm, leaving but little space for a moderate number of mitochondria and thin bundles of filaments. The nucleus is located toward the apex of the cell, being separated from it by a small Golgi apparatus. The plasma membrane at the base of the cell is repeatedly invaginated, but the basal labyrinth is not as complex as in nonpigmented cells.

The ciliary epithelium is exceptional among actively transporting epithelia because it consists of two layers of cells, both provided with a basal labyrinth of interdigitating processes. These structural specializations suggest that the ciliary epithelium represents a unique biological device, consisting of two pumps working in series. This might result in a considerable amplification of the transport efficiency, but it requires accurate synchronization of the cells' activity. Gap junctions probably ensure such a precise coordination of the function of the myriad independent cell units; they connect adjacent pigmented cells, adjacent nonpigmented cells, and the confronted apices of the pigmented and nonpigmented cells. Furthermore, the lateral surfaces of the nonpigmented cells are connected to each other by an elaborate zonula occludens, a zonula adherens, and a few desmosomes.

Aqueous Humor and the Blood-Aqueous Barrier

Proper eye functioning requires a precise spatial arrangement of the retina with respect to the refractive media and a special chemical composition of the intraocular fluids, optimally adjusted to the metabolic needs of the retina, lens, and cornea. The aqueous humor subserves both of these functions. An accurate balance between its rates of production and reabsorption is responsible for maintenance of the intraocular pressure, which confers mechanical stability upon the ocular structures. Its specific composition, differing from plasma and somewhat resembling cerebrospinal fluid, cooperates with the blood-retinal barrier in generating an extracellular environment best suited to the functional requirements of the cells of the retina, lens, and cornea. Finally, it nourishes the lens, which lacks a blood supply. The aqueous humor is a clear, watery fluid of slightly alkaline reaction with an index of refraction of 1.33, contained in the anterior and posterior chambers of the eye. In its chemical composition, the aqueous humor differs from blood plasma in its lower content of proteins, higher content of ascorbate, pyruvate, and lactate, and lower content of urea and glucose. Also, its electrolyte content is slightly different from that of the plasma. Continuously secreted by the ciliary epithelium, probably through a process of active transport, it fills the posterior chamber, nourishes the lens, and permeates the vitreous body. From the posterior chamber, it flows into the anterior chamber through the pupil and is finally drained through the trabecular meshwork and canal of Schlemm. The flow of the aqueous humor is determined by the difference in pressure between the fluids within the eye (about 20 mm. Hg) and the pressure in the episcleral veins (about 13 mm. Hg); in turn, the intraocular pressure is generated by an accurate adjustment of the rate of aqueous humor secretion by the ciliary epithelium and its rate of reabsorption at the limbus. When this balance is disrupted, as in glaucoma, the intraocular pressure increases, with devastating effects on the function of the eye.

Secretion of a fluid with a composition different from that of the plasma, such as the

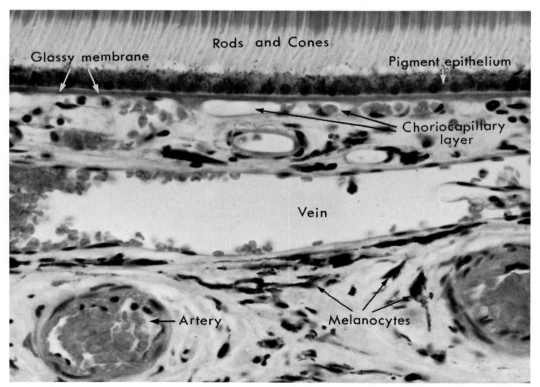

Figure 35–14 Photomicrograph of choroid and outermost layers of the retina. (After T. Kuwabara, *in* R.O. Greep, ed.: Histology. 2nd ed. New York, McGraw-Hill Book Co., 1966.)

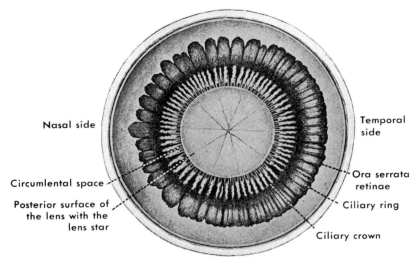

Nasal side

Temporal side

Circumlental space

Posterior surface of the lens with the lens star

Ora serrata retinae

Ciliary ring

Ciliary crown

Figure 35–15 Anterior half of the right eye, seen from within. × 3. (After Salzmann.)

aqueous humor, is possible only if free diffusion of solutes between blood and the chambers of the eye is prevented. This is the role of the so-called *blood-aqueous barrier,* the peculiar physiological mechanism which limits the exchange of materials between the vascular compartment and the interior of the eye. When an ultrastructural tracer, such as horseradish peroxidase, is injected into the bloodstream, it rapidly diffuses across the permeable walls of the vessels of the ciliary body, permeates the stroma underlying the ciliary epithelium, and is finally blocked by the tight junctions which connect the apices of the nonpigmented cells (Fig. 35–16). These junctions, which limit free movement of molecules between ciliary body stroma and posterior chamber, are therefore believed to represent the major anatomical site of the blood-aqueous barrier.

Iris

The posterior surface of the iris near the pupil rests upon the anterior surface of the lens; in this way the iris separates the anterior chamber from the posterior chamber. The margin of the iris connected with the ciliary body is called the *ciliary margin,* or the root of the iris. The pupil is surrounded by the *pupillary margin of the iris.* The iris diminishes in thickness toward both margins. Besides its individually varying color, the anterior surface of the iris presents certain distinct mark-

ings. About 1.5 mm. from the pupillary margin, a jagged line concentric with the pupillary margin separates the anterior surface into a *pupillary zone* and a wider *ciliary zone.* Near the pupillary and the ciliary margins the anterior surface has many irregular excavations, the *crypts,* which may extend deep into the tissue. In addition, there are oblique, irregularly arranged contraction furrows, which are especially marked when the pupil is dilated.

The main mass of the iris consists of a loose, pigmented, highly vascular connective tissue. The anterior surface of the stroma is said to be lined with a discontinuous layer of fibroblasts and melanocytes. A thin layer of stroma immediately beneath this cell investment, the *anterior stromal sheet* or lamella, is devoid of blood vessels. Deep to this is a layer containing numerous vessels, which have walls unusually thick for their diameter. The posterior surface of the iris is covered with a double layer of heavily pigmented epithelium, the iridial portion of the retina (Figs. 35–9 and 35–18).

The anterior stromal sheet or lamella contains a few collagenous fibers and many fibroblasts and melanocytes in a homogeneous ground substance. The color of the iris depends on the quantity and the arrangement of the pigment and on the thickness of the lamella. If this layer is thin and its cells contain little or no pigment, the black pigment epithelium on the posterior surface, as seen through the colorless tissue, gives the iris a blue color (Fig. 35–19). An increasing amount of pigment brings about the different shades of gray and greenish hues. Large amounts of dark pigment cause the brown color of the iris. In albinos, the pigment is absent or scanty, and the iris is pink because of its rich vascularity.

The epithelial pigment layer on the posterior surface of the iris is a direct continuation of the ciliary portion of the retina and, like it, originally consists of two layers of epithelium. The inner, nonpigmented layer of the ciliary portion of the retina becomes heavily pigmented in the iridial region with dark brown melanin granules that obscure the cell outlines. The posterior or inner surface is covered by the *limiting membrane of the iris*, a typical basal lamina. The outer or anterior pigmented layer becomes less pigmented. These outer epithelial cells derived from the outer wall of the embryonic optic cup undergo a remarkable transformation into contractile elements—the myoepithelium of the dilator pupillae.

Being an adjustable diaphragm, the iris contains two muscles that keep the membrane stretched and hold it against the surface of the lens. The contraction of the circular sphincter of the pupil reduces the diameter of the pupil. It is a thin, flat ring surrounding the margin of the pupil. Its breadth changes, according to the contraction of the iris, from 0.6 to 1.2 mm. Its smooth muscle fibers are arranged in thin, circumferentially oriented bundles. The dilator of the pupil opens the pupil and consists of radially arranged myoepithelial elements, which form a thin membrane between the vessel layer and the pigment epithelium (Fig. 35–20).

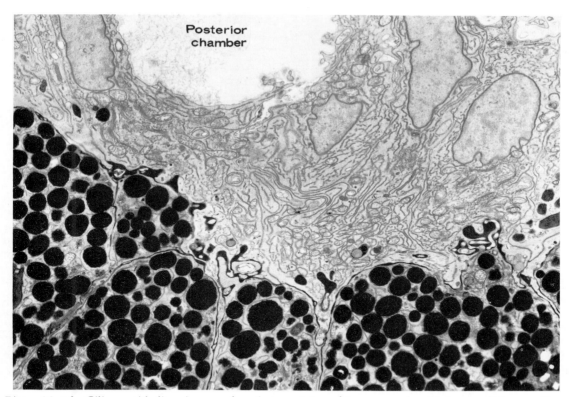

Figure 35–16 Ciliary epithelium in a monkey that was injected intravenously with horseradish peroxidase. The ciliary epithelium consists of two cell layers, one nonpigmented (above), which bounds the posterior chamber; the other pigmented (below), which rests on the stroma of the ciliary body. The tracer escaped through the permeable walls of the vessels of the ciliary body and has permeated the intercellular clefts between pigmented and nonpigmented cells, but its further progression toward the posterior chamber is blocked by an impermeable tight junction, which connects the apices of the nonpigmented cells. × 6400. (From Raviola, G., Invest. Ophthalm., *13*:828, 1974.)

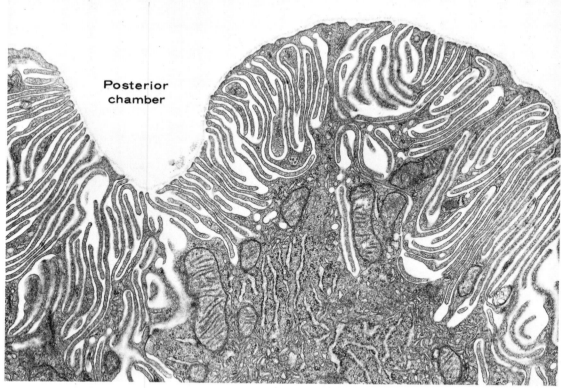

Posterior chamber

Figure 35–17 Electron micrograph of the ciliary epithelium of a rabbit. The base of the nonpigmented cells is occupied by a complex labyrinth of interdigitating processes. The basal lamina which separates the ciliary epithelium from the content of the posterior chamber is barely visible. × 18,000. (Courtesy of G. Raviola.)

The innervation of the two muscles is quite different. The dilator is innervated by sympathetic postganglionic neurons located in the superior cervical ganglion. Their axons pass to the gasserian ganglion, thence into the ophthalmic branch of the latter, and finally reach the dilator muscle through the long ciliary nerves. The sphincter muscle is innervated by parasympathetic fibers from postganglionic neurons located in the ciliary ganglion, and their axons reach the sphincter with the short ciliary nerves. The sympathetic and parasympathetic divisions of the autonomic nervous system thus have opposite effects upon the pupil. On the other hand, the sphincter and the ciliary muscles, which are both innervated by the short ciliary nerves, work in concert. When the eye accommodates for near vision by contraction of the ciliary muscle, there is always a simultaneous contraction of the pupillary sphincter.

In electron micrographs, the axons among the contractile elements of the sphincter pupillae are seen to be packed with agranular "synaptic" vesicles typical of cholinergic axons. Axons associated with the dilator muscle contain a mixture of granular and agranular vesicles typical of the endings of adrenergic sympathetic nerve fibers.

An accurate adjustment of the size of the pupil modifies the amount of light entering the eye, thus permitting useful vision over a wide range of light intensities. Furthermore, as the pupil constricts in brilliant light, the depth of focus of the dioptric media is increased, and aberrations are minimized.

REFRACTIVE MEDIA OF THE EYE

The cornea and the anterior and posterior chambers of the eye have been described.

The other components of the refractive apparatus of the eye are the crystalline lens and vitreous body.

Lens

The lens is a transparent, biconvex body situated immediately behind the pupil. Its shape changes during the process of accommodation. Its outer form varies somewhat in different persons and also with age. Its diameter ranges from 7 mm. in a newborn to 10 mm. in an adult. Its thickness is approximately 3.7 to 4 mm., increasing during accommodation to 4.5 mm. and more. The posterior surface or pole is more convex than the anterior, the respective radii of curvature being 6.9 and 10 mm. The index of refraction is 1.36 in the peripheral layers and 1.4 in the inner zone. The lens weighs 0.2 gm. and is slightly yellow.

The lens is covered with a homogeneous, highly refractive *capsule*, an 11 to 18 μm. carbohydrate-rich coating on the outer surface of the layer of flattened or cuboidal cells comprising the epithelium of the lens (Figs. 35–21 and 35–22). Toward the equator of the lens these cells approach a columnar form and become arranged in meridional rows. Becoming progressively elongated, the cells at the equator are transformed into *lens fibers* that constitute the bulk of the substance of the lens. In this transition or *nuclear zone* the cells have a characteristic arrangement. The epithelial cells are of prime importance for the normal metabolism of the lens. The capsule covering the posterior pole has no underlying epithelium.

In the human lens, each fiber is a six-sided prism, 7 to 10 mm. long, 8 to 12 μm. wide, and only 2 μm. thick (Fig. 35–23). In the region of the nucleus the thickness may reach 5 μm. The prismatic fibers of the cortical zone of the lens are hexagonal in cross section, when the closely apposed cell surfaces are quite straight. It was formerly thought that a cementing substance between the lens fibers acted as a lubricant, permitting movement of the fibers with respect to one another during accommodation. No appreciable intercellular space is found, however, in electron micrographs. The cell surfaces are about 150 Å apart and attached by numerous gap junctions. The cells of the lens epithelium and the fibers of the equatorial region both exhibit complex interdigitations of their surfaces. This is particularly marked at the "sutures," where cortical fibers from opposite sectors of the lens converge (Fig. 35–23). Since these interdigitations occur principally in the anterior curvature, periaxial zone, and equator—those regions that undergo the greatest dimensional changes—it has been suggested that their presence may be associated with changes of fiber shape in the mechanism of intracapsular accommodation (Wanko and Gavin).

The lens fibers have a finely granular cytoplasm, with a few small vesicles scattered through the ectoplasmic region of the cell and occasional mitochondria in the vicinity of the sutures, but in general the organelles and inclusions are exceedingly sparse (Fig. 35–24).

The lens is held in position by a system of fibers constituting the *ciliary zonule*. The zon-

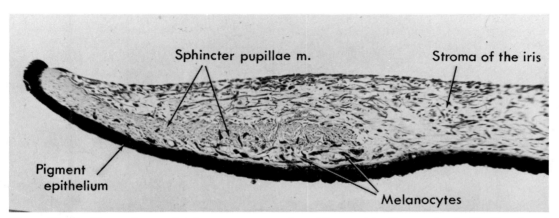

Figure 35–18 Photomicrograph of a transverse section of human iris. (Preparation by T. Kuwabara.)

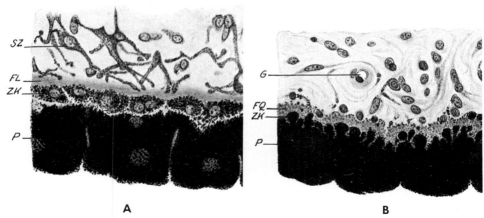

A　　　　　　　　　　　　　　　**B**

Figure 35-19　Sections of human iris. *A*, Posterior part of a radial (meridional) section of a dark human iris, from an enucleated eyeball. *FL*, Fibrillae of the dilator muscle in longitudinal section; *P*, pigment epithelium of the inner (posterior) layer of the iridial portion of the retina; *SZ*, pigment-containing connective tissue cells (melanocytes) of the vascular layer; *ZK*, pigment-containing cell bodies of the dilator muscle (outer or anterior layer of the iridial portion of the retina). *B*, Tangential section of a light human iris. *FQ*, Fibers of the dilator muscle in cross section; *G*, blood vessel in the stroma; other symbols as in *A*. × 380. (After Schaffer.)

ule fibers (Fig. 35–8) arise from the epithelium of the ciliary portion of the retina. Near the ciliary crown they fuse into thicker fibers and finally form about 140 bundles. At the anterior margin of the ciliary processes they leave the surface of the ciliary body and radiate toward the equator of the lens. The larger ones are straight and reach the capsule in front of the equator of the lens *(anterior zonular sheet)*. The thinner fibers assume a slightly curved course and are attached to the posterior surface of the lens *(posterior zonular sheet)*. All zonular fibers break up into a multitude of finer fibers, which fuse with the substance of the outermost layer of the capsule (Fig. 35–22). With the electron microscope, the zonular fibers appear as bundles or sheets of exceedingly fine filaments, 110 to 120 Å in diameter, which have a hollow appearance in cross section (Fig. 35–25). They are digested with elastase, but not by collagenase, and have an amino acid composition different from collagen. They are probably identical to the microfibrils embedded in the elastic fibers of other organs. Where the vitreous body touches the lens capsule, it forms the *hyaloideocapsular ligament*.

The radii of curvature of the surfaces of the several dioptric media of the normal eye, especially of the lens, and their indices of refraction are such that light rays coming from a remote point form an inverted and real image of the object in the layer of the photoreceptive cones and rods in the retina. If the object is approaching, the light rays diverge more and more, and the image moves backward. A change of position of an object from infinite distance to about 5 meters causes the image to shift about 60 μm. backward in the retina. Since this image is still within the outer segments of the rods and cones, accommodation is not needed. For nearer distances, accommodation is necessary.

In a camera the focusing of objects that move nearer to the lens is effected by moving the ground glass plate away from the lens. In the higher vertebrates and in man, the curvature of the lens is changed. When the eye is at rest, the lens is kept stretched by the ciliary zonule in the plane vertical to the optic axis. When the eye has to focus on a near object, the ciliary muscle contracts—its meridional fibers pull the choroid and the ciliary body forward, whereas its circular fibers, acting as a sphincter, move the ciliary body toward the axis of the eye. This relieves the tension on the zonule; the lens gets thicker, and its surface, especially at the anterior pole, becomes more convex. This increases the refractive power of the lens and keeps the focus within the photoreceptor layer.

Vitreous Body

The vitreous body fills the vitreal cavity between the lens and the retina. It adheres everywhere to the optical portion of the retina, and the connection is especially firm at the ora serrata. Farther forward, it gradually recedes from the surface of the ciliary portion of the retina.

The fresh vitreous body is a colorless, structureless, gelatinous mass with a glasslike transparency. Its index of refraction is 1.334. Nearly 99 per cent of the vitreous body consists of water. A liquid and a solid phase can be distinguished in it; the liquid phase contains hyaluronic acid in the form of long, coiled molecules enclosing large amounts of water; the solid phase is collagen in the form of thin fibrils that lack the usual 640 Å periodicity, and are arranged in a random network. The hyaluronate of the liquid phase is joined to the collagen network by weak bonds. The peripheral region of the vitreous body or cortex has more collagen fibrils and hyaluronate than the central region and contains cells, called *hyalocytes*, which may be concerned with the synthesis of collagen and hyaluronic acid. Macrophages are also occasionally found.

Extending through the vitreous body from the papilla of the optic nerve to the posterior surface of the lens is the *hyaloid canal* (canal of Cloquet). It is a residue remaining after the resorption of the embryonic hyaloid artery. It has a diameter of 1 mm. and is filled with liquid. In the living, especially in young persons, it is visible with the help of the slit lamp microscope.

THE RETINA

The retina (Fig. 35–26) is the innermost of the three coats of the eyeball and is the photoreceptor organ. It arises in early embryonic development from a bilateral evagination of the prosencephalon, the *primary optic vesicle*. Later it is transformed by local invagination into the *secondary optic vesicle*. Each optic cup remains connected with the brain by a stalk, the future optic nerve. In the adult, the derivatives of the bilaminar secondary optic vesicle consist of an outer, pigmented epithelial layer, the *pigment epithelium*, and an inner sheet, the *neural retina* or *retina proper*. The latter contains elements similar to those of the brain, and it may be considered to be a specially differentiated part of the brain.

The *optical* or *functioning portion of the retina* lines the inner surface of the choroid and extends from the papilla of the optic nerve to the ora serrata anteriorly. At the papilla, where the retina continues into the tissue of the nerve, and at the ora serrata, the retina is firmly connected with the choroid. In the retina, exclusive of the fovea, the papilla, and the ora serrata, 10 parallel layers can be distinguished from outside inward (Figs. 35–27 and 35–28): (1) the pigment epithelium; (2) the layer of rods and cones (bacillary layer); (3) the outer limiting membrane; (4) the outer nuclear layer; (5) the outer plexiform layer; (6) the inner nuclear layer; (7) the inner plexiform layer; (8) the layer of ganglion cells; (9) the layer of optic nerve fibers; and (10) the inner limiting membrane. About 2.5 mm. lateral to the border of the optic papilla, the inner surface of the retina shows a shallow, round depression, the fovea

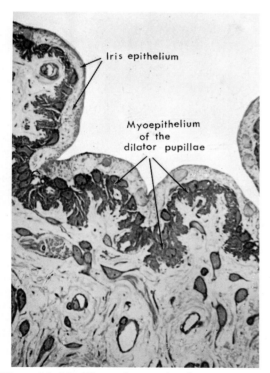

Figure 35–20 Photomicrograph of transverse section through the posterior surface of albino rabbit iris, showing the pale cuboidal iris epithelium and the underlying dark-staining myoepithelium of the dilator pupillae muscle. × 480. (After K. C. Richardson, Am. J. Anat., *114*:173, 1964.)

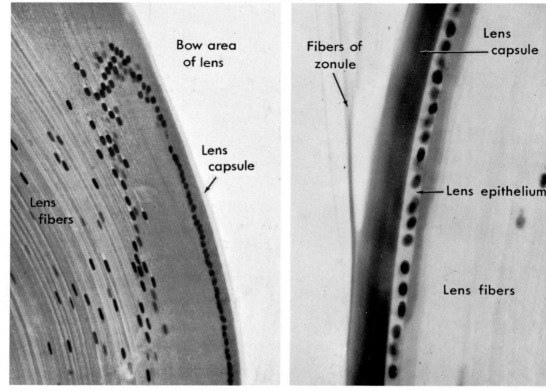

Figure 35–21

Figure 35–22

Figure 35–21 Photomicrograph of the bow area of the human lens, where the epithelial cells become greatly elongated to form lens fibers. (Courtesy of T. Kuwabara.)

Figure 35–22 Photomicrograph at higher magnification of human lens stained with the periodic acid–Schiff reaction. The lens capsule overlying the epithelium stains strongly. Zonule fibers merge with the capsule. (Preparation by T. Kuwabara.)

(Figs. 35–26 and 35–44). This is surrounded by the *central area,* distinguished by the great number of ganglion cells and by the general refinement and even distribution of the structural elements, especially of the rods and cones. The smallest and most precisely ordered sensory elements are in the fovea, where they are accumulated in greatest numbers. In the retinal periphery, the elements are fewer, larger, and less evenly distributed.

When detached from the pigment epithelium, the fresh retina is almost perfectly transparent. It has a distinctly red color because of the presence in its rod cells of *visual purple,* or *rhodopsin.* Light rapidly bleaches the visual purple; in darkness the color gradually reappears. The fovea and its immediate vicinity contain yellow pigment and are called the *macula lutea.* Large blood vessels circle above

and below the central fovea, whereas only fine arteries and veins and capillaries are present in it. In the very center of the fovea, in an area measuring 0.5 mm. across, even the capillaries are absent, greatly increasing its transparency.

Only the portion of the image of an external object that falls upon the fovea is seen sharply. Accordingly, the eyes are moved so as to bring the object of special attention into this central part of the visual field. Photoreceptors are absent from the optic papilla. This is the "blind spot" of the visual field.

Pigment Epithelium

This sheet of heavily pigmented epithelial cells is derived from the outer layer of the cuplike outgrowth of the embryonic nervous system that gives rise to the retina, and it has traditionally been included as one of the layers of the retina (Figs. 35–27 and 35–29). Bruch's membrane, on the other hand, has been considered part of the choroid. The demonstration that this latter structure includes the basal lamina of the pigment epithelium makes it illogical to assign the pigment epithelium to the retina and its basal lamina to the choroid. Some authors therefore prefer to consider the pigment epithelium as a component of the choroid. Although the cells of this layer extend processes that interdigitate with the retinal rods and cones, there is no actual anatomical connection between the photosensitive and the pigmented layer, except at the head of the optic nerve and at the ora serrata. An artifactitious separation is found between the two layers in most histological preparations, and in the "retinal detachment" that is a common cause of partial blindness, the separation occurs along this plane of cleavage between the photosensitive elements of the retina and the pigment epithelium.

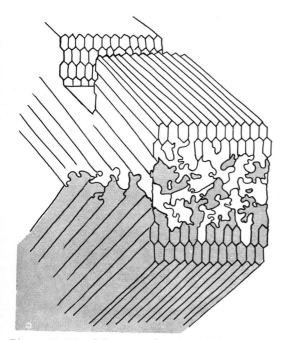

Figure 35–23 Schematic drawing of the arrangement of lens fibers in rows and their prevailing hexagonal cross sectional form, except in the suture area, where there may be considerable irregularities and interdigitation of fibers converging from opposite sectors of the lens. (After T. Wanko and M. Gavin: The Structure of the Eye. New York Academic Press, 1961.)

Pigment epithelial cells have a remarkably regular shape, appearing as hexagonal prisms about 14 μm. wide and 10 to 14 μm. tall; toward the ora serrata, they increase in diameter. The cell base, which rests on Bruch's membrane, displays the labyrinth of interdigitating processes typical of actively transporting epithelia, whereas the lateral cell surface has only a slightly undulating course. Adjacent cells are connected to each other by a junctional complex consisting of apical gap junctions, followed by an elaborate tight junction and a zonula adherens. The cell apex, which faces the rods and cones, gives rise to two sorts of processes: cylindrical sheaths which invest the tip of the photoreceptor outer segments, and slender microvilli, which occupy the interstices between the photoreceptors. The cell nucleus is displaced toward the cell base, and numerous mitochondria intervene between the nucleus and basal labyrinth of interdigitating processes. The most prominent feature of the apical cytoplasm is the presence of numerous melanin granules, elliptical or rounded in shape. A second important component of the apical cytoplasm consists of residual bodies filled with lamellar debris, which represents the partially digested residue of the phagocytized tips of the rod outer segments. Another prominent feature of the cytoplasm of these cells is a highly developed agranular endoplasmic reticulum in the form of a rich network of branching and anastomosing tubules which permeate the interstices among the melanin granules and residual bodies. Cisternae of the granular endoplasmic reticulum and a supranuclear Golgi apparatus complete the list of the cytoplasmic organelles.

The pigment epithelium has many important functions. The tight junctions which seal the intercellular spaces between adjoining epithelial cells protect the retina proper from undesirable metabolites that may be present in the stroma of the choroid. The pigment granules absorb light after it has traversed the photoreceptor layer, thus preventing its reflection from the external ocular tunics. In retinas of lower vertebrates, it has been shown that the pigment granules migrate among the photoreceptors upon illumination, thus effectively screening scattered light and they return to the cell body in the dark. The pigment epithelial cells participate in the turnover of the photoreceptors, continuously engulfing and digesting the growing

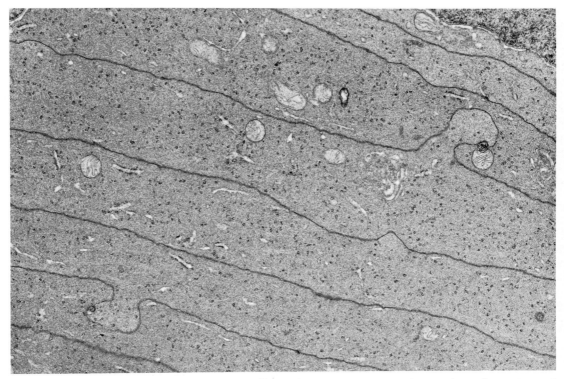

Figure 35-24 Electron micrograph of cortical fibers of the human lens. A few profiles of granular endoplasmic reticulum, occasional mitochondria, and numerous polyribosomes are distributed in an otherwise homogeneous and concentrated cytoplasmic matrix. (Courtesy of T. Kuwabara.)

tips of the rod outer segments. Finally, regeneration of rhodopsin after exposure to light occurs only if photoreceptors maintain an intimate relationship with the pigment epithelium. Vitamin A, a precursor of rhodopsin and one of the products of rhodopsin degradation upon light absorption, moves to the pigment epithelium after maximal light adaptation and returns to the photoreceptors during dark adaptation. Vitamin A is a fat-soluble hydrocarbon and may be stored in the membranes of the agranular endoplasmic reticulum found throughout the cytoplasm of the cells of the pigment epithelium.

Neural Retina

The retina proper contains six types of neurons: (1) *rod photoreceptor cells* and (2) *cone photoreceptor cells*, (3) *horizontal cells*, (4) *bipolar cells*, (5) *amacrine cells*, and (6) *ganglion cells*. Photoreceptor, horizontal, and bipolar cells synapse with each other in the *outer plexiform layer*; bipolar, amacrine, and ganglion cells synapse with each other in the *inner plexiform layer*. The axons of the ganglion cells leave the retina to become fibers of the optic nerve. The retinal neurons are supported by neuroglial elements called *radial cells of Müller*.

Photoreceptor Cells

There are two kinds of visual cells, the rod cells and the cone cells. Their outer segments are the parts sensitive to light, and the light rays, before reaching them, must first penetrate most of the retina.

Rod Cells. The rod cell is a long, slender, highly specialized cell with its outer portion vertical to the retinal layers (Figs. 35-29, 35-30, and 35-31). The parallel arrangement of these elements is responsible for the regular striation of the layer of rods and cones. The scleral part of the rod cell, the *rod proper*, is situated between the outer limiting membrane and the pigment epithelium, its outward third being embedded in the pigment-containing processes of the pigment epithelial cells. The vitreal end of the rod proper extends through the so-called outer limiting membrane into the outer nuclear layer. The rods are fairly uniform in appearance, although their dimensions vary somewhat from region to region. Their thickness in the central area is 1 to 1.5 μm. gradually increasing to 2.5 or 3 μm. near the ora serrata. Their length decreases from approximately 60 μm. near the fovea to 40 μm. in the far periphery. Each rod proper consists of an outer and an inner segment. The *outer segment* is a slender cylinder of uniform thickness, which appears homogeneous in the fresh condition. It possesses a peculiarly brilliant refractility and is positively birefringent in polarized light. The *inner segment* contains the usual complement of cytoplasmic organelles.

The finer structure of the rod cells has been greatly clarified by electron microscopy.

The outer segment in longitudinal section is seen to be composed of a very large number of parallel lamellae oriented transverse to the axis of the rod (Figs. 35–32*A* and 35–33). Each lamella is in fact a closed, membrane limited sac flattened into a disk approximately 2 μm. in diameter and about 140 Å thick. In section, therefore, the profile of each lamella or disk appears as a pair of parallel membranes continuous with one another at the ends and enclosing an exceedingly narrow cavity about 80 Å across. The outer segment is joined to the inner segment by a slender stalk, which contains nine longitudinally oriented fibrils terminating in a centriole or basal body in the distal end of the inner segment. In transverse sections, the stalk has the appearance of a defective cilium, having the nine peripheral doublets but lacking the central pair of fibrils. Studies on the development of the photoreceptors have shown that the outer segments of the rods do in fact de-

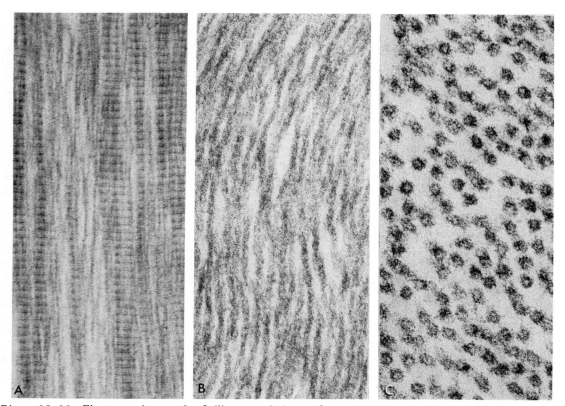

Figure 35–25 Electron micrograph of ciliary zonule in monkeys. *A, B,* Zonular fibers, which consist of exceedingly fine fibrils, 110 to 120 Å in diameter. When fibrils are tightly packed (*A*), the zonular fibers display a cross striation. *A,* × 40,000; *B,* × 160,000. *C,* In cross section, the fibrils have a hollow appearance. *C,* × 200,000. (From Raviola, G., Invest. Ophthalm., *10*:851, 1971.)

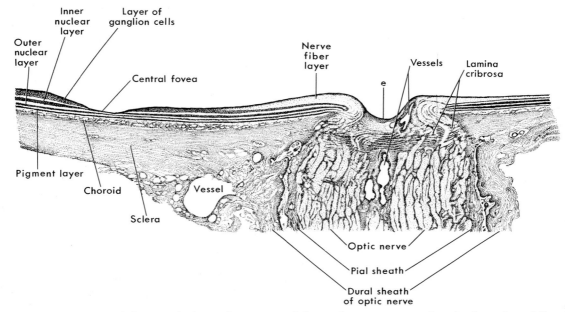

Figure 35-26 Central fovea and place of entrance of the optic nerve as seen in a horizontal meridional section of an enucleated human eye. *e,* Excavation. × 18. (Redrawn and slightly modified from Schaffer.)

velop by modification of cilia. The inner segment consists of two portions, the *ellipsoid* toward the sclera and the *myoid* toward the vitreous. The ellipsoid contains a great number of mitochondria. Cross-striated fibrous rootlets may extend downward from the basal body of the rod outer segment among the mitochondria. The myoid contains the Golgi apparatus, free ribosomes, and cisternae of both agranular and granular endoplasmic reticulum. Microtubules are abundant throughout the rod inner segment.

Autoradiographic studies with the light and electron microscopes demonstrate that the outer segments of rod cells are being renewed constantly. Protein is first synthesized on the ribosomes of the myoid; after moving through the Golgi apparatus, it migrates to the base of the outer segment, where it is used in the assembly of the membranous discs. As new discs are continously added at the vitreal end of the outer segments, the old ones move sclerally toward the tip of the rods till they are phagocytized and destroyed by the cells of the pigment epithelium (Fig. 35–34). In the rat, rod outer segments are totally renewed in about 10 days.

The rest of the rod cell is made up of the *outer fiber,* the *cell body,* the *inner fiber,* and the rod synaptic ending or *spherule.* The rod outer fiber is a slender protoplasmic process, 1 μm. or less in thickness, that extends from the base of the inner segment of the rod proper deep into the outer nuclear layer. Here it joins a small spherical cell body containing the rod nucleus, which is smaller and stains more intensely than the cone nucleus. The rod nuclei represent the majority of the nuclei of the outer nuclear layer in all retinal regions except in the fovea, where rods are few, and in its center, where they are absent. The rod inner fiber, rich in microtubules, connects the body to a pear-shaped spherule, rich in synaptic vesicles, which is located in the outer plexiform layer. In the central area, the rod inner fibers assume a slanting to horizontal course, while in the more peripheral retinal regions they are vertical. The rod proper along with the outer fiber is the homologue of a dendrite of a neuron; the inner rod fiber corresponds to the axon, and through its terminal spherule this fiber is connected to bipolar and horizontal cells.

All rod cells, except those in a zone 3 to 4 mm. wide at the ora serrata, contain visual purple or rhodopsin, the substance responsible for absorption of light. The rhodopsin molecules are localized in the interior of the membrane of the outer segment discs, where they appear as intramembranous particles in freeze-fractured specimens (Fig. 35–35).

As there are only a few rods in the periphery of the fovea and none in its center, this area appears devoid of rhodopsin. When the retina is exposed to light, rhodopsin breaks down, but it is constantly produced anew. This regeneration occurs only as long as the close relation of the rods with the pigment epithelium is preserved.

Cone Cells. These neurons (Figs. 35–29, 35–30, and 35–31) are made up of essentially the same parts as the rod cells, but they differ in certain details. There is no visual purple in the cones but instead there are different types of pigments sensitive to blue, green, and red light. Instead of a slender cylinder, the cone outer segment is a long, conical structure, considerably wider than a rod at its base and tapering down to a blunt rounded tip. As in the rod, the outer segment is made up of a large number of discs stacked

one above the other. Each of these consists of a pair of membranes. In most of the discs the two membranes are continuous at their margins and enclose a narrow space. In the discs close to the inner segment, the two membranes are continuous with the plasma membrane, and the narrow cleft between them is open to the extracellular space (Fig. 35–32B). This appears to be a consistent and possibly a significant difference between rods and cones.

The cone outer segment is also connected to the inner segment by an eccentrically placed modified cilium, terminating in a basal body set in the distal end of the inner segment. The other member of the diplosome is usually oriented at a right angle to the basal body, and striated rootlets extend from it downward among the longitudinally oriented mitochondria that crowd the ellipsoid. Cone inner segments resemble in fine structure those of rod cells (Figs. 35–36 and 35–37).

The cones vary considerably in different

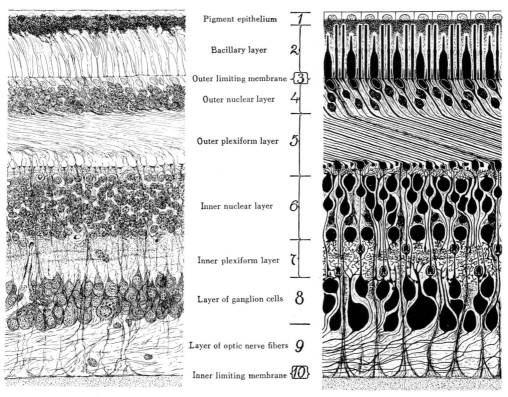

Pigment epithelium — 1
Bacillary layer — 2
Outer limiting membrane — {3}
Outer nuclear layer — 4
Outer plexiform layer — 5
Inner nuclear layer — 6
Inner plexiform layer — 7
Layer of ganglion cells — 8
Layer of optic nerve fibers — 9
Inner limiting membrane — {10}

Figure 35–27 Layers of adult human retina. Left half of the figure stained routinely, about 400 ×. The right half of the figure is a schematic reconstruction from sections stained with Golgi's method. (Slightly modified from Polyak.)

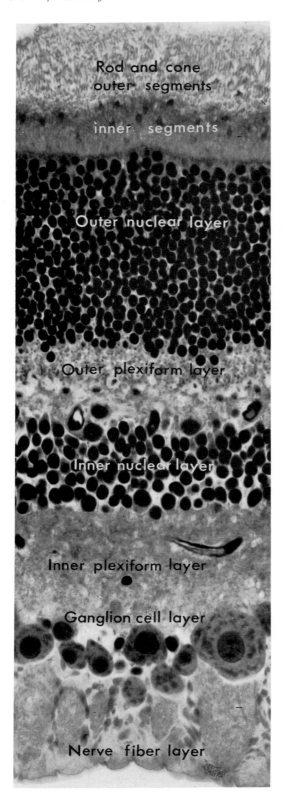

Rod and cone
outer segments

inner segments

Outer nuclear layer

Outer plexiform layer

Inner nuclear layer

Inner plexiform layer

Ganglion cell layer

Nerve fiber layer

regions of the retina. In the central fovea they measure 75 μm. or more in length and from 1 to 1.5 μm. in thickness. Their length gradually decreases to 45 μm. in the periphery. The relative length of the outer and the inner segments is usually 3:4. In the fovea the two segments are approximately the same length. The proximal end of the inner cone segment occupies an opening in the "outer limiting membrane," and protrudes slightly into the fourth layer.

In teleostean fishes and amphibians the inner cone segment is contractile. It shortens in bright light and stretches in dim light or darkness. The displacement of these cones is, accordingly, opposite in direction to that of the rods. It is not definitely established whether human cones are contractile.

In contrast to rods, the turnover of cone outer segments does not involve continuous movement of the discs toward the pigment epithelium nor phagocytosis of the growing tips by the pigment epithelium cells. Proteins found in the inner segment are inserted randomly into the disc membrane throughout the outer segment. The reason for this difference is not clear.

Proximal to the outer limiting membrane, the inner cone segment merges with its *body*, containing a nucleus, which is larger and paler staining than the rod nucleus. The bodies and nuclei of the cones, in contrast to those of the rods, are arranged in a single row immediately beneath the outer limiting membrane. Exceptional in this regard are the cones in the outer fovea, whose nuclei are accumulated in several rows. Only in this region do the cones have an *outer fiber*. But from the body of all cones, a stout, smooth *inner fiber* descends to the middle zone of the outer plexiform layer, where it terminates with a thick triangular or clubshaped synaptic ending, the *cone pedicle*. Up to a dozen short, barb-like processes emanate from the base of each pedicle, except in the fovea, where there are usually none. These outgrowths are deployed horizontally in the outer plexiform layer. The length and course of the inner cone fibers may vary considerably, depending on the region, the longest (600 μm.) and

Figure 35–28 Photomicrograph of cat retina. (Courtesy of A. J. Ladman.)

CH

PE

OS

IS

OLM

ONL

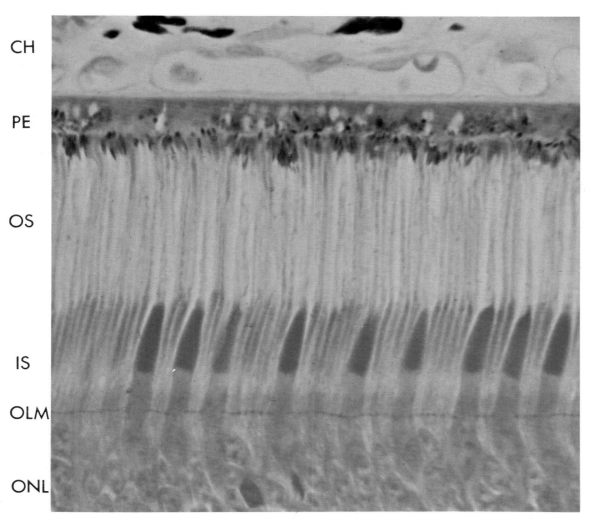

Figure 35-29 Light micrograph of the outermost retinal layers in monkey. Cones are easily distinguished from rods, for their inner segment is larger and the ellipsoid intensely stained. *CH*, choroid; *PE*, pigment epithelium; *OS*, outer segments; *IS*, inner segments; *OLM*, outer limiting membrane; *ONL*, outer nuclear layer. (Courtesy of J. Rostgaard.)

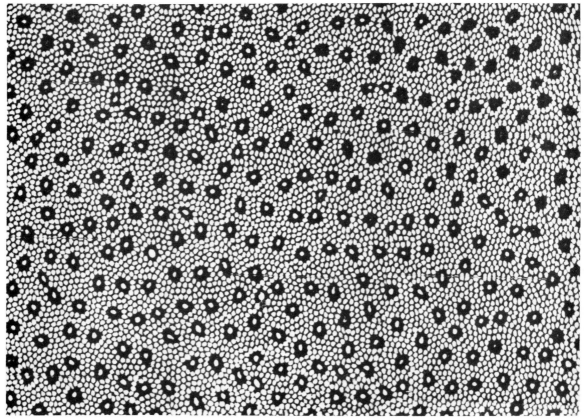

Figure 35–30 Light micrograph of a cross section through the outer segments of the photoreceptor cells in the retinal periphery of a monkey. The large diameter of cone inner segments keeps the rods at a distance from cone outer segments. Toluidine blue, printed as a negative. × 800. (Courtesy of E. Raviola.)

most nearly horizontally placed being those in the central area, where the inner rod and cone fibers form a thick fiber layer at the boundary between outer nuclear and outer plexiform layers, called the *outer fiber layer of Henle.* The inner cone fibers have all the characteristics of an axon, while the cone pedicle has those of the telodendron of a neuron and makes synapses with bipolar and horizontal cells.

The number of cones in the human retina is estimated at six to seven millions (Østerberg). The ratio of the number of nerve fibers of the optic nerve (438,000) to the number of cones of one eye is 1:6 or 1:7.

The relative number and distribution of the rods and cones in different vertebrates present great variations, depending on the mode of life. In diurnal birds the cones are more numerous than the rods. In most diur-

nal reptiles rods are exceedingly rare. In many nocturnal vertebrates only rods are present, although in others a few rudimentary cones can be found among numerous rods. On similar comparative data M. Schultze (1866) based his assumption that there is a difference in the function of the two kinds of photoreceptors (duplicity theory).

Outer Limiting Membrane. The dense staining line traditionally called the *outer limiting membrane* is not a membrane at all. Instead it is found in electron micrographs to be a row of dense junctional complexes where the photoreceptor cells are attached to the Müller cells, which surround and support all of the neural elements (Fig. 35–38). Distal to this row of junctional complexes, tufts of microvilli project from the free surface of the Müller cells into interstices between the rod and cone inner segments.

Horizontal Cells

These cells are typical neurons whose bodies form the uppermost one or two rows of the inner nuclear layer. From the scleral end of the body arise short dendritic twigs, which produce several tufts deployed in the outer plexiform layer. Each dendritic tuft is connected to a single cone pedicle. The axon takes a horizontal course in the outer plexiform layer and its terminal twigs come into contact with rod spherules (Fig. 35–39).

Bipolar Cells

These neurons extend from the outer to the inner plexiform layer and therefore stand approximately upright with respect to the retinal layers (Figs. 35–39 and 35–40). Their body is located in the inner nuclear layer and gives rise to one or more primary dendrites, which ascend to the outer plexiform layer, where they branch and connect with the photoreceptor cell terminals. The single, inwardly directed axon of the bipolar cells ramifies in the inner plexiform layer, where it is synaptically related to ganglion and amacrine cells. Four types of bipolar cells can be distinguished in the primate retina: (1) *rod bipolar cells,* which connect to rod cells; (2) and (3) *invaginating midget bipolar cells* and *flat midget bipolar cells,* each synapsing with a single cone pedicle, and (4) *flat* or *diffuse cone bipolar cells,* connected to many cone pedicles. The precise synaptic relationships of the axonal terminals of the four types of bipolar cells with the amacrine and ganglion cells are poorly understood.

Outer Plexiform Layer

This is the region of synaptic interplay between photoreceptor, bipolar, and horizontal cells. The synaptic terminals of cone cells or pedicles are large pyramidal endings containing synaptic vesicles and mitochondria, whose flattened base is invaginated at many points to enclose the tips of the dendrites of the horizontal and invaginating midget bipolar cells. The remaining, free surface of the base of the pedicle makes hundreds of superficial contacts with the dendrites of the flat midget and diffuse cone bipolars. With a high degree of consistency and geometrical order, each of the 12 to 25 synaptic invaginations of a cone pedicle contains the tip of two horizontal cell dendrites and one dendrite of an invaginating midget bipolar cell ("*a triad*"). The horizontal cell dendrites contain synaptic vesicles, are deeply inserted and lie on either side of a wedge-shaped projection of the pedicle, called the *synaptic ridge.* The dendrite of the invaginating midget bipolar cell lies centrally and more superficially, separated from the apex of the ridge by the cleft intervening between adjoining horizontal cell dendrites. The synaptic ridge is bisected by a dense lamella or synaptic ribbon, surrounded by a halo of synaptic vesicles; the ribbon sits at a right angle to the apex of the ridge, separated from the pedicle membrane by a trough-shaped body, the arciform density (Fig. 35–41*B*). The significance of the synaptic ribbon is poorly understood, but it is prob-

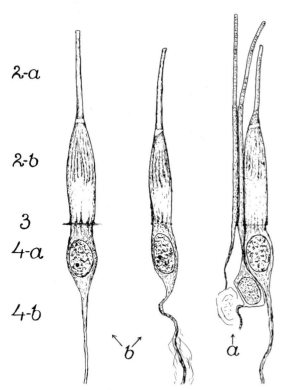

Figure 35–31 Rods (*a*) and cones (*b*) from an osmic acid-fixed, unstained, teased preparation of retina of a rhesus monkey (preparation of G. W. Bartelmez). *2-a,* Outer rod and cone segments; *2-b,* inner segments; *3,* outer limiting membrane; *4-a,* cone cell bodies with nuclei; *4-b,* rod cell bodies with nuclei. (Courtesy of S. Polyak.)

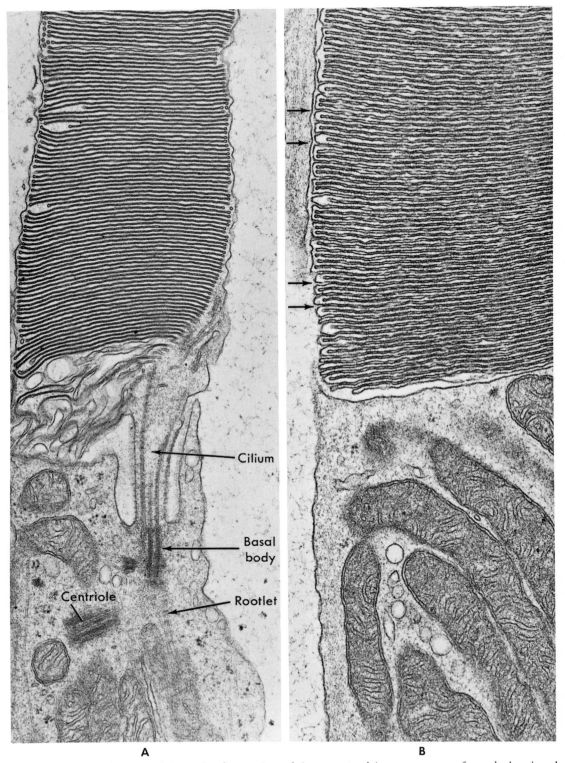

A **B**

Figure 35–32 A, Electron micrograph of a portion of the outer and inner segment of a rod, showing the connection of the two by a modified cilium. *B,* Corresponding region of a cone. Notice that some of the discs are open to the extracellular space (arrows). (Courtesy of T. Kuwabara.)

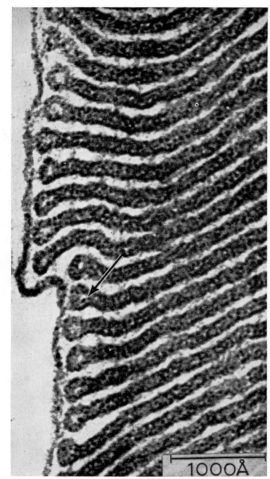

Figure 35-33 Electron micrograph showing profiles of the membranous discs of the outer segment of a rod cell from frog retina. They exhibit a compact granular fine structure (arrow) when prepared with very low temperature and osmium fixation (osmium-cryofixation), low-temperature dehydration, and embedding. (Courtesy of H. Fernández-Morán.)

ably instrumental in the mechanism of transmitter release by the photoreceptor ending. The superficial or basal contacts of cone pedicles do not display prominent junctional specializations; the synaptic cleft is slightly enlarged and the adjoining membranes of the pedicle and bipolar dendrites bear a layer of fluffy cytoplasmic material.

Rod spherules have a single synaptic invagination and no superficial contacts. In their invaginating synapse, two deeply inserted axonal endings of the horizontal cells lie on either side of a ridge containing a ribbon and vesicles (Fig. 35–41*A*). The tips of 1 to 4 dendrites belonging to the rod bipolar cells lie centrally and less deeply inserted. The axonal endings of the horizontal cells usually contain synaptic vesicles.

Using Golgi's chromo-argentic impregnation and electron microscopy, the neural interconnections in the outer plexiform layer of the primate retina have been worked out in great detail. Both invaginating and flat midget bipolars are "private" cone bipolars; that is, each of them is contacted by a single cone pedicle. The invaginating variety, however, sends its dendrites to the invaginating synapses, whereas the flat variety makes superficial contacts with the cone pedicles. The diffuse cone bipolars, on the other hand, touch about six cone pedicles at superficial contacts. The rod bipolar cells connect exclusively with rod cells; their dendritic terminals end as slightly inserted processes in the invaginations of numerous spherules. Horizontal cells contact cone cells with their dendrites and rod cells with their axon; both dendritic and axonal terminals of these cells end as deeply inserted processes in the invaginating synapses(Fig. 35–42).

Amacrine Cells

These neurons have numerous dendrites, but lack an axon (Fig. 35–39). Their body lies in the vitreal part of the inner nuclear layer and their dendrites spread in the inner plexiform layer. They connect with each other, with the axonal endings of the bipolar cells, and with the dendrites of the ganglion cells. The primate retina contains numerous varieties of amacrine cells; these are classified as *diffuse* and *stratified*. Diffuse amacrine cells send their dendritic branches throughout the thickness of the inner plexiform layer, whereas the ramifications of the stratified amacrine cells are confined to one or two horizontal levels of the inner plexiform layer.

Ganglion Cells

Ganglion cells represent the terminal link of the neural networks of the retina. With their dendrites, they connect with bipolar endings and amacrine dendrites in the inner plexiform layer; their body is located in the ganglion cell layer; their axon, which

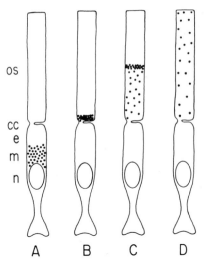

Figure 35–34 Diagram illustrating the turnover of rod outer segments. After injection of a radioactive amino acid, electron microscope autoradiography shows that the label is first concentrated in the myoid of rod cells (*A*), where ribosomes and the Golgi apparatus are contained. Later, labeled protein moves to the membranous discs at the base of the outer segments (*B*) and ascends progressively toward the tip of the rods (*C*). Finally it disappears from rod cells (*D*) and becomes localized in the residual bodies contained in the cytoplasm of the pigment epithelium cells. *OS*, outer segments; *CC*, connecting cilium; *e*, ellipsoid; *m*, myoid; *n*, nucleus. (From Young, R. W., and D. Bok, J. Cell Biol., *42*:392, 1969.)

becomes a fiber of the optic nerve, conducts to the brain the results of the complex neural activity which takes place in the retina (Fig. 35–39). The primate retina contains numerous varieties of ganglion cells, classified according to the shape of their dendritic tree and the mode of distribution of their dendritic branches in the inner plexiform layer. In the central area the most common type of ganglion cell is represented by the *midget ganglion cell*, characterized by a single dendritic shaft which ascends into the inner plexiform layer, where it ends with a minute basket of short secondary and tertiary dendrites. *Diffuse ganglion cells* send their dendrites throughout the thickness of the inner plexiform layer, whereas *stratified ganglion cells* have their dendritic arborization confined to one or more levels of the inner plexiform layer. Intermediate forms between diffuse and stratified ganglion cells were also described.

Inner Plexiform Layer

This is the region of synaptic interplay between bipolar, amacrine, and ganglion cells. Two kinds of synaptic contacts are found in this layer: the ribbon synapse, characterized by a dense lamella, surrounded by a halo of vesicles in the presynaptic process, and a more conventional type of synaptic contact, which lacks ribbon and is characterized by clustering of vesicles against the presynaptic membrane (Fig. 35–43). At ribbon synapses, the axonal endings of the bipolar cells are presynaptic to amacrine and ganglion cell dendrites. Amacrine cell dendrites, in turn, make conventional synapses with bipolar endings, ganglion cell dendrites, and dendrites of other amacrine cells. Reciprocal synapses between bipolar terminals and amacrine dendrites frequently occur in this layer, with the bipolar contacting the amacrine cell as the presynaptic element of a ribbon synapse, and the amacrine cell returning a conventional feedback synapse onto the bipolar. Thus, amacrine cell dendrites have the unusual property of containing synaptic vesicles and behaving as presynaptic elements of *dendroaxonic* and *dendro-dendritic* synapses. The existence of dendro-dendritic synapses was originally described in the olfactory bulb, where the granule cells, which lack an axon, establish reciprocal dendro-dendritic synapses with the dendrites of the mitral cells.

The precise pattern of neural interconnections in the inner plexiform layer is poorly understood. Sublayers can be distinguished in it, for the axonal arborizations of the bipolar cells and the dendritic expansions of the stratified amacrine and ganglion cells are distributed at different levels within the layer. This and recent findings in nonprimate retinas suggest that the various types of bipolar, amacrine, and ganglion cells establish specific synaptic connections with each other. However, the details of their "wiring" have not yet been worked out for the primate retina.

Optic Nerve Fibers in the Primate Retina

Because of the presence of the central fovea, the optic nerve fibers have a special course. In general they converge radially toward the optic papilla. However, those originating in the upper temporal quadrant of the retina circle above the central area, while those originating in the lower temporal quadrant circle below it on their way to the papilla. They follow the larger retinal vessels fairly closely. A line connecting the fovea with the temporal circumference of the retina separates the optic nerve fibers of the upper from those of the lower temporal quadrant. This separation is preserved along the central visual pathway as far as the cortex.

In primates each retina is divided into two halves along the vertical meridian passing through the center of the fovea. The fibers from the nasal half cross in the optic chiasma and pass to the optic tract of the opposite side; those from the temporal half enter the tract on the same side. Each optic tract is, therefore, composed of fibers from the temporal half of the retina of the same side and the nasal half of the retina of the opposite

eye. This arrangement remains in the visual radiation in the occipital lobes of the brain. It accounts for the blindness in the opposite halves of the two fields of view (homonymous hemianopsia) when the optic tract or the visual radiation of one side is interrupted.

Inner Limiting Membrane

This traditional term is no longer appropriate. It is not a membrane but merely the basal lamina of the Müller cells. It separates their inner conical ends from the vitreous body.

Supporting, or Neuroglial, Elements of the Retina

The retina, being a modified part of the brain, contains supporting elements of neuroglial character. The most important are the radial cells of Müller. These are present throughout the central area, including the fovea, as well as in the periphery.

Their oval nuclei lie in the middle zone of the inner nuclear layer. The cell body is a slender fiber or pillar which extends radially from the outer to the inner limiting membrane. In the two plexiform layers the radial fibers give off many branches, which form a dense neuroglial network in whose meshes are lodged the ramifications of the neurons described earlier.

The cell bodies of Müller cells are beset with excavations, which envelop the bodies of the retinal neurons.

At the limit between the outer nuclear layer and the layer of the rods and cones, Müller cells, as described, have prominent junctional complexes that produce the linear density formerly interpreted as an outer limiting membrane.

Central Area and Fovea ("Macula")

Slightly lateral to the papilla is the place of most distinct vision. This region, the central area, is characterized by the presence of cones and other nervous elements in numbers greater than elsewhere and by their structural specialization and synaptic perfection. In the center of this area, the layers inward to the outer nuclear layer are displaced laterally, producing a shallow depression on the vitreal surface of the retina, called the central fovea.

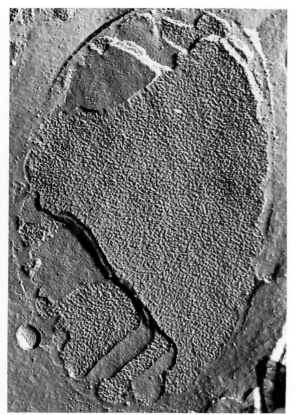

Figure 35–35 Freeze-fracture appearance of a rod outer segment in a monkey. The membranes of the discs contain a large number of particles, which probably are rhodopsin. × 82,500. (Courtesy of E. Raviola.)

Figure 35–36

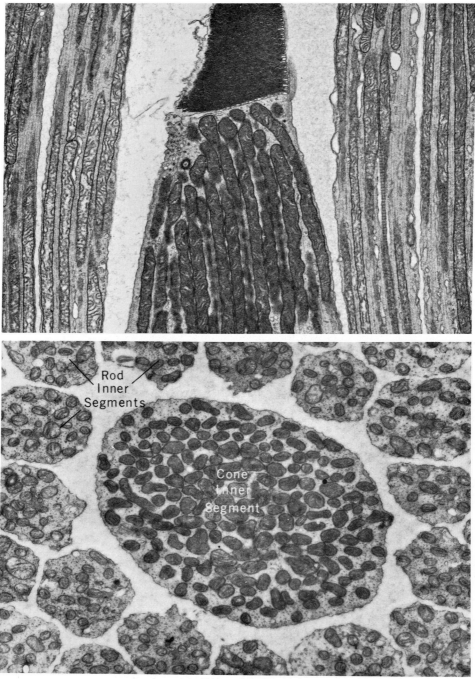

Figure 35–37

Figure 35–36 Vertical section of the inner segments of a cone and several neighboring rods in the human retina, illustrating the larger size of the cone and the high concentration of longitudinally oriented mitochondria in the ellipsoid. (Courtesy of T. Kuwabara.)

Figure 35–37 Horizontal section through the inner segments of the photoreceptor elements in rat retina. Notice the larger size of the cone ellipsoid and its great number of mitochondria. (After Marchesi, Sears, and Barrnett, Invest. Ophthalm., 3:1, 1964.)

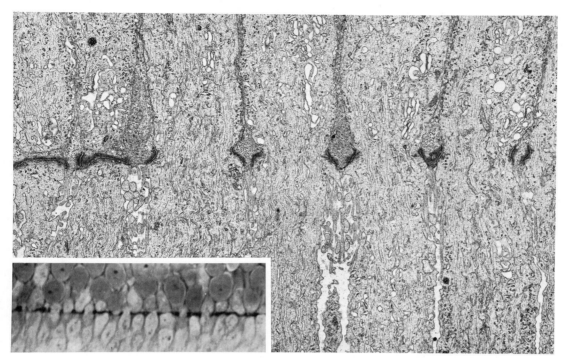

Figure 35–38 Electron micrograph of the region of the "outer limiting membrane" of the retina, showing that it is not a membrane, as it appears to be with the light microscope (see inset), but a row of junctional complexes between the rod and cone cells and the surrounding Müller cells. (Courtesy of T. Kuwabara.)

This permits an almost free passage of rays of light to the layer of photoreceptors, and it is here that the visual axis touches the retina.

The central fovea is a shallow bowl with its concavity toward the vitreous (Fig. 35–44). It is in the center of the central area, 2 to 2.5 mm. on the temporal side of the papilla. In its center a *floor* or *fundus* can be distinguished, with the *slopes* and a *margin of the fovea*. The width of the entire foveal depression measures 1.5 mm.

In the fundus of the central fovea, the cones are thinner and longer than elsewhere in the retina. This area, the *outer fovea*, contains 20,000 to 25,000 cones. This region, measuring about 400 μm. across, corresponds to the portion of the field of view in which vision is most discriminating. The *rod-free* area, where only cones are present, measures 500 to 550 μm. in diameter and contains up to 30,000 cones.

Capillaries are present in the foveal slopes to the very edge of the foveal floor, or 275 μm. from the very center. The *avascular central territory* is almost as large as the rodless area (500 to 500 μm.).

HISTOPHYSIOLOGY OF THE RETINA

The eye is essentially a camera obscura provided with dioptric media: the cornea, the aqueous humor, and the adjustable crystalline lens. The inner surface of this dark chamber is lined with the photosensitive retina. The rays of light emanating from each point of an illuminated object impinging on the cornea are refracted by it and converge on the lens. In the lens, the rays are further refracted and focused in the photosensitive layer of the retina. In relation to the object, the retinal image is inverted (because of the crossing of the rays in the pupil's aperture); it is a real image, and it is very much reduced in size.

In the retina, the quanta of incident light are converted or transduced by the photoreceptor cells into nerve signals; these are elaborated by the networks of retinal neurons and finally translated into a code of nerve impulses, which is conducted to the brain by the fibers of the optic nerve.

The transduction process can be conveniently subdivided into primary and secondary steps. The primary step is a photochemical reaction and consists in the absorption of a quantum of light by one of the visual pigments contained in the discs of the photoreceptor outer segments, and a subsequent configurational change in the absorbing molecule. The secondary step presumably consists of a series of reactions that ultimately lead to a hyperpolarization of the receptor cell membrane. The molecular basis of the primary photochemical absorption is well understood for the rod pigment, but little is known of the secondary reactions that result in hyperpolarization of the cell membrane.

Rod and cone cells differ in their sensitivity to intensity and wavelength of light. Rod cells are active in dim illumination (scotopic vision) and contain a single visual pigment, rhodopsin, which absorbs light of various wavelengths, although most efficiently in the blue-green. In the human retina there are three types of cones, containing different visual pigments that absorb maximally red, blue, or green light; furthermore, cone cells are active under the conditions of diurnal illumination (photopic vision).

Visual pigments consist of a combination of vitamin A aldehyde, known as *retinal*, with a protein of the class called *opsins*. Opsins are hydrophobic proteins with one retinal group per molecule, a carbohydrate side chain, no phospholipid, and a molecular weight of about 27,000 daltons. They are buried within the membrane of the discs of the photoreceptor outer segments. When retinal is combined with opsin in the dark-adapted retina, it has a bent and twisted form (*11-cis*). When the pigment molecule absorbs a quantum of light, the retinal shape becomes straight (*all-trans*) and separates from opsin, which in turn undergoes a conformational change. This leads, in some unknown way, to hyperpolarization of the photoreceptor cell membrane. Meanwhile the cell is recombining retinal and opsin into the light-absorbing form of the pigment molecule.

Most of the present knowledge on the electrophysiology of retinal neurons stems from intracellular recordings in nonprimate retinas. In fact, only ganglion cells have been successfully penetrated with microelectrodes in monkeys. Stripped of many important details, the complex story of the interneuronal relationships in the retina is as follows. Most retinal neurons generate slow, graded potentials; spikes first appear in amacrine cells and are especially typical of the ganglion cell response. The photosensitive rod and cone cells are depolarized and probably release transmitter in the dark; they hyperpolarize upon

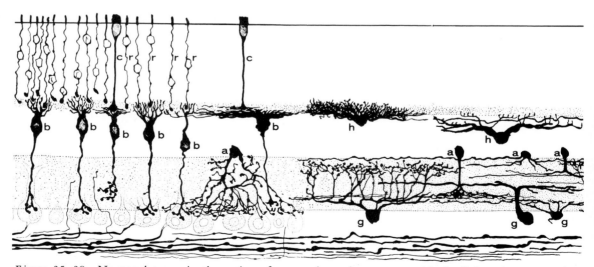

Figure 35-39 Neuronal types in the retina of mammals as they appear with the light microscope after Golgi's chromo-argentic impregnation. *r,* Rod cells (dog); *c,* cone cells (dog); *b,* bipolar cells (dog); *h,* horizontal cells (dog); *a,* amacrine cells (dog and ox); *g,* ganglion cells (ox). In rod and cone cells, the photoreceptor proper is not represented. (After Cajal, 1893, modified.)

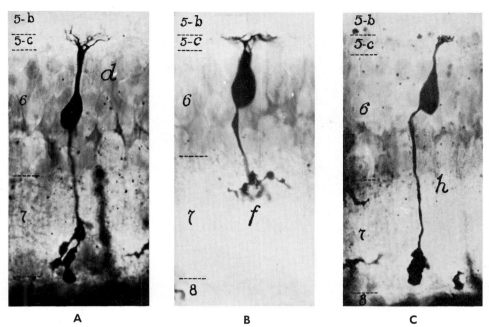

Figure 35–40 Photomicrographs of bipolar cells of retina of rhesus monkey. *A,* Rod bipolar; *B,* diffuse cone bipolar; *C,* invaginating midget bipolar. Method of Golgi. (Courtesy of S. Polyak.)

illumination. There are two physiological classes of horizontal cells: *luminosity* horizontal cells, which respond to illumination of the photoreceptors by hyperpolarization, and *chromaticity* horizontal cells, which may hyperpolarize or depolarize, depending on the wavelength of the stimulating light. In the retina of the turtle, the hyperpolarization of luminosity horizontal cells causes depolarization of cone cells; it has therefore been suggested that cones and horizontal cells are connected by a reciprocal synapse. In fishes, amphibians, and reptiles, there are also two physiological classes of bipolar cells, one depolarizing, the other hyperpolarizing, upon light stimulation. Bipolar cells are the first elements in the chain of retinal neurons which show a "center-and-surround" organization of their receptive field; that is, the cell response to stimulation of neighboring photoreceptors is antagonized by the stimulation of distant photoreceptors. Furthermore, some bipolars are color-coded; that is, they respond to light of specific wavelength. The neuronal circuitry which underlies the bipolar activity is not well understood; the response of bipolars to stimulation of the photoreceptors in the center of their receptive field may be mediated by a photoreceptor-to-bipolar synapse, at least insofar as hyperpo-

larizing bipolars are concerned. The "surround effect" is certainly due to the activity of the horizontal cells, which are activated by the photoreceptors and in turn inhibit the bipolar response. The precise mechanism of this inhibitory interaction, however, is unknown. In the turtle, horizontal cells feed back onto photoreceptors, but in other species, a direct horizontal-to-bipolar cell synapse has also been postulated. Thus, the function of the synapses in the outer plexiform layer is to signal intensity and color of the retinal image and at the same time to accentuate its contrast through the activity of the horizontal cells.

The signals of bipolar cells are further processed in the inner plexiform layer by the amacrine and ganglion cells before their transmittal to the brain in the form of changes in the frequency of the nerve impulses traveling along the fibers of the optic nerve.

The function of the amacrine cells is poorly understood. In nonmammalian retinas, amacrine cells were identified which respond with transient depolarization at both onset and cessation of retinal illumination, with spikes superimposed on the slow potential. In the monkey retina, two main types of ganglion cells were identified by intracellular recordings, one responding to the onset, the

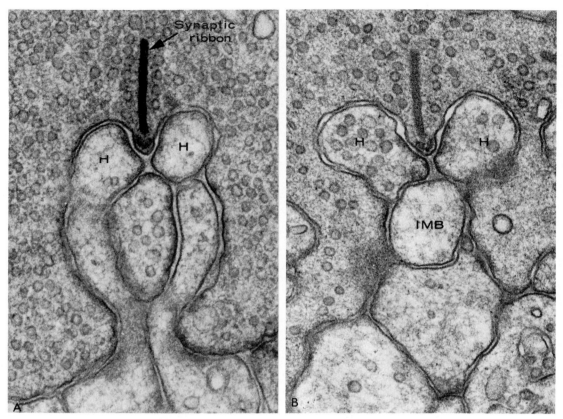

Figure 35–41   A, Electron micrograph of the invaginating synapse of a rod spherule in the retina of a rabbit. Two deeply inserted processes (*H*), probably arising from the axon of the horizontal cells, lie on either side of a wedge-shaped projection of the spherule (synaptic ridge) which contains the synaptic ribbon, surrounded by a halo of synaptic vesicles, and the arciform density. The dendrites of the rod bipolar cells can not be identified in this micrograph. × 65,000. (Courtesy of E. Raviola.) *B,* Invaginating synapse of a cone pedicle in the retina of a monkey. A typical "triad" consists of two deeply invaginated dendrites of the horizontal cells (*H*) and a slightly inserted, centrally positioned dendrite of an invaginating midget bipolar cell (*IMB*). Notice the synaptic vesicles in the horizontal cell dendrites. × 65,000. From Raviola, E., and N. B. Gilula, J. Cell Biol. (in press).

other to the cessation, of a light stimulus applied to the center of their receptive field; the response was inverted upon stimulation of the periphery of their receptive field. Among the on-center cells, some are not color-coded and phasic—that is, they discharge transiently to maintained stimuli of any wavelength; others are color-coded and tonic—that is, they discharge continuously to maintained stimuli of either green or red light. The tonic cells are thought to correspond to the midget ganglion cells. It has been speculated that the neural interactions in the inner plexiform layer may be concerned with codification of the dynamic or temporal aspects of the visual image, but much work remains to be done before the significance of the synaptic interactions between bipolar, amacrine, and ganglion cells is fully elucidated.

BLOOD VESSELS OF THE EYE

These arise from the ophthalmic artery and can be subdivided into two groups, which are almost completely independent and anastomose with each other only in the region of the entrance of the optic nerve. The first group, the *retinal system,* represented by the central artery and vein, supplies a part of the optic nerve and the retina. The second, the *ciliary system*, is destined mainly for the uveal tunic.

LYMPH SPACES OF THE EYE

True lymph capillaries and lymph vessels are present only in the scleral conjunctiva. In the eyeball they are absent.

A mass injected into the space between the choroid and sclera penetrates along the walls of the vortex veins into the space of Tenon. The latter continues as the *supravaginal space* along the outer surface of the dural sheath of the optic nerve to the optic foramen. Again, it is possible to inject into Tenon's space from the subarachnoid space of the brain. From the anterior chamber the injected liquid passes into the posterior chamber and also into Schlemm's canal. All these spaces cannot, however, be regarded as belonging to the lymphatic system.

NERVES OF THE EYE

These are the optic nerve, originating from the retina, and the ciliary nerves, supplying the eyeball with motor, sensory, and sympathetic fibers.

The optic nerve, an evagination of the prosencephalon, is not a peripheral nerve like the other cranial nerves, but is a tract of the central nervous system. It consists of about 1200 bundles of nerve fibers whose myelin sheaths are produced by oligodendroglial cells.

The meninges and the intermeningeal spaces of the brain continue into the optic nerve. The outer sheath of the nerve is formed by the dura, which continues toward the eyeball and fuses with the sclera. The pia mater forms a connective tissue layer which is closely adherent to the surface of the nerve and fuses with the sclera at the entrance of the optic nerve. This pial layer sends connective tissue partitions and blood vessels into the nerve. Inflammatory processes can extend from the eyeball toward the meningeal spaces of the brain through the spaces between the sheaths.

The optic nerve leaves the posterior pole of the eyeball in a slightly oblique direction and continues into the entrance canal of the optic nerve. Just after leaving the eye through the openings in the lamina cribrosa, the fibers acquire their myelin sheaths. The central artery and central vein reach the eyeball through the optic nerve; they penetrate the nerve on its lower side at a distance from the eyeball varying from 5 to 20 mm., but usually being 6 to 8 mm.

ACCESSORY ORGANS OF THE EYE

In an early stage of embryonic development the anterior segment of the eyeball projects freely on the surface. Later a circular fold of integument encircles the cornea. From its upper and lower parts the upper and lower lids grow toward each other over the surface of the cornea. In this way, the conjunctival sac is formed, which protects and moistens the free surface of the eye, especially the cornea. The part lining the inner surface of the lids is the *palpebral conjunctiva*, and that covering the eyeball is the *bulbar conjunctiva*. The reflection of the palpebral onto the bulbar conjunctiva forms deep recesses between the lids and the eyeball, the *superior* and the *inferior fornices*.

Eyelids

The outermost layer is the skin. It is thin and provided with a few papillae and many small hairs with sebaceous and small sweat

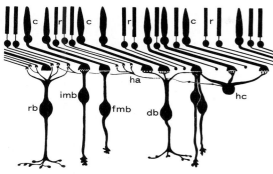

Figure 35–42   Diagram of the synaptic connections in the outer plexiform layer of the primate retina. For explanation, see text. *c*, Cone cells; *r*, rod cells; *rb*, rod bipolar cell; *imb*, invaginating midget bipolar cell; *fmb*, flat midget bipolar cell; *db*, diffuse cone bipolar cell; *ha*, horizontal cell axon; *hc*, horizontal cell. (From Kolb, H., Phil. Trans. Roy. Soc. Lond. B, 258:261, 1970.)

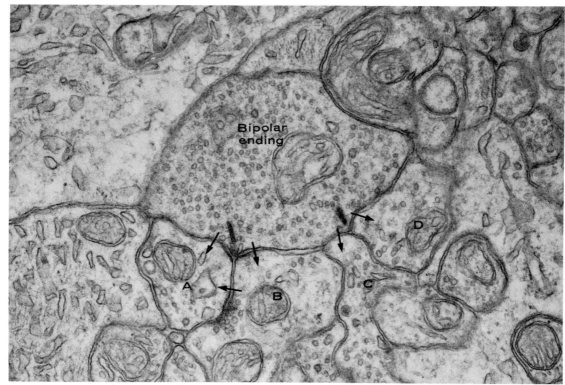

Figure 35–43 Electron micrograph of a portion of the inner plexiform layer in the retina of a monkey. An axonal ending of a bipolar cell makes two ribbon synapses with four processes, labeled *A, B, C, D*. Processes *B, C,* and *D* contain synaptic vesicles and may represent dendrites of amacrine cells. Process *B* makes a conventional type of synaptic contact with process *A,* whose identity is unknown. The arrows indicate the direction of the synaptic influences. × 38,400. (Courtesy of E. Raviola.)

glands (Fig. 35–45). The dermis contains a varying number of pigment cells with yellow or brown granules. The loose subcutaneous layer is rich in fine elastic fibers, and in Caucasians is almost completely devoid of fat. Toward the edge of the lid the dermis becomes denser and has higher papillae.

The *eyelashes* are large hairs obliquely inserted in three or four rows along the edge of the lid. With their follicles they penetrate deeply into the tissue. The sebaceous glands connected with the eyelashes are small, and arrector muscles are missing. The eyelashes are replaced every 100 to 150 days.

Between and behind the follicles of the eyelashes are peculiar sweat glands, the *glands of Moll.* Unlike ordinary sweat glands, the terminal portion here is generally straight or only slightly coiled. The ducts open, as a rule, into the follicles of the eyelashes. The epithe-

lium of the terminal portions consists of an indistinct, outer myoepithelial layer and an inner layer of pyramidal, apocrine glandular elements. The lumen is often considerably dilated, and the glandular cells are flattened. In the ducts the epithelium consists of two distinct cell layers. The nature of the secretion of these glands is not known.

The next layer inward consists of the thin, pale, striated fibers of the palpebral portion of the ring muscle of the eye *(orbicularis oculi).* The part behind the follicles of the eyelashes or behind the ducts of the meibomian glands is the *ciliary muscle of Riolan.*

Deep to the orbicular muscle is a layer of connective tissue, the palpebral fascia, a continuation of the tendon of the palpebral levator *(levator palpebrae)* muscle. In the upper part of the upper lid, strands of smooth muscle, the *superior tarsal muscle of Müller,* are attached to the edge of the *tarsus,* a plate of dense connective tissue that forms the skeleton of the lid. In the upper lid its breadth is about 10 mm., in the lower only 5 mm. The *glands of Meibom* are embedded in its substance. They are elongated and arranged in one layer, parallel to one another and perpendicular to the length of the tarsal plate. Their openings form a single row immediately in front of the inner free edge of the lid, at the line of transition from the skin into the conjunctiva.

The meibomian glands are sebaceous but have lobated alveolar terminal portions. They are connected by short lateral ducts with a long central excretory duct lined with stratified squamous epithelium.

The innermost layer of the lid is the *conjunctiva.* At the inner edge of the margin of the lid the epidermis continues into the inner surface of the lid. Here the superficial cells become thicker, the number of layers decreases, mucous cells appear, and the epithelium assumes a stratified columnar character, which is typical of the whole conjunctiva and varies only in thickness in different places. The superficial cells have a short prismatic form. Goblet cells are scattered between them.

At the upper edge of the tarsus the epithelium is sometimes reduced to two cell layers, and its surface presents many irregular invaginations. Some of them are lined with mucous cells and are described as glands. In the conjunctiva of the fornix, the epithelium is thicker.

The lamina propria of the conjunctiva is dense connective tissue. In the region of the fornix it is very loosely attached to the intraorbital fat tissue, permitting the free motion of the eyeball in the conjunctival sac.

In the region of the corneal limbus the epithelium of the conjunctiva assumes a stratified squamous character and continues as such onto the surface of the cornea. It may still contain a few scattered mucous cells.

The rudimentary *third eyelid,* or *semilunar fold* (the homologue of the nictitating membrane of the lower vertebrates), is formed by the scleral conjunctiva at the inner palpebral commissure, lateral to the lacrimal caruncle. It consists of connective tissue that contains smooth muscle fibers and is covered with conjunctival epithelium, which, on the outer surface, contains many mucous cells.

Lacrimal Gland

In connection with the conjunctival space there is a system of glands whose secretion moistens, lubricates, and flushes the surface of the eyeball and of the lids. Of these glands, only the lacrimal gland reaches a high degree of development. It has the size and shape of an almond and is lodged beneath the conjunctiva at the lateral upper side of the eyeball. It consists of a group of separate glandular bodies and sends out 6 to 12 excretory ducts, which open along the upper and lateral surfaces of the superior conjunctival fornix.

The lacrimal gland is of the tubuloalveo-

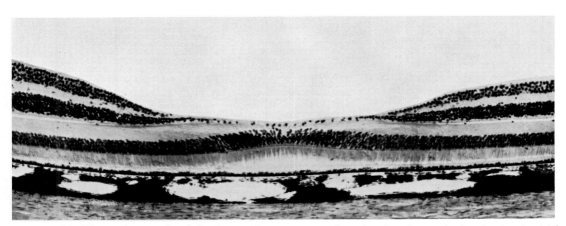

Figure 35-44 Photomicrograph of the fovea of a macaque retina, showing the marked reduction in thickness in this area of maximum visual acuity. (Courtesy of H. Mizoguchi.)

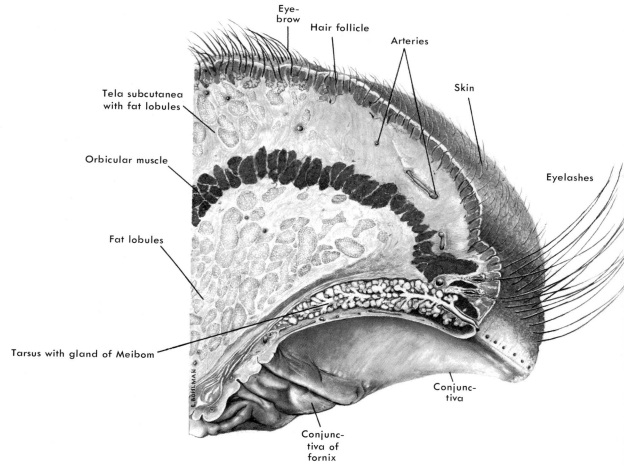

Figure 35–45 Camera lucida drawing of a slice of the upper eyelid of a newborn infant. Stained with hematoxylin. × 12.

lar type. Its terminal portions are provided with a relatively large lumen and with irregular, saccular outpocketings. The basal lamina is lined with glandular cells resembling those of the serous salivary type. They have, however, a narrower columnar shape and contain, in addition to small fat droplets, large, pale secretion granules whose number changes according to the functional conditions.

These cells are provided with secretory canaliculi. Between their bases and the basal lamina are well developed basket (myoepithelial) cells. The smallest intralobular ducts are lined with a layer of low columnar or cuboidal cells and have a few myoepithelial cells. The larger intralobular ducts have a two layered epithelium.

On the inner surface of the lids, especially the upper one, near the upper edge of the tarsus, there are a varying number of small accessory lacrimal glands—the *tarsal lacrimal glands*.

After having washed the conjunctival cavity, the secretion of the lacrimal gland (the tears, a sterile liquid) reaches the region of the inner palpebral commissure (internal canthus). Here the two eyelids are separated by a triangular space, the *lacrimal lake*, in which the secretion accumulates temporarily. From here it passes through two tiny orifices called *lacrimal points*, one on the margin of each eyelid, into the *lacrimal ducts*. The latter converge medially into the lacrimal sac, whence the *nasolacrimal duct* leads into the inferior meatus of the nasal fossae.

The wall of the excretory lacrimal passages is formed by connective tissue lined with epithelium. The epithelium of the lacrimal ducts is stratified squamous. The lacrimal sac and the nasolacrimal duct are lined with a pseudostratified, tall columnar epithelium.

From the bottom of the lacrimal lake, between the two lacrimal ducts, there bulges a small, soft mass of tissue, the *lacrimal caruncle*. The top is covered with a thick, squamous epithelium in which only the uppermost layers are flattened, although not cornified. It contains mucous cells, and gradually merges into the conjunctival epithelium. The lamina propria contains bundles of striated muscles, sweat glands, abortive lacrimal glands, and tiny hairs with sebaceous glands. These are the source of the whitish secretion that often collects in the region of the inner palpebral commissure.

Blood and Lymph Vessels of the Eyelids

The arteries in each lid form two arch-like anastomoses, which run in front of the tarsus, one near the free margin of the lid, the other near the other margin of the tarsus. The palpebral conjunctiva is provided with dense, subepithelial capillary networks which can be easily studied in living condition with the aid of the slit-lamp microscope. Branches of the blood vessels in the scleral conjunctiva anastomose with the marginal blood vessels of the cornea and with the branches of the anterior ciliary arteries.

The lymphatics form a dense plexus in the conjunctiva behind the tarsus. In front of the latter there is another, thinner, pretarsal net. A third net can be distinguished in the skin and the subcutis. All these networks communicate with one another. The lymphatic capillaries of the scleral conjunctiva end blindly near the corneal margin.

The abundant supply of the conjunctiva with blood and lymph capillaries accounts for the rapid absorption of solutions introduced into the conjunctival sac.

HISTOGENESIS OF THE EYE

The stalk of the optic vesicle growing out of the brain is transformed into the optic nerve (Fig. 35–46). The double walled vesicle gives rise to the retina. Where the optic vesicle touches the ectoderm, the latter forms an invagination with a greatly thickened bottom, the *primordium of the lens*. It apparently develops as the result of inductive stimulation of the ectoderm by the optic vesicle. In amphibian larvae, after excision of the optic vesicle, the lens is not formed. The lens primordium comes to lie in the invagination of the optic vesicle. Simultaneously, mesenchyme and blood vessels grow into the choroidal fissure, in the lower part of the optic vesicle. These vessels give rise to the hyaloid and retinal vascular systems. The opposite margins of the fissure, which received the vessels, soon grow together, and the secondary optic vesicle assumes the form of a double walled cup, while the stalk is transformed into a solid strand, the optic nerve.

The lens primordium soon becomes detached from the ectoderm, and the space between the two is filled by a layer of mesen-

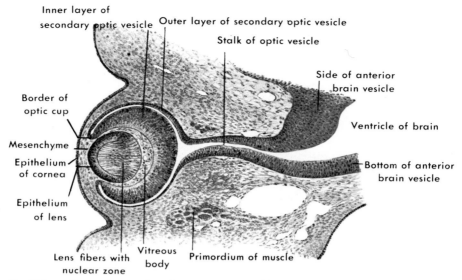

Inner layer of
secondary optic vesicle
Outer layer of secondary optic vesicle
Stalk of optic vesicle
Side of anterior brain vesicle
Ventricle of brain
Bottom of anterior brain vesicle
Border of optic cup
Mesenchyme
Epithelium of cornea
Epithelium of lens
Lens fibers with nuclear zone
Vitreous body
Primordium of muscle

Figure 35-46 Primordium of eye of an 8 mm. mouse embryo. The cavity of the primary optic vesicle is reduced to a thin cleft. × 70. (After Schaffer.)

chyme—the primordium of the substantia propria of the cornea and of the connective tissue of the iris. The lens, surrounded by vascular mesenchyme, acquires a solid, spherical form, while the original cavity disappears. The inner, thicker sheet of the double wall of the optic cup differentiates into the retina proper. It remains permanently in direct continuation with the optic nerve. The outer sheet of the cup is transformed into the pigment epithelium. The surrounding mesenchyme comes into close relation with the optic cup and gives rise to the two outer tunics of the eyeball, the uveal and fibrous tunics. The structural differentiation of the retina proceeds in a way similar to that of the wall of the neural tube. The eyeball attains full size toward the end of the first decade. The structure of the retina, including the central fovea, matures toward the end of the first year.

REFERENCES

Arey, L. B.: Retina, choroid and sclera. *In* Cowdry, E. V. (ed.): Special Cytology. New York, Paul B. Hoeber, Inc., 1932, Vol. III, p. 1213.

Berliner, M. L.: Biomicroscopy of the Eye. New York, Paul B. Hoeber, Inc., 1949.

Boycott, B. B., and J. E. Dowling: Organization of the primate retina: light microscopy. Phil. Trans. Roy. Soc. Lond. B, *255*:109, 1969.

Davson, H.: The Physiology of the Eye. New York, Academic Press, 1972.

De Robertis, E.: Electron microscope observations on the submicroscopic organization of the retinal rods. J. Biophys. Biochem. Cytol., *2*:319, 1956.

De Robertis, E., and C. M. Franchi: Electron microscope observations on synaptic vesicles in synapses of the retinal rods and cones. J. Biophys. Biochem. Cytol., *2*:307, 1956.

Dowling, J. E.: Organization of vertebrate retinas. Invest. Ophth., *9*:655, 1970.

Dowling, J. E., and B. B. Boycott: Organization of the primate retina: electron microscopy. Proc. Roy. Soc. B, *116*:80, 1966.

Duke-Elder, S.: System of Ophthalmology. St. Louis, C. V. Mosby Co., 1961.

Fernández-Morán, H.: The fine structure of vertebrate and invertebrate photoreceptors as revealed by low-temperature electron microscopy. *In* Smelzer, H. (ed.): The Structure of the Eye. New York, Academic Press, 1961, p. 521.

Fernández-Morán, H.: Lamellar systems in myelin and photoreceptors as revealed by high-resolution electron microscopy. *In* Edds, M. V., Jr. (ed.): Macromolecular Complexes. New York, Ronald Press, 1961, p. 113.

Friedenwald, J. S.: The formation of the intraocular fluid. Am. J. Ophth., *32*:9, 1949.

Fuortes, M. G. F. (ed.): Physiology of Photoreceptor Organs. Handbook of Sensory Physiology, Vol. VII/2. Berlin, Springer-Verlag, 1972.

Granit, R.: Receptors and Sensory Perception; A Discussion of Aims, Means, and Results of Electrophysiological Research into the Process of Reception. New Haven, Yale University Press, 1955.

Hartline, H. K.: Receptor mechanisms and the integration

of sensory information in the eye. *In* Oncley, J. L., et al. (eds.): Biophysical Science—A Study Program. New York, John Wiley & Sons, 1959, p. 515.

Hecht, S.: Rods, cones, and the chemical basis of vision. Physiol. Rev., *17*:239, 1937.

Hecht, S., S. Shlaer, and M. H. Pirenne: Energy, quanta, and vision. J. Gen. Physiol., *25*:819, 1942.

Hogan, M. Y., Y. A. Alvarado, and J. E. Weddell: Histology of the Human Eye. An Atlas and Textbook. Philadelphia, W. B. Saunders Co., 1971.

Hubbard, R., and A. Kropf: The action of light on rhodopsin. Proc. Nat. Acad. Sci., *44*:130, 1958.

Hubbard, R., and A. Kropf: Molecular aspects of visual excitation. Ann. N. Y. Acad. Sci., *81*:388, 1959.

Ishikawa, T.: Fine structure of the human ciliary muscle. Invest. Opth., *1*:587, 1962.

Jakus, M. A.: Studies on the cornea. II. The fine structure of Descemet's membrane. J. Biophys. Biochem. Cytol. (Suppl.), *2*:243, 1956.

Kolb, H.: Organization of the outer plexiform layer of the primate retina: electron microscopy of Golgi-impregnated cells. Phil. Trans. Roy. Soc. Lond. B, *258*:261, 1970.

Kolmer, W., and H. Lauber: Auge. *In* von Möllendorff, W., and W. Bargmann (eds.): Handbuch der mikroskopischen Anatomie des Menschen. Berlin, Julius Springer, 1936, Vol. 3, Part 2.

Ladman, A. J.: The fine structure of the rod-bipolar cell synapse in the retina of the albino rat. J. Biophys. Biochem. Cytol., *4*:459, 1958.

Lasansky, A.: The pathway between hyaloid blood and retinal neurons in the toad. Structural observations and permeability to tracer substances. J. Cell Biol., *34*:617, 1967.

Mann, I. C.: The Development of the Human Eye. New York, Macmillan Co., 1937.

Polyak, S.: The Retina. Chicago, University of Chicago Press, 1941.

Polyak, S.: The Vertebrate Visual System. Chicago, University of Chicago Press, 1957.

Raviola, G.: The fine structure of the ciliary zonule and ciliary epithelium. Invest. Opth., *10*:851, 1971.

Raviola, G.: Effects of paracentesis on the blood-aqueous barrier: an electron microscope study on *Macaca mulatta* using horseradish peroxidase as a tracer. Invest. Ophthalm., *13*:828, 1974.

Raviola, G., and E. Raviola: Light and electron microscopic observations on the inner plexiform layer of the rabbit retina. Am. J. Anat., *120*:403, 1967.

Richardson, K. C.: The fine structure of the albino rabbit iris with special reference to the identification of adrenergic and cholinergic nerves and nerve endings in its intrinsic muscles. Am. J. Anat., *114*:173, 1964.

Rohen, J. W.: Das Auge und seine Hilforsorgane. *In* von Möllendorf, W., and W. Bargmann (eds.): Handbuch der mikroskopischen Anatomie des Menschen. Berlin, Springer-Verlag, 1964, Vol. 3, Part 4.

Salzmann, M.: The Anatomy and Histology of the Human Eyeball in the Normal State (translated by E. V. L. Brown). Chicago, University of Chicago Press, 1912.

Sjöstrand, F. S.: An electron microscope study of the retinal rods of the guinea pig eye. J. Cell. Comp. Physiol., *33*:383, 1949.

Sjöstrand, F. S.: The ultrastructure of the outer segments of rods and cones of the eye as revealed by the electron microscope. J. Cell. Comp. Physiol., *43*:15, 1953.

Sjöstrand, F. S.: Ultrastructure of retinal rod synapses of the guinea pig eye as revealed by three-dimensional reconstructions from serial sections. J. Ultrastr. Res., *2*:112, 1958.

Smelzer, G. K. (ed.): The Structure of the Eye (A Symposium). New York, Academic Press, 1961.

Tormey, J. McD.: Fine structure of the ciliary epithelium of the rabbit with particular reference to "infolded membranes," "vesicles" and the effects of Diamox. J. Cell. Biol., *17*:641, 1963.

Wald, G.: The photoreceptor process in vision. Am. J. Ophth., *40*:18, 1955.

Wald, G.: The molecular organization of visual systems. *In* McElroy, W. D., and B. Glass (eds.): Light and Life. Baltimore, The Johns Hopkins Press, 1960, p. 724.

Walls, G. L.: The Vertebrate Eye and Its Adaptive Radiation. Bloomfield Hills, Mich., Cranbrook Press, 1943.

Wanko, T., and M. A. Gavin: Electron microscopic study of lens fibers. J. Biophys. Biochem. Cytol., *6*:97, 1959.

Wislocki, G. B., and A. J. Ladman: The demonstration of a blood-ocular barrier in the albino rat by means of the intravitam deposition of silver. J. Biophys. Biochem. Cytol., *1*:501, 1955.

Young, R. W., and B. Droz: The renewal of protein in retinal rods and cones. J. Cell Biol., *39*:169, 1968.

Young, R. W., and D. Bok: Participation of the retinal pigment epithelium in the rod outer segment renewal process. J. Cell Biol., *42*:392, 1969.

36

The Ear

The organ of hearing is divisible into three parts, each of which differs from the others not only in its gross anatomy but also in its histology and in the functions that it subserves in the translation of sound waves into meaningful information that can be processed in the central nervous system. The first part, the *external ear*, receives the sound waves. In the second part, the *middle ear*, the waves are transformed into the mechanical vibrations of bony *auditory ossicles.* These, in turn, by impinging upon the fluid-filled spaces of the third part, the *internal ear* (or labyrinth), generate specific nerve impulses that are conveyed by the acoustic nerve to the central nervous system. In addition to organs for analysis of sound, the internal ear contains vestibular organs, which are concerned chiefly with the function of maintaining equilibrium.

EXTERNAL EAR

The external ear includes the auricle and the external auditory meatus (Fig. 36–1).

Auricle

The *auricle*, or *pinna*, consists of a single, highly irregular plate of elastic cartilage, 0.5 to 1 mm. thick, overlain by a flexible perichondrium containing abundant elastic fibers. The covering skin has a distinct subcutaneous layer only on the posterior surface of the auricle and is provided with a few small hairs and associated sebaceous glands, the latter sometimes being of considerable size. In old age, especially in men, large stiff hairs develop on the dorsal edge of the auricle and on the ear lobe. Sweat glands are scarce, and, when present, are small.

External Auditory Meatus

The outer portion of the external auditory meatus is a medial continuation of the auricular cartilage, and the inner portion is a canal in the temporal bone (Fig. 36–1). It forms an S-shaped curve coursing for about 2.5 cm. medially and inferiorly and is bounded at its medial end by the ear drum or *tympanic membrane.* The skin lining the meatus is thin and devoid of papillae, and is firmly attached to the underlying perichondrium and periosteum. Numerous hairs in the lining of the cartilaginous portion of the meatus tend to prevent entrance of foreign bodies. In old age these hairs enlarge considerably, as do those on the auricle. Sebaceous glands connected with the hair follicles are exceptionally large. In the bony portion of the meatus, small hairs and sebaceous glands are found only along the upper wall. No eccrine sweat glands are present in the meatus.

The external meatus contains *cerumen,* a brown, waxy secretion that protects the skin from desiccation and presumably from invasion by insects. It is a mixture of the secretion of the sebaceous and *ceruminous glands* of the skin of the meatus. Ceruminous glands are a special variety of coiled tubular apocrine sweat gland. In cross section, they appear to be aggregated into discrete lobules invested by connective tissue. Each glandular tubule is surrounded by a thin network of myoepithelial cells. In the resting state, the gland lumen is large and the epithelial cells lining it are cuboidal. In the active state, however, the cells are columnar and the lumen is constricted. Ducts of ceruminous glands open either onto the free surface of the skin or, with the sebaceous glands, into the necks of hair follicles.

964

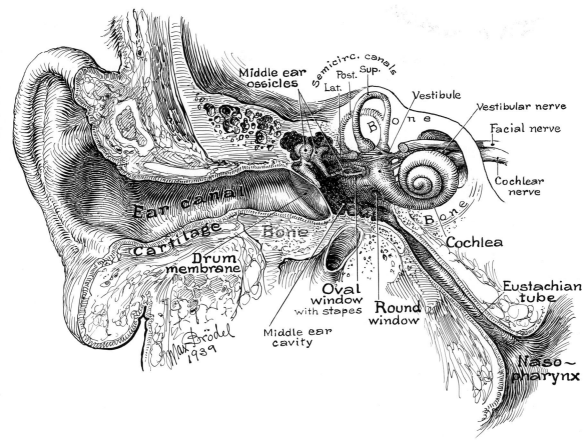

Figure 36-1 Schematic representation of the anatomic relations of the various parts of the human ear. (After M. Brödel, *in* Malone, Guild, and Crowe, Three Unpublished Drawings of the Human Ear. Philadelphia, W. B. Saunders Co., 1946.)

MIDDLE EAR

The middle ear comprises the *tympanic cavity* and its contents (the *auditory ossicles*), the *auditory* or *eustachian tube*, and the *tympanic membrane*, which closes the tympanic cavity externally.

TYMPANIC CAVITY

The tympanic cavity is an irregular, air-filled space in the temporal bone. Its lateral wall is formed largely by the tympanic membrane and its medial wall by the lateral aspect of the bony wall of the internal ear (Fig. 36–2). Anteriorly it continues into the *auditory tube* and posteriorly it is connected, through the tympanic antrum, with air-filled cavities, or "cells," in the mastoid process of the temporal bone. The cavity contains the *auditory ossicles*, the tendons of two small muscles (the *tensor tympani* and the *stapedius*), connected with the ossicles, the *chorda tympani nerve*, and connective tissue (Fig. 36–2).

The epithelium lining the tympanic cavity is generally of the simple squamous type, but near the opening of the auditory tube and near the edge of the tympanic membrane it is cuboidal or columnar and provided with cilia. The presence of glands is generally denied, although detailed study of the mucous membrane here has not been undertaken.

Auditory Ossicles

Three small bones—the *malleus*, the *incus*, and the *stapes*—extend from the attachment of the malleus to the tympanic membrane on

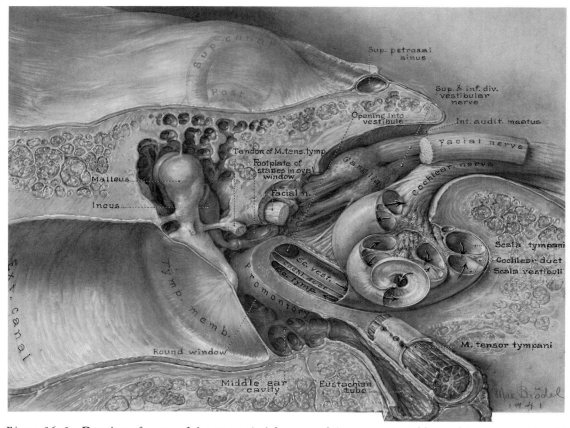

Figure 36–2 Drawing of some of the anatomical features of the external, middle, and inner ear. (After M. Brödel, *in* Malone, Guild, and Crowe, Three Unpublished Drawings of the Human Ear. Philadelphia, W. B. Saunders Co., 1946.)

the one hand, to the medial wall of the tympanic cavity on the other, where the footplate of the stapes fits into the *fenestra vestibuli* or oval window, a hiatus in the wall of the osseous labyrinth (Figs. 36–1 and 36–2). The footplate is maintained in the fenestra by means of an annular fibrous ligament. The three bones are connected to one another by means of typical diarthrodial joints and are supported in the cavity by minute connective tissue ligaments. Small patches of hyaline cartilage are usually found on the manubrium of the malleus and on the footplate of the stapes. The mucosa lining the tympanic cavity is reflected over the ossicles and is firmly attached to their periosteum.

TYMPANIC MEMBRANE

This oval, semitransparent membrane is shaped like a very flat cone with its apex directed medially (Figs. 36–1 to 36–3). Its conical form is maintained by the insertion, onto its inner surface, of the manubrium of the malleus, which tends to pull the center of the membrane medially. The tympanic membrane is formed of two layers of collagenous fibers and fibroblasts similar to those of a flat tendon (Fig. 36–3). However, there is a flaccid portion in its anterosuperior quadrant (Shrapnell's membrane) that is devoid of collagenous fibers. In the outer layer of the membrane the collagen fibers have a radial arrangement, whereas those in the inner layer are disposed circularly. There are also thin networks of elastic fibers, located mainly in the central and peripheral parts of the membrane. Externally the membrane is covered by a thin (50 to 60 μm.) layer of skin devoid of hairs and other appendages. Its inner surface is lined by the mucosa of the tympanic cavity, here only 20 to 40 μm. thick and consisting of simple squamous epithelium overlying a lamina propria of sparse collagenous fibers and capillaries. Over the manubrium of the malleus is a layer of connective tissue through which vessels and nerves reach the center of the membrane.

AUDITORY TUBE

From its origin in the anterior wall of the tympanic cavity, the auditory tube extends anteromedially and inferiorly for about 4 cm. to an opening on the posterolateral wall of the nasopharynx. The rostral two thirds of the tube is supported medially by cartilage, and the portion toward the tympanic cavity is supported by bone.

The cartilage supporting the auditory tube lies mainly medial to the lumen, but a ridge of cartilage running longitudinally for most of the length of the tube curves superolaterally, so that in cross section the cartilage has the appearance of a shepherd's crook (Fig. 36–4). The cartilage is elastic throughout most of its length, but at the isthmus it loses its elastic fibers and becomes hyaline. The lumen of the tube, flattened in the vertical plane, is largest at its pharyngeal end, decreases to a mere slit at the junction of the

cartilaginous and bony portions (isthmus), and then expands again in its course through the temporal bone. The tube is lined by a mucosa, of variable thickness, thrown into folds (rugae) at both the pharyngeal and tympanic ends. In the bony portion of the auditory tube, it is relatively thin and is composed of low columnar ciliated epithelium resting upon a thin lamina propria firmly bound to the periosteum. The epithelium in the cartilaginous portion of the tube is pseudostratified and composed of tall columnar cells, many of which are ciliated. The underlying lamina propria is much more complex here than in the bony portion. Toward the pharyngeal orifice, it contains many compound tubuloalveolar glands that secrete mucus via ducts opening into the tubal lumen. In this vicinity, also, goblet cells are interspersed among the columnar epithelial cells.

There is considerable individual variation in number and distribution of ciliated cells and goblet cells, and in the degree of development of the glandular elements. Throughout the lamina propria, in both portions of the tube, a great many lymphocytes can be found, the number varying with age and from one individual to another. Near the pharyngeal opening there are often discrete

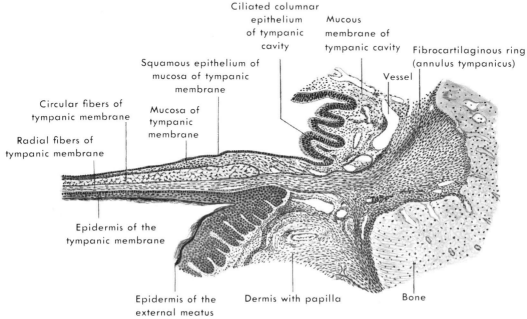

Ciliated columnar epithelium of tympanic cavity

Mucous membrane of tympanic cavity

Fibrocartilaginous ring (annulus tympanicus)

Squamous epithelium of mucosa of tympanic membrane

Vessel

Circular fibers of tympanic membrane

Mucosa of tympanic membrane

Radial fibers of tympanic membrane

Epidermis of the tympanic membrane

Epidermis of the external meatus

Dermis with papilla

Bone

Figure 36–3   Cross section of edge of tympanic membrane of a child. (Redrawn from von Ebner.)

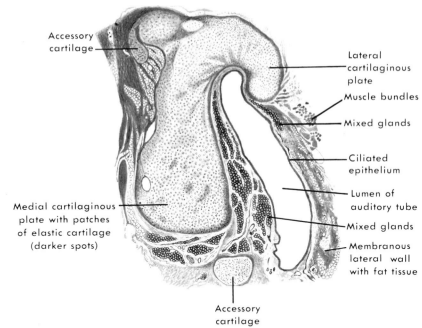

Accessory cartilage

Lateral cartilaginous plate

Muscle bundles

Mixed glands

Ciliated epithelium

Lumen of auditory tube

Mixed glands

Medial cartilaginous plate with patches of elastic cartilage (darker spots)

Membranous lateral wall with fat tissue

Accessory cartilage

Figure 36–4 Transection of cartilaginous portion of the auditory tube near its opening into the pharynx. × 11. (Redrawn from von Ebner.)

collections of lymphoid tissue forming the *tubal tonsils* (of Gerlach). Usually the auditory tube is closed. During the acts of swallowing and yawning, the lumen is opened for a short interval, allowing the pressure in the tympanic cavity to equalize with that outside.

INTERNAL EAR

The internal ear, called the labyrinth because of its complex structure, is composed of a series of fluid-filled sacs and tubules suspended in cavities of corresponding form in the petrous portion of the temporal bone (Fig. 36–5).

The canals and cavities in the bone constitute the bony or *osseous labyrinth*. Suspended within this system of cavities are the thin-walled, fluid-filled tubules and saccules of the *membranous labyrinth*, which constitute the *endolymphatic system*. This is surrounded by the cells and fluid of the *perilymphatic system*.

THE BONY LABYRINTH

There are two major cavities in the bony labyrinth: the *vestibule*, which houses the *sac-*

cule and *utricle*, and anteromedial to it, the spirally coiled *cochlea*, which contains the *organ of Corti* (Figs. 36–1 and 36–2).

The Vestibule

The vestibule is an irregularly ovoid cavity located medial to the tympanic cavity. Its wall facing the tympanic cavity is penetrated by the fenestra vestibuli, and certain recesses in its wall produce characteristic bony protrusions on the medial wall of the tympanic cavity in relationship to the fenestra. For a more detailed description, the student is referred to a textbook of gross anatomy. Three *semicircular canals* arise from recesses in the wall of the vestibule and return to it. According to their position, they are named the superior, posterior, and lateral semicircular canals. Two of the recesses located anterosuperiorly accommodate the dilated *ampullae* of the superior and lateral *semicircular ducts* of the membranous labyrinth, and posteriorly a third recess houses the *posterior ampulla*. Given off from these recesses are the superior (or anterior), the lateral, and the posterior *semicircular canals*. The lateral canal curves laterally around the vestibule and rejoins it behind the posterior ampullary recess. The superior and posterior canals join each other superior to the vestibule in the recess for the *crus commune*, which opens into the medial part of the vestibule. From the medial wall of the vestibule a thin canal, the *vestibular aqueduct*, extends to the posterior surface of the petrous portion of the temporal bone.

The Cochlea

The bony cochlea is anteromedial to the vestibule (Figs. 36–1, 36–2 and 36–5). It consists of a complex bony canal that makes two and three quarter-spiral turns around an axis formed by the conical pillar of spongy bone called the *modiolus*. The base of the modiolus forms the deep end of the *internal acoustic meatus*. Blood vessels and the central processes of nerve fibers belonging to the cochlear division of the eighth cranial nerve pass through numerous openings into the bony substance of the modiolus. The cell bodies of these bipolar afferent neurons are found in the *spiral ganglion*, which courses spirally within the modiolus along the inner wall of

the cochlear canal (Fig. 36–11). Their peripheral processes traverse the remaining distance to the cochlear hair cells which they innervate.

The lumen of the canal of the osseous cochlea (about 3 mm. in diameter) is divided along its whole course (about 35 mm. in man) into an upper and a lower section by the *spiral lamina*. The lamina is divided into two zones: an inner zone containing bone (the *osseous spiral lamina*) and a fibrous outer zone (the *membranous spiral lamina*). The latter is also called the *basilar membrane* (Figs. 36–11, 36–13 and 36–14). At the attachment of the basilar membrane to the outer wall of the cochlea, the periosteum is thickened and forms a distinct structure that has been called the *spiral ligament*, although histologically it does not have the characteristics of a ligament. The cochlear canal is further subdivided by a thin membrane, the *vestibular membrane (Reissner's membrane)*, which extends obliquely from the spiral lamina to the outer wall of the bony cochlea (Fig. 36–11). Thus, a cross section of the bony cochlea will show

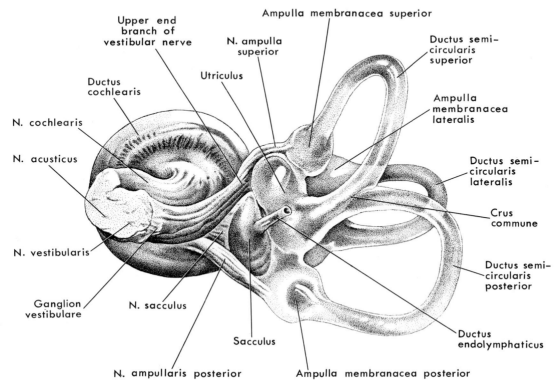

Figure 36-5 Right membranous labyrinth of an adult; medial and posterior aspects. About × 5. (Redrawn and modified from Spalteholz.)

three compartments: an upper cavity, the *scala vestibuli;* a lower cavity, the *scala tympani;* and an intermediate cavity, the *scala media* (Fig. 36–11). The latter is the *cochlear duct,* a portion of the endolymphatic system that connects with the vestibular part of the membranous labyrinth by way of the small *ductus reuniens.*

The scala tympani and scala vestibuli are perilymphatic spaces. The scala vestibuli extends into and through the perilymphatic cistern of the vestibule and reaches the inner surface of the *fenestra ovalis.* The scala tympani ends at the *fenestra rotundum.* At the apex of the cochlea the two scalae communicate through a small opening, the *helicotrema.*

THE MEMBRANOUS (OR ENDOLYMPHATIC) LABYRINTH

The fluid-filled sacs of the membranous labyrinth arise embryologically from a single otic vesicle of ectodermal origin, and, although the semicircular ducts are derived from the utricle, and the cochlear duct and the endolymphatic sac are derived from the saccule, all of these parts of the labyrinth are in communication and all are filled with *endolymph.*

Utricle, Saccule, and Ampullae

In the vestibule, the oblong utricle lies superior and then posterior to the roughly spherical saccule and communicates via five orifices with the three semicircular ducts and their ampullae (Fig. 36–5). The semicircular

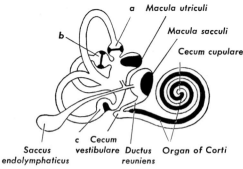

Figure 36-6 Diagram of membranous labyrinth with neuroepithelial areas in black. *a, b,* and *c* respectively designate the ampullae of the superior, lateral, and posterior semicircular canals. (Modified from von Ebner.)

ducts are eccentrically placed in the bony canals and are lined by a simple squamous epithelium. Each ampulla has a flattened floor and a hemispherical roof bulging on the concave side of the duct. Both the saccule and utricle give off ducts medially, which join and form the slender *endolymphatic duct* (Fig. 36–5), which in turn courses under the utricle and then medially through the vestibular aqueduct to end on the posterior surface of the petrous portion of the temporal bone as a small dilation, the *endolymphatic sac.* The sac is located between layers of the meninges and is richly surrounded by blood vessels and connective tissue.

The epithelium lining the membranous structures in the vestibule is of simple squamous type, similar to that found in the semicircular ducts except in the immediate vicinity of sensory areas. The sensory areas and cells just peripheral to them, however, are specialized and, in many respects, highly complex.

Crista Ampullaris and Maculae. The epithelium in the floor of the three ampullae is raised into a transverse ridge, the *crista,* which is covered with the sensory epithelium and is bounded at either end by cells of the *planum semilunatum* (Figs. 36–8 and 36–9). The latter are perpendicular to the long axis of the crista.

Sensory epithelium on the cristae is histologically the same as that composing the *maculae* of the utricle and saccule, with variation apparently only in the relative number of different cell types. Classically, sensory epithelia in the vestibular portion of the internal ear are described as possessing two cell types, *hair cells* and *supporting cells.* Recent investigations have shown, however, that among the hair cells two morphological types can be distinguished.

HAIR CELLS. Hair cells of type I are flask-shaped cells with a rounded base and constricted neck region (Fig. 36–9). The round nucleus is located basally and surrounded by a more or less dense population of mitochondria. Mitochondria also are found congregated at the apex of the cell immediately beneath the free surface, which bears specialized microvilli, or hairs, of considerable length, and a single cilium. From its constricted neck inferiorly the hair cell is enclosed in a chalice-like nerve terminal.

Hair cells of type II are simple columnar cells innervated by numerous small synaptic

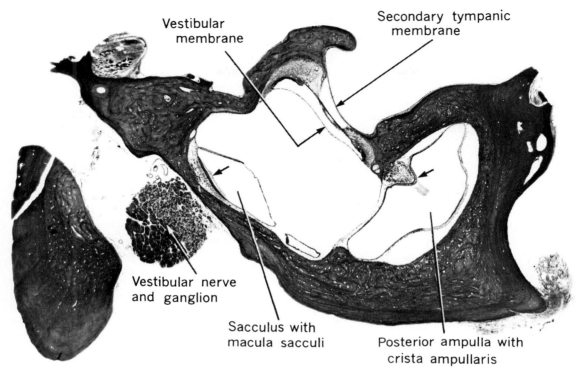

Vestibular membrane

Secondary tympanic membrane

Vestibular nerve and ganglion

Sacculus with macula sacculi

Posterior ampulla with crista ampullaris

Figure 36-7 Photomicrograph of a section of a rhesus monkey inner ear, including the sacculus with the macula sacculi (at arrow) and the posterior ampulla with the crista ampullaris (at arrow). (Courtesy of H. Mizoguchi.)

endings that are difficult to see with the light microscope (Fig. 36–9). Nuclei of type II hair cells are round and regular in outline, like those of type I hair cells. They can be found at various levels in the cell but usually form a row at a higher level in the epithelium than those of the type I hair cells and the supporting cells.

Seen with the electron microscope, the luminal border of both type I and type II hair cells is characterized by the presence of a single cilium and 50 to 110 straight hairs. These are actually highly specialized microvilli and, in the belief that they are nonmotile, have been described as *stereocilia.* The hairs are covered by plasma membrane and are noticeably constricted at their bases. Their substance appears to be fibrillar and they have a denser axial core, which is composed of longitudinally arranged fine filaments. This core continues downward from the narrow base of the hair and is embedded in the thickened terminal web, which extends across the cell immediately below its specialized free border. The hairs are arranged upon the cell surface

in regular hexagonal array and in successive rows show a progressive increase of length from less than 1 μm. on one side to 100 μm. on the other side, the longest hairs being located at the side of the cell bearing the cilium (Fig. 36–20). The cilium originates from a basal body located in a terminal web-free area of the apical cytoplasm. The cilium has the typical nine outer doublet tubules and two central tubules found in cilia elsewhere, although the central tubules end shortly after leaving the basal body. A rootlet extends from the basal body into the cytoplasm on the side opposite the stereocilia aggregate. Although the cilium is considered to be nonmotile, it is commonly called a *kinocilium.* The existence of a gradient of stereocilia length, the eccentric location of the kinocilium, and the arrangement of the rootlet result in a morphological polarization of the hair cell, which is reflected in the physiological responses of the hair cell to stimuli. Both sensory cell types have a very dense terminal web or *cuticular plate* just below the apical plasmalemma. This structure may extend 0.5 μm. or more into

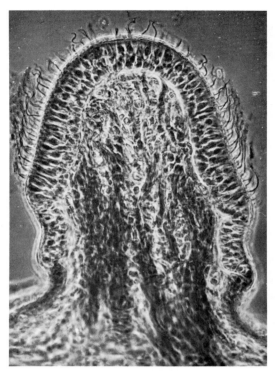

Figure 36–8 Phase contrast photomicrograph of an unstained section in plastic of guinea pig crista ampullaris, showing the hairs projecting from the hair cells of the neuroepithelium. (Courtesy of H. Engström.)

the cell cytoplasm, but is discontinuous in the area of the basal body.

In both types of hair cells there are scattered profiles of granular endoplasmic reticulum, but smooth surfaced tubules and vesicles are more abundant. Vesicles about 200 Å in diameter are present in greatest profusion in the type II hair cells. The supranuclear Golgi complex is also more extensively developed in this type. Characteristic of the type I cell is the occurrence of a great many microtubules, mostly concentrated in the apical cytoplasm just beneath the terminal web.

The nature of the synaptic contact between the two types of hair cells and the terminations of the vestibular nerve fibers is quite different (Fig. 36–9). In the case of type I, the afferent nerve envelops the hair cell in a cuplike ending. At the base of the cell, the intercellular space between the plasmalemma and the axolemma is about 300 Å wide. Dense linear structures with an associated halo of small vesicles (resembling the so-called *synaptic ribbons* found at the junction of

the rod axon and bipolar cell dendrite in the retina) are found in varying numbers in the hair cell cytoplasm immediately opposite the nerve calyx. These specializations are considered indicative of chemical synapses. Additionally there are certain discrete areas where the intercellular substance is lacking and the membranes are only about 50 Å apart. These specializations exhibit the same morphological characteristics as low resistance contacts found at electrical synapses. At present, however, there are no physiological data relevant to this question. Nearer the rim of the cuplike ending around the upper part of the hair cell, no obvious junctional specializations of the kind usually found at synapses are observed, but there are in the axoplasm large numbers of vesicles 500 to 2000 Å in diameter, some with dense cores.

The type II hair cell is not enveloped by a chalice-like ending, but a large number of separate terminal *boutons* impinge upon its surface. Synaptic ribbons are often found in the hair cell opposite sparsely granulated boutons, and the bouton membrane may also be thickened at such presumably synaptic points. A second type of bouton is distinguished by its dense packing of small synaptic vesicles. Lesion and histochemical studies strongly suggest that these boutons are efferent in nature. In addition to contacting type II hair cell bases directly, such boutons also contact type I nerve chalices, other afferent boutons and passing nerve fibers. However, the pre- and postsynaptic membrane thickenings traditionally considered indicative of synapses are only rarely noted at points of apposition between vesiculated boutons and hair cells. They are more common where the vesiculated efferents contact other neural structures. It is clear that the synaptic relationships are far more complicated than was imagined from light microscope studies, and their exact nature remains unsettled.

The effective stimulus for vestibular hair cells is movement of the head in one or another plane. This, in turn, presumably sets up movement of the endolymph, which acts in some manner to trigger an impulse in the afferent vestibular nerve. The transducers of the original mechanical stimulus into electrical signals are presumably the hair-bearing surfaces of the hair cells. Exactly how a receptor potential is set up in the hair cell and how it, in turn, influences the afferent nerve are problems that are only now being investigated. Recent evidence seems to indicate that bending of the hairs initiates the process, but so little is known of their physiological properties that no more can be said at present.

SUPPORTING CELLS. The supporting cells have their nuclei near the base of the sensory epithelium and extend to its free surface, but their cell bodies are so irregularly contorted that the full extent of any given cell can never be seen in a single section (Fig. 36–

9). One usually sees a mosaic of sections of many cells cut at different levels. With the light microscope little can be resolved in their cytoplasm, but in electron micrographs they are found to possess a cytoskeleton of bundles of microtubules running from the basal cytoplasm to the dense terminal web, which is far more elaborately developed in these cells than in the hair cells. They have a prominent Golgi complex and the cytoplasm is crowded with membrane limited granules resembling

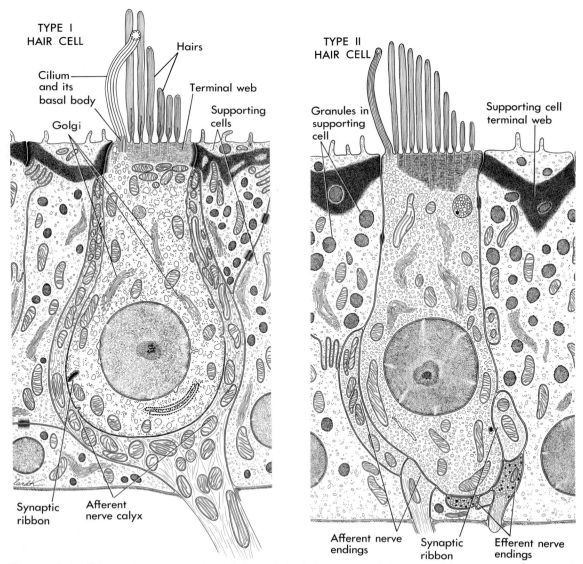

Figure 36–9 Schematic representation of the principal ultrastructural features of the vestibular type I and type II hair cells and their supporting cells. (Drawn by Sylvia Colard Keene.)

secretory granules. Little is known about the function of the supporting cells. They may contribute to the nutrition of the hair cells or may be involved in some way in the metabolism of the endolymph. Toward the periphery of the sensory region there is a gradual transition to the cells comprising the *planum semilunatum.*

The planum semilunatum is generally composed of columnar cells with slightly infolded lateral membranes. Investigations using ^{35}S and colloidal iron implicate these cells in the elaboration and secretion of sulfated mucopolysaccharide components of the cupula.

On the sloping sides of the crista ampullaris are very complex cells with highly infolded basal membranes and a dense cytoplasmic matrix with large vacuoles containing a flocculent material. These "dark" cells are reminiscent of other cells known to be involved in ion movement, and it has been speculated that they maintain the high K^+ level in endolymph.

CUPULAE AND OTOLITHS. Overlying the hairs in maculae are a multitude of minute (3 to 5 μm.) crystalline bodies, *otoliths.* These are a mixture of calcium carbonate and a protein. In life, they are suspended within the jellylike mucopolysaccharide substance that surrounds the sensory areas of the maculae.

The *cupulae* are gelatinous bodies located above the cristae. In life, these too are composed of glycoprotein that is evidently much more viscous than the rest of the endolymph. When fixed, the structure is often lost or deformed, and indeed this fact has, in the past, led some otologists to question its reality. That a cupula does exist is no longer doubted, but there is very little substantial information about its origin.

Endolymphatic Sac

The cell types encountered in different parts of the vestibular system are basically similar from one region to the other. In the endolymphatic sac, however, one finds cells that appear to be specialized for an absorptive function, and these are structurally different from other cells in the vestibular membranous labyrinth. Unlike the other membranous sacs, the endolymphatic sac usually contains cellular debris of one sort or another. The electrolyte concentration in its endolymph also differs from that elsewhere in the inner ear.

Histologically, there is a transition from the squamocuboidal cells of the endolymphatic duct to tall columnar cells in the sac. The latter have been variously described as covering protruding papillae or occupying crypts. Whichever is the case, there are two distinct columnar cell types present. One is a dense cell with a large irregularly shaped nucleus, a relatively unspecialized free surface, and a cell base with slightly infolded membranes. The other is a less dense cell characterized by long microvilli on its surface and many pinocytotic vesicles and vacuoles. Basally the cell membrane is smooth, but laterally it interdigitates extensively with other cells. There is good evidence that the endolymphatic sac acts as a site for absorption of endolymph and that free phagocytic cells, which appear to be macrophages and neutrophils, may cross the epithelium here to engulf and digest cellular debris and foreign material that may gain access to the endolymph.

The Cochlear Duct

The cochlear duct is a highly specialized diverticulum of the saccule. It contains the *organ of Corti*—the effective organ of hearing—and a number of other specialized areas subserving different functions and having their own special histological characteristics. This is a very complex area, and in order to facilitate understanding, the different regions will be described individually in the following order: *vestibular membrane, stria vascularis, spiral prominence, organ of Corti,* and *tectorial membrane.* It can be seen in Figure 36–11 that this order of descriptions proceeds in a counterclockwise direction around the circumference of the cochlear duct.

Vestibular Membrane. The vestibular membrane is a delicate bilaminar structure extending across the cochlea from medial to lateral. Its inner surface is lined by cells that are differentiated in a manner suggesting that they may be involved in water and electrolyte transport. The bulging perinuclear region of the cell is readily apparent in the light microscope, but peripherally, the cell body is highly attenuated. The surface of these cells (toward the scala media) bears many short, clavate microvilli similar to those found on cells in the choroid plexus (see Chapter 12). At the basal surface, the membranes are highly infolded and interdigitate extensively with those of neighboring cells. A distinct basal lamina is found along this basal surface. Directly apposed to these cells, with little or no intervening collagen, is a layer of squamous perilymphatic cells of the scala vestibuli, so attenuated that they can scarcely be seen in well fixed material.

Stria Vascularis. The epithelial covering of the vestibular membrane becomes continuous, at the outer wall of the cochlea, with the basal layer of cells in the specialized band of stratified epithelium called the *stria vascularis* (Figs. 36–10 to 36–12). With the light microscope it is possible to distinguish two cell types in this epithelium—a layer of light-staining *basal cells* and a darker-staining superficial layer of marginal cells possessing numerous mitochondria. In electron micrographs some workers have identified a third cell type, the *intermediate cells.* Although these latter are intermediate between marginal and basal cells in their location, they are difficult to distinguish cytologically from basal cells. The convex free surface of the marginal cells apparently varies with the species and may be smooth or have microvilli, as it does in the human. The basal portion of these cells is divided by deep infoldings of the plasmalemma into a labyrinthine system of narrow compartments occupied by numerous mitochondria. The intermediate and basal cells have relatively few mitochondria and numerous processes which interdigitate with each other and with the marginal cells. Ascending processes of the basal cells form cuplike structures surrounding and partially isolating each marginal cell from neighboring areas of the epithelium (Fig. 36–12). Capillaries penetrate into the stria vascularis and course longitudinally within the epithelium, surrounded by processes of the intermediate and marginal cells. The stria vascularis is presumed to be involved in the secretion of the endolymph, and the resemblance of the elaborate basal compartmentation of the marginal cells to similar basal specializations of other cells involved in ion transport has led to the suggestion that these cells may help maintain the unusual ionic composition of the endolymph.

Spiral Prominence. The stria vascularis ends inferiorly, and its basal cell layer is continuous with the cells overlying the *spiral prominence* (Fig. 36–13). This prominence extends the whole length of the cochlear duct and rests upon a very richly vascularized thickening of the underlying periosteum.

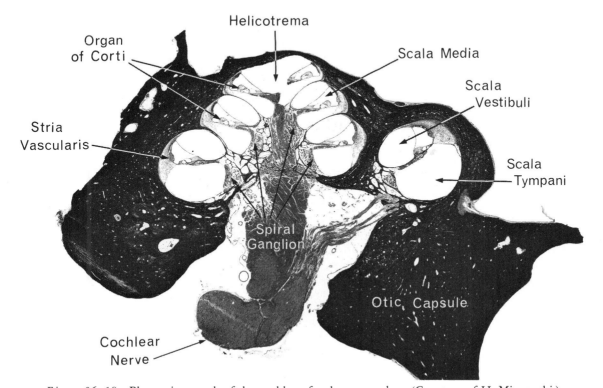

Figure 36–10 Photomicrograph of the cochlea of a rhesus monkey. (Courtesy of H. Mizoguchi.)

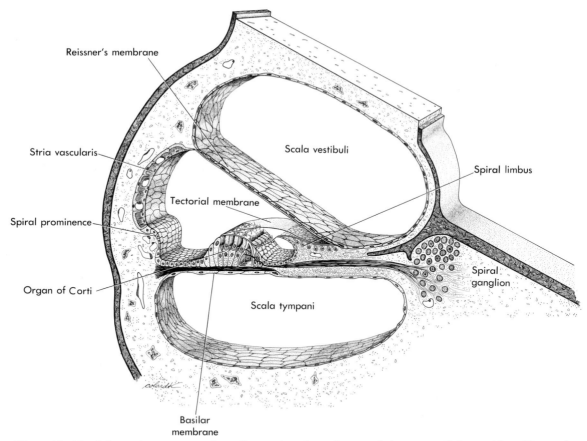

Figure 36-11 Schematic representation of a section through one of the turns of the cochlea. (Drawn by Sylvia Colard Keene.)

The epithelium of the spiral prominence continues downward and is reflected from the outer wall of the cochlea onto the basilar membrane, forming at its line of reflection the *external spiral sulcus*. The cells here take on a cuboidal shape, and those continuing onto the pars pectinata of the basilar membrane are known as the *cells of Claudius*. In the basal coil of the cochlea small groups of polyhedral cells *(cells of Boettcher)* are interposed between the basilar membrane and the cells of Claudius (Fig. 36–14). These cells have large spherical nuclei, and their cytoplasm is denser than that of the adjoining cells of Claudius. The plasma membrane of the lower half of these cells gives rise to numerous microvilli, which may either interdigitate extensively with those of adjacent cells, or protrude into the intercellular space. Such specializations suggest that the Boettcher cells have a secretory or absorptive

function. The reason for their exclusive localization in the cochlear basal coil is unclear at present.

Organ of Corti

Over the pars pectinata and pars arcuata the cells become columnar and bulge into the cochlear duct, forming the epithelial ridge called the *organ of Corti* (Figs. 36–10, 36–11, and 36–13). This highly specialized complex of epithelial cells extends throughout the length of the cochlea and is composed of *hair cells*, the receptors of stimuli produced by sound, and various *supporting cells.*

Supporting Cells. The several types of supporting cells have certain characteristics in common. They are tall, slender cells extending from the basilar membrane to the free surface of the organ of Corti, and they contain conspicuous tonofibrils. Although the cells are separated by large intercellular spaces, their upper surfaces are in contact with each other and with the hair cells to form a continuous free surface for the organ. This surface is called the *reticular membrane*. The supporting cells include *inner* and *outer pillars*, *inner* and *outer phalangeal cells*, *border cells*, and *cells of Hensen*.

Within the organ of Corti is the *inner tunnel*, a canal extending the length of the cochlea and bounded below by extensions of the pillar cells, which lie on top of the basilar membrane, and above by the bodies of the inner and outer pillar cells. The bodies of the pillars are separated by clefts through which the tunnel communicates with the other intercellular cavities in the organ of Corti, including the *outer tunnel* or *space of Nuel*.

INNER PILLARS. The inner pillars have a broad base that rests on the basilar membrane and a conical cell body with its apex extending upward (Figs. 36–14 and 36–16). The cytoplasm of the pillar cell contains the nucleus at the inner angle of the roughly tri-angular tunnel. The most distinctive feature of these cells is the darkly staining tonofibrils that course from the cell base through the cylindrical body of the pillar to end in the junctional complexes at the apex, where the cell expands into a flat flange to contact neighboring pillar cells and the inner hair cells. The contact between inner and outer pillar cells is of particularly large area and forms a structurally sound supporting mechanism. What appear to be tonofibrils with the light microscope are found in electron micrographs to be a highly organized array of tubules, with an outside diameter of 275 Å and a wall thickness of about 60 Å. Interspersed among these "tubular tonofilaments" are 60 Å microfilaments (Fig. 36–25). This array runs from the base of the pillar cell to the apex of the cell at the top of the organ of Corti.

OUTER PILLARS. The outer pillars are longer than the inner ones (Figs. 36–14 and 36–16). Their base is situated on the basilar membrane at the junction of the pars pec-

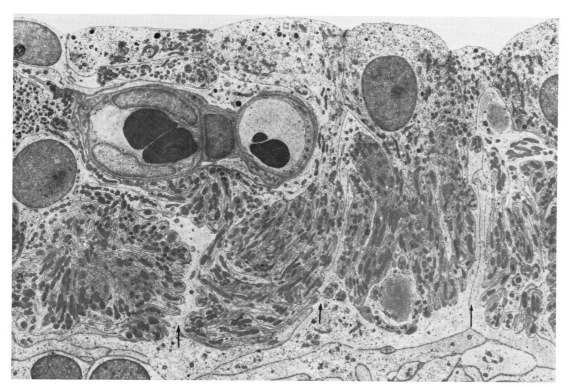

Figure 36–12 Electron micrograph of the stria vascularis of the cat inner ear, illustrating the intraepithelial capillaries, the ascending process of the basal cells (at arrows), and the elaborately infolded bases of the marginal cells. (After R. Hinojosa and E. Rodriguez-Echandia, Am. J. Anat., *118*:631, 1966.)

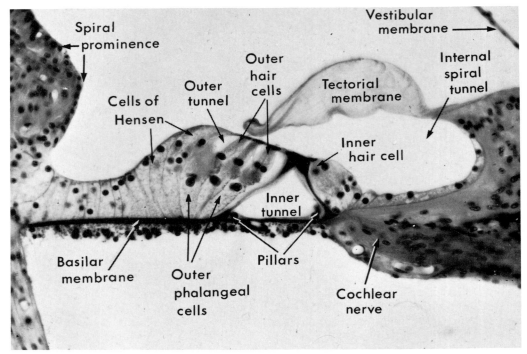

Figure 36-13 Photomicrograph of the organ of Corti of a cat. The tectorial membrane has been lifted away from the inner hair cells in specimen preparation. (Courtesy of H. Engström.)

tinata and pars arcuata, adjoining the base of the inner pillar. The cell body is similar to that of the inner pillar, but the free surface of the cell has a somewhat different shape. The head of the outer pillar abuts the head of the inner pillar and sends out a phalangeal process that forms a junction with the outer hair cells. The outer pillars, in fact, form the first row of phalanges.

The inner pillars number approximately 5600, the outer ones 3800. On an average, three inner pillars are connected with two outer pillars.

INNER PHALANGEAL CELLS. These cells are arranged in a row on the inner surface of the inner pillars and completely surround the inner hair cells. In contradistinction to the outer phalangeal cells there is no enlarged extracellular space between the supporting cells and the hair cells. Afferent and efferent nerve fibers travel through and are supported by the inner phalangeal cells. The relationship between supporting cells and inner hair cells is completely analogous to that of the supporting and hair cells of the vestibular system.

OUTER PHALANGEAL CELLS (OF DEITERS). The outer phalangeal cells act as supporting elements for the three to four rows of outer hair cells (Figs. 36–17, 36–18, and 36–19). These phalangeal cells are columnar, with their bases resting on the basilar membrane. Apically they surround the inferior third of the outer hair cell and also enclose the afferent and efferent nerve bundles traveling to the hair cell base. This portion of the cell does not reach the free surface of the organ of Corti, but on the side of the cell away from the outer pillar cells, it gives off a slender finger-like process internally reinforced by a bundle of microtubules. This phalanx expands at the surface of the organ of Corti to form a flat apical plate joined at its edges to the hair cell that it is supporting and to the hair cell in the row next to it. The plate-like expansion at the surface also contains abundant supporting microtubules.

The upper two thirds of the outer hair cells are not surrounded by other cells but are exposed within a fluid-filled space (the space of Nuel) that is in communication with the inner tunnel through the clefts between the pillars. The fluid that bathes the hair cells and occupies the space of Nuel and inner tunnel is apparently separated from the endolymphatic or perilymphatic spaces and thus may be of different composition than either perilymph or endolymph.

BORDER CELLS. The inner phalangeal cells continue into a row of slender cells, termed border cells, that delimit the inner boundary of the organ of Corti (Fig. 36–14). There is a gradual transition in height from these to the squamous cells lining the inner spiral sulcus.

CELLS OF HENSEN. Adjacent to the last row of outer phalangeal cells are the tall cells of Hensen that constitute the outer border of the organ of Corti. They are arranged in several rows decreasing rapidly in height and laterally abutting the cells of Claudius.

Cochlear Hair Cells. In the cochlea, as in the vestibule, two types of hair cells are present (Figs. 36–11, 36–13, and 36–19). The *inner hair cells* are arranged in a single row along the whole length of the cochlea. The *outer hair cells* form three rows and are lodged between the outer pillars and the outer phalangeal cells. In the human, a fourth and sometimes a fifth row of outer hair cells may appear toward the apex, though these supernumerary rows may not be as regular as the first three.

Inner hair cells resemble type I cells in

the vestibular labyrinth in many respects. They are relatively short, goblet-shaped cells with a slightly constricted neck region. The surface of the cell bears hairs, similar in structure to those on vestibular hair cells, but in the adult there is no associated cilium. However, a basal body and an associated typical centriole persist as the only remnants of the ciliary apparatus. The hairs are arranged on the cell surface in the form of a letter W or U, with the base of the letter directed toward the centrioles (Fig. 36–23). The rootlets of the hairs extend down into, and at times through, the dense terminal web or cuticular plate. The cell body contains scattered ribosomes and 200 Å vesicles interspersed among larger vesicular profiles, presumably representing the smooth endoplasmic reticulum. Mitochondria are aggregated under the terminal web and at the cell base but are scattered in smaller numbers throughout the cytoplasm. The synaptic area of the inner hair cell extends from the base of the cell to the level of the nucleus. The vast majority of the endings contacting the inner hair cell are sparsely vesiculated and are considered to be endings of the cochlear nerve. Many of these run beside the hair cell up to the level of its nucleus, though not all the area of apposition is synaptic. Pre- and postsynaptic membrane thickenings and synaptic ribbons are consid-

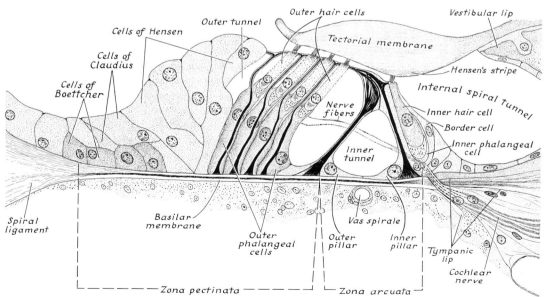

Figure 36–14 Radial transection of the organ of Corti, from the upper part of the first coil of human cochlea. (Slightly modified from Held.)

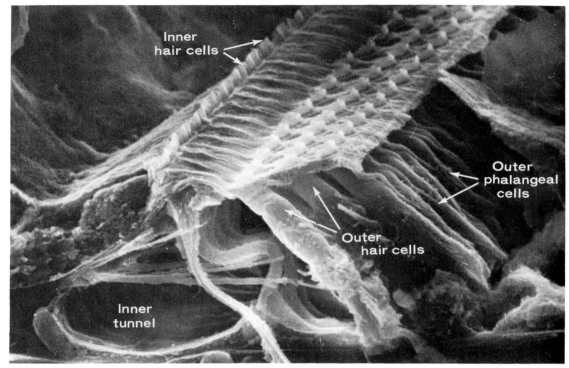

Figure 36-15 Scanning electron micrograph of guinea pig organ of Corti. For further orientation, see Figure 36-14. (Micrograph courtesy of H. Engström.)

ered to demarcate sites of synaptic transmission. In addition, small neuronal profiles containing many synaptic vesicles, some of which are dense-cored, make contact with inner hair cells, though this is rather rare. More often contacts with pre- and postsynaptic membrane thickenings are seen between these heavily vesiculated fibers and the afferent fibers just before the latter make contact with the inner hair cell. Many such vesiculated fibers are found beneath the inner hair cell, and they are considered efferent in nature.

Outer hair cells have a different structure from inner hair cells and this has led to speculations that the two cell types have different functions. Outer hair cells, as previously stated, are supported on the apices of outer phalangeal cells and receive innervation from the cochlear nerve at their bases (Figs. 36–14 and 36–27). The hairs on the apex of these cells form a distinctive W similar to that of the inner hair cells, but here there are more rows of hairs, and the length

of the hairs varies from long at the periphery to short centrally (Figs. 36–20 and 36–24). Again, no cilium is present, although a basal body can be found at the base of the W. Immediately deep to the terminal web are dense lipid-like inclusions interspersed with elongated, highly convoluted elements of the granular endoplasmic reticulum. Mitochondria are generally aggregated in the basal cytoplasm and line up along the sides of the cell in relation to one or more rows of smooth surfaced vesicles that are aligned parallel to the plasmalemma. A single row of such smooth surfaced vesicles is also found along the nonsynaptic plasmalemma of the inner hair cell. At present the function of these vesicular aggregates is unknown.

The basal part of the outer hair cell receives synapses from both efferent and afferent nerve fibers. Here, however, the afferent fibers from the cochlear nerve frequently give rise to the smaller endings. Such synapses exhibit pre- and postsynaptic membrane thickenings and, in some species, synaptic ribbons, but they are not heavily vesiculated. The efferent endings on the outer hair cells are larger than those of the afferent fibers and contain many densely packed vesicles. In the hair cell cytoplasm, parallel to the plasmalemma and extending the entire length of the efferent synapse, is found a single continuous flattened cisterna, the "subsynaptic cisterna."

Spiral Limbus. In the inner angle of the scala media, the periosteal connective tissue of the upper surface of the osseous spiral lamina bulges into the scala media as the *spiral limbus* (Figs. 36–11, 36–13, and 36–14). Its edge overhangs the internal spiral sulcus (or tunnel). The two margins of the sulcus are the *vestibular lip* and *tympanic lip*. The collagenous fibers of the limbus continue laterally, via the tympanic lip, into the pars arcuata of the basilar membrane. Within the body of the limbus the fibers are arranged vertically to produce the distinctive *auditory teeth* (of Huschke). Between these collagenous fibers are stellate fibroblasts. Uniformly spaced along the upper margin of the limbus, between the auditory teeth, are the so-called *interdental cells*, which secrete the tectorial membrane. The bases of interdental cells are firmly embedded in the connective tissue of the limbus, but their apices spread out over the upper surface of the limbus, interdigitating and joined by junctional complexes. These form a continuous sheet over the upper surface of the limbus and complete the cellular investment of the cochlear duct.

Tectorial Membrane. The tectorial membrane is secreted from the luminal surfaces of the interdental cells and overlies these cells as a cuticle. It extends laterally beyond the vestibular lip of the limbus to overlie the hairs on the hair cells of the organ of Corti (Figs. 36–11 and 36–13). Recent evidence indicates that the tips of the hairs are embedded within or are firmly bound to the membrane. If this is so, then micrographs showing a space between the hairs and the cuticle must be artifactitious. The tectorial membrane is composed primarily of a protein having a number of similarities to epidermal keratin. In fixed preparations numerous fibrils are observed within it, forming patterns suggesting a highly ordered structure.

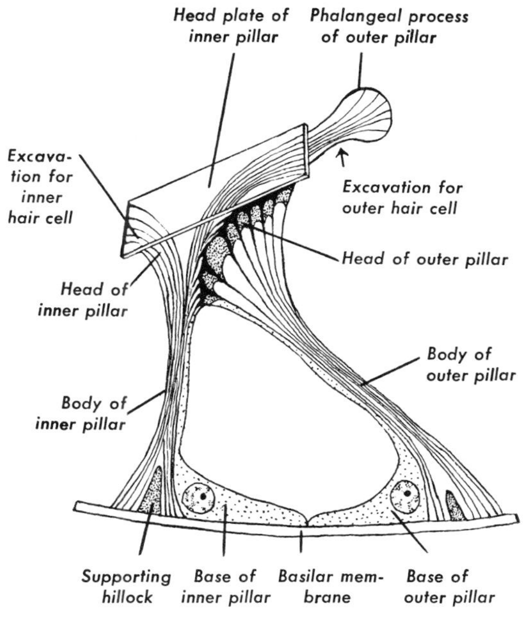

THE PERILYMPHATIC LABYRINTH

The perilymphatic system surrounds the whole of the membranous labyrinth and provides support for its epithelium lining. The distinct scalae vestibuli and tympani in the cochlea have been mentioned, but it must be remembered that similar, though less specialized, perilymphatic spaces surround the structures in the vestibule.

Histologically the perilymphatic tissue is described as a reticulum, and close examination with the electron microscope shows that this reticulum is composed primarily of highly attenuated processes of many stellate cells. Except close to the periosteum of the bony labyrinth and to the membranous labyrinth, there are few extracellular fibers associated with these reticular cells. Immediately surrounding the membranous labyrinth, however, extracellular fibers are elaborated and, in some species, form a relatively dense, stable sheath 1 or 2 μm. thick, composed of multitudes of short fibers. In the vicinity of the fibrocytes of the perilymphatic system, both in the cochlea and in the vestibule, are

Figure 36–16 Diagram of inner and outer pillars of organ of Corti. (Modified from Kolmer.)

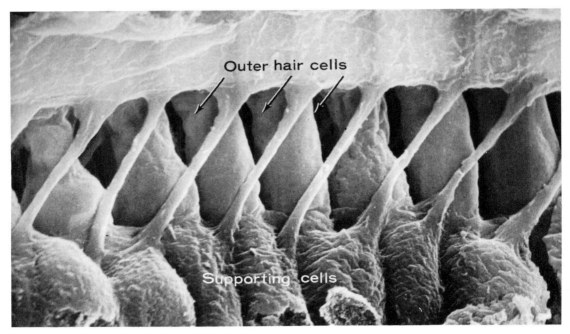

Figure 36-17 Scanning electron micrograph of outer hair cells and slender processes of supporting cells of Deiter. For orientation, see Figure 36-18. (Micrograph courtesy of H. Engström.)

fiber bundles that have a characteristic form different from that of any other known extracellular fiber. The fiber bundles are composed of a variable number of dense 100 Å fibers, which can be shown to be composed of four 50 Å subunits that appear to be helically wound around one another. The dense fibers that form the bundles are embedded in an amorphous filamentous matrix.

Numerous blood capillaries course throughout the perilymphatic tissue destined to supply the metabolic needs of the labyrinthine epithelium.

Scala Vestibuli and Scala Tympani

The cells that line these two scalae are usually extremely attenuated squamous cells with very little obvious cellular differentiation. At times, however, especially in the vicinity of the basilar membrane, the cells do become somewhat cuboidal, although they possess few structural features of note.

The Basilar Membrane. The most elaborate specialization of perilymphatic tissue is the basilar membrane, which provides a supporting base for the cells of the organ of Corti and which by its movement presumably transmits vibrations to the hair cells. The basilar membrane is a highly organized layer of collagen-like fibers. There is some indication that the perilymphatic cells may actively secrete the basilar membrane, but this has not been clearly established. It is divided into two distinct zones: one, running from the osseous spiral lamina approximately one third of the way to the outer cochlear wall, is termed the *pars arcuata (tecta);* the other, comprising approximately two thirds of the width of the basilar membrane, is termed the *pars pectinata* and contains, as can be seen even at the light microscope level, distinct parallel striations termed the *auditory strings.* In fact, both portions of the membrane are composed of transversely oriented filaments (80 to 100 Å thick) embedded in an amorphous matrix. In the pars pectinata the filaments are aggregated into bundles that run in two strata: one immediately beneath the organ of Corti, composed of small bundles, and another situated more deeply in the lamina, composed of larger bundles. At the outer wall of the cochlea, these two layers again merge, to pass into the connective tissue of the spiral ligament.

Blood vessels penetrate into the pars arcuata but not into the pars pectinata.

The term *spiral ligament* is an unfortunate designation for the lateral insertion of the basilar membrane, because this component does not have the histological structure of ligaments found elsewhere in the body (Fig. 36–11). It is merely a local differentiation of periosteal connective tissue containing numerous fibroblasts and blood vessels. A better term would be *spiral crest*.

ENDOLYMPH AND PERILYMPH

The spaces delimited by the membranous labyrinth are filled with the viscous fluid called endolymph, and the labyrinth is surrounded by the perilymph, which occupies the perilymphatic spaces. The two fluids are amazingly different in their chemical composition. The most striking difference is in their electrolyte composition. Whereas perilymph to some degree resembles extracellular fluid in general, endolymph has the characteristics of intracellular fluid in having high K^+ and low Na^+ concentrations (Table 36–1).

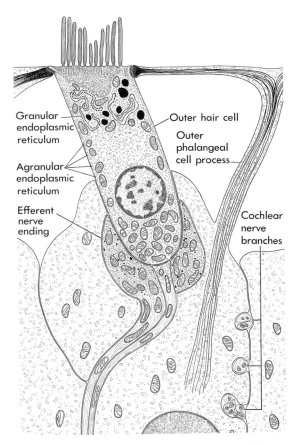

Figure 36–19 Schematic representation of the relationship of the outer hair cells to the outer phalangeal cells, as revealed in electron micrographs. (Drawn by Sylvia Colard Keene.)

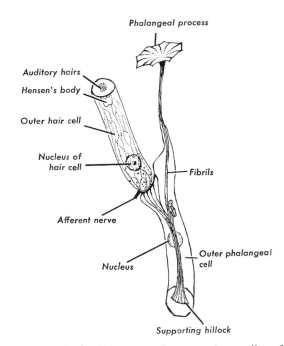

Figure 36–18 Diagram of supporting cells of Deiters and the associated outer hair cell. (Modified from Kolmer.)

It was recognized early in this century that endolymph was a product of secretion, although the actual site or sites of its elaboration were not known. It was supposed that the stria vascularis, the spiral prominence, and the extrasensory cells around the maculae and cristae were primarily responsible. Recent evidence would indicate that these areas do indeed take part in elaboration of endolymph, but the electron microscope has made it clear that many of the cells lining the membranous labyrinth have cytological characteristics compatible with synthetic and secretory activity and might therefore participate in endolymph metabolism. Specifically, autoradiographic studies have implicated the planum semilunatum in elaboration of sulfated mucopolysaccharides, and measure-

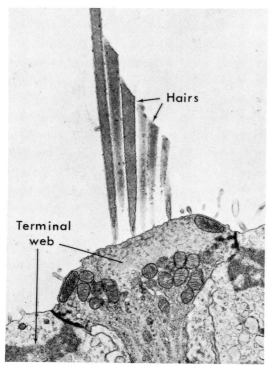

Figure 36-20 Electron micrograph showing the hairs on a hair cell. Notice their narrow base and the continuation of their fibrous core into the terminal web. (Courtesy of D. Hamilton.)

ment with microelectrodes has shown that the high DC potential of the scala media is produced in the vicinity of the stria vascularis, which would indicate that some sort of ion secretion is taking place there.

The site of absorption of endolymph has been thought to be the endolymphatic sac. Recent evidence is compatible with this interpretation. Again, however, electron micrographs of cells of the membranous labyrinth show many instances of micropinocytotic activity, which would suggest that absorption may be going on in many areas of the labyrinth.

Although it is well established that endolymph is a secretion, the genesis of perilymph is still being debated. Some feel that it is an ultrafiltrate of plasma, others that it is derived from cerebrospinal fluid. There is no doubt that the perilymphatic spaces are functionally connected to the subarachnoid space, but the exact functional significance of this relationship is not yet clear.

NERVES OF THE LABYRINTH

The eighth cranial nerve supplies the sensory areas of the labyrinth. It consists of two parts of quite different functional nature and central connections—the *vestibular* and the *cochlear* nerves (Figs. 36–5 and 36–28). Each is composed of primary afferent fibers from the sense organs and efferent feedback fibers from the central nervous system. The cell bodies of the afferent fibers are bipolar cells and form two peripheral ganglia, the *spiral* or *cochlear ganglion* in the modiolus and the *vestibular* or *Scarpa's ganglion* in the internal auditory meatus of the temporal bone.

The vestibular nerve divides into a superior and an inferior branch. The superior branch supplies the horizontal crista ampullaris, the superior crista ampullaris, the macula utriculi, and a small part of the macula sacculi. The inferior branch supplies the posterior crista ampullaris and the major portion of the macula sacculi, and it sends a small anastomosing branch to the cochlear nerve.

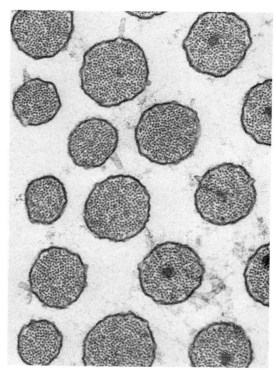

Figure 36-21 Transverse sections through the hairs on a guinea pig outer hair cell, showing the large number of filaments in their interior. (Micrograph courtesy of H. Engström.)

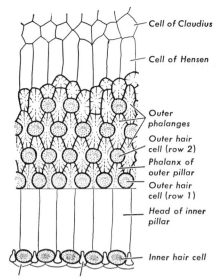

Cell of Claudius

Cell of Hensen

Outer phalanges

Outer hair cell (row 2)

Phalanx of outer pillar

Outer hair cell (row 1)

Head of inner pillar

Inner hair cell

Border cell   Inner phalanx

Figure 36-22 Diagram of the organ of Corti viewed from above, showing the relationship of the phalanges of the supporting cells to the hair cells. (Modified from Retzius, Kolmer, Schaffer.)

The bipolar cell bodies, both in the vestibular ganglion and in the cochlear ganglion, are invested by a thin layer of myelin, and this continues onto the axons. The axons of the cochlear nerve lose their myelin as they run through the openings of the osseous spiral lamina beneath the inner hair cells. In the vestibular nerve, myelin persists until the nerve enters the sensory area.

The cochlear nerve contains two morphological kinds of afferent nerve fibers. The more numerous ones radiate from the spiral ganglion in parallel bundles to the nearest segments of the organ of Corti. Because of their course they are called the radial *acoustic fibers.* The second category of fibers, usually thicker and fewer than the first, are also arranged radially at the outset, but after reaching the outer hair cells of the organ of Corti, they turn sharply and follow a spiral course. These are the *spiral fibers* (Fig. 36–26).

The functional implications of these two patterns of distributions are not clear. Although the relationship between the peripheral receptors and acoustic neurons is not as individualized as the monosynaptic relationship of the foveal cones, it is sufficiently restricted to permit the reception of local-ized stimuli impinging upon small segments of the cochlea.

The vestibular nerve terminates centrally in the reflex centers of the medulla oblongata and cerebellum. Its cortical connections are unknown, although it mediates reflex movements of the eyes through its thalamic connections. The cochlear nerve synapses in the cochlear nucleus, whence fibers ascend in the lateral lemniscus to the medial geniculate body of the thalamus and thence to the temporal lobe gyri of the cortex.

Both the vestibular and cochlear divisions of the eighth cranial nerve contain appreciable numbers of efferent fibers (of Rasmussen) that originate bilaterally from the vicinity of the superior olive. Initially these fibers travel in the vestibular nerve, but within the internal auditory meatus some efferent fibers reach the cochlear nerve by way of the anastomosis between the vestibular and cochlear nerves. The peripheral terminations of the efferent component are presumably at the hair cells, but incontrovertible evidence for the position and mode of ending of these fibers is still lacking. Stimulation of the efferent bundle results in suppression of auditory nerve activity, and anatomical evidence derived from sectioning the bundle indicates that the "granulated" endings are efferent, for they apparently degenerate after sectioning (Figs. 36–9 and 36–19).

BLOOD VESSELS OF THE LABYRINTH

The labyrinthine artery is a branch of the inferior cerebellar artery. It enters the internal auditory meatus and divides into two branches, the *vestibular* artery and the *common cochlear* artery. The latter divides into the *vestibulocochlear* artery and the *cochlear* artery proper.

The vestibular artery supplies the upper and lateral parts of the utricle and saccule and parts of the superior and lateral semicircular ducts. It forms dense networks of capillaries in the region of the maculae; in the thin perilymphatic tissue of these structures, the capillary networks are relatively loose.

The vestibulocochlear artery supplies, with its vestibular branch, the lower and medial parts of the utricle and saccule, the crus commune, and the posterior semicircular

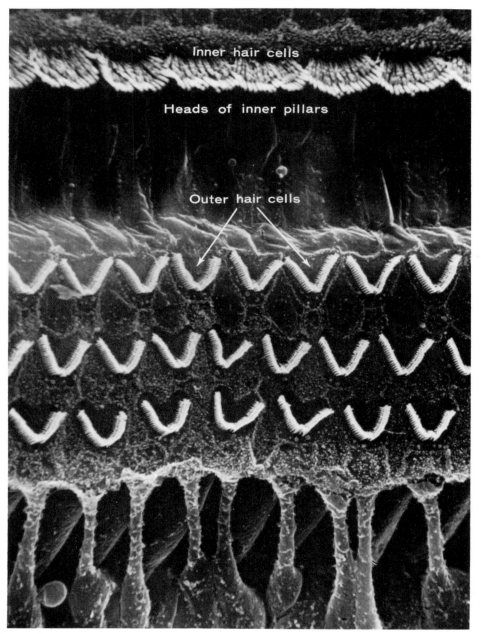

Figure 36-23 Scanning micrograph of guinea pig organ of Corti, middle turn, seen from above. For orientation, see Figure 36-22. (Micrograph courtesy of H. Engström.)

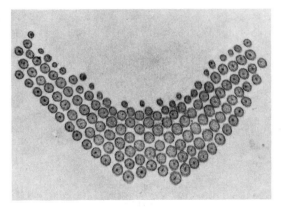

Figure 36–24 Electron micrograph of the W configuration of the hairs or stereocilia on the outer sensory cells of the human organ of Corti. × 10,500. (Courtesy of R. Kimura.)

duct. Its cochlear branch supplies the lowest part of the first cochlear coil.

The cochlear artery proper penetrates the cavities of the modiolus, where its tortuous branches run spirally to the apex. This is the so-called "spiral modiolar artery." From it, branches go to the spiral ganglion and, through the periosteum of the scala vestibuli and the osseous spiral lamina, to the inner parts of the basilar membrane. Here the capillaries are arranged in arcades in the tympanic covering layer under the tunnel and the limbus; from them arise the *vas spirale*. The vascular stria and the spiral crest receive their blood through branches of the spiral modiolar artery, which run in the roof of the scala vestibuli. They do not form connections with the vessels of the basilar membrane. The lower wall of the scala tympani receives its own small arteries from the same source.

The course of the veins of the labyrinth is quite different from that of the arteries. There are three main venous drainage channels. In the cochlea, veins originate in the region of the spiral prominence and run downward and inward through the periosteum of the scala tympani to the spiral vein, which is found under the spiral ganglion. Upper and lower spiral veins, belonging to the corresponding coils of the cochlea, receive branches from the osseous spiral lamina and the spiral ganglion. Above the spiral vein is the small vein of the spiral lamina, which receives a part of the blood from the spiral lamina and spiral ganglion and is connected by anastomoses with the spiral vein. These

cochlear veins form a plexus in the modiolus, which empties the blood partly into the internal auditory vein and partly into the vein of the cochlear aqueduct, which drains into the jugular vein. The veins of the vestibule empty into the veins of the vestibular and cochlear aqueducts.

This arrangement of the vessels in the internal ear seems to ensure the best possible protection of the sound receptors from the arterial pulse wave. The arteries are arranged for the most part in the wall of the scala vestibuli, while the wall of the scala tympani contains the veins. The course of the spiral arteries in the modiolus probably also contributes to the damping of pulsations. In certain mammals the coiling of these arteries is so prominent that the convoluted regions suggest glomeruli.

True lymphatics are absent from the labyrinth. Instead the fluid is drained into the perilymphatic spaces, which are connected with the subarachnoid space. A certain amount of drainage may be effected through perivascular and perineural connective tissue sheaths.

EMBRYOLOGICAL DEVELOPMENT OF THE EAR

External and Middle Ears

The tympanic cavity and the auditory tube are derivatives of the first branchial pouch. The external auditory meatus develops through an invagination of the integument directed toward the tympanic cavity. The tissue layer remaining between this invagination and the tympanic cavity becomes the tympanic membrane.

Internal Ear

The primordium of the labyrinth develops as a shallow groove of thickened ectoderm, dorsal to the first branchial groove, on both sides of the brain, between the myelencephalon and the metencephalon (human embryo of eight somites). The groove is invaginated into the subjacent mesenchyme and becomes the *otic vesicle*. In the human embryo of 2.8 mm., it separates from the ectoderm by constriction and is surrounded by mesenchyme. The vesicle is lined by tall,

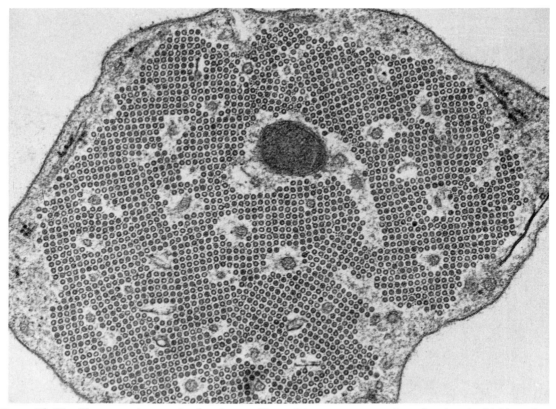

Figure 36-25 Electron micrograph of an inner pillar cell in transverse section, showing the highly ordered bundle of thick walled microtubules and microfilaments. (Electron micrograph courtesy of H. Engström.)

pseudostratified epithelium, which secretes the endolymph filling it. From its earliest stages, the otic vesicle comes into contact with the large acoustic ganglion, which later divides into vestibular and cochlear ganglia. Unequal proliferation in places in the wall of the otic vesicle transforms it into an extremely complex system of saccular and tubular cavities. Soon after its isolation from the ectoderm, the otic vesicle sends out a dorsal evagination, which is the primordium of the endolymphatic duct. Then a larger, dorsal part of the vesicle becomes distinct from a smaller, ventral part. The first, or vestibular, portion gives rise to the semicircular ducts and the utricle. The second, the cochlear portion, forms the saccule and cochlea.

On the wall of the vestibular portion, three evaginations appear and develop into the three semicircular ducts and their ampullae. What remains of the vestibular portion is now the utricle. The cochlear portion sends out a curved outer-pocketing—the primordium of the cochlea. It gradually gains in length, coils as it grows, and becomes separated from the saccule by a deep constriction. In a human embryo of 22 mm. the form of the labyrinth corresponds to that in the adult.

Maculae, Cristae, and Organ of Corti. The maculae and cristae develop earlier than the organ of Corti. On its medial side, where the acoustic ganglion is located, the epithelium of the wall of the otic vesicle develops a thickened area, the *macula communis*, which later divides into an upper and a lower epithelial pad. The first gives rise to the macula of the utricle and to the upper and lateral cristae. A small part of the second thickening forms the crista of the posterior ampulla; the rest of the second part divides into the macula sacculi and the primordium of the organ of Corti, which gradually extends into the growing cochlea.

The differentiation of the organ of Corti

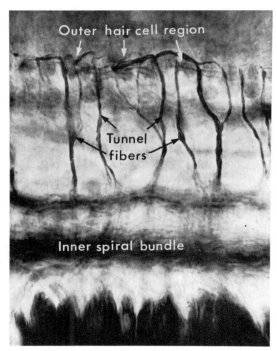

Figure 36-26 Optical section of guinea pig organ of Corti viewed from above, showing nerve fibers traversing the tunnel to reach the region of outer hair cells. Modified Maillet nerve stain using zinc iodide and osmium tetroxide. (From Engström, Ades, and Andersson, 1966.)

tiates, the mesenchyme surrounding it develops into a layer of cartilage, which remains separated from the epithelium by a layer of mesenchyme. This later condenses into a fibrous layer around the membranous labyrinth to form a supporting structure for the epithelium. Between the wall and the cartilaginous capsule, the mesenchyme loosens, and its meshes enlarge into the perilymphatic spaces. The mesenchymal cells which remain on the surface of the trabeculae and of the labyrinthine wall and perichondrium become mesenchymal epithelium.

In anuran tadpoles, if the otic vesicle is transplanted into another area, it becomes surrounded by cartilage arising from local mesenchyme.

The cochlea receives its perilymphatic spaces through extension of the perilymphatic cisterna surrounding the saccule and utricle in the vestibule. The scala tympani appears in the region of the cochlea fenestra in embryos of 43 mm., and the scala vestibuli appears at the 50 mm. stage. They gradually grow and coil with the cochlear duct, remaining attached to its upper and lower walls. At the outer aspect of the cochlear duct, as well as at its inner edge, the wall of the duct remains connected with the cartilaginous capsule. Later, ossification occurs and gives rise to the modiolus and the bony cochlea.

proceeds from the basal coil of the growing cochlea to its apex. The epithelium extends along the basal wall of the canal as a long ridge, which divides longitudinally into a large inner ridge and small outer one. In the former, connective tissue penetrates the epithelium and separates it into radial rows of flask-shaped cells embedded in the connective tissue. This region develops into the spiral limbus. In the outer part of the ridge, the tall cells gradually involute, leaving a squamous epithelium that lines the inner spiral sulcus.

The small outer ridge, the primordium of the organ of Corti, at first consists of uniform cells. Then, flask-shaped inner and outer hair cells appear among them. The remaining elements elaborate tonofilaments and differentiate into the supporting cells.

The surface of both epithelial ridges is covered from the beginning by the future tectorial membrane.

While the otic vesicle grows and differen-

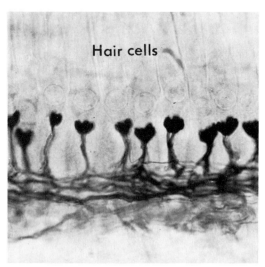

Figure 36-27 Longitudinal section of the organ of Corti, showing the efferent nerve fibers ending about bases of the outer hair cells. (Micrograph courtesy of H. Engström.)

TABLE 36–1 ELECTROLYTE COMPOSITION
OF BODY FLUIDS (mEq./l.)*

	PLASMA	C.S.F.	PERILYMPH	ENDOLYMPH
Protein	6000–8000	10–38	75–100	10
K	20	12–17	15	140
Na	140	150	148	26
Cl	600	750	120	110
Sugar	70–120	40–80		
Mg	1.0–3.0	2.0	2.0	0.9
Ca	7.0	3.0	3.0	3.0

*From F. C. Ormerod.

FUNCTIONAL CONSIDERATIONS

Functions of the various structural components of the ear have already been mentioned briefly in the descriptions under specific headings. It is impossible, of course, to consider in detail the functioning of the ear in a textbook of histology, but there are certain physiological considerations that suggest new problems and approaches to research on this organ.

The external and middle ears lend themselves quite well to physiological research and have been intensively studied for some time. The vibrations of the tympanic membrane are transmitted through the chain of auditory ossicles to the fenestra ovalis and thence to the perilymph filling the scala tympani. The organ of Corti is the receptor for sound stimuli, but this function depends to a large degree upon the properties of the basilar membrane. This membrane may be compared to an unstressed gelatinous plate with varying resistance to displacement related to its uniformly varying width. The deformation of this membrane produced by movement of the stapes resembles a traveling wave. Regions of observed maximum displacement change with frequency, but are rather broad. As the stimulus frequency rises, the length of the basilar membrane responding becomes shorter, and progressively more of the distal area becomes inactive. The pitch discriminating ability of the ear is only partly due to this physical separation of the responding areas along the basilar membrane.

Nerve impulses elicited by stimulation of the maculae and the cristae play an important role in the regulation and coordination of the movements of equilibrium and locomotion. The stimuli to the vestibular end organs are *angular acceleration for the semicircular ducts* and *linear acceleration* for the maculae. These impulses exert their influences upon coordinated muscular contraction, upon muscular tonus, and upon eye movement through the brainstem and cerebellum.

The ear is essentially a biological transducer. The transduction in the external and middle ears is relatively easily monitored.

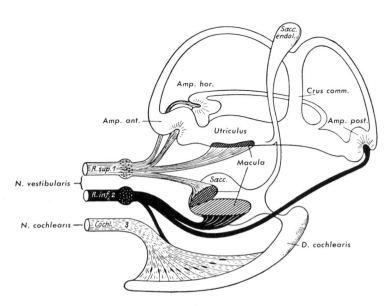

Figure 36–28 Diagram of distribution of nerves in the membranous labyrinth of the rabbit. (After deBurlet, from Kolmer.)

The extreme anatomical complexity of the internal ear, however, has hindered attempts at understanding the transducer phenomenon by which mechanical energy (the stimulus) is transferred into electrical energy (the nerve impulse). It is generally believed that the transduction process takes place in the apex of the hair cells. Indications are that the mechanism in vestibular and cochlear hair cells probably does not differ significantly, even though there are considerable anatomical differences in the cells.

It has been possible to show very clearly in the ampulla of Lorenzini in fish, where the sensory cells are in many respects anatomically similar to vestibular hair cells, that bending of the hairs toward the kinocilium results in depolarization of the cell. Bending in the opposite direction hyperpolarizes the cell, while bending normal to these directions has no appreciable ionic effect. Since mammalian vestibular hair cells are morphologically polarized, the same functional responses to stimuli which bend the hair cells toward or away from the kinocilium would probably occur. The polarization of the hair cells of the maculae varies regularly from one part of these organs to the other, covering within each organ a full 360 degrees. Thus, a movement of the head in any direction will be a sufficient stimulus to excite some of the hair cells and inhibit others. Furthermore, the stepwise lengthening of the hairs may provide a built-in biological amplifier. How the transduction process takes place remains unexplained, however, for the hairs extend into the endolymph with its highly unusual ionic composition. Thus, with equal K^+ and Na^+ inside and outside the cell, the $Na^+ = K^+$ movements that are known to be involved in excitation in other excitable cells would not take place. Nevertheless, it has been shown that a nerve cell membrane put into the same ionic conditions as the hairs responds to pressure changes by transient potential changes across the membrane, and although the mechanism for this is equally unclear, it is possible that this experimental system is analogous to the hairs. In the near future it may help to explain how hair cells function.

REFERENCES

Ades, H. W., and H. Engström: Inner ear studies. Acta Otolaryng., Suppl. 301, 1972.

Alexander, G.: Zur Histologie der Mittelohrschleimhaut. Monatschr. Ohrenh., *61*:446, 1927.

Alexander, G., and O. Marburg: Handbuch der Neurologie des Ohres. Vienna and Berlin, 1921–1926.

Bast, T. H.: Ossification of the otic capsule in human fetuses. Carnegie Contributions to Embryol., *21*:53, 1930.

Bast, T. H., and B. J. Anson: The Temporal Bone and the Ear. Springfield, Ill., Charles C Thomas, 1949.

von Békésy, G.: Experiments in Hearing. New York, McGraw-Hill Book Co., 1960.

Bredberg, G.: Cellular pattern and nerve supply of the human organ of Corti. Acta Otolaryng., Suppl. 236, p. 1, 1968.

deBurlet, H. M.: Vergleichende Anatomie des stato-akustischen Organs. *In* Bolk, et al. (eds.): Handbuch der Vergleichenden Anatomie der Wirbelthiere. Berlin and Vienna, Urban und Schwarzenberg, 1934, Vol. 2, p. 1293.

Citron, L., D. Exley, and C. S. Hallpike: Formation, circulation and chemical properties of the labyrinthine fluids. Brit. Med. Bull., *12*:101, 1956.

Carlström, D., H. Engström, and S. Hjorth: Electron microscopic and x-ray diffraction studies of statoconia. Laryngoscope, *63*:1052, 1953.

Davis, H.: Mechanisms of the inner ear. Ann. Otol., *77*:644, 1968.

Engström, H.: The cortilymph, the third lymph of the inner ear. Acta Morph. Nederlandoscandinavica, *3*:195, 1960.

Engström, H., H. W. Ades, and A. Andersson: Structural Pattern of the Organ of Corti. Stockholm, Almqvist and Wiksell, 1966.

Engström, H.: The first-order vestibular neuron. In U.S. National Aeronautics and Space Administration, *Fourth Symposium on the Role of the Vestibular Organs in Space Exploration,* 1968, pp. 123–134.

Engström, H., H. Ades, and J. Hawkins: Structure and function of the sensory hairs of the inner ear. J. Acoust. Soc. Amer., *34*:1356, 1962.

Fernandez, C.: The innervation of the cochlea (guinea pig). Laryngoscope, *51*:1152, 1951.

Fex, J.: Auditory activity in centrifugal and centripetal cochlear fibers in the cat. Acta Physiol. Scandinav., *55*(Suppl.):189, 1962.

Flock, A.: The ultrastructure of the macula utriculi with special reference to directional interplay of sensory response as revealed by morphological polarization. J. Cell Biol., *22*:413, 1964.

Flock, A.: Transducing mechanisms in lateral line canal organ receptors. Cold Spring Harbor Symposium on Quantitative Biology, Vol. 30, Sensory Receptors, 1965, p. 133.

Flock, A., and J. Wersäll: A study of the orientation of the sensory hairs of the receptor cells in the lateral line organ of fish with special reference to the function of the receptors. J. Cell Biol., *15*:19, 1962.

Foley, J. O.: The cytological processes involved in the formation of the scalae of the internal ear. Anat. Rec., *49*:1, 1931.

Granit, R.: Receptors and Sensory Perception; A Discussion of the Aims, Means and Results of Electrophysiological Research into the Process of Reception. New Haven, Conn., Yale University Press, 1955.

Graves, G. O., and L. F. Edwards: The eustachian tube. A review of its descriptive, microscopic, topographic and clinical anatomy. Arch. Otolaryngol., *39*:359, 1944.

Guild, S. R.: Observations upon the structure and normal contents of the ductus and saccus endolymphatic in the guinea pig (Cavia cobaya). Am. J. Anat., *39*:1, 1927.

Guild, S. R.: Circulation of the endolymph. Am. J. Anat., *39*:57, 1927.

Hamilton, D. W.: The calyceal synapse of type I vestibular hair cells. J. Ultrastr. Res., 23:98, 1968.

Held. H.: Die Cochlea der Sauger und der Vögel, Entwicklung und ihr Bau. Handbuch der normale und pathologische Physiologie. Berlin, Julius Springer, 1926, Vol. 11, p. 467.

Hinojosa, R., and E. L. Rodriguez-Echandia: The fine structure of the stria vascularis of the cat inner ear. Am. J. Anat., 188:631, 1966.

Ishiyama, E., R. A. Cutt, and E. W. Keels: Distribution and ultrastructure of Boettcher's cells in mammals. Ann. Otol. Rhin. Laryng., 79:54, 1970.

Iurato, S.: Submicroscopic structure of the membranous labyrinth. 1. The tectorial membrane. 2. The epithelium of Corti's organ. 3. The supporting structure of Corti's organ (basilar membrane, limbus spiralis and spiral ligament). Zeitschr. f. Zellforsch., 52:105, 1960; 53:259, 1961; 56:40, 1962.

Iurato, S.: Submicroscopic Structure of the Inner Ear. New York, Pergamon Press, 1967.

Iurato, S., L. Luciano, E. Pannese, and E. Reale: Histochemical localization of acetylcholinesterase (ACLE) activity in the inner ear. Acta Otolaryng., Suppl. 279, 1971.

Kimura, R. S.: Hairs of the cochlear sensory cells and their attachment to the tectorial membrane. Acta Otolaryng., 61:55, 1966.

Kimura, R. S., P.-G. Lundquist, and J. Wersäll: Secretory epithelial linings in the ampullae of the guinea pig labyrinth. Acta Otolaryngol., 57:517, 1964.

Kimura, R. S., H. F. Schuknecht, and I. Sundo: Fine morphology of the sensory cells in the organ of Corti in man. Acta Otolaryngol., 58:390, 1965.

Kimura, R. S., and J. Wersäll: Termination of the olivocochlear bundle in relation to the outer hair cells of the organ of Corti in guinea pig. Acta Otolaryngol., 55:1, 1962.

Kimura, R. S., and H. F. Schuknecht: The ultrastructure of the human stria vascularis. Part I. Acta Otolaryng., 69:415, 1970.

Kolmer, W.: Gehörorgan. In von Möllendorff, W., and W. Bargmann (eds.): Handbuch der mikroskopischen Anatomie des Menschen. Berlin, Julius Springer, 1927, Vol. 3, p. 250.

Ladman, A. J., and A. J. Mitchell: The topographical relations and histological characteristics of the tubuloacinar glands of the eustachian tube in mice. Anat. Rec., 121:167, 1955.

Lawrence, M.: In vivo studies of the microcirculation. Advances in Oto-Rhino-Laryngology. Vol. 20, pp. 244-255. Basel, Karger, 1973.

Lindeman, H. H.: Studies on the morphology of the sensory regions of the vestibular apparatus. Ergeb. der Anat. u. Entwick-gesch., 42:1, 1969.

Lindeman, H. H.: Anatomy of the otolith organs. Advances in Oto-Rhino-Laryngology. Vol. 20, pp. 405-433. Basel, Karger, 1973.

Lorente de Nó, R.: Études sur l'anatomie et la physiologie du labyrinthe de l'oreille et du Ville nerf. Trabajos (Travaux) Invest. Biol. Madrid, 24:53, 1926.

Lorente de Nó, R.: Anatomy of the eighth nerve. Laryngoscope, 43:3, 1933.

Lundquist, P.-G.: The endolymphatic duct and sac in the guinea pig. Acta Otolaryngol., Suppl. 201, 1965.

Lundquist, P.-G., R. Kimura, and J. Wersäll: Ultrastructural organization of the epithelial lining in the endolymphatic duct and sac in the guinea pig. Acta Otolaryngol., 57:65, 1963.

Ormerod, F. C.: The physiology of the endolymph. J. Laryngol. Otol., 74:659, 1960.

Perry, E. T.: The Human Ear Canal. Springfield, Ill., Charles C Thomas, 1957.

Polyak, S.: Über den allgemeinen Bauplan des Gehör-systems und über seine Bedeutung fur die Physiologie, für die Klinik und für die Psychologie. Zeitschr. f. d. ges. Neurol. u. Psychiat., 110:1, 1927.

Polyak, S., G. McHugh, and D. K. Judd, Jr.: The Human Ear in Anatomical Transparencies. New York, T. H. McKenna, Inc., 1946.

Ramón y Cajal, S.: Histologie du Système Nerveux de l'Homme et des Vertébrés. 2 vols. Paris, A. Maloine, 1909-1911.

Rasmussen, G., and W. F. Windle, eds.: Neural Mechanisms of the Auditory and Vestibular Systems. Springfield, Ill., Charles C Thomas, 1961.

DeReuck, A. V. S., and J. Knight (eds.): Myototic, Kinesthetic and Vestibular Mechanisms. Ciba Foundation Symposium. Boston, Little, Brown and Company, 1966.

Rodriguez-Echandia, E. L., and M. H. Burgos: The fine structure of the stria vascularis of the guinea-pig inner ear. Zeitschr. f. Zellforsch., 67:600, 1965.

Smith, C. A.: Structure of the stria vascularis and spiral prominence. Ann. Otol. Rhin. Laryngol., 66:521, 1957.

Smith, C. A., O. H. Lowry, and M. L. Wu: The electrolytes of the labyrinthine fluids. Laryngoscope, 64:141, 1954.

Smith, C. A.: Ultrastructure of the organ of Corti. Advance. Sci., 24:419, 1968.

Smith, C. A.: The extrasensory cells of the vestibule. In Paparella, M. M. (ed.): Biochemical Mechanisms in Hearing and Deafness. Springfield, Ill., Charles C Thomas, 1970, pp. 171-185.

Smith, C. A.: The efferent neural supply to the vertebrate ear. Advances in Oto-Rhino-Laryngology. Vo. 20, pp. 296-310. Basel, Karger, 1973.

Smith, C. A., and G. L. Rasmussen: Nerve endings in the maculae and cristae of the chinchilla vestibule, with a special reference to the efferents. U.S. Nat. Aeronautics and Space Administration, Third Symposium on the Role of the Vestibular Organs in Space Exploration, 1967, pp. 183-200.

Sophian, L. H., and B. H. Senturia: Anatomy and histology of the external ear in relation to the histogenesis of external otitis. Laryngoscope, 64:772, 1954.

Spoendlin, H.: Innervation patterns in the organ of Corti of the cat. Acta Oto-Laryngol., 67:239, 1969.

Spoendlin, H.: Degeneration behavior of the cochlear nerve. Arch. klin. exp. Ohr.-Nar.-u Kehlk. Heilk., 200:275, 1971.

Spoendlin, H.: Innervation densities of the cochlea. Acta Otolaryng., 73:235, 1972.

Wersäll, J.: Studies on the structure and innervation of the sensory epithelium of the cristae ampullares in the guinea pig. Acta Otolaryngol., Suppl. 126, 1956.

Wersäll, J., and A. Flock: Physiological aspects on the structure of vestibular end organs. Acta Otolaryngol., Suppl. 192, 1964, p. 85.

Wersäll, J., A. Flock, and P.-G. Lundquist: Structural basis for directional sensitivity in cochlear and vestibular sensory receptors. Cold Spring Harbor Symposium on Quantitative Biology, Vol. 30, Sensory Receptors, 1965, p. 133.

Wislocki, G. B., and A. J. Ladman: Selective and histochemical staining of the otolithic membranes, cupulae and tectorial membrane of the inner ear. J. Anat., 89:3, 1955.

Wolff, D., R. J. Belucci, and A. A. Eggston: Microscopic Anatomy of the Temporal Bone. Baltimore, Williams & Wilkins Co., 1957.

Index

Page numbers in *italics* refer to illustrations; (t) indicates table.

A bands, of cardiac myofibrils, 316
  of skeletal myofibrils, 299, *299–301, 305, 307–309*
Absorption, intestinal, histophysiology of, 676–680
Absorptive cell, intestinal, 659
  absorptive mechanism of, 676–680, *678, 679*
Accidental involution, of thymus, *458,* 465
Acetylcholine, 123, 313, 371
  in motor end plates, acetylthiocholine staining, *313*
Acetylcholinesterase, 371
Acetylthiocholine staining, for cholinesterase, *313*
Acid fuchsin, 162
Acid hydrolases, 49
Acid orcein staining, of valve of vein, *415*
Acid phosphatase reaction, of epinephrine storing cells, 544
  of monocytes, 153
  of myelocytes, 228
  of neutrophilic leukocyte, *148*
  of sheathed capillaries, 494
  of vas deferens lysosomes, *50*
Acidophilic cells, of hypophysis, 505, *506, 507, 508–511*
Acinar cells, of pancreas, 726, *728–733*
Acinus(i), of liver, 691, *695*
  of pancreas, 726, *728, 729*
    duct system and, *738*
Acridine orange, 50
Acromegaly, 513
Acrosomal cap. See *Acrosome.*
Acrosomal granule, 823
Acrosomal vesicle, 823, *825*
Acrosome, of spermatozoon, 812, 814, *814, 815, 821,* 826
  formation of, *825, 826*
Acrosome reactions, 815
ACTH. See *Adrenocorticotropic hormone.*
ACTH-RF. See *Adrenocorticotropic hormone releasing factor.*
Actin, 660
  filaments of, 58
    in blood platelets, 141
    in skeletal muscle, 304, *306*
    subunits of, *306,* 307, *311*
  in smooth muscle, 294
Action potential, of neuron, 343
Addison's disease, 518, 551
Adenohypophysis, 503, *503,* 505–518

Adenohypophysis (*Continued*)
  as master gland, 515
  divisions of, *503*
  pars distalis of, 505–516, *506*
  pars intermedia of, 516–518
  pars tuberalis of, 518
Adenomyosis, 888
Adenosine monophosphate, cyclic. See *Cyclic AMP.*
Adenosine triphosphate, 545
Adenosine triphosphatase reaction, of bile canaliculi, *713*
Adenyl cyclase, 134
ADH. See *Hormones, antidiuretic.*
Adipokinetic hormone, 202
Adipose cells, 172, *176, 177.* See also *Adipose tissue.*
  in parathyroid, *537*
Adipose tissue, 196–207
  brown, 196, 199, *202–204*
    after prolonged fasting, *204*
    after prolonged fasting and refeeding, *206*
    as a heat generator, 205
    blood supply of, 199, *204*
    distribution of, 200
    during hibernation, *203*
  effect of autonomic nervous system on, 204
  histogenesis of, 201, *205*
  histological characteristics of, 196
  histophysiology of, 202
  hormonal influences on, 202
  ordinary. See *Adipose tissue, white.*
  perineural, *359*
  white, 196, *196,* 197, *197, 204*
    after prolonged fasting and refeeding, *206*
    distribution of, 198
Adrenal glands, 540–553
  blood supply of, 546, *550*
  chromaffin tissue of, 540
  cortex of, 540–543, *542*
    blood supply of, 546, *550*
    cell renewal and regeneration in, 553
    fetal, *130,* 552
    histophysiology of, 549–551
    permanent, 552
    X zone of, 553
    zones of, 540, *542*
  histogenesis of, 552
  interrenal tissue of, 540
  lymphatic drainage of, 546

Adrenal glands (*Continued*)
  medulla of, 543–546, *548, 549*
    blood supply of, 546, *550*
    histophysiology of, 551
    hyperfunction of, 552
    sympathetic ganglion cells of, 546
  nerves of, 548
  phylogeny of, 553
Adrenalectomy, effects of, 551
Adrenocorticotropic hormone, 513(t), 515, 548, 912
Adrenocorticotropic hormone releasing factor, in stress, 133, *133*
Adrenogenital syndrome, 551
A-face, of erythrocyte, *30*
  of liver cell membrane, *715*
  of plasma membrane, *40*, 92, *94*
    intramembranous particles of, *40, 97*
Agammaglobulinemia, 182
Age involution, of thymus, *458*, 465
Albinism, 573
Albumin, 155
  serum, liver and, 715
Alcian blue staining, of capillary membrane, 388
  of mucus, 662
Aldehyde-fuchsin staining, of elastic fibers in arteries, 400, *402*
Aldosterone, 549, 550, 784
Aldosterone stimulating factor, 548
Alizarin, 7
Alkaline phosphatase, Gomori-Takamatsu staining for, 18
Alkaline phosphatase reaction, of osteoblasts, 255
Allogeneic, 441
Alloxan, 741
Alpha cells, of hypophysis, 505, *506*, 507, *508–511*
  of islet of Langerhans, 730, *734, 735*
Alpha motor neurons, 361
Alveolar cells, lamellar bodies of, 757, *760*
Alveolar bone, *621, 623*, 631, *632*
Alveolar ducts, of lung, 749, 752, *751–753*
  of breast, 907, *912*
Alveolar pores, 755, *756*
Alveolar sacs, 749, *752, 753, 753*
Alveoli, of lung, 749, 753, *753, 755*
  lining of, 755, *756, 757*
  of mammary gland, 907, *910–913, 915*
  of mandible, 621
Alveolocapillary membrane, *758*
Amacrine cells, 343
  of retina, 949, *954*
Ameloblasts, 625, 632, *636, 637*
  secretory, enamel matrix and, *636, 637*
  Tomes' processes of, *637*
Amido black staining, of intestinal absorptive cell, 659
α-Aminobutyric acid, as transmitter substance, 371
Amnion, *896, 897*
Amniotic cavity, *895, 898*
AMP, cyclic. See *Cyclic AMP.*
Ampulla(e), of bile canaliculi, 711
  of inner ear, 968, *969*, 970, *971*
  of oviduct, 881, *882*
  of Vater, 721

Amylase, 606
Anaphase, meiotic, 74
  in spermatogenesis, 822
  mitotic, 70, *71, 72*
Anaphylaxis, 428
Anastomoses, arteriovenous, 414
Anemia, macrocytic, 139
  microcytic, 139
  pernicious, 654
  sickle cell, 139
Aneuploidy, 75
Angiotensin I, 782
Angiotensin II, 782
Angiotensinogen, 782
Aniline-acid fuchsin staining, of oxyphilic cells, 536
  of ovarian follicle, *864*
  of thyroid follicles, 528
Aniline blue, 162
Aniline blue staining, of colloid, 525
Anisocytosis, 139
Annulate lamellae, 54, *57*
Annuli fibrosi, 417
Annulospiral endings, of sensory nerve fibers, 361
Annulus, of nuclear pore, 69
  of spermatozoon 817, *818, 821*
    anlage of, *827*
Antibody(ies), 149, 155, 428
  anti-immunoglobulin, labeling of B lymphocytes with, *438–440*
  eosinophils and, 183
  production of, by plasma cells, 181
Antidiuretic hormone, 520, *521*, 794
Antigen, 149, 427, 468
  response of T lymphocytes to, 436, *437–440*
  theta, 436, 468
Antigen presentation, 443
Antigen processing, 444
Antigen recognition, 437
Antigenic determinant, 427
Anti-pernicious anemia factor, 655
Antisphering substance, 138
Antrum, of ovarian follicles, *862, 864, 869, 870*
Anus, and rectal columns of Morgagni, 675
Aorta, 401, *406, 407*
  arch of, wall of, *405*
  descending, wall of, *406*
  thoracic, wall of, *405*
  tunica media of, *407*
    fenestrated elastic membranes of, *407*
Aortic body, 415
Aortic valves, 418
Apatite crystals, formation of, in mineralization of bone, 271, *271*
Apertures, numerical, of microscope lenses, 22
Apical foramina, 621
Aponeuroses, 188
Appendices epiploicae, 675
Appendix, vermiform, 673, *674*
Aqueduct, vestibular, 969
Aqueous humor, of eye, 918
  blood-aqueous barrier and, 930
  outflow system of, *928*
Arachnoid membrane, 375, *375, 376*

Arachnoid trabecula, *375, 376*
Arachnoid villi, *376,* 380
Arantius, nodule of, 418
Area cribrosa, 767
Areola, of breast, 907, 908
Areolar glands, of Montgomery, 908
Areolar tissue, 158. See also
 Connective tissue, loose.
Argentaffin cells, of gastric glands, 651, *655*
 of intestinal epithelium, 663, *669*
Argentaffin reaction, of norepinephrine
 storing cells, 544
Argentaffinomas, 665
Argyrophilic cells, 651, 664
Arrector pili muscle, 586
Arterioles, *387,* 397, *397,* 398, *398, 399,* 408
 permeability of, to peroxidase, *399*
 precapillary, 398
 smooth muscle of, *398, 399, 400*
 tunicae of, 398, *398, 408*
 vasoconstriction and vasodilation of, *408*
Arteriosclerosis, 407
Arteriovenous anastomoses, 414
Artery(ies), 396–408
 axillary, 915
 basilar, 381
 bronchial, 760
 carotid, 381
 celiac, 735
 central, of spleen, *488,* 492, *493*
 cerebral, anterior, wall of, *405*
 changes in with age, 406
 cochlear, 985
 components of, 396
 conducting, 397
 coronary, 419
 cortical, of adrenal, 546
 cystic, 720
 distributing, 397, *399*
 efferent, 414
 elastic, 397, *405, 406*
  large, 401, *406, 407*
  walls of, *405*
 elasticity of, 404
 femoral, wall of, *405*
 hardening of, 406
 helicine, 853, 880
 hepatic, 692, *694,* 735
 hybrid type, 403
 hypophyseal, 511
 inferior cerebellar, 985
 innominate, wall of, *405*
 intercostal, 915
 internal mammary, 915
 internal spermatic, 835
 labyrinthine, 985
 large, blood supply of, 402
 laryngeal, 747
 layers of, 396
 mixed type, 402
 muscular, 397, 399, *402, 403, 405*
  elastica interna of, 399, *401–403*
  smooth muscle of, *403, 404*
  walls of, *405*
 of adrenal cortex, 546
 of penis, 853
 of spleen, 492, 735
 ophthalmic, 956

Artery(ies) (*Continued*)
 ovarian, 880
 pancreaticoduodenal, 735
 placental, 902
 pulmonary, 759
 pulp, of spleen, 493
 radial, wall of, *405*
 radicular, 381
 reactive hyperemia of, 406
 renal, 784, *791*
 small, 397, *397,* 398, *400*
  tunicae of, 398, *400, 403, 410*
 special types of, 402
 spinal, 381
 splenic, lymphoid sheaths of, 487, *488, 493*
 structure of, physiology and, 403
 superior mesenteric, 735
 suprarenal, 546
 thyroid, 747
 transitional types, 402
 tunicae of, 396
 umbilical, 403, 902
 vasoconstriction of, agonal, *409*
 vasoconstriction and vasodilatation of, 404,
  408
 vestibular, 985
 walls of, physiological implications of, 403
Arthus reaction, 428
Artifacts, fixation, 10
Aryepiglottic folds, 747
Aryl-sulfatase reaction of, monocytes, 153
Arytenoid cartilage, 747
Astrocytes, fibrous, 368, *368*
 plasmatofibrous, 368
 protoplasmic, 367, *368*
Atherosclerosis, 407
ATP. See *Adenosine triphosphate.*
Atresia, of ovarian follicles, 873, *881*
Atrial granules, in atrial muscle fibers, 324,
 326
Atrioventricular bundle, 324, *327, 328, 329,*
 419
 cell junction in, *329*
 innervation of, *328*
Atrioventricular node, 324
Atrium, 416
 of alveolus, 749, *753*
Atrophy, 244
Auditory meatus, external, 964, *965*
 internal, 969
Auditory ossicles, 965, *965, 966*
Auditory strings, 982
Auditory teeth, of Huschke, 981
Auditory tube, 965, 967, *968*
Auerbach, myenteric plexus of, 682, *684, 685*
Auricle, 964, *965*
Autonomic nervous system. See *Nervous
 system, autonomic.*
Autophagy, 50
 lysosomes and, *51*
Autoradiography, 19
 in study of chromosomes, *23, 24*
Autosomes, 822
Axis cylinder, of neurons, 334. See also
 Axon.
Axoaxonic synapses, 369, *370*
Axodendritic synapses, 369, *370*
Axolemma, 352

Axon, 334, *334, 335, 338, 339,* 343. See also
  Nerve fiber.
  boutons terminaux of, 370, *371*
  collaterals of, 334, *334*
  myelin sheath of, 343, 353, *354, 355, 357*
  primary degeneration of, 382
  reinnervation of, after injury, 382
  unmyelinated, 343, 351, *354, 355*
Axon collaterals, 334, *334*
Axon endings, 359
Axon hillock, 339, *340*
Axonal reaction, 383
Axoneme, *104*
  of cilium, 100
  of spermatozoon, 817, *818, 828*
    formation of, 827, *828*
Axosomatic synapses, 369, *370*
Azocarmine staining, of catecholamine
    storing cells, 544
  of mammatropes, 507
Azurophil granules, in lymphocyte, *152*
  in monocytes, *153*
  in promyelocytes, 224, *225, 226*
  of neutrophils, 144, *148*

B lymphocytes, 429, *436–440,* 482, 498
Balbiani ring, *24*
Band of Bungner, 382
Bar, terminal, 92, *92*
Barr body, 77, *77*
Bartholin, glands of, 904, *904*
Basal bodies, 57, 99
  origin of, in ciliogenesis, *105*
Basal cells, of epididymis, 844
  myoepithelial, of glands of oral cavity, 609
  of olfactory epithelium, 744, *746*
  of taste bud, 604
Basal granular cells, of intestine, 663
Basal lamina, 97
Basement membrane. See *Basal lamina.*
Basic fuchsin staining, 16
Basilar membrane, of cochlea, 969, *978, 979,
  981*
Basket cells, of glands of oral cavity, 609
  myoepithelial, of mammary gland, 907,
    915
Basophilic bodies, of liver, *705, 706 ·*
Basophilic cells, of hypophysis, 505, 509, *512*
Basophils. See *Leukocytes, basophilic.*
Bellini, papillary ducts of, 781, *788*
Berlin blue staining, of liver, *691*
Best's carmine staining, for glycogen, 62
Beta cells, of hypophysis, 505, 509, *512*
  of islets of Langerhans, 730, *734, 736, 741*
Beta globulins, 155
BF. See *Blastogenic factor.*
B-face, of cardiac muscle fiber, *30*
  of plasma membrane, 40, 92, *94, 97*
Bielschowsky silver staining, 162
Bielschowsky staining, of bone marrow, *213*
  of corpus luteum, *876*
  of myenteric plexus, *684*
  of pituicyte pigment granules, 519
Bielschowsky-Foot staining, of colon, *676*
  of reticular fibers, *170*

Bile, 688
  function of, in digestion, 676
  mechanism of concentration of, 720
  storage of, 721
Bile canaliculi, of liver, *694, 696, 704,* 708,
  713, 714
Bile ducts, *690–694,* 717, *717*
  common, 717
Bilirubin, excretion of, by liver, 716
Billroth, cords of, 487
Bipolar cells, of retina, 947, *954–958*
Bladder, urinary, 794, *794, 795*
  internal sphincter of, 798
  transitional epithelium of, *796*
Blandin, gland of, 612
Blast cells, 430
Blastogenic factor, 438
Blood, 136–156. See also *Hemopoiesis.*
  albumin of, 155
  clotting of. See *Clotting.*
  erythrocytes of. See *Erythrocytes.*
  formed elements of, 137–153
  globulins of, 155
  leukocytes of. See *Leukocytes.*
  lymphoid elements of, 209
  myeloid elements of, 209
  plasma of, 153
  platelets of. See *Platelets.*
  serum lipoproteins of, 156
Blood-air barrier, *758*
Blood-aqueous barrier, of eye, 930
Blood-brain barrier, 381, 395, 839
Blood calcium levels, thyroid and, 532
Blood cells, formation of, 209–231. See also
    *Erythrocytes; Erythropoiesis; Leukocytes;
    Platelets.*
Blood clotting. See *Clotting.*
Blood islands, embryonic, and hemopoiesis,
  210
Blood-ocular barrier, 396
Blood-testis barrier, 839
  Sertoli cell and, 841, *843*
Blood-thymus barrier, 396, 463, *466*
Blood vascular system, 386–420. See also
    Arteries; Capillaries; Heart; Veins.
  ancillary organs of, 415
  portal systems of, 413
Blood vessels, histogenesis of, 420
Bodian staining, of parathyroid principal
    cells, 536
Body, aortic, 415
  Barr, 77, *77*
  basal, 57, 99
    origin of, in ciliogenesis, *105*
  Call-Exner, 864, *866, 867*
  carotid, 415
  chromatoid, of spermatozoon, 827
  ciliary, of eye, 917, *919, 925,* 927
  coccygeal, 415
  Hassall-Henle, 922
  Hassall's, 458, *459, 460, 464*
  Herring, 518, *519*
  malpighian, of spleen, 487
  multilamellar, of alveolar cells, 757, *760*
  multivesicular, 51, *52*
    in lymphocytes, *433*
  pineal. See *Pineal body.*
  polar, in maturing ovum, 869, *873, 874*

Body (*Continued*)
  residual, 49
    of Regnaud, 828
  Russell, in plasma cells, 433
    of stomach wall, 652
  ultimobranchial, 527
  vitreous, of eye, 918, *918, 919, 925*, 937
Body fluids, electrolyte composition of, 990(t)
Boettcher, cells of, 976
  crystals of, in semen, 856
Bone(s), 244–285
  absorption cavities in, 275
  alveolar, *621, 623,* 631, *632*
  as store of mobilizable calcium, 279
  calcification of, 269, *269–271*
  canaliculi of, 247, *249, 250*
  cancellous, 245, *245, 246*
    lamellae of, 249
  cartilage, 264
  cells of, 254–261
  collagen of, 253
  compact, 245, *245, 246*
    lamellae of, 247, *247–252*
  diaphysis of, *244,* 245
  effects of endocrine hormones on, 280
  effects of nutrition on, 281
  endosteum of, 246
  epiphyses of, *244,* 245
  flat, of skull, 246
  formation of, 256. See also *Ossification.*
    ectopic, 262, 277
    inductor substance and, 279
    secondary, 275
  ground substance of, 253
  haversian systems of, 247, *247–252*
  histogenesis of, 262–279. See also *Ossification.*
  histophysiology of, 279
  inorganic salts of, 254
  internal reorganization of, 275
  interstitial systems of, 247, *247, 248*
  lacunae of, 247, *250*
  lamellae of, 246
  lamellar, 263, *265*
    rate of formation of, 276
  long, 245
    development of, *266–270*
    epiphyseal plate of, *244,* 245
    growth in diameter of, *266,* 273, *275*
    growth in length of, *266,* 271, *275*
    intramembranous ossification in, 273
    metaphysis of, 245
  macroscopic structure of, 244, *244–246*
  matrix of, 246
    submicroscopic structure and composition of, 253
  medullary cavity of, 245
  membrane, *241,* 263
  metabolic, 280
  microscopic structure of, 246, *247, 248, 250*
  mineral content of, 254
  organic matrix of, 253
  osteons of. See *Bone, haversian systems of.*
  parathyroid hormone and, 257, 259, 280
  periosteum of, 245
  repair of, 277
  resorption of, 257
  resorption cavities of, 275, *279*

Bone(s) (*Continued*)
  sesamoid, 277
  spongy, 245, *245, 246*
  structural, 280
  surface remodeling of, 273, *275*
  trabeculae of, 245, *246*
  transplants of, 278
  woven, 263, *265*
Bone marrow, 209–231, 245
  erythropoiesis in, 216–220, *218*
  fatty, *210*
  granulopoiesis in, 224–229
  hemopoiesis in, *210,* 211, 213–231
  hemopoietic cell lineages in, 213, *215, 217*
  histological organization of, 212, *213, 214*
  lymphopoiesis in, 231
  monopoiesis in, 230
  stem cells of, 213, *217, 218*
  thrombopoiesis in, 221–224
Border, brush. See *Brush border.*
  ruffled, of osteoclasts, 258, *261, 262*
  striated, of intestinal absorptive cells, 659,
    664, 666, 668, 673
Border cells, of organ of Corti, 979, *979*
Bouin fixation, 11
Boutons, terminal, 370, *371*
  of hair cells, 972
Bowman, capsule of, 768, *771*
  membrane of, 921, *921*
  olfactory gland of, *745,* 746
  space of, 770, *775, 789*
Brain, and blood-brain barrier, 381
  blood supply of, 381
  choroid plexus of, 378, *378–310*
  cisternae of, 377
  connective tissue sheaths of, 376, *376*
  cytoarchitecture of, 373
  granule cells of, 350
  gray matter of, 347, *349, 350*
  membranes of, 375, *376*
  meningeal spaces of, 377
  nerve fibers of, 356
  pia-arachnoid of, *375,* 377
  ventricles of, 378
  white matter of, 347, *349*
Brain sand, *557,* 558
Breast. See *Gland, mammary.*
Bridges, intercellular, between spermatids,
  822, *823*
Broad ligament, of uterus, *887*
Bronchioles, 749
  respiratory, 749, 751, *751–753*
Bronchus(i), 749, *749*
Brown fat. See *Adipose tissue, brown.*
Bruch's membrane, 926, *931*
Brücke's muscle, of ciliary body, 928
Brunner's glands, of intestine, *660, 661, 663,*
  671
  secretion of, 672
Brush border, epithelial, 98, *98*
  of intestinal absorptive cells, 659, *664, 666,*
  668, 673
Buccal glands, 611
Buds, taste. See *Taste buds.*
Bulbourethral glands, 850, *854*
Bulbs, terminal, of Krause, 364
Bundle, atrioventricular, 324, *327–329,* 419
  of His, 324, *327–329*

Bungner, band of, 382
Bursa, of Fabricius, 429, 451, 671
Bursa analogue, 429, 451

C cells, of islets of Langerhans, 731
  of thyroid, 526, 533
Cajal's silver nitrate staining, of parafollicular
  cells, 527, 530
Calcification, of bone, 269, 269–271. See also
    Ossification.
  of cartilage, 241
  of dentin, 623, 633
    provisional, zone of, 242
  of teeth, 634
Calcitonin, 281, 528, 532
  effect of on osteoclast, 260
  role of in bone metabolism, 259
Calcium, in bone, x-ray determination of, 19,
    21
  interchange of, between blood and bone,
    279
  plasma concentration of, bone and, 279
    parathyroid hormone and, 280
    regulation of, 538
  skeletal muscle contraction and, 308, 311
  storage of in bone, 254, 279
Calcium phosphate, of bone, 254
Call-Exner bodies, of ovarian follicle, 864,
    866, 867
Callus, bony, 277
  fibrocartilaginous, 277
Calyces, of kidneys, 766, 767
Canal(s), haversian, 247, 248, 248. See also
    Haversian systems.
  hyaloid, 937
  of Cloquet, 937
  of Hering, 694
  of Schlemm, 918, 924, 925, 926, 927, 928,
    930
  semicircular, of ear, 965, 968, 969, 970
  Volkmann's, 248
Canaliculi, apical, of proximal tubule, 775,
    780
  bile, of liver, 694, 696, 704, 708, 713, 714
  intercellular, of sweat gland, 593
  intracellular, of exocrine glands, 119
  of bone, 247, 249, 250
  secretory, of gastric parietal cell, 648, 653,
    654
  of multicellular exocrine glands, 118
Cap, acrosomal. See Acrosome.
Capillaries, blood, 386–396, 387–389
  and blood-brain permeability barrier, 395
  caveolae of, 390, 390
  continuous, 388, 393
  fenestrated, 391, 393, 394
    pores of, 394, 395
  marginal fold of, 390, 391
  of spleen, 493
  pericytes of, 388, 388
  permeability of, structural basis of, 393
  pinocytosis by, 393, 396
  pore systems of, 394, 395
  vesicular inpocketings of, 390, 390
  cross section of, 389, 393
  endothelial cell junction of, 389–392

Capillaries (Continued)
  fenestrated, pores of, 394
  glomerular, 775–777
    pores in, 776–778
  lymph, 420, 421, 422, 423
    of heart, 419
  of thymus, 466
  of thyroid follicle, 527
  sheathed, of spleen, 493, 494
Capsule, Bowman's, 768, 771
  Glisson's, 711
  of encapsulated sensory nerve endings, 363
  of lymph nodes, 471–473, 478
  of spleen, 487, 488
  of Tenon, 920
Carbohydrates, cellular, identification of, 12,
    17, 17
Carbonic anhydrase, 764
Carboxypeptidase, 738
Carcinoid tumors, 665
Cardia, of stomach, 644
Cardiac glands, esophageal, 640
  of stomach, 645, 652. See also Glands,
    gastric.
Carmine staining, of dermoepidermal junc-
    tions, 580
Carotene, 571
Carotid body, 415
  cells of, 415
Carrier proteins, 134
Cartilage, 233–243. See also Fibrocartilage.
  appositional growth of, 235
  articular, of long bones, 245
  arytenoid, 747
  calcification of, 241, 241
  cells of, 234, 235–237
  corniculate, 747
  cricoid, 747
  cuneiform, 747
  elastic, 239, 239
  histogenesis of, 234
  histophysiology of, 242
  hyaline, 233, 234–238
    histogenesis of, 234, 234, 235
    of trachea, 748, 748
  interstitial growth of, 235
  matrix of, 233, 233, 236, 237
    capsular, 233, 238
    interterritorial, 238
    secretion of components of, 238, 238
  matrix vesicles of, 242
  nutritional deficiencies and, 242
  perichondrium of, 234
  regeneration of, 241
  regressive changes in, 241
  special types of, 240
  thyroid, 747
  transformation of into bone, 262, 264
  zones of development of, 237
Castration, effect of on hypophyseal cells,
    506
Castration cells, 506, 515
Catalase, 706
Catecholamines, 543, 551, 665. See also
    Epinephrine; Norepinephrine.
  storage granules of, 544, 549
    in paraganglia, 554
Caveolae, of blood capillaries, 390, 390

Cavity, tympanic, 965, *965*, *966*
Cell(s), 35–77
  absorptive, of intestines, 659
  acidophilic, of hypophysis, 505, *506*, 507, *508–511*
  acinar, of pancreas, *109*, *110*, 726, *728–733*
  actions of hormones on, 134, *134*
  adipose, 172, *176*, *177*, *198–201*. See also *Adipose Tissue.*
    in parathyroid, *537*
  alpha, of islet of Langerhans, 730, *734*, *735*
  alveolar, 756, *756*, *757*, *759*, *760*
  amacrine, 343
    of retina, 949, *954*
  antibody producing, 484
  argentaffin, of gastric glands, 651, *655*
    of intestinal epithelium, 663, *669*
  argyrophilic, 651, 664
  band, 142
  basal, of epididymis, 844
    of olfactory epithelium, 744, *746*
    of taste bud, 604
  basal granular, of intestine, 663
  basal myoepithelial, of glands of oral cavity, 609
  basket, of glands of oral cavity, 609
    of mammary gland, *915*
  basophilic (beta), of hypophysis, 505, 509, *512*
  beta, of islets of Langerhans, 730, *734*, *736*, *741*
  bipolar, of retina, 947, *954–958*
  blast, 430
  blood. See specific types, such as *Erythrocyte, Leukocyte.*
    formation of, 209–231
  Boettcher's, 976
  bone. See *Osteoblasts; Osteoclasts; Osteocytes.*
  border, of organ of Corti, 979, *979*
  C, of thyroid, 526, 533
  cartilage. See *Chondrocytes.*
  castration, *506*, 515
  centroacinar, of pancreas, *729*, *733*, *738*, *739*
  chief, of gastric glands, 647, *648*, 651, 652
    of paraganglia, *554*
    of parathyroids, 536, *536*
    of pineal body, 556
  chromaffin, 543
  chromophobic, 510
  Claudius's, 976
  clear, of sweat glands, 590, *593*
  cone, of retina, 943–946, *945–948*, *952*, *954*, *957*
  corticotropes, *508*, 511
  cytoplasmic inclusions of, 61–63
  cytoplasmic matrix of, 37
  cytoplasmic organelles of, 37–58
  culture of, 4
  cuticle, of hairs, *584*
  decidual, of ovary, 876
  Deiters's, 978, *978–980*, *982*, *983*
  delta, of islets of Langerhans, 731, *734*, *737*
  dendritic, of germinal center, 448
  dust, 758, *761*, *762*
  effector, 427
  endocrine, 664

Cell(s) (*Continued*)
  endocrine, protein or polypeptide producing, 125, *126*
    relation of to blood and lymph vascular systems, 130
    steroid secreting, cytology of, 126, *131*
  endothelial, composing capillary, *389*, *391*
  enterochromaffin, 651, 663
  epithelial, follicular, of thyroid, 524, *525*, *526*, *529*, *531*
    pulmonary, 756
  epithelioid, 177
  fat, 172, *176*, *177*
  fat-storing, of liver, 700, *700*, *701*
  fixed, of connective tissue, 171
  follicular, of ovarian follicle, 859, *863*, *870*
  fractionation of, *12*
  ganglion, of retina, 949, *954*
  giant, foreign body, 177
  glial. See *Neuroglia.*
  glomus, of carotid body, 415
  goblet, 117,*119*
    of respiratory epithelium, *749*
  granule, of brain, 350
  granulosa, of ovarian follicle, 862, *865*, *866*, *868*
  granulosa lutein, of corpus luteum, 871, *876*, *877*, *879*
  ground substance of, 37
  hair, of crista ampullaris, 970, *972*, *973*
    of organ of Corti, *978*, *979*, *979–989*
  Hensen's, *978*, *979*, *979*, *985*
  hilus, of ovary, 878
  horizontal, of retina, 947, *954*, 955, *956*, *957*
  inclusions of, 36, *36*
  interdental, of ear, 981
  interstitial, 684
    of liver, 700, *700*, *701*
    of ovary, 876
    of pineal body, 556, *559*
    of testis, 806
  islet, of pancreas, *729–733*, *735–737*, *741*
  juxtaglomerular, 782, *789*
  Kupffer, 695, 698, *700*
  Langerhans, 565
    of epidermis, 574, *576–578*
  Leydig, 806, *808*, 833, *838–842*
  light, 526
  littoral, of bone, marrow sinusoids, *213*
  liver. See *Hepatocytes.*
  living, differential centrifugation of, 8
    direct observation of, 2–8
    micromanipulation of, 6, *9*
  lutein, 871, *876–879*
  malpighian, cytomorphosis of, 565
  mammatropes, 507, *508*, *510*, 511
  mast, *176*, *177*, 184, *185*, *186*
  matrix, of hair follicle, 582, *585*
    of hairs, 582
  matrix components of, 58–61
  memory, 427
  Merkel, 565
    of epidermis, 576, *579*, *580*
  mesangial, 772
  mesenchymal, 171, 172
    formation of cartilage from, *234*, *235*
  mesothelial, of serous exudate, 187

Cell(s) (*Continued*)
  micromanipulation of, 6
  mucoid, of sweat glands, 590, *593*
  mucous, 117, *119*, 607, 608
    neck, of gastric glands, 649
  muscle. See *Muscle fibers.*
  myoepithelial, of mammary gland, 907,
    915
    of salivary glands, 609
    of sweat glands, 590, *591, 593*
  myoepithelioid, 782
  myoid, of testis, 807
    of thymus, 462
  neck mucous, of gastric glands, 649
  nerve. See *Neuroglia; Neurons.*
  neuroepithelial, of taste bud, 603
  neuroglial. See *Neuroglia.*
  nuclear organelles of, 63–70
  olfactory, 744, *745*
  organelles of, 36, *36*
  osteoprogenitor, 255
  oxyntic, of gastric glands, 648, *648, 653,
    654*
  oxyphilic, of parathyroid glands, 536, *536*
  Paneth, of crypt of Lieberkühn, 667, *669,
    670*
  parafollicular, 526, *530, 531*, 532
  parenchymal, of liver. See *Hepatocytes.*
  parietal, of gastric glands, 648, *648, 653,
    654*
  peripheral, of sweat glands, *594*
    of tongue, 604
  peritubular contractile, of testis, 807
  phalangeal, of organ of Corti, 978, *978–
    980, 982, 983*
  photoreceptor, 940–946. See also *Cone
    cells; Rod cells.*
  pigment epithelial, 939
  plasma, *143*, 427, 432, *434*
    of connective tissue, 180, *182, 183, 184*
  principal, of epididymis, 844
    of parathyroids, 536, *536*
    of thyroid, 528
  prolactin, 507
  Purkinje, of cerebellar cortex, *338*, 343,
    344, 345
  pyramidal, of cerebral cortex, *338*
  pyroninophilic, 430
  radial, of Müller, 940, 951, *953*
  reserve, of hypophysis, 510
  reticular, 446
    of lymph node, *448*
    of spleen, *489, 490, 491*
  rhagiocrine, 175
  rod, of retina, 940, *945–951, 954, 957*
  Rouget, 387
  satellite, of neurons, *339*, 349
    of peripheral ganglia, 366
    of skeletal muscle, 297, 329
  Schwann, 349
  sebaceous, *590*
  septal, of alveoli, 756, *756, 757*
  serous, 607, 608, *610–613, 616*
  Sertoli, 807, *809–813, 836, 843*
    relationship of to spermatogenic cells,
      813
  somatotropes, 507, *508, 509*
  specializations of for attachment and
    communication, 91

Cell(s) (*Continued*)
  spermatogenic, 807, *809–812*. See also
    Spermatozoa.
  staining of. See *Staining.*
  stellate, of liver, 700, *700, 701*
    of pineal, *559*
  stem, of blood, 212, *218*
    of bone marrow, 213, *217, 218*
  superficial, of sweat glands, *594*
  supporting, of inner ear, 973, *973*
    of olfactory epithelium, 744, *746*
    of organ of Corti, 976–979, *979, 980–
      983, 985*
    of seminiferous epithelium, 807, *809–
      813, 836, 843*
    of taste bud, 603
  surface mucous, of stomach, 646, *646, 649,
    650*
  sustentacular, of olfactory epithelium, *745*
    of seminiferous epithelium. See *Sertoli
      cells.*
  synovial, 282
  thecal, of antral follicle, 872
  theca lutein, of corpus luteum, 871, *876–
    878*
  thyroidectomy, 515
  trophoblast, 897
  ultimobranchial, 526
  unit membrane of, 38, *38, 39*
  ventricular, 374
  visual, of retina, 940–946, *945–950*
  wandering, mononuclear, 175
    of connective tissue, 171
  zymogenic, of gastric glands, 647, *648, 651,
    652*
Cell axis, of epithelia, 91
Cell center, 54
Cell cycle, 73
  diplosome and, *59*
Cell division, 70–77. See also *Meiosis;
  Mitosis.*
  centrioles and, 57
  chromatin and, 63, 70, 77
  nucleoli and, 69
  stages of, 73
Cell membrane, 37, *38*, 40
Cell protein. See *Protein, cellular.*
Cell wall, 40
Cement, intercellular, 91, 386
Cement lines, 276
  of compact bone, 247, *247, 248*
Cementicles, 630
Cementoalveolar fibers, of periodontal
  membrane, 630
Cementocytes, 628
Cementum, 623, 628
  hyperplasia of, 628
  of teeth, acellular, *622*, 628
    cellular, *622*, 628
Central arteries, of spleen, *488, 492, 493*
Central fovea, of retina. See *Fovea.*
Central nervous system. See *Nervous sys-
  tem, central.*
Central veins, of liver lobules, 688, *689, 691,
  694, 695*
Centrifugation, density gradient, 9
  differential, of living cells, 8
Centrioles, *36*, 54, *58, 433*
  cross section of, *58*

Centrioles (*Continued*)
  of spermatozoa, 817, *827, 828*
Centroacinar cells, of pancreas, *729, 738, 739*
Centromere, 69, 70
Centrosome, 54, *58*
  of neurons, 340
Centrosphere, 54
Cerebellum. See also *Brain.*
  cortex of, distribution of neurons in, *349*
Cerebrospinal fluid, *376*, 379
  electrolyte composition of, 990(t)
Cerebrum. See also *Brain.*
  cortex of, distribution of neurons in, *350*
Ceruloplasmin, 155
Cerumen, 591, 964
Ceruminous glands, 591, 964
Cervix, of tooth, 621
  uterine, 884, 893
    histophysiology of, 895
Chamber, transparent, for studying living
  tissues, *2, 3, 3, 4, 5*
Channels, platelet demarcation, in mega-
  karyocytes, 223, *223*
Charcot-Böttcher, crystalloids of, 811
Cheek, glands of, 611
Chiasmata, 74
Chief cells, of gastric glands, 647, *648, 651,
  652*
  of paraganglia, *554*
  of parathyroids, 536, *536*
  of pineal body, 556
Chloasma, 574
Cholangioles, 710
Cholecystokinin, 721, 738
Choledochoduodenal junction, 718
Chondrification, centers of, 234
Chondrocytes, 233, 234, 235, *236*
Chondroid tissue, 240
  of heart, 417
Chondroitin sulfate, 168, 252
Chondromucoprotein, 238
Chorda tympani nerve, 965
Choriocapillary layer, of eye, 926, *931*
Chorion, *896, 897, 898, 898*
Chorion frondosum, *896*, 900
Chorion laeve, 900
Choroid of eye, 917, *918, 919*, 926, *942*
  layers of, 926, *931*
Choroid plexus, 378, *378, 379, 380*
Chromaffin reaction, 543
  in paraganglia, 553
Chromaffin system, 553
Chromaffin tissue, 540. See also *Adrenal
  medulla.*
Chromaticity horizontal cells, of retina, 955,
  956
Chromatids, 70, 822
Chromatin, 63
  in interphase nuclei, *66*
  nucleolus associated, 66
  sex, 77, *77*
Chromatoid body, of spermatozoon, 827
Chromatolysis, retrograde, of nerve cell
  body, 383
Chrome alum-hematoxylin staining, of
  Herring bodies, 518
Chrome alum-hematoxylin-phloxine
  staining, of epithelium, *87*

Chromidial substance, 40. See also *Endoplasmic reticulum, granular.*
Chromium shadowing, in study of collagen,
  164
Chromogranin, 545
Chromomere, of blood platelet, 140
Chromophilic substance, of neurons. See
  Nissl substance.
Chromophobes, 510
Chromosomes, 63
  aneuploidy of, 75
  crossing over of, 822
  deletion of, 75
  diploid, 74
  haploid, 74
  human, 74
    metaphase, *76*
  metaphase, study of, by ultraviolet light,
    11, 12
  polyploidy of, 75
  sex, 822
  translocations of, 76
Chyle, 681, 688
Chylomicra, 156, 661, *678, 681, 682*
Chyme, 643
Chymotrypsin, 738
CIF. See *Cloning inhibiting factor.*
Cilia, 99, *101, 103*
  axoneme of, 100, *104*
  cross sections of, *103*
  genesis of, and origin of basal bodies, *105*
  isochronal rhythm of, 100
  metachronal rhythm of, 100
  of retinal rod cell, *948*
  olfactory, 744
  sliding filament theory of, *104*
Ciliary body of eye, 917, *919, 925*, 927
  ciliary epithelium of, 929, *933, 934*
Ciliary zonule, of eye, 918, *918, 925*, 935, *941*
Circle of Willis, 381
Circulatory system, 386–424. See also
  Artery(ies); Capillaries; Heart; Vein(s).
Circumpulpar dentin, 623
Circumvallate papillae, of tongue, *601, 602,
  603, 605*
Cisterna(e), of brain, 377
  of endoplasmic reticulum, 41, *41, 111,
    112, 113*
  perinuclear, 70
  terminal, of skeletal myofibrils, 303, *305*
Cisterna cerebellomedullaris, 377
Cisterna magna, 377
Clasmatocytes, 175
Claudius, cells of, 976
Clear cells, of sweat glands, 590, *593*
Cleft(s), of Schmidt-Lanterman, 352, *352,
  353, 357*
  synaptic, 370, *371, 372*
  of skeletal muscle, 312, *312*
Clitoris, 904
Clonal expansion, 427
Clonal selection theory, 427
Cloning inhibiting factor, 438
Cloquet, canal of, 937
Clotting, blood, 140
Club hair, 582, *582, 586*
Coat, surface, on intestinal brush border,
  659, *667, 668*

Coccygeal body, 415
Cochlea, *965, 966,* 969, *975, 976.* See also
    Organ of Corti.
  hair cells of, *978,* 979, *979–989*
Cochlear duct, *966, 969,* 974
Cochlear nerve, *965, 966, 975, 978,* 984
Cohnheim's fields, of myofibrils, *296,* 298
Colchicine, 60
Collagen, 160, *162–164.* See also *Collagenous
    fibers.*
  amounts of in various types of connective
    tissue, *189, 192*
  and smooth muscle, *291*
  arrangement of molecules in, and calcifica-
    tion of bone, *271*
  associated with capillary, *389*
  calcification of, in formation of bone, 263,
    264, *265–271*
  fibers of. See *Collagenous fibers.*
  fibrous long spacing, 161, *164*
  formation of, *162,* 169, *170, 173, 174*
  metabolism of, disturbances of, 193
  molecules of, alpha units of, 162
  of bone, 253
  of endoneurium, *354, 355*
  segment long spacing, 161, *164*
Collagenase, 192
Collagenous fibers, 159–162, *159, 160.* See
    also *Collagen.*
  breaking point of, 160
  formation of, 168–169, *170*
  in intramembranous ossification, 263
  of adrenal glands, 546
  of bone, 253
  of connective tissue, functions of, 191
  of dense connective tissue, 188
  of hypophysis, 505
  of periodontal membrane, 630
  of synovial membranes, 284
  submicroscopic fibrils of, 160
  structure of, *172*
Collateral ganglia, 364
Collaterals, axon, 334, *334*
Colliculus seminalis, 799, 846, *850, 852*
Colloid, of thyroid, *129,* 524, *525, 526*
Colon, 675–677. See also *Intestines.*
Colostrum, 908
Complement, 428
Concanavalin A, 444
Concretions, pineal, *557,* 558
Conductivity, of nerve fibers, 333
Cone cells, 943–946, *945–948, 952, 954, 957*
  bipolar, 947, *955, 957*
Coni vasculosi, *806,* 842
Conical papilla, of tongue, *602*
Conjunctiva, 957, 959, *960*
  bulbar, *925,* 957
Connective tissue, 158–193
  adipose cells of, 172–173
  blood as, 136
  amounts of collagen in, *189, 192*
  cells of, 171–186
    osteogenic potencies of, 277
  classification of, 158
  collagenous fibers of, 159, *159–164.* See
    also *Collagen; Collagenous fibers.*
  dense, irregular, 188, *189*
    regular, 188, *189, 192*
  effect of hormones on, 192

Connective tissue (*Continued*)
  elastic, 189
  elastic fibers of, 162, *165, 166*
  eosinophilic cells of, 182–184
  fibroblasts of, 171–172
  fixed cellular elements of, 171
  formation of fibers of, 168
  ground substance of, 167
  histiocytes of, 173–175
  histophysiology of, 190
  inflammation and, 191
  loose, 158–188, *159*
    cells of, *176, 185*
    extracellular components of, 159
    serous membranes and, 186
  lymphocytes of, 179–180
  macrophages of, 173–175
  mast cells of, 184–186
  mesenchymal cells of, 172
  metaplasia of, 241
  monocytes of, 175–178
  mononuclear wandering cells of, 175–186
  mucous, 189
  nerve endings in, 363
  normal functions of, 190
  of central nervous system, 375–381
  of nerves, 356, *359, 360*
  of skeletal muscle, 295, *295*
  phagocytosis in, 174
  plasma cells of, 180–182
  repair and, 192
  reticular, 190
  reticular fibers of, 165, *167*
  special types of, 189
  tissue fluid of, 158
  types of, 136, 158
  undifferentiated cells of, 172
Contraction, of skeletal muscle, coupling of
    excitation with, 310
  sliding filament mechanism, *308,* 309
Cord(s), medullary, of lymph nodes, 473, *474*
  of Billroth, of spleen, 487
  spermatic, 806
  vocal, 747, *747*
Corium, 563. See also *Dermis.*
Cornea, 917, *918, 919,* 920, *921, 922*
  Bowman's membrane of, 921, *921*
  dense regular connective tissue in, *192*
  Descemet's membrane of, *921,* 922, *923,
    924*
  endothelium of, *921,* 922, *923*
  epithelium of, 920, *921*
  histophysiology of, 923
  keratocytes in, 921, *922*
  stroma of, 921, *921, 922*
Corneoscleral coat, 917
Corona, of germinal center, 448, *449*
Corona radiata, 865
Corpora arenacea, of pineal, *557,* 558
Corpora cavernosa penis, 851, *855*
Corpus, of stomach, 644
Corpus albicans, 872, *880*
Corpus cavernosum urethrae, 851, *855*
Corpus luteum, *860,* 871, *875*
  formation of, 871
  granulosa lutein cells of, 871, *876, 877, 879*
  of menstruation, 872, *875, 877*
  of pregnancy, 872, *876–879*
  theca lutein cells of, 871, *876–878*

Corpus luteum atretica, 875
Corpus uteri, 884
Corpuscle(s), blood. See *Erythrocytes; Leukocytes.*
　genital, 364, *364*, 855
　Hassall's, 458, *459, 460, 464*
　lingual, *364*
　meconium, 686
　Meissner's, 364, *365, 366*
　　in penis, 855
　of Golgi-Mazzoni, 364
　of Vater-Pacini, 363, *363*, 855
　pacchionian, 381
　renal. See *Kidney, renal corpuscle of.*
　salivary, 606, 616
　thymic, 458, *459, 460, 464*
Cortex, adrenal. See *Adrenal glands, cortex of.*
Cortex cerebri, of brain, *375, 376*
Corti, organ of, *970, 974, 976, 975–981*
Corticosterone, 549
Corticotropes, *508*, 511
Corticotropin. See *Adrenocorticotropic hormone.*
Cortisol, 549
Cortisone, 549
Cotyledons, placental, 902
Cowper's glands, 850, *854*
Craniosacral nerves, 364
Creatinine, 790
Cremaster muscle, 846
Crenation, of erythrocytes, 138, *138, 140*
Cresyl blue, 217
Cresyl violet staining, of gastric pyloric glands, 652
　of Nissl bodies, 339
Cretinism, 531
Crevice, gingival, 630
CRF, 551
Crinophagy, 508
Crista(e), mitochondrial, 45, *45, 46*
Crista ampullaris, 970, *971*
　hair cells of, 970, *972, 973*
　supporting cells of, 973, *973*
Crossing over, chromosomal, 74
Crown, of tooth, 621
Crus commune, 969, *969*
Crypt(s), of Lieberkühn, of colon, *677*
　　of small intestines, 659, *661, 663*, 665, *669, 671*
　　　Paneth cells of, 667, *669, 670*
　of lingual tonsil, *602, 603*
Cryptorchidism, 832
Crystals, of Böttcher, in semen, 856
　of Reinke, in Leydig cells, 838, *840, 841*
Cumulus oophorus, *859, 864, 869, 870*
Cupulae, of inner ear, 974
Cushing's disease, 551
Cuticle, enamel, 627, 634
　of hair, 582, *584, 585, 587*
Cuticular border, of superficial cells of sweat gland, 591, *594*
Cyclic AMP, 134
　as second messenger, 134, *134*
　role of in hormone action, 134, *134*
Cyst(s), Nabothian, 894
　Rathke's, 517
Cystic duct, 717
Cytochalasin B, 129
Cytochrome *c*, and blood-thymus barrier, *466*

Cytokinesis, 70, 822
Cytology, methods of, 1–33
Cytolysosome, 50
Cytoplasm, 35
　matrix components of, 58
Cytoplasmic matrix. See *Matrix.*
Cytoskeleton, 91
Cytotoxic lymphocytes, 428
Cytotrophoblast, *892, 894, 898, 899*

Da Fano technique, of osmium impregnation, *54*
Decidua basalis, *897, 899*, 900
Decidua capsularis, *897, 899*, 900
Decidua vera, *897, 899*, 900
Decidual cells, of ovary, 876
Decidualization, of endometrium, 889
Degeneration, primary, of nerve, 382
　transneuronal, 371
　Wallerian, of nerve, 382
Deiters, cells of, 978, *978–980, 982, 983*
Deletion, chromosomal, 75
Delta cells, of hypophysis, 509, *512*
　of islets of Langerhans, 731, *734, 737*
Demilunes, serous, 121, *125*
　of Giannuzzi, 609, *610, 611*, 612
Dendrites, 334, *335, 338*, 342, *344–346*
　electrical potential of, 347
　gemmules of, *338*, 343
　spines of, *338*, 343, *344, 370, 371*
Dendritic cells, of germinal center, 448, *450*
Dendrodendritic synapses, 343, 369, *370*
Dental lamina, 631, *633*
Dental sac, 631
Dentin, 622, *622, 623*
　calcification of, 623
　circumpulpar, 623
　mantle, 623
　relationship of odontoblasts to, 624
Dentinal tubules, 622, *623*
Dentinoenamel junction, 627, 628, *628*
Deoxycorticosterone, 549
Deoxyribonuclease, secretion of, 738
Deoxyribonucleic acid, cell division and, 73
　Feulgen reaction for, *11*, 18
　in chromatin, 63
　in mitochondria, 47, 48, *49*
　in nucleus, 63
　labeling of, 18, 64–65
　staining for, *15*, 16
　structure of, 65
　synthesis of, 73
　synthesis of cell protein and, 109
Dermal papilla, of hair follicle, 582, *582, 585*
Dermatan sulfate, 168
Dermatosparaxis, 193
Dermis, *564, 565, 566, 573*, 577–579
　blood supply of, *595*
　layers of, 577
　papillae of, 563
Dermoepidermal junctions, *580*
Descemet's membrane, *921*, 922, *923, 924*
Desmosine, 164
Desmosomes, 59, 92, 94, *95*
　between epidermal cells, 567, *569, 570, 572*
　half. See *Hemidesmosomes.*
　in atrioventricular bundle, *329*

Desmosomes (*Continued*)
in intercalated disc, *323*
in stratum corneum, *572*
of esophageal epithelium, *642*
of Purkinje cells, 327
of reticular cells and thymus, 458, *462,
463,* 464
Determinant, antigenic, 427
Deuterosomes, 102, *105*
Diabetes insipidus, 521
Diabetes mellitus, 740
Diaphragma sellae, 504, *504*
Diaphysis, of long bones, *244,* 245
Diarthroses, 282
Diastole, 404
Dictyate stage, of meiosis, chromosomes in,
863
Diffraction, x-ray, 31–33
myoglobin pattern in, *32*
Digestion, intracellular, 49, *51*
Digestive system, 598. See also listings of
specific organs, e.g., *Intestines; Stomach;*
etc.
general organization of, 598, *599*
1,3,4-Dihydroxyphenylalanine, in study of
melanocytes, 572, *574*
Diiodotyrosine, 529
Dioptric media, of eye, 918, 953
Diploë, of flat bones, 246
Diplosome, 57, *58*
cell cycle of, *59*
Diplotene stage, of meiosis, 74
Discs, intercalated, of cardiac muscle, 315,
316, 320, *323*
membranous, of retinal rod and cone cells,
948, 949
freeze fractured, *951*
Disse, space of, 698, 701, *702–704*
Division, cell, 70–74. See also *Meiosis; Mitosis.*
DNA. See *Deoxyribonucleic acid.*
Dopamine, 543
Down's syndrome, 74
Drug tolerance, liver and, 716
"Drumstick" appendage, in neutrophilic
leukocytes, 144, *145*
Duct(s). See also *Ductus.*
alveolar, of lung, 749, 752, *751–753*
of mammary gland, 907, *912*
Bellini's, 781, *788*
bile, *690–694,* 717, *717*
cochlear, *966, 969, 974*
ejaculatory, 799, 846
Gartner's, 879
intercalated, of glands of oral cavity, 607,
610, 614
lactiferous, 907, *909*
lymphatic, 420, 424
of Luschka, 720
of pancreas, 733, *738, 739, 740*
of testis, 841–846
papillary, of Bellini, 781, *788*
salivary, 607, *610,* 611, *614, 615*
Santorini's, 733
Stensen's, 611
striated, of oral cavity, 607, *614, 615*
thoracic, 424
Wharton's, 611
Wirsung's, 733

Duct system, of compound tubuloacinar
gland, *126*
of mixed mucous and serous glands, 121,
125
Ductuli efferentes, *806,* 842
Ductus choledochus, 717
Ductus deferens, 806, *806,* 844, 846, *848, 849*
Ductus ejaculatorius, 799
Ductus epididymidis, *806,* 843
epithelium of, *846, 847*
Ductus reuniens, 970
Duodenum, 658, *660, 661, 663.* See also
Intestines, small.
Brunner's glands of, *660, 661, 663,* 671
Dura mater, 246, 375, 376, *376*
Dust cells, 758, *761, 762*
from nonsmoker, *761*
from smoker, *762*
Dwarfism, 513
Dyes. See *Staining* and listings of specific
stains.
Dynein, 101

Ear, 964–991, *965, 966*
external, 964, *965*
functional considerations, 990–991
histogenesis of, 987–989
internal, *965, 966,* 968–987. See also
Labyrinth, of ear; Organ of Corti.
middle, 965–968, *965, 966*
structure of, *964, 965*
Eardrum. See *Tympanic membrane.*
Edema, 421
Effector cells, 427
Effector organs, 334
Ehlers-Danlos syndrome, 193
Ehrlich's hematoxylin staining, of para-
follicular cells, *530*
Ejaculatory ducts, 799, 846
Elastase, 164, 738
Elastic connective tissue, 189
Elastic fibers, 162, *165, 166*
in walls of arteries, *405*
Elastic fiber staining, of descending aorta,
406
of spleen, 492
Elastic lamina. See *Elastica externa; Elastica
interna.*
Elastic membranes, fenestrated, of aorta, *407*
Elastica externa, of arteries, 397, *402, 404,
406*
Elastica interna, of arteries, 397, *399, 400,
401–404,* 408
of muscular arteries, 399, *401–403*
of small muscular artery, *403, 404*
Elastin, 163
Electromagnetic spectrum, *31*
Electron microprobe analysis, 19, *22*
Electron microscopy, scanning, 27, *28*
specimen preparation for, 27
transmission, 26, *29*
Ellipsoid, of retinal rod and cone cells, 942,
945, 950, 952
Embedding, of tissues, 10
Embryo, implantation of in endometrium,
892–895

Embryo (*Continued*)
  of 40 days, *896*
Emperipolesis, 437
Enamel, of teeth, *622, 623, 625, 627, 629, 630, 632*
    lines of Retzius, *622, 627, 627*
    lines of Schreger, *622, 627*
    matrix of, calcification of, 633
    rods of, 626, *627, 629, 630*
    secretion of by ameloblasts, 625, *636, 637*
Enamel cuticle, 627, 634
Enamel knot, 631
Enamel lamellae, 628
Enamel organ, 631, *632, 633*
Enamel prisms, 626, *627, 629, 630*
Enamel spindles, 628
Enamel sheath, 626
Enamel tufts, 628
End plate, motor See *Motor end plate.*
Endocardium, 416, *417*
  subendocardial layer of, 416
  subendothelial layer of, 416
Endochondral ossification, 241, *241*
Endocrine glands. See *Glands, endocrine,* and name of specific gland.
Endolymph, of ear, 970, 983
  electrolyte composition of, 990(t)
Endolymphatic sac, *970, 974*
  of inner ear, 970
Endometrium, 887–893, *887*
  blood supply of, 888
  changes in during menstrual cycle, *888–890*
  implantation of embryo in, *892–895*
Endomysium, 295
Endoneurium, 357, *359, 360*
Endopeptidases, 738
Endoplasmic reticulum, agranular, 43, *44*
  cisternae of, 41, *41*
  granular, *36, 40, 41*
    relationship of microsomes and ribosomes to, 42, *43*
    with spiral and rosette polyribosomes, *112, 113*
  relationship of to Golgi complex, *56*
Endosteum, 246
Endothelial cells, of hepatic sinusoids, 696, *697, 698*
Endothelium, 84
Enterochromaffin cells, 651, 663
Enterochromaffin system, 664
Enteroglucagon, 652, 665
Envelope, nuclear, *67, 69*
Enzymes, cellular, identification of, 19, *19, 20*
    in lysosomes, 48
    in microbodies, 52
    in mitochondria, 48
    pancreatic, synthesis of, 738
Eosin, 16
Eosin-azure staining, of endochondral ossification, *267, 268*
  of hyaline cartilage, *235*
  of intramembranous ossification, *263*
Eosinophils. See *Leukocytes, eosinophilic.*
Ependyma, 366
Epicardium, 417
Epidermal ridges, 563
Epidermis, 563–577

Epidermis (*Continued*)
  fine structure of, 569
  keratinization of, 569–571
  keratohyalin granules of, 567, *576*
  Langerhans cells of, 574, *576–578*
  layers of, 565
  melanosomes of, 572, *575*
  Merkel cell of, 576, *579, 580*
  of body, 569, *573*
  of palms and soles, 565, *566, 567, 568*
  specializations of, 563
  stratum basale of, 565
  stratum corneum of, 566, *566, 567, 571–573*
  stratum disjunctum of, *566,* 569
  stratum germinativum of, 565, *568*
  stratum granulosum of, 566, *566, 570, 573, 576*
  stratum lucidum of, 566, *566*
  stratum malpighii of, 565, *566, 568, 573, 575, 576*
  stratum spinosum of, 566
  structure of, 565, *566*
Epididymis, 806, *806*
Epiglottis, 747
Epimysium, 295
Epinephrine, 543
  actions of, 551
  as first messenger, 134
  storage of in adrenal medulla, 544, *549*
Epineurium, 356, *359*
Epiphyseal plate, of long bones, *244,* 245
Epiphysis, closure of, 272
  of long bones, *244,* 245
Epiphysis cerebri, 556
Epithelial cells. See also *Epithelium.*
  cilia of, 89, 99–102, *101, 103, 104*
  flagella of, 102–103
  microvilli of, 98, *98, 99, 102*
  pulmonary, 756
  specializations of for cell attachment, 91–97
  specializations of free surface, 98–103
  stereocilia of, 98–99, *100*
  structure of, *93*
Epithelial sheath, of Hertwig, 637
Epithelial tissue, nerve endings in, 362–363
Epithelioid cells, 177
Epithelium, 83–106. See also *Epithelial cells.*
  basal lamina of, 96–97
  basal surface of, 96
  blood supply of, 104
  brush border of, 98, *98, 99, 102*
  ciliary, of retina, 929, *933, 934*
  ciliated, 84, *87, 88*
  classification of, 84, *85*
  distribution of, 83
  esophageal, *641–644*
  extraneous cells of, 105–106
  false, 83
  freeze-fractured, zonula occludens of, *94*
  germinal, of ovary, 859, *861*
  glands of, 118
  ground substance of, 97
  intestinal, 659, *666, 668*
  junctional complex of, *93*
  metaplasia of, 90
  nerve endings in, 362
  nerve supply of, 105

Epithelium (*Continued*)
  olfactory, 743, *744–746*
  organization and distribution of, 83
  pigment, of eye, *931, 932, 935, 936, 938, 942, 943, 945*
  pseudostratified ciliated, *101*
  pseudostratified columnar, *85*, 89
    stereocilia of, *100*
  renewal and regeneration of, 106
  seminiferous, 807–811, *809–813*
    cell associations in, *831–836*
    cells of. See *Sertoli cells; Spermatozoa.*
    cycle of, 828, *831–836*
    degeneration and regeneration of, 830
    first meiotic division in, *810*
    second meiotic division in, *811*
    wave of, 829
  sensory, of inner ear, 970
  simple columnar, 84, *85, 87*
  simple cuboidal, 84, *85*
  simple squamous, 84, *85*
  specializations of, 90
    for attachment and communication, 91
  specializations of free surface of, 98
  stratified columnar, *85, 87*, 88, *90*
  stratified squamous, 86, *87*
    keratinized, 84, *87*, 88
    nonkeratinized, *87*, 88
    of esophagus, *641, 643, 644*
  striated border of, 98, *98, 99, 102*
  transitional, 89, *91*
    of bladder, *796*
      cell membrane of, *797*
  types of, *85, 87*
Eponychium, 587, *588*
Epoöphoron, 879
Equational division, in meiosis, 74
Equatorial plate, 70
Ergastoplasm. See *Endoplasmic reticulum, granular.*
Erythroblasts, 214
  acidophilic, 216
  basophilic, 216, *218*
  definitive, 210
  orthochromatic, 216, *220*
  polychromatophilic, 216, *219*
    definitive, *211, 212*
  primitive, 210, *211*
Erythrocytes, 137, *138–140*
  crenation of, 138, *138, 140*
  development of in bone marrow, *218*
  extrusion of nucleus of, *220*
  formation of, 216–220
  ghost of, 138
  hypochromic, 139
  normochromic, 139
  polychromatophilic, 139, 219
  rouleau formation by, 137, *138*
Erythropoiesis, 216–220
  control of, 219
  sequence of, *221*
Erythropoiesis stimulating factor, 219
Erythropoietin, 219, 766
Erythrosin staining, of mammatropes, 507
Esophagogastric junction, *644*
Esophagus, 639–643, *640*
  epithelium of, *641–644*
  glands of, 640, *643*
  histological organization of, 639, *630, 643*

Esophagus (*Continued*)
  histophysiology of, 641
  junction of with stomach, *644*
  wall of, *643*
Estradiol, 897
Estrogens, 281, 866, 897
Estrone, 897
Euchromatin, 64, *66*
Eustachian tube, 967
  cartilage of, 239
Excretion, 108
Exocoelom, 898
Exocrine glands. See *Glands, exocrine.*
Exocytosis, 112, 129
Exopeptidases, 738
Exophthalmic goiter, 532
Exteriorization, in study of organs, 2
Exteroceptive system, 333
Exudate, serous, 186
  free cells of, 187
Eye, 917–962, *918, 919.* See also *Cornea; Retina.*
  accessory organs of, 957
  anterior chamber of, 918, *918, 919*, 925–927
    as medium for study of living tissues, 3, 5
  axes of, 918
  blood supply of, 957
  cornea of. See *Cornea.*
  fibrous tunic of, 920–925
  focusing of, 928
  histogenesis of, 961, *962*
  lymph spaces of, 957
  muscles of, 917, 928
  nerves of, 957
  planes of, 918
  posterior chamber of, 918, *918, 919*, 925–927
  refractive media of, 934–937
  retina of. See *Retina.*
  structure of, 917, *918, 919*
  vascular tunic of, 926–934
Eyelashes, 958, *960*
Eyelids, 957, *960*
  blood and lymph supply of, 961
  meibomian glands of, 588
  Moll's glands of, 591

Fab fragments of IgG, 428
Fabricius, bursa of, 451, 671
F-actin, filaments of, *306*, 307, *311*
Factor(s), aldosterone stimulating, 548
  blastogenic, 438
  cloning inhibiting, 438
  growth, nerve, 374
  lymphocyte transforming, 438
  migration inhibiting, 438
  proliferation inhibiting, 438
  releasing, 512, 515
  transfer, 438
Fallopian tube, 880–883, *882, 883*
  blood supply of, 883
  epithelium of, 883, *884, 885*
    effect of hormones on, *886*
  mucosa of, 883
  structure of, 881, *882, 883*
Falx cerebri, of brain, *376*

Fascia(e), 188
Fascia adherens, 321, *323*. See also *Intercalated discs.*
Fascicles, of skeletal muscle, 295, *295*
Fasciculi longitudinales, 718
Fat. See also *Adipose tissue; Lipids.*
    absorption of, intestinal, 677–680, *678–682*
    fetal, 197. See also *Adipose tissue, brown.*
Fat cells, 172, *176, 177*
    multilocular, 197
    unilocular, 197
Fat storing cells, of liver, 700, *700, 701*
Fauces, 615
Fc fragments, of IgG, 428
Feedback mechanism, endocrine, simple, *132*
    in response to stress, *133*
    in suckling reflex, *133, 521*
    negative, 132
    simple, of pancreas, *132*
Fenestra ovalis, *965, 966,* 970
Fenestra rotundum, *965, 966,* 970
Fenestra vestibuli, *966, 966*
Ferric chloride staining, of adrenal medulla, 543
Ferritin, 62, 220
    in study of ligands, 445
    in study of plasma cells, 433
    uptake of, by Langerhans cells, 575
Ferritin labeling, in study of T lymphocytes, 436
Fertilization, of ovum, 869
Feulgen reaction, 16
    for deoxyribonucleic acid, 18, 64
    of spermatozoa, *814*
Fibers, cementoalveolar, of periodontal membrane, 630
    collagenous, 159, *159–164*. See also
        Collagen.
        development of from fibroblasts, *173, 174*
        development of in tissue culture, 169, *170*
        in tunica media of aorta, *407*
    connective tissue, development of, 168
    elastic, 162, *165, 166*
        in elastic cartilage, 239, *239*
        microfibrils of, 163
    extrafusal, of annulospiral endings, 361
    gamma, of neuromuscular spindles, 361
    intrafusal, of muscle spindle, *313, 314, 314,* 361
    Korff's, 633
        of tooth pulp, 629, *637*
    muscle. See *Muscle fibers.*
    nerve. See *Nerve fibers.*
    perforating, of bone, 252
    Purkinje, of heart, 325, *326, 327, 328*
    reticular, 165, *166*
        compared to collagen fibers, 172
        of lymph node, *448*
        of spleen, *489, 490, 491*
    Sharpey's, of bone, 252, *253*
    Tomes', 623, *623, 637*
Fibrin, 140
Fibrinogen, 140, 155, 156
Fibroblasts, 158, *161,* 171, *173, 175*
    development of adipose cells from, *205*
    in cornea, 921, *922*
    of developing connective tissue, *173*
    pericryptal, 667
    tissue culture of, *6, 7, 8*
Fibrocartilage, 239, *240*

Fibrocyte, 171
Fibrohyaline tissue, 240
Fibrous long spacing collagen, 161, *164*
Fibrous sheath, of spermatozoon, 818, *818, 821*
Fields, Cohnheim's, *296,* 298
Fila olfactoria, 744
Filaments, actin, 58
    cytoplasmic, 58, *60*
    F-actin, *306,* 307, *311*
    lymphatic anchoring, 421
    myosin, 58
    of lipid droplet, 198, *201*
Filiform papillae, of tongue, *601, 602, 603, 604*
Filtrate, glomerular, 769
Filtration barrier, of glomerulus, 772
Filtration slits, of renal corpuscles, 770, *772–774, 777*
Fimbriae, of oviduct, 881
    ciliation of, *885*
Final common pathway, 372
    of central nervous system, 351, 372
Fixation, of tissues, 10, 11
    artifacts of, 10
Flagella, 102
Flower-spray endings, of sensory nerve fibers, 361
Fluid, cerebrospinal. See *Cerebrospinal fluid.*
Fluorescein, 20
Fluorescein isothiocyanate, in study of B lymphocytes, *437*
Fluorescence microscopy, *21,* 26
Fluorescent antibody staining, for plasma cells, *184*
    of connective tissue eosinophils, 184
Fluorescent antibody technique, 20, *25*
Foliate papillae, of tongue, 603, *606*
Follicle(s), hair, 579, *580–582, 586, 587*
    growing, 582, *582*
    keratogenous zone of, 582
    number of per square centimeter of skin, *594*
    quiescent, 582, *582*
    sebaceous glands and, 586
    ovarian, 858–866, *859–872*
        antral, *862, 864, 869, 870*
        atretic, *859, 860, 873, 881*
        graafian, *859, 864, 871*
        primary, *860, 862, 864–866*
        primordial, 859, *862, 863*
        secondary, *862, 864, 869, 870*
        stigma of, 867, *872*
        unilaminar, 859
    thyroid, 524, *525, 527, 530*
Follicle stimulating hormone, 510, 513, 513(t), 895
Follicular cells, of ovarian follicle, 859, *863, 870*
    effect of on seminiferous tubules, *839*
Foot processes, of podocytes, 770, *771–774, 776, 777*
Foramen(ina), apical, 621
    arterial, 417
    atrioventricular, 417
    of Luschka, 377
    of Magendie, 377
Foramen caecum, 601
Foreign body giant cells, 177
Formalin fixation, 11
Fornices, of eye, 957, *960*

Fossa, implantation, of spermatozoon, 816, 827, 828
Fossa navicularis, 800
Fovea, 918, 920, 938, 942, 951, 959
Foveolae gastricae, 644, 645, 646, 647
Fractionation, of cells, 12, 13
Fractions, cell, from homogenization, 12, 13
Freeze-cleaving, 29, 30
Freeze-drying, 11
Freeze-etching, 29, 30
Freeze-substitution, 11
FSH, 510, 513, 513(t), 895
Fuchsin staining, of bone, 247, 248
Fundus, of stomach, 644
Fungiform papillae, of tongue, 601, 602, 603, 605

GABA, 371
G-actin, units of, 306, 307
Gairn's gold chloride staining, of Langerhans cells, 576
Galactopoiesis, 911
Gallbladder, 718–723
  blood supply of, 720
  concentration of bile in, 720
  concentration of solutes in, 721, 722
  histology of, 718
  histophysiology of, 721
  mucosal folds of, 722
  nerves of, 721
  wall of, 719, 721–723
Gamma-aminobutyric acid, 371
Gamma fibers, of neuromuscular spindles, 361
Gamma globulins, 155
Gamma motor neurons, 361
Ganglia, cochlear, 984
  collateral, 364
  inferior cervical, 761
  of autonomic nervous system, 364, 367
  of myenteric plexus, 684
  prevertebral, 364, 367
  Scarpa's, 984
  spiral, of ear, 969, 975, 976
  terminal, 364
  thoracic, 761
  vertebral, 364, 367
  vestibular, 984
Ganglion cells, of retina, 949, 954
  sympathetic, of adrenal medulla, 546
Gap junction, 93, 95, 97. See also Nexus.
  in cardiac muscle, 322, 324, 325, 329
  intramembranous particles of, 715
  of neurons, 371
  of osteocytes, 257
  of smooth muscle fibers, 294
Gartner, duct of, 879
Gastric anti-pernicious anemia factor, 655
Gastric glands. See Glands, gastric.
Gastric intrinsic factor, 654
Gastric pits, of stomach, 644, 645–647
Gastrin, 651, 655, 665, 738
Gastrointestinal tract, blood supply of, 680, 683, 684
  general organization of, 598, 599
  lymph vessels of, 681, 683
Gelatin, from collagen, 160
Gemmules, of dendrites, 338, 343, 344

Genital corpuscle, 364, 364, 855
Genitalia, female, 904–905. See also Reproductive system, female.
  male, 805–856
Genitourinary system. See Reproductive system; Urinary system.
Gerlach, tubal tonsils of, 968
Germ, tooth, 621, 631
Germinal center, of lymphoid tissue, 448, 449, 450, 474, 478, 479
  cap of, 448, 449
  capsule of, 449
Germinal epithelium, of ovary, 859, 861
Ghost, erythrocyte, 138
Giannuzzi, serous demilunes of, 609, 610, 611, 612
Giemsa staining, of blood cells, 145
  for chromosomes, 75
  of gastric pyloric glands, 652
Gigantism, 613
Gingiva, 621, 622, 623, 630, 634
Gingival crevice, 630
Gland(s), 108–134
  accessory, of male reproductive tract, 847–851
  acinar, 120, 121
  adrenal. See Adrenal glands.
  areolar, of Montgomery, 908
  Bartholin's, 904, 904
  Blandin's, 612
  blood vessels of, 121
  Bowman's, 745, 746
  Brunner's, intestinal, 660, 661, 663, 671
    of small intestines, secretion of, 672
  buccal, 611
  bulbourethral, 850, 854
  cardiac, esophageal, 640
    of stomach, 645. See also Glands, gastric.
  ceruminous, 591, 964
  Cowper's, 850, 854
  duodenal, 660, 661, 663, 671
  endocrine, 123–134
    control mechanisms and interrelationships of, 132, 132, 133
    cytology of, 125, 126
  esophageal, 640, 643
  exocrine, 108
    classification of, 117–121
    compound, acinar, 120, 121
      mixed mucous and serous, 120, 125
        duct system of, 121, 125
      mucous, 120, 124
      saccular, 120
      serous, 120, 124
      tubular, 120, 121
      tubuloacinar, 120, 121, 123
        duct system of, 126
    diagram of typical cell, 109
    duct system of, 122
    histological organization of, 121
    intraepithelial, 118
    multicellular, 118, 119
    simple, acinar, 120, 121
      branched acinar, 120, 121
      branched tubular, 119, 121, 122
      coiled tubular, 119, 121
      tubular, 119, 121
    unicellular, 117, 119

Gland(s) (*Continued*)
  fundic, of stomach, 645, *645, 647, 648.*
    See also *Glands, gastric.*
  gastric, 645, 647–652
    argentaffin cells of, 651, *655*
    chief cells of, 647, *648, 651, 652*
    neck mucous cells of, 649
    oxyntic cells of, 648, *648, 653, 654*
    parietal cells of, 648, *648, 653, 654*
    zymogenic cells of, 647, *648, 651, 652*
  glossopalatine, 612
  histological organization of, 121
  intermediate, of stomach, 645
  interstitial, of ovary, 878
  labial, *610,* 611
  lacrimal, 959
  Lieberkuhn's, 665, 675, *675–677*
  lingual, anterior, 612
  Littre's, 800, *801*
  mammary, 907–916
    active, 908, *910–913*
    blood and lymph supply of, 915
    endocrine control of, 911
    in pregnancy, *910*
    innervation of, 915
    involution of, 915
    lactating, *911–913*
    merocrine secretion by, 910, *914*
    regression of, 914
    resting, 907–908
  meibomian, 588, 959, 960
  mixed, of oral cavity, 606, 608, *610–615*
  mixed endocrine and exocrine, 124
  Moll's, 958
    of eyelids, 591
  mucous, of bronchi, 750
    of oral cavity, 606, 607, *610, 616*
    of tongue, 613
  multicellular, 118–121
  nerve endings in, 363
  nerves of, 121
  Nuhn's, 612
  of digestive tract, 605–619, 640, 645
  of esophagus, 640, *643*
  of fundus of stomach, 645. See also
    Glands, gastric.
  of intestine, 665, 671
  of oral cavity, 605–619
    ducts of, 606
  of pharynx, 618
  of skin, 588–592
  of stomach, 647–652. See also *Glands,*
    gastric.
  of tongue, *602,* 603
  olfactory, of Bowman, *745,* 746
  palatine, 613
  parathyroid. See *Parathyroid glands.*
  parotid, 606, 611, *615*
  pituitary. See *Hypophysis.*
  preen, of birds, 589
  prostate. See *Prostate gland.*
  protein secreting, 108
  pyloric, of stomach, 645, *656.* See also
    Glands, gastric.
  salivary, 605–614
  sebaceous, *590*
    of glans penis, 853
    of hair follicles, 586
    of skin, 588, *590*
  serous, of oral cavity, 606, 607, *616*

Gland(s) (*Continued*)
  steroid secreting, 126
  sublingual, 606, 612, *616*
  submandibular, 606, 611, *610–615*
    cell types in, *614*
    serous demilunes of, *125*
  submaxillary. See *Glands, submandibular.*
  suprarenal. See *Adrenal glands.*
  sweat, 589–592, *590–594*
  thyroid. See *Thyroid.*
  tubular, 119, 120, *121*
  Tyson's. 853
  unicellular, 117–118
  urethral, *801*
  uropygial, 589
  uterine, 887
  vestibular, 904
  von Ebner's, *602,* 603, *605,* 613
Glans clitoridis, 904
Glans penis, *805,* 851, 852
Glassy membrane, of atretic follicle, 875
  of eye, 926, *931*
  of hairs, *585, 587*
Glaucoma, 925
Glia, 366–369. See also *Neuroglia.*
Glisson's capsule, 711
Globular leukocyte, 670
Globulin, plasma, 155
Glomerular filtrate, 769
Glomerulus, 768, *771–774, 778, 787, 789*
  filtration barrier of, 772
  histophysiology of, 788
  podocytes of, 770, *771–775*
Glomus, 414
Glomus cell, of carotid body, 415
Glossopalatine glands, 612
Glottis, frontal section of, *747*
Glucagon, 741
Glucocorticoids, 549
Glucose, blood concentration of, liver and,
  713
  Tm of, 790
Glutaraldehyde fixation, of adipose tissue,
  200
Glycocalyx, 40
  of gastric parietal cells, 648
  of gastric surface mucous cells, *650*
Glycogen, alpha particles of, 62, *64*
  beta particles of, 62
  cytoplasmic deposits of, 62, *64*
  in adipose tissue, *206*
  in cardiac muscle fiber, 319, *321, 322*
  in Purkinje fibers, *326*
  of parathyroid principal cells, 536
  of vaginal epithelium, *17*
  storage of in liver, 703, *709, 710*
Glycogenesis, 713
Glycogenolysis, 713
Glycopeptide, 167
Glycoprotein, 167
Glycosaminoglycans, 167
Glycosaminolipids, 167
Goblet cell, 117, *119*
  of colon, *677*
  of intestine, 661, *664, 665*
  of respiratory epithelium, *749*
Goiter, 531
  colloid, 532
  exophthalmic, 532
Goitrogen, 531

Gold chloride staining, of fat-storing cells, 700, *700, 701*
  of Kupffer cells, 698, *700*
  of Langerhans cells, 574, *576*
  of nerve ending of muscle spindle, *315*
Golgi chromo-argentic impregnation, of retinal neurons, 949, *954, 955*
Golgi complex, 36, 52, *54, 55*
  condensing vacuoles of, 111, *115*
  in osteocyte, *258*
  of neurons, 339, *341*
  relationship of to endoplasmic reticulum, 56
  role of in elaboration of collagen, *174*
  role of in exocrine gland secretion, 111, *114*
Golgi-Mazzoni, corpuscles of, 364
Golgi staining, in study of interrelationships of neurons, 372
  of neurons of central nervous system, *335, 338*
  of Purkinje cell, *345*
  of retina, *943*
Golgi Type I neurons, 347, 350
Golgi Type II neurons, 347
Gomori-Takamatsu reaction, for alkaline phosphatase, 18
Gonadotropes, 509, *512*
Gonadotropic hormones. See *Hormones, gonadotropic.*
Gottlieb, epithelial attachment of, of gum, 630
Graafian follicle, *859*, 864, *871*
Granule, acrosomal, 823
  alpha, of platelets, 140
    of pancreatic cells, *735*
  atrial, in atrial muscle fibers, 324, *326*
  azurophilic, in lymphocyte, *152*
    in promyelocytes, 224, *225, 226*
    of neutrophils, 144, *148*
  beta, of pancreatic cells, *736*
  delta, of pancreatic cells, 737
  dense, of gastric parietal cell, 649, *653*
    of Merkel cell, 576, *579, 580*
    of protein and polypeptide secreting endocrine glands, *128*
  eosinophilic, with crystals, 145, *149*
  keratohyalin, 567, *570*
    in Hassall's corpuscle, 461
    in stratum granulosum, *576*
  lipofuscin, in neurons, 342
    of cardiac muscle, *13*
  matrix, mitochondrial, *46*, 47
  melanin, of hairs, 584, *584*
    in neurons, 342
  membrane-coating, 570
  mucigen, of gastric surface mucous cells, 646, *649, 650*
  neurosecretory, 519, *520*
  of basophils, 147, *150, 151*
  perichromatin, of liver cells, 702
  pigment of, 61, *62*
  proacrosomal, 823
  sand, of pineal, *557, 558*
  secretion, *36*
  secretory, *115*
    of acidophilic cell, *509, 510, 511*
    of adrenal medulla, *549*
    of basophilic cells, *512*

Granule (*Continued*)
  secretory, of neutrophilic leukocytes, 144, *146, 147*
    of Paneth cell, *670*
    of serous cells of submandibular gland, *613*
    of thyroid parafollicular cells, *531, 532*
  trichohyalin, of hair follicles, 582
  vermiform, of Langerhans cells, 575, *578*
  zymogen, 114, *118*
    of gastric zymogenic cells, *652*
    of pancreatic acinar cells, 726, *729, 731–733*
Granule cells, of brain, 350
Granulomere, of blood platelet, 140
Granulopoiesis, 224–229
  regulation of, 228
Granulosa cells, of ovarian follicle, 862, *866, 868*
Granulosa lutein cells, of corpus luteum, 871, *876, 877, 879*
Graves' disease, 532
Gray column, intermediolateral, of spinal cord, 365
Gray matter, of central nervous system, 347, *348, 349, 350*
  of cerebral cortex, cytoarchitecture of, 373
    motor areas of, 373
    somatosensory areas of, 373
Ground substance, 97
  cellular, 37
  of connective tissue, 167
Growth factors, nerve, 374
Growth hormone, 281, 507, 512, 513(t)
  effect of on cartilage, 242
Gum. See *Gingiva.*

H band, of skeletal myofibril, 299, *306, 307, 308*
Hair(s), 579–586
  club, 582
  follicle of, 579, *580–582, 586, 587*
    active and quiescent, 582, *582*
    nerve endings in, 363
    sebaceous glands and, 586
  of hair cells of ear, *984, 987*
  resting, 582, *582, 586*
  root of, *581*
  shaft of, 582, *583*
Hair cells, of crista ampullaris, 970, *972, 973*
  of organ of Corti, *978*, 979, *979–989*
  hairs of, *984, 987*
Hair shaft, 582, *583*
Halmi's aldehyde fuchsin stain, 163
Hammar's myoid cells, of thymus, 462
Harris hematoxylin staining, of tissue culture fibroblasts, *7, 175*
Hassall-Henle bodies, of cornea, 922
Hassall's bodies, of thymus, 458, *459, 460, 464*
Haversian canals, *247*, 248, *248*
Haversian systems, *21*, 247, *247–252*
  by four optical methods, *251, 278*
  definitive, 275
  primitive, 275
  stages in formation of, *277, 278, 279*
Heart, 416–419. See also *Muscle, cardiac; Muscle fibers, cardiac.*
  annuli fibrosi of, 417

Heart (*Continued*)
  blood vessels of, 419
  chondroid of, 417
  connective tissue of, 418
  endocardium of, 416, *417*
  epicardium of, 417
  impulse conducting system of, 418
  lymphatics of, 419
  muscle of, 315–330. See also *Muscle,*
    cardiac; Muscle fibers, cardiac.
  myocardium of, 416
  nerves of, 419
  pacemaker of, 325, 418
  Purkinje fibers of, 419
  septum membranaceum of, 417
  skeleton of, 417
  specialized conducting tissue of, 324
  trigona fibrosa of, 417
  valves of, 416, 418, *418*
  wall of, layers of, 416
Heavy meromyosin, 59, 660
Heidenhain's azan staining, 16
  of epithelium, *87*
Heidenhain's azan trichrome staining, of
  mammatropes, 507
Heidenhain's iron-hematoxylin staining, 11
  of nucleus in mitosis, *71*
  of pineal, *559*
Heister, spiral valve of, 720
Helicotrema, 970, *975*
Hemal nodes, 485
Hematoencephalic barrier, 381
Hematoxylin, 11
Hematoxylin and eosin staining, 11, *87*
  of elastic cartilage, *239*
  of fibrocartilage, *240*
  of hyaline cartilage, *233, 234, 237*
Hematoxylin-eosin-azure II staining, 12
  of bone marrow, *214*
  of decalcified bone, *270*
  of hemopoietic cells, *211, 212*
  of loose connective tissue, 185
  of lymph node, *432, 476*
  of omentum, *187*
  of palatine tonsil, 618
  of plasma cells, *182*
  of spleen, *490*
  of tendon, *191*
Hemidesmosomes, *60, 95, 96.* See also
  Desmosomes.
Hemocytoblasts, *211, 215,* 430
Hemocyanin, in study of ligands, 445
Hemocyanin reaction, of B lymphocyte, *439,*
  440
Hemoglobin, 62, 137
  concentration of in erythrocytes, *221*
  fetal, 138
Hemoglobin A, 138
Hemolysis, 138
Hemopoiesis, 209
  during embryonic development, 210, *211*
  hepatic phase, 210, *211*
  mesoblastic phase, 210, *211*
  monophyletic school of, 214, *215*
  myeloid phase, 210
  polyphyletic school of, 213
  theories of cell lineages, 213, *214, 215, 218*
Hemosiderin, 62, 758

Henle, layer of, of hair follicle, 582, *585, 587*
  loop of. See *Loop of Henle.*
  outer fiber layer of, 946
Hensen, cells of, *978,* 979, *979, 985*
Heparin, 184
Hepatic duct, 717
Hepatocytes, *702–708, 710*
  cytology of, 701, *704*
  microbodies of, 705, *707, 711, 712*
Hering, canals of, 694
Herring bodies, 518, *519*
Hertwig's epithelial root sheath, *621,* 628,
  630, 637
Heterochromatin, *66*
Heterophagy, 49
  role of lysosomes in, *51*
Heterophils. See *Leukocytes, neutrophilic.*
Hibernation, role of brown adipose tissue
  in, 205, *207*
Hilus, of lymph nodes, 471
Hilus cells, of ovary, 878
His, bundle of, 324, *327–329*
Histamine, 184, 192, 410
Histiocytes, 173
Histology, methods of, 1–33
Historadiography, 19, *21*
Holmes staining, of tissue culture neurons,
  336
Homogenization, of cells, *12, 13*
Horizontal cells, of retina, 947, *954–957*
Hormones, 123
  adipokinetic, 202
  adrenal cortical, effect of on adipose
    tissue, 203
  adrenocorticotropic, 513(t), 514, 912
  antidiuretic, 520, *521*
  carrier proteins and, 134
  effects of on adipose tissue, 202
  effects of on bone, 280
  effects of on connective tissue, 192
  follicle stimulating, 510, 513, 513(t)
    effect of on seminiferous tubules, *839*
  gonadotropic, 513
    mammary gland and, 912
    testis and, 838
  growth, 281, 507, 512, 513(t)
    effect of on bone, 281
    effect of on cartilage, 242
    secretion of, 513(t)
  hypophyseotropic, 512
  interstitial cell stimulating, 838
  lactogenic, 513(t), 514
    action of on Leydig cells, *839*
  luteinizing, 513(t), 514
  mechanism of action on target cells, 134,
    134
  melanocyte stimulating, 517
  neurohypophyseal, 127
  of nervous system, 333
  parathyroid, 257, 259, 280
  releasing, 512, 515
  sex, 837
  sex, effect of on adipose tissue, 203
    effect of on bone, 281
  smooth muscle and, 294
  somatotropic. See *Hormones, growth.*
  steroid, synthesis of, 126
  storage and secretion of, 127

Hormones (Continued)
  synthesis of, 127
    agranular endoplasmic reticulum and, 45
  thyroid, 524, 525
  thyroid stimulating, 530
  thyrotropic, 513(t), 515, 912
Horseradish peroxidase, as protein tracer, 773
  in study of ciliary epithelium of retina, 933
Hortega's stain, for pituicyte pigment granules, 519
Howship's lacunae, 257
Humor, aqueous, of eye, 918
    blood-aqueous barrier and, 930
     outflow system of, 928
  vitreous, of eye, 918, 918, 919, 925, 937
Humoral immune response, 149
Huschke, auditory teeth of, 981
Huxley's layer, of hair follicle, 582, 585, 587
Hyaline cartilage, of trachea, 748, 748
Hyalocytes, 937
Hyaloid canal, 937
Hyaloideocapsular ligament, 936
Hyalomere, of blood platelet, 140
Hyaluronic acid, 168, 253
Hyaluronidase, 168
Hydatid, of Morgagni, 879
Hydroxyapatite, 254, 622
Hydroxyapatite crystal, of tooth enamel, 629
Hydroxyindole-O-methyl transferase, 561
5-Hydroxytryptamine, 140, 186, 543, 651, 664. See also Serotonin.
Hymen, 902
Hyperadrenocorticism, 551
Hyperbilirubinemia, 716
Hyperemia, reactive, of arteries, 406
Hyperglobulinemia, 182
Hyperparathyroidism, 281, 539
Hyperplasia, of cementum, 628
Hyperthyroidism, 532
Hypertrophy, 244
Hypoadrenocorticism, 551
Hypodermis, 578
Hyponychium, of nails, 588, 588
Hypophyseoportal system, 512
Hypophysis, 503–521. See also Adenohypophysis; Neurohypophysis.
  acidophilic (alpha) cells of, 505, 506, 507, 508–511
  anterior lobe of. See Pars distalis.
  basophilic (beta) cells of, 505, 509, 512
  blood supply of, 511, 514, 515
  chromophobic cells of, 510
  control of male reproduction by, 839
  histophysiological correlations of, 515
  pars distalis of, 505–516, 506
    histophysiology of, 512–515
  pars intermedia of, 516–518
    histophysiology of, 517
  pars nervosa of, 518–521
  pars tuberalis of, 518
  relationship of to hypothalamus, 505
  relationship of to sella turcica, 504, 504
  reserve cells of, 510
  subdivisions of, 503, 503
Hypothalamohypophyseal tract, 518, 520
Hypothalamus, relationship of hypophysis to, 505
Hypothyroidism, 531

I bands, of skeletal myofibrils, 299, 299–301, 305, 307–310
ICSH, 838
IgA. See Immunoglobulins A.
IgG. See Immunoglobulins G.
IgM. See Immunoglobulins M.
Ileum, 658. See also Intestines, small.
  microvilli of, 667
  Peyer's patches of, 670, 671
Immune globulins, 155
Immune response, 427
  cell mediated, 428, 429
    mechanism of, 484
    mediators of, 438
    role of thymus in, 467, 468
  humoral, 428
  primary, 427
  role of lymph nodes in, 482
  role of macrophages in, 443
  role of spleen in, 500
  secondary, 428
Immune system, 427–454
  cells of, 430–446
    cytology of, 430
    histophysiology of, 434–446
  histophysiology of, 451
Immunity, and cell mediated response, 151
  and humoral immune response, 149
  cellular, 151
  lymphocytes and, 149
  primary response of, 149
  secondary response of, 149
Immunoblasts, 430
Immunoglobulins, 428
  human, sites of origin of, 184, 184
  production of by plasma cells, 669
Immunoglobulins A, plasma cells and, 432
  secretory, 429, 669
Immunoglobulins D, 429
Immunoglobulins E, 429
Immunoglobulins G, 428
  fragments of, 428
Immunoglobulins M, 429
  production of by B lymphocytes, 439
Immunohistochemistry, 20, 25
Implantation, of ovum, 892, 897
Implantation fossa, of spermatozoon, 816, 827, 828
Inborn lysosomal diseases, 53(t)
Incisures, of Schmidt-Lanterman, 352, 352, 353, 357
Inclusions, cellular, 36
  cytoplasmic, 61
Incus, 965, 966
India ink, in study of blood supply of adipose tissue, 204
  in study of bone marrow, 214
  in study of blood supply of hypophysis, 514, 515
  in study of blood supply of intestinal villi, 684
  in study of blood supply of parathyroid, 538
  in study of Kupffer cells, 699, 699
Indium staining, of perichromatin granules of liver cells, 702
Inflammation, role of connective tissue in, 191
Infundibulum, of oviduct, 881

Insulin, 125
    effect of on adipose tissue, 203, *206*
    feedback mechanism of, *132*
    secretion of, 739
Intercalated discs, of cardiac muscle, 315, *316*, 320, *323*
Intercellular bridges, 92
    between spermatids, 822, *823*
    of stratum germinativum, 566, *568*
Intercellular cement, 91, 386
Intercristal space, of mitochondria, 45, *47*
Interdental cells, of ear, 981
Interendothelial junctions, of thymic capillary, *466*
Interfacial canals, 92
Interference microscopy, 25
Interneurons, of central nervous system, 351
Interphase, mitotic, 70
    chromatin in, *66*
Interoceptive system, 333, 364
Interrenal tissue, 540. See also *Adrenal cortex.*
Interstitial glands, of ovary, 878
Interstitial cells, 684
    of ovary, 876
    of pineal body, 556, *559*
    of testis, 806, 833, *838–842*
        lipid in, *838*
        lipochrome pigment in, 834, *840*
Interstitial cell stimulating hormone, 838
Interstitial tissue, of bone, 247, *247, 248*
        composition and structure of, 253–254
    of cancellous bone, 249
    of cartilage, 234
    of ovary, 876
    of testis, 833, *837*
Intestinal juice, 676
Intestines, 658–686
    absorption by, histophysiology of, 676–680
    blood supply of, 680, *683, 684*
    Brunner's glands of, *660, 661, 663,* 671
    glands of, 665, 671
    histogenesis of, 686
    large, 674–675, *675–677*
        glands of Lieberkühn of, 674, *675–677*
        taeniae coli of, 675
    lymph vessels of, 681, *683*
    microvilli of, cross section of, *39*
    nerve supply of, 682–685, *684, 685*
    small, 658–673
        crypts of Lieberkühn of, 659, *661, 663, 665, 669, 671*
        epithelium of, 659, *666, 668*
        lymphoid tissue of, 659, 670, *671, 672*
        mucosa of, 658, *659–661, 663*
        mucosa of, lamina propria of, 668
        muscularis of, 673
        muscularis mucosae of, 671
        Peyer's patches of, 670, *671*
        plicae circulares of, 658, *659, 660*
        serosa of, 673
        submucosa of, 671
        valves of Kerckring of, 658, *659, 660*
        villi of, 658, *659–663, 665*
            surface coat of, 659, *667, 668*
Intracristal space, mitochondrial, 45
Inulin, 789
Inulin clearance, as test of kidney function, *789*

Iris, 917, *918, 919, 925,* 932–934, *935–937*
    crypts of, 932
    epithelium of, 933, *934–936*
Iron, storage of, 220
Iron-hematoxylin staining, of epithelium, *92*
    of fibroblasts, 171
    of pineal, *559*
    of skeletal muscle fibers, *299*
    of testis, *810, 812*
Iron-hematoxylin-azan staining, of jejunum, *664*
Iron oxide, uptake of, by capillary endothelium, *396*
Irritability, of nerve fibers, 333
Islets of Langerhans, *728,* 729–733, *734*
    alpha cells of, 730, *734, 735*
    beta cells of, 730, *734, 736, 741*
    delta cells of, 731, *734, 737*
Isochromosomes, 76
Isodesmosine, 164
Isoelectric point, 16
Isotopes, bone seeking, 254
Isthmus, of oviduct, 881, *882*

Janus green, 8, 11, 152
Jaundice, 716
Jejunum, 658, *662, 664, 665.* See also *Intestines, small.*
Joints, 282–285, *283, 284*
Junction, choledochoduodenal, 718
    dentinoenamel, *627, 628, 628*
    dermoepidermal, *580*
    esophagogastric, *644*
    gap. See *Gap junction.*
    interendothelial, of thymic capillary, *466*
    mucocutaneous, 576, *580*
    myoneural, 311, *312, 313*
    occluding, between Sertoli cells, *843*
    sclerocorneal, 923, *925, 926*
    tight. See *Tight junction.*
Junctional complex. See *Tight junction.*
Juxtaglomerular cells, 782, *789*
Juxtaglomerular complex, 782

Karyokinesis, 70, 822
Karyolymph, 64
Karyoplasm, 35
Karyosomes, 63
Karyotype, 75
Keith and Flack, node of, 324
Keratan sulfate, 168, 253
Keratin, 84
Keratinization, mechanism of, 569
Keratinizing system, 563
Keratinocyte, melanosome complexes in, 574, *575*
Keratinosomes, 570
Keratocytes, in cornea, 921, *922*
Keratogenous zone, of hair follicle, 582
Keratohyalin granules, 567, *570*
    in stratum granulosum, *576*
Kerckring, valves of, 658, *659, 660*
Kidneys, 766–794
    blood supply of, 784, *791, 792, 793*
    excretory function of, 787

Kidneys (Continued)
  function of, clinical evaluation of, 790
  glomeruli of, 768, 771, 778
    capillaries of, 771–778
    function of, clinical evaluation of, 788
  histophysiology of, 787
  juxtaglomerular complex of, 782
  lymphatic supply of, 786
  medulla of, zones of, 767, 778
  nephrons of. See Nephrons.
  nerves of, 787
  renal corpuscle of, 768, 769, 771, 775,
    787, 789, 790
    macula densa of, 780, 787, 790
    podocytes of, 770, 771–775
  structure of, 766, 767–769
  tubules of, 767–781. See also Nephron.
    collecting, 767, 770, 781, 784, 785, 788,
      791, 793
    convoluted, distal, 768, 770, 779, 785,
      786
      proximal, 768, 770, 779–783
        excretory capacity of, 792
        filtration by, 782
        histophysiology of, 790
    distal, 779, 785, 787
      histophysiology of, 792
    proximal, 768, 780, 783
    straight, 781
Killer lymphocytes, 428
Kinases, 134
Kinetochore, 69, 70
Kinetosomes, 57
Kinocilium, of hair cells, 971
Klinefelter's syndrome, 76
Kluver-Barrera staining, for nerve cells and
  myelin sheaths, 337, 351
Korff's fibers, 629, 633, 637
Krause, terminal bulbs of, 364
Kupffer cells, 695, 698, 700
  peroxidase reaction of, 700
Kupffer's gold impregnation method, 700,
  701

Labia majora, 904
Labia minora, 904, 905
Labial glands, 610, 611
Labyrinth, of ear, blood supply of, 985
  bony, 968–970
  endolymphatic, 970
  membranous, 969, 970, 971
  nerves of, 984, 990
  osseous, 968–970
  perilymphatic, 981–983
Lacrimal glands, 959
Lactase, 676
Lacteals, 681
  of intestinal villus, 669
Lactiferous ducts, 907, 909
Lactogenesis, 911
Lacunae, Howship's, 257
  of bone, 247, 249, 250
  of cartilage, 234, 235
  of Morgagni, 800
Lamellae, annulate, of cell, 54, 57
  enamel, 628
  of bone, 246
    circumferential, 248, 252

Lamellar bodies, of alveolar cells, 757, 760
Lamina, basal, 97
  dental, 631, 632
Lamina cribrosa, 942
Lamina dura, 631
Lamina epithelialis, 378
Lamina propria, of gastrointestinal tract,
    598, 599, 618
  of intestinal mucosa, 668
  of stomach wall, 652
Langerhans, islets of. See Islets of
  Langerhans.
Langerhans cells, 565
  of epidermis, 574, 576–578
  vermiform granules of, 575, 578
Larynx, 746–747, 747
  blood, lymph, and nerve supply of, 747
  muscles of, 747
Lasers, for study of living cells, 7
Lathyrism, 165, 193
LDL. See Lipoproteins, low density.
Lectins, 444
Lens, of eye, 918, 918, 919, 935–936, 938
  fibers of, 935, 938–940
Lens fibers, of eye, 935, 938, 940
  arrangement of, 939
Lenticular papillae, of tongue, 602
Leptomeninges, 375
Leptotene stage, of meiosis, 74
  in spermatogenesis, 821
Leucine aminopeptidase, 676
Leukocytes, 141
  basophilic, 143, 146, 147, 150, 151
    granules of, 147, 150, 151
  circulating pool of, 229
  classification of, 144
  eosinophilic, 143, 145, 146, 149
    granules of, 145, 149
    of connective tissue, 182
  formation of, 221–231
  globular, 670
  granular, 141, 144
  marginated pool of, 155, 229
  mononuclear, 141
  neutrophilic, 142, 143
    band forms, 142
    "drumstick" appendage in, 144, 145
    phagocytosis by, 154
    timing of events of differentiation, 230
  nongranular, 141, 144. See also Lympho-
    cytes; Monocytes.
  polymorphonuclear, 141, 142. See also
    Leukocytes, neutrophilic.
Leukocyte count, 141
  differential, 142
Leukopoietin, 229
Leukorrhea, 895
Leydig cells, 806, 808, 838–842
  crystals of Reinke in, 834, 840, 841
  effect of LH on, 839
  lipochrome pigment in, 834, 840
LH. See Hormone, luteinizing.
Lids, eye. See Eyelids.
Lieberkühn, crypts of, of small intestine,
    659, 661, 663, 665, 669, 671
  Paneth cells of, 667, 669, 670
  glands of, of large intestine, 674,
    675–677
Ligaments, 188
  hyaloideocapsular, 936

Ligands, 444
Light cells, of thyroid, 526
Light green staining, 16
Light meromyosin, 59
Limbus, of eye, 923, *925–927*
    trabecular meshwork of, 924, *926–929*
    spiral, of cochlea, *976,* 981
Lines of Retzius, of enamel, *622,* 627, *627*
Lines of Schreger, of enamel, *622,* 627
Lingual corpuscle, *364*
Lingual glands, anterior, 612
Lip, glands of, *600, 610,* 611
    of newborn, 600, *600*
Lipid, absorption of, in intestine, 677–680,
    678–682
    bimolecular layer of, 37, *38, 39*
    blood concentration of, liver and, 714
    cytoplasmic storage of, 63, *65*
    droplets of, in adipose cells, *199–201*
    in interstitial cells of testis, *838*
    in lactating mammary gland, *912–914*
    in neurons, 342
    in protoplasm, *36*
    intracellular, 63
    metabolism of, agranular endoplasmic
        reticulum and, 45
    molecular structure of, 37, *38, 39*
    staining for, *15*
Lipoblasts, *205*
Lipochrome pigment, in Leydig cells, 834,
    840
    in zona fasciculata of adrenal, 542
Lipocytes, of liver, 700
Lipofuscin, granules of, in cardiac muscle, *13*
    in neurons, 342
Lipofuscin pigment, 50, 62, *63*
    in zona reticularis of adrenal, 543
Lipoma, 201
Lipoproteins, beta, 156
    plasma, liver and, 714
    serum, 156
        low density, 156
        very low density, 156, 703, *707*
            synthesis and release of, *718*
Liquor folliculi, 864
Lithium carmine, in study of phagocytosis,
    174, *176, 481*
    uptake of, by bone marrow, *214*
Lithium carmine staining, of Kupffer cells,
    699
Littoral cells, of bone marrow, *213*
Littre, glands of, 800, *801*
Liver, 688–716, *689, 693*
    acinus of, 691, *695*
    bile canaliculi of, *694, 696, 704,* 708,
        713, 714
    bile capillaries of, *689*
    bile ducts of, *690–694,* 717, *717*
    bilirubin uptake and excretion by, 716
    blood supply of, *689,* 692, *692, 694, 717*
    capsule of, 711
    central veins of, 688, *689, 691, 694, 695*
    connective tissue of, 711
    drug metabolism in, 715
    fat-storing cells of, 700, *700, 701*
    functional unit of, 691, *695,* 710
    functions of, 713
    glycogenesis in, 713
    glycogenolysis in, 713

Liver (*Continued*)
    histological organization of, 688–712,
        689, 693
    histophysiology of, 713
    lipoprotein formation in, 714, *718*
    lobules of, 689, *689–693*
        zonation within, 706
    lymph production by, 711
    lymph spaces of, 711
    lymphatic supply of, *717*
    parenchymal cells of. See *Hepatocytes.*
    plates of cells of, *702*
    portal canal of, 689, *690*
    regeneration of, 712
    sinusoids of, 688, *689,* 694, 695,
        696–698, 702–704, 714
    veins of, 688, *689, 690*
Lobules, of liver, 689, *689–693*
    of lung, 749
    of testis, 805
Lobuli testis, 805
Long-acting thyroid stimulator, 532
Loop of Henle, 768, *770,* 776, *783*
    histophysiology of, 792
    junction of proximal tubule and thin limb
        in, *783*
LT. See *Lymphotoxin.*
LTF. See *Lymphocyte transforming factor.*
LTH. See *Prolactin.*
Luminosity horizontal cells, of retina, 955
Lungs, 748–764. See also *Bronchus.*
    alveolar ducts of, 749, *751–753*
    alveolar sacs of, 749, *752,* 753, *753*
    alveoli of, 749, 753, *753*
    blood supply of, 759
    fetal, *763*
    histogenesis of, 762
    histophysiology of, 764
    lobes of, 748
    lobules of, 749, *754*
    lymphatic system of, 760
    nerves of, 761
    pleura of, 761
    repair of, 764
    respiratory unit of, 750, *753*
Lunula, of nails, 587
Luschka, ducts of, 720
    foramina of, 377
Lutein cells, 871, *876–879*
Luteinizing hormone, 513(t), 514
Luteotropes, 507
Luteotropin, 507
Lymph, 420
    as ultrafiltrate of blood plasma, 421
Lymph nodes, 421, 471–485
    blood supply of, *473,* 478
    capsule of, 471, *472, 473,* 478
    cortex of, 472, 475, *478, 479*
    functions of, 481
    germinal center of, *449, 450, 474, 478, 479*
    hilus of, 471
    histogenesis of, 480
    histological organization of, 471–480
    histophysiology of, 481
    in antigenic challenge, 483
    lymphatic vessels of, 471
    medulla of, 472, *476,* 478
    medullary cords of, 473, *474*
    nerves of, 478

Lymph nodes (*Continued*)
  phagocytosis in, 481, *481*
  postcapillary venules of, lymphocyte
    migration through, 479, *479, 480*
  reticular cells and fibers of, *448*
  role of in immune defenses, 481
  sinuses of, 471, 472, *473–475, 477*
  trabeculae of, 471, *473*, 478
  types of lymphocytes in, *432*
Lymphatic nodules, of tongue, *601, 602*, 603
Lymphatic vessels, 420–424, *422–424*
  afferent, 421
  innervation of, 423
  nerve supply of, 423
  of heart, 419
  valves of, 423
  walls of, 422, *422*
Lymphoblasts, 214, 430
Lymphocytes, *143, 146*, 148, 151, *152*
  activated, 427
  antibody secreting, *441, 442*
  azurophilic granules of, 148
  B, 429
    development of, *453*, 457
    memory, 442
    microvilli of, 434, *436*
    response of to antigen, 439
    surface properties of, 434, *436*
  bursa dependent, 429, 434, *436–440*
  circulation of, 451, *453*
  cytotoxic, 428
  depletion of, 452
  differentiation of, *453*
  formation of, tonsils and, 617
  functional types of, 149, 430
  hemolytic plaque-forming, 441
  in blood, migration of, 187
  killer, 428
  migration of through lymph node
    venule, *479, 480*
  nonspecific stimulation of, 444
  of immune system, 430, *431–433*
  of thymus, *459–462*
  peripolesis of, 437
  production of, by thymus, 465
  recirculation of, 452, *453*
  T, 429, 440
    development of, *453*, 457
    microvilli of, 434, *435*
    response of to antigen, 436, *437–440*
    surface properties of, 434, *435*
  thymus dependent, 429, 434, *435*
  transformation of into lymphoblasts, *431*
  types of, in lymph node, *432*
  wandering, of loose connective tissue, 179
Lymphocyte transforming factor, 438
Lymphoid nodules, 447, 475
Lymphoid organs, 209, *215*
Lymphoid tissue, 446–451
  diffuse, 446
    reticular fibers of, 446
  germinal center of, 448, *449, 450*
  of small intestine, *659, 670, 671, 672*
  thymus dependent, 454
  thymus independent, 454
Lymphokines, 437, 445
Lymphopoiesis, 209
  in bone marrow, 231

Lymphotoxin, 438
Lysis, of erythrocytes, by antibody producing
  lymphocytes, 440, *441*
Lysosomal diseases, inborn, 51, 53(t)
Lysosomes, 49, *50*
  and inborn storage diseases, 51, 53(t)
  of neurons, *341*
  role of in heterophagy and autophagy, *51*
Lysozyme, 146
  of Paneth cells, 668

M band, of muscle myofibrils, 299, *305,
  307*, 316
Macrocytes, 139
Macroglia, 367, *368*
Macrophage(s), alveolar, from nonsmoker,
  761
    from smoker, *762*
  coalescence of, 177
  development of from monocytes in tissue
    culture, *179*
  fixed, 173
  free, 174, 178
    of lung, 758, *761, 762*
  histogenous, 191
  processing of antigens by, 669
  role of in immune response, 443
Macrophage system, 178, *180*
Macula, 951. See also *Fovea*.
  of inner ear, 970, *971*
Macula adherens, 92, *92, 94*. See also
  Desmosome.
Macula densa, 782
  of distal tubule of kidney, 780, *787, 790*
Macula lutea, of retina, 938
Macula pellucida, 867, *872*
Magendie, foramen of, 377
Maillet nerve stain, for nerve fibers of
  organ of Corti, *989*
Malleus, 965, *966*
Mallory-azan staining, of adrenal glands,
  541
  of collagenous and reticular fibers, *170*
  of colon, *676*
  of epithelium, *87*
  of hypophysis, *506*
  of lung, *755*
  of pancreas, 730, *734*
  of parathyroid gland, *536*
  of reticular cells of lymph node, *448*
Mallory's connective tissue staining, of tooth
  primordium, *633*
Mallory's stain, 162, 168
  of kidney, *769*
Mallory's trichrome staining, 16
  of epithelium, *87*
  of hypophyseal cells, 509
Malpighian bodies, of spleen, 487
Malpighian cell, cytomorphosis of, 565
Malpighian system, 563
Maltase, 676
Mammary gland, 907–916. See also *Gland,
  mammary*.
Mammary papilla. See *Nipple*.
Mammatropes, 507, *508, 510*
  secretory pathway of, *511*

Mammogenesis, 911
Manchette, *829*
  of spermatozoon, 826
Mantle, of germinal center, 448, *449*
Mantle dentin, 623
Marginal fold, of capillaries, 390, *391*
Marrow, bone. See *Bone marrow.*
Masson's stain, 16
  of olfactory epithelium, *745*
Mast cells, *176, 177, 184, 185, 186*
  of thymus, 461
Matrix, bone, 246
    submicroscopic structure and composition of, 253
  cartilage, secretion of, 238, *238*
  cytoplasmic, *36, 37*
    components of, 58
  mitochondrial, 46, *46*
Matrix cells, of hair follicle, 582, *585*
  of hairs, 582
Matrix granules, mitochondrial, *46,* 47
Matrix vesicles, of cartilage, 242
May-Grünwald-Giemsa staining, of blood vessels of mesentery, *411*
  of capillary, *388*
  of mesentery, *86*
  of thoracic duct lymphocytes, *431*
  of tissue culture monocytes, *179*
Meatus, auditory, external, 964, *965*
  internal, 969
Meconium corpuscles, 686
Mediastinum testis, 805, 841
Mediators, of cell mediated immune response, 437
Medulla, adrenal, 543–546. See also *Adrenal glands, medulla of.*
Megakaryoblast, 222
Megakaryocytes, 221, *222*
  platelet demarcation channels in, 223, *223*
  platelet forming, 222, *223*
  reserve, 222
Meibomian glands, 588, 959, *960*
Meiosis, 74
  in spermatogenesis, *810, 811,* 819
  stages of, 74
Meissner's corpuscles, 364, *365, 366*
  in penis, 855
Meissner's plexus, 679, 682, *683*
Melanin, 61, 571
  in neurons, 342
  of hairs, 584, *584*
Melanocytes, 61, *62,* 565, 571, *574*
  numbers of, in various types of mammalian skin, *574*
    per square centimeter of skin, *594*
  of hair follicles, 584, *586*
  of iris, 932, *935, 936*
Melanocyte stimulating hormone, 517
Melanocyte system, 571–576
Melanosomes, 61, *62,* 572, *576*
  complexes of, in keratocytes, 574, *575*
  developing, fine structure of, *575*
Melatonin, 560
Membrana perforata, 632
Membrane(s), alveolocapillary, *758*
  arachnoid, 375, *375, 376*
  basement. See *Basal lamina.*
  basilar, of perilymphatic labyrinth, 982
  Bowman's, 921, *921*
  Bruch's, 926, *931*

Membrane(s) (*Continued*)
  cell, schematic interpretations of, *38, 39*
  choroid, 917, *918, 919, 926, 931*
  Descemet's, *921,* 922, *923, 924*
  fenestrated, 190
  fetal, *898*
  glassy, of atretic follicles, 875
    of eye, 926, *931*
    of hairs, *585, 587*
  mitochondrial, 45, *47*
  Nasmyth's, 627, 635
  of brain and spinal cord, 375, *376*
    nerves of, 377
  periodontal, 621, *623,* 629
  plasma, *36, 37, 38, 39*
    freeze cleaved, *40*
  platelet demarcation, in megakaryocytes, 223, *223*
  serous, 186
  Shrapnell's, 966
  synovial, 282–285, *285*
  tectorial, *976, 978, 979, 981*
  tympanic, 964, *965, 966, 966, 967*
  vestibular, 969, *971, 974, 976*
    of cochlear duct, 974
Membrane-coating granules, 570
Membrane space, mitochondrial, 45, *47*
Membranous labyrinth, of ear. See *Labyrinth.*
Memory cells, 427
Meninges, 375–377, *375, 376*
  nerves of, 377
  spaces of, 377
Menopause, 887
Menstrual cycle, changes in sweat glands in, 591, *592*
Menstruation, 887
  hormonal control of, *888*
Merkel cells, 565
  dense granules of, 576, *579, 580*
  of epidermis, 576, *579, 580*
Meromyosin, heavy, 59, *306,* 308, *311*
    in intestinal microvilli, 660
  light, 59, *306,* 308
Mesangial cells, 772
Mesaxon, 352, *355*
Mesenchymal cells, 171, 172
  in formation of cartilage, *234, 235*
Mesenchyme, blood vessels and, 420
  cartilage and, 234, *234, 235*
  hemopoiesis and, 210
  intramembranous ossification and, 263
  loose connective tissue and, 158
  smooth muscle and, 330
Mesothelium, 84
  simple squamous, *86*
Mesovarium, 858
Messenger RNA. See *Ribonucleic acid, messenger.*
Metabolic rate, control of by thyroid, 531
Metabolism, collagen, disturbances of, 193
Metamyelocyte, *224,* 224
Metaphase, meiotic, 74
    in oocyte, *874*
    in spermatogenesis, 822
  mitotic, 70, *71, 72*
    human chromosomes in, *76*
Metaphysis, of long bones, 245
Metaplasia, myeloid, 491
  squamous, 90

Methylene blue staining, 16
of axons, 351
of mast cells, 184
of Meissner's corpuscle, *366*
of tendon, *190*
Microanalyzer, electron probe, *22*
Microbeam, ultraviolet, in study of living
cells, 6, *10, 11, 12*
Microbodies, 52
of hepatocytes, *705, 707, 711, 712*
Microglia, *368*, 369
Micromanipulation, of living cells, 6, *9*
Microprobe, electron, 19, *22*
Microscopes, compound, 21
electron, scanning, 27, *28*
transmission, 26, *29*
fluorescence, *21*, 26
interference, 25
light, 22
magnification of, 22
numerical apertures of, 22
phase contrast, 24
polarizing, 26
principles of, 21–31
projection x-ray, 19
resolving power of, 22
ultraviolet, 26
Microsomes, *13*, 42
relationship of to endoplasmic reticulum,
42, *43*
Microspectrophotometry, ultraviolet, 18, *20*
Microtubules, cytoplasmic, 59, *61*
in blood platelets, *142*
of cilium, 100
of diplosome, *58*
of neurons, 339
Microvilli, 98, *98, 99, 102*
intestinal, cross section of, *39*
of B lymphocytes, *436*
of cells of choroid plexus, 378, *380*
of hepatic cells, *703, 704*
of intestinal absorptive cells, 659, *666–668*
of secretory canaliculus in gastric parietal
cell, 648, *653, 654*
of sensory cells of taste buds, *608*
of T lymphocytes, *435*
of thyroid epithelial cells, *529*
of zymogenic cells, 648
Midget bipolar cells, of retina, 947, *955, 957*
MIF. See *Migration inhibiting factor.*
Migration inhibiting factor, of cell mediated
immune response, 438
Milk ejection reflex, *133*, 520, *521*
Mineralization, of dentin, 623, 633
Mineralocorticoids, 549
Mitochondria, *36*, 45, *45, 46*
DNA in, 47, *48, 49*
in adipose cell during hibernation, *203*
in cardiac muscle, *318, 319*
in Purkinje fibers of heart, *328*
in various types of skeletal muscle fibers,
300, *302*
liver cell, *13*
of neurons, 340, *371*
of synapses, *371, 372*
Mitochondrial sheath, of spermatozoon,
816, 817, *817, 821, 828*
Mitogens, 444

Mitosis, 70
nuclear changes in, *71, 72*
phases of, 70, 73
Mitotic spindle, *59, 60*, 70
Mitral valve, 416, *418*
Mixed glands, of oral cavity, 606, 608,
610–615
Modiolus, 969
Moll, glands of, of eyelid, 591, 958
Monoblasts, 214, 230
Monocytes, *143, 146*, 152, *153*, 175
azurophil granules in, 153
in connective tissue, 175
Monoiodotyrosine, 529
Mononuclear phagocyte system, 178, *180*
Kupffer cells and, 700
Mononuclear wandering cells, of connective
tissue, 175
Monophyletic school, of hemopoiesis, 214,
215
Monopoiesis, 230
Montgomery, areolar glands of, 908
Morgagni, hydatid of, 879
lacunae of, 800
rectal columns of, 675
Motor end plate, 311, *312, 313*, 359, *361*
Motor unit, 359
Mucicarmine staining, of mucigen granules
of gastric mucous cells, 646
of neck mucous cells, 650
Mucigen, 117
of gastric epithelial cells, 646, *649, 650*
Mucihematein staining, of neck mucous cells,
650
Mucin, 117
Mucin reaction, of esophageal cardiac
glands, 640
Mucocutaneous junctions, 576, *580*
Mucoid cells, of sweat glands, 590, *593*
Mucoprotein 167
Mucopolysaccharides, 167
Mucosa, of gastrointestinal tract, 598,
599, 600, 617
respiratory, of nose, *744*
Mucous cells, 607, 608, *610, 611, 616*
neck, of gastric glands, 649
surface, of stomach, 646, *646, 649, 650*
Mucous connective tissue, 189
Mucous glands, of oral cavity, 606, *607,
610, 616*
of tongue, 613
Mucus, 117
secretion of by goblet cell, 662
Müller, radial cells of, 940, 951, *953*
Müller's muscle, of ciliary body, 928
Multilamellar bodies, of alveolar cells, 757,
760
Multivesicular body, 51, 52
in lymphocyte, *433*
Muscle(s), 288–330. See also *Muscle fibers.*
arrector pili, 586
Brücke's, 928
cardiac, 315–328, *316–318*
blood supply of, *318*
cytology of, 316
differences between atrial and ventricular
fibers, 322
histogenesis of, 329

Muscle(s) (*Continued*)
  cardiac, regeneration of, 330
  ciliary, 928
    of Riolan, 958
  connective tissue of, 295, *295*
  constrictor, of pupil, 917
  cremaster, 846
  dilator, of pupil, 917
  heart, freeze-etched, *30*
  histogenesis of, 328
  Müller's, 928
  of iris, 933
  of uterus, 884
  regeneration of, 330
  relaxing factor in, 311
  skeletal, 295–315, *295*
    atrophy of disuse of, 296
    band patterns of, 298, *300, 301, 305, 307, 310*
    blood supply of, 295, *297*
    histogenesis of, 328
    histological organization of, 295, *295*
    hypertrophy of use, 296
    regeneration of, 330
    sarcomere of, 299, *305, 307*
    sarcoplasmic reticulum of, 298, *303, 305*
    structural organization of, *306*
    tonic, 317
    twitch, 319
    types of fibers of, 300
  smooth, 288–295, *290–293*
    cell to cell relations in, *290, 291,* 293
    contractile mechanism of, 294
    histogenesis of, 328
    physiological properties of, 294
    regeneration of, 330
    vascular, *293,* 294
    visceral, 294
  striated. See *Muscle, cardiac; Muscle, skeletal.*
  tone of, 294
  types of, 288
Muscle fibers, cardiac, 315–328, *316–318*
    atrial, and atrial granules, 324, *326*
    differences in atrium and ventricle, 322
    nerve endings in, 359
  skeletal, 295, *296, 298*
    blood supply of, 295, *296*
    cytological differences in, 300
    cytology of, 296
    in thymus, 462
    intermediate, 300, *302, 303*
    motor nerve endings in, 359, *361.* See also *Motor end plate.*
    myofibrils of, 296, *299, 301, 305, 307.* See also *Myofibrils.*
    red, 300, *302, 303*
    sarcolemma of, 296
    sensory nerve endings in, 360, *362.* See also *Spindle, neuromuscular.*
    white, 300, *302, 303*
  smooth, 288, *289, 292, 293*
    associations of, 289, *290*
    cell to cell relations of, *290, 291,* 293
    fine structure of, 291, *291, 292*
    nerve endings in, 359
    of arteriole, *398–400*
    of wall of vena cava, *414*
    vascular, *293,* 294
  structure of, *296*

Muscle spindle, 313, *313,* 360, *362*
  innervation of, *314*
  primary nerve ending in, 315
Muscular tissue. See *Muscle(s); Muscle fibers.*
Muscularis externa, of esophagus, 639
  of gastrointestinal tract, 598, *599*
  of stomach, 653
Muscularis mucosae, of esophagus, 639, *640*
  of gastrointestinal tract, 598, *599*
  of small intestines, 671
  of stomach, 652
Myelin, 343, 347
Myelin sheaths, *337,* 343, 351, 353, *353, 354, 357*
  development of, 353, *355*
Myelinization, 353, *355, 356*
Myeloblasts, 214, 224
Myelocyte, basophilic, 228
  eosinophilic, 227, *228, 229*
  neutrophilic, *224,* 226
Myeloid metaplasia, 491
Myeloperoxidase, as protein tracer, 773
Myelopoiesis, 209
  timing of events of differentiation in, *230*
Myoblasts, 328
Myocardium, 416. See also *Muscle, cardiac; Muscle fibers, cardiac.*
  innervation of, 327
Myoepithelial cells, of mammary gland, 907, *915*
  of sweat glands, 590, *591, 593*
Myoepithelium, of iris, *937*
Myofibrils, Cohnheim's fields of, *296,* 298
  of skeletal muscle, 296, *299, 301, 305, 307*
  substructure of, 303, *306, 308, 309*
Myofilaments, of cardiac muscle, *319*
  of skeletal myofibrils, 303, *306, 308, 309.* See also *Actin; Myosin.*
Myoglobin, 298
  in various types of skeletal muscle fibers, 300, *302, 303*
  x-ray diffraction pattern of, *32*
Myoglobin reaction, of muscle fibers, *303*
Myoid, of retinal rod and cone cells, 942, *945, 950*
Myoid cells, Hammar's, of thymus, 462
  of testis, 807
Myometrium, 884, *887*
  histophysiology of, 885
Myoneural junction, 311, *312, 313,* 359, 361. See also *Motor end plate.*
Myosin, filaments of, 58
  in blood platelets, 141
  in skeletal muscle, 303, *306*
  in smooth muscle, 294
  molecular fragments of, *306,* 308, *311.* See also *Meromyosin.*
Myxedema, 531

Nabothian cysts, 894
Nails, 587–588, *588, 589*
Nasmyth's membrane, 627, 635
Neck, of tooth, 621
Neck mucous cells, of gastric glands, 649
Nephron, 767, 768, *770, 791, 793*
  blood supply of, *793*
  tubules of. See *Kidney, tubules of.*

Nerve(s). See also *Nerve fibers*.
  cell body of, retrograde chromatolysis of, 383
  chorda tympani, 965
  ciliary, 957
  cochlear, 984
  degeneration of, Wallerian, 382
  fusimotor, 314
  laryngeal, 747
  of heart, 419
  of meninges of central nervous system, 377
  olfactory, 745
  optic, 917, *919, 942*, 957
  response of to injury, 382
  splanchnic, 364
  vagus, 748, 761
  vestibular, 984
  visceral, 364, *367*
Nerve cells. See *Neuroglia; Neurons.*
Nerve endings, in connective tissue, 363
  in epithelial tissue, 362
  in smooth and cardiac muscle, 359
  motor, on striated muscle, 359, *361*. See also *Motor end plate.*
  sensory, encapsulated, 363, *363–366*
    in tendons, 315, 362
    on skeletal muscle, 360, *362*
      epilemmal, 360
      interstitial, 360
Nerve fibers, 351–364
  afferent pathways of, 358
  classification of, 357
  efferent pathways of, 358
  impulse transmission in, 357
  myelinated, *360*
    motor endings of, 359, *361*. See also *Motor end plate.*
    sensory endings of, 360, *362*. See also *Spindle, neuromuscular.*
  optic, of retina, 950
  peripheral, endings of, 358
  pilomotor, 365
  preganglionic, 365, *367*
  Rasmussen's, 985
  sensory, encapsulated endings of, 363, *363–366*
  spinal roots of, 358
  sudomotor, 365
  unmyelinated, *360*
    endings of, 359
  vasomotor, 365
Nerve tracts, 347
Nervous system, autonomic, 364–366
    parasympathetic division, 364
    sympathetic division, 364
    sympathetic trunk of, 364, *367*
  central, 333
Nervous system, central, blood vessels of, 381
    connective tissue of, 375, *376*
    final common pathway of, 351, 372
    gray matter of, 347, *348–350*
    interneurons of, 351
    limiting membranes of, 367
    neurons of, *335*, 347
    non-nervous elements of, 366. See also *Ependyma; Neuroglia.*
    parts of, 333
    white matter of, 347, *348–350*
  craniosacral, 364

Nervous system (*Continued*)
  parasympathetic, 364
  peripheral, 333
    nerve endings in, 358–364
    nerve fibers of, 356, *357*
  somatic, *367*
  supportive elements of, 366
  thoracolumbar, 364
  visceral, *367*
Nervous tissue, 333–383. See also *Nerve(s); Nerve fibers; Nervous system.*
  development of, 373
Neumann, sheath of, 622, *623*
Neural crests, 373
Neural tube, 373
Neuraxis, 333. See also *Nervous system, central.*
Neurilemma, 352
Neurobiotaxis, 374
Neuroblasts, 374
Neuroendocrine feedback mechanisms, in pancreas, *132*
  in response to stress, *133*
  in suckling reflex, *133*
Neuroepithelial cells, of taste bud, 603
Neurofilaments, 338, *346, 372*
Neuroglia, 333, 337, 366
  peripheral, 366
  types of, 367, *368*
Neurohormones, 333
Neurohumor, 552
Neurohypophysis, 503, *503*, 518–521, *519, 520*
  Herring bodies of, 518, *519*
  histophysiology of, 520
  posterior lobe of, 503, *503*
Neurokeratin, *353*, 358
Neuromotor systems, 334
Neuromuscular spindles, 313, *313–315*, 360, *362*
Neuron(s), 333
  action potential of, 343
  alpha motor, 361
  autonomic, 365
  axis cylinder of, 334
  axon of, 333, *334*, 342, 347
  bipolar, 347, *684*
    olfactory, *746*
  cell bodies of, 334, *335, 337*
  chromatophilic substance of, 339, *340, 342*
  conductile portion of, *334*
  degeneration of, 371
  dendrites of. See *Dendrites.*
  development of, 373
  distribution of, 347
  effector portion of, *334*
  forms of, *335, 338*, 347–351
  gamma motor, 361
  Golgi complex of, 339, *341*
  Golgi Type I, 347, 350
  Golgi Type II, 347
  inclusions of, 340
  integrator, 351
  interrelationships of, 372
  mitochondria of, 340, *371*
  motor, 351, 361, 365
    somatic, *334*
  multipolar, *336, 684*
  myelin sheaths of. See *Myelin sheaths.*
  myelinated, of spinal cord, *348*

Neuron(s) (*Continued*)
  neurofibrils of, *336*, 338, *340*
  Nissl bodies of, 339, *340–342*
  nucleus of, 336, *337, 341*
  perikaryon of, 334, 338–347, *341*
  pigment granules of, 340
  postganglionic, 365
  preganglionic, 365
  processes of, 342. See also *Axon; Dendrites.*
  pseudounipolar, 348
  pyramidal, 350
  receptor portion of, *334*
  relationships of, 369–373, *370, 372.* See
    also *Synapses.*
  response of to injury, 382
  retinal, 940–950, *954–958*
  satellite cells of, *339*, 349
  sensory, 351
  star-shaped, 349
  structural divisions of, *334*
  structure of, 336–347
  synapses of, 369. See also *Synapses.*
  transmitter substance of, 371
  unipolar, 347
  unmyelinated, *354, 355*
  varieties of, 347
    of central nervous system, *335, 338*
  visceral sensory, 359, 364
Neuron doctrine, 334, 370
Neurophysins, 127, 520
Neuropil, 351
Neurosecretions, 552
Neurotendinal spindles, 362
Neurotubules, 339
  of dendrites, *345, 346*
Neutral red, 8, 152
Neutral red staining, of loose connective
  tissue, *185*
Neutrophils. See *Leukocytes, neutrophilic.*
Nexus, *93*, 95, 97. See also *Gap junction.*
  in cardiac muscle, 322, *324, 325, 329*
  of osteocytes, *257*
  of smooth muscle fibers, 294
Nile blue staining, 16
Nipple, 907, 908, *909*
Nissl substance, 339, *340–342*
  of hypophysis, 519
Node, atrioventricular, 324, 418
Node(s), hemal, 485
  lymph. See *Lymph nodes.*
  of Ranvier, 352, *353, 357, 358*
  sinoatrial, 324, 418
Nodules, lymphoid, 447
Nodulus Arantii, 418
Nomarski optics, 25
Norepinephrine, 204, 543
  actions of, 552
  and vasoconstriction of arteries, 404, *408*
  as neurohumor, 552
  effect of on adipose tissue, *206*
  storage of in adrenal medulla, 544, *549*
Normoblasts, 216, *220*
Nose, 743–746
  histophysiology of, 746
  paranasal sinuses of, 746
Notochord, 240
Nuclear bag, of muscle spindle, 314, 361
Nuclear chain, 361

Nuclear envelope, *36, 67,* 69
  fibrous lamina of, *67,* 69
Nuclear pores, 69
Nuclear sap, 64
Nucleation, heterogenous, in crystallization
  of minerals, 269
Nucleoid, of hepatocyte peroxisomes, 706,
  707, 712
  of peroxisomes, 52
Nucleolonema, 66, *68*
Nucleolus, *36*, 64, 65, 67
  liver cell, *13*
Nucleoplasm, 35
Nucleus, 35, *67*
  cellular, organelles of, 63
  extrusion of, in erythropoiesis, *220*
  "drumstick" appendage of, in neutrophilic
    leukocytes, 144, *145*
  in mitosis, *71, 72*
  interphase, chromatin in, *66*
  liver cell, *13*
  of nerve cell bodies in gray matter, 347
  of spermatozoon, 815, *815, 825, 826*
    relationship of acrosome to, *815*
  paraventricular, 518
  supraoptic, 518·
Nucleus pulposus, *265*
Nuel, space of, 977, *978*
Nuhn, gland of, 612
Nutrition, deficiencies of, effects of on
  bone, 281

Occluding junction, between Sertoli cells, 843
Oddi, sphincter of, 718
Odontoblasts, 623, *624, 626*
  processes of, *624, 625, 625*
  relationship of to predentin and dentin,
    624, 625, 626
Olfaction, organ of, 743
Olfactory epithelium, 743, *744–746*
Olfactory rods, *745*
Olfactory vesicle, 744
Oligodendrocytes, 368, *368*
Omentum, 186
  human, *187*
Oocyte, 858, *859, 862–866, 869, 870, 874.*
  See also *Ovum.*
Oolemma, 862
Opsins, *954*
Opsonization, 428, 444
Optic diaphragm, 917
Optic nerve, 917, *919, 942, 957*
Ora serrata, of eye, 917, *918, 919, 925, 927*
Ora terminalis, 927
Oral cavity, 598–617
  glands of, 605–614
    blood and lymph supply of, 613
    innervation of, 613
  mucosa of, 599
Orange G staining, 16
  of Paneth cells, 668
  of somatotropes, 507
Orbicularis oculi, 958, *960*
Orcein staining, of elastic tissue of arteries,
  401
Orcein-hematoxylin staining, of tunica media
  of aorta, *407*

Organ(s), 35
  culture of, 4, 5
  exteriorization and transillumination of, 2
Organ of Corti, *970*, 974, *975–981*, 976
  hair cells of, *978*, 979, *979–989*
  pillars of, 977, *978*, *979*, *981*
  supporting cells of, 976–979, *979–983*, 985
Organ system, 35
Organelles, cellular, 36. See also listings of
    specific organelles, e.g., *Golgi complex.*
  cytoplasmic, 37
    role of in secretion, *117*
  nuclear, 63
Orthochromatic erythroblasts, 216, *220*
Osmic acid staining, of lipid, *200*
  in lactating mammary gland, *913*
Osmium-cryofixation, in study of retinal
    photoreceptor cells, *949*
Osmium fixation, for lipid, 63, *65*, *176*
  of dense regular connective tissue, 192
Osmium-lead staining, of adrenal cortex lyso-
    somes, *50*
Osmium staining, of Golgi complex, *54*
Osmium tetroxide fixation, for electron
    microscopy, 28
  in study of fat absorption, 677, *682*
Osmium tetroxide staining, of myelin, 351,
    352, *353*
Ossicles, auditory, 965, *965*, *966*
Ossification, ectopic, 262, 277
  endochondral, 241, *241*, 262, 264
    centers of ossification in, 264, *265*, 268
    mechanism of calcification in, 269,
        269–271
    of long bones, *266–270*
    stages of, *265–270*
  intramembranous, 262, *263*
    of shaft of long bone, 273
    pattern of trabeculae in, *264*
Osteitis fibrosa, 281
Osteoblasts, 249, 255, *256*
Osteoclasts, 221, 257, *261*, *262*
  origin of, 260
  ruffled border of, 258, *261*, *262*
Osteocytes, 247, 256, *257*, *258*, *259*
  process of, *260*
Osteoid, 272
Osteolathyrism, 165
Osteolysis, 257
Osteomalacia, 254, 272, 280, 282
Osteons. See *Haversian systems.*
Osteoprogenitor cells, 255
Otoliths, 974
Oval window, of inner ear, *965*, *966*, 970
Ovary(ies), 858–880, *858–863*
  blood supply of, 880
  changes in during menstrual cycles, *888*
  corpus luteum of. See *Corpus luteum.*
  cortex of, 858
  epithelium of, 859
  follicles of. See *Follicles, ovarian.*
  germinal epithelium of, 859, *861*
  interstitial tissue of, 876
  lymphatic vessels of, 880
  medulla of, 858
  nerves of, 880
  rat, transplanted to mouse anterior
    chamber, 5
  vestigial organs associated with, 879

Ovary(ies) (*Continued*)
  zones of, 858
Oviduct, 880–883, *882*, *883*
  blood supply of, 883
  effect of ovariectomy on, 883, *884*,
  epithelium of, *884*
    effect of hormones on, *886*
  mucosa of, *883*
  structure of, 881, *882*, *883*
Ovulation, 866
  hormonal control of, 867, *888*
Ovum, *865*, 886. See also *Oocyte.*
  fertilization of, 869
  implantation of, *892*, 897
  maturation of, 868, *873*
  two-cell stage, *891*
Owen, contour lines of, of teeth, 623
  interglobular layer of, *622*
Oxyhemoglobin, 571
Oxyntic cells, of gastric glands, 648, *648*, *653*,
  654
Oxyphilic cells, of parathyroid, 536, *536*
Oxytocin, 127, 294, 552, 886, 914
  role of in suckling reflex, 520, *521*

Pacchionian corpuscles, 381
Pacemaker, of heart, 325, 418
Pachymeninx, 375. See *Dura mater.*
Pachytene stage, of meiosis, 74
  in spermatogenesis, 822
Palate, soft, 600
Palatine glands, 613
Palatine tonsils, *601*, 615, *617*, *618*
Palms, epidermis of, 565, *567*, *568*
Pampiniform plexus, 835
Pancreas, 726–742
  acinar cell of, *109*, *110*
  acinar tissue of, 726, *728*, *729*
  alpha cells of, dense granules of, *128*
  as compound tubuloacinar gland, 123
  beta cells of, 730, *734*, *736*, *741*
  blood supply of, 735
  centroacinar cells of, 726, *729–733*, *738–
    740*
  delta cells of, 731, *734*, *737*
  duct system of, 733
  endocrine, 729–733
    histophysiology of, 739
  enzymes secreted by, 738
  exocrine, 726–729
    histophysiology of, 737
  feedback mechanism of, *132*
  function of nervous system and, 736
  islet cells of, 729–733, *735–737*, *741*
  islets of. See *Islets of Langerhans.*
  lymph supply of, 735
  nerve supply of, 735, *740*, *741*
  regeneration of, 737
  relation of upper abdominal viscera to, *727*
  structure of, 726
  zymogen and, 726, *729*, *731–733*
Pancreatitis, acute, 739
Pancreozymin, 123, 736, 737
Paneth cells, of crypts of Lieberkühn, 667,
  669, *670*

Panniculus adiposus, 198
Panniculus carnosus, 578
Papilla(e), dermal, 563
 of hair follicle, 582, *582, 585*
 mammary. See *Nipple.*
 of hair follicles, 582, *582, 585*
 of optic nerve, 917, *918, 919*
Paps' silver staining, of collagen fibers, *160, 162*
 of reticular fibers of liver, *716*
Parafollicular cells, of thyroid, 526, *530, 531, 532*
 secretion of calcitonin by, 528, 532
 secretory granules of, *531, 532*
Paraganglia, 553–555
 "achromaffin," 554
 chief cells of, *554*
Paranasal sinuses, 746
Parapineal organ, 558
Parasympathetic nervous system, 364
Parathormone, 257, 259, 280, 538
 effects of, 538
 effect of on osteoclast, 260
Parathyroid glands, 535–539, *535–537*
 adipose cells in, *537*
 blood supply of, *538*
 cells of, 536–538, *536, 537*
 changes in with age, *537*
 chief cells of, 536, *536*
 effect of graft on bone, *538*
 histophysiology of, 538
 oxyphilic cells of, 536, *536*
 principal cells of, 536, *536*
Paraventricular nucleus, 518
Parietal cells, of gastric glands, 648, *648, 653, 654*
Paroöphoron, 88
Parotid glands, 606, 611, *615*
Pars amorpha, of nucleolus, 66
Pars distalis, of hypophysis, 505–516, *506*
 acidophilic (alpha) cells of, 505, *506, 507, 508–511*
 histophysiology of, 512–515
Pars fibrosa, of nucleolus, 66
Pars granulosa, of nucleolus, 66
Pars infundibularis, 518
Pars intermedia, of hypophysis, 516–518
 histophysiology of, 517
Pars interstitialis, of oviduct, 881, *882*
Pars membranacea, of urethra, 800
Pars prostatica, of urethra, 799
Pars spongiosa, of urethra, 800
Pars tuberalis, of hypophysis, 518
Particles, intramembranous, of cell membrane, 39, *40, 97*
PAS staining. See *Periodic acid–Schiff reaction.*
Patches, Peyer's. See *Peyer's patches.*
Pedicels, of podocytes, 770, *771–774, 776, 777*
Penis, 851–855, *855*
 blood supply of, 853
 lymphatic supply of, 854
 nerve supply of, 855
Pepsin, 654
Pepsinogen, 648, 654
Periaxial space, of muscle spindle, 314
Pericardium, 186
Perichondrium, 234
 in endochondral ossification, 267

Pericranium, 246
Pericryptal fibroblasts, 667
Pericyte, 388, *388, 393*
Perikaryon, of neurons, 334, 338–347, *341*
Perilymph, 983
 electrolyte composition of, 990(t)
Perimysium, 295
Perineurium, 356, *359, 360*
Perineuronal space, nerve cells in, *375*
Perinuclear cisterna, 70
Perinuclear space, 69
Periodate-leukofuchsin reaction, 16
Periodic acid–Schiff-hematoxylin staining, of epithelium, *87*
Periodic acid–Schiff reaction, 12, 18
 for basal lamina, 96
 for carbohydrates, of vagina, *17*
 for glycogen, 62
 for intracellular cement, 91
 for mucigen of gastric mucous cells, 646
 of bone ground substance, 253
 of cartilage ground substance, 237
 of connective tissue ground substance, 167
 of fibroblast granules, 171
 of goblet cells, *677*
 of hypophyseal cells, 506, 513(t)
 of lens of eye, *938*
 of mucus, 662
 of neck mucous cells, 650
 of osteoblasts, 255
 of smooth muscle, 290, *290*
 of thymic macrophages, 461
 of thyroid colloid, 525
 of tunica media of muscular arteries, 399, *400*
Periodontal membrane, 621, *623, 629*
Periosteal collar, 267, 273
Periosteum, 245
Peripheral cells, of taste bud, 604
Peripolesis, 437
Perisinusoidal space, of liver, 701, *702, 703, 704*
Peritoneum, 186, 598
Peritubular contractile cells, of testis, 807
Permeability, capillary, 393
Pernicious anemia, 654
Peroxidase, 182, 183
Peroxidase reaction, in azurophil granules, 226, *226, 227*
 in choroid plexus, 379
 in myelocytes, 226, *226, 227, 227, 229*
 in study of blood-thymus barrier, *466*
 in study of capillary permeability, 394
 of arteriole, *399*
 of chromophobic hypophyseal cells, 511
 of Kupffer cells, 699, *700*
 of liver, *711*
 of lymphocytes, 150
 of monocytes, 153
 of plasma cells, *434*
 of thyroid cells, 529
Peroxisomes, 52
 of hepatocytes, 705, *707, 711, 712*
Peyer's patches, 446, 670, *671*
 and bursa of Fabricius, 671
Phagocytes, alveolar, 758, *761, 762*
 of reticuloendothelial system, *180*
Phagocytins, 144

Phagocytosis, 51
  by neutrophilic leukocyte, 154
  in lymph nodes, 481, 481
  lysosomes and, 49
  study of by vital dyes, 8
Phagosomes, 49
Phalangeal cells, of organ of Corti, 978, 978–980, 982, 983
Pharyngeal tonsils, 616
Pharyngoesophageal "sphincter," 641
Pharynx, 617, 618
Phase contrast microscopy, 24
Phosphatase reaction, in duodenum, 19
Phosphomolybdic acid staining, of intestinal absorptive cell, 659
Phosphotungstic acid-hematoxylin staining, of collagen, 164
Phosphovitellin, 281
Photoreceptor cells, 940–946. See also Cone cells; Rod cells.
Phytohemagglutinin, 444
Pia-arachnoid, 375, 377
Pia mater, 367, 375, 375, 376, 376
Picrocarmine staining, of nerve fibers, 352
PIF. See Proliferation inhibiting factor.
Pigment, lipochrome, in Leydig cells, 834, 840
  lipofuscin, 50
  visual, 954. See also Rhodopsin.
Pigment epithelium, of eye, 931, 932, 935, 936, 938, 942, 943, 945
Pigment granules, cytoplasmic, 61, 62
  of neurons, 340
Pigmentation, skin, 571–576
Pillars, of organ of Corti, 977, 978, 979, 981
  microtubules of, 988
Pilomotor fibers, 365
Pineal body, 556–561, 557–561
  antigonadotropic effect of, 560
  chief cells of, 556
  corpora arenacea of, 557, 558
  histogenesis of, 558
  histophysiology of, 560
  innervation of, 558
  interlobular tissue of, 560
  interstitial cells of, 556, 559
  melatonin in, 560
  metabolic activity of, 560
  neuroendocrine function of, 561
  sand granules of, 557, 558
Pineal sand, 557, 558
Pineal system, of lower vertebrates, 558
Pinealocytes, 556, 559
  vesicles of, 561
Pinna, 964, 965
Pinocytosis, by capillary endothelial cells, 393
Pits, gastric, of stomach, 644, 645–647
Pituicytes, 518, 519
Pituitary. See Hypophysis.
Placenta, 898–902
  circulation of, 901, 902
  formation and structure of, 897, 898, 899, 901
  hemochorial, 902
Planum semilunatum, 970, 974
Plasma, blood, 137, 153
  electrolyte composition of, 990(t)
  seminal, 856
Plasma cell, 143, 427

Plasma cell (Continued)
  fluorescent antibody staining of, 184
  fluorescent anti-immunoglobulin reaction of, 437
  immunoglobulins A and, 432
  of connective tissue, 180, 182, 183, 184
  of thymus, 461
  production of antibodies by, 669
  Russell bodies in, 181, 182, 433
Plasma membrane, 36, 37, 38, 39
  freeze cleaved, 40
Plasmablasts, 434
Plasmacytes, 432
Plasmalemma, 36, 37, 38, 39
  of capillaries, vesicles of, 390, 390
Plate(s), epiphyseal, of long bones, 244, 245
  motor end. See Motor end plate.
  of liver cells, 694, 695, 702
Platelets, 139, 141, 142
  alpha granules of, 140
  and platelet forming megakaryocytes, 222, 223
  circulating, 141
  granulomere of, 140
  role of in blood clotting, 140
Platelet demarcation channels, in megakaryocyte, 223, 223
Platelet thrombus, 140
Pleura, 186, 762
  visceral, 748
Plexus, choroid, 378, 378, 379, 380
  Meissner's, 679, 682, 683
  myenteric, of Auerbach, 682, 684, 685
    of small intestine, 673
  pampiniform, 835
Plexus vesicalis, 799
Plicae circulares, 658, 659, 660
Plicae palmatae, 894
Plutonium, as bone seeking isotope, 254
Pneumonocytes, 756
Pneumothorax, 764
Podocytes, of renal corpuscles, 770, 771–775
  foot processes of, 770, 771–774, 776, 777
Poietins, 216
Poikilocytosis, 139
Polar bodies, in maturing ovum, 869, 873, 874
Polarization, of epithelial cells, 90
Polarizing microscopy, 26
Polydipsia, 521
Polykaryocytes, 221
Polyphyletic school, of hemopoiesis, 213
Polyploidy, 75
Polyribosomes, 42, 111, 112
  in polychromatophilic erythroblast, 219
  in polychromatophilic erythroblast, 219
Polysaccharides, cell membrane and, 38, 40
Polysomes, 42, 111, 112
Polyuria, 521
Pores, alveolar, 755, 756
  nuclear, 69
  of capillary walls, 394, 394, 395
  slit, of podocytes, 770, 773, 774
  taste. See Taste pore.
Portal canal, of liver, 689, 690
Portal systems, of blood vessels, 413
Portio vaginalis, of uterus, 884
Postacrosomal region, of spermatozoon, 814, 815, 816

Potassium bichromate staining, of adrenal medulla, 543
  of chromaffin tissue, 543
  of norepinephrine storing cells, 544
Predentin, *624–626*, 633
  relationship of odontoblast to, *624–626*
Preen glands, of birds, 589
Preganglionic fibers, 365, *367*
Pregnancy, stages of, *897*
Prepuce, 853
Presentation, antigen, 443
Preverterbral ganglia, 364, *367*
Principal cells, of epididymis, 844
Prismatic rod sheath, of enamel, 626
Prisms, enamel, 626, *627, 629, 630*
Proacrosomal granules, 823
Probes, radiation, in study of living cells, 6, *10, 11, 12*
Procentriole, 57
Procentriole organizers, 102, *105*
Processes, odontoblast, *624, 625, 625*
  Tomes', 623, *623, 637*
Processing, antigen, 444
Procollagen, 169
Procollagen peptidase, 193
Proerythroblasts, 216
Progesterone, 897
  secretion of, 872
Progranulocyte, 224
Proinsulin, 741
Prolactin, 507, 513(t), 514, 912
Prolactin cell, 507
Proliferation inhibiting factor, 438
Promegakaryocyte, 222
Promonocytes, 153
Promyelocyte, 224, *224–226*
  polymorphonuclear, 226, *226, 227*
Prophase, meiotic, in spermatogenesis, 822
  stages of, 74
  mitotic, 70, *71, 72*
Proplasmacytes, 434
Proprioceptive system, 333
Prostaglandins, 886
Prostate gland, 846, 848, *850, 852*
  benign nodular hyperplasia of, 849
  concretions in, 849, *853*
  epithelium of, *853*
Proteins, carrier, transportation of hormones by, 134
  cellular, synthesis of, 42
  deficiency of, effect of on cartilage, 242
  formation of collagen fibrils by, 161
  intestinal absorption of, 676, *679*
  isoelectric point of, 16
  molecular composition of, 32, *32, 38, 39*
  plasma, synthesis of in liver, 714
  synthesis of, 53
  synthesis of, in liver, 714
Prothrombin, 140, 156
Protochondral tissue, 234
Protoplasm, 35
  amphoteric constituents of, 16
Prussian blue reaction, of splenic macrophages, 491
Pseudocartilage, 240
Pseudoeosinophils, 144
Pulmonic valves, 418

Pulp, of tooth, 622, *623,* 628, *632, 635, 637*
  and zone of Weil, 629
    Korff's fibers of, 629, *637*
  red, of spleen, 487, *489,* 490
  white, of spleen, 487, *488, 493*
Pulp arteries, of spleen, 493
Pulp cavity, of tooth, 621, *622*
Pulp veins, of spleen, 496
Pupil, 917
Purkinje cell, of cerebellar cortex, *338,* 343, *344, 345,* 350
Purkinje fibers, of heart, 325, *326–328*
Purple, visual, 938
Pus, 145
Pylorus, 644

Quinacrine mustard staining, for chromosomes, 75

Radiation probes, for study of living cells, 6, *10, 11, 12*
Rami communicantes, 364
Ranvier, node of, 352, *353, 357, 358*
Rathke's cysts, 517
Reabsorption of glucose, tubular maximum, 790
Reaction, Arthus, 428
Receptors, sensory, 333, 359
Recirculation, of lymphocytes, 452, *453*
Reconstitution, of thymus, 467
Rectum, 674
  and rectal columns of Morgagni, 675
Red blood cells. See *Erythrocytes.*
Reductional division, in meiosis, 74
Reflex, milk ejection, *133,* 520, *521*
Regeneration, of adrenal cortex, 553
  of cartilage, 241
  of epithelium, 106
  of liver, 712
  of muscular tissue, 330
  of pancreas, 737
Regnaud, residual body of, 828
Reinke, crystal of, in Leydig cell, 838, *840, 841*
Reissner's membrane, 969, *976*
Relaxin, 886
Relaxing factor, in muscle, 311
Releasing factors, 512, 515
Renal corpuscle. See *Kidney, renal corpuscle of.*
Renin, 766, 782
Repair, of tissues, role of connective tissue in, 192
Reproductive system, female, 858–905. See also *Ovaries; Uterus; Vagina.*
  endocrine regulation of, 895
  male, 805–856, *805.* See also *Penis; Testis.*
  accessory glands of, 847–851
Reserpine, 545
Residual bodies, of intracellular digestion, 49, *51*
  of Regnaud, 828
Resorcin fuchsin staining, of elastic fibers, 163, *165,* 400
  of hypophyseal cells, 509

Resorption cavities, and internal reorganization of bone, 275, *279*
Respiratory distress syndrome, 758
Respiratory system, 743–764. See also *Lung(s).*
Response, immune, 427
    cell mediated, 428, 429
        humoral, 428
        primary, 427
        secondary, 428
Rete cutaneum, *595*
Rete mirabile, 785, *793*
Rete subpapillare, *595*
Rete testis, 806, *806*, 841, *844*
Retia mirabilia. See *Rete mirabile.*
Reticular cells, 446
    of lymph node, *448*
    of spleen, *489*, 490, *491*
    of thymus, tonofilaments of, 463
    primitive, of hemopoietic tissue, 212, *213*, *215*
    squamous, in Hassall's body, *464*
Reticular connective tissue, 190
Reticular fibers, 165
    compared to collagen fibers, *172*
    development of in tissue culture, *170*
    of adrenal cortex, *167*
    of spleen, *167*
Reticulocytes, 139, 219
Reticulocyte count, 139
Reticuloendothelial system, 178, *180*
    Kupffer cells and, 699
    relationships between cells of, *181*
Reticulum, endoplasmic. See *Endoplasmic reticulum.*
    sarcoplasmic. See *Sarcoplasmic reticulum.*
Retina, 917, *918, 919*, 937–956
    bipolar cells of, 947, *954, 955, 957*
    ciliary epithelium of, 929, *933, 934*
    cone cells of. See *Cone cells.*
    fovea of. See *Fovea.*
    ganglion cells of, 949
    histogenesis of, 937
    histophysiology of, 953
    image formation on, 953
    inner plexiform layer of, *943, 944*, 950, *958*
    layers of, *931*, 937, *943–945*
    neuroglia of, 951
    neurons of, 940–950, *954–958*. See also *Cone cells; Rod cells.*
    optic nerve fibers in, 950
    outer limiting membrane of, *943, 946, 947, 953*
    outer plexiform layer of, *943, 944, 947, 956*
        synaptic connections in, *957*
    photoreceptor cells of, 940–946. See also *Cone cells; Rod cells.*
    pigment epithelium of, 938, *943*
    supporting cells of, 951
    veins of, 956
    visual cells of, 940–946
Retinal, 954
Retroannular recess, of spermatozoon, *818*
Retzius, lines of, of enamel, *622*, 627, *627*
Rhagiocrine cells, 175
Rhodopsin, 938
    particles of, in retinal rod cell, *951*

Ribonucleic acid, in mitochondria, 47
    in nucleolus, 64, 68
    messenger, 42, 110
    ribosomal, 110
    staining for, *15*
    synthesis of cell protein and, 110
    transfer, 42, 110
    types of, 42, 47, 68, 110
Ribonucleoprotein, 41
    in mitochondria, *48*
Ribosomes, *13*, 41
    and microsomes, 42, *43*
    in pancreatic acinar cell, 110
    mechanism of protein synthesis on, 109, *113*
    on cisternae of endoplasmic reticulum, 110
    on Nissl bodies, 339, *342*
Rickets, 272, 282, 539
Ridges, epidermal, 563
Riolan, ciliary muscle, 958
Rod(s), enamel, 626, *627, 629, 630*
Rod cells, of retina, 940, *945–951, 954, 957*
    bipolar, 947, *955, 957*
        inner segment of, 941, *945, 947, 948*
        outer segments of, 941, *947–950, 951*
        turnover of, *950*
Rokitansky-Aschoff sinuses, 720
Romanowsky staining, 216
Romanowsky staining, for blood cells, 140, *146*. See also *Wright's stain.*
Root, of tooth, 621
Rouget cells, 387
Rouleaux, of erythrocytes, 137, *138*
Round window, of inner ear, *965, 966*, 970
Ruffled border, of osteoclasts, 258, *261, 262*
Rugae, of stomach, 644
Russell bodies, 433
    in plasma cells, 181, *182*
    of stomach wall, 652
Ruthenium red staining, of capillary membrane, 388

Sac(s), alveolar, 749, *752, 753, 753*
    endolymphatic, 970, *970, 974*
Saccule, of ear, 970
Saliva, 606
Salivary corpuscles, 606, 616
Salivary glands, 605–614
    basal cells of, 609
    basket cells of, 609
    blood supply of, 613
    cell types in, 606
    ducts of, 606, 611
    mixed, cells of, 608
    mucous cells of, 606, 607, *610*
    myoepithelial cells of, 609
    nerves of, 613
    serous cells of, 606, 607, *610–613*
Sand granules, of pineal, *557, 558*
Santorini, duct of, 733
Sarcolemma, of skeletal muscle fibers, 296
Sarcomere, of skeletal muscle, 299
Sarcoplasm, 289, 296
    of skeletal muscle, fine structure of, 302, *304, 305, 307*
    submicroscopic structure of, 317

Sarcoplasmic reticulum, of cardiac muscle, 319, *320, 321*
  of skeletal muscle, 298, *303, 304, 305*
Sarcosomes, 298
Sarcotubules, of skeletal muscle fibers, 303, *304, 305*. See also *T tubules.*
Satellite(s), of centrioles, 59
Satellite cells, of neurons, *339,* 349
  of peripheral ganglia, 366
  of skeletal muscle, 297, 329
Scala media, 970, *975*
Scala tympani, *966,* 970, *975, 976, 982*
Scala vestibuli, *966,* 970, *975, 976, 982*
Scarpa's ganglion, 984
Schlemm, canal of, *918,* 924, *925–928, 930*
Schmidt-Lantermann, incisures of, 352, *352, 353, 357*
Schreger, lines of, of enamel, *622,* 627
Schwann, sheath of, 351, *352.* See also *Schwann cells.*
Schwann cells, 349, 351, *353–357*
  as peripheral neuroglia, 366
Schweigger-Seidel sheath, of spleen, 493, *494*
Sclera, 917, *918, 919, 920, 925*
Sclerocorneal junction, 923, *925, 926*
Scorbutus, 193, 242, 282
Scurvy, 193, 242, 282
Sebaceous glands, of hair follicles, 586
  of skin, 588, *590*
"Second messenger" concept, of hormone action on cells, 134, *134*
Secretin, 736, 737
Secretion(s), 108–134, *116*
  apocrine, 116, 910
  cytocrine, 572
  endocrine, 123–134
    feedback mechanisms of, 132
  exocrine, 108–123
    control of, 122
  holocrine, 117, 909
  merocrine, 116, 909
    of mammary gland, *914*
  of cartilage matrix, 238, *238*
  of thyroglobulin, *129, 532*
  polypeptide, 125
  protein, 125
  protein rich, synthesis, storage, and release of, 108
  role of various cell organelles in, *117*
  steroid, 126
Secretion granules, *36*
Secretory canaliculus, of gastric parietal cell, 648, *653, 654*
Secretory granules, *115*
Secretory IgA, 669
Sectioning, of tissues, 10
Segment long spacing collagen, 161, *164*
Sella turcica, and hypophysis, 504, *504*
Semen, 855
  crystals of Böttcher of, 856
Semicircular canals, of ear, *965,* 968, *969, 970*
Semilunar valves, 416
Seminal plasma, 856
Seminal vesicles. See *Vesicles, seminal.*
Seminiferous tubules. See *Tubules, seminiferous.*
Septal cells, 756, *756, 757*
Septula testis, 805
Septum membranaceum, 417

Serosa, of gastrointestinal tract, 598, *599*
  of small intestines, 673
Serotonin, 140, 186, 410, 664
  permeability of venules to, *413*
  synthesis and storage of, 651
Serous cells, 607, 608, *610–613, 616*
Serous demilunes, of Giannuzzi, 609, *610, 611,* 612
Serous exudate, 186
  free cells of, 187
Serous glands, of oral cavity, 606, 607, *616*
Serous membranes, 186
Sertoli cells, 807, *809–813, 836, 843*
  blood-testis barrier and, 841, *843*
  relationship of to spermatogenic cells, *813*
Sex chromatin, 77, *77*
Sharpey's fibers, of bone, 252, *253*
Sheath, enamel, 626
  endoneurial, 353
  fibrous, of spermatozoon, 818, *818, 821*
  Hertwig's epithelial, of root of tooth, *621,* 628, 630, 637
  mitochondrial, of spermatozoon, *816,* 817, *817, 821, 828*
  myelin, *337, 343, 353, 353–355, 357*
  neurilemmal, 351, *352*
  of Neumann, 622, *623*
  of Schwann, 351, *352.* See also *Schwann cells.*
  periarterial, around splenic arteries, 487, *488, 493*
  prismatic rod, of enamel, 626
  Schweigger-Seidel, of spleen, 493, *494*
Shrapnell's membrane, 966
Sickle cell anemia, 139
Silver impregnation, for Korff's fibers of tooth pulp, 629, *637*
  in study of Auerbach's plexus, *685*
  of basal lamina, 96
  of pineal, 556, *560*
  of spleen, *489*
Silver nitrate staining, of capillaries, 386
  of parafollicular cells, 527, *530*
Silver staining, 162
  of adipose tissue, 197
  of argentaffin cells, 651
  of bone salt, 269
  of dendritic cells of germinal center, 448
  of encapsulated sensory nerve endings, *364, 366*
  of mammary gland alveoli, *915*
  of Meissner's corpuscle, *366*
  of neurofibrils, 338, *340*
  of reticular fibers, 166, *167, 171,* 190
Sinoatrial node, 324, 418
Sinus(es), lymph, 472, *473–475,* 477
  of valves, 412
  paranasal, 746
  Rokitansky-Aschoff, 720
  superior sagittal, *376*
  venous, of spleen, 494, *495, 496*
Sinus lactiferus, 907
Sinusoids, 392
  discontinuous, 392
  fenestrated, 392
  hepatic, 688, *689,* 694, 695, *696–698, 702, 714*
    fenestrated lining of, 696, *697, 698*
Skeleton, cardiac, 417

Skin, 563–596, *564, 565.* See also *Dermis; Epidermis.*
  blood supply of, 592–593
  functions of, 563
  glands of, 588–592. See also *Glands, sebaceous; Glands, sweat.*
  histogenesis of, 594–596
  Langerhans cells of, 574, *576–578*
  lymphatic vessels of, 593
  melanocyte system of, 571–576
  Merkel cell of, 576, *579, 580*
  mucocutaneous junctions and, 576, *580*
  nerve endings in, 593
  nerves of, 593
  pigmentary system of, 565
  pigmentation of, 571–576
  tanning of, 574
Sliding filament theory, of ciliary binding, 101, *104*
  of muscle contraction, *308,* 309
Slit pores, of podocytes, 770, *773, 774*
Soft palate, 600
Soles, epidermis of, 565, *566*
Somatotropes, 507, *508, 509*
Somatotropin, 281, 507, 512, *513,* 912
Space(s), Bowman's, 770, *775, 789*
  of Disse, 698, 701, *702–704*
  of Nuel, 977, *978*
  of Tenon, 920, 957
  perisinusoidal, of liver, 701, *702–704*
  supravaginal, of eye, 957
Specific granules, of myelocytes, 226, *227, 229*
  of neutrophilic leukocytes, 144, *146, 147*
Spectrum, electromagnetic, *31*
Spermatic cord, 806
Spermatids, 807, *809–813*
  intercellular bridges between, 822, *823*
  stages in differentiation of, *829, 830*
Spermatocytes, 807, *809–813*
Spermatocytogenesis, 819
Spermatogenesis, 819–828, *809–813*
  cell associations in, *831–836*
  cycle of, 828, *831–836*
  guinea pig, stage I of, *832*
    stage VII of, *833*
  stages of, *831*
Spermatogonia, 807, *809–812*
  type A, 820, *832, 836*
  type B, 820, *836*
Spermatozoa, 807, 811–828, *814, 821*
  clonal nature of, *824*
  nucleus of, 815, *815, 825, 826*
  release of, *830*
  stages in differentiation of, *829, 830*
Spermiogenesis, 820, 823
  phases of, 824
Sphincter, internal, of bladder, 798
  of Oddi, 718
  pharyngoesophageal, 641
Sphincter ampullae, 718
Sphincter choledochus, 718
Sphincter pancreaticus, 718
Sphincter pupillae, 934, *935*
Spinal cord. See also *Nervous system, central.*
  intermediolateral gray column of, 365
  membranes of, 375, *376*
  nerve fibers of, 356
  somatic nerves in, *367*
  white and gray matter of, *356*

Spinal roots, of peripheral nervous system, 358
Spindle(s), enamel, 628
  mitotic, *59, 60,* 70
  muscle, 313, *313*
  neuromuscular, 313, *313–315,* 360, *362*
  neurotendinal, 362
Spindle apparatus, *59, 60, 61,* 70
Spine, dendritic, *370, 371*
Spiral ganglion, of ear, 969, *975, 976*
Spiral limbus, *976, 981*
Spiral prominence, of cochlear duct, 975, *976, 978*
Spiral valve, of Heister, 720
Spleen, 487–501
  accessory, 499
  arteries of, 492–494, *493*
  blood supply of, 492–498, *493–497*
  capsule of, 487, *488*
  central arteries of, *488,* 492, *493*
  "closed circulation" theory of, *493,* 497, *497,* 499
  connective tissue of, 487
  cords of, cross section, *490, 491*
  cords of Billroth of, 487
  destruction of erythrocytes by, 499
  functions of, 487
  histogenesis of, 498
  histological organization of, 487–498
  histophysiology of, 499
  lymphatic tissue of, 488
  lymphatic vessels of, 498
  marginal zone of, 491
  myeloid metaplasia of, 491
  nerves of, 498
  "open circulation" theory of, 497, *497,* 499
  penicillar arteries of, 493
  pulp veins of, 496
  red pulp of, 487, *489, 490*
  regeneration of, 498
  removal of, 499
  Schweigger-Seidel sheath of, 493, *494*
  sheathed capillaries of, 493, *494*
  T lymphocytes of, 498
  trabeculae of, 487, *488,* 492, *492*
  venous sinuses of, 487, *494, 495, 496*
  white pulp of, 487, *488, 493*
Splenectomy, effects of, 499
Staining, of tissues, 11
  chemical basis of, 16
  histological and cytochemical procedures of, 16
  methods of, *14, 15*
  supravital, 7
  vital, 7
Stapedius, 965
Stapes, 965, *966*
Stellate cells, of liver, 700, *700, 701*
Stellate reticulum, of enamel pulp, *621,* 632, *635*
Stem cells, of blood, 212
  of bone marrow, 213
    pluripotential, 213, *217*
    unipotential, 213, *217*
Stensen's duct, 611
Stereocilia, 98, *100*
  of epididymal epithelium, 844, *846*
  of hair cells of ear, 971, *972*
STH, 912. See also *Hormone, growth.*
Stigma, of ovarian follicle, 867, *872*

Stomach, 643–657
blood supply of, 680
cardiac glands of, 645, 652
cell renewal and regeneration in, 655, *657*
fundic glands of, 645, *645, 647, 648.* See
also *Glands, gastric.*
gastric pits of, 644, *645–647*
histophysiology of, 654
intermediate glands of, 645
junction of with esophagus, *644*
lamina propria of, 652
lymph vessels of, 681
mucosa of, effect of aspirin or alcohol on,
656
muscularis externa of, 653
muscularis mucosae of, 652
protective permeability barrier of, *656*
pyloric glands of, 645, 652, *656*
regions of, 644
rugae of, 644
Russell's bodies of, 652
secretory activity of, 654
submucous layer of, 653
surface epithelium of, *644,* 645, *646, 647*
Stratum corneum, of epidermis, 566, *566,
567, 571–573*
Stratum disjunctum, of epidermis, *566,* 569
Stratum germinativum, of epidermis, 565,
568
of epidermis, "intercellular bridges" of,
566, *568*
Stratum granulosum, of epidermis, 566, *566,
570, 573, 576*
Stratum lucidum, of epidermis, 566, *566*
Stratum malpighii, of epidermis, 565, *566,
568, 573, 575, 576*
Stratum spinosum, of epidermis, 566
Stress, responses to, neuroendocrine rela-
tionships in, *133*
Stria vascularis, of cochlear duct, 975, *975–
977*
Striated border, epithelial, 98, *98*
Stroma, of erythrocytes, 138
Stromatin, 138
Strontium, as bone seeking isotope, 254
Subarachnoid space, of brain, *375, 376,* 377
Subdural space, of brain, *376,* 377
Sublingual glands, 606, 612, *616*
Submandibular glands, *125,* 606, *610–615,*
611
cell types in, *614*
Submaxillary glands. See *Submandibular glands.*
Submucosa, of esophagus, 639, *640, 643*
of gastrointestinal tract, 598, *599*
of small intestines, 671
of stomach, 653
Subneural apparatus, of skeletal muscle, 312,
312
Substantia compacta, of bone, 245
Substantia spongiosa, of bone, 245
Succedaneous teeth, 621
Succinic dehydrogenase reaction, for mito-
chondria of muscle fibers, *302*
of liver, *18*
of pancreas, *18*
Succus entericus, 676
Suckling reflex, *133,* 520, *521*
neuroendocrine relationships in, *133*

Sucrase, 676
Sudan black staining, 16
of adipose tissue, *197*
Sudomotor fibers, 365
Supporting cells, of olfactory epithelium,
744, *746*
of taste bud, 603
Suprachoroidal lamina, 920
Supraoptic nucleus, 518
Suprarenal glands. See *Adrenal glands.*
Supravaginal space, of eye, 957
Surface coat, of intestinal brush border, 659
667, 668
Surfactant, 758
Sweat glands, apocrine, 589, *590, 591*
changes in during menstrual cycle, 591,
592
clear cells of, 590, *593*
eccrine, 589, *592–594*
mucoid cells of, 590, *593*
myoepithelial cells of, 590, *591, 593*
number of per square centimeter of skin,
594
special types of, 591
Sympathetic nervous system, 364
Sympathetic trunk, of autonomic nervous
system, 364, *367*
Sympathicotropic hilus gland, 878
Synapses, axoaxonic, 369, *370*
axondendritic, *344,* 369, *370*
axosomatic, 369, *370*
between nerve cells, 334, 369–373, *370*
chemical, in peripheral nervous system,
361
dendrodendritic, 343, 369
en passant, 370
Synaptic cleft, 370, *371, 372*
Synaptic ribbons, of hair cells, 972, *973*
Synaptic trough, of skeletal muscle fibers,
312, *312*
Synaptic vesicles, 370, *371, 372*
of motor end plate, 312, *312,* 360, *361*
Synaptonemal complex, of leptotene chromo-
somes, 821
Synarthroses, 282
Synchondroses, 282
Syncytiotrophoblast, *892, 894,* 898
Syngeneic, 441
Synostosis, 282
Synovial membranes, 282–285, *285*
Systole, 404

T lymphocytes, 429, 434, *435,* 482
of spleen, 498
T system, of cardiac muscle, 319, *320*
of muscle fiber, 303
T tubules, of cardiac muscle, 319, *320, 322*
of skeletal muscle fiber, 303, *304, 305*
Taeniae coli, 675
Tannic acid staining, of intestinal absorptive
cell, 659
Tanning, of skin, 574
Taste buds, of tongue, 602, *603, 605, 607–
609*
Taste pore, 603, *607–609*

Tectorial membrane, *976, 978, 979,* 981
Teeth, 621–637
    auditory, of Huschke, 981
    deciduous, 621, *621, 632*
        life cycle of, *632*
    germ of, *621,* 631
    histogenesis of, 631, *632*
    parts of, 621
    permanent, 621, *621*
    primordia of, *621, 632–634*
    succedaneous, 621
Tela choroidea, 378
Teloglia, 311
Telophase, meiotic, 74
        in spermatogenesis, 822
    mitotic, 70, *71, 72*
Tendon(s), 188, *190*
    connective tissue of, 188, *190, 191*
    cross section of, *191*
    fibrocartilage and, *240*
    sensory nerve endings in, 315, 362
    sheaths of, 188
    structure of, 188
Tendon organs, 315
Tenon, capsule of, 920
    space of, 920, 957
Tensor tympani, 965, *966*
Terminal bars, 92, *92*
Terminal cisternae, of skeletal myofibrils,
    303, *305*
Terminal ganglia, 364
Terminal web, 91, 94
    of intestinal absorptive cell, 659, *666*
Testes, 805–811, *806,* 830–846
    blood supply of, 835, *842*
    duct system of, *806*
    endocrine function of, 837
    excretory ducts of, 841–846
    exocrine function of, 838
    failure of descent of, 832
    histophysiology of, 837–841
    interstitial tissue of, 833, *837.* See also
        Leydig cells.
    lymphatics of, 835, *842*
    seminiferous tubules of. See *Epithelium,
        seminiferous; Tubules, seminiferous.*
Testosterone, 837
Tetraiodothyronine. See *Thyroxin.*
TF. See *Transfer factor.*
Thalassemia, 138
Theca externa, of ovarian follicle, 863
Theca folliculi, 863
Theca interna, of atretic ovarian follicle, *881*
    of ovarian follicle, 863
Theca lutein cells, of corpus luteum, 871,
    876–878
Thermography, in study of brown adipose
    tissue, 207, *207*
Theta antigens, 436, 468
Thiamine pyrophosphatase, 53
Thiazin red staining, of cardiac muscle, *316*
Thionine staining, of basophilic leukocyte,
    146
    of mast cells, 184
    of neurons, *348, 349*
    of Nissl bodies, 339
Thiouracil, 532
Thoracolumbar nerves, 364

Thrombin, 140, 156
Thrombocytes, 140
Thrombocytopenia, 224
Thromboplastin, 140, 156
Thrombopoiesis, 221–224
Thrombopoietin, 224
Thrombosthenin, 140
Thrombus, platelet, 140
Thymocytes, 457
Thymosin, 468
Thymus, 457–468
    adipose tissue of, 465
    as primary lymphoid organ, 429, 457
    blood barrier of, 463, *466*
    blood supply of, 462
    cells of, 467
    connective tissue septa of, *459, 461*
    cortex of, 457, 458, *459, 460,* 462
    functions of, 465–468
    Hammar's myoid cells of, 462
    Hassall's bodies of, 458, *459, 460, 464*
    histogenesis of, 464
    histological organization of, 457
    histophysiology of, 465
    hormone of, 468
    innervation of, 462
    involution of, accidental, *458,* 465
        age, *458,* 465
    medulla of, 457, *459, 460,* 461, *463*
    nerve supply of, 462
    reconstitution of, 467
    striated muscle fibers in, 462
    structure of, 457
Thyrocalcitonin, 281, 532
Thyroglobulin, 126, 525
    hydrolysis of, 530
    mechanism of secretion, *532*
    synthesis of, 528, *532*
Thyroid, 524–533
    blood supply of, 527
    colloid of, 524, *525, 526*
    control of metabolic rate by, 531
    epithelial cells of, *525, 526*
    follicles of, 524, *525, 527, 530*
    follicular epithelial cells of, 524, *525, 526,
        529, 531*
    histological organization of, 524–528
    histophysiology of, 528–533
    hormone of, 524, 525
    iodine concentration by, 525
    nerve supply of, 524
    parafollicular cells of, 526, *530, 531,* 532
    principal cells of, 528
    regulation of blood calcium levels by, 532
Thyroid stimulating hormone, 530
Thyroidectomy cells, 515
Thyrotropes, 509
Thyrotropic hormone, 509, 513(t), 515, 912
Thyrotropin, 509, 513(t), 515, 912
Thyroxin, 242, 525
    formation and secretion of, *129*
Tight junction, 92, *92*
    of thymic capillary, and blood-thymus
        barrier, *466*
Tissue(s), 35
    adipose, 196–207. See also *Adipose tissue;
        Cells, adipose.*
    chondroid, 240

Tissue(s) (*Continued*)
  connective. See *Connective tissue.*
  culture of, 4. See also *Tissue culture.*
    of fibroblasts, *6–8*
  fibrohyaline, 240
  fixation, embedding, and sectioning of, 10
  fractionation of, *12*
  histological staining of, 11
  homogenization of, *12*
  living, direct observation of, 2–8
  muscular. See *Muscle(s); Muscle fibers.*
  preparation and examination of, 9–16
  protochondral, 234
  vesicular supporting, 240
Tissue culture, 4
  development of macrophages from mono-
    cytes in, *179*
  in study of fibroblasts, *6–8, 170, 175*
  of lymphocytes, peripolesis of, 437
TL antigens, 468
Tm, 790, 792
Toluidine blue staining, 12
  of cardiac muscle, *316*
  of cartilage ground substance, 238
  of connective tissue ground substance, 167
  of lymph node venule, *479*
  of mucus, 662
  of Nissl bodies, 339
  of olfactory epithelium, *745*
  of pancreas, *729*
  of retina, *946*
  of thymus, *459*
Tomes, fibers of, of tooth, 623, *623, 637*
  granular layer of, of dentin, 622, 623
  processes of, of ameloblasts, *637*
Tongue, 601–605, *601, 602*
  innervation of, 604
  lingual follicles of, *602,* 603
  mucous glands of, 613
  papillae of, 601, *602, 604–606*
  taste buds of, 602, *603,* 605, *607–609*
  taste pore of, 603, *607–609*
Tonofibrils, 59, *60,* 91
  of stratum malpighii, 567
Tonofilaments, *96*
  of stratum malpighii, 570
  of thymic reticular cells, 463
Tonsils, 615–617
  crypts of, 615, *617*
  lingual, *601, 602,* 603
  palatine, *601,* 615, *617, 618*
  pharyngeal, 616
  tubal, of Gerlach, 968
Tonus, muscle, 294, 404
Tooth germ, *621,* 631
Trabecula(e), arachnoid, *375, 376*
  of bone, 245, *246*
  of lymph nodes, 471, *473, 478*
  of spleen, 487, *488,* 492, *492*
Trabeculae carneae, 416
Trachea, 748, *748*
Transfer factor, 438
Transfer RNA. See *Ribonucleic acid, transfer.*
Transferrin, 155, 220
Transillumination, in study of organs, 2
Translation, of genetic code, 42
Translocations, chromosomal, 76

Transneuronal degeneration, 371
Transparent chamber, for studying living
    tissues, *2,* 3, *3–5*
Triad, of retinal neurons, 947, *956*
  of skeletal muscle, 303, *304, 305*
  portal, of liver, *692*
Trichohyalin granules, of hair follicles, 582
Trichrome staining, in study of hypophyseal
    cells, 506
  Mallory's, for hypophyseal cells, 509
Tricuspid valve, 416
Trigona fibrosa, 417
Triiodothyronine, 525, 529
Trophoblast, *892, 894, 898*
Tropocollagen, 160, *163*
  of ground substance, 168
Tropoelastin, 164
Tropomyosin, 307
Troponin, 308
Trough, synaptic, of skeletal muscle, 312,
    312
Trypan blue staining, of Kupffer cells, 699
Trypan blue uptake, by fibroblasts, 172
  by macrophages, 174, 178
  of choroid plexus, 378
Trypsin, 738
TSH, 913. See also *Thyrotropic hormone.*
Tube, auditory, 965, 967, *968*
  fallopian. See *Fallopian tube.*
Tubule(s), dentinal, 622, *623*
  seminiferous, 805, *806,* 807–811, *808–812*
    cell associations in, *831–836*
      effect of FSH on, *839*
    epithelium of. See *Epithelium, seminiferous.*
    lamina propria of, 807
  T, of cardiac muscle, 319, *320, 322*
    of skeletal muscle fiber, 303, *304, 305.*
      See also *Sarcotubules.*
  transverse, 303, *304, 305*
  uriniferous, 767–781. See also *Kidney,
    tubules of.*
Tubuli recti, 806, *806,* 841
Tufts, enamel, 628
Tumors, carcinoid, 665
Tunica adventitia, of arteries, 396, *401, 402,*
    405, 406, 408
  of arterioles, 398, *408*
  of esophagus, 640
  of small muscular artery, *404*
  of vena cava, *414*
Tunica albuginea, 805, 852
  of ovary, 859, *862*
Tunica intima, fibrous plaque of, in athero-
    sclerosis, 408
  of arteries, 396, *401, 406, 408*
  of arterioles, 398, *408*
  of medium caliber veins, 410
Tunica media, of aorta, *407*
  of arteries, 396, *401, 402, 406, 408*
  of arterioles, 398, *408*
  of small muscular artery, *404*
Tunica vaginalis propria testis, 807
Tunica vasculosa testis, 806
Turner's syndrome, 76
Tympanic cavity, 965, *965, 966*
Tympanic membrane, 964, *965,* 966, *966,*
    967

Type I cells, of carotid body, 415
Type II cells, of carotid body, 415
Tyson, glands of, 853

Ultimobranchial bodies, 527
Ultimobranchial cells, 526
Ultraviolet light, microbeam of, in study of living cells, 6, *10–12*
Ultraviolet microscopy, 26
Ultraviolet microspectrophotometry, 18, *20*
Unit membrane, of cells, 38, *39*
Uranyl acetate staining, of perichromatin granules of liver cells, 702
Urea, 790
Ureters, 794, *798*
Urethra, 799–802, *800*, 851, *855*
    female, 800, *802*
    male, 799, *799*
        gland of Littre of, *801*
Uretz microbeam, in study of metaphase chromosomes, *11*
Uric acid, 790
Urinary system, 766–802. See also *Kidneys; Urethra.*
Urine, 769
    passages for excretion of, 794–799
Urobilinogens, 716
Uropygial glands, of birds, 589
Uterine glands, 887
Uterus, *858*, 883–895
    cervix of, 893
    endometrium of. See *Endometrium.*
Uterus, glands of, 887
    isthmus of, 893
    myometrium of, 884, *887*
    regions of, 884
    smooth muscle of, 884
    wall of, *887*
Utricle, of ear, *969, 970*
Utriculus, of ear. See *Utricle.*
Utriculus masculinus, 846
Utriculus prostaticus, 799, 849, *850*
Uvea, 917, 926–934

Vacuoles, condensing, of Golgi complex, 111, *115*
Vagina, 902–904, *903*
Valve(s), aortic, 418
    atrioventricular, 418
    cardiac, 418, *418*
    mitral, 416, *418*
    of heart, 416, 418, *418*
    of lymphatic vessels, 423
    of Kerckring, 658, *659, 660*
    of veins, 412, *415*
        walls of, *415*
    pulmonic, 418
    semilunar, 416
    sinus of, 412
    spiral, of Heister, 720
    tricuspid, 416
van Gieson's stain, 162, 168
Varicocoele, 835
Vasa recta, of kidneys, 769, *784*, 785, *793*

Vasa vasorum, 402
Vasoconstriction, agonal, of small artery, *409*
    of arteries, 404, *408*
Vasodilatation, of arteries, 404, *408*
Vasomotor fibers, 365
Vasopressin, 127, 552
    role of in regulating body fluids, 520, *521*
Vater, ampulla of, 721
Vater-Pancini, corpuscle of, 363, *363*, 855
Veins, 409–413, *410*
    arcuate, 785
    bronchial, 760
    caliber of, 409–411
    cardiac, 419
    cochlear, 987
    collecting, of liver, 694
    hepatic, 695
    large caliber, 411
    laryngeal, 747
    medium caliber, 410, *414*
    of spleen, 494, *495, 496*
    portal, 413
    pulp, of spleen, *491*, 496
    renal, 785, *791*
    small caliber, 409
    special types of, 411
    spiral, 987
    stellate, of kidneys, 785
    suprarenal, 547
    thyroid, 747
    tunicae of, 409
    umbilical, 902
    valves of, 412, *415*
    walls of, *410, 414, 415*
Vena cava, wall of, *414*
Ventricles, of brain, 378
    of heart, 416
Ventricular cell, 374
Venule, *387*, 409, *411, 412*
    permeability of to serotonin, 413
    postcapillary, of lymph node, lymphocyte migration through, 479, *479, 480*
    wall of, 412
Verhoeff's stain, 163
Vermiform granules, of Langerhans cells, 575, *578*
Vertebral ganglia, 364, *367*
Verumontanum, 799, 846, *850, 852*
Vesicle(s), acrosomal, 823, *825*
    coated, of Golgi complex, 53
    matrix, of cartilage, 242
    olfactory, 744
    plasmalemmal, of capillary, 390, *390*
    seminal, 846, 847, *851*
    synaptic, 370, *371, 372*
        of motor end plate, 312, *312*, 360, *361*
    transitional, of Golgi complex, 53
    transport, of Golgi complex, 111
Vesicular supporting tissue, 240
Vessels, blood, 386–420. See also *Arteries; Capillaries; Veins.*
    lymphatic. See *Lymphatic vessels.*
Vestibule, of ear, *965*, 968
Villus(i). See also *Microvilli.*
Villus(i), arachnoid, *376*, 380
    chorionic, *895, 896, 898, 899*
    of small intestine, 658, *659–663, 665*
Vinblastin, 60

Vincristin, 60
Viscera, upper abdominal, *727*
Visual purple, 938
Vitamin A, deficiency of, effect of on bones, 282
Vitamin A aldehyde, 954
Vitamin B$_{12}$, 654
Vitamin C, deficiency of, and scurvy, 193, 242, 282
Vitamin D, deficiency of, and rickets, 242, 282
Vitreous body, of eye, 918, *918, 919, 925,* 937
Vitreous humor, of eye. See *Vitreous body.*
VLDL. See *Lipoproteins, very low density.*
Vocal cords, 747, *747*
Volkmann's canals, 248
von Ebner, glands of, *602,* 603, *605,* 613
von Kóssa's silver staining, in study of calcification, *241, 270, 272*
von Recklinghausen's disease, 281

Wall, capillary, structural basis of exchange across, 393
    cell, 40
Wandering cells, mononuclear, 175
    of connective tissue, 171
    resting, 175
Web, terminal, 91
    of intestinal absorptive cell, 659, *666*
Weigert's resorcin fuchsin stain, 163
Weigert-Weil staining, for myelinated fibers, *348, 349,* 351
Weil, zone of, of tooth pulp, 629
Wharton's duct, 611
Wharton's jelly, 189
White blood cells. See *Leukocytes.*
White matter, of central nervous system, 347, *348, 349*
    distribution of, 373
Willis, circle of, 381
Wilson's disease, 155
Wirsung, duct of, 733
Wright's stain, *218*
    for blood cells, 139, 140, *143, 146*

X-ray diffraction, myoglobin pattern in, *32*
    principles of, 31–33

Yolk sac, of embryo, *895, 896,* 898

Z bands, of muscle myofibrils, 299, *300,* 302, *305,* 307, *307, 310,* 316
Z band, of skeletal muscle, arrangement of filaments in, *310*
Z disc, 307, *310*
    Z filaments of, 307
Z disc matrix, 307
Z lines, of skeletal myofibrils, 299, *300, 301,* 304, *305, 307, 310*
Zenker-acetic acid fixation, 11
Zenker-formol fixation, 11
Zona fasciculata, of adrenal cortex, 540, *542, 544*
    secretion of glucocorticoids by, 549
Zona glomerulosa, of adrenal cortex, 540, *542, 543*
    secretion of mineralocorticoids by, 549
Zona intermedia, 542
Zona pellucida, of ovarian follicles, 863, *866, 868, 870, 874*
Zona reticularis, of adrenal cortex, 540, *542, 548*
    secretion of glucocorticoids by, 549
Zone of Weil, of tooth pulp, 629
Zonula adherens, 92, *92,* 93
Zonula occludens, 92, *93*
    freeze-fractured preparation of, *94*
Zonule, ciliary, of eye, 918, *918, 925,* 935, *941*
Zygotene stage, of meiosis, 74
    in spermatogenesis, 821
Zymogen granules, 114, *118*
    of gastric glands, 647, *648, 651, 652*
    of gastric zymogenic cells, *652*
    of pancreatic acinar cells, 726, *729, 731–733*
Zymosan particles, phagocytosis of, by leukocyte, *154*